Quick Reference to Occupational Therapy

Quick Reference to Occupational Therapy

FOURTH EDITION

Kathlyn L. Reed

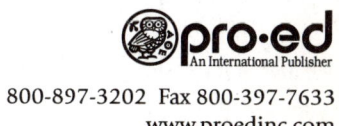

800-897-3202 Fax 800-397-7633
www.proedinc.com

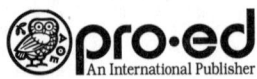

© 2024, 2014, 2001 by PRO-ED, Inc.
1301 W. 25th St., Suite 300
Austin, TX 78705-4248
800-897-3202 Fax 800-397-7633
www.proedinc.com

Library of Congress Cataloging-in-Publication Data

Names: Reed, Kathlyn L., author.
Title: Quick reference to occupational therapy / Kathlyn L. Reed.
Description: Fourth edition. | Austin, TX : PRO-ED, Inc., [2023] | Includes
    bibliographical references.
Identifiers: LCCN 2022019129 (print) | LCCN 2022019130 (ebook) | ISBN
    9781416412175 (paperback) | ISBN 9781416412182 (ebook)
Subjects: LCSH: Occupational therapy--Handbooks, manuals, etc.
Classification: LCC RM735.3 .R42 2023 (print) | LCC RM735.3 (ebook) | DDC
    615.8/515--dc23/eng/20220512
LC record available at https://lccn.loc.gov/2022019129
LC ebook record available at https://lccn.loc.gov/2022019130

Art Director: Jason Crosier
Designer: Sandy Salinas
This book is designed in Giovanni and Myriad.

Printed in the United States of America

1 2 3 4 5 6 7 8 9 10   32 31 30 29 28 27 26 25 24 23

Contents

Section 7: Musculoskeletal Disorders   625

Section 8: Systemic Disorders   685

Section 9: Immunologic and Infection Diseases   723

Section 10: Skin Disorders   761

Section 11: Cognitive-Perceptual Disorders   793

Appendices available online: www.proedinc.com, search "Quick Reference"

Appendix A: Instruments Developed by Occupational Therapy Personnel
Appendix B. Instruments Developed by Other Professionals and Used by Occupational
      Therapy Personnel

Introduction

The fourth edition of the *Quick Reference to Occupational Therapy* covers articles, chapters, books, manuals, or official association documents published from 2010 through 2019, with some articles published in 2020 that were uploaded in prepublication form in 2018 or 2019. A total of 158 diagnoses are covered in detail in 13 categories, and another 71 diagnoses are identified as having at least one reference. The outline of the chapters is based on the *Occupational Therapy Practice Frameworks III* and *IV* (*OTPF*; American Occupational Therapy Association [AOTA], 2014, 2020) but is condensed to save space. The new occupation in the *OTPF-IV*, Health Maintenance, is covered under Activities of Daily Living and Instrumental Activities of Daily Living because the occupation was not a separate category when the outline for the *Quick Reference* was set in 2019. Another space saver is to list the names of the assessment instruments in each chapter, but summarize the source information in two appendices—one for assessments authored exclusively or in part by occupational therapy personnel (Appendix A) and one for assessments authored by other professionals but used by occupational therapy personnel (Appendix B). The assessment instruments are divided because those created exclusively or in part by occupational therapy personnel are more likely to provide information that can be directly translated into goals related to occupational performance typically addressed in occupational therapy. Assessment instruments developed by other professionals may require translation or additional analysis to be useful in developing and implementing goals related to occupational performance.

To provide a consistent source of diagnostic information, two sources were used primarily, the *Diagnostic and Statistical Manual of Mental Disorders* (5th ed.; *DSM-5*; American Psychiatric Association [APA], 2013) and *The Merck Manual of Diagnosis and Therapy* (20th ed.; Porter, 2018). For some diagnoses, the best diagnostic information was provided in one or two articles. Supplemental information was obtained from a medical and nursing dictionary (O'Toole, 2017), *Stedman's Medical Dictionary* (2011), and the *Quick Reference Dictionary for Occupational Therapy* (Jacobs & Simon, 2015).

The primary sources were journal articles, indexes in databases, books and book chapters, published manuals, or official documents of associations or governmental agencies. The inclusion criteria were one or more of the following:

- Occupational-therapy-focused journal, textbook, manual, or document.
- Occupational-therapy-authored (at least one of the authors) article, chapter, book, manual, or official association document.
- Occupational therapy subject or topic data included with other disciplines or diagnoses (e.g., number of client visits or discharges, length of intervention, number of occupational therapy personnel on staff, cost analysis).
- Occupational therapy association, department, division, discipline, program, clinic, or service identified as a source of information or data.
- Content published or copyrighted between the years 2010 and 2019.
- Content published in English or summarized in detail in an abstract published in English. A total of 35 occupational-therapy-focused journal or serial publications printed in English were identified as available online.

Specific subjects or topics identified and selected for analysis are one or more of the following:

- Evaluation or assessment of clients.
- Assessment instrument developed in whole or in part by occupational therapy personnel (already published, newly published, or revised).
- Assessment instruments developed by other professionals but used by occupational therapy personnel in practice or research (already published, newly published, or revised).
- Theoretical basis or rationale for referral and/or intervention, including name of theory or model if identified.

- Intervention program description including length (number of sessions, number of days or weeks) and type (remedial or compensatory) of intervention, objectives, and goals.
- Media, methods, approaches, techniques, procedures, protocols, or modalities used or considered for use.
- Intervention team members (interdisciplinary, multidisciplinary, health-care team).
- Delivery sites (home, hospital, clinic, rehabilitation facility, telerehabilitation, or other distance platform).
- Precautions, safety issues, or considerations observed or recommended for observation.
- Results or outcomes short-term and/or long-term obtained.
- Cost effectiveness and efficiency to society.
- Benefit, value, or satisfaction to client.

Items excluded from inclusion in the search and selection process include the following:

- Articles on student education, training, fieldwork, or standards unless part of systematic review or meta-analysis.
- Articles that can only be accessed through a subscription or membership fee and do not appear to be indexed in any of the databases searched.
- Student papers, theses, dissertations, or capstone projects published on the college or university online platform but not published in article, chapter, book, manual, or official document format.
- PowerPoint presentations, lecture notes, and conference note summaries.
- Brochures or pamphlets designed for client education or advertising about available services.
- Surveys of practitioner knowledge of or attitude toward a disorder, disease, injury, or condition (exception if survey includes questions about assessment or intervention).
- Clinical trial protocols (study not yet completed or published).
- Research on animals or using animal models.
- Pharmaceutical or drug trials (unless specifically related to occupational therapy assessment or intervention).
- Surgery protocols (unless specifically related to occupational therapy assessment or intervention).
- Assessments being normed on typically developing children or healthy adults only.
- Methods of conducting research projects or preparing research protocols.
- Articles in occupational-therapy-focused journals written by other professionals (no occupational therapy author) unless content is directed toward occupational therapy assessment or intervention.
- Meta-analyses, scoping reviews, literature reviews, mapping reviews, systematic reviews (unless relevant to specific types of assessment, intervention, or outcome).
- Descriptions of developing or revising service programs in hospitals, clinics, communities, or countries (unless specific information related to assessment and intervention is included).
- Descriptions of occupational therapy professional or student associations or activities of an association.
- General descriptions of "how to treat" a particular disorder, disease, injury, or condition that mentions occupational therapy briefly in one or two sentences but provides no detail.
- Data-mining articles summarizing use of occupational therapy services (usually with data from other services included but providing no explanation of how the services are used).
- Articles on the value or purpose of continuing education or continuing professional development of practitioners.
- Issues related to credentialing practitioners (registration, certification, or licensure).
- Articles in which the profession of the author could not be determined because the department, discipline, or service is listed as including two or three professions (such as the Department of Occupational Therapy and Social Work, or Occupational, Speech, and Physical Therapy Services).

- Articles on translating an assessment instrument from English into another language.
- Pre- and posttests for continuing education credit or professional development units.
- Content published or copyrighted before 2010, except to identify source of assessment instruments.
- Data studies on the frequency or type of a disorder in a particular country.
- Commentaries about a group of articles in a special issue of a journal.
- Editorials, letters to the editor, or author replies (unless specific content is included related to assessment, intervention, or outcome).
- Audiovisual-type materials published online (such as YouTube; a few audiovisual aids are listed in the Bibliography sections).
- Blogs or other types of web pages maintained by individuals with or without professional credentials.
- Social media of all types (Facebook, Twitter, Instagram, etc.).
- Contributions of occupational therapy or credentials of occupational therapy contributors that could not be clearly established.

Databases searched with names of vendors, if known, include the following:[*]

- Academic Search Complete (EBSCO)
- APA PsycArticles (EBSCO)
- CINAHL (Cumulative Index to Nursing and Allied Health Literature; EBSCO)
- ERIC (Education Resource Information Clearinghouse)
- Google
- Google Scholar
- Health Source: Nursing/Academic Edition (EBSCO)
- MEDLINE (National Library of Medicine; EBSCO)
- NeuroBITE
- Nursing & Allied Health Database (ProQuest)
- OT Search (AOTA)
- OTseeker (Australia)
- Psychology and Behavioral Sciences Collection (EBSCO)
- PsycInfo
- PubMed (National Library of Medicine)
- SocINDEX (EBSCO)
- Web of Science
- Women's Studies International (EBSCO)
- Yahoo!
- Author names of researchers who published in specific diagnostic areas

Several additions or new chapters were added that did not appear in the third edition of the *Quick Reference to Occupational Therapy*. Inclusion was possible because at least three articles focused on the diagnosis were identified and located for analysis, including the following:

- Borderline Personality Disorder
- Celiac Disease
- Concussion
- Conversion Disorder
- Disaster Management
- Driving Cessation
- Frailty and Frail Conditions
- Frontotemporal Dementia

---

[*] Diagnoses were searched through databases that cover the subject or topic area, so not every diagnosis was searched through every database.

- Lesbian, Gay, Bisexual, Transgender, and Queer (LGBTQ) Population
- High- or At-Risk Infant or Child
- Hoarding
- Inflammatory Arthritis
- Motor Neuron Diseases
- Obsessive-Compulsive Disorder
- Older Adults
- Pediatric Acute-onset Neuropsychiatric Syndrome (PANS) and Pediatric Autoimmune Neuropsychiatric Disorders Associated with Streptococcal infections (PANDAS)
- Polytrauma
- Poverty
- Psoriatic Arthritis
- Retirement
- Serious Mental Illness
- Sickle Cell Disease
- Sjögren Syndrome
- Somatosensory Dysfunction or Impairment or Disorders
- Vegetative and Minimally Conscious States

Some diagnoses appearing as separate chapters in the third edition were combined or renamed in the fourth edition:

- Asperger's Syndrome. Combined with Autism Spectrum Disorder in accordance with the *Diagnostic and Statistical Manual of Mental Disorders* (5th ed.; *DSM-5*; American Psychiatric Association, 2013).
- Boutonniere Deformity. Combined with Osteoarthritis of the Hand.
- Burns of the Hand. Combined with Burns: Adults.
- Dyspraxia, Gravitational Insecurity, Intolerance or Adverse Response to Movement, Tactile Defensiveness, and Vestibular Bilateral Disorder. Combined into Sensory Integrative Dysfunction.
- Learning Disabilities. Renamed Specific Learning Disorders.
- Mental Retardation. Renamed Intellectual Disability.
- Swan Neck Deformity. Combined with Rheumatoid Arthritis.

The major reason for a diagnosis covered in the third edition but not covered in the fourth edition was lack of articles, chapters, books, manuals, or official association documents describing or discussing the diagnosis. Many of the diagnoses dropped from chapter status do appear in the section on Single- or Two-Article Disorders.

The top 10 diagnoses covered in the fourth edition (those with the most articles, chapters, books, or manuals that were identified based on the diagnosis) include the following:*

- Stroke (acute, chronic, hemiplegia)
- Driving Fitness/Cessation
- Cerebral Palsy (all types)
- Autism Spectrum Disorder (including Asperger's Syndrome)
- Sensory Processing Disorders (all types)
- Cancer (breast, child, adult)
- Dementia (Alzheimer's, general, frontotemporal dementia)
- Brain Injuries (acute, traumatic)
- Spinal Cord Injuries (complete/incomplete)
- Multiple Sclerosis (all types)

---

*If mental disorders were grouped by major mental disorders (schizophrenia, severe mental illness, bipolar disorders, and major depression), the total number of articles would rank above Brain Injuries.

The most cited assessments authored by occupational therapy personnel were the Canadian Occupational Performance Measure (COPM), Assessment of Motor and Process Skills (AMPS), Nine Hole Peg Test, and Box and Block Test. The assessments authored by other professions but widely used by occupational therapy personnel include the Functional Independence Measure (FIM) and Disabilities of the Arm, Shoulder, and Hand (DASH) and QuickDASH.

All publications have limitations, and the current text is no exception. Access to publications, especially articles, was restricted during manuscript development due to the COVID-19 pandemic, which caused libraries to close, limiting access to interlibrary loan services. Some journal articles may have been missed because they were not accessible for review and analysis. Other articles may have been overlooked in database searches due to limitations in database indexing. Articles authored by occupational therapy personnel may not be indexed under the terms "occupational therapy" or "occupational therapist" because the text of the article does not specifically mention occupational therapy or an occupational therapy practitioner. If the terms do not appear in the text itself, even a text word search will not identify the article. Still other articles were excluded because it could not be determined whether at least one of the article authors was an educated or credentialed occupational therapy practitioner, or that occupational therapy services were being cited separately from rehabilitation or physical therapy services in data summary tables. Finally, readers may be disappointed to find that some chapters lack information in various occupational areas or other parts of the outline. The lack of information is a direct result of lack of data in the literature cited for the diagnosis. For example, several of the disabilities related to hand function are missing information about occupational performance areas and the psychological impact of hand disability in daily life. The authors of the literature did not provide information about certain areas of occupational performance, and no attempt was made to "fill in the blanks." Articles about the impact of occupational dysfunction and psychosocial response to hand disability do exist, but they tend not to be associated with a specific hand disorder. Thus, the chapters on hand disorders may be missing information useful to the reader. The focus of the *Quick Reference to Occupational Therapy* is to summarize and organize existing literature, but not to ad-lib where information is not provided in the literature or is unclearly related to a specific diagnosis.

REFERENCES

American Occupational Therapy Association (AOTA). (2014). *Occupational therapy practice framework: Domain and process* (3rd ed.). Also *American Journal of Occupational Therapy, 68*(Suppl. 1), S1–S48. https://doi.org/10.5014/ajot.2014.682006

American Occupational Therapy Association (AOTA). (2020). *Occupational therapy practice framework: Domain and process* (4th ed.). Also *American Journal of Occupational Therapy, 74*(Suppl. 2), Article 7412410010. https://doi.org/10.5014/ajot.2020.74s2001

American Psychiatric Association. (2013). *Diagnostic and statistical manual of mental disorders* (5th ed.). https://doi.org/10.1176/appi.books.9780890425596

Jacobs, K., & Simon, L. (2015). *Quick reference dictionary for occupational therapy* (6th ed.). Slack.

O'Toole, M. T. (Ed.). (2017). *Mosby's dictionary of medicine, nursing & health professions* (10th ed.). Elsevier.

Porter, R. S. (Ed.). (2018). *The Merck manual of diagnosis and therapy* (20th ed.). Merck Sharp & Dohme.

Stedman's medical dictionary for the health professions and nursing (7th ed.). (2011). Wolters Kluwer.

Developmental Disorders

Arthrogryposis Multiplex Congenita

Description

Arthrogryposis multiplex congenita (AMC) refers to a group of nonprogressive conditions that are present at birth and involve fibrous stiffness of one or more joints resulting in limitation of movement. Muscles may be incompletely developed, smaller than normal, reduced in size, and replaced by fibrous tissue. The most common or classic type is amyoplasia, in which contractures occur symmetrically in multiple joints (Lake & Oishi, 2015; O'Toole, 2017; Porter, 2018). A consensus-based definition includes the following concepts: The term *arthrogryposis multiplex congenita* describes a group of congenital conditions characterized by joint contractures in two or more body areas. The precise cause may be unknown for some individuals but includes genetic, parental, and environmental factors as well as abnormalities during fetal development. Individuals with AMC have limited joint movement, with or without muscle weakness in the involved body areas. Contractures vary in distribution and severity, do not progress to previously unaffected joints, but may change over time due to growth and treatment. Spinal deformities may be present at birth or develop throughout childhood and adolescence. Depending on the underlying diagnosis, other body systems, such as the central nervous system (CNS), respiratory, gastrointestinal, and genitourinary systems, may be affected. Cognition may be affected if the CNS in involved; sensation is usually intact. The impact on mobility, activities of daily living (ADLs), and participation is variable (Cachecho et al., 2019; Dahan-Oliel, Cachecho, et al., 2019; Dahan-Oliel, van Bosse, et al., 2019).

Cause

Multiple causes have been suggested, including physical limitation of movement in the uterus, maternal disorders such as multiple sclerosis, or genetic disorder affecting the nervous, muscular, or vascular systems (Gagnon et al., 2019; Porter, 2018).

Evaluation/Assessment

Areas
- Activities of Daily Living/Instrumental ADL: eating, bathing, dressing (including managing socks, shoes, and fasteners), grooming, mobility, transfers, toileting, housekeeping, shopping, driving/transportation
- Education/Work: school and work accessibility, academic performance, work skills
- Play/Leisure: interests, abilities, choices
- Rest/Sleep: sleep disturbance
- Social Participation: home, school, community activities
- Sensorimotor: contractures, endurance, gross and fine motor skills, muscle strength, positioning of head and trunk, positioning of upper and lower extremities, range of motion, tendon reflexes, scoliosis, plagiocephaly, torticollis, pain (sensation is usually normal)
- Cognitive/Perceptual: generally, cognition and perception are within normal range
- Psychosocial: anxiety, body image, roles and role performance
- Context/Environment: family/caregivers, assistive devices, mobility devices, services available
- Development (Infant, Child, Adolescent only): developmental milestones, changes due to growth factors such as contractures and pain
- Comorbidities: CNS, respiratory, gastrointestinal, genitourinary systems (effect is variable from no involvement to severe)

Instruments
Instruments Developed by Occupational Therapy Personnel
- None identified

Instruments Developed by Other Professionals and Used by Occupational Therapy Personnel
- Alberta Infant Motor Scale (AIMS; Piper & Darrah, 1994)
- Bayley Scales of Infant and Toddler Development (4th ed.; Bayley-4; Bayley & Aylward, 2019)
- Face, Legs, Activity, Cry, and Consolability Pain Scale (FLACC Pain Scale; Merkel et al., 1997)
- Joint range of motion (goniometry; Shurtleff & Kaskutas, 2018)
- Patient Specific Functional Scale (PSFS; Strafford et al., 1995)
- Peabody Developmental Motor Scales (3rd ed.; PDMS-3; Folio & Fewell, 2023)

Problems/Issues

Activities of Daily Living/Instrumental ADL
- Infant/Toddler will have difficulty performing all self-care tasks, starting with self-feeding.
- Child will have difficulty performing some self-care tasks depending on the limitations of movement and strength (Joubert & Franzsen, 2016).
- All ages may have difficulty with mobility and transportation, including driving.

Education/Work
- Child may have difficulty performing school tasks.
- Child may have difficulty moving about the classroom and school facilities.
- Person may have difficulty with work skills that require dexterity and coordination.

Play/Leisure
- Infant/toddler may have difficulty manipulating toys and other objects.
- Child/adolescent may have difficulty engaging successfully in activities favored by siblings and friends, especially those with high movement demands.

Rest/Sleep
- Rest and sleep may be disturbed due to pain.
- Sleep may be disturbed due to lack of bed mobility, such as ability to roll over.

Social Participation
- Child/adolescent may have difficulty participating in activities favored by friends.
- Child/adolescent may feel excluded and left out of activities being enjoyed by others.
- Adult may self-exclude due to pain or lack of mobility.

Sensorimotor
- Infant will have limited range of motion with a firm, inelastic end point and lack of normal skin creases.
- Infant's head may be turned primarily to the right or left.
- Infant may have positional plagiocephaly (asymmetrical head shape).
- Infant may have diminished or absent deep tendon reflexes.
- Infant's upper extremities may present with adducted, internally rotated shoulders; extended or flexed elbows; pronated forearms; flexed wrists with ulnar deviation; fingers tend to be rigidly flexed and thumbs adducted (Azbell & Dannemiller, 2015).
- Infant may have poor strength in the biceps and brachialis muscles.
- Infant's lower extremities may present with variable positioning (some have flexed and dislocated hips and extended knees, others have abducted hips and abducted and externally rotated hips with flexed knees, and most will have clubfeet; Azbell & Dannemiller, 2015).
- Infant may have scoliosis of the spine.
- Infant may have torticollis.
- Child/adolescent may have poor endurance and experience fatigue.
- Child/adolescent/adult may experience contractures, especially in the knee joint.
- Child/adolescent/adult may experience musculoskeletal pain (Cirillo et al., 2019).
- Sensation (tactile, deep pressure) should be normal, but deep tendon reflexes may be diminished or absent.

Cognitive/Perceptual
- Should be within normal limits.

Psychosocial
- Child may experience anger and frustration at not being able to "keep up" with others.
- Child/adolescent may express concern about body image and being "different" than others.
- Adult may be limited in role performance.

Context/Environment
- Family may express difficulty in managing disabled child who requires frequent doctor visits and multiple surgeries.
- Family and friends may have limited or no knowledge about AMC.
- All ages: assistive and mobility devices may be needed; include access to resources, training, and care.
- All ages: information about community and internet resources may be needed.

Development
- Infant will be behind in attaining normal movement milestones, such as head up, rolling, crawling, and walking; static motor positions such as sitting and standing may be less delayed.
- Infant may have congenital heart disease
- Infant may have respiratory problems due to contractures in the rib cage or weak muscles of respiration.

Intervention/Treatment

Intervention for infants begins with remedial techniques focused on increasing joint range of motion, muscle strength, and endurance (biomechanical model; Azbell & Dannemiller, 2015). For the child and adolescent, compensatory and adapted techniques should be added to increase function and performance (Dalton & Hoyt-Hallett, 2013; Elfassy et al., 2019; Joubert & Franzsen, 2016). Most infants and children will require multiple orthopedic surgeries for upper and lower extremities to better align joints. Intervention after surgery should address facilitating function performance of the repositioned joint or joints (Lake & Oishi, 2015; Wall et al., 2017). Team members include physicians, orthopedic surgeons, plastic surgeons, nursing personnel, physical therapists, dentists, educators, family members, and occupational therapy personnel (Dahan-Oliel & Hall, 2019). Goals include preventing contractures, maintaining good body positions (especially elbows, wrists, knees, and feet), maintaining or increasing range of motion, improving hand function (reach, grasp, manipulate, release), and facilitating functional performance in ADLs.

Activities of Daily Living/Instrumental ADL
- Infant: Encourage participation in eating and self-feeding if elbow flexion to about 90 degrees can be obtained. Move to other self-care activities as range of motion permits.
- Child/Adolescent: Encourage performance of self-care activities. Try out compensatory techniques and assistive devices as child or adolescent is willing to accept. (Note: Children and adolescents are often creative in finding their own ways of completing self-care activities.)

Education/Work
- Assist school personnel and child in identifying problems that interfere with performing school activities in the classroom or building, such as limited joint range of motion, muscle weakness, pain, fatigue, lack of mobility, and barriers to access or other issues. Suggest and try out possible solutions.
- Assist child and adolescent to explore volunteer and potential work activities that are within their physical abilities.

Play/Leisure
- Assist in adapting toys and play activities to enable engagement. Remote controls may be useful.
- Assist child and adolescent to explore leisure activities that are within their ability, capacity, and interest.

Rest/Sleep
- Assist in identifying issues that interfere with sleep and make recommendations for changes, such as changes in position.

Social Participation
- Explore with child or adolescent what home, school, and community activities are available that are within the individual's ability, capacity, and interest.
- Assist the child or adolescent to practice participation if the individual requests.

Sensorimotor
- Strengthen postural muscles.
- Provide opportunity to practice fine motor activities.
- Maximize mobility for age-appropriate activities.
- Provide active range-of-motion exercises.
- Facilitate attainment of elbow flexion to 90 degrees by stretching, splinting, or surgical capsular release and triceps lengthening to allow performance of most self-care activities.
- Use hand splints to position finger–thumb opposition.
- Serial casting may assist in realigning ankles and wrists.
- Initiate a pain management program if pain is an issue.
- Initiate a fatigue management program, such as pacing alternate cycles of activity and rest.

Cognitive/Perceptual
- Encourage child or adolescent to engage in finding and trying out solutions to identified problems.

Psychosocial
- Focus on increasing/improving occupational performance.
- Allow child or adolescent to discuss concerns about "being different" and "being disabled."
- Suggest possible outlets for anger and frustration.

Context/Environment
- Provide a home program that includes directions for skin care, scar care, splint use and care, and home exercise program (see samples for elbow release and triceps transfer for elbow flexion in Lake & Oishi, 2015, p. 224).
- Provide information to family members and caregivers about AMC.

Precautions/Safety Considerations
No specific precautions or safety considerations were mentioned. However, contractures that limit mobility, especially in the knees, continue to be an ongoing problem, and musculoskeletal chronic pain is more often reported in adults (Cirillo et al., 2019).

Prognosis and Outcome
Most clients will be able to walk short distances, but may require mobility equipment to travel longer distances. Most can live in the community. Some may require home modification (Porter, 2018).

REFERENCES

Azbell, K., & Dannemiller, L. (2015). A case report of an infant with arthrogryposis. *Pediatric Physical Therapy*, *27*, 293–301. https://doi.org/10.1097/PEP.0000000000000148

Cachecho, S., Elfassy, C., Hamdy, R., Rosenbaum, P., & Dahan-Oliel, N. (2019). Arthrogryposis multiplex congenita definition: Update using an international consensus-based approach. *American Journal of Medical Genetics Part C: Seminars in Medical Genetics*, *181*(3), 280–287. https://doi.org/10.1002/ajmg.c.31739

Cirillo, A., Collins, J., Sawatzky, B., Hamdy, R., & Dahan-Oliel, N. (2019). Pain among children and adults living with arthrogryposis multiplex congenita: A scoping review. *American Journal of Medical Genetics Part C: Seminars in Medical Genetics*, *181*(3), 436–453. https://doi.org/10.1002/ajmg.c.31725

Dahan-Oliel, N., Cachecho, S., Barnes, D., Bedard, T., Davison, A. M., Dieterich, K., Donohoe, M., Fąfara, A., Hamdy, R., Hjartarson, H. T., Hoffman, N. S., Kimber, E., Komolkin, I., Lester, R., Pontén, E., van Bosse, H. J. P., & Hall, J. G. (2019). International multidisciplinary collaboration toward an annotated definition of arthrogryposis multiplex congenita. *American Journal of Medical Genetics Part C: Seminars in Medical Genetics*, *181*(3), 288–299. https://doi.org/10.1002/ajmg.c.31721

Dahan-Oliel, N., & Hall, J. G. (2019). Collaborating to advance interdisciplinary care for individuals with arthrogryposis. *American Journal of Medical Genetics Part C: Seminars in Medical Genetics*, *181*(3), 273–276. https://doi.org/10.1002/ajmg.c.31741

Dahan-Oliel, N., van Bosse, H. J. P., Bedard, T., Darsaklis, V. B., Hall, J. G., & Hamdy, R. C. (2019). Research platform for children with arthrogryposis multiplex congenita: Findings from the pilot registry. *American Journal of Medical Genetics Part C: Seminars in Medical Genetics*, *181*(3), 427–435. https://doi.org/10.1002/ajmg.c.31724

Dalton, C., & Hoyt-Hallett, G. (2013). Enablement through provision of assistive technology: Case reports of two children with physical disabilities. *British Journal of Occupational Therapy*, *76*(2), 108–111. https://doi.org/10.4276/030802213X13603244419356

Elfassy, C., Darsaklis, V. B., Snider, L., Gagnon, C., Hamdy, R., & Dahan-Oliel, N. (2019). Rehabilitation needs of youth with arthrogryposis multiplex congenita: Perspectives from key stakeholders. *Disability and Rehabilitation*, *42*(16), 2318–2324. https://doi.org/10.1080/09638288.2018.1559364

Gagnon, M., Caporuscio, K., Veilleux, L. N., Hamdy, R., & Dahan-Oliel, N. (2019). Muscle and joint function in children living with arthrogryposis multiplex congenita: A scoping review. *American Journal of Medical Genetics Part C: Seminars in Medical Genetics*, *181*(3), 410–426. https://doi.org/10.1002/ajmg.c.31726

Joubert, F., & Franzsen, D. (2016). Self-care of children with arthrogryposis in Gauteng, South Africa. *British Journal of Occupational Therapy*, *79*(1), 35–41. https://doi.org/10.1177/0308022615580327

Lake, A. L., & Oishi, S. N. (2015). Hand therapy following elbow release for passive elbow flexion and long head of the triceps transfer for active elbow flexion in children with amyoplasia. *Journal of Hand Therapy*, *28*(2), 222–227. https://doi.org/10.1016/j.jht.2014.10.007

O'Toole, M. T. (Ed.). (2017). *Mosby's dictionary of medicine, nursing & health professions* (10th ed.). Elsevier.

Porter, R. S. (Ed.). (2018). *The Merck manual of diagnosis and therapy* (20th ed.). Merck Sharp & Dohme.

Wall, L. B., Calhoun, V., Roberts, S., & Goldfarb, C. A. (2017). Distal humerus external rotation osteotomy for hand position in arthrogryposis. *Journal of Hand Surgery*, *42*(6), 473.E1–473.E7. https://doi.org/10.1016/j.jhsa.2017.03.002

Yang, S. S., Dahan-Oliel, N., Montpetit, K., & Hamdy, R. C. (2010). Ambulation gains after knee surgery in children with arthrogryposis. *Journal of Pediatric Orthopaedics*, *30*(8), 863–869. https://doi.org/10.1097/BPO.0b013e3181f5a0c8

Attention-Deficit/Hyperactivity Disorder
Also called ADHD, attention-deficit disorder (without hyperactivity),
minimal brain dysfunction, hyperkinesis.

Description

Attention-deficit/hyperactivity disorder (ADHD) is a syndrome of inattention, hyperactivity, and impulsivity. There are three types of ADHD—predominantly inattentive, predominantly hyperactive/impulsive, and combined. Attention-deficit/hyperactivity disorder is considered a neurodevelopmental disorder. Neurodevelopmental disorders are neurologically based conditions that appear early in childhood, typically before school entry, and impair development of personal, social, academic, and/or occupational functioning (Porter, 2018). ADHD is characterized by short attention span, hyperactivity, and poor concentration. Other symptoms may include impairment in perception, conceptualization, language, memory, and motor skills, along with increased impulsivity and emotional lability (O'Toole, 2017). Sensory overresponsivity and difficulty with sensory modulation have also been documented in both children and adults (Clince et al., 2016; Lane et al., 2012; Lane et al., 2010; Mimouni-Bloch et al., 2018; Mazor-Karsenty et al., 2015; Mazor-Karsenty et al., 2018; Yochman et al., 2013).

Cause

No single cause is known. Potential causes include genetic, biochemical, sensorimotor, physiological, and behavioral factors (Porter, 2018). Hypotheses include cortical activation dysregulation, cerebellar dysfunction, and delayed white matter maturation (Brossard-Racine et al., 2011). Formal criteria for a diagnosis of ADHD are listed in the *Diagnostic and Statistical Manual of Mental Disorders* (5th ed.; *DSM-5*; American Psychiatric Association, 2013).

Evaluation/Assessment

Areas

- Activities of Daily Living/Instrumental ADL: performing basic ADLs at age-appropriate level, functional mobility, communication skills
- Education/Work: academic performance (coloring, writing), classroom and school behavior (social interactions, toileting, hygiene)
- Play/Leisure: types of interests, location, frequency
- Rest/Sleep: sleep disturbances, sleep apnea
- Social Participation: type, location, frequency, with whom
- Sensorimotor: gross motor skills, fine motor skills, motor control (speed, accuracy), sensory processing
- Cognitive/Perceptual: attention, memory, executive function (mental flexibility)
- Psychosocial: hyperactivity, emotional and self-regulation (inhibition, impulsivity, irritability), depression, anxiety, quality of life
- Context/Environment: parent knowledge, social support, resources
- Development (Infant, Child, Adolescent only): developmental delay
- Comorbidities: learning disabilities, conduct disorder, neurofibromatosis 1, fragile X syndrome

Instruments

Instruments Developed by Occupational Therapy Personnel

- Assessment of Time Management Skills (ATMS; White et al., 2013)
- Canadian Occupational Performance Measure (5th ed.; COPM-5; Law et al., 2014)
- Children Activity Scales for Parents (ChAS-P; Rosenblum, 2006)
- Children's Assessment of Participation and Enjoyment (CAPE; King et al., 2004)
- Do-Eat (D-E; Josman et al., 2010; see Rosenblum et al., 2015, in References)
- Evaluation of Sensory Processing Questionnaire (ESP; Parham & Johnson-Ecker, 2002)
- KaTid–Child (Janeslätt et al., 2008)

- KaTid–Youth (Janeslätt, 2012)
- Participation in Childhood Occupations Questionnaire (PICO-Q; Bar-Shalita et al., 2009; see Bar-Ilan et al., 2018, in References)
- Pictorial Interview of Children's Metacognition and Executive Functions (PIC-ME; Maeir et al., 2014)
- Sensory Over-Responsivity Inventory (SensOR; Schoen et al., 2008)
- Sensory Processing Measure–Preschool (SPM-P; Miller Kuhaneck et al., 2010)
- Sensory Profile (2nd ed.; SP-2; Dunn, 2014)
- Teacher Social Validity Scale (TSVS; Fedewa & Erwin, 2011)
- Test of Playfulness (Version 4.2; ToP 4.2; Bundy, 2010)
- Time Self-Rating Scale (Time-S; Sköld & Janeslätt, 2017, in References)

Instruments Developed by Other Professionals and Used by Occupational Therapy Personnel

- ADHD Rating Scale-IV (ADHD-RS; DuPaul et al., 1998)
- Behavior Assessment System for Children (3rd ed., Preschool & Child; BASC-3; Reynolds & Kamphaus, 2015)
- Behavior Rating Inventory of Executive Function–Adult Version (BRIEF-A; Roth et al., 2005)
- Behavior Rating Inventory of Executive Function (2nd ed.; BRIEF-2; Gioia et al., 2015)
- Behavioural Assessment of the Dysexecutive Syndrome in Children (BADS-C; Emslie et al., 2003)
- Bruininks-Oseretsky Test of Motor Proficiency (BOT-2; Bruininks & Bruininks, 2005)
- Children's Color Trails Test (CCTT; Llorente et al., 2003)
- Cognitive Assessment System (2nd ed.; CAS2; Naglieri et al., 2014)
- Cognitive-Functional Evaluation (CFE) Battery (Stern & Maier, 2014, in References)
- Conners' Continuous Performance Test (3rd ed.; CCPT 3; Conners, 2014)
- Conners' Parent Rating Scale–Revised (CPRS-R; Conners et al., 1998)
- Disruptive Behavior Disorders Rating Scale (DBDRS; Silva et al., 2005)
- Fabric Prickliness Test (FPT; Garnsworthy et al., 1988)
- Goal Attainment Scaling (GAS; Kiresuk & Sherman, 1968)
- Movement Assessment Battery for Children (2nd ed.; M-ABC-2; Henderson et al., 2007)
- NEPSY: Developmental Neuropsychological Assessment (2nd ed.; NEPSY-II; Korkman et al., 2007)
- Pediatric Quality of Life Inventory (PedsQL 4.0; Varni et al., 2001)
- Physical and Neurological Examination for Soft Signs (PANESS; Werry & Aman, 1976)
- Pursuit Test (PT; Huijbregts et al., 2003)
- Raven's Progressive Matrices and Vocabulary Scales (RPMVS; Raven et al., 1998)
- Revised Childhood Manifest Anxiety Scale (2nd ed.; RCMAS-2; Reynolds & Richmond, 2008)
- Service for Children and Adolescents–Parent Interview (SCAPI; Jensen et al., 2004)
- Test of Everyday Attention for Children (2nd ed.; TEA-Ch2; Manly et al., 2016)
- Tool to Measure Parenting Self-Efficacy (TOPSE; Bloomfield et al., 2010)
- Tower of London (ToL; Shallice, 1982)
- Von Frey filaments (pinprick pain test; Smith & Nephew Rolyan, Inc.)
- Wechsler Intelligence Scale for Children (5th ed.; WISC-V; Wechsler, 2014)
- Weiss Functional Impairment Rating Scale (WFIRS; Weiss, 2000)
- World Health Organization Adult ADHD Self-Report Scale (ASRS; Kessler et al., 2005)

Problems/Issues

Activities of Daily Living/Instrumental ADL

- Child may need more assistance to complete basic ADLs than other children the same age (fasteners, orienting clothing for back or front, left or right, inside or outside).
- Adolescent or adult may experience difficulty learning driving skills (Almberg et al., 2017; Classen & Monahan, 2013; Poulsen et al., 2010).

Education/Work
- Child may have difficulty completing assignments.
- Child may have difficulty remaining seated during class.
- Child may talk excessively and may have difficulty being quiet in the classroom.
- Child may interrupt others during classroom discussions.
- Child may resist work (assignments) that requires effort (are not easy for child to do).
- Adolescents or adults may experience challenges in complying with job demands (Schreuer & Dorot, 2017).
- Adolescents or adults may have difficulty reading the "social map" (hierarchy, rules, and expectations) in the workplace (Schreuer & Dorot, 2017).

Play/Leisure
- Child may have difficulty playing quietly.
- Child may have difficulty engaging in cooperative play activities that require taking turns (waiting his or her turn).
- Child may try to dominate play activity to control others and toys or equipment.

Rest/Sleep
- Child may have sleep disturbances: difficulty going to and staying asleep.

Social Participation
- Child may have difficulty participating appropriately in social activities with peers.

Sensorimotor
- Child may be delayed in motor development (gross and fine motor skills; de Oliveira et al., 2018; Lavasani & Stagnitti, 2011; Pila-Nemutandani et al., 2018).
- Child may demonstrate difficulty with motor control (I. C. Lee et al., 2010).
- Child, adolescent, or adult may have difficulty with sensory processing, especially with strong auditory or visual stimuli (oversensitivity).

Cognitive/Perceptual
- Child may have difficulty maintaining attention.
- Child may be disorganized (messy, sloppy).
- Child may be easily distracted.
- Child may be "accident prone" due to accelerated movement without adequate cognitive judgment of safety.
- Child may act before thinking of possible consequences of action.
- Child may be forgetful (leaving tasks undone or jackets and sweaters at school).
- Child may have difficulty listening to and remembering instructions.
- Child may have difficulty with cognitive and mental flexibility (changing from one task to another in rapid succession or from one environment to another).
- Child may have difficulty paying attention to details.
- Child may have difficulty with time management.
- Child may have difficulty with organization skills.
- Child may have difficulty with metacognition (Shimoni et al., 2012).

Psychosocial
- Child may demonstrate fidgeting especially when seated or waiting in line.
- Child, adolescent, or adult may demonstrate difficulty with emotional and self-regulation (Schreuer & Dorot, 2017; Shimoni et al., 2012).
- Child may be easily frustrated and quit trying if performing task is not easy to do.
- Child may become depressed and anxious.
- Child may have decreased quality of life (Boojari et al., 2016).

- Adolescent or adult may experience difficulty achieving occupational identity and sense of competence (Altit et al., 2019).
- Adolescent or adult may have decreased self-identity.

Context/Environment
- Parents may lack knowledge about ADHD and its management.
- Parents may lack information about resources available in the school, community, or internet.
- Parents or caregivers may lack knowledge of child behavior and management techniques.

Intervention/Treatment

Four categories of intervention appear in the literature: cognition, motor, play, and sensory (Nielsen et al., 2017). Models and programs developed by occupational therapy personnel include Cognitive-Functional (Cog-Fun) Dyadic Intervention (Hahn-Markowitz et al., 2017; Hahn-Markowitz et al., 2018; Hahn-Markowitz et al., 2011; Maeir et al., 2014; Rosenberg et al., 2015), Cognitive Orientation to Daily Occupational Performance (CO-OP; Gharebaghy et al., 2015), cognitive rehabilitation (Cermak, 2018), home-based sensorimotor program (Kim, 2018), metronome training (Park & Choi, 2017), play-based program (Allan et al., 2018; Cantrill et al., 2015; Cordier et al., 2010a, 2010b; Wilkes et al., 2011; Wilkes-Gillan et al., 2014a, 2014b), sensory diet (Sahoo & Senapati, 2014), time management (Sköld & Janeslätt, 2017; Wennberg et al., 2018), and weighted vests (Buckle et al., 2011; Lin et al., 2014). Models and programs developed by other professionals but used by occupational therapy personnel include cognitive assistive technology (Lindstedt & Umb-Carlsson, 2013), mindfulness (C. S. C. Lee et al., 2017), Montessori classroom (Luborsky, 2017), play-based intervention (Wilkes-Gillan et al., 2016), and stability balls (Fedewa & Erwin, 2011). Team members include physicians, psychologists, educators, parents and caregivers, physical therapy personnel, and occupational therapy personnel. The goal is to improve the ability to participate successfully in home, school, work, and community life.

Activities of Daily Living/Instrumental ADL
- Consider simplifying dressing tasks by reducing use of fasteners, including buttons, zippers, tying shoelaces, and snaps. Recommend clothing without fasteners or use Velcro-type fasteners to reduce frustration and time in dressing.
- Suggest laying out or selecting clothes the night before to reduce time in selection in the morning.
- Suggest using a handheld shower rather than bathing to reduce time and effort during the week (bathing on weekends may be possible when the schedule is less tight).
- Pictures and a checklist of what to wear may help focus attention.

Education/Work
- Assist teacher to determine which techniques may be most useful: sensory modification, time management, environmental modification, classroom organization, modified curriculum, and increased use of support prompts (human and symbolic).
- Use of pictures and time schedules of daily classroom and school activities can help focus attention and reduce anxiety.
- Explore different types of prompts to focus attention to specific tasks (different colors, horizontal or vertical line markers, geometric symbols, verbal reminders, computer and smartphone apps).
- Explore use of work simplification and activity analysis to break down tasks into manageable units to increase performance.
- Use environmental modifications to control sensory input, including seating arrangements that reduce extraneous stimuli and provide ready access for teacher or teacher's aide to assist when needed.

Play/Leisure
- Structure play activities such as use of play and amusement centers.
- Provide supervised play situations.
- Support development of leisure occupations.

Rest/Sleep
- Develop sleep habits and routine (specific bedtime hour, specific tasks to do before going to bed).
- Consider sleep environment: type of bedding; type of sleepwear; sensory control of light, sound, temperature, and location of other sleepers, including children and adults.

Social Participation
- Provide supervised and structured social activities.
- Assist parents and caregivers in providing structured social activity experiences.

Sensorimotor
- Increase opportunity to engage in physical motor activities at home, school, and in the community (scheduled time may be needed for focus on gross motor and fine motor activities).
- Consider sensory modification techniques.
  - ▶ Visual: Decrease distractors, increase use of walls or dividers to reduce visual input, decrease overhead lighting, use more focused lighting, provide visual cues and reminders of lesson assignments.
  - ▶ Auditory: Decrease extraneous noise, use noise-canceling headphones, place workspace in quietest place in room.
  - ▶ Proprioception: Increase input through use of weighted-ball activities, using a rolling pin, walking a line carrying a weighted tray, water activities, working with modeling clay, indoor or outdoor gardening tasks.

Cognitive/Perceptual
- Provide a daily schedule using pictures or photos and labels.
- Use time management strategies, including verbal or auditory signals when events are about to change.
- Make sure child knows the purpose and conditions of each task or activity.
- Assist client to identify activities that are fun, inspiring, and demanding (Ek & Isaksson, 2013).
- Assist client to set achievable goals and steps to attain the goal.

Psychosocial
- Fidget items (bracelets, spinners, tops) may help reduce anxiety.
- Reward success and achievement based on rewards selected by the child.

Context/Environment
- Provide parents and caregivers with information on ADHD and its management.
- Provide family and caregivers with access to school, community, and internet resources.
- Encourage family, caregivers, teachers, supervisors, and others to provide social support.
- Consider environmental organization at home, school, and the community (designate study space; specify places and spaces for different types of toys, games, bikes, etc.; designate times to cleanup and organize, such as before dinner or as part of a bedtime routine).

Precautions/Safety Considerations
Child may need additional monitoring to prevent accidents.

Prognosis and Outcome
There is no known cure. Symptoms may subside or disappear in some children but can continue into adolescence and adulthood.

Cost Effectiveness

In Germany, occupational therapy services are a major cost item for the treatment of ADHD (Braun et al., 2013). A study in New York City found no benefit of rehabilitation services (Mlodnicka et al., 2016).

REFERENCES
Child

Allan, N., Wilkes-Gillan, S., Bundy, A., Cordier, R., & Volkert, A. (2018). Parents' perspectives of the long-term appropriateness of psychosocial intervention for children with attention deficit hyperactivity disorder. *Australian Occupational Therapy Journal, 65*(4), 259–267. https://doi.org/10.1111/1440-1630.12460

American Psychiatric Association. (2013). *Diagnostic and statistical manual of mental disorders* (5th ed.). https://doi.org/10.1176/appi.books.9780890425596

Bar-Ilan, R. T., Cohen, N., & Maeir, A. (2018). Comparison of children with and without ADHD on a new pictorial self-assessment of executive functions. *American Journal of Occupational Therapy, 72*(3), Article 7203205040. https://doi.org/10.5014/ajot.2018.021485

Boojari, S., Haghgoo, H., Rostami, R., Ghanbari, S., & Nematollahi, S. (2016). Relationship between quality of life and cognitive function in school aged children with attention deficit and hyperactivity disorder. *Journal of Research & Health, 6*(3), 345–354. https://doi.org/10.7508/jrh.2016.03.008

Braun, S., Zeidler, J., Linder, R., Engel, S., Verheyen, F., & Greiner, W. (2013). Treatment costs of attention deficit hyperactivity disorder in Germany. *European Journal of Health Economics, 14*, 939–945. https://doi.org/10.1007/s10198-012-0440-5

Brossard-Racine, M., Majnemer, A., & Shevell, M. I. (2011). Exploring the neural mechanisms that underlie motor difficulties in children with attention deficit hyperactivity disorder. *Developmental Neurorehabilitation, 14*(2), 101–111. https://doi.org/10.3109/17518423.2010.547545

Buckle, F., Franzsen, D., & Bester, J. (2011). The effect of the wearing of weighted vests on the sensory behavior of learners diagnosed with attention deficit hyperactivity disorder within a school context. *South African Journal of Occupational Therapy, 41*(3), 36–42.

Cantrill, A., Wilkes-Gillan, S., Bundy, A., Cordier, R., & Wilson, N. J. (2015). An eighteen-month follow-up of a pilot parent-delivered play-based intervention to improve the social play skills of children with attention deficit hyperactivity disorder and their playmates. *Australian Occupational Therapy Journal, 62*, 197–207. https://doi.org/10.1111/1440-1630.12203

Cermak, S. A. (2018). Cognitive rehabilitation of children and adults with attention deficit hyperactivity disorder. In N. Katz & J. Toglia (Eds.), *Cognition, occupation, and participation across the lifespan* (4th ed., pp. 189–217). AOTA Press. https://doi.org/10.7139/2017.978-1-56900-479-1

Cordier, R., Bundy, A., Hocking, C., & Einfeld, S. (2010a). Comparison of the play of children with attention deficit hyperactivity disorder by subtypes. *Australian Occupational Therapy Journal, 57*, 137–145. https://doi.org/10.1111/j.1440-1630.2009.00821.x

Cordier, R., Bundy, A., Hocking, C., & Einfeld, S. (2010b). Playing with a child with ADHD: A focus on the playmates. *Scandinavian Journal of Occupational Therapy, 17*(3), 191–199. https://doi.org/10.3109/11038120903156619

de Oliveira, C. C., Neto, J. L. C., & Palhares, M. S. (2018). Motor characteristics of students with attention deficit hyperactivity disorder. *Cadernos de Brasileiros Terapia Ocupacional, 26*(3), 590–600.

Fedewa, A., & Erwin, H. E. (2011). Stability balls and students with attention and hyperactivity concerns: Implications for on-task and in-seat behavior. *American Journal of Occupational Therapy, 65*(4), 393–399. https://doi.org/10.5014/ajot.2011.000554

Gharebaghy, S., Rassafiani, M., & Cameron, D. (2015). Effect of cognitive intervention on children with ADHD. *Physical & Occupational Therapy in Pediatrics, 35*(1), 13–23. https://doi.org/10.3109/01942638.2014.957428

Hahn-Markowitz, J., Berger, I., Manor, I., & Maeir, A. (2017). Impact of the cognitive-functional (Cog-Fun) intervention on executive functions and participation among children with attention deficit hyperactivity disorder: A randomized controlled trial. *American Journal of Occupational Therapy, 71*(5), Article 7105220010p1–7105220010p9. https://doi.org/10.5014/ajot.2017.022053

Hahn-Markowitz, J., Berger, I., Manor, I., & Maeir, A. (2018). Cognitive-functional (Cog-Fun) dyadic intervention for children with ADHD and their parents: Impact on parenting self-efficacy. *Physical & Occupational Therapy in Pediatrics, 38*(4), 444–456. https://doi.org/10.1080/01942638.2018.1441939

Hahn-Markowitz, J., Manor, I., & Maeir, A. (2011). Effectiveness of cognitive-functional (Cog-Fun) intervention with children with attention deficit hyperactivity disorder: A pilot study. *American Journal of Occupational Therapy, 65*(4), 384–392. https://doi.org/10.5014/ajot.2011.000901

Kim, J.-K. (2018). The effects of a home-based sensorimotor program on executive and motor functions in children with ADHD: A case series. *Journal of Physical Therapy Science, 30*(8), 1138–1140. https://doi.org/10.1589/jpts.30.1138

Lane, S. J., Reynolds, S., & Dumenci, L. (2012). Sensory overresponsivity and anxiety in typically developing children and with autism and attention deficit hyperactivity disorder: Cause or coexistence? *American Journal of Occupational Therapy, 66*(5), 595–603. https://doi.org/10.5014/ajot.2012.004523

Lane, S. J., Reynolds, S., & Thacker, L. (2010). Sensory over-responsivity and ADHD: Differentiating using electrodermal responses, cortisol, and anxiety. *Frontiers in Integrative Neuroscience, 4*, Article 8. https://doi.org/10.3389/fnint.2010.00008

Lavasani, M. N., & Stagnitti, K. (2011). A study on fine motor skills of Iranian children with attention deficit/hyperactivity disorder aged from 6 to 11 years. *Occupational Therapy International, 18*, 106–114. https://doi.org/10.1002/oti.306

Lee, I.-C., Hung, C.-C., Yang, W.-H., Chen-Sea, M.-J., & Tsai, C.-L. (2010). The pursuit flexibility of children with attention-deficit/hyperactive disorder. *Medical and Health Science Journal, 4*, 8–17.

Lin, H.-Y., Lee, P., Chang, W.-D., & Hong, F.-Y. (2014). Effects of weighted vests on attention, impulse control, and on-task behavior in children with attention deficit hyperactivity disorder. *American Journal of Occupational Therapy, 68*(2), 149–158. https://doi.org/10.5014/ajot.2014.009365

Luborsky, B. (2017). Helping children with attentional challenges in a Montessori classroom: The role of the occupational therapist. *NAMTA Journal, 42*(2), 287–352.

Maeir, A., Fisher, O., Bar-Ilan, R. T., Boas, N., Berger, I., & Landau, Y. E. (2014). Effectiveness of cognitive-functional (Cog-Fun) occupational therapy intervention for young children with attention deficit hyperactivity disorder: A controlled study. *American Journal of Occupational Therapy, 68*(3), 260–267. https://doi.org/10.5014/ajot.2014.011700

Mimouni-Bloch, A., Offek, H., Rosenblum, S., Posener, I., Silman, Z., & Engel-Yeger, B. (2018). Association between sensory modulation and daily activity function of children with attention deficit/hyperactivity disorder and children with typical development. *Research in Developmental Disabilities, 83*, 69–76. https://doi.org/10.1016/j.ridd.2018.08.002

Mlodnicka, A. E., O'Neill, S., Marks, D. J., Rajendran, K., Bedard, A. C. V., Schneiderman, R. L., Basu, B., & Halperin, J. M. (2016). Impact of occupation, physical, and speech and language therapy in preschoolers with hyperactive/inattention symptoms: A naturalistic 2-year follow-up study. *Children's Health Care, 45*(1), 67–83. https://doi.org/10.1080/02739615.2014.979918

Nielsen, S. K., Kelsch, K., & Miller, K. (2017). Occupational therapy interventions for children with attention deficit hyperactivity disorder: A systematic review. *Occupational Therapy in Mental Health, 33*(1), 70–80. https://doi.org/10.1080/0164212X.2016.1211060

O'Toole, M. T. (Ed.). (2017). *Mosby's dictionary of medicine, nursing & health professions* (10th ed.). Elsevier.

Park, Y.-Y., & Choi, Y.-J. (2017). Effects of interactive metronome training on timing, attention, working memory, and processing speed in children with ADHD: A case study of two children. *Journal of Physical Therapy Science, 29*(12), 2165–2167. https://doi.org/10.1589/jpts.29.2165

Pila-Nemutandani, G. R., Pillay, B. J., & Meyer, A. (2018). Gross motor skills in children with attention deficit hyperactivity disorder. *South African Journal of Occupational Therapy, 48*(3), 19–23. http://dx.doi.org/10.17159/2310-3833/2017/vol48n3a4

Porter, R. S. (Ed.). (2018). *The Merck manual of diagnosis and therapy* (20th ed.). Merck Sharp & Dohme.

Rosenberg, L., Maier, A., Yochman, A., Dahan, I., & Hirsch, I. (2015). Effectiveness of a cognitive-functional group intervention among preschoolers with attention deficit hyperactivity disorder: A pilot study. *American Journal of Occupational Therapy, 69*(3), Article 6903220040. https://doi.org/10.5014/ajot.2015.014795

Rosenblum, S., Frisch, C., Deutsh-Castel, T., & Josman, N. (2015). Daily functioning profile of children with attention deficit hyperactive disorder: A pilot study using an ecological assessment. *Neuropsychological Rehabilitation, 25*(3), 402–418. https://doi.org/10.1080/09602011.2014.940980

Sahoo, S. K., & Senapati, A. (2014). Effect of sensory diet through outdoor play on functional behavior in children with ADHD. *Indian Journal of Occupational Therapy, 46*(2), 49–54.

Shimoni, M., Engel-Yeger, G., & Tirosh, E. (2012). Executive dysfunctions among boys with attention deficit hyperactivity disorder (ADHD): Performance-based test and parents report. *Research in Developmental Disabilities, 33*(3), 858–865. https://doi.org/10.1016/j.ridd.2011.12.014

Sköld, A., & Janeslätt, G. K. (2017). Self-rating of daily time management in children: Psychometric properties of the Time-S. *Scandinavian Journal of Occupational Therapy, 24*(3), 178–186. https://doi.org/10.1080/11038128.2016.1185465

Wennberg, B., Janeslätt, G., Kjellberg, A., & Gustafsson, P. A. (2018). Effectiveness of time-related interventions in children with ADHD aged 9-15 years: A randomized controlled study. *European Child & Adolescent Psychiatry, 27*, 329–342. https://doi.org/10.1007/s00787-017-1052-5

Wilkes, S., Cordier, R., Bundy, A., Docking, K., & Munro, N. (2011). A play-based intervention for children with ADHD: A pilot study. *Australian Occupational Therapy Journal, 58*(4), 231–240. https://doi.org/10.1111/j.1440-1630.2011.00928.x

Wilkes-Gillan, S., Bundy, A., Cordier, R., & Lincoln, M. (2014a). Eighteen-month follow-up of a play-based intervention to improve the social play skills of children with attention deficit hyperactivity disorder. *Australian Occupational Therapy Journal, 61*(5), 299–307. https://doi.org/10.1111/1440-1630.12124

Wilkes-Gillan, S., Bundy, A., Cordier, R., & Lincoln, M. (2014b). Evaluation of a pilot parent-delivered play-based intervention for children with attention deficit hyperactivity disorder. *American Journal of Occupational Therapy, 68*(6), 700–798. https://doi.org/10.5014/ajot.2014.012450

Wilkes-Gillan, S., Bundy, A., Cordier, R., Lincoln, M., & Chen, Y.-W. (2016). A randomised controlled trail of a play-based intervention to improve the social play skills of children with attention deficit hyperactivity disorder (ADHD). *PLOS ONE, 11*(8), Article e0160228. https://doi.org/10.1371/journal.pone.0160558

Yochman, A., Alon-Beery, O., Sribman, A., & Parush, S. (2013). Differential diagnosis of sensory modulation disorder (SMD) and attention deficit hyperactivity disorder (ADHD): Participation, sensation, and attention. *Frontiers in Human Neuroscience, 7*, Article 862. https://doi.org/10.3389/fnhum.2013.00862

Adolescent and Adult

Almberg, M., Selander, H., Falkmer, M., Vaz, S., Ciccarelli, M., & Falkmer. T. (2017). Experiences of facilitators or barriers in driving education from learner and novice drivers with ADHD or ASD and their driving instructors. *Developmental Neurorehabilitation, 20*(2), 59–67. https://doi.org/10.3109/17518423.2015.1058299

Altit, T. P., Shor, R., & Maeir, A. (2019). Occupational identity, competence, and environments among adults with and without attention deficit hyperactivity disorder. *Occupational Therapy in Mental Health, 35*(2), 205–215. https://doi.org/10.1080/0164212X.2019.1588833

Cermak, S. A. (2018). Cognitive rehabilitation of children and adults with attention deficit hyperactivity disorder. In N. Katz & J. Toglia (Eds.), *Cognition, occupation, and participation across the lifespan* (4th ed., pp. 189–217). AOTA Press.

Classen, S., & Monahan, M. (2013). Evidence-based review on interventions and determinants of driving performance in teens with attention deficit hyperactivity disorder or autism spectrum disorder. *Traffic Injury Prevention, 14*(2), 188–193. https://doi.org/10.1080/15389588.2012.700747

Clince, M., Connolly, L., & Nolan, C. (2016). Comparing and exploring the sensory processing patterns of higher education students with attention deficit hyperactivity disorder and autism spectrum disorder. *American Journal of Occupational Therapy, 70*(2), Article 7002250010. https://doi.org/10.5014/ajot.2016.016816

Ek, A., & Isaksson, G. (2013). How adults with ADHD get engaged in and perform everyday activities. *Scandinavian Journal of Occupational Therapy, 20*(4), 282–291. https://doi.org/10.3109/11038128.2013.799226

Lee, C. S. C., Ma, M.-T., Ho, H.-Y., Tsang, K.-K., Zheng, Y.-Y., & Wu, Z.-Y. (2017). The effectiveness of mindfulness-based intervention in attention on individuals with ADHD: A systematic review. *Hong Kong Journal of Occupational Therapy, 30*(1), 33–41. https://doi.org/10.1016/j.hkjot.2017.05.001

Lindstedt, H., & Umb-Carlsson, Ö. (2013). Cognitive assistive technology and professional support in everyday life for adults with ADHD. *Disability and Rehabilitation: Assistive Technology, 8*(5), 402–408. https://doi.org/10.3109/17483107.2013.769120

Mazor-Karsenty, T., Parush, S., Bonneh, Y., & Shalev, L. (2015). Comparing the executive attention of adult females with ADHD to that of females with sensory modulation disorder (SMD) under aversive and non-aversive auditory conditions. *Research in Developmental Disabilities, 37*(1), 17–30. https://doi.org/10.1016/j.ridd.2014.10.041

Mazor-Karsenty, T., Shalev, L., Parush, S., & Bonneh, Y. (2018). Perception of aversive auditory stimuli is different in sensory modulation disorders and attention deficit hyperactivity disorder. *American Journal of Occupational Therapy, 72*(6), Article 7206205020. https://doi.org/10.5014/ajot.2018.022327

Poulsen, A. A., Horswill, M. S., Wetton, M. A., Hill, A., & Lim, S. M. (2010). A brief office-based hazard perception intervention for drivers with ADHD symptoms. *Australian and New Zealand Journal of Psychiatry, 44*(6), 528–534. https://doi.org/10.3109/00048671003596048

Schreuer, N., & Dorot, R. (2017). Experiences of employed women with attention deficit hyperactive disorder: A phenomenological study. *Work, 56*(3), 429–441. https://doi.org/10.3233/WOR-172509

Stern, A., & Maeir, A. (2014). Validating the measurement of executive functions in an occupational context for adults with attention deficit hyperactivity disorder. *American Journal of Occupational Therapy, 68*(6), 719–728. https://doi.org/10.5014/ajot.2014.012419

BIBLIOGRAPHY

Frolek Clark, G. (2019). Best practices in supporting students with attention deficit hyperactivity disorder. In G. Frolek Clark, J. E. Rioux, & B. E. Chandler (Eds.). *Best practices for occupational therapy in schools* (2nd ed., pp. 227–235). AOTA Press. https://doi.org/10.7139/2019.978-1-56900-591-0

Janeslätt, G. K., Holmqvist, K. L., White, S., & Holmefur, M. (2018). Assessment of time management skills: Psychometric properties of the Swedish version. *Scandinavian Journal of Occupational Therapy, 25*(3), 153–161. https://doi.org/10.1080/11038128.2017.1375009

Linder, N., Kroyzer, N., Maeir, A., Wertman-Elad, R., & Pollak, Y. (2010). Do ADHD and executive dysfunctions, measured by the Hebrew version of Behavior Rating Inventory of Executive Functions (BRIEF), completely overlap? *Child Neuropsychology, 16*(5), 494–502. https://doi.org/10.1080/09297041003781884

Mulligan, S. (2017). Attention deficit disorder. In B. J. Atchison & D. P. Dirette (Eds.), *Conditions in occupational therapy* (5th ed., pp. 83–100). Kluwer.

Pfeifer, L. I., Terra, L. N., dos Santos, J. L. F., Stagnitti, K. E., & Panúncio-Pinto, M. P. (2011). Play preference of children with ADHD and typically developing children in Brazil: A pilot study. *Australian Occupational Therapy Journal, 58*(6), 419–428. https://doi.org/10.1111/j.1440-1630.2011.00973.x

Poulsen, A. A. (2011). Children with attention deficit hyperactivity disorder, developmental coordination disorder, and learning disabilities. In S. Bazyk (Ed.), *Mental health promotion, prevention, and intervention with children and youth* (pp. 231–266). AOTA Press.

Rosenblum, S., & Yom-Tov, E. (2017). Seeking web-based information about attention deficit hyperactivity disorder: Where, what, and when. *Journal of Medical Internet Research, 19*(4), Article e126. https://doi.org/10.2196/jmir.6579

Autism Spectrum Disorder (ASD): Adolescent and Adult

Description

Autism spectrum disorder (ASD) is a neurodevelopmental disorder characterized by persistent deficits in social communication and interaction; restricted, repetitive patterns of behaviors, interests, or activities; and uneven intellectual development (American Psychiatric Association, 2013; Porter, 2018).

Cause

The specific cause in most cases is unknown, but a genetic component appears to be involved (Porter, 2018).

Evaluation/Assessment

Areas

- Activities of Daily Living/Instrumental ADL: communication skills, medication management, driving
- Education/Work: work history, work habits and style
- Play/Leisure: interests, frequency, type
- Rest/Sleep: sleep habits and routines
- Social Participation: social interactions, types of social activities, frequency, location
- Sensorimotor: sensory responsiveness
- Cognitive/Perceptual: executive functions, visual acuity and perception
- Psychosocial: stereotypical, repetitive behaviors
- Context/Environment: social support, family and caregiver knowledge, community and internet resources
- Comorbidities: seizure or epilepsy disorders, diabetes, bowel disorders and diseases, depression, anxiety, psychosis, obsessive-compulsive disorder, intellectual disability, and attention-deficit/hyperactivity disorder

Instruments

Instruments Developed by Occupational Therapy Personnel

- Adolescent/Adult Sensory Profile (AASP; Brown & Dunn, 2002)
- Assessment of Communication and Interaction Skills (Version 4.0; ACIS; Forsyth et al., 1998)
- Assessment of Motor and Process Skills (8th ed.; AMPS-8; Fisher & Bray Jones, 2016)
- Autism Work Skills Questionnaire (AWSQ; Gal et al., 2013, in References)
- Integrated Employment Success Tool (IEST; Scott et al., 2018, in References)

Instruments Developed by Other Professionals and Used by Occupational Therapy Personnel

- 2 Meter 2000 Series Revised ETDRS Chart (visual acuity; Precision Vision, n.d.)
- Autism Quotient Short Form (AQ-S; Hoekstra et al., 2011)
- Behavior Problem Inventory (BPI; Rojahn et al., 2013)
- Continuous Performance Test (CPT; Rosvold et al., 1956)
- Environmental Job Assessment Measure (E-JAM; Waintrup & Kelley, 1999)
- Leisure Satisfaction Scale (LSS; Beard & Ragheb, 1980)
- Life Assessment Scale for the Mentally Ill (LASMI; Iwasaki et al., 1994)
- Patient Health Questionnaire-9 (PHQ-9; Löwe et al., 2004)
- Schizophrenia Cognition Rating Scale (SCoRS; Keefe et al., 2006)
- Severity Measure for Generalized Anxiety Disorder–Adult (Craske et al., 2013)
- Social Responsiveness Scale (2nd ed.; SRS-2; Constantino, 2012)
- Wisconsin Card Sort Test (WCST; Heaton et al., 1993)

Problems/Issues

Activities of Daily Living/Instrumental ADL

- Person may have difficulty fitting clothing to weather situation or to requirements for work assignments.
- Person may eat substances with no nutritional value or may be diagnosed with pica.
- Person may have difficulty with money management.
- Person may have difficulty managing sexual expression.
- Person may have difficulty using public transportation.
- Person may have difficulty getting a driver's license because of difficulty performing in multi-tasking and complex driving tasks, consistently maintaining a safe speed, decreased maneuvering ability, and increased response time to traffic hazards (Chee et al., 2017, 2019; Classen & Monahan, 2013).

Education/Work

- Person may have difficulty gaining or maintaining employment (Harmuth et al., 2018).
- Person may require constant supervision and thus may not be able to work independently.
- Person may have difficulty following directions regarding work assignments.
- Person may have difficulty adjusting to changes at work such as changes in job assignment.
- Person may need to develop work habits and routines.
- Person may have difficulty cooperating with colleagues in work environment.

Play/Leisure

- Person usually has a restricted repertoire of interests and activities.
- Person may engage primarily in solitary leisure activities (Stacey et al., 2019).

Rest/Sleep

- Person may have sleep disturbances.

Social Participation

- Person may avoid social situations due to overstimulation, which may limit social participation.
- Person may avoid visiting family or friends, attending sporting or cultural events, or using social media.

Sensorimotor

- Person may have poor postural control that results in poor postural responses to maintain body balance required for the task or environmental demands.
- Person may be overresponsive or under-responsive to sensory stimuli including sound, vision, touch, movement, taste, and smell.
- Person may have difficulty prioritizing visual information in the central visual field over visual information in the peripheral visual field, especially in unfamiliar environments (Lim et al., 2018a, 2018b).
- Person may be under-responsive to pain.
- Person may engage in self-stimulating behavior.

Cognitive/Perceptual

- Person may have difficulty maintaining attention and concentration.
- Person may have difficulty with time management.
- Person may have difficulty judging issues of safety.

Psychosocial

- Person may display aggressive behavior.
- Person may experience depression.
- Person may have tantrums or "meltdowns."
- Person may incur self-injury.
- Person may experience loneliness and social isolation.

Context/Environment

- Person may lack social support.
- Person may lack access to or be unfamiliar with community resources.
- Person may avoid certain environments due to hypersensitivity.
- Person may display inappropriate behavior in public such as touching genitals.
- Person may experience discrimination in hiring due to diagnosis and lack of knowledge of employers about ASD even though the person has excellent technical and vocational skills. Advocacy may be needed.
- Family members may complain that they are unable to control the person's behavior.

Intervention/Treatment

Models of practice and programs developed by occupational therapy personnel include CO-OP approach (Wilson et al., 2018), deep pressure (Bestbier & Williams, 2017), Dunn's model of sensory processing (Metz et al., 2019), Integrated Employment Success Tool (IEST; Scott et al., 2018; Scott et al., 2015), patient passport program (Francis, 2019), PhotoVoice program (Krutt et al., 2018), and sensory motorway program (Keeble, 2014). Models of practice programs developed by other professionals but used by occupational therapy personnel include autistic spectrum conditions team (Gasson, 2018a, 2018b). Better OutcOmes & Successful Transitions for Autism (BOOST-A; Hatfield, Falkmer, et al., 2017, 2018; Hatfield, Murray, et al., 2017), behavior approaches (Koegel et al., 2014), driver education (Almberg et al., 2017), frontal executive program (Miyajima et al., 2018), and transition planning and programming (Swami-nathan, 2015; Thompson et al., 2018a, 2018b; Turcotte et al., 2015). Team members include physicians, nursing personnel, social workers, psychologists, vocational rehabilitation counsel-ors, and occupational therapy personnel. Goals include assisting adolescents to transition to adulthood, focus on employment, and gain independent living skills.

Activities of Daily Living/Instrumental ADL

- Assist client to develop daily living skills including management of food intake and diet, dressing and undressing self, bathing and showering regularly, management of bowel and bladder, and for females, management of menstrual period.

- Improve communication skills (examples include simplifying language, leaving pauses and waiting for a reply, communicating one idea at a time, speaking in a normal tone of voice, avoiding ambiguous language or words, determining whether written or verbal communication style would be best, considering using multiple formats).
- Provide training in tactical skills as part of a driver education program.

Education/Work
- Assist adolescents with career planning and exploration.
- On-site coaching can help person gain and maintain work skills.
- Advocate and facilitate workplace accommodation including modification of the work. environment, job adjustments, and behavioral management.
- Providing information about ASD to employers can increase acceptance of clients in work settings.
- A successful work environment depends on clear descriptions of job requirements, a shared understanding of the time in which tasks need to be completed, appropriate training, necessary resources, and a supportive workplace culture (Scott et al., 2015).

Play/Leisure
- Encourage exploration and engagement in leisure activities such as puzzles and board games.

Rest/Sleep
- See Sleep–Wake Disorders in Section 13: Lifestyle Conditions.

Social Participation
- Encourage client to participate in social activities, which might begin by going for group walks.

Sensorimotor
- Clients may benefit from reducing visual distractions, avoiding fluorescent lighting, dimming overhead lights.
- Clients may benefit from reducing auditory distractions or use noise-canceling headphones.

Cognitive/Perceptual
- Role playing with discussion can be used to practice working memory and promote cognitive flexibility, problem solving, and planning ahead.
- Use visual schedules to assist client to learn time use and time management skills including checking schedule to determine "what's next?"

Psychosocial
- Assist client to develop a positive self-image based on neurodiversity rather than deficit or disease model.
- Assist client to increase self-regulation behavior by identifying types of items that aid in calming such as tactile or weighted items, deep-breathing exercises, listening to a certain type of music or rhythm.
- Assist client in achieving self-determination through increased opportunity to choose options.
- Assist client to increase self-esteem by participating in activity groups such as games and puzzles, horticulture, healthy living, kitchen skills, community skills, or social club.

Context/Environment
- Work with caregivers to reduce their stress and increase knowledge about working with adults with ASD.
- Assist with referring client, family, or other caregivers to other resources as warranted such as vision specialists.
- Consider if lighting such as florescent lights can be avoided or if noisy areas can be avoided.
- A brief notebook (passport) may be helpful that includes information about the client, which can quickly inform service providers of presenting characteristics, communication preferences, and environmental needs.

- Providing information about ASD to community residents can increase acceptance of adults with ASD within the community.
- Instruct family, in behavior modification techniques, to control behavior, including self-regulation, offering choices, and talking about problem solving when person is no longer upset.
- Provide knowledge to community members about adults with ASD to increase comfort with adults living in the community (Jacoby et al., 2019).

Precautions/Safety Considerations

- Be aware of possible adverse effects of medication due to symptoms of ASD, in addition to side effects associated with the medication, as listed for each medication in the online Physician's Desk Reference (PDR.net).
- Person is at risk for suicide and suicidal ideation (Hedley et al., 2018).
- Note there is no evidence of "eagle-eyed" vision (Falkmer et al., 2011).

Prognosis and Outcome

ASD is a chronic, lifelong condition. Health and behavioral problems change as the client ages and should be reevaluated regularly. Social, emotional, and psychological support will continue to be needed (Hwang et al., 2017; Hwang et al., 2019).

Cost Effectiveness

An article by Jacob et al. (2015) stated that enhancing the opportunities for adults with ASD to participate in the workforce is beneficial from both the societal perspective and the economic standpoint because supported employment services reduced the cost compared with providing standard care and provides better outcomes. However, no cost figures were supplied. The article also noted that providing vocational rehabilitation services to the ASD population is expensive but that services have a strong chance of leading to employment. A study reported by Scott et al. (2017) states that employment benefits adults with ASD and does result in incurring additional costs to employers.

REFERENCES

Almberg, M., Selander, H., Falkmer, M., Vaz, S., Ciccarelli, M., & Falkmer, T. (2017). Experiences of facilitators or barriers in driving education from learner and novice drivers with ADHD or ASD and their driving instructors. *Developmental Neurorehabilitation, 20*(2), 59–67. https://doi.org/10.3109/17518423.2015.1058299

American Psychiatric Association. (2013). *Diagnostic and statistical manual of mental disorders* (5th ed.). https://doi.org/10.1176/appi.books.9780890425596

Bestbier, L., & Williams, T. I. (2017). The immediate effects of deep pressure on young people with autism and severe intellectual difficulties: Demonstrating individual differences. *Occupational Therapy International, 2017*, Article 7534972. https://doi.org/10.1155/2017/7534972

Chee, D. Y., Lee, H. C., Patomella, A.-H., & Falkmer, T. (2017). Driving behavior profile of drivers with autism spectrum disorder (ASD). *Journal of Autism and Developmental Disorders, 47*(9), 2658–2670. https://doi.org/10.1007/s10803-017-3178-1

Chee, D. Y. T., Lee, H. C. Y., Patomella, A.-H., & Falkmer, T. (2019). Investigating the driving performance of drivers with and without autism spectrum disorders under complex driving conditions. *Disability and Rehabilitation, 41*(1), 1–8. https://doi.org/10.1080/09638288.2017.1370498

Classen, S., & Monahan, M. (2013). Evidence-based review on interventions and determinants of driving performance in teens with attention deficit hyperactivity disorder or autism spectrum disorder. *Traffic Injury Prevention, 14*(2), 188–193. https://doi.org/10.1080/15389588.2012.700747

Falkmer, M., Stuart, G. W., Danielsson, H., Bram, S., Lönebrink, M., & Falkmer, T. (2011). Visual acuity in adults with Asperger's syndrome: No evidence for "eagle-eyed" vision. *Biological Psychiatry, 70*(9), 812–816. https://doi.org/10.1016/j.biopsych.2011.07.025

Francis, E. (2019). Specialist intervention for self-management. *OT News, 27*(3), 20–21.

Gal, E., Meir, A. B., & Katz, N. (2013). Developmental and reliability of the Autism Work Skills Questionnaire (AWSQ). *American Journal of Occupational Therapy, 67*(1), e1–e5. https://doi.org/10.5014/ajot.2013.005066

Gasson, S. (2018a). An occupational therapy-led enablement intervention. In M. Bushell, S. Gasson, & U. Vann (Eds.), *Autism and enablement: Occupational therapy approaches to promote independence for adults with autism* (pp. 62–99). Jessica Kingsley.

Gasson, S. (2018b). Prevention and early intervention. *OT News, 26*(12), 20–21.

Harmuth, E., Silletta, E., Bailey, A., Adams, T., Beck, C., & Barbic, S. P. (2018). Barriers and facilitators to employment for adults with autism: A scoping review. *Annals of International Occupational Therapy, 1*(1), 31–40. https://doi.org/10.3928/24761222-20180212-01

Hatfield, M., Falkmer, M., Falkmer, T., & Ciccarelli, M. (2017). Effectiveness of the BOOST-A online transition planning program for adolescents on the autism spectrum: A quasi-randomized controlled trial. *Child and Adolescent Psychiatry and Mental Health, 11,* Article 54. https://doi.org/10.1186/s13034-017-0191-2

Hatfield, M., Falkmer, M., Falkmer, T., & Ciccarelli, M. (2018). Process evaluation of the BOOST-A transition planning program for adolescents on the autism spectrum: A strengths-based approach. *Journal of Autism and Developmental Disorders, 48*(2), 377–388. https://doi.org/10.1007/s10803-017-3317-8

Hatfield, M., Murray, N., Ciccarelli, M., Falkmer, T., & Falkmer, M. (2017). Pilot of the BOOST-A: An online transition planning program for adolescents with autism. *Australian Occupational Therapy Journal, 64*(6), 448–456. https://doi.org/10.1111/1440-1630.12410

Hedley, D., Uljarević M., Foley, K.-R., Richdale, A., & Trollor, J. (2018). Risk and protective factors underlying depression and suicidal ideation in autism spectrum disorder. *Depression and Anxiety, 35*(7), 648–657. https://doi.org/10.1002/da.22759

Hwang, Y. I. J., Foley, K.-R., & Trollor, J. N. (2017). Aging well on the autism spectrum: The perspectives of autistic adults and carers. *International Psychogeriatrics, 29*(12), 2033–2046. https://doi.org/10.1017/S1041610217001521

Hwang, Y. I. J., Srasuebkul, P., Foley, K.-R., Arnold, S., & Trollor, J. N. (2019). Mortality and cause of death of Australians on the autism spectrum. *Autism Research, 12*(5), 806–815. https://doi.org/10.1002/aur.2086

Jacob, A., Scott, M., Falkmer, M., & Falkmer, T. (2015). The costs and benefits of employing an adult with autism spectrum disorder: A systematic review. *PLOS ONE, 10*(10), Article e0139896. https://doi.org/10.1371/journal.pone.0139896

Jacoby, E. C., Walton, K., & Guada, J. (2019). Community perspectives on adults with autism spectrum disorder. *Occupational Therapy in Mental Health, 35*(1), 72–91. https://doi.org/10.1080/0164212X.2018.1507774

Keeble, M. (2014). Finding the therapeutic key to engage with people with autism. *OT News, 22*(2), 38–39.

Koegel, L., Detar, W., Koegel, R. L., & Ashbaugh, K. (2014). Behavioral approaches for adults with autism and related intellectual disabilities. In K. Haertle (Ed.), *Adults with intellectual and developmental disabilities* (pp. 187–204). AOTA Press.

Krutt, H., Dyer, L., Arora, A., Rollman, J., & Jozkowski, A. C. (2018). PhotoVoice is a feasible method of program evaluation at a center serving adults with autism. *Evaluation and Program Planning, 68,* 74–80. https://doi.org/10.1016/j.evalprogplan.2018.02.003

Lim, Y. H., Lee, H. C., Falkmer, T., Allison, G. T., Tan, T., Lee, W. L., & Morris, S. L. (2018a). Effect of visual information on postural control in adults with autism spectrum disorder. *Journal of Autism and Development Disorders, 49*(12), 4731–4739. https://doi.org/10.1007/s10803-018-3634-6

Lim, Y. H., Lee, H. C., Falkmer, T., Allison, G. T., Tan, T., Lee, W. L., & Morris, S. L. (2018b). Effect of optic flow on postural control in children and adults with autism spectrum disorder. *Neuroscience, 393*, 138–149. https://doi.org/10.1016/j.neuroscience.2018.09.047

Metz, A. E., Boling, D., DeVore, A., Holladay, H., Liao, J. F., & Vander Vlutch, K. (2019). Dunn's model of sensory processing: An investigation of the axes of the four-quadrant model in healthy adults. *Brain Sciences, 9*(2), 35. https://doi.org/10.3390/brainsci9020035

Miyajima, M., Omiya, H., Yamashita, K., Yambe, K., Matsui, M., & Denda, K. (2018). Therapeutic responses to a frontal/executive programme in autism spectrum disorder: Comparison with schizophrenia. *Hong Kong Journal of Occupational Therapy, 31*(2), 69–75. https://doi .org/10.1177/1569186118808217

Porter, R. S. (Ed.). (2018). *The Merck manual of diagnosis and therapy* (20th ed.). Merck Sharp & Dohme.

Scott, M., Falkmer, M., Falkmer, T., & Girdler, S. (2018). Evaluating the effectiveness of an autism-specific workplace tool for employers: A randomised controlled trial. *Journal of Autism and Developmental Disorders, 48*(10), 3377–3392. https://doi.org/10.1007/s10803-018-3611-0

Scott, M., Falkmer, M., Girdler, S., & Falkmer, T. (2015). Viewpoints on factors for successful employment for adults with autism spectrum disorder. *PLOS ONE, 10*(10), Article e0139281. https://doi.org/10.1371/journal.pone.0139281 (See figure correction in *PLOS ONE, 10*(11), Article e0143674. https://doi.org/10.1371/journal.pone.0139281)

Scott, M., Jacob, A., Hendrie, D., Parsons, R., Girdler, S., Falkmer, T., & Falkmer. M. (2017). Employers' perception of the costs and the benefits of hiring individuals with autism spectrum disorder in open employment in Australia. *PLOS ONE, 12*(5), Article e0177607. https://doi .org/10.1371/journal.pone.0177607

Stacey, T.-L., Froude, E. H., Trollor, J., & Foley, K.-R. (2019). Leisure participation and satisfaction in autistic adults and neurotypical adults. *Autism, 23*(4), 993–1004. https://doi.org/10 .1177/1362361318791275

Swaminathan, A. (2015). Transition planning in adolescents with low functioning autism. *Indian Journal of Occupational Therapy, 47*(3), 67–71.

Thompson, C., Bölte, S., Falkmer, T., & Girdier, S. (2018a). To be understood: Transitioning to adult life for people with autism spectrum disorder. *PLOS ONE, 13*(3), Article e0194758. https://doi.org/10.1371/journal.pone.0194758

Thompson, C., Bölte, S., Falkmer, T., & Girdier, S. (2018b). Viewpoints on how students with autism can best navigate university. *Scandinavian Journal of Occupational Therapy, 26*(4), 294–305. https://doi.org/10.1080/11038128.2018.1495761

Turcotte, P. L., Côté, C., Coulombe, K., Richard, M., Larivière, N., & Couture, M. (2015). Social participation during transition to adult life among young adults with high-functioning autism spectrum disorders: Experiences from an exploratory multiple case study. *Occupational Therapy in Mental Health, 31*(3), 234–252. https://doi.org/10.1080/0164212X.2015 .1051641

Wilson, J., Mandich, A., Magalhaes, L., & Gain, K. (2018). Concept mapping and the CO-OP approach with adolescents with autism spectrum disorder: Exploring participant experiences. *Open Journal of Occupational Therapy, 6*(4), Article 3. https://doi.org/10.15453/2168 -6408.1455

BIBLIOGRAPHY

American Occupational Therapy Association. (2015). Scope of occupational therapy services for individuals with autism spectrum disorder across the life course. *American Journal of Occupational Therapy, 69*(Suppl. 3), Article 6913410054. https://doi.org/10.5014/ajot.2015.696S18

Arnold, S., Foley, K.-R., Hwang, Y. I., Richdale, A. L., Uljarević, M., Lawson, L. P., Cai, R. Y., Falkmer, T., Falkmer, M., Lennox, N. G., Urbanowicz, A., & Trollor, J. (2019). Cohort profile: The Australian Longitudinal Study of Adults with Autism (ALSAA). *BMJ Open, 9*, Article e3030798. https://doi.org/10.1136/bmjopen-2019-030798

Bushell, M., Gasson, S., & Vann, U. (Eds.). (2018). *Autism and enablement: Occupational therapy approaches to promote independence for adults with autism.* Jessica Kingsley.

Bushell, M., Gasson, S., & Vann, U. (2018). Key learning and recommendations. In M. Bushell, S. Gasson, & U. Vann (Eds.), *Autism and enablement: Occupational therapy approaches to promote independence for adults with autism* (pp. 143–176). Jessica Kingsley.

Cai, R. Y., Richdale, A. L., Foley, K.-R., Troller, J., & Uljarević, M. (2018). Brief report: Cross-sectional interactions between expressive suppression and cognitive reappraisal and its relation to depressive symptoms in autism spectrum disorder. *Research in Autism Spectrum Disorders, 45,* 1–8. https://doi.org/10.1016/j.rasd.2017.10.002

Chee, D. Y.-T., Lee, H. C.-Y., Falkmer, M., Barnett, T., Falkmer, O., Siljehav, J., & Falkmer, T. (2015). Viewpoints on driving of individuals with and without autism spectrum disorder. *Developmental Neurorehabilitation, 18*(1), 26–36. https://doi.org/10.3109/17518423.2014.964377

Cvejic, R. C., Arnold, S. R. C., Foley, K.-R., & Trollor, J. N. (2018). Neuropsychiatric profile and psychotropic medication use in adults with autism spectrum disorders: Results from the Australian Longitudinal Study of Adults with Autism. *BJPsych Open, 4*(6), 461–466. https://doi.org/10.1192/bjo.2018.64

Diaz-Stransky, A., Tierney, E., & López-Arvizu, C. (2014). Adults with autism spectrum disorders: A psychiatry perspective. In K. Haertl (Ed.). *Adults with intellectual and developmental disabilities* (pp. 127–144). AOTA Press.

Ee, D., Hwang, Y.-I., Reppermund, S., Srasuebkul, P., Trollor, J. N., Foley, K.-R., & Arnold, S. R. C. (2019). Loneliness in adults on the autism spectrum. *Autism in Adulthood, 1*(3), 182–193. https://doi.org/10.1089/aut.2018.0038

Foley, K.-R., & Trollor, J. (2015). Management of mental ill health in people with autism spectrum disorder. *Australian Family Physician, 44*(11), 784–790.

Haertl, K., Callahan, D., Markovics, J., & Sheppard, S. S. (2013). Perspectives of adults living with autism spectrum disorder: Psychosocial and occupational implications. *Occupational Therapy in Mental Health, 29*(1), 27–41. https://doi.org/10.1080/0164212X.2012.760303

Hwang, Y. I., Foley, K.-R., & Trollor, J. N. (2018). Aging well on the autism spectrum: An examination of the dominant model of successful aging. *Journal of Autism and Developmental Disorders.* Advance online publication. https://doi.org/10.1007/s10803-018-3596-8

Syu, Y.-C., & Lin, L.-Y. (2018). Sensory overresponsivity, loneliness, and anxiety in Taiwanese adults with autism spectrum disorder. *Occupational Therapy International, 2018.* Article 9165978. https://doi.org/10.1155/2018/9165978

Vann, U., & Gasson, S. (2018). Specialist enablement research results and analysis. In M. Bushell, S. Gasson, & U. Vann (Eds.), *Autism and enablement: Occupational therapy approaches to promote independence for adults with autism* (pp. 100–142). Jessica Kingsley.

Wilson, N. J., Lee, H. C., Vaz, S., Vindin, P., & Cordier, R. (2018). Scoping review of the driving behaviour of and driver training programs for people on the autism spectrum. *Behavioral Neurology, 2018,* Article 6842306. https://doi.org/10.1155/2018/6842306

Autism Spectrum Disorder (ASD): Child

Previous terms now encompassed under ASD include Asperger's syndrome, childhood disintegrative disorder, and pervasive developmental disorder (Porter, 2018).

Also called infantile autism, Kanner's syndrome, autism spectrum conditions (ASC).

See also Sensory Processing Disorders, Sensory Integrative Dysfunction, Sensory Modulation Disorders, Sensory Over-Responsivity, Feeding Disorders in Children.

Description

Autism spectrum disorder (ASD) is a neurodevelopmental disorder characterized by impaired social interaction and communication, repetitive and stereotyped patterns of behavior, and uneven intellectual development, often with intellectual disability (Porter, 2018).

Cause

The specific cause in most cases is unknown, but a genetic component appears to be involved. However, some cases have occurred with congenital rubella syndrome, cytomegalic inclusion disease, phenylketonuria, or fragile X spectrum disorder (Porter, 2018).

Evaluation/Assessment

Areas

- Activities of Daily Living/Instrumental ADL: communication skills
- Education/Work: academic skills, handwriting
- Play/Leisure: type, interests, frequency, location, value
- Rest/Sleep: sleep disturbance, sleep habits and routine
- Social Participation: frequency, type, location, with whom
- Sensorimotor: gross and fine motor skills, sensory responsiveness, sensory sensitivities
- Cognitive/Perceptual: attention, perception, memory, executive functions
- Psychosocial: social skills, role performance
- Context/Environment: family and social support, community resources
- Development (Infant, Child, Adolescent only): developmental milestones
- Comorbidities: obsessive behaviors, seizures or epilepsy

Instruments

Instruments Developed by Occupational Therapy Personnel

- Assessment of Communication and Interaction Skills (Version 4.0; ACIS; Forsyth et al., 1998)
- Assessment of Motor and Process Skills (8th ed.; AMPS-8; Fisher & Bray Jones, 2016)
- Autism Work Skills Questionnaire (AWSQ; Gal et al., 2013; in References)
- Children's Assessment of Participation and Enjoyment and Preferences for Activities of Children (CAPE/PAC; King et al, 2004; see Potvin et al., 2013, in References)
- Developmental Concerns Questionnaire (DCQ; Reznick et al., 2005)
- Eating Profile (EP; Nadon, 2007; Nadon et al., 2010, 2011, in References)
- First Year Inventory (v3.1; FYI; Turner-Brown et al., 2012, in References)
- Infant/Toddler Sensory Profile (ITSP; Dunn, 2002)
- Let's Eat (LE; Little & Wallisch, 2018, in References)
- McDonald Play Inventory (MPI; McDonald & Vigen, 2012, in References)
- Modified Interest Checklist (MIC; Kielhofner & Neville, 1983)
- Occupational Performance Questionnaire (OPQ; Wallace et al., 2016, in References)
- Pediatric Evaluation of Disability Inventory–Computer Adaptive Test (PEDI-CAT; Kramer et al., 2016, in References)
- Sensory Experiences Questionnaire 3.0 (SEQ-3; Baranek, 1999; Baranek et al., 2006; see also Ausderau & Baranek, 2013; Ausderau et al., 2014; and Little et al., 2011, in References)
- Sensory Integration and Praxis Tests (SIPT; Ayres, 1989)
- Sensory Over-Responsivity (SensOR) Scales (Schoen et al., 2008)
- Sensory Processing Assessment (SPA; Baranek, 1999)
- Sensory Processing Measure (SPM) Home Form (SPM-HF; Parham & Ecker, 2007)
- Sensory Processing Measure (SPM) Main Classroom and School Environments Forms (Miller Kuhaneck et al., 2010)
- Sensory Processing Measure–Preschool (SPM-P; Miller Kuhaneck et al., 2010)
- Sensory Processing Measure–Preschool: Home Form (SPM-P-HF; Ecker & Parham, 2010)
- Sensory Processing Scale Inventory (SPSI; Schoen et al., 2017)
- Sensory Profile (2nd ed.; SP-2; Dunn, 2014; see also van der Linde et al., 2013, in References)
- Short Child Occupational Profile (Version 2.2; SCOPE; Bowyer et al., 2008)
- Short Sensory Profile (SSP; McIntosh et al., 1999)
- Tactile Defensiveness and Discrimination Test–Revised (TDDT-R; Baranek, 2010; see also Watling, 2013)

Instruments Developed by Other Professionals and Used by Occupational Therapy Personnel
- Auditory Behavior Questionnaire (ABQ; Egelhoff et al., 2013)
- Autism Diagnostic Interview–Revised (ADI-R; Rutter et al., 2003)
- Autism Diagnostic Observation Schedule (2nd ed.; ADOS-2; Lord et al., 2012)
- Autism Spectrum Quotient (AQ; Allison et al., 2012)
- Autism Quotient Short Form (AQ-S; Hoekstra et al., 2011)
- Beck Depression Inventory (2nd ed.; BDI-II; Beck et al., 1996)
- Childhood Autism Rating Scale (2nd ed.; CARS-2; Schopler et al., 2010)
- Empathy Quotient–Child (EQ-C; Auyeung et al., 2009)
- Goal Attainment Scaling (GAS; example in Shrivastav, 2014, in References)
- Home and Community Activities Scale (HCAS; Dunst et al., 2000)
- Leisure Satisfaction Scale (LSS; Beard & Ragheb, 1980)
- Modified Checklist for Autism in Toddlers (M-CHAT; Robins et al., 2001)
- Mullen Scales of Early Learning (MSEL; Mullen, 1995)
- Repetitive Behavior Scales–Revised (RBS-R; Bodfish et al., 1999)
- Social Communication Questionnaire (SCQ; Rutter et al., 2003)
- Social Responsiveness Scale (2nd ed.; SRS-2; Constantino, 2012)
- Vineland Adaptive Behavior Scales (3rd ed.; Vineland-3; Sparrow et al., 2016)
- World Health Organization Quality of Life–BREF (WHOQOL-BREF; The WHOQOL Group, 1998)

Problems/Issues

Activities of Daily Living/Instrumental ADL
- Child may be a picky eater, selecting only a limited number of foods to eat.
- Child may wear only certain garments and refuse to dress in any other items of clothing.
- Child usually has difficulty with communication skills.

Education/Work
- Child may have difficulty performing academic tasks, including reading, math, and writing.

Play/Leisure
- Child may display limited play skills, lack of cooperative play skills.
- Child may have few or limited leisure skills, focused on solitary interests rather than social.

Rest/Sleep
- Child may have sleep disturbances.

Social Participation
- Child usually has difficulty with social relationships including peer interactions.

Sensorimotor
- Child may have difficulty performing advanced motor skills such as hopping, jumping, or skipping.
- Child may have poor fine motor skills such as using scissors or holding a pencil or brush.
- Child may have stereotypical motor movements such as rocking or hand flapping.
- Child may be hyposensitive to pain.
- Child may have sensory hypersensitivity to noise or tactile stimuli.
- Child may attempt to avoid certain sensory input related to hypersensitivity (refuse to wear certain clothing, put hands over ears to avoid certain noises, refusing to eat certain foods).
- Child may limit visual gaze and fixation thus reducing amount of visual cues received.

Cognitive/Perceptual
- Child usually has difficulty paying attention, especially shifting attention.
- Child may have difficulty remembering previously learned skills.

- Child may display executive dysfunction.
- Child may have poor facial recognition due to reduced eye tracking and gaze fixation.

Psychosocial

- Child may express or display symptoms of anxiety and depression.
- Child may display oppositional behavior, aggressive behavior.
- Child may display obsessive compulsive behavior.
- Child may display repetitive stereotypical behavior.

Context/Environment

- Family may have little knowledge of ASD or its management in the home.
- Family may live in a school district that has no special programs for ASD.
- Family may experience a decreased quality of life due to having a child with ASD.
- Mothers of children with ASD may express symptoms of depression.

Intervention/Treatment

Models and programs developed by occupational therapy personnel include Ayres Sensory Integration (Watling & Hauer, 2015), case examples and studies (Gutman et al., 2010; Parham et al., 2019), Cognitive Orientation to daily Occupational Performance (CO-OP; Czmowski et al., 2014), deep pressure stimulation (McGinnis et al., 2013), noise-attenuating/canceling headphones program (Ikuta et al., 2016; Pfeiffer et al., 2019), occupational therapy intervention program for mothers (Khanum & Begum, 2018; Shrivastav, 2014), play-based intervention (Henning et al., 2016), Proloquo2Go (Apple application communication) program (Collette et al., 2019), sensory diet (Reinson, 2012), sensory integration therapy (Kashefimehr et al., 2018; Mishra & Senapati, 2015), time processing aids (Janeslätt et al., 2014), and vestibular and tactile stimulation (Ghanavati et al., 2013). Models and programs developed by other professionals but used by occupational therapy personnel include adapted responsive teaching (Baranek et al., 2015), craniosacral therapy (Mishra & Senapati, 2015), eating program (Miyajima et al., 2017), emotional regulation (Parkinson & Sivyer, 2017), floor time (Dionne & Martini, 2011), information communication technology (Parsons et al., 2019), keyboarding (Ashburner et al., 2012), parent-mediated intervention training (Parsons et al., 2017), social interaction skills (Gokhale & Sawant, 2014), therapy cushions (Umeda & Deitz, 2011), Therapy Outcomes by You (TOBY; Rogerson et al., 2019), and virtual reality program (Ghanouni et al., 2019). Team members may include educators, psychologists, physicians, social workers, and occupational therapy personnel. Goal is to plan and implement strategies to help compensate for specific deficits in motor function, motor planning, and sensory processing (Porter, 2018).

Activities of Daily Living/Instrumental ADL

- Photographic instructions may facilitate performance of basic ADLs, such as brushing teeth, getting dressed.
- Use of differential reinforcement of alternate behavior (behavior modification method reinforcing positive behaviors) may be useful to change eating behavior.
- Visual personalized instruction may facilitate meal preparation.
- Use of phone apps may be useful to assist in following medication schedules, recipes, finding local transportation, dressing for outside weather.

Education/Work

- Photo-based visual aids outlining step-by-step task performance may assist learning academic tasks or following work assignments.
- To date, use of cushions or balls in classroom seats has not improved in-seat or on-task behavior.

Play/Leisure

- Assist client to explore and engage in leisure interests involving others.

Rest/Sleep
- Weighted blankets may assist client to relax and go to sleep.

Social Participation
- Encourage participation in social activities.

Sensorimotor
- Weighted vests and blankets may reduce anxiety (increase sense of calmness) for some clients.
- Client may benefit from use of noise-canceling headphones in situations where large numbers of people and noise are present (shopping centers, airport terminals, festivals, fairs, sporting events).

Cognitive/Perceptual
- Encourage child to focus attention on task (reduce distractions when possible).
- Assist client to learn time use and time management skills.

Psychosocial
- Provide stress management techniques to parents and caregivers.
- Use of deep pressure stimulation (mats, pillows, beanbag chairs, mattresses, trampolines, trapeze bars, chin-up bars, "squeeze machines," and climbing structures) may provide a calming effect on the body and reduce levels of anxiety.

Context/Environment
- Telerehabilitation or telecare may be useful to provide assistance to families and children with ASD.

Precautions/Safety Considerations

Children with ASD are at increased risk of suicidal behavior and self-injury.

Prognosis and Outcome

ASD is a lifelong chronic condition (Rodger et al., 2010). Management of symptoms is the primary goal.

Cost Effectiveness

Cost of care for a medium-income family in Australia in 2014 was AU$34,900 per annum (about US$25,000). Almost 90% of the sum (AU$29,200) was due to loss of income from employment (about US$20,000; Horlin et al., 2014).

REFERENCES

Ashburner, J., Ziviani, J., & Pennington, A. (2012). The introduction of keyboarding to children with autism spectrum disorders with handwriting difficulties: A help or a hindrance? *Australasian Journal of Special Education, 36*(1), 32–61. https://doi.org/10.1017/jse.2012.6

Ausderau, K. K., & Baranek, G. T. (2013). Sensory Experiences Questionnaire. In F. R. Volkmar (Ed.), *Encyclopedia of autism spectrum disorders* (pp. 2770–2774). Springer. https://doi.org/10.1007/978-1-4419-1698-3_1192

Ausderau, K., Sideris, J., Furlong, M., Little, L. M., Bulluck, J., & Baranek, G. T. (2014). National survey of sensory features in children with ASD: Factor structure of the Sensory Experience Questionnaire (3.0). *Journal of Autism and Developmental Disorders, 44*, 915–925. https://doi.org/10.1007/s10803-013-1945-1

Baranek, G. T., Watson, L. R., Turner-Brown, L., Field, S. H., Crais, E. R., Wakeford, L., Little, L. M., & Reznick, J. S. (2015). Preliminary efficacy of adapted responsive teaching for infants at risk of autism spectrum disorder in a community sample. *Autism Research and Treatment, 2015*, Article 386951. https://doi.org/10.1155/2015/386951

Collette, D., Brix, A., Brennan, P., DeRoma, N., & Muir, B. C. (2019). Proloquo2Go enhances classroom performance in children with autism spectrum disorder. *OTJR: Occupation, Participation and Health, 39*(3), 143–150. https://doi.org/10.1177/1539449218799451

Czmowski, G. M., Willert, S. L., & Nielsen, S. K. (2014). Addressing social, emotional, and organization goals for a child with an autism spectrum disorder (ASD) using the Cognitive Orientation to daily Occupational Performance (CO-OP) approach. *Journal of Special Education Apprenticeship, 3*(1), 1–15.

Dionne, M., & Martini, R. (2011). Floor time play with a child with autism: A single-subject study. *Canadian Journal of Occupational Therapy, 78*(3), 196–203. https://doi.org/10.2182/cjot.2011.78.3.8

Egelhoff, K., & Lane, A. E. (2013). Brief report: Preliminary reliability, construct validity and standardization of the Auditory Behavior Questionnaire (ABQ) for children with autism spectrum disorders. *Journal of Autism and Developmental Disorders, 43*, 978–984. https://doi.org/10.1007/s10803-012-1626-5

Gal, E., Meir, A. B., & Katz, N. (2013). Development and reliability of the Autism Work Skills Questionnaire (AWSQ). *American Journal of Occupational Therapy, 67*(1), e1–e5. https://doi.org/10.5014/ajot.2013.005066

Ghanavati, E., Zarbakhsh, M., & Haghgoo, H. (2013). Effects of vestibular and tactile stimulation on behavioral disorders due to sensory processing deficiency in 3–13 years old Iranian autistic children. *Iranian Rehabilitation Journal, 11*(1), 52–57. http://irj.uswr.ac.ir/article-1-371-en.html

Ghanouni, P., Jarus, T., Zwicker, J. G., Lucyshyn, J., Mow, K., & Ledingham, A. (2019). Social stories for children with autism spectrum disorder: Validating the content of a virtual reality program. *Journal of Autism and Developmental Disorders, 49*(2), 660–668. https://doi.org/10.1007/s10803-018-3737-0

Gokhale, P. S., & Sawant, P. (2014). Intervention on social interaction skills in children with mild autism spectrum disorder. *Indian Journal of Physiotherapy and Occupational Therapy, 9*(4), 229–234.

Gutman, S. A., Raphael, E. I., Ceder, L. M., Khan, A., Timp, K. M., & Salvant, S. (2010). High-functioning autism: Two single-subject design cases. *Occupational Therapy International, 17*(4), 188–197.

Henning, B., Cordier, R., Wilkes-Gillan, S., & Falkmer, T. (2016). A pilot play-based intervention to improve the social play interactions of children with autism spectrum disorder and their typically developing playmates. *Australian Occupational Therapy Journal, 63*(4), 223–232. https://doi.org/10.1111/1440-1630.12285

Horlin, C., Falkmer, M., Parsons, R., Albrecht, M. A., & Falkmer, T. (2014). The cost of autism spectrum disorders. *PLOS ONE, 9*(9), Article e106552. https://doi.org/10.1371/journal.pone.0106552

Ikuta, N., Iwanaga, R., Tokunaga, A., Nakane, H., Tanaka, K., & Tanaka, G. (2016). Effectiveness of earmuffs and noise-cancelling headphones for coping with hyper-reactivity to auditory stimuli in children with autism spectrum disorder: A preliminary study. *Hong Kong Journal of Occupational Therapy, 28*, 24–32. https://doi.org/10.1016/j.hkjot.2016.09.001

Janeslätt, G., Kottorp, A., & Granlund, M. (2014). Evaluating intervention using time aids in children with disabilities. *Scandinavian Journal of Occupational Therapy, 21*(3), 181–190. https://doi.org/10.3109/11038128.2013.870225

Kashefimehr, B., Kayihan, H., & Huri, M. (2018). The effect of sensory integration therapy on occupational performance in children with autism. *OTJR: Occupation, Participation and Health, 38*(2), 75–83. https://doi.org/10.1177/1539449217743456

Khanum, S., & Begum, R. (2018). Effectiveness of occupational therapy interventions on depression and quality of life of mothers with autistic children. *Indian Journal of Physiotherapy and Occupational Therapy, 12*(4), 120–125.

Kramer, J. M., Liljenquist, K., & Coster, W. J. (2016). Validity, reliability, and usability of the Pediatric Evaluation of Disability Inventory–Computer Adaptive Test for autism spectrum disorders. *Development Medicine and Child Neurology, 58*(3), 255–261. https://doi.org/10.1111/dmcn.12837

Little, L. M., Freuler, A. C., Houser, M. B., Guckian, L., Carbine, K., David, F. J., & Baranek, G. T. (2011). Psychometric validation of the Sensory Experiences Questionnaire. *American Journal of Occupational Therapy, 65*, 207–210. https://doi.org/10.5014/ajot.2011.000844

Little, L. M., & Wallisch, A. (2018). Let's Eat: Development and reliability of an eating behavior assessment for children with autism spectrum disorders. *Annals of International Occupational Therapy, 1*(1), 24–30. https://doi.org/10.3928/24761222-20180212-03

McDonald, A. E., & Vigen, C. (2012). Reliability and validity of the McDonald Play Inventory. *American Journal of Occupational Therapy, 66*(4), e52–e60. https://doi.org/10.5014/ajot.2012.002493

McGinnis, A. A., Blakely, E. Q., Harvey, A. C., Hodges, A. C., & Rickards, J. B. (2013). The behavioral effects of a procedure used by pediatric occupational therapists. *Behavioral Interventions, 28*(1), 48–57. https://doi.org/10.1002/bin.1355

Mishra, D. P., & Senapati, A. (2015). Effectiveness of combined approach of craniosacral therapy (CST) and sensory integration therapy (SIT) on reducing features in children with autism. *Indian Journal of Occupational Therapy, 47*(1), 3–8.

Miyajima, A., Tateyama, K., Fuji, S., Nakaoka, K., Hirao, K., & Higaki, K. (2017). Development of an intervention programme for selective eating in children with autism spectrum disorder. *Hong Kong Journal of Occupational Therapy, 30*(1), 22–32. https://doi.org/10.1016/j.hkjot.2017.10.001

Nadon, G., Ehrmann Feldman, D., Dunn, W., & Gisel, E. (2010). Mealtime problems in children with autism spectrum disorder and their typically developing siblings: A comparison study. *Autism, 15*(1), 198–113. https://doi.org/10.1177/1362361309348943

Nadon, G., Ehrmann Feldman, D., Dunn, W., & Gisel, E. (2011). Association of sensory processing and eating problems in children with autism spectrum disorders. *Autism Research and Treatment, 2011,* Article 541926. https://doi.org/10.1155/2011/541926

Parham, L. D., Clark, G. F., Watling, R., & Schaaf, R. (2019). Occupational therapy interventions for children and youth with challenges in sensory integration and sensory processing: A clinic-based practice case example. *American Journal of Occupational Therapy, 73*(1), Article 7301395010. https://doi.org/10.5014/ajot.2019.731002

Parkinson, S., & Sivyer, S. (2017). A joined approach to emotional regulation. *OT News, 25*(4), 34–35.

Parsons, D., Cordier, R., Lee, H., Falkmer, T., & Vaz, S. (2019). A randomised controlled trial of an information communication technology delivered intervention for children with autism spectrum disorder living in regional Australia. *Journal of Autism and Developmental Disorders, 49*(2), 569–581. https://doi.org/10.1007/s10803-018-3734-3

Parsons, D., Cordier, R., Vaz, S., & Lee, H. C. (2017). Parent-mediated intervention training delivered remotely for children with autism spectrum disorder living outside of urban areas: Systematic review. *Journal of Medicine and Internet Research, 19*(8), Article e198. https://doi.org/10.2196/jmir.6651

Pfeiffer, B., Erb, S. R., & Slugg, L. (2019). Impact of noise-attenuating headphones on participation in the home, community, and school for children with autism spectrum disorder. *Physical & Occupational Therapy in Pediatrics, 39*(1), 60–76. https://doi.org/10.1080/01942638.2018.1496963

Porter, R. S. (Ed.). (2018). *The Merck manual of diagnosis and therapy* (20th ed.). Merck Sharp & Dohme.

Potvin, M.-C., Snider, L., Prelock, P., Kehayia, E., & Wood-Dauphinee, S. (2013). Children's Assessment of Participation and Enjoyment/Preference for Activities of Children: Psychometric properties in a population with high-functioning autism. *American Journal of Occupational Therapy, 67,* 209–217. https://doi.org/10.5014/ajot.2013.006288

Reinson, C. (2012). A collaborative decision tree system for designing a sensory diet curriculum of children with autism in the classroom setting. *Journal of Occupational Therapy, Schools & Early Intervention, 5*(1), 61–72. https://doi.org/10.1080/19411243.2012.673327

Rodger, S., Ashburner, J., Cartmill, L., & Bourke-Taylor, H. (2010). Helping children with autism spectrum disorders and their families: Are we losing our occupation-centred focus? *Australian Occupational Therapy Journal, 57*(4), 276–280. https://doi.org/10.1111/j.1440-1630.20 10.00877.x

Rogerson, J., Falkmer, M., Cuomo, B., Falkmer, T., Whitehouse, A. J. O., Granich, J., & Vaz, S. (2019). Parental experiences using the Therapy Outcomes by You (TOBY) application to deliver early intervention to their child with autism. *Developmental Neurorehabilitation, 22*(4), 219–227. https://doi.org/10.1080/17518423.2018.1440259

Shrivastav, N. K. (2014). Occupational therapy intervention to combat stress level of mothers of children with autism. *Indian Journal of Occupational Therapy, 46*(2), 55–60.

Turner-Brown, L. M., Baranek, G. T., Reznick, J. S., Watson, L. R., & Crais, E. R. (2012). The First Year Inventory: A longitudinal follow-up of 12-month-old to 3-year-old children. *Autism, 17*(5), 527–540. https://doi.org/10.1177/1362361312439633

Umeda, C., & Deitz, J. (2011). Effects of therapy cushions on classroom behavior of children with autism spectrum disorder. *American Journal of Occupational Therapy, 65,* 152–159. https://doi.org/10.5014/ajot.2011.000760

van der Linde, J., Franzsen, D., & Barnard-Ashton, P. (2013). The sensory profile: Comparative analysis of children with specific language impairment, ADHD and autism. *South African Journal of Occupational Therapy, 43*(3), 34–40.

Wallace, K., Franzsen, D., & Potterton, J. (2016). Development of an Occupational Performance Questionnaire for preschool children with autistic spectrum disorder. *South African Journal of Occupational Therapy, 46*(2), 23–30. https://doi.org/10.17159/2310-3833/2016/v46n2a5

Watling, R., & Hauer, S. (2015). Effectiveness of Ayres Sensory Integration and sensory-based interventions for people with autism spectrum disorder: A systematic review. *American Journal of Occupational Therapy, 69,* Article 6905180030. https://doi.org/10.5014/ajot.2015.018051

BIBLIOGRAPHY

Abelenda, J., Mailloux, Z., & Smith Roley, S. (2015). Dyspraxia in autism spectrum disorders: Evidence and implication. *Sensory Integration Special Interest Section Quarterly, 38*(3), 1–3.

Abu-Dahab, S. M. N., Skidmore, E. R., Holm, M. B., Rogers, J. C., & Minshew, N. J. (2013). Motor and tactile-perceptual skill differences between individuals with high-functioning autism and typically developing individuals ages 5–21. *Journal of Autism and Developmental Disorders, 43,* 2241–2248. https://doi.org/10.1007/s10803-011-1439-y

Albrecht, M. A., Stuart, G. W., Falkmer, M., Ordqvist, A., Leung, D., Foster, J. K., & Falkmer, T. (2014). Brief report: Visual acuity in children with autism spectrum disorders. *Journal of Autism and Developmental Disorders, 44*(9), 2369–2374. https://doi.org/10.1007/s10803-014 -2086-x

Ashburner, J. K., Bennett, L., Rodger, S., & Ziviani, J. M. (2013). Understanding the sensory experiences of young people with autism spectrum disorder: A preliminary investigation. *Australian Occupational Therapy Journal, 60*(3), 171–180. https://doi.org/10.1111/1440-1630 .12025

Ashburner, J. K., Rodger, S. A., Ziviani, J. M., & Hinder, E. A. (2014). Optimizing participation of children with autism spectrum disorder experiencing sensory challenges: A clinical reasoning framework. *Canadian Journal of Occupational Therapy, 81*(1), 29–38. https://doi .org/10.1177/0008417413520440

Ashburner, J., Rodger, S., Ziviani, J., & Jones, J. (2014). Occupational therapy services for people with autism spectrum disorders: Current state of play, use of evidence and future learning priorities. *Australian Occupational Therapy Journal, 61*(2), 110–120. https://doi.org/10.1111/1440-1630.12083

Ashburner, J., Ziviani, J., & Rodger, S. (2010). Surviving in the mainstream: Capacity of children with autism spectrum disorders to perform academically and regulate their emotions and behavior at school. *Research in Autism Spectrum Disorders, 4*(1), 18–27. https://doi.org/10.1016/j.rasd.2009.07.002

Ausderau, K. K., Furlong, M., Sideris, J., Bulluck, J., Little, L. M., Watson, L. R., Boyd, B. A., Belger, A., Dickie, V. A., & Baranek, G. T. (2014). Sensory subtypes in children with autism spectrum disorder: Latent profile transition analysis using a national survey of sensory features. *Journal of Child Psychology & Psychiatry, 55*(8), 935–944. https://doi.org/10.1111/jcpp.12219

Baranek, G. T., Carlson, M., Sideris, J., Kirby, A. V., Watson, L. R., Williams, K. L., & Bullock, J. (2019). Longitudinal assessment of stability of sensory features in children with autism spectrum disorders or other developmental disabilities. *Autism Research, 12*(1), 100–111. https://doi.org/10.1002/aur.2008

Baranek, G. T., Little, L. M., Parham, D., Ausderau, K. K., & Sabatos-DeVito, M. G. (2014). Sensory features in autism spectrum disorders. In F. R. Volkmar, S. J. Rogers., R. Paul, & K. A. Pelphrey (Eds.), *Handbook of autism and pervasive developmental disorders: Diagnosis, development, and brain mechanisms* (pp. 378–407). Wiley.

Baranek, G. T., Watson, L. R., Boyd, B. A., Poe, M. D., David, F. J., & McGuire, L. (2013). Hyporesponsivenss to social and nonsocial sensory stimuli in children with autism, children with developmental delays, and typically developing children. *Development and Psychopathology, 25*(2), 307–320. https://doi.org/10.1017/S0954579412001071

Baranek, G. T., Woynaroski, T. G., Nowell, S., Turner-Brown, L., DuBay, M., Crais, E. R., & Watson, L. R. (2018). Cascading effects of attention disengagement and sensory seeking on social symptoms in a community sample of infants at-risk for a future diagnosis of autism spectrum disorder. *Developmental Cognitive Neuroscience, 29*, 30–40. https://doi.org/10.1016/j.dcn.2017.08.006

Benevides, T. W., Carretta, H. J., & Lane, S. J. (2015). Unmet need for therapy among children with autism spectrum disorder: Results from the 2005–2006 and 2009–2010 National Survey of Children with Special Health Care Needs. *Maternal and Child Health Journal, 20*, 878–888. https://doi.org/10.1007/s10995-015-1876-x

Bestbier, L., & Williams, T. I. (2017). The immediate effects of deep pressure on young people with autism and severe intellectual difficulties: Demonstrating individual differences. *Occupational Therapy International, 2017*, Article 7534972. https://doi.org/10.1155/2017/7534972

Birch, R. C., Foley, K.-R., Pollack, A., Britt, H., Lennox, N., & Trollor, J. N. (2018). Problems managed and medications prescribed during encounters with people with autism spectrum disorder in Australian general practice. *Autism, 22*(8), 995–1004. https://doi.org/10.1177/1362361317714588

Black, M. H., Chen, N. T. M., Iyer, K. K., Lipp, O. V., Bölte, S., Falkmer, M., Tan, T., & Girdler, S. (2017). Mechanisms of facial emotion recognition in autism spectrum disorders: Insights form eye tracking and electroencephalography. *Neuroscience & Biobehavioral Reviews, 80*, 488–515. https://doi.org/10.1016/j.neubiorev.2017.06.016

Bölte, S., Girdler, S., & Marschik, P. B. (2019). The contribution of environmental exposure to the etiology of autism spectrum disorder. *Cell and Molecular Life Sciences, 76*(7), 1275–1297. https://doi.org/10.1007/s00018-018-2988-4

Boyd, B. A., Baranek, G. T., Sideris, J., Poe, M. D., Watson, L. R., Patten, E., & Miller, H. (2010). Sensory features and repetitive behaviors in children with autism and developmental delays. *Autism Research, 3*(2), 78–87. https://doi.org/10.1002/aur.124

Boyd, B. A., McDonough, S. G., & Bodfish, J. W. (2012). Evidence-based behavioral interventions for repetitive behaviors in autism. *Journal of Autism and Developmental Disorders, 42,* 1236–1248. https://doi.org/10.1007/s10803-011-1284-z

Brock, M. E., Freuler, A., Baranek, G. T., Watson, L. R., Poe, M. D., & Sabatino, A. (2012). Temperament and sensory features of children with autism. *Journal of Autism and Developmental Disorders, 42*(22), 2271–2284. https://doi.org/10.1007/s10803-012-1472-5

Cascio, C. J., Lorenzi, J., & Baranek, G. T. (2016). Self-reported pleasantness ratings and examiner-coded defensiveness in response to touch in children with ASD: Effects of stimulus material and bodily location. *Journal of Autism and Developmental Disorders, 46,* 1528–1537. https://doi.org/10.1007/s10803-013-1961-1

Chan, P.-C., Chen, C.-T., Feng, H., Lee, Y.-C., & Chen, K.-L. (2016). Theory of mind deficit is associated with pretend play performance, but not playfulness, in children with autism spectrum disorder. *Hong Kong Journal of Occupational Therapy, 28,* 43–52. https://doi.org/10.1016/j.hkjot.2016.09.002

Chiang, W.-C., Tseng, M.-H. Fu, C.-P., Chuang, I.-C., Lu, L., & Shieh, J.-Y. (2019). Exploring sensory processing dysfunction, parenting stress, and problem behaviors in children with autism spectrum disorder. *American Journal of Occupational Therapy, 73*(1), Article 7301205130. https://doi.org/10.5014/ajot.2019.027607

Crabtree, L., & DeLany, J. V. (2011). Autism: Promoting social and participation and mental health. In S. Bazyk, (Ed.), *Mental health promotion, prevention, and intervention with children and youth: A guiding framework for occupational therapy* (pp. 163–188). AOTA Press.

Crais, E. R., McComish, C. S., Humphreys, B. P., Watson, L. R., Baranek, G. T., Reznick, J. S., Christian, R. B., & Earls, M. (2014). Pediatric healthcare professionals' views on autism spectrum disorder screening at 12–18 months. *Journal of Autism and Developmental Disorders, 44,* 2311–2328. https://doi.org/10.1007/s10803-014-2101-2

Cuomo, B. M., Vaz, S., Lee, E. A. L., Thompson, C., Rogerson, J. M., & Falkmer, T. (2017). Effectiveness of sleep-based interventions for children with autism spectrum disorder: A meta-synthesis. *Pharmacotherapy, 37*(5), 555–578. https://doi.org/10.1002/phar.1920

Donkers, F. C. L., Schipul, S. E., Baranek, G. T., Cleary, K. M., Willoughby, M. T., Evans, A. M., Bulluck, J. C., Lovmo, J. E., & Belger, A. (2015). Attenuated auditory event-related potential and associations with atypical sensory response patterns in children with autism. *Journal of Autism and Developmental Disorders, 45,* 506–523. https://doi.org/10.1007/s10803-013-1948-y

Dumont, C. (2013). Mobile technologies and individuals with an autism spectrum disorder: A list of applications and reflections on their use. *Occupational Therapy Now, 15*(6), 14–15.

Eschenfelder, V. G., & Gavalas, C. M. (2017). Joint attention and occupations for children and families living with autism spectrum disorder: A scoping review. *Open Journal of Occupational Therapy, 5*(4), Article 5. https://doi.org/10.15453/2168-6408.1349

Falkmer, M., Black, M., Tang, J., Fitzgerald, P., Girdler, S., Leung, D., Ordqvist, A., Tan, T., Jahan, I., & Falkmer, T. (2016). Local visual perception bias in children with high-functioning autism spectrum disorders; do we have the whole picture? *Developmental Neurorehabilitation, 19*(2), 117–122. https://doi.org/10.3109/17518423.2014.928387

Falkmer, M., Granlund, M., Nilholm, C., & Falkmer, T. (2012). From my perspective—Perceived participation in mainstream schools in students with autism spectrum conditions. *Developmental Neurorehabilitation, 15*(3), 191–201. https://doi.org/10.3109/17518423.2012.671382

Falkmer, M., Oehlers, K., Granlund, M., & Falkmer, T. (2015). Can you see it too? Observed and self-rated participation in mainstream schools in students with and without autism spectrum disorders. *Developmental Neurorehabilitation, 18*(6), 365–374. https://doi.org/10.3109/17518423.2013.850751

Falkmer, T., Anderson, K., Falkmer, M., & Horlin, C. (2013). Diagnostic procedures in autism spectrum disorders: A systematic literature review. *European Child and Adolescent Psychiatry, 22,* 329–340. https://doi.org/10.1007/s00787-013-0375-0

Flanagan, J. E., Landa, R., Bhat, A., & Bauman, M. (2012). Head lag in infants at risk for autism: A preliminary study. *American Journal of Occupational Therapy, 66*(5), 577–585. https://doi.org/10.5014/ajot.2012.004192

Foley, K. R., Pollack, A. J., Britt, H. C., Lennox, N. G., & Trollor, J. N. (2018). General practice encounters for young patients with autism spectrum disorder in Australia. *Autism, 22*(7), 784–793. https://doi.org/10.1177/1362361317702560

Freuler, A., Baranek, G. T., Watson, L. R., Boyd, B. A., & Bulluck, J. C. (2012). Brief report—Precursors and trajectories of sensory features: Qualitative analysis of infant home videos. *American Journal of Occupational Therapy, 66*, e81–e84. https://doi.org/10.5014/ajot.2012.004465

Gee, B. M., Nwora, A., & Peterson, T. W. (2018). Occupational therapy's role in the treatment of children with autism spectrum disorders. In M. Huri (Ed.), *Occupational therapy: Therapeutic and creative use of activity* (pp. 3–27). IntechOpen.

Ghanizadeh, A. (2011). Can tactile sensory processing differentiate between children with autistic disorder and Asperger's disorder? *Innovations in Clinical Neuroscience, 8*(5), 25–30.

Hand, B. N., Dennis, S., & Lane, A. E. (2017). Latent constructs underlying sensory subtypes in children with autism: A preliminary study. *Autism Research, 10*(8), 1364–1371. ttps://doi.org/10.1002/aur.1787

Harris, B., & d'Abo, V. (2018). Achieving the best outcomes for children, young people and their families. *OT News, 26*(1), 36–38.

Hazen, E. P., Stornelli, J. L., O'Rourke, J. A., Koesterer, K., & McDougle, C. J. (2014). Sensory symptoms in autism spectrum disorders. *Harvard Review of Psychiatry, 22*(2), 112–124. https://doi.org/10.1097/01.HRP.0000445143.08773.58

Hébert, M. L. J., Kehayia, E., Prelock, P., Wood-Dauphinee, S., & Snider, L. (2012). Communication and occupation: New avenues for autism. *Occupational Therapy Now, 14*(2), 22–23.

Higashionna, T., Iwanaga, R., Tokunaga, A., Nakai, A., Tanaka, K., Nakane, H., & Tanaka, G. (2017). Relationship between motor coordination, cognitive abilities, and academic achievement in Japanese children with neurodevelopmental disorders. *Hong Kong Journal of Occupational Therapy, 30*, 49–55. https://doi.org/10.1016/j.hkjot.2017.10.002

Hilton, C. L., Harper, J. D., Kueker, R. H., Lang, A. R., Abbacchi, A. M., Todorov, A., & LaVesser, P. D. (2010). Sensory responsiveness as a predictor of social severity in children with high functioning autism spectrum disorders. *Journal of Autism and Developmental Disorders, 40*(8), 937–945. https://doi.org/10.1007/s10803-010-0944-8

Hilton, C. L., Ratcliff, K., Collins, D. M., Flanagan, J., & Hong, I. (2019). Flourishing in children with autism spectrum disorders. *Autism Research, 12*(6), 952–966. https://doi.org/10.1002/aur.2097

Horlin, C., Black, M., Falkmer, M., & Falkmer, T. (2015). Proficiency of individuals with autism spectrum disorder at disembedding figures: A systematic review. *Developmental Neurorehabilitation, 19*(1), 54–63. https://doi.org/10.3109/17518423.2014.888102

Jones, J., Rodger, S., Walpole, A., & Bobir, N. (2019). Holding the cards: Empowering families through an ASD family goal setting tool. *Topics in Early Childhood Special Education, 39*(2), 117–130. https://doi.org/10.1177/0271121418766240

Joosten, A., & Bundy, A. C. (2010). Sensory processing and stereotypical and repetitive behavior in children with autism and intellectual disability. *Australian Occupational Therapy Journal, 57*(6), 366–372. https://doi.org/10.1111/j.1440-1630.2009.00835.x

Joosten, A., Girdler, S., Albrecht, M. A., Horlin, C., Falkmer, M., Leung, D., Ordqvist, A., Fleischer, H., & Falkmer, T. (2016). Gaze and visual search strategies of children with Asperger syndrome/high functioning autism viewing a magic trick. *Developmental Neurorehabilitation, 19*(2), 95–102. https://doi.org/10.3109/17518423.2014.913081

Kuhaneck, H., & Watling, R. (2019). Best practices in supporting students with autism. In G. Frolek Clark, J. E. Rioux, & B. E. Chandler (Eds.), *Best practices for occupational therapy in schools* (2nd ed., pp. 235–342). AOTA Press.

Lane, A. E., Young, R. L., Baker, A. E. Z., & Angley, M. T. (2010). Sensory processing subtypes in autism: Association with adaptive behavior. *Journal of Autism and Developmental Disabilities*, *40*, 112–122. https://doi.org/10.1007/s10803-009-0840-2

Little, L. M., Ausderau, K., Sideris, J., & Baranek, G. T. (2014). Activity participation and sensory features among children with autism spectrum disorders. *Journal of Autism and Developmental Disorders*, *45*, 2981–2990. https://doi.org/10.1007/s10803-015-2460-3

Little, L. M., Rojas, J. P., Bard, A., Luo, Y., Irvin, D., & Rous, B. (2019). Automated measures to understand communication opportunities for young children with autism in the community: A pilot study. *OTJR: Occupational, Participation and Health*, *39*(2), 124–131. https://doi.org/10.1177/1539449219834911

Little, L. M., Sideris, J., Ausderau, K., & Baranek, G. T. (2014). Activity participation among children with autism spectrum disorder. *American Journal of Occupational Therapy*, *68*(2), 177–185. https://doi.org/10.5014/ajot.2014.009894

Matsushima, K., & Kato, T. (2013). Social interaction and atypical sensory processing in children with autism spectrum disorders. *Hong Kong Journal of Occupational Therapy*, *23*, 89–96. https://doi.org/10.1016/j.hkjot.2013.11.003

McAuliffe, T., Cordier, R., Vaz, S., Thomas, Y., & Falkmer. T. (2017). Quality of life coping styles, stress levels, and time use in mothers of children with autism spectrum disorders: Comparing single versus coupled household. *Journal of Autism and Developmental Disorders*, *47*(10), 3189–3203. https://doi.org/10.1007/s10803-017 3240-z

McAuliffe, T., Thomas, Y., Vaz, S., Falkmer, T., & Cordier, R. (2019). The experiences of mothers of children with autism spectrum disorder: Managing family routines and mothers' health and wellbeing. *Australian Occupational Therapy Journal*, *66*(1), 68–76. https://doi.org/10.1111/1440-1630.12524

McAuliffe, T., Vaz, S., Falkmer, T., & Cordier, R. (2017). A comparison of families of children with autism spectrum disorders in family daily routines, service usage, and stress levels by regionality. *Developmental Neurorehabilitation*, *20*(8), 483–490. https://doi.org/10.1080/17518423.2016.1236844

McNamee, T., & Patton, S. (2018). Teachers' perspectives on handwriting and collaborative intervention for children with autistic spectrum disorder. *Irish Journal of Occupational Therapy*, *46*(1), 46–58. https://doi.org/10.1108/IJOT-12-2017-0026

Miller-Kuhaneck, H. (2015). Autism spectrum disorder. In J. Case-Smith & J. C. O'Brien (Eds.), *Occupational therapy for children and adolescents* (7th ed., pp. 766–792). Mosby.

Morris, S. L., Foster, C. J., Parsons, R., Falkmer, M., Falkmer, T., & Rosalie, S. M. (2015). Differences in the use of vision and proprioception for postural control in autism spectrum disorder. *Neuroscience*, *307*, 273–280. https://doi.org/10.1016/j.neuroscience.2015.08.040

Nadon, G., Feldman, D., & Gisel, E. (2013). Feeding issues associated with the autism spectrum disorders. In M. Fitzgerald (Ed.), *Recent advances in autism spectrum disorders* (Vol. 1, pp. 599–632). IntechOpen. https://doi.org/10.5772/53644

Reinoso, G., Carsone, B., Weldon, S., Powers, J., & Bellare, N. (2018). Food selectivity and sensitivity in children with autism spectrum disorder: A systematic review defining the issue and evaluating intervention. *New Zealand Journal of Occupational Therapy*, *65*(1), 36–42.

Rekoutis, P. A. (2019). Providing occupational therapy for individuals with autism. In B. A. Boyt Schell & G. Gillen (Eds.), *Willard & Spackman's occupational therapy* (13th ed., pp. 1011–1023). Wolters Kluwer.

Repetto, L. P., Jasmin, E., Fombonne, E., Gisel, E., & Couture, M. (2017). Longitudinal study of sensory features in children with autism spectrum disorder. *Autism Research and Treatment*, *2017*, Article 1934701. https://doi.org/10.1155/2017/1934701

Reszka, S. S., Boyd, B. A., McBee, M., Hume, K. A., & Odom, S. L. (2014). Brief report: Concurrent validity of autism symptom severity measures. *Journal of Autism and Developmental Disorders*, *44*, 446–470. https://doi.org/10.1007/s10803-013-1879-7

Reynolds, S., Bendixen, R. M., Lawrence, T., & Lane, S. J. (2011). A pilot study examining activity participation, sensory responsiveness and competence in children with high functioning autism spectrum disorder. *Journal of Autism and Developmental Disorders, 41,* 1496–1506. https://doi.org/10.1007/s10803-010-1173-x

Ricon, T., Sorek, R., & Engle-Yeger, B. (2017). Association between sensory processing by children with high functioning autism spectrum disorder and their daily routines. *Open Journal of Occupational Therapy, 5*(4), Article 3. https://doi.org/10.15453/2168-6408.1337

Rodger, S., & Polatajko, H. J. (2014). Occupational therapy for children with autism. In V. B. Patel, V. R. Preedy, & C. R. Martin (Eds.), *Comprehensive guide to autism* (pp. 2297–2314). Springer.

Rodger, S., & Ziviani, J. (2014). Autism spectrum disorders. In S. J. Lane & A. C. Bundy (Eds.), *Kids can be kids: A childhood occupations approach* (pp. 483–524). F. A. Davis.

Saggers, B., Klug, D., Harper-Hill, K., Ashburner, J., Costley, D., Clark, T., Bruck, S., Trembath, D., Webster, A. A., & Carrington, S. (2016). *Australian autism education needs analysis—What are the needs of schools, parents and students on the autism spectrum?* Autism CRC.

Schaaf, R. C., & Lane, A. E. (2015). Toward a best-practice protocol for assessment of sensory features in ASD. *Journal of Autism and Developmental Disorders, 45,* 1380–1395. https://doi.org/10.1007/s10803-014-2299-z

Schaaf, R. C., Toth-Cohen, S., Johnson, S. L., Outten, G., & Benevides, T. W. (2011). The everyday routines of families of children with autism: Examining the impact of sensory processing difficulties on the family. *Autism, 15*(3), 373–389. https://doi.org/10.1177/1362361310386505

Shah, S. P., Joshi, A., & Kulkami, V. (2015). Prevalence of sensory processing dysfunction and patterns on sensory profile of children with autism spectrum disorder in Mumbai: A pilot study. *Indian Journal of Occupational Therapy, 47*(2), 52–57.

Sim, A., Cordier, R., Vaz, S., Netto, J., & Falkmer, T. (2017). Factors associated with negative co-parenting experiences in families of a child with autism spectrum disorder. *Developmental Neurorehabilitation, 20*(2), 83–91. https://doi.org/10.3109/17518423.2015.1069414

Sim, A., Cordier, R., Vaz, S., Parson, R., & Falkmer, T. (2017). Relationship satisfaction and dyadic coping in couples with a child with autism spectrum disorder. *Journal of Autism and Developmental Disorders, 47*(11), 3562–3573. https://doi.org/10.1007/s10803-017-3275-1

Sim, A., Vaz, S., Cordier, R., Joosten, A., Parson, D., Smith, C., & Falkmer, T. (2018). Factors associated with stress in families of children with autism spectrum disorder. *Developmental Neurorehabilitation, 21*(3), 155–165. https://doi.org/10.1080/17518423.2017.1326185

Swami, P. R., & Vaidya, P. M. (2015). Correlation of self-injurious behavior, stereotyped movements and aggressive/destructive behavior with sensory processing disorder in children with autism and mental retardation. *Indian Journal of Occupational Therapy 47*(3), 81–88.

Suarez, M. A., Nelson, N. W., & Curtis, A. B. (2014). Longitudinal follow-up of factors associated with food selectivity in children with autism spectrum disorders. *Autism, 18*(8), 924–932. https://doi.org/10.1177/1362361313499457

Tang, J., Falkmer, M., Horlin, C., Tan, T., Vaz, S., & Falkmer, T. (2015). Face recognition and visual search strategies in autism spectrum disorders: Amending and extending a recent review by Weigelt et al. *PLOS ONE, 10*(8), Article e0134439. https://doi.org/10.1371/journal.pone.0134439

Tavassoli, T., Miller, L. J., Schoen, S. A., Brout, J. J., Sullivan, J., & Baron-Cohen, S. (2018). Sensory reactivity, empathizing and systemizing in autism spectrum conditions and sensory processing disorder. *Developmental Cognitive Neuroscience, 29,* 72–77. https://doi.org/10.1016/j.dcn.2017.05.005

Watson, L. R., Roberts, J. E., Baranek, G. T., Mandulak, K. C., & Dalton, J. C. (2012). Behavioral and physiological responses to child-directed speech of children with autism spectrum disorders or typical development. *Journal of Autism and Developmental Disorders, 42,* 1616–1629. https://doi.org/10.1007/s10803-011-1401-z

Welch, C., Polatajko, H., Rigby P., & Fitch, M. (2019). Autism inside out: Lessons from the memoirs of three minimally verbal youths. *Disability and Rehabilitation, 41*(19), 2308–2316. https://doi.org/10.1080/09638288.2018.1465133

Wigston, C., Falkmer, M., Vaz, S., Parsons, R., & Falkmer, T. (2017). Participation in extracurricular activities for children with and without siblings with autism spectrum disorder. *Developmental Neurorehabilitation, 20*(1), 25–39. https://doi.org/10.3109/17518423.2015.1046091

Williams, K. L., Kirby, A. V., Watson, L. R., Sideris, J., Bulluck, J., & Baranek, G. T. (2018). Sensory features as predictors of adaptive behaviors: A comparative longitudinal study of children with autism spectrum disorder and other developmental disabilities. *Research in Developmental Disabilities, 81*, 103–112. https://doi.org/10.1016/j.ridd.2018.07.002

Brachial Plexus Birth Injury

Also called BPBI, brachial plexus injury at birth, obstetrical brachial plexus injury, brachial plexus birth palsy, obstetrical brachial plexus palsy, perinatal brachial plexus injury, Erb-Duchenne paralysis, Déjérine-Klumpke's paralysis.

Description

Brachial plexus birth injury or palsy involves injury to any nerve of the brachial plexus, usually during birth. Injuries may involve the following:

- Upper brachial plexus (C5 to C7, Erb's palsy): Affects shoulder and elbow muscles, causing adduction and internal rotation of the shoulder and pronation of the forearm. Biceps reflex may be absent, and Moro reflex is asymmetrical. Muscle atrophy may be present. Sensory loss usually occurs. Ipsilateral paralysis of the diaphragm may occur due to injury to the phrenic nerve.
- Lower plexus (C8 to T1, Klumpke palsy): Primarily affects muscles of the forearm and hand, causing weakness or paralysis of the hand and wrist. Grasp reflex is usually absent. Horner syndrome may occur if T1 fibers are involved, causing miosis, ptosis, and facial anhidrosis.
- Entire brachial plexus (global injury, total plexus palsy): Affects entire upper extremity and often sympathetic fibers of T1. Upper extremity if flaccid with little or no movement, absent reflexes, and usually sensory loss (O'Toole, 2017; Porter, 2018).

Cause

Lateral stretching of the neck during delivery caused by shoulder dystocia (a birth emergency), breech extraction, or hyperabduction of the neck in cephalic presentation. Injuries can be due to simple stretching of the nerve, hemorrhage with a nerve, tearing of the nerve or root, or avulsion of the roots with accompanying cervical cord injury (Porter, 2018).

Raimondi Grading System for Hand Function (adapted from Mulcahey et al., 2012)

- Complete paralysis or slight finger flexion of no functional use; no thumb pinch or opposition; no or some sensation
- Limited active flexion of fingers, no extension of wrist or fingers; passive lateral pinch of thumb; supinated forearm
- Active extension of wrist gives passive flexion of fingers (tenodesis); passive lateral pinch of thumb; pronated forearm
- Complete active flexion of wrist and fingers; mobile thumb with partial abduction and opposition; some intrinsic balance; no active pronation and supination; good sensation
- Complete active flexion of wrist and fingers; active wrist extension; weak or absent

finger extension; good thumb opposition with active intrinsic function; partial active pronation and supination

- Function as stated above plus active finger extension and near complete pronation and supination

---

Evaluation/Assessment

Areas

- Activities of Daily Living/Instrumental ADL: age-appropriate basic ADLs
- Education/Work: age-appropriate classroom skills and behavior
- Play/Leisure: age-appropriate play skills and leisure occupations
- Rest/Sleep: age-appropriate sleep habits and routine
- Social Participation: age-appropriate social activities
- Sensorimotor: postural reflexes (primitive, righting, equilibrium), muscle atrophy (deltoid, biceps, brachialis), muscle strength, joint range of motion, hand functions, positioning, sensation (pain, proprioception, tactile, temperature)
- Cognitive/Perceptual: age-appropriate cognition and perception
- Psychosocial: emotional regulation, anxiety, age-appropriate peer relations, parent–child relations, self-esteem, self-efficacy, quality of life
- Context/Environment: social support, adapted devices including splints
- Development (Infant, Child, Adolescent only): developmental milestones, development delay, parent knowledge of normal development
- Comorbidities: limb length difference

Instruments

Instruments Developed by Occupational Therapy Personnel

- Activity Item Bank (list of items; Mulcahey et al., 2012, and Mulcahey et al., 2013, in References)
- Assisting Hand Assessment (AHA; Krumlinde-Sundholm & Eliasson, 2003)
- Box and Block Test (BBT; Holser & Fuchs, 1957; Mathiowetz et al., 1985, norms for children)
- Brachial Plexus Outcome Measure (BPOM; Ho et al., 2012, in References)
- Upper Extremity Item Bank (list of items; Mulcahey et al., 2012, and Mulcahey et al., 2013, in References)

Instruments Developed by Other Professionals and Used by Occupational Therapy Personnel

- Active Movement Scale (AMS; Clark & Curtis, 1995)
- Adolescent Pediatric Pain Tool (APPT; Jacob et al., 2014)
- Behavior Assessment System for Children, Parent Rating Scales (2nd ed.; BASC-2 PRS; Reynolds & Kamphaus, 2004)
- Draw A Person: Screening Procedure for Emotional Disturbance (DAP SPED; Naglieri et al., 1991)
- Faces Pain Scale–Revised (FPS-R; Hicks et al., 2001)
- Modified Mallet (MM; Bae et al., 2003)
- Piers-Harris Children's Self-Concept Scale (2nd ed.; Piers-Harris 3; Piers & Herzberg, 2002)
- Weinstein Enhanced Sensory Test (WEST; Commercially available from multiple sources)

Problems/Issues

Activities of Daily Living/Instrumental ADL

- Child may have difficulty performing ADLs that require two hands and finger dexterity such as fasteners (buttons, zippers, snaps).
- Child may have difficulty reaching to back of head to brush and comb hair.
- Child/adolescent may have difficulty reaching into back pocket.
- Child/adolescent may have difficulty reaching overhead to put dishes away or retrieve them.

Education/Work
- Infant/child with fixed forearm supination contracture cannot position hand optimally (in pronation) for activities on a desk such as writing and keyboarding.

Play/Leisure
- Infant/child may be delayed or have difficulty in developing two-handed play activities.
- Child/adolescent may have difficulty performing leisure occupations that require upper extremity coordination, such as playing the piano, playing drums, swinging a bat.

Rest/Sleep
- Not discussed.

Social Participation
- Child/adolescent may experience social isolation due to disability.

Sensorimotor
- Infant/child may demonstrate delayed integration of primitive reflexes.
- Infant/child usually has limited range of motion in shoulder external rotation and forearm supination.
- Infant/child usually positions limb in shoulder internal rotation and forearm pronation.
- Infant/child usually has a compensatory scapular winging.
- Infant/child may have tightness or contractures in shoulder musculature (glenohumeral joint) primarily affecting adduction, horizontal adduction, and internal rotation (Gharbaoui et al., 2015).
- Infant/child may have contractures in elbow joint limiting extension (Ho, Kim, et al., 2019; Ho, Zuccaro, et al., 2019; Ho, Klar, et al., 2019).
- Infant/child may have contractures in the forearm limiting pronation (Gladstein et al., 2017).
- Infant/child may have muscle weakness in deltoid, biceps, and brachialis.
- Infant/child may have difficulty abducting the thumb to oppose fingers for cylinder grasp.
- Infant/child may have difficulty using thumb to oppose fingers for pinch grasp.
- Infant/child may have limb length differences (Bain et al., 2012).
- Infant/child usually has decreased or loss of sensation (proprioception, tactile, stereognosis, pressure, temperature).
- Infant/child may experience pain, especially after surgical procedures (Ho et al., 2015).

Cognitive/Perceptual
- Injury does not directly affected cognition.
- Tactile perception is involved.

Psychosocial
- Child/adolescent may be noncompliant with intervention, especially in treatment of elbow flexion contracture.
- Child/adolescent may experience increased anxiety, especially females (Belfiore et al., 2016).
- Child/adolescent may have poor self-concept or sense of self-efficacy.
- Child/adolescent may have reduced quality of life.

Context/Environment
- Family members may lack information about brachial plexus birth palsy and its management.
- Family members may need instruction in proper positioning and carrying of an infant.
- Family may lack knowledge about available resources.

Intervention/Treatment

Models and programs developed by occupational therapy personnel include management protocol for Erb's palsy (Singh & Kolamala, 2015) and scapular stabilizer brace (Daftary & Jywant, 2012). Models and programs developed by other professionals but used by occupational therapy personnel include constraint-induced movement therapy (CIMT; Berggren & Baker, 2015; Vaz et al., 2010), education day for families (Ho & Ulster, 2011), electrical stimulation (Berggren & Baker, 2015; Justice et al., 2018), International Classification of Functioning, Disability, and Health (ICF) model (Duff & DeMatteo, 2015), stretching (Russo et al., 2019), serial casting and splinting (Ho et al., 2010), Sup-ER Orthosis (Durlacher et al., 2014), and therapeutic taping (Russo et al., 2016; Russo et al., 2018). Team members include physicians, pediatricians, surgeons, nursing personnel, physical therapy personnel, and occupational therapy personnel. Goals are to use splinting to prevent contractures, strengthen muscles, stimulate sensory nerves, and encourage the achievement of normal developmental milestones.

Activities of Daily Living/Instrumental ADL
- Compensatory techniques should be taught to facilitate performance of basic ADLs (e.g., elbow can be placed on a tabletop and head lowered to permit child to reach over and behind head to comb and brush hair).

Education/Work
- Child may need modification of some classroom tasks that normally require two hands, such as cutting with scissors, stringing beads, unscrewing paint-jar lids.

Play/Leisure
- Assist child to develop age-appropriate play skills.
- Assist child/adolescent to develop leisure occupations that are within the child's or adolescent's functional skills level.

Rest/Sleep
- Not discussed.

Social Participation
- Encourage child/adolescent to participate in social activities with peers. Provide assistance with modifications as needed.

Sensorimotor
- Gentle stretching of the shoulder girdle muscles and inferior scapula-humeral angle (ISHA) should begin early and continue to prevent contracture (Berggren & Baker, 2015). Note that scapular stabilization may be detrimental to passive stretching of the glenohumeral joint (Russo et al., 2019).
- Focus on maximizing hand and arm function.

Cognitive/Perceptual
- Not discussed.

Psychosocial
- Explore with client approaches and actions to improve self-concept.
- Explore with client methods to reduce anxiety such as deep breathing, mindfulness, yoga, guided imagery.

Context/Environment
- Serial casting or splinting can assist in reducing elbow flexion contracture.
- Splinting or casting may be needed to facilitate supination.
- Body cast or shoulder positioning splint may be needed to maintain shoulder position.
- Hand splints may be needed to facilitate opposition.
- Provide instruction on positioning and carrying. Infant should be carried so injured arm is free, not trapped against adult's body, and available to encourage exploration of environment.
- Provide family with information about managing brachial plexus birth injury.
- Provide family with access to resources.

Precautions/Safety Considerations

Child/adolescent is at risk for injury due to reduced sensory awareness. Infant should not be positioned such that the involved upper extremity movement is restricted by external environment.

Prognosis and Outcome

About 92% of infants show partial or full recovery in the first 3 months. Infants with global injury and a positive Horner's sign usually do not recover by 3 months and have a worse prognosis (Berggren & Baker, 2015). Sensory outcomes in children following microsurgery were generally good (Ho, Davidge, et al., 2019).

REFERENCES

Bain, J. R., DeMatteo, C., Gjertsen, D., Packham, T., Galea, V., & Harper, J. A. (2012). Limb length differences after obstetrical brachial plexus injury: A growing concern. *Plastic and Reconstructive Surgery, 130*(4), Article 558e-571e. https://doi.org/10.1097/PRS.0b013e318262f26b

Belfiore, L. A., Rosen, C., Sarshalom, R., Grossman, L., Sala, D. A., & Grossman, J. A. I. (2016). Evaluation of self-concept and emotional-behavioral functioning of children with brachial plexus birth injury. *Journal of Brachial Plexus and Peripheral Nerve Injury, 11*(1), e42–e47. https://doi.org/10.1055/s-0036-1593440

Berggren, J., & Baker, L. L. (2015). Therapeutic application of electrical stimulation and constraint induced movement therapy in perinatal brachial plexus injury: A case report. *Journal of Hand Therapy, 28*(2), 217–221. https://doi.org/10.1016/j.jht.2014.12.006

Daftary, R., & Jywant, S. (2012). To study the effectiveness of a scapular stabilizer brace on shoulder functions of a child with the brachial plexus injury. *Indian Journal of Occupational Therapy, 44*(3), 3–10.

Duff, S. V., & DeMatteo, C. (2015). Clinical assessment of the infant and child following perinatal brachial plexus injury. *Journal of Hand Therapy, 28,* 126–134. https://doi.org/10.1016/j.jht.2015.01.001

Durlacher, K. M., Bellows, D., & Verchere, C. (2014). Sup-ER orthosis: An innovative treatment for infants with birth related brachial plexus injury. *Journal of Hand Therapy, 27,* 335–340. https://doi.org/10.1016/j.jht.2014.06.001

Gharbaoui, I. S., Gogola, G. R., Aaron, D. H., & Kozin, S. H. (2015). Perspectives on glenohumeral joint contractures and shoulder dysfunction in children with perinatal brachial plexus palsy. *Journal of Hand Therapy, 28*(2), 176–184. https://doi.org/10.1016/j.jht.2014.12.001

Gladstein, A. Z., Sachleben, B., Ho, E. S., Anthony, A., Clarke, H. M., & Hopyan, S. (2017). Forearm pronation osteotomy for supination contracture secondary to obstetrical brachial plexus palsy: A retrospective cohort study. *Journal of Pediatric Orthopaedics, 37*(6), e357–e363. https://doi.org/10.1097/BPO.0000000000001053

Ho, E. S., Curtis, C. G., & Clarke, H. M. (2012). The Brachial Plexus Outcome Measure: Developmental, internal consistency, and construct validity. *Journal of Hand Therapy, 25*(4), 406–417. https://doi.org/10.1016/j.jht.2012.05.002

Ho, E. S., Curtis, C. G., & Clarke, H. M. (2015). Pain in children following microsurgical reconstruction for obstetrical brachial plexus palsy. *Journal of Hand Surgery American, 40*(6), 1177–1183. https://doi.org/10.1016/j.jhsa.2015.02.003

Ho, E. S., Davidge, K., Curtis, C. G., & Clarke, H. M. (2019). Sensory outcome in children following microsurgery for brachial plexus birth injury. *Journal of Hand Surgery American, 44*(2), 159.e1–159.e8. https://doi.org/10.1016/j.jhsa.2018.05.009

Ho, E. S., Kim, D., Klar, K., Anthony, A., Davidge, K., Borschel, G. H., Hopyan, S., Clarke, H. M., & Wright, F. V. (2019). Prevalence and ethology of elbow flexion contractures in brachial plexus birth injury: A scoping review. *Journal of Pediatric Rehabilitation Medicine, 12*(1), 75–86. https://doi.org/10.3233/PRM-180535

Ho, E. S., Klar, K., Klar, E., Davidge, K., Hopyan, S., & Clarke, H. M. (2019). Elbow flexion contractures in brachial plexus birth injury: Function and appearance related factors. *Disability and Rehabilitation, 41*(22), 2648–2652. https://doi.org/10.1080/09638288.2018.1473512

Ho, E. S., Roy, T., Stephens, D., & Clarke, H. M. (2010). Serial casting and splinting of elbow contractures in children with obstetric brachial plexus palsy. *Journal of Hand Surgery, 35*(1), 84–91. https://doi.org/10.1016/j.jhsa.2009.09.014

Ho, E. S., & Ulster, A. A. (2011). Evaluation of an education day for families of children with obstetrical brachial plexus palsy. *Families, Systems, and Health, 29*(3), 206–214. https://doi.org/10.1037/a0025105

Ho, E. S., Zuccaro, J., Klar, K., Anthony, A., Davidge, K., Borschel, G. H., Hopyan, S., Clarke, H. M., & Wright, F. V. (2019). Effectiveness of non-surgical and surgical interventions for elbow flexion contracture in brachial plexus birth injury: A systematic review. *Journal of Pediatric Rehabilitation Medicine, 12*(1), 87–100. https://doi.org/10.3233/PRM-180563

Justice, D., Awori, J., Carlson, S., Chang, K. W.-C., & Yang, L. J.-S. (2018). Use of neuromuscular electrical stimulation in the treatment of neonatal brachial plexus palsy: A literature review. *Open Journal of Occupational Therapy, 6*(3), Article 10. https://doi.org/10.15453/2168-6408.1431

Mulcahey, M. J., Kozin, S., Merenda, L., Gaughan, J., Tian, F., Gogola, G., James, M. A., & Ni, P. (2012). Evaluation of the Box and Blocks Test, stereognosis and item banks of activity and upper extremity function in youths with brachial plexus birth palsy. *Journal of Pediatric Orthopaedics, 32*(Suppl. 2), S114–S122. https://doi.org/10.1097/bpo.0b013e3182595423

Mulcahey, M. J., Merenda, L., Tian, F., Kozin, S., James, M., Gogola, J., & Ni, P. (2013). Computer adaptive test approach to the assessment of children and youth with brachial plexus birth palsy. *American Journal of Occupational Therapy, 67*(5), 524–533. https://doi.org/10.5014/ajot.2013.008037

O'Toole, M. T. (Ed.). (2017). *Mosby's Dictionary of medicine, nursing & health professions* (10th ed.). Elsevier.

Porter, R. S. (Ed.). (2018). *The Merck manual of diagnosis and therapy* (20th ed.). Merck Sharp & Dohme.

Russo, S. A., Killelea, C. M., Zlotolow, D. A, Kozin, S. H., Rodriguez, L. M., Chafetz, R. S., & Richards, J. G. (2019). Scapular stabilization limits glenohumeral stretching in children with brachial plexus injuries. *Journal of Hand Surgery American, 44*(1), 63.e1–63.e9. https://doi.org/10.1016/j.jhsa.2018.04.025

Russo, S. A., Rodriguez, L. M., Kozin, S. H., Zlotolow, D. A., Chafetz, R. S., Killelia, C. M., Nicholson, K. F., & Richards, J. G. (2016). Therapeutic taping for scapular stabilization in children with brachial plexus birth palsy. *American Journal of Occupational Therapy, 70*(5), Article 7995229939. https://doi.org/10.5014/ajot.2016.018903

Russo, S. A., Zlotolow, D. A., Chafetz, R. S., Rodriquez, L. M., Kelly, D., Linamen, H., Richards, J. G., Lubahn, J. D., & Kozin, S. H. (2018). Efficacy of therapeutic taping configurations for children with brachial plexus birth palsy. *Journal of Hand Therapy, 31*(3), 357–370. https://doi.org/10.1016/j.jht.2017.03.001

Singh, P. P., & Kolamala, K. (2015). Development of a protocol for the management of obstetric Erb's palsy. *Indian Journal of Occupational Therapy, 47*(1), 14–19.

Vaz, D. V., Mancini, M. C., do Amaral, M. F., de Brito Brandão, M., de França Drummond, A., & da Fonsca, S. T. (2010). Clinical changes during an intervention based on constraint-induced movement therapy principles on use of the affected arm of a child with obstetric brachial plexus injury: A case report. *Occupational Therapy International, 17*, 159–167. https://doi.org/10.1002/oti.295

BIBLIOGRAPHY

Ridgway, E., Valicenti-McDermott, M., Kornhaber, L., Kathirthamby, D. R., & Wieder, H. (2013). Effects from birth brachial plexus injury and postural control. *Journal of Pediatrics, 162*(5), 1065–1067. https://doi.org/10.1016/j.jpeds.2012.12.073

Tanta, K. J., Gunsolus, K., Harley, N., Grosvenor, K., Garcia, J., & Jirikowic, T. (2012). Protocol development for infants with orthopedic complications in the neonatal intensive care unit: Brachial plexus injuries and clubfoot. *Journal of Occupational Therapy, Schools, & Early Intervention, 5*(3/4), 275–292. https://doi.org/10.1080/19411243.2012.750544

Verchere, C., Durlacher, K. I., Bellows, D., Pike, J., & Bucevska, M. (2014). An early shoulder repositioning program in birth-related brachial plexus injury: A pilot study of the sup-ER protocol. *Hand, 9*(2), 187–195. https://doi.org/10.1007/s11552-014-9625-y

Yasukawa, A., & Uronis, J. (2014). Effectiveness of the dynamic movement orthosis glove for a child with cerebral palsy hemiplegia and obstetric brachial plexus palsy. *JPO: Journal of Prosthetics and Orthotics, 26*(2), 107–112. https://doi.org/10.1097/jpo.0000000000000022

Cerebral Palsy: Adolescent and Adult

Description

Cerebral palsy is a nonprogressive lesion. However, the pattern of motor impairment changes as the person develops throughout life, affecting all daily occupations. In addition, there may be disturbances in sensation, perception, cognition, and communication, which manifest as different types of problems as the person is expected to perform occupations and roles associated with adolescence and adulthood (Coker-Bolt et al., 2015).

Cause

In part, the cause is the result of neurophysiological changes in the brain. Other "causes" relate to changing expectations for occupational performance coinciding with social and cultural norms.

Evaluation/Assessment

Areas

- Activities of Daily Living/Instrumental ADL: self-maintenance skills (dressing, grooming, bathing, toileting, mobility), independent living (home management, meal preparation and nutrition, financial management, shopping, transportation), fitness (general health), sexuality
- Education/Work: educational achievement, work skills, seeking work (paid, volunteer)
- Play/Leisure: interests, values, frequency
- Rest/Sleep: no information identified
- Social Participation: type, location, frequency, with whom
- Sensorimotor: range of motion, muscle tone, muscle strength, balance reactions, contractures, fatigue, pain, visual loss
- Cognitive/Perceptual: memory loss, executive skills (time management)
- Psychosocial: sense of autonomy, anxiety, quality of life, self-awareness, self-confidence, self-determination, self-esteem, social and personal interaction skills
- Context/Environment: adapted devices, assistive technology, home adaptation, social support (family, friends), caregiver needs (personal attendant/provider), service animals, community resources, community accessibility and safety
- Comorbidities: seizures, intellectual disability, vision or hearing impairment, obesity, sarcopenia (loss of skeletal muscle mass)

Instruments

Instruments Developed by Occupational Therapy Personnel

- Assisting Hand Assessment for Adolescents (Ad-AHA; Louwers et al., 2016, and Louwers et al., 2017, in References)
- Canadian Occupational Performance Measure (5th ed.; COPM-5; Law et al., 2014)

- Manual Ability Classification System (MACS; Eliasson et al., 2006)
- Parent Stress Measure (PSM; Crowe et al., 2019, in References)
- Pediatric Evaluation of Disability Inventory (PEDI; Haley et al., 1992)

Instruments Developed by Other Professionals and Used by Occupational Therapy Personnel
- Barthel Index (BI; Mahoney & Barthel, 1965)
- Gross Motor Function Classification System–Expanded & Revised (GMFCS; Palisano et al., 2008)
- Jebsen-Taylor Hand Function Test (JTHFT; Jebsen et al., 1969)
- Multidimensional Scale of Perceived Social Support (MSPSS; Zimet et al., 1988)
- Parenting Stress Index (4th ed.; PSI-4; Abidin, 2012)
- Rosenberg Self-Esteem Scale (RSES; Rosenberg, 1965)
- Store Social Interaction and Behaviors Outcome Measure (SSIBOM; Harrop & Daniels, 1986)
- Strengths and Difficulties Questionnaire (SDQ; Goodman, 1997)
- Transitional Behaviors Outcome Measure (TBOM; Harrop & Daniels, 1986)
- Vineland Adaptive Behavior Scales (3rd ed.; Vineland-3; Sparrow et al., 2016)

Problems/Issues
Activities of Daily Living/Instrumental ADL
- Person may have difficulty performing self-maintenance skills due to spasticity or contractures.
- Person may lack knowledge, training, and practice in independent living skills (finding housing, maintaining a home including cleaning and doing laundry, shopping for groceries, planning and preparing meals).

Education/Work
- Person may lack job training skills.

Play/Leisure
- Person may have difficulty engaging in valued or preferred leisure occupations (Shikako-Thomas et al., 2015).

Rest/Sleep
- No information identified.

Social Participation
- Person may lack opportunities to participate in social occupations.

Sensorimotor
- Person may have limited range of motion in certain joints.
- Person may have hypertonicity (spasticity) or hypotonicity.
- Person may have weak muscle strength.
- Person may have poor balance reactions.
- Person may have contractures.
- Person may experience pain due to muscle spasms, contractures, or positioning especially in lower back, hips, and legs.
- Person may have reduced sensation.

Cognitive/Perceptual
- Person may have cognitive impairments, such as memory loss.
- Person may be intellectually disabled.
- Person may have difficulty scheduling and managing time, including creating a daily schedule and managing free time.

Psychosocial
- Person may lack self-awareness.
- Person may lack self-confidence and self-esteem.

- Person may lack self-determination and self-efficacy.
- Person may lack social interaction and social interpersonal skills.
- Person may experience social isolation.
- Person may demonstrate behavioral difficulties (Brossard-Racine et al., 2013).

Context/Environment
- Person may experience architectural barriers in community settings (lack of accessible routes to get into buildings and lack of access to services, such as no sidewalks, uneven sidewalks, stairs, narrow doors, no elevator, narrow aisles in stores, items placed out of reach; Dahan-Oliel et al., 2016).
- Person may be unfamiliar with or lack experience in finding their way about the community, including walking, driving, or using public transportation.
- Person may lack knowledge about community resources.
- Person may have limited social support.

Intervention/Treatment

Models and programs developed by occupational therapy personnel include the Cognitive Orientation to daily Occupational Performance (CO-OP) approach (Peny-Dahlstrand et al., 2018). Models and programs developed by other professionals but used by occupational therapy personnel include eye-gaze control technology (Karlsson et al., 2018), haptic exploratory procedures (Taylor et al., 2019), independence program (Kingsnorth et al., 2015), and service dog partnership (Crowe et al., 2019). Team members include physicians, psychologists, physical therapists, dieticians or nutritionists, animal behaviorists or trainers, and occupational therapy personnel. Goal is to facilitate maximum occupational performance in self-maintenance, independent living skills, work, and leisure consistent with client's abilities, needs, and limitations. More severe levels of gross and fine motor dysfunction tend to result in lower levels of self-care, mobility, and social function while increasing the level of caregiver assistance needed (Phipps & Roberts, 2012).

Activities of Daily Living/Instrumental ADL
- Provide opportunity to learn and practice meal planning, preparation, and cleanup.
- Provide opportunity to practice creating a budget, writing checks or entering amounts online to pay bills, balancing an account, applying for a checking account.
- Provide opportunity to create a shopping and shop for groceries or clothing.
- Nutrition program may be needed to manage weight.

Education/Work
- Provide opportunity to explore possible job or career opportunities (paid or unpaid).
- Provide opportunity to practice applying for a job/career opportunity, including completing an application and interviewing.
- Assist client in determining whether additional education and training would be useful, and if so, assist with application process.

Play/Leisure
- Assist person to develop and plan leisure occupations (activities, outings, options).
- Examples of favorite leisure activities were computer or video games, going to movies, watching TV or renting a movie, hanging out, and listening to music (Shikako-Thomas et al., 2015).

Rest/Sleep
- No information identified.

Social Participation
- Provide opportunity to participate in planned and guided social events (parties, outings, field trips).
- Provide opportunity to participate in unplanned and spontaneous social situations.

Sensorimotor
- Pain management program may be useful (see Pain and Chronic Pain in Section 2: Sensory Disorders).
- Fatigue management program may be needed as physical and psychological energy are reduced.

Cognitive/Perceptual
- Provide memory assist options, such as using a calendar or smartphone reminder.
- Provide opportunity to practice creating and following a daily schedule, including planning activities for free time.

Psychosocial
- Provide opportunity for client to try out activities on his or her own (sense of autonomy) and discuss what went right and what went wrong.
- Provide opportunity to increase self-awareness, self-efficacy, and self-identity (Who am I?; Bergqvist et al., 2019).
- Provide opportunity to increase self-determination and sense of self-efficacy (What can I do?).
- Provide opportunity to increase self-confidence (What am I good at?).
- Provide opportunity to participate in situations that require interaction with others (role-playing, practice trips to a store, shopping at a mall).
- Assist client in reducing anxiety through repeated practice and successful results.

Context/Environment
- Consider if telerehabilitation may be useful in addition to or instead of on-site visits for intervention services.
- Assist client to plan community-based activities and trips to reduce incidence of encountering physical and social barriers.
- Assist client to explore transportation alternatives (unassisted or assisted for disabled).
- Assist client on how to inform and educate others about condition as an adolescent or adult with physical and sensory limitations but also strengths and abilities.
- Assist client, family, and caregivers to explore and become familiar with information and community resources available to educate them about functioning as an adult with a disability (housing, work, leisure, medical care, insurance, financial resources, volunteer agencies).
- Person may need direct referral for vision or hearing services.
- Person, therapists, and family can be advocates for a more accessible community.

Precautions/Safety Considerations
Person may be at risk for falls due to poor balance reactions or visual impairment. Person may be at risk for seizures due to epilepsy.

Prognosis and Outcome
Prognosis is dependent on client's ability to learn skills, manage behaviors, and make use of available resources needed to fulfill requirements of life situation and make adaptations necessary as personal or environment situation changes (independent living, group or family living). Outcome is a dynamic target since life situation and means to meet goals will change as the person progresses through life.

REFERENCES
Bergqvist, L., Öhrvall, A.-M., Himmelmann, K., & Peny-Dahlstrand, M. (2019). When I do, I become someone: Experiences of occupational performance in young adults with cerebral palsy. *Disability and Rehabilitation*, 41(3), 341–347. https://doi.org/10.1080/09638288.2017.1390696

Brossard-Racine, M., Waknin, J., Shikako-Thomas, K., Shevell, M., Paulin, C., Lach, L., Law, M., Schmitz, N., QUALA Group, & Majnemer, A. (2013). Behavioral difficulties in adolescents with cerebral palsy. *Journal of Child Neurology, 28*(1), 27–33. https://doi.org/10.1177/0883 073812461942

Coker-Bolt, P. C., Garcia T., & Naber, E. (2015). Neuromotor: Cerebral palsy. In J. Case-Smith & J. C. O'Brien (Eds.), *Occupational therapy for children and adolescents* (7th ed., pp. 793–811). Elsevier-Mosby.

Crowe, T. K., Dietz, J. C., Winkle, M., Nelson, R. A., & Woolf, J. (2019). Effects of partnerships between adolescents with developmental disabilities and service dogs. *Open Journal of Occupational Therapy, 7*(1), Article 3. https://doi.org/10.15453/2168-6408.1520

Dahan-Oliel, N., Shikako-Thomas, K., Mazer, B., & Majnemer, A. (2016). Adolescents with disabilities participate in the shopping mall: Facilitators and barriers framed according to the ICF. *Disability and Rehabilitation, 38*(21), 2101–2113. https://doi.org/10.3109/09638288.2 015.1114033

Karlsson, P., Allsop, A., Dee-Price, B.-J., & Wallen, M. (2018). Eye-gaze control technology for children, adolescents and adults with cerebral palsy with significant physical disability: Findings from a systematic review. *Developmental Neurorehabilitation, 21*(8), 497–505. https://doi.org/10.1080/17518423.2017.1362057

Kingsnorth, S., King, G., McPherson, A., & Jones-Galley, K. (2015). A retrospective study of past graduates of a residential life skills program for youth with physical disabilities. *Child: Care, Health and Development, 41*(3), 374–383. https://doi.org/10.1111/cch.12196

Louwers, A., Beelen, A., Holmefur, M., & Krumlinde-Sundholm L. (2016). Development of the Assisting Hand Assessment for adolescents (Ad-AHA) and validation of the AHA from 18 months to 18 years. *Developmental Medicine & Child Neurology, 58*(12), 1303–1309. https://doi.org/10.1111/dmcn.13168

Louwers, A., Krumlinde-Sundhom, L., Boescholten, K., & Beelen, A. (2017). Reliability of the Assisting Hand Assessment in adolescents. *Developmental Medicine & Child Neurology, 59*(9), 926–932. https://doi.org/10.1111/dmcn.13465

Peny-Dahlstrand, M., Bergqvist, L., Hofgren, C., Himmelmann, K., & Öhrvall, A.-M. (2018). Potential benefits of the cognitive orientation to daily occupational performance approach in young adults with spina bifida or cerebral palsy: A feasibility study. *Disability and Rehabilitation, 42*(2), 228–239. https://doi.org/10.1080/09638288.2018.1496152

Phipps, S., & Roberts, P. (2012). Predicting the effects of cerebral palsy severity on self-care, mobility, and social function. *American Journal of Occupational Therapy, 66*, 422–429. https://doi.org/10.5014/ajot.2012.003921

Shikako-Thomas, K. I., Shevell, M., Lach, L., Law, M., Schmitz, N., Poulin, C., Majnemer, A., & QUALA Group. (2015). Are you doing what you want to do? Leisure preferences of adolescents with cerebral palsy. *Developmental Neurorehabilitation, 18*(4), 234–240. https://doi.org/10.3109/17518423.2013.794166

Taylor, S., Girdler, S., McCutcheon, S., McLean, B., Parsons, R., Falkmer, T., Jacoby, P., Carey, L., & Elliott, C. (2019). Haptic exploratory procedures of children and youth with and without cerebral palsy. *Physical & Occupational Therapy in Pediatrics, 39*(3), 337–351. https://doi.org/10.1080/01942638.2018.1477228

BIBLIOGRAPHY

Chikwanha, T. M., Chidhakwa, S., & Dangarembizi, N. (2015). Occupational therapy needs of adolescents and young adults with cerebral palsy in Zimbabwe: Caregivers' perspectives. *Central African Journal of Medicine, 61*(5/8), 38–44.

Espin-Tello, S. M., Dickinson, H. O., Bueno-Lozano, M., Jiménez-Bernadó, M. T., & Caballero-Navarro, A. L. (2018). Functional capacity and self-esteem of people with cerebral palsy.

American Journal of Occupational Therapy, 72, Article 203295120. https://doi.org/10.5014/ajot.2018.025940

Golomb, M. R., McDonald, B. C., Warden, S. J., Yonkman, J., Saykin, A. J., Shirley, B., Huber, M., Rabin, B., AbdelBaky, M., Nwosu, M. E., Barkat-Masih, M., & Burdea, G. C. (2010). In-home virtual reality videogame telerehabilitation in adolescents with hemiplegic cerebral palsy. *Archives of Physical Medicine and Rehabilitation, 91*(1), 1–8.e1. https://doi.org/10.1016/j.apmr.2009.08.153

Hirsh, A. T., Gallegos, J. C., Gertz, K. J., Engle, J. M., & Jensen, M. P. (2010). Symptom burden in individuals with cerebral palsy. *Journal of Rehabilitation Research & Development, 47*(9), 863–876. https://doi.org/10.1682/jrrd.2010.03.0024

Hirsh, A. T., Kratz, A. L., Engle, J. M., & Jensen, M. P. (2011). Survey results of pain treatments in adults with cerebral palsy. *American Journal of Physical Medicine & Rehabilitation, 90*(3), 207–216. https://doi.org/10.1097/PHM.0b013e3182063bc9

James, S., Ziviani, J., & Boyd, R. (2014). A systematic review of activities of daily living measures for children and adolescents with cerebral palsy. *Developmental Medicine & Child Neurology, 56,* 233–244. https://doi.org/10.1111/dmcn.12226

King, G., Imms, C., Palisano, R., Majnemer, A., Chiarello, L., Orlin, M., Law, M., & Avery, L. (2013). Geographical patterns in the recreation and leisure participation of children and youth with cerebral palsy: A CAPE international collaborative network study. *Developmental Neurorehabilitation, 16*(3), 196–206. https://doi.org/10.3109/17518423.2013.773102

Lindsay, S. (2016). Child and youth experiences and perspectives of cerebral palsy: A qualitative systematic review. *Child: Care, Health and Development, 42*(2), 153–175. https://doi.org/10.1111/cch.12309

Livingston, M. H., Stewart, D., Rosenbaum, P. L., & Russell, D. J. (2011). Exploring issues of participation among adolescents with cerebral palsy: What's important to them? *Physical & Occupational Therapy in Pediatrics, 31*(3), 275–287. https://doi.org/10.3109/01942638.2011.565866

Majnemer, A., Shikako-Thomas, K., Shevell, M., Poulin, C., Lach, L., Law, M., Schmitz, N., & QUALA Group. (2013). The relationship between manual ability and ambulation in adolescents with cerebral palsy. *Physical & Occupational Therapy in Pediatrics, 33*(2), 243–252. https://doi.org/10.3109/01942638.2012.754394

Nordstrand, L., & Eliasson, A. C. (2013). Six years after a modified constraint induced movement therapy (CIMT) program—What happens when the children have become young adults? *Physical & Occupational Therapy in Pediatrics, 33*(2), 163–169. https://doi.org/10.3109/01942638.2013.757157

Cerebral Palsy: Infant and Child

Description

Cerebral palsy (CP) is a group of nonprogressive syndromes characterized by impaired voluntary movement or posture which results from prenatal developmental malformation or perinatal or postnatal central nervous system (CNS) damage. Syndromes manifesting before age 2 years may include spasticity, ataxia, or involuntary movements (Porter, 2018). Categories or types of CP syndromes are spastic syndromes (hemiplegic or unilateral, quadriplegic or tetraplegic), athetoid or dyskinetic syndromes, ataxic syndromes, and mixed.

Cause

Etiology is multifactorial, and a specific cause may be difficult to determine. Prematurity, in utero disorders, neonatal encephalopathy, and kernicterus often contribute. Prenatal factors such as perinatal asphyxia, stroke, or CNS infections probably cause 15% to 20% of cases (Porter, 2018).

Evaluation/Assessment

Areas
- Activities of Daily Living/Instrumental ADL: eating and swallowing, dressing and undressing, bathing, toileting, transfers, bowel and bladder function, self-maintenance, transition skills to independent living
- Education/Work: academic achievement, handwriting
- Play/Leisure: interests, type, frequency, location
- Rest/Sleep: sleep disturbance, sleep disorders
- Social Participation: type frequency, location, with whom
- Sensorimotor: abnormal muscle tone including muscle weakness (hypotonia), muscle tightness (hypertonia) spasticity, and fluctuating muscle tone; persistent primitive reflexes, atypical righting, equilibrium, and protective responses; joint hypermobility or stiffness, joint contractures; gait; balance; posture; involuntary movements; fine motor skills (opposition, object manipulation); gross motor skills (sitting, standing, walking); impaired sensation (visual, hearing)
- Cognitive/Perceptual: intellectual ability, specific learning disability, visual perception
- Psychosocial: interpersonal skills, quality of life, self-efficacy
- Context/Environment: adapted equipment, information and resources
- Development (Infant, Child, Adolescent only): developmental delay
- Comorbidity: seizures (epilepsy), intellectual disability, pressure sores, osteoporosis

Instruments
Instruments Developed by Occupational Therapy Personnel
- Assessment of Motor and Process Skills (8th ed.; AMPS-8; Fisher & Bray Jones, 2016)
- Assisting Hand Assessment (AHA; Krumlinde-Sundholm & Eliasson, 2003; see also Krumlinde-Sundholm, 2012, and Ryll et al., 2017, in References)
- Assisting Hand Assessment (Kids AHA 5.0; Holmefur & Krumlinde-Sundholm, 2016, in References)
- Bimanual Fine Motor Function (BFMF) Classification (Elvrum et al., 2016, in References)
- Both Hands Assessment (BoHA; Elvrum et al., 2018, in References)
- Canadian Occupational Performance Measure (5th ed., COPM-5; Law et al., 2014)
- Children's Assessment of Participation and Enjoyment (CAPE; King et al., 2004)
- Children's Hand-use Experience Question (CHEQ; Sköld et al., 2011; see also Amer et al., 2016; Ryll et al., 2017; Ryll et al., 2019, in References)
- Grasp and Reach Assessment of Brisbane (GRAB; Perez et al., 2016, in References)
- Hand Assessment for Infants (HAI; Krumlinde-Sundholm et al., 2017, in References; see also Wallen, 2019, in References)
- Klein-Bell ADL Scale (KB-ADL; Klein & Bell, 1982)
- Leiter International Performance Scale (3rd ed.; Leiter-3; Roid et al., 2013)
- Manual Ability Classification System (MACS; Eliasson et al., 2006; see also Burgess et al., 2019; Öhrvall & Eliasson, 2010; Öhrvall et al., 2013; and Öhrvall et al., 2014, in References)
- Mini-Assisting Hand Assessment (Mini-AHA; Greaves et al., 2013, in References)
- Mini-MACS (Eliasson et al., 2017, in References)
- Neurological Hand Deformity Classification (2nd ed.; NHDC-2; Garbellini & Wilton, 2000; see also Georgiades et al., 2014, in References)
- Pediatric Evaluation of Disability Inventory (PEDI; Haley et al., 1992)
- Posture and Fine Motor Assessment of Infants (PFMAI; Case-Smith & Bigsby, 2001)
- Quality of Upper Extremity Skills Test (QUEST; DeMatteo et al., 1993)
- Revised Knox Preschool Play Scale (RKPPS; Knox, 2008)
- School Function Assessment (SFA; Coster et al., 1998; see also Li et al., 2015, in References)
- Stereognosis (Tyler, 1972)
- Tactile Object Recognition Test (TORT; Taylor et al., 2018, in References)
- Toddler and Infant Motor Evaluation (T.I.M.E.; Miller & Roid, 1994)

Instruments Developed by Other Professionals and Used by Occupational Therapy Personnel
- ABILHAND-Kids (Arnould et al., 2004)
- ACQUIREc Motor Activity Log (AMAL; DeLuca et al., 2010)
- Bayley Scales of Infant and Toddler Development (4th ed.; Bayley-4; Bayley & Aylward, 2019)
- Beery-Buktenica Developmental Test of Visual-Motor Integration (6th ed.; Beery VMI-6; Beery et al., 2010)
- Bimanual Fine Moor Function (BFMF; Beckung & Hagberg, 2002)
- Bruininks-Oseretsky Test of Motor Proficiency (2nd ed.; BOT-2; Bruininks & Bruininks, 2005)
- Cerebral Palsy Quality of Life–Child (CP QOL-Child; Waters et al., 2013)
- Cerebral Palsy Quality of Life–Teen (CP QOL-Teen; Davis et al., 2013)
- Childhood Health Assessment Questionnaire (CHAQ; Singh et al., 1994; see also Chae et al., 2018, in References)
- Communication Function Classification System (CFCS; Cooley Hidecker et al., 2011)
- Developmental Test of Visual Perception (3rd ed.; DTVP-3; Hammill et al., 2014)
- Dimensions of Mastery Questionnaire 18 (DMQ-18; Morgan et al., 2017; see also Miller et al., 2014, in References)
- Functional Independence Measure for Children (Version 5.01; WeeFIM; Uniform Data System for Medical Rehabilitation, 1998)
- Gross Motor Function Classification System–Expanded & Revised (GMFCS; Palisano et al., 2008)
- Gross Motor Function Measure (GMFM; Gémus et al., 2001)
- Impact on Family Scale (IOFS; Stein & Riessman, 1980)
- Infant Motor Profile (IMP; Heineman et al., 2008)
- Jebsen-Taylor Hand Function Test (JTHFT; Jebsen et al., 1969)
- Joint range of motion (goniometry; Shurlett & Kaskutuas, 2018)
- Kinematic Measurement (Schneiberg, McKinley, Gisel, et al., 2010, in References)
- Melbourne Assessment of Unilateral Upper Limb Function (MAUUL; Randall et al., 1999; see also Spirtos et al., 2011, in References)
- Modified Ashworth Scale (MAS; Bohannon & Smith, 1987)
- Movement Assessment Battery for Children (2nd ed.; M-ABC-2; Henderson et al., 2007)
- Movement Assessment of Infants (MAI; Harris et al., 1984)
- Patient-Reported Outcome Measures (PROMIS; Upper Limb Measures; Food and Drug Administration, 2009; see also Mulcahey et al., 2018, in References)
- Peabody Developmental Motor Scales (3rd ed.; PDMS-3; Folio & Fewell, 2023)
- Pediatric Motor Activity Log (Pediatric MAL; Taub et al., 2007; see also Wallen & Ziviani, 2013, in References)
- Semmes-Weinstein Monofilaments (SWMs; Bell-Krotoski, 2011; see also Patterson Medical Supply)
- Surveillance of Cerebral Palsy in Europe (SCPE; Surveillance of Cerebral Palsy in Europe, 2000)
- Two-Point Discrimination Test (TPDT; Disk-Criminator or Boley Gauge; Patterson Medical Supply)
- Vineland Adaptive Behavior Scales (3rd ed.; Vineland-3; Sparrow et al., 2016)
- WeeFIM (see Function Independence Measure for Children)

Problems/Issues

Activities of Daily Living/Instrumental ADL
- Child usually has difficulty with mobility: rolling over, crawling, walking, jumping, hopping, running.
- Child may have difficulty eating and swallowing.
- Child may have difficulty with self-maintenance skills: feeding, dressing and undressing, bathing, toileting, brushing teeth, transfers.
- Child may have difficulty with functional communication.

Education/Work
- Child may have difficulty with handwriting.
- Child may have specific learning disabilities (see chapter on Specific Learning Disorders).

Play/Leisure
- Child may have difficulty manipulating objects and managing movements in space needed to engage in a specific type of play (playing in a sandbox with toys, riding a tricycle, playing kickball, running a footrace).
- Child may have difficulty engaging in the functions of play such as taking roles and following rules integral to sports and games.
- Child may miss out on the meaning of play experiences including use of intrinsic motivation to play due to inability to manipulate objects or management movements needed in space.
- Child may be unable to engage in hobbies that require manipulation of objects such as model building, baseball card collecting, or coin collecting.

Rest/Sleep
- Child may have sleep disturbances due to muscle spasms, lack of bed mobility, or side effects of medications.

Social Participation
- Child may have limited opportunity for social interaction with peers due to physical limitations in manipulating objects or movement in space.

Sensorimotor
- Child may have hypertonia in some muscle groups and hypotonia in others.
- Child may have difficulty maintaining trunk (core) stability and strength.
- Child may have difficulty with and delay in development of gross motor skills.
- Child may have difficulty with upper extremity coordination and dexterity, especially use of bimanual (bilateral) skills.
- Child may have difficulty with fine motor skills involving grasp, pinch, and in-hand manipulation.
- Child may have difficulty with visual motor skills (eye–hand coordination).

Cognitive/Perceptual
- Child may have intellectual disability.
- Child may have difficulty with visual perception.

Psychosocial
- Child may have behavioral disorders.
- Child may have reduced quality of life.
- Child may have poor sense of self-efficacy.

Context/Environment
- Family or caregivers may have limited information about CP and its management.
- Family may have limited access to community resources.
- Family or caregivers may have limited knowledge of normal child development, including how to manage behavior and engage in play activities.

Intervention/Treatment

(Note: Because of volume of literature available, only samples of intervention are mentioned.) Useful reviews include Anaby et al. (2017), Dodd et al. (2010), Gilmore, Sakzewski, & Boyd (2010), Hoare et al. (2019), James et al. (2014), Krumlinde-Sundholm et al. (2015), Novak et al. (2013), and Sakzewski et al. (2014).

Models and programs developed by occupational therapy personnel include Cognitive Orientation to daily Occupational Performance (CO-OP; Cameron et al., 2017), context-focused intervention (Darrah et al., 2011), orthoses and splints (Hughes et al., 2017; Jackman et al., 2014; Jackman et al., 2019; Kumar & Senapati, 2012), task-oriented intervention (Schneiberg, McKinley, Sveistrup, et al., 2010), and time management (Sköld & Janeslätt, 2017).

Models and programs developed by other professionals but used by occupational therapy personnel include bimanual upper extremity training (Green et al., 2013), botulinum toxin injection (Copeland et al., 2014; Edwards et al., 2015; Fehlings et al., 2010; Hoare et al., 2013; Lidman et al., 2015; Lin et al., 2015; Olesch et al., 2010), conductive education (Schenker et al., 2016), constraint-induced movement therapy (CIMT; Case-Smith et al., 2012; Chen et al., 2013; Chen et al., 2014; Eliasson et al., 2018; Eliasson et al., 2011; Hamer-Rohrer et al., 2012; Rich et al., 2017), CIMT adapted/modified (de Brito Brandão et al., 2010; Gilmore, Ziviani, et al., 2010; Wallen et al., 2011; Wu et al., 2013), CIMT plus bimanual training (Chamudot et al., 2018; Hoare et al., 2010; Sakzewski et al., 2011), eye-gaze control (Karlsson et al., 2018; Karlsson et al., 2019; Karlsson & Wallen, 2017), family-centered care (Wiart et al., 2010), functional electrical stimulation (Xu et al., 2015), game theory (de Silva Dias et al., 2017), goal-directed training (Branjerdporn et al., 2018), home program (Saleh & Abu, 2011), magic-themed program (Hines, Bundy, Black, et al., 2019; Hines, Bundy, Haertsch, et al., 2019; Shetty et al., 2014), neurodevelopmental therapy (NDT; Camacho et al., 2016), play (Graham et al., 2015), parent/caregiver education (Jahagirdar, 2012), positioning (Batra et al., 2010; Costigan & Light, 2010), repetitive transcranial magnetic stimulation (Rich et al., 2017), rhizotomy (Ailon et al., 2015), sensory training (McLean et al., 2019; McLean et al., 2017), splinting/orthoses (Chhawchhria et al., 2014; Hughes et al., 2017), virtual reality (Do et al., 2016; Snider et al., 2010), visual perception (Ramkumar & Gupta, 2016), web-based (James et al., 2015), and Windmill-task (Zielinski et al., 2018). Team members include physicians, nursing personnel, psychologists, physical therapists, social workers, and occupational therapy personnel. Goal of intervention is to promote functional performance and independence.

Activities of Daily Living/Instrumental ADL
Fitness training/aerobic training
- Purpose: Maintain cardiovascular function, control body weight, and preserve bone mass.
- Technique: Any activity that increases heart rate to a level sufficient to result in physiological changes.
- Examples: Group exercises, swimming, cycling, walking.

Education/Work
- Provide opportunity to practice handwriting, including use of assistive devices.
- Assist in developing computer skills, including use of software programs such as word prediction or use of head stick rather than figures.
- Assist teachers/instructors to modify lessons to enable child to complete assigned work.

Play/Leisure
- Play learning
  - Form: Provide play that involves managing objects and space for solitary (play by self), passive onlooker (watching others), and engaged play session (parallel play in which others are present but not interacting, or cooperative-interactive play in which children must share objects such as toys or tools, and/or plan together to complete a project).
  - Function: Provide purposeful play that facilitates development of cognitive and motor skills and social roles.
  - Meaning: Provide play opportunities that are meaningful to the child to demonstrate enjoyment and experience intrinsic motivation.
  - Types: Provide opportunities for child to experience pretend play, symbolic play, object interaction play, and social cooperative play.
- Games (simple to complex) including card games, board games, or computer-based games

Rest/Sleep

- Assist in establishing a sleep routine and sleep habits.

Social Participation

- Assist in promoting participation in social occupations (parties, play dates, trips to parks, eating out, shopping, going to concerts or museums).

Sensorimotor (Dodd et al., 2010)

Bimanual upper extremity training: Hand Arm Bimanual Intensive Training (HABIT)

- Purpose: Improve child's ability to use both hands together to perform a task.
- Technique: Involves providing intensive practice (6 hours per day) of bimanual activities. Selection of activities used in practice sessions is dependent on child's movement deficits. Training includes part-task or movement practice as well as whole-task practice.

Constraint-induced movement training

- Purpose: Promote functional use of hemiplegic or motor impaired upper extremity (UE) based on idea of counteracting learned dis-use (non-use in adults and developmental disregard in children) of the impaired UE, and shaping effective (forced) use through controlled practice.
- Technique: Nonimpaired UE is restricted from movement using a sling or glove, and tasks are presented that must be performed by impaired UE for a given length of time that varies with the specific protocol.

Functional electrical stimulation (FES)

- Purpose: Stimulate muscles lacking neurological control to improve motor performance.
- Technique: Select stimulation of a certain muscle or muscle group to obtain a given muscle action, such as stimulating wrist extensors to improve hand function.

Neurodevelopmental therapy (NDT, Bobath)

- Purpose: Normalize muscle tone and practice moving in more normal movement patterns to promote optimal participation and independence.
- Technique includes handling (placing hands on body parts to facilitate stability and normalized movement), positioning (putting body parts in correct position for desired movement), and guiding or facilitating movement toward normalized muscle tone and optimal movement pattern.

Positioning and handling

- Purpose: Increase parent or caregiver's ability to engage safely and successfully in everyday tasks.
- Technique: Positioning requires analyzing client's posture and movement deficits and then recommending to parent or caregiver best posture for client that optimizes ability to perform everyday activities. Handling requires analyzing and recommending to child, parents, and caregivers the best methods to move, transfer, or maintain a functional posture.

Sensory processing and modulation

- Purpose: Improve client's ability to receive, organize, and interpret sensory input from the client's body and external environment through proprioception, smell, taste, touch, vestibular, and vision based on whether client's response is hyporesponsive or hyperresponsive (over-responsive).
- Technique: Adapt environment by removing or reducing stimuli, adapt responses by giving client ways to reduce or enhance stimuli (noise-canceling headphones, sack of fidget materials, quiet space).

Sensory retraining

- Purpose: Improve ability to retrieve, analyze, and interpret proprioception, two-point discrimination, stereognosis, and haptic/tactile perception.
- Technique: Provide practice in handling objects of different texture, weight, shape, and size.

Strength training (progressive resisted exercise)
- Purpose: Increase muscle's ability to generate force aimed at addressing muscle weakness.
- Technique: Lift weights against gravity, gradually increasing the number of repetitions and amount of weight.

Taping and strapping
- Purpose:
  - ▶ Rigid tape: Limit movement around a joint or protect a joint during movement.
  - ▶ Kinesio Tape: Increase stimulation to cutaneous mechanoreceptors to facilitate muscle contraction or inhibition to support a weakened muscle, improve circulation, reduce pain, and improve joint alignment.
- Technique: Tape is applied directly to the skin over areas of mechanoreceptors that correspond to desired result.

Visual skills training
- Purpose: Improve visual, visual-attention, visual-discrimination, visual-memory, visual-motor, and visual-perceptual skills.
- Technique: Visual attention may be improved by modulating lighting, color, movement, novel stimuli presentation, decreasing distracting stimuli, grading the complexity of task, or providing more or less visual cues. Visual memory may be improved by ascribing meaning to stimuli and associating new information with old. Visual perception involves improving ability to recognize, match, categorize, and detect relationship between shapes, color, and size of objects (see also Visual Impairment in Children and Adolescents in Section 2: Sensory Disorders).

Cognitive/Perceptual
Learning approaches
- Conductive education
  - ▶ Purpose: Promote independence by learning correct movements.
  - ▶ Technique: Imitate movements made by conductor/therapist, practice movements, and participate in daily activities.
- Cognitive orientation to daily occupational performance
  - ▶ Purpose: Help child learn and use cognitive strategies that are meaningful but not task-dependent.
  - ▶ Technique: Assist client to learn the four strategies. Goal (what do I want to achieve?), Plan (how will I do it?), Do (execute my plan), Check (did I follow my plan, and did it work?).
  - ▶ Technique assists: Verbal self-guidance (talking self through task), positioning body to prepare for doing task, and feeling the movement (attending to sensation of movements required).
- Goal-directed training
  - ▶ Purpose: Teach four components of goal-directed training (select meaningful goal, analyze baseline performance, practice regimen/intervention, evaluate outcome).
  - ▶ Technique: Practice is structured using motor learning principles—task structure, feedback, and results.

Perception: See Visual Skills Training, above

Psychosocial
Behavior management
- Provide clear and specific praise describing desired behavior and degree of successful performance.
- Plan intervention session in detail, especially transition from one task to another.
- Reward success, ignore failure, redirect attention.
- Be sure activities are "just right challenges"—not too easy or too hard.

Context/Environment

Adaptive devices, equipment

- Purpose: Facilitate movement and function by widening base of support, providing stability, improving body alignment, increasing safe mobility.
- Technique: Evaluate use of different mobility aids (walkers, crutches, wheelchairs, strollers, ankle-foot orthosis [AFO]). More than one may be useful at any given time.

Assistive technology

- Purpose: Provide communication, play/leisure activities, social interaction, and environmental control.
- Technique: Single switch-operated or joystick operated toys. Environmental control switches or joysticks (lights, doors, temperature, TV, radio).

Casts

- Purpose: Provide stretch on muscles to lengthen them.
- Technique
  - ▶ Time: Usually applied for 2–6 weeks.
  - ▶ Serial casting: Removal of cast periodically to adjust and increase tension.

Context-focused therapy

- Purpose: Change task or environment, not child, to promote successful task performance.
- Technique: Focus on client's strengths and abilities, including use of movements considered abnormal but effective for client in obtaining desired results. Work toward finding solutions that yield success at obtaining goal or completing a task.

Family/parent/caregiver education and training

- Purpose: Provide information and instruction for management of client's physical, psychological, social, and educational needs.
- Technique: Provide verbal and written information about services. Encourage partnership between parents and service providers. Provide opportunity for supervised practice.

Home program

- Purpose: Designed to provide therapeutic activities in the home environment supervised by parents or caregivers to maximize therapy effects or to take the place of therapy if access and resources are limited.
- Technique: Develop a collaborative relationship, set mutually agreed upon goals, select therapeutic activities, support implementation, and evaluate outcomes.

Splints

- Purpose:
  - ▶ Biomechanical: Promote joint alignment, maintain muscle stretch, prevent soft tissue contractures, promote and facilitate functional ability (grip, grasp).
  - ▶ Neurophysiological: Reduce muscle tone (spasticity), inhibit unwanted movement (hyperkinesis).
- Technique: Practice making various splints. Work with management team to determine which, if any, splint might be useful in managing joint and muscle action and position.

Precautions/Safety Considerations

Person is at risk for falls due to movement disorders and poor balance reactions. Person is at risk for contractures due to lack of movement and poor positioning. Person is at risk for osteoporosis due to lack of joint compression, which may be remediated with medication. Person is at risk for cardiomyopathy due to lack of fitness training and exercise.

Prognosis and Outcome

Cerebral palsy is a lifelong condition. Specific needs, problems, and solutions change as person grows and ages. Effective intervention must change and adjust as person progresses through life cycle.

Cost Effectiveness

Comans et al. (2017) found a web-based multimodal therapy program to be cost effective.

REFERENCES

Ailon, T., Beauchamp, R., Miller, S., Mortenson, P., Kerr, J. M., Hengel, A. R., & Steinbok, P. (2015). Long-term outcome after selective dorsal rhizotomy in children with spastic cerebral palsy. *Child's Nervous System, 31*(3), 415–423. https://doi.org/10.1007/s00381-015-2614-9

Amer, A., Eliasson, A. C., Peny-Dahlstrand, M., & Hermansson, L. (2016). Validity and test–retest reliability of Children's Hand-use Experience Questionnaire in children with unilateral cerebral palsy. *Developmental Medicine & Child Neurology, 58*(7), 743–749. https://doi.org/10.1111/dmcn.12991

Anaby, D., Korner-Bitensky, N., Steven, E., Tremblay, S., Snider, L., Avery, L., & Law, M. (2017). Current rehabilitation practices for children with cerebral palsy: Focus and gaps. *Physical & Occupational Therapy in Pediatrics, 37*(1), 1–15. https://doi.org/10.3109/01942638.2015.11 26880

Batra, M., Batra, V., & Sharma, V. P. (2010). Multi-Variant Tone Influencing Positioning System (MV-TIPS) to maximize task specific functional abilities in cerebral palsy. *Indian Journal of Occupational Therapy, 42*(2), 15–16.

Branjerdporn, N., Ziviani, J., & Sakzewski, L. (2018). Goal-directed occupational therapy for children with unilateral cerebral palsy: Categorising and quantifying session content. *British Journal of Occupational Therapy, 81*(3), 138–146. https://doi.org/10.1177/0308022617743458

Burgess, A., Boyd, R., Ziviani, J., Chatfield, M. D., Ware, R. S., & Sakzewski, L. (2019). Stability of the Manual Ability Classification System in young children with cerebral palsy. *Developmental Medicine and Child Neurology, 61*(7), 798–804. https://doi.org/10.1111/dmcn.14143

Camacho, R., McCauley, B., & Szczech Moser, C. (2016). Pediatric neurodevelopmental treatment. *Journal of Occupational Therapy, Schools & Early Intervention, 9*(4), 305–320. https://doi.org/10.1080/19411243.2016.1244995

Cameron, D., Craig, T., Edwards, B., Missiuna, C., Schwellnus, H., & Polatajko, H. J. (2017). Cognitive orientation to daily occupational performance (CO-OP): A new approach for children with cerebral palsy. *Physical & Occupational Therapy in Pediatrics, 37*(2), 183–198. https://doi.org/10.1080/01942638.2016.1185500

Case-Smith, J., DeLuca, S. C., Stevenson, R., & Ramey, S. L. (2012). Multicenter randomized controlled trial of pediatric constraint-induced movement therapy: 6-month follow-up. *American Journal of Occupational Therapy, 66*(1), 15–23. https://doi.org/10.5014/ajot.2012.002386

Chae, S., Park, E. Y., & Choi, Y. I. (2018). The psychometric properties of the Childhood Health Assessment Questionnaire (CHAQ) in children with cerebral palsy. *BMC Neurology, 18*, Article 151. https://doi.org/10.1186/s12883-018-1154-9

Chamudot, R., Parush, S., Rigbi, A., Horovitz, R., & Gross-Tsur, V. (2018). Effectiveness of modified constraint-induced movement therapy compared with bimanual therapy home programs for infants with hemiplegia: A randomized controlled trial. *American Journal of Occupational Therapy, 72*(6), Article 7206206010. https://doi.org/10.5014/ajot.2018.025981

Chen, C.-L., Kang, L.-J., Hong, W.-H., Chen, F.-C., Chen, H.-C., & Wu, C.-Y. (2013). Effect of therapist-based constraint-induced therapy at home on motor control, motor performance and daily function in children with cerebral palsy: A randomized controlled study. *Clinical Rehabilitation, 27*(3), 236–245. https://doi.org/10.1177/0269215512455652

Chen, C.-L., Lin, K.-C., Kang, L.-J., Wu, C.-Y., Chen, H.-C., & Hsieh, Y.-W. (2014). Potential predictors of functional outcomes after home-based constraint-induced therapy for children with cerebral palsy. *American Journal of Occupational Therapy, 68*(2), 159–166. https://doi.org/10.5014/ajot.2014.009860

Chhawchhria, Y., Gupta, A., & Ganatra, N. (2014). Comparison between above elbow wrist hand orthosis and combination of elbow gutter with below elbow wrist hand orthosis in children with spastic cerebral palsy. *Indian Journal of Occupational Therapy, 46*(3), 83–89.

Comans, T., Mihala, G., Sakzewski, L., Boyd, R. N., & Scuffham, P. (2017). The cost-effectiveness of a web-based multimodal therapy for unilateral cerebral palsy: The Mitii randomized controlled trial. *Developmental Medicine and Child Neurology, 59*(7), 756–761. https://doi.org/10.1111/dmcn.13414

Copeland, L., Edwards, P., Thorley, M., Donaghey, S., Gascoigne-Pees, L., Kentish, M., Lindsley, J., McLennan, K., Sakzewski, L., & Boyd, R. N. (2014). Botulinum toxin A for nonambulatory children with cerebral palsy: A double blind randomized controlled trial. *Journal of Pediatrics, 165*(1), 140–146. https://doi.org/10.1016/j.jpeds.2014.01.050

Costigan, F. A., & Light, J. (2010). Effect of seated position on upper-extremity access to augmentative communication for children with cerebral palsy: Preliminary investigation. *American Journal of Occupational Therapy, 64*(4), 596–604. https://doi.org/10.5014/ajot.2010.09013

Darrah, J., Law, M. C., Pollock, N., Wilson, B., Russell, D. J., Walter, S. D., Rosenbaum, P., & Galuppi, B. (2011). Context therapy: A new intervention approach for children with cerebral palsy. *Developmental Medicine & Child Neurology, 53*(7), 615–620. https://doi.org/10.1111/j.1469-8749.2011.03959.x

de Brito Brandão, M., Mancini, M. C., Vaz, D. V., de Melo, A. P. P., & Fonseca, S. T. (2010). Adapted version of constraint-induced movement therapy promotes functioning in children with cerebral palsy: A randomized controlled trial. *Clinical Rehabilitation, 24*(7), 639–647. https://doi.org/10.1177/0269215510367974

de Silva Dias, T., da Conceição, K. F., de Oliveira, A. I. A., & da Silva, R. L. M. (2017). The contributions of game therapy concerning motor performance of individuals with cerebral palsy. *Cadernos Brasileiros Terapia Ocupacional* Sān Carlos, *25*(3), 575–584. https://doi.org/10.4322/2526-8910.ctoAO0934

Do, J.-H., Yoo, E.-Y., Jung, M.-Y., & Park, H. Y. (2016). The effects of virtual reality-based bilateral arm training on hemiplegic children's upper limb motor skills. *NeuroRehabilitation, 38*(2), 115–127. https://doi.org/10.3233/NRE-161302

Dodd, K. J., Imms, C., & Taylor, N. F. (2010). *Physiotherapy and occupational therapy for people with cerebral palsy: A problem-based approach to assessment and management.* Mac Keith Press.

Edwards, P., Sakzewski, L., Copeland, L., Gascoigne-Pees, L., McLennan, K., Thorley, M., Kentish, M., Ware, R., & Boyd, R. N. (2015). Safety of botulinum toxin type A for children with nonambulatory cerebral palsy. *Pediatrics, 136*(5), 895–904. https://doi.org/10.1542/peds.2015-0749

Eliasson, A. C., Nordstrand, L., Ek, L., Lennartsson, F., Sjöstrand, L., Tedroff, K., & Krumlinde-Sundholm, L. (2018). The effectiveness of Baby-CIMT in infants younger than 12 months with clinical signs of unilateral-cerebral palsy: An explorative study with randomized design. *Research in Developmental Disabilities, 72*, 191–201. https://doi.org/10.1016/j.ridd.2017.11.006

Eliasson, A. C., Shaw, K., Berg, E., & Krumlinde-Sundholm, L. (2011). An ecological approach of Constraint Induced Movement Therapy for 2–3-year-old children: A randomized control trial. *Research in Developmental Disabilities, 32*(6), 2820–2828. https://doi.org/10.1016/j.ridd.2011.05.024

Eliasson, A. C., Ullenhag, A., Wahlström, U., & Krumlinde-Sundholm. L. (2017). Mini-MACS: Development of the Manual Ability Classification System for children younger than 4 years of age with signs of cerebral palsy. *Developmental Medicine and Child Neurology, 59*(1), 72–78. https://doi.org/10.1111/dmcn.13162

Elvrum, A.-K. G., Andersen, G. L., Himmelmann, K., Beckung, E., Öhrvall, A.-M., Lydersen, S., & Vik, T. (2016). Bimanual fine motor function (BFMF) classification in children with cerebral palsy: Aspects of construct and content validity. *Physical & Occupational Therapy in Pediatrics, 36*(1), 1–16. https://doi.org/10.3109/01942638.2014.975314

Elvrum, A.-K. G., Zethræus, B.-M., Vik, T., & Krumlinde-Sundholm, L. (2018). Development and validation of the Both Hands Assessment for children with bilateral cerebral palsy. *Physical and Occupational Therapy in Pediatrics, 38*(2), 113–126. https://doi.org/10.1080/01942638.2017.1318431

Fehlings, D., Novak, I., Berweck, S., Hoare, B., Stott, N. S., Russo, R. N., & the Cerebral Palsy Institute. (2010). Botulinum toxin assessment, intervention and follow-up for paediatric upper limb hypertonicity: International consensus statement. *European Journal of Neurology, 17*(Suppl. 2), 38–56. https://doi.org/10.1111/j.1468-1331.2010.03127.x

Georgiades, M., Elliott, C., Wilton, J., Blair, E., Blackmore, M., & Garbellini, S. (2014). The Neurological Hand Deformity Classification for children with cerebral palsy. *Australian Occupational Therapy Journal, 61*(6), 394–402. https://doi.org/10.1111/1440-1630.12150

Gilmore, R., Sakzewski, L., & Boyd, R. (2010). Upper limb activity measures for 5- to 16-year-old children with congenital hemiplegia: A systematic review. *Developmental Medicine & Child Neurology, 52*(1), 14–21. https://doi.org/10.1111/j.1469-8749.2009.03369.x

Gilmore, R., Ziviani, J., Sakzewski, L., Shields, N., & Boyd, R. (2010). A balancing act: Children's experience of modified constraint-induced movement therapy. *Developmental Neurorehabilitation, 13*(2), 88–94. https://doi.org/10.3109/17518420903386161

Graham, N. E., Truman, J., & Holgate, H. (2015). Parents' understanding of play for children with cerebral palsy. *American Journal of Occupational Therapy, 69*(3), Article 6903220050. https://doi.org/10.5014/ajot.2015.015263

Greaves, S., Imms, C., Dodd, K., & Krumlinde-Sundholm, L. (2013). Development of the Mini-Assisting Hand Assessment: Evidence for content and internal scale validity. *Developmental Medicine & Child Neurology, 55*(11), 1030–1037. https://doi.org/10.1111/dmcn.12212

Green, D., Schertz, M., Gordon, A. M., Moore, A., Schejter Margalit, T., Farquharson, Y., Ben Bashat, D., Weinstein, M., Lin, J.-P., & Fattal-Valevski, A. (2013). A multi-site study of functional outcomes following a themed approach to hand-arm bimanual intensive therapy for children with hemiplegia. *Developmental Medicine & Child Neurology, 55*(6), 527–533. https://doi.org/10.1111/dmcn.12113

Hamer-Rohrer, U., Smit, N., & Burger, M. (2012). The effect of a repeated course of constraint-induced movement therapy, implemented in the home environment, on the functional skills of a young child with cerebral palsy. *South African Journal of Occupational Therapy, 42*(3), 2–6.

Hines, A., Bundy, A. C., Black, D., Haertsch, M., & Wallen, M. (2019). Upper limb function of children with unilateral cerebral palsy after a magic-themed HABIT: A pre-post-study with 3- and 6-month follow-up. *Physical & Occupational Therapy in Pediatrics, 39*(4), 404–419. https://doi.org/10.1080/01942638.2018.1505802

Hines, A., Bundy, A. C., Haertsch, M., & Wallen, M. (2019). A magic-themed upper limb intervention for children with unilateral cerebral palsy: The perspectives of parents. *Developmental Neurorehabilitation, 22*(2), 104–110. https://doi.org/10.1080/17518423.2018.1442372

Hoare, B. J., Imms, C., Rawicki, H. B., & Carey, L. (2010). Modified constraint-induced movement therapy or bimanual occupational therapy following injection of Botulinum toxin-A to improve bimanual performance in young children with hemiplegic cerebral palsy: A randomised controlled trial methods paper. *BMC Neurology, 10*, Article 58. https://doi.org/10.1186/1471-2377-10-58

Hoare, B., Imms, C., Villanueva, E., Rawicki, H. B., Matyas, T., & Carey, L. (2013). Intensive therapy following upper limb botulinum toxin A injection in young children with unilateral cerebral palsy: A randomized trial. *Developmental Medicine & Child Neurology, 55*(3), 238–247. https://doi.org/10.1111/dmcn.12054

Hoare, B. J., Wallen, M. A., Thorley, M. N., Jackman, M. L., Carey, L. M., & Imms, C. (2019). Constraint-induced movement therapy in children with unilateral cerebral palsy. *Cochrane Database of Systematic Reviews, 4,* Article CD004149. https://doi.org/10.1002/14651858.CD 004149.pub3

Holmefur, M. M., & Krumlinde-Sundholm, L. (2016). Psychometric properties of a revised version of the Assisting Hand Assessment (Kids-AHA 5.0). *Developmental Medicine and Child Neurology, 58*(6), 618–624. https://doi.org/10.1111/dmcn.12939

Hughes, A. A., Franzsen, D., & Freeme, J. (2017). The effect of neoprene thumb abduction splints on upper limb function in children with cerebral palsy. *South African Journal of Occupational Therapy, 47*(3), 3–10. https://doi.org/10.17159/2310-3833/2017/v47n3a2

Jackman, M., Novak, I., & Lannin, N. (2014). Effectiveness of hand splints in children with cerebral palsy: A systematic review with meta-analysis. *Developmental Medicine & Child Neurology, 56*(2), 138–147. https://doi.org/10.1111/dmcn.12205

Jackman, M., Novak, I., Lannin, N., & Galea, C. (2019). Immediate effect of a functional wrist orthosis for children with cerebral palsy or brain injury: A randomized controlled trial. *Journal of Hand Therapy, 32*(1), 10–16. https://doi.org/10.1016/j.jht.2017.09.006

Jahagirdar, S. (2012). Occupational therapy psycho-education group: Empowering caregivers of children with cerebral palsy. *Indian Journal of Occupational Therapy, 44*(2), 15–23.

James, S., Ziviani, J., & Boyd, R. (2014). A systematic review of activities of daily living measures for children and adolescents with cerebral palsy. *Developmental Medicine & Child Neurology, 56*(3), 233–244. https://doi.org/10.1111/dmcn.12226

James, S., Ziviani, J., Ware, R. S., & Boyd, R. N. (2015). Randomized controlled trial of web-based multimodal therapy for unilateral cerebral palsy to improve occupational performance. *Developmental Neurology & Child Neurology, 57*(6), 530–538. https://doi.org/10.1111/dmcn .12705

Karlsson, P., Allsop, A., Dee-Price, B. J., & Wallen, M. (2018). Eye-gaze control technology for children, adolescents and adults with cerebral palsy with significant physical disability: Findings from a systematic review. *Developmental Neurorehabilitation, 21*(8), 497–505. https:// doi.org/10.1080/17518423.2017.1362057

Karlsson, P., Bech, A., Stone, H., Vale, C., Griffin, S., Monbaliu, E., & Wallen, M. (2019). Eyes on communication: Trailling eye-gaze control technology in young children with dyskinetic cerebral palsy. *Developmental Neurorehabilitation, 22*(2), 134–140. https://doi.org/10.1080/ 17518423.2018.1519609

Karlsson, P., & Wallen, M. (2017). Parent perception of two eye-gaze control technology systems in young children with cerebral palsy: Pilot study. *Studies in Health Technology and Informatics, 242,* 1095–1102.

Krumlinde-Sundholm, L. (2012). Reporting outcomes of the Assisting Hand Assessment: What scale should be used? *Developmental Medicine & Child Neurology, 54*(9), 807–808. https:// doi.org/10.1111/j.1469-8749.2012.04361.x

Krumlinde-Sundholm, L., Ek, L., & Eliasson, A. C. (2015). What assessments evaluate use of hands in infants? A literature review. *Developmental Medicine and Child Neurology, 57*(Suppl. 2), 37–41. https://doi.org/10.1111/dmcn.12684

Krumlinde-Sundholm, L., Ek, L., Sicola, E., Sjöstrand, L., Guzzetta, A., Sgandurra, G., Cioni, G., & Eliasson, A. C. (2017). Development of the Hand Assessment for Infants: Evidence of internal scale validity. *Developmental Medicine & Child Neurology, 59*(12), 1276–1283. https:// doi.org/10.1111/dmcn.13585

Kumar, A., & Senapati, A. (2012). Effect of soft splinting for upper extremity, on manual ability in children with spastic cerebral palsy. *Indian Journal of Occupational Therapy, 44*(1), 30–33.

Li, X.-L., Dong, V. A.-Q., & Fong, K. N. K. (2015). Reliability and validity of School Function Assessment for children with cerebral palsy in Guangzhou, China. *Hong Kong Journal of Occupational Therapy, 26*(1), 43–50. https://doi.org/10.1016/j.hkjot.2015.12.001

Lidman, G., Nachemson, A., Peny-Dahlstrand, M., & Himmelmann, K. (2015). Botulinum toxin A injections and occupational therapy in children with unilateral spastic cerebral palsy: A randomized controlled trial. *Developmental Medicine & Child Neurology, 57*(8), 754–761. https://doi.org/10.1111/dmcn.12739

Lin, Y.-C., Huang, C.-Y., Lin, I.-L., Shieh, J.-Y., Chung, Y.-T., & Chen, K.-L. (2015). Evaluating functional outcomes of botulinum toxin type A injection combined with occupational therapy in the upper limbs of children with cerebral palsy: A 9-month follow-up from the perspectives of both child and caregiver. *PLOS ONE, 10*(11), Article e0142769. https://doi.org/10.1371/journal.pone.0142769

McLean, B., Girdler, S., Taylor, S., Valentine, J., Carey, L., & Elliott, C. (2019). Experience of engagement in a somatosensory discrimination intervention for children with hemiplegic cerebral palsy: A qualitative investigation. *Developmental Neurorehabilitation, 22*(5), 348–358. https://doi.org/10.1080/17518423.2018.1503620

McLean, B., Taylor, S., Blair, E., Valentine, J., Carey, L., & Elliott, C. (2017). Somatosensory discrimination improves body position sense and motor performance in children with hemiplegia cerebral palsy. *American Journal of Occupational Therapy, 71*(3), Article 7103190060. https://doi.org/10.5014/ajot.2016.024968

Miller, L., Marnane, K., Ziviani, J., & Boyd, R. N. (2014). The Dimensions of Mastery Questionnaire in school-aged children with congenital hemiplegia: Test–retest reproducibility and parent–child concordance. *Physical & Occupational Therapy in Pediatrics, 34*(2), 168–184. https://doi.org/10.3109/01942638.2013.806978

Mulcahey, M. J., Slavin, M. D., Pengsheng, N., Kratz, A., Kisala, P. A., Tulsky, D. S., & Jette, A. M. (2018). Examination of psychometric properties of PROMIS®: Pediatric upper limb measures in youth with cerebral palsy. *British Journal of Occupational Therapy, 81*(7), 393–401. https://doi.org/10.1177/0308022618757961

Novak, I., McIntyre, S., Morgan, C., Campbell, L., Dark, L., Morton, N., Stumbles, E., Wilson, S.-A., & Goldsmith, S. (2013). A systematic review of interventions for children with cerebral palsy: State of the evidence. *Developmental Medicine & Child Neurology, 55*(10), 885–910. https://doi.org/10.1111/dmcn.12246

Öhrvall, A. M., & Eliasson, A. C. (2010). Parents' and therapists' perceptions of the content of the Manual Ability Classification System, MACS. *Scandinavian Journal of Occupational Therapy, 17*(3), 209–216. https://doi.org/10.3109/11038120903125101

Öhrvall, A. M., Krumlinde-Sundholm, L., & Eliasson, A. C. (2013). Exploration of the relationship between the Manual Ability Classification System and hand-function measures of capacity and performance. *Disability and Rehabilitation, 35*(11), 913–918. https://doi.org/10.3109/09638288.2012.714051

Öhrvall, A. M., Krumlinde-Sundholm, L., & Eliasson, A. C. (2014). The stability of the Manual Ability Classification System over time. *Developmental Medicine & Child Neurology, 56*(2), 185–189. https://doi.org/10.1111/dmcn.12348

Olesch, C. A., Greaves, S., Imms, C., Reid, S. M., & Graham, H. K. (2010). Repeat botulinum toxin-A injections in the upper limb of children with hemiplegia: A randomized controlled trial. *Developmental Medicine & Child Neurology, 52*(1), 79–86. https://doi.org/10.1111/j.1469-8749.2009.03387.x

Perez, M., Ziviani, J., Guzzetta, A., Ware, R. S., Tealdi, G., Burzi, V., & Boyd, R. N. (2016). Development, and construct validity and internal consistency of the Grasp and Reach Assessment of Brisbane (GRAB) for infants with asymmetric brain injury. *Infant Behavior and Development, 45*(Part A), 110–123. https://doi.org/10.1016/j.infbeh.2016.10.004

Porter, R. S. (Ed.). (2018). *The Merck manual of diagnosis and therapy* (20th ed.). Merck Sharp & Dohme.

Ramkumar, S., & Gupta, A. (2016). A study on effect of occupational therapy intervention program using cognitive-perceptual and perceptual-motor activities on visual perceptual skills in children with cerebral palsy. *Indian Journal of Physiotherapy and Occupational Therapy, 10*(3), 60–68.

Rich, T., Cassidy, J., Menk, J., Van Heest, A., Krach, L., Carey, J., & Gillick, B. T. (2017). Stability of stereognosis after pediatric repetitive transcranial magnetic stimulation and constraint-induced movement therapy clinical trial. *Developmental Neurorehabilitation, 20*(3), 169–172. https://doi.org/10.3109/17518423.2016.1139008

Ryll, U. C., Bastiaenen, C. H., & Eliasson, A. C. (2017). Assisting Hand Assessment and Children's Hand-Use Experience Questionnaire—Observed versus perceived bimanual performance in children with unilateral cerebral palsy. *Physical & Occupational Therapy in Pediatrics 37*(2), 199–209. https://doi.org/10.1080/01942638.2016.1185498

Ryll, U. C., Eliasson, A. C., Bastiaenen, C. H., & Green, D. (2019). To explore the validity of change scores of the Children's Hand-use Experience Questionnaire (CHEQ) in children with unilateral cerebral palsy. *Physical & Occupational Therapy in Pediatrics, 39*(2), 168–180. https://doi.org/10.1080/01942638.2018.1438554

Sakzewski, L., Ziviani, J., Abbott, D. F., Macdonell, R. A., Jackson, G. D., & Boyd, R. N. (2011). Randomized trial of constraint-induced movement therapy and bimanual training on activity outcomes for children with congenital hemiplegia. *Developmental Medicine and Child Neurology, 53*(4), 313–320. https://doi.org/10.1111/j.1469-8749.2010.03859.x

Sakzewski, L., Ziviani, J., & Boyd, R. N. (2014). Efficacy of upper limb therapies for unilateral cerebral palsy: A meta-analysis. *Pediatrics, 133*(1), e175–e204. https://doi.org/10.1542/peds.2013-0675

Saleh, A. O., & Abu, T. H. (2011). Home based constraint-induced therapy for children with hemiplegic cerebral palsy: A pilot study. *Indian Journal of Physiotherapy and Occupational Therapy, 5*(1), 100–102.

Schenker, R., Parush, S., Rosenbaum, P., Rigbi, A., & Yochman, A. (2016). Is a family-centred initiative a family-centred service? A case of a Conductive Education setting for children with cerebral palsy. *Child: Care, Health and Development, 42*(6), 909–917. https://doi.org/10.1111/cch.12354

Schneiberg, S., McKinley, P., Gisel, E., Sveistrup, H., & Levin, M. F. (2010). Reliability of kinematic measures of functional reaching in children with cerebral palsy. *Developmental Medicine & Child Neurology, 52*, e167–e173. https://doi.org/10.1111/j.1469-8749.2010.03635.x

Schneiberg, S., McKinley, P. A., Sveistrup, H., Gisel, E., Mayo, N. E., & Levin, M. F. (2010). The effectiveness of task-oriented intervention and trunk restraint on upper limb movement quality in children with cerebral palsy. *Developmental Medicine & Child Neurology, 52*(11), e245–e253. https://doi.org/10.1111/j.1469-8749.2010.03768.x

Shetty, R., Joshi, A., & Shibila, J. (2014). The magical pouch program: A case study of modified constraint induced movement therapy with bimanual training on a child with unilateral spastic cerebral palsy. *Indian Journal of Occupational Therapy, 46*(1), 3–9.

Sköld, A., Hermansson, L. N., Krumlinde-Sundholm, L., & Eliasson, A. C. (2011). Development and evidence of validity for the Children's Hand-use Experience Questionnaire (CHEQ). *Developmental Medicine and Child Neurology, 53*(5), 436–442. https://doi.org/10.1111/j.1469-8749.2010.03896.x

Sköld, A., & Janeslätt, G. K. (2017). Self-rating of daily time management in children: Psychometric properties of the Time-S. *Scandinavian Journal of Occupational Therapy, 24*(3), 178–186. https://doi.org/10.1080/11038128.2016.1185465

Snider, L., Majnemer, A., & Darsaklis, V. (2010). Virtual reality as a therapeutic modality for children with cerebral palsy. *Developmental Neurorehabilitation, 13*(2), 120–128. https://doi.org/10.3109/17518420903357753

Spirtos, M., O'Mahony, P., & Malone, J. (2011). Interrater reliability of the Melbourne Assessment of Unilateral Upper Limb Function for children with hemiplegic cerebral palsy. *American Journal of Occupational Therapy, 65*, 378–383. https://doi.org/10.5014/ajot.2011.001222

Taylor, S., Girdler, S., Parsons, R., McLean, B., Falkmer, T., Carey, L., Blair, E., & Elliott, C. (2018). Construct validity and responsiveness of the functional Tactile Object Recognition Test for children with cerebral palsy. *Australian Occupational Therapy Journal 65*(5), 420–430. https://doi.org/10.1111/1440-1630.12508

Wiart, L., Ray, L., Darrah, J., & Magill-Evans, J. (2010). Parents' perspectives on occupational therapy and physical therapy goals for children with cerebral palsy. *Disability & Rehabilitation, 32*(3), 248–258. https://doi.org/10.3109/09638280903095890

Wallen, M. (2019). The Hand Assessment for Infants at risk for cerebral palsy. *Developmental Medicine & Child Neurology, 61*(9), 999. https://doi.org/10.1111/dmcn.14183

Wallen, M., & Ziviani, J. (2013). Caution regarding the Pediatric Motor Activity Log to measure upper limb intervention outcomes for children with unilateral cerebral palsy. *Developmental Medicine & Child Neurology, 55*(6), 497–498. https://doi.org/10.1111/dmcn.12057

Wallen, M., Ziviani, J., Naylor, O., Evans, R., Novak, I., & Herbert, R. D. (2011). Modified constraint-induced therapy for children with hemiplegic cerebral palsy: A randomized trial. *Developmental Medicine & Child Neurology, 53*(12), 1091–1099. https://doi.org/10.1111/j.1469-8749.2011.04086.x

Wu, W.-C., Hung, J.-W., Tseng, C.-Y., & Huang, Y.-C. (2013). Group constraint-induced movement therapy for children with hemiplegic cerebral palsy: A pilot study. *American Journal of Occupational Therapy, 67*(2), 201–208. https://doi.org/10.5014/ajot.2013.004374

Xu, K., He, L., Mai, J., Yan, X., & Chen, Y. (2015). Muscle recruitment and coordination following constraint-induced movement therapy with electrical stimulation on children with hemiplegic cerebral palsy: A randomized controlled trial. *PLOS ONE, 10*(10), Article e0138608. https://doi.org/10.1371/journal.pone.0138608

Zielinski, I. M., Steenbergen, B., Schmidt, A., Klingels, K., Simon Martinez, C., de Water, P., & Hoare, B. (2018). Windmill-task as a new quantitative and objective assessment for mirror movements in unilateral cerebral palsy: A pilot study. *Archives of Physical Medicine and Rehabilitation, 99*(8), 1547–1552. https://doi.org/10.1016/j.apmr.2018.01.035

BIBLIOGRAPHY

Almasri, N. A., Saleh, M., Abu-Dahab, S., Malkawi, S. H., & Nordmark, E. (2018). Functional profiles of children with cerebral palsy in Jordon based on the association between gross motor function and manual ability. *BMC Pediatrics, 18*, Article 276. https://doi.org/10.1186/s12887-018-1257-x

Angelin, A. C., Sposito, A. M. P., & Pfeifer, L. I. (2018). Influence of functional mobility and manual function on play in preschool children with cerebral palsy. *Hong Kong Journal of Occupational Therapy, 31*(1), 46–53. https://doi.org/10.1177/1569186118783889

Brossard-Racine, M., Hall, N., Majnemer, A., Shevell, M. I., Law, M., Poulin, C., & Rosenbaum, P. (2012). Behavioural problems in school age children with cerebral palsy. *European Journal of Paediatric Neurology, 16*(1), 35–41. https://doi.org/10.1016/j.ejpn.2011.10.001

Burgess, A., Boyd, R. N., Ziviani, J., Ware, R. S., & Sakzewski, L. (2019). Self-care and manual ability in preschool children with cerebral palsy: A longitudinal study. *Developmental Medicine and Child Neurology, 61*(5), 570–578. https://doi.org/10.1111/dmcn.14049

Calley, A., Williams, S., Reid, S., Blair, E., Valentine, J., Girdler, S., & Elliott, C. (2012). A comparison of activity, participation and quality of life in children with and without spastic diplegia cerebral palsy. *Disability & Rehabilitation, 34*(14), 1306–1310. https://doi.org/10.3109/09638288.2011.641662

Carlon, S., Shields, N., Yong, K., Gilmore, R., Sakzewski, L., & Boyd, R. (2010). A systematic review of the psychometric properties of Quality of Life measures for school aged children with cerebral palsy. *BMC Pediatrics, 10*, Article 81. https://doi.org/10.1186/1471-2431-10-81

Chamudot, R., Parush, S., Rigbi, A., & Gross-Tsur, V. (2018). Brain lesions as a predictor of therapeutic outcomes of hand function in infants with unilateral cerebral palsy. *Journal of Child Neurology, 33*(14), 918–924. https://doi.org/10.1177/0883073818801632

Coker-Bolt, P. C., Garcia T., & Naber, E. (2015). Neuromotor: Cerebral Palsy. In J. Case-Smith & J. C. O'Brien (Eds.), *Occupational therapy for children and adolescents* (7th ed., pp. 793–811). Mosby.

Diaz Heijtz, R., Almeida, R., Eliasson, A. C., & Forssberg, H. (2018). Genetic variation in the dopamine system influences intervention outcome in children with cerebral palsy. *EBioMedicine, 28*, 162–167. https://doi.org/10.1016/j.ebiom.2017.12.028

Duff, S. V., & Wolff, A. L. (2018). Fine motor skill development in children and youth with unilateral cerebral palsy. In F. Miller, S. Bachrach, N. Lennon, & M. O'Neil (Eds.), *Cerebral palsy*. Springer Nature. https://doi.org/10.1007/978-3-319-50592-3_170-1

Ek, L., Eliasson, A. C., Sicola, E., Sjöstrand, L., Guzzetta, A., Sgandurra, G., Cioni, G., & Krumlinde-Sundholm, L. (2019). Hand Assessment for Infants: Normative reference values. *Developmental Medicine & Child Neurology, 61*(9), 1087–1092. https://doi.org/10.1111/dmcn.14163

Eliasson, A. C. (2015). What can be learned from reporting no-treatment effect of distribution of upper limb training? *Developmental Medicine & Child Neurology, 57*(6), 498. https://doi.org/10.1111/dmcn.12706

Eliasson, A. C., & Holmefur, M. (2015). The influence of early modified constraint-induced movement therapy training on the longitudinal development of hand function in children with unilateral cerebral palsy. *Developmental Medicine & Child Neurology, 57*(1), 89–94. https://doi.org/10.1111/dmcn.12589

Eliasson, A. C., Krumlinde-Sundholm, L., Gordon, A. M., Feys, H., Klingels, K., Aarts, P. B. M., Rameckers, E., Autti-Rämö, I., & Hoare, B. (2014). Guidelines for future research in constraint-induced movement therapy for children with unilateral cerebral palsy: An expert consensus. *Development Medicine & Child Neurology, 56*(2), 125–137. https://doi.org/10.1111/dmcn.12273

Forsman, L., & Eliasson, A. C. (2016). Strengths and challenges faced by school-aged children with unilateral CP described by the Five to Fifteen parental questionnaire. *Developmental Neurorehabilitation, 19*(6), 380–388. https://doi.org/10.3109/17518423.2015.1017662

Greaves, S., Imms, C., Dodd, K., & Krumlinde-Sundholm, L. (2010). Assessing bimanual performance in young children with hemiplegic cerebral palsy: A systematic review. *Developmental Medicine & Child Neurology, 52*(5), 413–421. https://doi.org/10.1111/j.1469-8749.2009.03561.x

Greaves, S., Imms, C., Krumlinde-Sundholm, L. Dodd, K., & Eliasson, A. C. (2012). Bimanual behaviours in children aged 8–18 months: A literature review to select toys that elicit the use of two hands. *Research in Developmental Disabilities, 33*(1), 240–250. https://doi.org/10.1016/j.ridd.2011.09.012

Hedberg-Graff, J., Granström, F., Arner, M., & Krumlinde-Sundholm, L. (2019). Upper-limb contracture development in children with cerebral palsy: A population-based study. *Developmental Medicine & Child Neurology, 61*(2), 204–211. https://doi.org/10.1111/dmcn.14006

Hoare, B. (2014). Rationale for using botulinum toxin A as an adjunct to upper limb rehabilitation in children with cerebral palsy. *Journal of Child Neurology, 29*(8) 1066–1076. https://doi.org/10.1177/0883073814533196

Hoare, B., & Eliasson, A. C. (2014). Evidence to practice commentary: Upper limb constraint in infants: Important perspectives on measurement and the potential for activity-dependent withdrawal of corticospinal projects. *Physical & Occupational Therapy in Pediatrics, 34*(1), 22–25. https://doi.org/10.3109/01942638.2014.868662

Hoare, B., & Greaves, S. (2017). Unimanual versus bimanual therapy in children with unilateral cerebral palsy: Same, same, but different. *Journal of Pediatric Rehabilitation Medicine, 10*(1), 47–59. https://doi.org/10.3233/PRM-170410

Hoare, B., Imms, C., Randall, M., & Carey, L. (2011). Linking cerebral palsy upper limb measures to the International Classification of Functioning, Disability and Health. *Journal of Rehabilitation Medicine, 43*(11), 987–996. https://doi.org/10.2340/16501977-0886

Holmefur, M., Kits, A., Bergström, J., Krumlinde-Sundholm, L., Flodmark, O., Forssberg, H., & Eliasson, A. C. (2013). Neuroradiology can predict the development of hand function in children with unilateral cerebral palsy. *Neurorehabilitation and Neural Repair, 27*(1), 72–78. https://doi.org/10.1177/1545968312446950

Holmström, L., Lennartsson, F., Eliasson, A. C., Flodmark, O., Clark, C., Tedroff, K., Forssberg, H., & Vollmer, B. (2011). Diffusion MRI in corticofugal fibers correlates with and function in unilateral cerebral palsy. *Neurology, 77*(8), 775–783. https://doi.org/10.1212/WNL.0b013e3 1822b0040

Islam, M., Gordon, A. M., Sköld, A., Forssberg, H., & Eliasson, A. C. (2011). Grip force coordination during bimanual tasks in unilateral cerebral palsy. *Developmental Medicine & Child Neurology, 53*(10), 920–926. https://doi.org/10.1111/j.1469-8749.2011.04040.x

Islam, M., Nordstrand, L., Holmström, L., Kits, A., Forssberg, H., & Eliasson, A. C. (2014). Is outcome of constraint-induced movement therapy in unilateral cerebral palsy dependent on corticomotor projection pattern and brain lesion characteristics? *Developmental Medicine & Child Neurology, 56*(3), 252–258. https://doi.org/10.1111/dmcn.12353

Keren-Capelovitch, T., Jarus, T., & Fattal-Valevski, A. (2010). Upper extremity function and occupational performance in children with spastic cerebral palsy following lower extremity botulinum toxin injections. *Journal of Child Neurology, 25*(6), 694–700. https://doi.org/10.1177/08 83073809344621

King, G., Imms, C., Palisano, R., Majnemer, A., Chiarello, L., Orlin, M., Law, M., & Avery, L. (2013). Geographical patterns in the recreation and leisure participation of children and youth with cerebral palsy: A CAPE international collaborative network study. *Developmental Neurorehabilitation, 16*(3), 196–206. https://doi.org/10.3109/17518423.2013.773102

Klevberg, G. L., Elvrum, A.-K. G., Zucknick, M., Elkjær, S., Østensjø, S., Krumlinde-Sundholm, L., Kjeken, I., & Jahnsen, R. (2018). Development of bimanual performance in young children with cerebral palsy. *Developmental Medicine and Child Neurology, 60*(5), 490–497. https://doi .org/10.1111/dmcn.13680

Klevberg, G. L. Østensjø, S., Krumlinde-Sundholm. L., Elkjær, S., & Jahnsen, R. B. (2017). Hand function in a population-based sample of young children with unilateral or bilateral cerebral palsy. *Physical & Occupational Therapy in Pediatrics, 37*(5), 528–540. https://doi.org/10 .1080/01942638.2017.1280873

Krajenbrink, H., Crichton, A., Steenbergen, B., & Hoare, B. (2019). The development of anticipatory action planning in children with unilateral cerebral palsy. *Research in Developmental Disabilities, 85*(1), 163–171. https://doi.org/10.1016/j.ridd.2018.12.002

Lam-Dami, S., Fay, L., Lockhart, J., & Hoffman, S. (2015). Moving constraint-induced movement therapy and bimanual therapy into practice. *Occupational Therapy Now, 17*(1), 14–16.

Law, M., & Darrah, J. (2014). Emerging therapy approaches: An emphasis on function. *Journal of Child Neurology, 29*(8), 1101–1107. https://doi.org/10.1177/0883073814533151

Law, M. C., Darrah, J., Pollock, N., Wilson, B., Russell, D. J., Walter, S. D., Rosenbaum, P., & Galuppi, B. (2011). Focus on function: A cluster, randomized controlled trial comparing child- versus context-focused intervention for young children with cerebral palsy. *Developmental Medicine & Child Neurology, 53*(7), 631–639. https://doi.org/10.1111/j.1469-8749.2011.03962.x

Lidman, G., Himmelmann, K., Gosman-Hedström, G., & Peny-Dahlstrand, M. (2018). How children with cerebral palsy master bimanual activities from a parental perspective. *Scandinavian Journal of Occupational Therapy, 25*(4), 252–259. https://doi.org/10.1080/11038128.20 17.1337807

Majnemer, A. (2012). *Measures for children with developmental disabilities: An ICF-CY approach.* Mac Keith Press.

Majnemer, A., Shevell, M., Hall, N., Poulin, C., & Law, M. (2010). Developmental and functional abilities in children with cerebral palsy as related to pattern and level of motor function. *Journal of Child Neurology, 25*(10), 1236–1241. https://doi.org/10.1177/0883073810363175

Majnemer, A., Shevell, M., Law, M., Poulin, C., & Rosenbaum, P. (2010). Level of motivation in mastering challenging tasks in children with cerebral palsy. *Developmental Medicine & Child Neurology, 52*(12), 1120–1126. https://doi.org/10.1111/j.1469-8749.2010.03732.x

Majnemer, A., Shikako-Thomas, K., Chokron, N., Law, M., Shevell, M., Chilingaryan, G., Poulin, C., & Rosenbaum, P. (2010). Leisure activity preferences for 6- to 12-year-old children with cerebral palsy. *Developmental Medicine & Child Neurology, 52*(2), 167–173. https://doi.org/10.1111/j.1469-8749.2009.03393.x

Manzini, M. G., Simóes Martinez, C. M., Lourenco, G. F., & de Brito Oliveira, B. (2017). Alternative communication training of interlocutors for children with cerebral palsy. *Cadernos Brasileiros Terapia Ocupacional São Carlos, 25*(3), 553–564. https://doi.org/10.4322/2526-8910.ctoAO1103

Nordstrand, L., & Eliasson, A. C. (2013). Six years after a modified constraint induced movement therapy (CIMT) program—What happens when the children have become young adults? *Physical & Occupational Therapy in Pediatrics, 33*(2), 163–169. https://doi.org/10.3109/0194 2638.2013.757157

Nordstrand, L., Eliasson, A. C., & Holmefur, M. (2016). Longitudinal development of hand function in children with unilateral spastic cerebral palsy aged 18 months to 12 years. *Developmental Medicine & Child Neurology, 58*(10), 1042–1048. https://doi.org/10.1111/dmcn.13106

Nordstrand, L., Holmefur, M., Kits, A., & Eliasson, A. C. (2015). Improvements in bimanual hand function after baby-CIMT in two-year old children with unilateral cerebral palsy: A retrospective study. *Research in Developmental Disabilities, 41–42*, 86–93. https://doi.org/10.1016/j.ridd.2015.05.003

Novak, I., & Honan, I. (2019). Effectiveness of paediatric occupational therapy for children with disabilities: A systematic review. *Australian Occupational Therapy Journal, 66*(3), 258–273. https://doi.org/10.1111/1440-1630.12573

Novak, I., Morgan, C., Adde, L., Blackman, J., Boyd, R. N., Brunstrom-Hernandez, J., Cioni, G., Damiano, D., Darrah, J., Eliasson, A. C., de Vries, L. S., Einspieler, C., Fahey, M., Fehlings, D., Ferriero, D. M., Fetters, L., Fiori, S., Forssberg, H., Gordon, A. M., & Badawi, N. (2017). Early, accurate diagnosis and early intervention in cerebral palsy: Advances in diagnosis and treatment. *JAMA Pediatrics, 171*(9), 897–907. https://doi.org/10.1001/jamapediatrics.2017.1689

Öhrvall, A. M., Eliasson, A. C. Löwing, K., Ödman, P., & Krumlinde-Sundholm, L. (2010). Self-care and mobility skills in children with cerebral palsy, related to their manual ability and gross motor function classifications. *Developmental Medicine and Child Neurology, 52*(11), 1048–1055. https://doi.org/10.1111/j.1469-8749.2010.03764.x

Pfeifer, L. I., Pacciulio, A. M., Abrão dos Santos, C., Lício dos Santos, J., & Stagnitti, K. E. (2011). Pretend play of children with cerebral palsy. *Physical & Occupational Therapy in Pediatrics, 31*(4), 390–402. https://doi.org/10.3109/01942638.2011.572149

Pihlar, A. (2012). From activity to participation—Occupational therapy intervention for CP children. *Eastern Journal of Medicine, 17*, 198–201.

Raji, P., Hassani Mehraban, A., Aliabadi, F., Ahmadi, M., & Schiariti, V. (2018). Content validity of the comprehensive ICF Core Set for children with cerebral palsy aged 0–6 years: Iranian occupational therapists perspective. *Iranian Journal of Child Neurology, 12*(3), 40–58.

Randall, M., Harvey, A., Imms, C., Reid, S., Lee, K. J., & Reddihough, D. (2013). Reliable classification of functional profiles and movement disorders of children with cerebral palsy. *Physical & Occupational Therapy in Pediatrics, 33*(3), 342–352. https://doi.org/10.3109/019 42638.2012.747584

Reedman, S., Boyd, R. N., & Sakzewski, L. (2017). The efficacy of interventions to increase physical activity participation of children with cerebral palsy: A systematic review and meta-analysis. *Developmental Medicine and Child Neurology, 59*(10), 1011–1018. https://doi.org/10.1111/dmcn.13413

Reedman, S. E., Boyd, R. N., Trost, S. G., Elliott, C., & Sakzewski, L. (2019). Efficacy of participation-focused therapy on performance of physical activity participation goals and habitual physical activity in children with cerebral palsy: A randomized controlled trial. *Archives of Physical Medicine and Rehabilitation, 100*(4), 676–686. https://doi.org/10.1016/j.apmr.2018.11.012

Rostami, H. R., & Malamiri, R. A. (2012). Effect of treatment environment on modified constraint-induced movement therapy results in children with spastic hemiplegic cerebral palsy:

A randomized controlled trial. *Disability and Rehabilitation, 34*(1), 40–44. https://doi.org/10
.3109/09638288.2011.585214

Russell, D. C., Scholtz, C., Greyling, P., Taljaard, M., Viljoen, E., & Very, C. (2018). A pilot
study on high dosage intervention of children with CP using combined therapy approaches.
South African Journal of Occupational Therapy, 48(2), 26–33. https://doi.org/10.17159/2310
-3833/2017/vol48n2a5

Ryll, U. C., Wagenaar, N., Verhage, C. H., Blennow, M., de Vries, L. S., & Eliasson, A. C. (2019).
Early prediction of unilateral cerebral palsy in infants with asymmetric perinatal brain injury—
Model development and internal validation. *European Journal of Paediatric Neurology, 23*(4),
621–628. https://doi.org/10.1016/j.ejpn.2019.04.004

Sakzewski, L., Carlon, S., Shields, N., Ziviani, J., Ware, R. S., & Boyd, R. N. (2012). Impact of
intensive upper limb rehabilitation on quality of life: A randomized trial in children with
unilateral cerebral palsy. *Developmental Medicine & Child Neurology, 54*(5), 415–423. https://
doi.org/10.1111/j.1469-8749.2012.04272.x

Sakzewski, L., Gordon, A., & Eliasson, A. C. (2014). The state of the evidence for intensive
upper limb therapy approaches for children with unilateral cerebral palsy. *Journal of Child
Neurology, 29*(8), 1077–1090. https://doi.org/10.1177/0883073814533150

Sakzewski, L., Reedman, S., & Hoffmann, T. (2016). Do we really know what they were testing? Incomplete reporting of interventions in randomised trials of upper limb therapies
in unilateral cerebral palsy. *Research in Developmental Disabilities, 59*, 417–427. https://doi
.org/10.1016/j.ridd.2016.09.018

Sakzewski, L., Miller, L., Ziviani, J., Abbott, D. F., Rose, S., Macdonell, R. A., & Boyd, R. N. (2015).
Randomized comparison trial of density and context of upper limb intensive group versus
individualized occupational therapy for children with unilateral cerebral palsy. *Developmental
Medicine & Child Neurology, 57*(6), 539–547. https://doi.org/10.1111/dmcn.12702

Sakzewski, L., Provan, K., Ziviani, J., & Boyd, R. N. (2015). Comparison of dosage of intensive upper limb therapy for children with unilateral cerebral palsy: How big should the
therapy pill be? *Research in Developmental Disabilities, 37*, 9–16. https://doi.org/10.1016/
j.ridd.2014.10.050

Sakzewski, L., Sicola, E., Verhage, C. H., Sgandurra, G., & Eliasson, A. C. (2019). Development of
hand function during the first year of life in children with unilateral cerebral palsy. *Developmental Medicine and Child Neurology, 61*(5), 563–569. https://doi.org/10.1111/dmcn.14091

Sakzewski, L., Ziviani, J., Abbott, D. F., Macdonell, R. A., Jackson, G. D., & Boyd, R. N. (2011a).
Equivalent retention of gains at 1 year after training with constraint-induced or bimanual
therapy in children with unilateral cerebral palsy. *Neurorehabilitation and Neural Repair, 25*(7),
664–671. https://doi.org/10.1177/1545968311400093

Sakzewski, L., Ziviani, J., Abbott, D. F., Macdonell, R. A., Jackson, G. D., & Boyd, R. N. (2011b).
Participation outcomes in a randomized trial of 2 models of upper-limb rehabilitation for
children with congenital hemiplegia. *Archives of Physical Medicine and Rehabilitation, 92*(4),
531–539. https://doi.org/10.1016/j.apmr.2010.11.022

Sakzewski, L., Ziviani, J., & Boyd, R. (2010). The relationship between unimanual capacity and
bimanual performance in children with congenital hemiplegia. *Developmental Medicine &
Child Neurology, 52*(9), 811–816. https://doi.org/10.1111/j.1469-8749.2009.03588.x

Sakzewski, L., Ziviani, J., & Boyd, R. N. (2011). Best responders after intensive upper-limb training for children with unilateral cerebral palsy. *Archives of Physical Medicine and Rehabilitation,
92*(4), 578–584. https://doi.org/10.1016/j.apmr.2010.12.003

Sakzewski, L., Ziviani, J., & Boyd, R. N. (2014). Delivering evidence-based upper limb rehabilitation for children with cerebral palsy: Barriers and enablers identified by three pediatric
teams. *Physical & Occupational Therapy in Pediatrics, 34*(4), 368–383. https://doi.org/10.310
9/01942638.2013.861890

Sakzewski, L., Ziviani, J., & Boyd, R. N. (2014). Efficacy of upper limb therapies for unilateral cerebral palsy: A meta-analysis. *Pediatrics, 133*(1), e175–e204. https://doi.org/10.1542/peds.2013-0675

Sakzewski, L., Ziviani, J., & Boyd, R. N. (2016). Translating evidence to increase quality and dose of upper limb therapy for children with unilateral cerebral palsy: A pilot study. *Physical & Occupational Therapy in Pediatrics, 36*(3), 305–329. https://doi.org/10.3109/01942638.2015.1127866

Saleh, E., Dahan-Oliel, N., Montpetit, K., Benaroch, T., Yap, R., Barakat, N. & Mulcahey, M. J. (2018). Functional gains in children with spastic hemiplegia following a tendon Achilles lengthening using computerized adaptive testing—A pilot study. *Child Neurology Open, 5.* https://doi.org/10.1177/2329048X18811452

Shikako-Thomas, K., Dahan-Oliel, N., Shevell, M., Law, M., Birnbaum, R., Rosenbaum, P., Poulin, C., & Majnemer, A. (2012). Play and be happy? Leisure participation and quality of life in school-aged children with cerebral palsy. *International Journal of Pediatrics, 2012*, Article 387280. https://doi.org/10.1155/2012/387280

Snider, L., Majnemer, A., & Darsaklis, V. (2011). Feeding interventions for children with cerebral palsy: A review of the evidence. *Physical & Occupational Therapy in Pediatrics, 31*(1), 58–77. https://doi.org/10.3109/01942638.2010.523397

Taylor, S., Girdler, S., McCutcheon, S., McLean, B., Parsons, R., Falkmer, T., Jacoby, P., Carey, L., & Elliott, C. (2019). Haptic exploratory procedures of children and youth with and without cerebral palsy. *Physical & Occupational Therapy in Pediatrics, 39*(3), 337–351. https://doi.org/10.1080/01942638.2018.1477228

Thorley, M., Donaghey, S., Edwards, P., Copeland, L., Kentish M., McLennan, K., Lindsley, J., Gascoigne-Pees, L., Sakzewski, L., & Boyd, R. N. (2012). Evaluation of the effects of botulinum toxin A injections when used to improve ease of care and comfort in children with cerebral palsy whom are non-ambulant: A double blind randomized controlled trial. *BMC Pediatrics, 12*, Article 120. https://doi.org/10.1186/1471-2431-12-120

Wallen, M., Imms, C., Hoare, B., & Greaves, S. (2017). Weak evidence supports intensive, task-oriented, early intervention with parent support for infants with, or at high risk of, cerebral palsy. *Australian Occupational Therapy Journal, 64*(5), 423–425. https://doi.org/10.1111/1440-1630.12426

Wallen, M., & Majnemer, A. (2014). No differences were observed between six months of context- versus child-focused intervention for young children with cerebral palsy on self-care, mobility, range-of-motion or participation. *Australian Occupational Therapy Journal, 61*(2), 126–127. https://doi.org/10.1111/1440-1630.12109

Wallen, M., & Stewart, K. (2016). Grading and quantification of upper extremity function in children with spasticity. *Seminars in Plastic Surgery, 30*(1), 5–13. https://doi.org/10.1055/s-0035-1571257

Wallen, M., & Stewart, K. (2015). Upper limb function in everyday life of children with cerebral palsy: Description and review of parent report measures. *Disability and Rehabilitation, 37*(15), 1353–1361. https://doi.org/10.3109/09638288.2014.963704

Walmsley, C., Taylor, S., Parkins, T., Carey, L., Girdler, S., & Elliott, C. (2018). What is the current practice of therapists in the measurement of somatosensation in children with cerebral palsy and other neurological disorders? *Australian Occupational Therapy Journal, 65*(2), 89–97. https://doi.org/10.1111/1440-1630.12431

Whalen, C. N., & Case-Smith, J. (2012). Therapeutic effects of horseback riding therapy on gross motor function in children with cerebral palsy: A systematic review. *Physical & Occupational Therapy in Pediatrics, 32*(3), 229–242. https://doi.org/10.3109/01942638.2011.619251

Wolff, A. L., Raghavan, P., Kaminski, T., Hillstrom, H. J., & Gordon, A. M. (2015). Differentiation of hand posture to object shape in children with unilateral spastic cerebral palsy. *Research in Developmental Disabilities, 45–46*, 422–430. https://doi.org/10.1016/j.ridd.2015.07.002

Childhood Trauma and Maltreatment

*Also called adverse childhood experiences, child abuse, abused and
neglected children, domestic abuse with children.*

*See also Posttraumatic Stress Disorder (PTSD),
Anxiety and General Anxiety Disorder, Polytrauma.*

Description

Trauma is defined as "a single event, multiple events, or a set of circumstances that is experienced by an individual as physically and emotionally harmful or threatening and that has lasting adverse effects on the individual's physical, social, emotional, or spiritual well-being" (Substance Abuse and Mental Health Services Administration [SAMHSA], 2012, as cited in SAMHSA, 2014, p. xix). Childhood trauma is described as a psychologically distressing event involving "exposure to actual or threatened death, serious injury, or sexual violence" (American Psychiatric Association, 2013, p. 261). Complex trauma is defined as "exposure to multiple, prolonged, or ongoing stressors" and usually includes repeated abuse, witnessing abuse, or prolonged neglect that occurs over time during the child's developmental years (Champagne, 2011, p. CE-1; Fraser et al., 2017). Developmental trauma results in a lack of scaffolding of learning and instrumental enrichment by a trusted caregiver (Ashcroft et al., 2019). Adverse childhood experiences include a set of defined, negative life experiences known to affect childhood development and to alter the trajectory of a child's life course (Ashcroft et al., 2019). Child maltreatment is behavior that is outside the norms of conduct toward a child and includes substantial risk of causing physical or emotional harm. Four types of abuse or maltreatment are recognized: physical, sexual, emotional (psychological), and neglect (Porter, 2018).

Cause

Etiology includes exposure to such events or experiences as abuse, bullying, displacement, food insecurity, life-threatening incidents, motor vehicle accidents, neglect, sexual assault, and terrorism violence.

Evaluation/Assessment

Areas

- Activities of Daily Living/Instrumental ADL: self-maintenance (eating, food hoarding, bathing and toileting hygiene)
- Education/Work: school attendance, behavior in school, academic performance, employment history (adolescent, adult)
- Play/Leisure: play skills, leisure activities and interests, frequency, location
- Rest/Sleep: sleep disturbances, bed-wetting
- Social Participation: social skills, opportunity to interact with peers, frequency, location
- Sensorimotor: delayed or lost gross and fine motor skills
- Cognitive/Perceptual: arousal, attention, executive functions
- Psychosocial: depression, anxiety, interpersonal relationships, affect, aggression, bullying, fear of failure, isolation and withdrawal
- Context/Environment: living environment, social support
- Development (Infant, Child, Adolescent only): developmental delay
- Comorbidity: posttraumatic seizures

Instruments

Instruments Developed by Occupational Therapy Personnel

- Sensory Integration and Praxis Tests (SIPT; Ayres, 1989)
- Sensory Profile (2nd ed.; SP-2; Dunn, 2014)

Instruments Developed by Other Professionals and Used by Occupational Therapy Personnel
- Child Stress Disorders Checklist 4.0 (CSDC-4.0; Saxe et al., 2003)
- Disturbances of Attachment Interview (DAI; Smyke & Zeanah, 1999)
- Pediatric Symptom Checklist (PSC; Jellinek et al., 1988)
- Trauma Symptom Checklist for Children (TSCC; Briere, 1996)

Problems/Issues
Activities of Daily Living/Instrumental ADL
- Child may have difficulty managing hygiene (bathing, toileting).
- Child may hoard food related to sense of food insecurity.
- Child may lack training in basic self-maintenance activities related to lack of parental or caregiver education and instruction.
- Child may have experienced abuse related to bedroom and bathroom tasks.

Education/Work
- Child's attendance at school may be erratic.
- Child may inconsistently complete homework assignments.
- Child's academic performance may be inconsistent.
- Child's teacher may wonder what is wrong with the child instead of asking what is happening to the child at home.
- Adolescent or adult may have difficulty attaining or maintaining employment related to poor hygiene habits or poor social interaction skills.

Play/Leisure
- Child may not initiate play activities.
- Child may be overaggressive and bully other children or isolate self (difficulty with appropriate peer interactions).
- Child may quit playing if he or she has minor difficulty performing the task.
- Child may not have been permitted to play or to have toys with which to play.
- Child may have no leisure activities or interests.

Rest/Sleep
- Child may have difficulty falling or staying asleep.
- Child may have nightmares or other sleep disturbances.
- Child may wet bed even after bladder and bowel control have been attained during the day.

Social Participation
- Child usually has impaired social skills when interacting with peers (fear of failure, teasing due to poor personal hygiene).
- Child usually has impaired interactions with adults (fear of authority, clinging for protection).
- Child may avoid participation related to fear of failure.

Sensorimotor
- Child may not have had opportunity to learn motor skills such as jumping, skipping, hopping, swinging, or have experienced playing on playground equipment.

Cognitive/Perceptual
- Child may have impairment in arousal regulation.
- Child may have difficulty concentrating on or paying attention to task.
- Child may have memory impairment and confusion.
- Child may demonstrate impairment in executive function, such as inability to envision a future or poor insight in situations.

Psychosocial
- Child may have symptoms of depression, anxiety, and emotional numbness (flat affect).

- Child may have overactive traumatic stress response and have difficulty managing emotions in stressful situations.
- Child may have poor interpersonal boundaries.
- Child may fear failure and have a hyperawareness of possible failure leading to reluctance to try new activities or situations.
- Child may withdraw from interactions with others.
- Child may have a history of isolation and lack of opportunity to play with peers or interact with others outside the family unit.

Context/Environment

- Child may experience physical and emotional abuse at home or other living environment.
- Child may experience physical and emotional neglect at home or other living environment.
- Child may experience isolation or separation (physical and temporal) from others as punishment for actions or lack of actions expected by adults.
- Child may lack basic training and education in eating and hygiene habits and routines at home or other living environment.
- Child may not be able to depend on adults to provide safety, shelter, or sustenance.

Intervention/Treatment

Occupational therapy can provide services in promoting awareness of childhood trauma, prevention, and intervention (American Occupational Therapy Association [AOTA], 2015b). Models and programs developed by occupational therapy personnel include occupation as therapy (Precin, 2011), person-environment-occupation (Champagne, 2019), and sensory integration (Denison et al., 2018). Models and programs developed by other professions include the Day Program (Holland et al., 2018), multidisciplinary model (Ryan et al., 2017; Suarez, 2017; Whiting, 2018), sensory approach (LeBel & Champagne, 2010, LeBel et al., 2010), Sensory Motor Arousal Regulation Treatment (SMART; Warner et al., 2014), social information processing model (Azar et al., 2017), trauma informed care model (Clark et al., 2015; Fette et al., 2019), trauma stress program (Snedden, 2012), therapeutic spiral model (Alers, 2010), and three-phase treatment model (Champagne, 2011). SAMHSA (2014) recommends six core concepts in a treatment program: safety; trustworthiness and transparency; peer support and mutual self-help; collaboration and mutuality; empowerment, voice, and choice; and addressing cultural, historical, and gender issues. Team members may include a physician, public health nurse, school nurse, social worker, psychologist, educator/teacher, speech–language pathologist or speech therapist, parents or foster parents, and occupational therapy personnel. The goal is to facilitate successful participation across various settings, including home, school, and community (AOTA, 2015a).

Activities of Daily Living/Instrumental ADL

- Assist child to master routine self-maintenance activities related to eating and hygiene activities.

Education/Work

- Assist child and teachers to address and understand what is happening at home and the relationship of home life to school life (academic and behavioral).

Play/Leisure

- Provide opportunities to play with a variety of objects to develop motivation and interests.
- Foster and support the child's interests in healthy and safe play and leisure interest.

Rest/Sleep

- See Sleep–Wake Disorders in Section 13: Lifestyle Conditions.

Social Participation

- Encourage participation in age-appropriate social activities.

Sensorimotor
- Use sensory approaches with cognitive approaches to teach self-regulation.

Cognitive/Perceptual
- Make activities and routines predictable so the child knows what is going to happen throughout the scheduled time.
- Provide opportunity to problem solve and make decisions.

Psychosocial
- Teach mindfulness strategies to reduce stress.
- Teach positive methods of interacting with others.
- Provide opportunities and situations designed to increase sense of mastery and self-efficacy.
- Provide group-based interventions focused on self-regulation, self-control, and sensory modulation.

Context/Environment
- Educate parents, caregivers, and teachers about healthy discipline and injury prevention.
- In the home, encourage predictable and routine activities including self-maintenance, play, and sleep.
- Promote family activities that support shelter, safety, and sustenance.
- Encourage family activities that promote normal child growth and development.

Precautions/Safety Considerations

Removal from the home environment may stop the immediate traumatic situations but placement in foster care may create additional trauma. Children with head injuries due to abuse have a higher frequency of posttraumatic seizures (Chen et al., 2019).

Prognosis and Outcome

Prognosis is tentative and outcome uncertain. Age, amount of trauma, and services received are all factors.

REFERENCES

Alers, V. (2010). Working with trauma survivors: From victim to trauma survivor to thriver. In V. Alers & R. Crouch (Eds.), *Occupational therapy: An African perspective* (pp. 268–285). Sarah Shorten.

American Occupational Therapy Association. (2015a). *Childhood trauma: School mental health toolkit.*

American Occupational Therapy Association. (2015b). *Information sheet: Occupational therapy's role in mental health promotion, prevention, & intervention with children & youth: Childhood trauma.* https://www.aota.org/~/media/Corporate/Files/Practice/Children/Childhood-Trauma-Info-Sheet-2015.pdf

American Psychiatric Association. (2013). *Diagnostic and statistical manual of mental disorders* (5th ed.). https://doi.org/10.1176/appi.books.9780890425596

Ashcroft, R., Lynch, A., & Tekell, L. (2019). Best practices in supporting students with childhood trauma. In G. Frolek Clark, J. E. Rioux, & B. E. Chandler (Eds.), *Best practices for occupational therapy in schools* (2nd ed., pp. 243–251). AOTA Press.

Azar, S. T., Miller, E. A., Stevenson, M. T., & Johnson, D. R. (2017). Social cognition, child neglect, and child injury risk: The contribution of maternal social information processing to maladaptive injury prevention beliefs within a high-risk sample. *Journal of Pediatric Psychology, 42*(7), 759–767. https://doi.org/10.1093/jpepsy/jsw067

Champagne, T. (2011). Attachment, trauma, and occupational therapy practice. *OT Practice, 16*(5), CE-1–CE-8.

Champagne, T. (2019). Trauma and stressor-related disorders. In C. Brown, V. C. Stoffel, & J. P. Muñoz (Eds.). *Occupational therapy in mental health* (2nd ed., pp. 211–224). Davis.

Chen, C.-C., Hsieh, P.-C., Chen, C. P. C., Hsieh, Y.-W., Chung, C.-Y., & Lin, K.-L. (2019). Clinical characteristics and predictors of poor hospital discharge outcome for young children with abusive head trauma. *Journal of Clinical Medicine, 8*(3). Advance online publication. https://doi.org/10.3390/jcm8030390

Clark, C., Classen, C. C., Fourt, A., & Shetty, M. (2015). *Treating the trauma survivor: An essential guide to trauma-informed care.* Routledge.

Denison, M., Gerney, A., Barbuti Van Leuken, J., & Conklin, J. (2018). The attitudes and knowledge of residential treatment center staff members working with adolescents who have experienced trauma. *Residential Treatment for Children & Youth, 35*(2), 114–138. https://doi.org/10.1080/0886571X.2018.1458689

Fette, C., Lambdin-Pattavina, C., & Weaver, L. L. (2019). Understanding and applying trauma-informed approaches across occupational therapy settings. *OT Practice, 24*(5), CE-1–CE-8. https://www.aota.org/-/media/Corporate/Files/Publications/CE-Articles/CE-Article-May-2019-Trauma.pdf

Fraser, K., MacKenzie, D., & Versnel, J. (2017). Complex trauma in children and youth: A scoping review of sensory-based interventions. *Occupational Therapy in Mental Health, 33*(3), 199–216. https://doi.org/10.1080/0164212X.2016.1265475

Holland, J., Begin, D., Orris, D., & Meyer, A. (2018). A descriptive analysis of the theory and processes of an innovative day program for young women with trauma-related symptoms. *Occupational Therapy in Mental Health, 34*(3), 228–241. https://doi.org/10.1080/0164212X2017.1393369

LeBel, J., & Champagne, T. (2010). Integrating sensory and trauma-informed interventions: A Massachusetts state initiative, Part 2. *Mental Health Special Interest Section Quarterly, 33*(2), 1–4.

LeBel, J., Champagne, T., Stromberg, N., & Coyle, R. (2010). Integrating sensory and trauma-informed interventions: A Massachusetts state initiative, Part 1. *Mental Health Special Interest Section Quarterly, 33*(1), 1–4.

Porter, R. S. (Ed.). (2018). *The Merck manual of diagnosis and therapy* (20th ed.). Merck Sharp & Dohme.

Precin, P. (2011). Occupation as therapy for traumatic recovery: A case study. *Work, 38,* 77–81. https://doi.org/10.3233/WOR-2011-1106

Ryan, K., Lane, S. J., & Powers, D. (2017). A multidisciplinary model for treating complex trauma in early childhood. *International Journal of Play Therapy, 26*(2), 111–123. https://doi.org/10.1037/pla0000044

Snedden, D. (2012). Trauma informed practice: An emerging role of occupational therapy. *Occupational Therapy Now, 14,* 26–28.

Suarez, M. A. (2017). They said: We are all in this together. *Open Journal of Occupational Therapy, 5*(3), Article 13. https://doi.org/10.15453/2168-6408.1435

Substance Abuse and Mental Health Services Administration. (2014). *Trauma-informed care in behavioral health services: Treatment Improvement Protocol (TIP) Series, No. 57* (HHS Publication No. [SMA] 13-4801). U.S. Department of Health and Human Services.

Warner, E., Spinazzola, J., Westcott, A., Gunn, C., & Hodgdon, H. (2014). The body can change the score: Empirical support for somatic regulation in the treatment of traumatized adolescents. *Journal of Child & Adolescent Trauma, 7*(4), 237–266. https://doi.org/10.1007/s40653-014-0030-z

Whiting, C. C. (2018). Trauma and the role of the school-based occupational therapist. *Journal of Occupational Therapy, Schools, & Early Intervention, 11*(3), 291–301. https://doi.org/10.1080/19411243.2018.1438327

BIBLIOGRAPHY

Alers, V. (2014). Trauma and its effects on children, adolescents and adults: The role of the occupational therapist. In R. Crouch & V. Alers (Eds.), *Occupational therapy in psychiatry and mental health* (5th ed., pp. 337–355). Wiley.

American Occupational Therapy Association. (2018). AOTA's societal statement on youth violence. *American Journal of Occupational Therapy, 72*(Suppl. 2), Article 7212410090. https://doi.org/10.5014/ajot.2018.72S209

Gabriel, L., James, H., Cronin-Davis, J., Tizro, A., Beetham, T., Hullock, A., & Raynar, A. (2017). Reflexive research with mothers and children victims of domestic violence. *Counseling & Psychotherapy Research, 17*(2), 157–165. https://doi.org/10.1002/capr.12117

Gabriel, L., Tizro, Z., James, H., Cronin-Davis, J., Beetham, T., Corbally, A., Lopez-Moreno, E., & Hill, S. (2018). "Give me some space": Exploring youth to parent aggression and violence. *Journal of Family Violence, 33*, 161–169. https://doi.org/10.1007/s10896-017-9928-1

Moore, K. M., & Balzarini-Leonhart, A. (2017, April 11–12). *Sensory connection to trauma and treatment in youth* [Conference session]. Trauma Informed Symposium of Wisconsin, Oshkosh, WI, United States.

Morkut, B. G., & Atchison, B. J. (2017). Complex trauma. In B. J. Atchison & D. P. Dirette (Eds.), *Conditions in occupational therapy: Effect on occupational performance* (5th ed., pp. 192–208). Wolters Kluwer.

Njelesani, J. (2019). "A child who is hidden has no rights": Responses to violence against children with disabilities. *Child Abuse & Neglect, 89*, 58–69. https://doi.org/10.1016/j.chiabu.2018.12.024

Oey, E., Tunningley, J., Brayman, T., Brokamp, K., & Lynch, D. (2019). Learning together in a community of practice to address pediatric trauma. *OT Practice, 24*(8), 20–25.

Pizur-Barnekow, K., & Erickson, S. (2011). Perinatal posttraumatic stress disorder: Implications for occupational therapy in early intervention practice. *Occupational Therapy in Mental Health, 27*(2), 126–139. https://doi.org/10.1080/0164212X.2011.566165

Developmental Coordination Disorder

Description

Developmental coordination disorder (DCD) is a neurodevelopmental condition that negatively affects a child's ability to perform the motor-based tasks required to complete self-care, academic, play, leisure, and social occupations. Children with DCD struggle to perform the everyday activities that most people are able to do with ease. As a result, parents become stressed, teachers often do not know how to help in the classroom, and children become frustrated and may exhibit behavioral symptoms. The motor difficulties are not due to any known neurological, sensory, or muscular disease (Campbell et al., 2012).

Cause

The exact cause is unknown. Formal criteria for a diagnosis of developmental coordination disorder are listed in the *Diagnostic and Statistical Manual of Mental Disorders* (5th ed.; *DSM-5*; American Psychiatric Association, 2013), and other criteria have been advanced (see Blank et al., 2012).

Evaluation/Assessment
Areas
- Activities of Daily Living/Instrumental ADL: self-care skills (eating, dressing, grooming, bathing, toileting, mobility, transfers, communication, physical fitness); independent living skills (meal preparation, homemaking, shopping, financial management, transportation)
- Education/Work: academic performance, school activities, vocational exploration, work skills
- Play/Leisure: play skills, interests, leisure occupations (type, frequency, location)
- Rest/Sleep: sleep habits
- Social Participation: type, frequency, location, with whom

- Sensorimotor: gross motor skills (walk, jump, climb, hop, skip), postural control, balance, fine motor skills (grasp, pinch, in-hand manipulation, release) upper extremity skills (throwing, catching)
- Cognitive/Perceptual: attention, memory, learning style, executive functions
- Psychosocial: self-confidence, self-competence, self-efficacy, self-esteem, interpersonal skills, quality of life
- Context/Environment: parent and educator education, community and internet resources
- Development (Infant, Child, Adolescent only): developmental milestones
- Comorbidities: attention-deficit/hyperactivity disorder, autism spectrum disorder, emotional and behavioral disorders, sensory processing dysfunction, specific learning disabilities

Instruments
Instruments Developed by Occupational Therapy Personnel
- Adolescents & Adults Coordination Questionnaire (AACQ; Tal-Saban, Ornoy, et al., 2012, in References)
- Canadian Little Developmental Coordination Disorder Questionnaire (CLDCDQ; Rihtman et al., 2011; Wilson et al., 2015, in References)
- Canadian Occupational Performance Measure 5th (COPM-5; Law et al., 2014)
- Children Activity Scales (ChAS-P/T; Rosenblum, 2006)
- Computerized Penmanship Evaluation Tool (ComPET; Rosenblum et al., 2003)
- Daily Life Functions Questionnaire (DLF-Q; Tal-Saban, Zarka, et al., 2012, in References)
- Developmental Coordination Disorder Questionnaire '07 (DCDQ '07; Wilson et al., 2012; see also de Souza Sarraff et al., 2018; Parmar et al., 2014; and Rivard et al., 2014, in References)
- Do-Eat (D-E; Josman et al., 2010)
- Handwriting Proficiency Screening Questionnaire (HPSQ; Rosenblum, 2008)
- Internal Factors Attributed to Success Questionnaire (IFASQ; Tal-Saban, Zarka, et al., 2012, in References)
- Life-Satisfaction Questionnaire (LISAT-9; Fugl-Meyer et al., 1991)
- Participation and Environment Measure–Children and Youth (PEM-CY; Coster et al., 2011)
- Participation in Every Day Activities of Life (PEDAL; Tal-Saban et al., 2014, in References)
- Performance Quality Rating Scale (PQRS; Martini et al., 2015)
- Participation in Physical Activity and Sedentary Behavior Questionnaire (PQ; Cermak, 2007; see also Beutum et al., 2013, in References)
- Problem Solving Questionnaire (PSQ; Tal-Saban, Zarka, et al., 2012, in References)
- Questionnaire for Assessing Students' Organizational Abilities–Teachers (QASA-T; Lifshitz & Josman, 2006; in Hebrew)
- Recent Emotional State Test (REST; Tal-Saban, Zarka, et al., 2012, in References)
- Sensory Integration and Praxis Tests (SIPT; Ayres, 1989)
- Southern California Sensory Integration Test (SCSIT; Ayres, 1980, out of print)

Instruments Developed by Other Professionals and Used by Occupational Therapy Personnel
- 6-Minute Walk Test (6MWT; American Thoracic Society, 2002)
- ActiGraph (GT3X Accelerometer, Pensacola, FL)
- Adult Developmental Coordination Disorder/Dyspraxia Checklist (ADC; Kirby & Rosenblum, 2008)
- Ages and Stages Questionnaires (3rd ed.; ASQ-3; Squires & Bricker, 2009; see also King-Dowling et al., 2016, in References)
- Arizona Social Support Interview Schedule (ASSIS; Barrera et al., 1981)
- Assessment of Life Habits for Children 5 to 13, 1.0 (Life-H-Children Short Form; Fougeyrollas et al., 2003)
- Beery-Buktenica Developmental Test of Visual-Motor Integration (6th ed.; Beery VMI-6; Beery et al., 2010)

- Behavior Assessment System for Children (3rd ed.; BASC-3; Reynolds & Kamphaus, 2015)
- Bruininks-Oseretsky Test of Motor Proficiency (2nd ed.; BOT-2; Bruininks & Bruininks, 2005)
- Child Behavior Checklist (CBCL; Achenbach, 2001)
- Children's Omni Scale of Perceived Exertion (COSPE; Robertson et al., 2000)
- Children's Perception of Motor Competence Scale (CPMCS; Ruiz Pérez & Graupera Sanz, 2005)
- Kaufman Brief Intelligence Test (2nd ed.; KBIT-2; Kaufman & Kaufman, 2004)
- KIDSCREEN 52 (KIDSCREEN Group Europe, 2006)
- Movement Assessment Battery for Children (2nd ed.; M-ABC-2; Henderson et al., 2007; see also Kwok et al., 2019, in References)
- Omni Scale of Perceived Exertion (OSPE)
- Parenting Stress Index (4th ed.; PSI-4; Abidin, 2012)
- Pictorial Scale of Perceived Competence and Social Acceptance (PSPCSA; Harter & Pike, 1984)
- Preschool Language Scales (5th ed.; PLS-5; Zimmerman et al., 2012)
- Strengths and Difficulties Questionnaire (SDQ; Goodman, 1997)
- Teacher Estimate of Activity Form (TEAF; Hay, 1992)
- Vineland Adaptive Behavior Scales (3rd ed.; Vineland-3; Sparrow et al., 2016)
- World Health Organization Quality of Life–BREF (WHOQOL-BREF; The WHOQOL Group, 1998)

Problems/Issues

Activities of Daily Living/Instrumental ADL
- Child has difficulty performing basic self-care skills appropriate to age level in spite of opportunity to practice, such as buttoning a shirt, using eating utensils, tying shoelaces.
- Child may require more assistance from adults to perform tasks peers are able to perform independently.
- Child or youth has difficulty performing independent living skills appropriate to age level in spite of opportunity to practice.

Education/Work
- Child's performance of academic tasks is below age and grade level.
- Child's ability to perform basic work skills is below age-appropriate level and performance is slower than other children doing the same task.
- Child's teacher may describe a significant discrepancy between oral (good) and written (poor) work.

Play/Leisure
- Child's play skills are below age-appropriate level.
- Child has limited leisure interests and skills.
- Child may have difficulty engaging in age-appropriate motor games and sports activities, such as playing tag, dodgeball, biking, swimming, playing hide-and-seek, running races, jumping or skipping rope, climbing a rope ladder, playing hopscotch, Simon Says, baseball, basketball, soccer, volleyball, bowling, football.
- Child prefers to watch peers play instead of joining in.

Rest/Sleep
- Not discussed.

Social Participation
- Child has difficulty participating with age-level peers in social activities.

Sensorimotor
- Child's ability to execute motor skills is below that expected of the child's age, such as printing, cutting, copying, opening containers, or completing puzzles.

- Child awkwardly grasps pencil either too tight or too loose with too much pressure or not enough.
- Child appears clumsy with objects and tools, frequently dropping them or using them incorrectly.
- Child has difficulty acquiring new motor skills.
- Child may appear to become fatigued more easily than other children or appear tired after little physical activity.
- Child may have difficulty maintaining a sitting posture (fidgets, is restless or constantly shifting weight).

Cognitive/Perceptual
- Child may have difficulty maintaining attention to task.
- Child may have difficulty with working memory.
- Child may have difficulty with external focus of attention (focusing on impact of movement on the environment) and an internal focus of attention (focusing on one's body movement using implicit [unconscious] and explicit [conscious] motor learning).
- Child may have difficulty performing executive functions, such as planning and problem solving.

Psychosocial
- Child may have low self-confidence and poor sense of self.
- Child may have low self-esteem due to repeated failure.
- Child does not improve performance through practice and repetition.
- Child may be easily frustrated or overwhelmed by what seems to be simple or basic tasks.
- Child may display behavioral problems (depression, frustration, withdrawal, passivity, anger, acting out, or aggression).
- Child may experience social isolation.
- Child may be bullied.
- Parents may express feelings of stress.

Context/Environment
- Parents and educators may lack information and resources to manage DCD.

Intervention/Treatment

Models and programs developed by occupational therapy personnel include the Cognitive Orientation to Occupational Performance (CO-OP) model (Araújo et al., 2019; Dawson et al., 2017; Scammell et al., 2016) and the MOSAIC program (Brammer et al., 2015). Models and programs developed by other professionals but used by occupational therapy personnel include the Apollo model (Camden et al., 2015), Partnering for Change (Missiuna et al., 2012), and summer camp (Zwicker et al., 2015). Team members include physicians, educators, psychologists, physical therapists, and occupational therapy personnel. Goals are to maximize child's participation in motor activities related to self-care, play, and school activities with the home, school, and community and increase social participation and motivation (Morgan & Long, 2012).

Activities of Daily Living/Instrumental ADL
- Provide opportunity to discuss, plan, and prepare healthy meals and snacks.
- Practice driving in a simulator or in an empty parking lot before on-road practice to reduce demands.

Education/Work
- Consider use of assistive technology, especially a computer, for academic tasks.
- Provide written instructions for completion of work tasks.

- Modify environment to reduce demands (more time, reduce number of items, early release to avoid crowds in hallways).

Play/Leisure
- Explore leisure occupations that are within skill level. Modify or simplify task demands.

Rest/Sleep
- No information identified.

Social Participation
- Assist client to select social activities that are less demanding (fewer people, less distance, shorter time period, with a trusted companion).

Sensorimotor
- Modify game or required actions to reduce demand for skill (use a balloon instead of a ball for volleyball), start with two actions (hands on head or jump) when playing Simon Says.

Cognitive/Perceptual
- Practice the Goal-Plan-Do-Check model. GOAL (select and decide what action, motion or movement is to be done), PLAN (instructions to determine how action, motion, or movement is to be done), DO (execute the action, motion, or movement), and CHECK (was the action, motion, or movement done correctly? What corrections need to be made?).
- Provide practice in using reminders (smartphone apps, checklists, time schedules).

Psychosocial
- Provide practice in using coping strategies and stress management (stretching exercises, mindfulness, deep breathing, yoga).

Context/Environment
- Provide information and resources online regarding issues and solutions for problems experienced by clients with DCD.
- Provide meet-and-greet sessions with clients and families to discuss.

Precautions/Safety Considerations
- None stated.

Prognosis and Outcome

DCD is a chronic health condition that is present throughout life that persists in all areas of life. Many of the motor and psychosocial difficulties continue into adulthood (Harris et al., 2015).

REFERENCES

American Psychiatric Association. (2013). *Diagnostic and statistical manual of mental disorders* (5th ed.). https://doi.org/10.1176/appi.books.9780890425596

Araújo, C. R. S., Cardosa, A. A., & Magalhães, L. C. (2019). Efficacy of the cognitive orientation to daily occupational performance with Brazilian children with developmental coordination disorder. *Scandinavian Journal of Occupational Therapy*, 26(1), 46–54. https://doi.org/10.1080/11038128.2017.1417476

Beutum, M. N., Cordier, R., & Bundy, A. (2013). Comparing activity patterns, biological and family factors in children with and without developmental coordination disorder. *Physical & Occupational Therapy in Pediatrics*, 33(2), 174–185. https://doi.org/10.3109/01942638.2012.747585

Blank, R., Smits-Engelsman, B., Polatajko, H., & Wilson, P. (2012). European Academy for Childhood Disability (EACD): Recommendations on the definition, diagnosis, and intervention of developmental coordination disorder (long version). *Developmental Medicine & Child Neurology, 54*(1), 54–93. https://doi.org/10.1111/j.1469-8749.2011.04171.x

Brammer, W., Malshuk, E., Robertson, L., Rubin, B., Rios, D., & Jirikowic, T. (2015). Improving functional motor skills and confidence. *OT Practice, 20*(18) 8–12.

Camden, C., Léger, F., Morel, J., & Missiuna, C. (2015). A service delivery model for children with DCD based on principles of best practice. *Physical & Occupational Therapy in Pediatrics, 35*(4), 412–425. https://doi.org/10.3109/01942638.2014.978932

Campbell, W. N., Missiuna, C., & Vaillancourt, T. (2012). Peer victimization and depression in children with and without motor coordination difficulties. *Psychology in the Schools, 49*(4) 328–341. https://doi.org/10.1002/pits.21600

Dawson, D. R., McEwen, S. E., & Polatajko, H. J. (Eds.). (2017). *Cognitive orientation to daily occupational performance in occupational therapy: Using the CO-OP approach to enable participation across the lifespan.* AOTA Press.

de Souza Sarraff, T. da F., Martinez, C. M. S., & Santos, J. L. F. (2018). Specificity and sensitivity of the DCDQ for children aged 8 to 1 years in Brazil. *Revista de Terapia Ocupacional da Unversidade de São Paulo, 29*(2), 135–143. https://doi.org/10.11606/issn.2238-6149.v29i2p135-143

Harris, S. R., Mickelson, E. C. R., & Zwicker, J. G. (2015). Diagnosis and management of developmental coordination disorder. *CMAJ, 187*(9), 659–665. https://doi.org/10.1503/cmaj.140994

King-Dowling, S., Rodriguez, M. C., Missiuna, C., & Cairney, J. (2016). Validity of the Ages and Stages Questionnaire to detect risk of developmental coordination disorder in preschoolers. *Child: Care, Health and Development, 42*(2), 188–194. https://doi.org/10.1111/cch.12314

Kwok, C., Mackay, M., Agnew, J. A., Synnes, A., & Zwicker, J. G. (2019). Does the Movement Assessment Battery for Children–2 at 3 years of age predict developmental coordination disorder at 4.5 years of age in children born very preterm? *Research in Developmental Disabilities, 84*, 36–42. https://doi.org/10.1016/j.ridd.2018.04.003

Missiuna, C. A., Pollock, N. A., Levac, D. E., Campbell, W. N., Sahagian Whalen, S. E., Bennett, S. M., Hecimovich, C. A., Gaines, B. R., Cairney, J., & Russell, D. J. (2012). Partnering for Change: An innovative school-based occupational therapy service delivery model for children with developmental coordination disorder. *Canadian Journal of Occupational Therapy, 79*(1), 41–50. https://doi.org/10.2182/cjot.2012.79.1.6

Morgan, R., & Long, T. (2012). The effectiveness of occupational therapy for children with developmental coordination disorder: A review of the qualitative literature. *British Journal of Occupational Therapy, 75*(1), 10–18. https://doi.org/10.4276/030802212X13261082051337

Parmar, A., Kwan, M., Rodriguez, C., Missiuna, C., & Cairney, J. (2014). Psychometric properties of the DCD-Q-07 in children ages to 4–6. *Research in Developmental Disabilities, 35*(2), 330–339. https://doi.org/10.1016/j.ridd.2013.10.030

Rihtman, T., Wilson, B. N., & Parush, S. (2011). Development of the Little Developmental Coordination Disorder Questionnaire for preschoolers and preliminary evidence of its psychometric properties in Israel. *Research in Developmental Disabilities, 32*(4), 1378–1387. https://doi.org/10.1016/j.ridd.2010.12.040

Rivard, L., Missiuna, C., McCauley, D., & Cairney, J. (2014). Descriptive and factor analysis of the Developmental Coordination Disorder Questionnaire (DCDQ'07) in a population-based sample of children with and without developmental coordination disorder. *Child: Care, Health and Development, 40*(1), 42–49. https://doi.org/10.1111/j.1365-2214.2012.01425.x

Scammell, E. M., Bates, S. V., Houldin, A., & Polatajko, H. J. (2016). The Cognitive Orientation to daily Occupational Performance (CO-OP): A scoping review. *Canadian Journal of Occupational Therapy, 83*(4), 216–225. https://doi.org/10.1177/0008417416651277

Tal-Saban, M., Ornoy, A., Grotto, I., & Parush, S. (2012). Adolescents and Adults Coordination Questionnaire: Development and psychometric properties. *American Journal of Occupational Therapy, 66*(4), 406–413. https://doi.org/10.5014/ajot.2012.003251

Tal-Saban, M., Ornoy, A., & Parush, S. (2014). Young adults with developmental coordination disorder: A longitudinal study. *American Journal of Occupational Therapy, 68*(3), 307–316. https://doi.org/10.5014/ajot.2014.009563

Tal-Saban, M., Zarka, S., Grotto, I., Ornoy, A., & Parush, S. (2012). The functional profile of young adults with suspected developmental coordination disorder (DCD). *Research in Developmental Disabilities, 33*(6), 2193–2202. https://doi.org/10.1016/j.ridd.2012.06.005

Wilson, B. N., & Crawford, S. G. (2012). *The Developmental Coordination Disorder Questionnaire 2007 (DCDQ '07): Administration manual for the DCDQ'07 with psychometric properties.* https://dcdq.ca/uploads/pdf/DCDQAdmin-Scoring-02-20-2012.pdf

Wilson, B. N., Creighton, D., Crawford, S. G., Heath, J. A., Semple, L., Tan, B., & Hansen, S. (2015). Psychometric properties of the Canadian Little Developmental Coordination Disorder Question for preschool children. *Physical & Occupational Therapy in Pediatrics, 35*(2), 116–135. https://doi.org/10.3109/01942638.2014.980928

Zwicker, J. G., Rehal, H., Sodhi, S., Karkling M., Paul, A., Hilliard, M., & Jarus, T. (2015). Effectiveness of a summer camp intervention for children with developmental coordination disorder. *Physical & Occupational Therapy in Pediatrics, 35*(2), 163–177. https://doi.org/10.3109/01942638.2014.957431

BIBLIOGRAPHY

Allen, S., & Casey, J. (2017). Developmental coordination disorders and sensory processing and integration: Incidence, associations and co-morbidities. *British Journal of Occupational Therapy, 80*(9), 549–557. https://doi.org/10.1177/0308022617709183

Armitage, S., Swallow, V., & Kolehmainen, N. (2017). Ingredients and change processes in occupational therapy for children. *Scandinavian Journal of Occupational Therapy, 24*(3), 208–213. https://doi.org/10.1080/11038128.2016.1201141

Batey, C. A., Missiuna, C. A., Timmons, B. W., Hay, J. A., Faught, B. E., & Cairney, J. (2014). Self-efficacy toward physical activity and the physical activity behavior of children with and without developmental coordination disorder. *Human Movement Science, 36*, 258–271. https://doi.org/10.1016/j.humov.2013.10.003

Brown-Lum, M., & Zwicker, J. G. (2017). Neuroimaging and occupational therapy: Bridging the gap to advance rehabilitation in developmental coordination disorder. *Journal of Motor Behavior, 49*(1), 98–110. https://doi.org/10.1080/00222895.2016.1271295

Cairney, J., Hay, J., Veldhuizen, S., Missiuna, C., Mahlberg, N., & Faught, B. E. (2010). Trajectories of relative weight and waist circumference among children with and without developmental coordination disorder. *CMAJ, 182*(11), 1167–1172. https://doi.org/10.1503/cmaj.091454

Camden, A., Couture, M., Pratte, G., Morin, M., Roberge, P., Poder, T., Maltais, D. B., Jasmin, E., Hurtubise, K., Ducreux, E., Léger, F., Zwicker, J., Berbari, J., Fallon, F., & Tousignant, M. (2019). Recruitment, use, and satisfaction with a web platform supporting families of children with suspected or diagnosed developmental coordination disorder: A randomized feasibility trial. *Developmental Neurorehabilitation, 22*(7), 470–478. https://doi.org/10.1080/17518423.2018.1523243

Camden, C., Foley, V., Anaby, D., Shikako-Thomas, K., Gauthier-Boudreault, C., Berbari, J., & Missiuna, C. (2016). Using an evidence-based online module to improve parents' ability to support their child with developmental coordination disorder. *Disability and Health Journal, 9*(3), 406–415. https://doi.org/10.1016/j.dhjo.2016.04.002

Camden, C., Wilson, B., Kirby, A., Sugden, D., & Missiuna, C. (2015). Best practice principles for management of children with developmental coordination disorder (DCD): Results of a scoping review. *Child: Care Health and Development, 41*(1), 147–159. https://doi.org/10.1111/cch.12128

Cermak, S. A., Katz, N., Weintraub, N., Steinhart, S., Raz-Silbiger, S., Munoz, M., & Lifshitz, N. (2015). Participation in physical activity, fitness, and risk for obesity in children with developmental coordination disorder: A cross-cultural study. *Occupational Therapy International, 22,* 163–173. https://doi.org/10.1002/oti.1393

Chung, A. (2015). *Clinical review: Developmental coordination disorder (Occupational therapy).* Cinahl Information Systems.

College of Occupational Therapists. (2013). *Practice briefing: Diagnosis of developmental coordination disorder.*

Darsaklis, V., Snider, L. M., Majnemer, A., & Mazer, B. (2013). Assessment used to diagnose developmental coordination disorder: Do their underlying constructs match the diagnostic criteria? *Physical & Occupational Therapy in Pediatrics, 32*(2), 186–198. https://doi.org/10.31 09/01942638.2012.739268

Elbasan, B., Kayihan, H., & Duzgun, I. (2012). Sensory integration and activities of daily living in children with developmental coordination disorder. *Italian Journal of Pediatrics, 38,* Article 14. https://doi.org/10.1186/1824-7288-38-14

Engel-Yeger, B., Sido, R., Mimouni-Bloch, A., & Weiss, P. L. (2017). Relationship between perceived competence and performance during real and virtual motor tasks by children with developmental coordination disorder. *Disability and Rehabilitation Assistive Technology, 12*(7), 752–757. https://doi.org/10.1080/17483107.2016.1261305

Gagnon-Roy, M., Jasmin, E., & Camden, C. (2016). Social participation of teenagers and young adults with developmental coordination disorder and strategies that could help them: Results from a scoping review. *Child: Care, Health and Development, 42*(6), 840–851. https://doi.org/10.1111/cch.12389

Hessell, S., Hocking, C., & Davies, S. G. (2010). Participation of boys with developmental coordination disorder in gymnastics. *New Zealand Journal of Occupational Therapy, 57,* 14–21.

Hsu, L.-Y., Jirikowic, T., Ciol, M. A., Clark, M., Kartin, D., & McCoy, S. W. (2018). Motor planning and gait coordination assessments for children with developmental coordination disorder. *Physical & Occupational Therapy in Pediatrics, 38*(5), 562–574. https://doi.org/10.1080/0194 2638.2018.1477226

Izadi-Najafabadi, S., Ryan, N., Ghafooripoor, G., Gill, K., & Zwicker, J. D. (2019). Participation of children with developmental coordination disorder. *Research in Developmental Disabilities, 84,* 75–84. https://doi.org/10.1016/j.ridd.2018.05.011

Jarus, T., Ghanouni, P., Abel, R. L., Fomenoff, S. L., Lundberg, J., Davidson, S., Caswell, S., Bickerton, L., & Zwicker, J. G. (2015). Effect of internal versus external focus of attention on implicit motor learning in children with developmental coordination disorder. *Research in Developmental Disabilities, 37,* 119–126. https://doi.org/10.1016/j.ridd.2014.11.009

Jarus, T., Lourie-Gelberg, Y., Engel-Yeger, B., & Bart, O. (2011). Participation patterns of school-aged children with and without DCD. *Research in Developmental Disabilities, 32*(4), 1323–1331. https://doi.org/10.1016/j.ridd.2011.01.033

Jasmin, E., Tétreault, S., & Joly, J. (2014). Ecosystemic needs assessment for children with developmental coordination disorder in elementary school: Multiple case studies. *Physical & Occupational Therapy in Pediatrics, 34*(4), 424–442. https://doi.org/10.3109/01942638.201 4.899284

Jasmin, E., Tétreault, S., Larivière, N., & Joly, J. (2018). Participation and needs of children with developmental coordination disorder at home and in the community: Perceptions of children and parents. *Research in Developmental Disabilities, 73,* 1–13. https://doi.org/10.1016/j.ri dd.2017.12.011

Joshi, D., Missiuna, C., Henna, S., Hay, J., Faught, B. E., & Cairney, J. (2015). Relationship between BMI, waist circumference, physical activity and probable developmental coordination disorder over time. *Human Movement Science, 40,* 237–247. https://doi.org/10.1016/j.hu mov.2014.12.011

Karkling, M., Paul, A., & Zwicker, J. G. (2017). Occupational therapists' awareness of guidelines for assessment and diagnosis of developmental coordination disorder. *Canadian Journal of Occupational Therapy, 84*(3), 148–157. https://doi.org/10.1177/0008417417700915

Karras, H. C., Morin, D. M., Gill, K., Izadi-Najafabadi, S., & Zwicker, J. G. (2019). Health-related quality of life of children with developmental coordination disorder. *Research in Developmental Disabilities, 84*, 85–95. https://doi.org/10.1016/j.ridd.2018.05.012

King-Dowling, S., Missiuna, C., Rodriquez, M. C., Greenway, M., & Cairney, J. (2015). Co-occurring motor, language and emotional-behavioral problems in children 3–6 years of age. *Human Movement Science, 39*, 101–108. https://doi.org/10.1016/j.humov.2014.10.010

King-Dowling, S., Rodriguez, C., Missiuna, C., Timmons, B. W., & Cairney, J. (2018). Health-related fitness in preschool children with and without motor delays. *Medicine & Science in Sports & Exercise, 50*(7), 1442–1448. https://doi.org/10.1249/MSS.0000000000001590

Lifshitz, N., Josman, N., & Tirosh, E. (2014). Disorganization as related to discoordination and attention deficit. *Journal of Child Neurology, 29*(1), 66–70. https://doi.org/10.1177/08830738 12469295

Magalhães, L. C., Cardoso, A. A., & Missiuna, C. (2011). Activities and participation in children with developmental coordination disorder: A systematic review. *Research in Developmental Disabilities, 32*(4), 1309–1316. https://doi.org/10.1016/j.ridd.2011.01.029

Margow, S. (2017, September). Developmental coordination disorder: The "hidden" facet of autism spectrum disorder. *Exceptional Parent Magazine, 47*, 46–48.

Missiuna, C., Cairney, J., Pollock, N., Campbell, W., Russell, D. J, Macdonald, K., Schmidt, L., Heath, N., Veldhuizen, S., & Cousins, M. (2014). Psychological distress in children with developmental coordination disorder and attention-deficit hyperactivity disorder. *Research in Developmental Disabilities, 35*(5), 1198–1207. https://doi.org/10.1016/j.ridd.2014.01.007

Missiuna, C., Cairney, J., Pollock, N., Russell, D., Macdonald, K., Cousins, M., Veldhuizen, S., & Schmidt, L. (2011). A staged approach for identifying children with developmental coordination disorder from the population. *Research in Developmental Disabilities, 32*(2), 549–559. https://doi.org/10.1016/j.ridd.2010.12.025

Montgomery, I., Glegg, S., Boniface, G., & Zwicker, J. G. (2018). *Management of developmental coordination disorder*. Health Centre for Children.

Neto, J. L. C., Zamunér, A. R., dos Santos Silva, R. A., Menegat, D., Silva, E., & Tudella, E. (2017). Effects of motor skills training program on the cardiac autonomic control in children with developmental coordination disorder: A preliminary study. *European Journal of Physiotherapy, 19*(Suppl. 1), 56–58. https://doi.org/10.1080/21679169.2017.1381314

O'Dea, Á., & Connell, A. (2016). Performance difficulties, activity limitations and participation restrictions of adolescents with developmental coordination disorder (DCD). *British Journal of Occupational Therapy, 79*(9), 540–549. https://doi.org/10.1177/0308022616643100

Prunty, M. M., Barnett, A. L., Wilmut, K., & Plumb, M. S. (2016). The impact of handwriting difficulties on compositional quality in children with developmental coordination disorder. *British Journal of Occupational Therapy, 79*(10), 591–597. https://doi.org/10.1177/03080226 16650903

Prunty, M. M., Barnett, A. L., Wilmut, K., & Plumb, M. (2016). Visual perceptual and handwriting skills in children with developmental coordination disorder. *Human Movement Science, 49*, 54–65. https://doi.org/10.1016/j.humov.2016.06.003

Raz-Silbiger, S., Lifshitz, N., Katz, N., Steinhart, S., Cermak, S. A., & Weintraub, N. (2015). Relationship between motor skills, participation in leisure activities and quality of life of children with developmental coordination disorder: Temporal aspects. *Research in Developmental Disabilities, 38*, 171–189. https://doi.org/10.1016/j.ridd.2014.12.012

Reynolds, J. E., Kerrigan, S., Elliott, C., Lay, B. S., & Licari, M. K. (2017). Poor imitative performance of unlearned gestures in children with probable developmental coordination disorder. *Journal of Motor Behavior, 49*(4), 378–387. https://doi.org/10.1080/00222895.2016.1219305

Rosenblum, S. (2015). Do motor ability and handwriting kinematic measures predict organizational ability among children with developmental coordination disorders? *Human Movement Science, 43,* 201–215. https://doi.org/10.1016/j.humov.2015.03.014

Rosenblum, S., & Engel-Yeger, B. (2015). Hypo-activity screening in school setting: Examining reliability and validity of the Teacher Estimation of Activity Form (TEAF). *Occupational Therapy International, 22*(2), 85–93. https://doi.org/10.1002/oti.1387

Rosenblum, S., Margieh, J. A., & Engel-Yeger, B. (2013). Handwriting features of children with developmental coordination disorder—Results of triangular evaluation. *Research in Developmental Disabilities, 34*(11), 4134–4141. https://doi.org/10.1016/j.ridd.2013.08.009

Saban, M. T., Ornoy, A., & Parush, S. (2014). Executive function and attention in young adults with and without developmental coordination disorder—A comparative study. *Research in Developmental Disabilities, 35*(11), 2644–2650. https://doi.org/10.1016/j.ridd.2014.07.002

Siaperas, P. (2012). Motor abilities, developmental movement disorders and the role of sensorimotor processing: Problems in terminology and interdisciplinary communication. *World Federation of Occupational Therapists Bulletin, 65*(1), 28–34. https://doi.org/10.1179/otb.2012.65.1.006

Smits-Engelsman, B. C. M., Blank, R., van der Kaay, A. C., Mosterd-Van Der Meijs, R., Vlugt-Van Den Brand, E., Polatajko, H., & Wilson, P. H. (2012). Efficacy of interventions to improve motor performance in children with developmental coordination disorder: A combined systematic review and meta-analysis. *Developmental Medicine & Child Neurology, 55*(3), 229–237. https://doi.org/10.1111/dmcn.12008

Szklut, S. E., & Philbert, D. B. (2013). Learning disabilities and developmental coordination disorder. In D. A. Umphred, G. U. Burton, R. T. Lazaro, & M. L. Roller (Eds.), *Umphred's neurological rehabilitation* (6th ed., pp. 379–418). Elsevier.

Tal-Saban, M., Ornoy, A., & Parush, S. (2014). Executive function and attention in young adults with and without developmental coordination disorder: A comparative study. *Research in Developmental Disabilities, 35*(11), 2644–2650. https://doi.org/10.1016/j.ridd.2014.07.002

Tokolahi, E. (2014). Developmental coordination disorder: The domain of child and adolescent mental health occupational therapists? *New Zealand Journal of Occupational Therapy, 61*(1), 21–25.

Withers, R., Tsang, Y., & Zwicker, J. G. (2017). Intervention and management of developmental coordination disorder: Are we providing evidence-based services? *Canadian Journal of Occupational Therapy, 84*(3), 158–167. https://doi.org/10.1177/0008417417712285

Zwicker, J. G., Harris, S. R., & Klassen, A. F. (2013). Quality of life domains affected in children with developmental coordination disorder: A systematic review. *Child: Care, Health and Development, 39*(4), 562–580. https://doi.org/10.1111/j.1365-2214.2012.01379.x

Zwicker, J. G., Missiuna, C., Harris, S. R., & Boyd, L. A. (2011). Brain activation associated with motor skills practice in children with developmental coordination disorder: An fMRI study. *International Journal of Developmental Neuroscience, 29*(2), 145–152. https://doi.org/10.1016/j.ijdevneu.2010.12.002

Zwicker, J. G., Missiuna, C., Harris, S. R., & Boyd, L. A. (2010). Brain activation of children with developmental coordination disorder is different than peers. *Pediatrics, 126*(3), e678–e686. https://doi.org/10.1542/peds.2010-0059

Zwicker, J. G., Missiuna, C., Harris, S. R., & Boyd, L. A. (2012). Developmental coordination disorder: A pilot diffusion tensor imaging study. *Pediatric Neurology, 46*(3), 162–167. https://doi.org/10.1016/j.pediatrneurol.2011.12.007

Zwicker, J. G., Missiuna, C., Harris, S. R., & Boyd, L. A. (2012). Developmental coordination disorder: A review and update. *European Journal of Paediatric Neurology, 16*(6), 573–581. https://doi.org/10.1016/j.ejpn.2012.05.005

Zwicker, J. G., Suto, M., Harris, S. R., Vlasakova, N., & Missiuna, C. (2018). Developmental coordination disorder is more than a motor problem: Children describe the impact of daily struggles on their quality of life. *British Journal Occupational Therapy, 81*(2), 65–73. https://doi.org/10.1177/0308022617735046

Zwicker, J. G., Yoon, S. W., MacKay, M., Petrie-Thomas, J., Rogers, M., & Synnes, A. R. (2013). Perinatal and neonatal predictors of developmental coordination disorder in very low birth-weight children. *Archives of Diseases in Childhood, 98*(2), 118–122. https://doi.org/10.1136/archdischild-2012-302268

Developmental Delay

See also Arthrogryposis Multiplex Congenita, Attention-Deficit/Hyperactivity Disorder, Cerebral Palsy, Congenital Heart Disease, Down Syndrome, Fetal Alcohol Spectrum Disorder, Intellectual Disability, Osteogenesis Imperfecta, Rett Syndrome, Sickle Cell Disease, Spina Bifida.

Description

Child is unable to accomplish the developmental tasks typical of his or her chronological age. Developmental delay may be observed and documented in a wide range of childhood disorders and environmental situations (K. Jacobs & Simon, 2015).

Cause

Prematurity (even with age corrected for preterm birth); arthrogryposis; attention deficit disorder; cerebral palsy; failure to thrive; genetic disorders; intellectual disability; international adoption; low family income (environment situations); HIV/AIDS infections; malnutrition; sensory processing difficulties; sickle cell disease; and younger, first-time mother who lacks parenting skills. Infants who required neonatal intensive care are more likely to demonstrate risk of developmental delay (Ballantyne et al., 2016). Internationally adopted children are at greater risk of demonstrating developmental delay (E. Jacobs et al., 2010).

Evaluation/Assessment

Areas

- Activities of Daily Living/Instrumental ADL: self-maintenance skills, communication (especially expressive)
- Education/Work: academic performance, school mobility
- Play/Leisure: play skills (especially symbolic play), leisure interests
- Rest/Sleep: no information identified
- Social Participation: type, frequency, location
- Sensorimotor: gross and fine motor skills, balance and coordination, postural (head and trunk) control, joint stability, muscle tone, sensory awareness, sensory responsiveness
- Cognitive/Perceptual: attention, memory, executive functions, visual perception, visual motor skills, visual spatial relations
- Psychosocial: interpersonal relations, emotional regulation
- Context/Environment: social support, adapted devices, community resources, family social economic status
- Development (Infant, Child, Adolescent only): developmental milestones—motor, sensory, cognition, perception, mental, emotions, social skills
- Comorbidities: prematurity, congenital disorder, genetic disorder

Instruments

Instruments Developed by Occupational Therapy Personnel

- Infant/Toddler Sensory Profile (ITSP; Dunn, 2002)

- School Function Assessment (SFA; Coster et al., 1998)
- Sensory Processing Measure (SPM) Home Form (SPM-HF; Parham & Ecker, 2007)

Instruments Developed by Other Professionals and Used by Occupational Therapy Personnel
- Ages and Stages Questionnaires (3rd ed.; ASQ-3; Squires & Bricker, 2009)
- Bayley Scales of Infant and Toddler Development (4th ed.; Bayley-4; Bayley & Aylward, 2019)
- Comprehensive Development Inventory of Infants and Toddlers–Diagnostic Test (CDIIT-D; Liao et al., 2005)
- Peabody Developmental Motor Scales (3rd ed.; PDMS-3; Folio & Fewell, 2023)
- Test of Visual Perception Skills (4th ed.; TVPS-4; Martin, 2017)
- Vineland Adaptive Behavior Scales (3rd ed.; Vineland-3; Sparrow et al., 2016)

Problems/Issues

Activities of Daily Living/Instrumental ADL
- Child may have delay in developing skills in self-feeding, dressing and undressing, toileting.
- Child may have delayed development of communication skills, especially gesture and expressive language.

Education/Work
- Child may have delay in academic performance, especially in reading.
- Child may have delay in motor skills and psychosocial behaviors expected in school environment.

Play/Leisure
- Child may have delay in development of play skills such as use of symbolic play.

Rest/Sleep
- Not discussed.

Social Participation
- Child may have delay in development of social interaction skills such as cooperative activities.

Sensorimotor
- Child may have delay in gross motor skills (rolling, creeping, crawling, standing, walking).
- Child may have delay in fine motor skills (ulnar-radial grasp, radial side grasp).
- Child may have delay in development of visual perception.
- Child may be hyporesponsive to sensory stimuli (Baranek et al., 2013).

Cognitive/Perceptual
- Child may have delay in development of attention/concentration (Leung et al., 2011).
- Child may have delay in development of visuomotor skills.

Psychosocial
- Child may have delayed emotional and behavioral control.
- Child may demonstrate hyperactivity (Leung et al., 2011).
- Child may be slow to respond to social stimuli (Baranek et al., 2013).

Context/Environment
- Family and caregivers may lack knowledge of parenting skills.
- Family and caregivers may lack knowledge of available community resources.

Intervention/Treatment

Models and programs developed by occupational therapy personnel include development support program (Shaikh & Valdya, 2013), games and play (Joaquim et al., 2018), and parent participation program (C. L. Lin et al., 2018). Models and programs developed by other professionals but used by occupational therapy personnel include BRIGHT coaching (Majnemer et al., 2019), home program (Tang et al., 2011), massage (Lu et al., 2019), outback services (Dew et al., 2014), rehabilitation intervention (Schurgers et al., 2010), and visual perception training (Chen et al., 2013; H.-C. Lin et al., 2017). Team members include physicians, nursing personnel, social workers, physical therapy personnel, psychologists, educators, parents and caregivers, and occupational therapy personnel. The goal is to facilitate the child's performance at the maximum level of function obtainable, which may include the use of adaptive devices and equipment.

Activities of Daily Living/Instrumental ADL
- Provide opportunity for parents and child to practice selected self-maintenance activities such as eating and dressing.
- Use games to promote gestures and oral expression.

Education/Work
- Consider whether adapted devices (assistive technology) may be useful to facilitate academic performance and school mobility.

Play/Leisure
- Promote play skills, especially symbolic play.

Rest/Sleep
- See Sleep–Wake Disorders in Section 13: Lifestyle Conditions.

Social Participation
- Provide opportunities to practice social interaction skills, such as learning to take turns or sharing supplies and equipment.

Sensorimotor
- Use games such as make-believe activities to promote motor and visuomotor skills.
- Consider whether infant massage may be useful in promoting motor and sensory development.
- Incorporate feet as well as hands in sensorimotor activities.

Cognitive/Perceptual
- Use multimedia approaches, such as computer-based programs, for visual perception training as opposed to pencil and paper approaches only.

Psychosocial
- Provide practice in emotional control using discussion and role playing.

Context/Environment
- Provide instruction and supervised practice for parents and caregivers in managing identified problems.
- Provide information on availability of community resources.

Precautions/Safety Considerations
- None stated.

Prognosis and Outcome

Variable. Severity of developmental delay and original diagnosis are factors in determining the degree of progress that is possible. Use of compensatory techniques and adapted devices and equipment may be indicated. Children with impaired motor performance in balance tasks, and those requiring help with cognitive and behavioral tasks at school are more likely to have global developmental delay (Dornelas et al., 2016). Early intervention services can improve gross and fine skills (L.-Y. Lin & Cheng, 2019).

REFERENCES

Ballantyne, M., Benzies, K. M., McDonald, S., Magill-Evans, J., & Tough, S. (2016). Risk of developmental delay: Comparison of late preterm and full term Canadian infants at age 12 months. *Early Human Development, 101*(1), 27–32. https://doi.org/10.1016/j.earlhumdev.2016.04.004

Baranek, G. T., Watson, L. R., Boyd, B. A., Poe, M. D., David, F. J., & McGuire, L. (2013). Hyporesponsiveness to social and nonsocial sensory stimuli in children with autism, children with developmental delays, and typically developing children. *Development and Psychopathology, 25*(2), 307–320. https://doi.org/10.1017/S0954579412001071

Chen, Y.-N., Lin, C.-K., Wei, T.-S., Liu, C.-H. & Wuang, Y.-P. (2013). The effectiveness of multimedia visual perceptual training groups for the preschool children with developmental delay. *Research in Developmental Disabilities, 34*(12), 4447–4454. https://doi.org/10.1016/j.ridd.2013.09.023

Dew, A., Bulkeley, K., Veitch, C., Bundy, A., Lincoln, M., Glenn, H., Gallego, G., & Brentnall, J. (2014). Local therapy facilitators working with children with developmental delay in rural and remote areas of western New South Wales, Australia: The "Outback" service delivery model. *Australian Journal of Social Issues, 49*(3), 309–328. https://doi.org/10.1002/j.1839-4655.2014.tb00315.x

Dornelas, L. F., Durarte, N. M. C., Morales, N. M. O., Pinto, R. M. C., Areújo, R. R. H., & Magolnães, L. C. (2016). Functional outcome of school children with history of global developmental delay. *Journal of Child Neurology, 31*, 1041–1051. https://doi.org/10.1177/0883073815536224

Jacobs, E., Miller, L. C., & Tirella, L. G. (2010). Developmental and behavioral performance of internationally adopted preschoolers: A pilot study. *Child Psychiatry and Human Development, 41*(1), 15–29. https://doi.org/10.1007/s10578-009-0149-6

Jacobs, K., & Simon, L. (Eds.). (2015). *Quick reference dictionary for occupational therapy.* Slack.

Joaquim, R. H. V. T., da Silva, F. R., & Lourenço, G. F. (2018). The make-believe and games as an intervention strategy for an infant with delay in child development. *Brazilian Journal of Occupational Therapy, 26*(1), 63–71. https://doi.org/10.4322/2526-8910.ctoAO1169

Leung, G. P. K., Chan, C. C. H., Chung, R. C. K., & Pang, M. Y. C. (2011). Determinants of activity and participation in preschoolers with developmental delay. *Research in Developmental Disabilities, 32*(1), 289–296. https://doi.org/10.1016/j.ridd.2010.10.005

Lin, C. L., Lin, C. K., & Yu, J. J. (2018). The effectiveness of parent participation in occupational therapy for children with developmental delay. *Neuropsychiatric Disease and Treatment, 14*, 623–630. https://doi.org/10.2147/NDT.S158688

Lin, H.-C., Chiu, Y.-H., Chen, Y. J., Wuang, Y.-P., Chen, C.-P., Wang, C.-C., Huang, C.-L., Wu, T.-M., & Ho, W.-H. (2017). Continued use of an interactive computer game-based visual perception learning system in children with developmental delay. *International Journal of Medical Informatics, 107*, 76–87. https://doi.org/10.1016/j.ijmedinf.2017.09.003

Lin, L.-Y., & Cherng, R.-J. (2019). Outcomes of utilizing early intervention services on the motor development of children with undefined developmental delay. *Journal of Occupational Therapy, Schools, & Early Intervention, 12*(2), 157–169. https://doi.org/10.1080/19411243.2018.1512437

Lu, W.-P., Tsai, W.-H., Lin, L.-Y., Hong R.-B., & Hwang, Y.-S. (2019). The beneficial effects of massage on motor development and sensory processing in young children with developmental delay: A randomized control trial study. *Developmental Neurorehabilitation, 22*(7), 487–495. https://doi.org/10.1080/17518423.2018.1537317

Majnemer, A., O'Donnell, M., Ogourtsova, T., Kasaai, B., Ballantyne, M., Cohen, E., Collett, J.-P., Dewan, T., Elsabbagh, M., Hanlon-Dearman, A., Filliter, J. H., Lach, L., McElroy, T., McGrath, P., McKellin, W., Miller, A., Patel, H., Rempel, G., Shevell, M., . . . The Parent-Panel (2019). BRIGHT Coaching: A randomized controlled trial on the effectiveness of a developmental coach system to empower families of children with emerging developmental delay. *Frontiers in Pediatrics, 7*, Article 332. https://doi.org/10.3389/fped.2019.00332

Schurgers, J., Sinyangwe, S., Burger, S., van Nieuwkerk, J., & Kamanga, E. (2010). Giving children with HIV and AIDS a future: The need for occupational therapy of HIV-positive children with developmental delay. *Medical Journal of Zambia, 37*(2), 93–98.

Shaikh, S. P., & Valdya, P. M. (2013). The effect of developmental support program (SDP) and play through feet on infants at risk for developmental delay. *Indian Journal of Occupational Therapy, 45*(3), 3–7.

Tang, M.-H., Lin, C.-K., Lin, W.-H., Chen, C.-H., Tsai, S.-W., & Chang, Y.-Y. (2011). The effect of adding a home program to weekly institutional-based therapy for children with undefined developmental delay: A pilot randomized clinical trial. *Journal of the Chinese Medical Association, 74*, 259–266. https://doi.org/10.1016/j.jcma.2011.04.005

BIBLIOGRAPHY

Drazen, C. H., Abel, R., Gabir, M., Farmer, G., & King A. A. (2016). Prevalence of developmental delay and contributing factors among children with sickle cell disease. *Pediatric Blood & Cancer, 63*(3), 504–510. https://doi.org/10.1002/pbc.25838

Kim, H.-J., & Shin, J.-I. (2015). A study of the correlation between BSID-III and KICDT for children with developmental delay. *Journal of Physical Therapy Science, 27*(1), 269–271. https://doi.org/10.1589/jpts.27.269

Lee, Y.-C., Chan, P.-C., Lin, S.-K., Chen, C.-T., Huang, C.-Y., & Chen, K.-L. (2016). Correlation patterns between pretend play and playfulness in children with autism spectrum disorder, developmental delay, and typical development. *Research in Autism Spectrum Disorders, 24*(1), 29–38. https://doi.org/10.1016/j.rasd.2016.01.006

Moreira, R. S., Magalnães, L. C. Siqueira, C. M., & Alves, C. R. L. (2018). "Survey of Wellbeing of Young Children (SWYC)": How does it fit for screening developmental delay in Brazilian children aged 4 to 58 months? *Research in Developmental Disabilities, 78*, 78–88. https://doi.org/10.1016/j.ridd.2018.05.003

Mwanjabe, T. T. (2010). Children with developmental delay. In V. Alers & R. Crouch (Eds.), *Occupational therapy: An African perspective* (pp. 190–205). Sarah Shorten.

Yu, T.-Y., Chen, K.-L., Chou, W., Yang, S.-H., Kung, S.-C., Lee, Y.-C., & Tung, L.-C. (2016). Intelligence quotient discrepancy indicates levels of motor competence in preschool children at risk for developmental delays. *Neuropsychiatric Disease and Treatment, 12*, 501–510. https://doi.org/10.2147/NDT.S101155

Developmental Disabilities

See also Autism Spectrum Disorder, Attention-Deficit/Hyperactivity Disorder, Cerebral Palsy, Congenital Heart Disease, Down Syndrome, Fetal Alcohol Spectrum Disorder, Intellectual Disability, Spina Bifida, Traumatic Brain Injury.

Description

Developmental disabilities are defined as severe, lifelong disabilities that are attributable to a mental and/or physical impairment, manifested before age 22. A developmental disability is an impairment caused by a neurologic or physical deficit beginning before age 22 that affects activities of daily living and significantly impairs the individual's general intellectual and/or adaptive functioning. Most developmental disabilities persist throughout life (O'Toole, 2017).

Cause

Causes include genetic disorders, trauma (especially trauma resulting in brain injury), infections (especially those affecting the central nervous system), and neurologic disorders (especially those affecting the central nervous system; Haertl, 2014a).

Evaluation/Assessment

Areas

- Activities of Daily Living/Instrumental ADL: basic ADLs (dressing, toileting), independent living skills (meal planning and preparation, shopping, driving or public transportation, financial management)
- Education/Work: academic performance, school behavior, work history, work skills
- Play/Leisure: interests, types, frequency, location
- Rest/Sleep: sleep habits
- Social Participation: type, location, frequency, with whom
- Sensorimotor: posture, positioning (standing, squatting, bending), mobility (walking, climbing), muscle strength (grip, pinch), eye–hand coordination, hand dexterity, endurance (activity tolerance), sensation
- Cognitive/Perceptual: attention, memory, executive functions (organization, problem solving, judgment of safety)
- Psychosocial: anxiety, stress, self-regulation, initiative and motivation, role performance, interpersonal relations, social skills, quality of life
- Context/Environment: social support (family, school, community), cultural and family values and beliefs, resources (legislation, community, internet), environmental modification, accessibility
- Comorbidities: autism spectrum disorder, attention-deficit/hyperactivity disorder, cerebral palsy, Down syndrome, spina bifida, traumatic brain injury

Instruments

Instruments Developed by Occupational Therapy Personnel

- Adolescent/Adult Sensory Profile (AASP; Brown & Dunn, 2002)
- Allen Cognitive Level Screen–5 (ACLS-5; Allen et al., 2007)
- Allen Diagnostic Module (2nd ed.; ADM-2; Earhart, 2006)
- Assessment of Communication and Interaction Skills (Version 4.0; ACIS; Forsyth et al., 1998)
- Assessment of Compared Qualities–Occupational Performance (ACQ-OP; Fisher, Griswold, & Kottorp, 2017; see Fisher, Griswold, Munkholm, et al., 2017, in References)
- Assessment of Compared Qualities–Social Interaction (3rd ed.; ACQ-SI; Fisher, Griswold, & Kottorp, 2017; see Fisher, Griswold, Munkholm, et al., 2017, in References)
- Assessment of Motor and Process Skills (8th ed.; AMPS-8; Fisher & Bray Jones, 2014)
- Canadian Occupational Performance Measure (5th ed.; COPM-5; Law et al., 2014)
- Dysphagia Evaluation Protocol (DEP; Avery-Smith et al., 1998)
- Evaluation of Social Interaction (3rd ed.; ESI-3; Fisher & Griswold, 2015)
- Feasibility Evaluation Checklist (FEC; Matheson, 1999)
- Irena Daily Activity Assessment (IDAA; Dychawy-Rosner & Eklund, 2003)
- Jacobs Prevocational Assessment (2nd ed.; JPA-2; Jacobs, 1991)
- Klein-Bell ADL Scale (KB-ADL; Klein & Bell, 1982)
- Occupational Circumstances Assessment Interview and Rating Scale (Version 4.0; OCAIRS; Forsyth et al., 2005)
- Occupational Performance History Interview (Version 2.1; OPHI-II; Kielhofner et al., 2004)
- Oral Function in Feeding Behavioral Scale (OFFBS) and Behavioral Assessment Scale of Oral Functions in Feeding (BASOFF; Stratton, 1981)
- Performance Assessment of Self-Care Skills (Version 4.1; PASS 4.1; Chisholm et al., 2016)
- Self-Care Skills Scale (for children; Shenai & Wadia, 2014)
- Sensory Integration Inventory–Revised (SII-R; Reisman & Hanschu, 1992)

Instruments Developed by Other Professionals and Used by Occupational Therapy Personnel

- AAMR Adaptive Behavior Scale–Residential and Community (Nihira et al., 1993)
- ADA (Americans With Disabilities Act) Checklist for Readily Achievable Barrier Removal (Adaptive Environments Center, 1995)

- Adaptive Behavior Assessment System (3rd ed.; ABAS-3; Harrison & Oakland, 2015)
- Child Behavior Checklist (CBCL; Achenbach, 2001)
- Functional Evaluation for Assistive Technology (FEAT; Raskind & Bryant, 2002)
- Functional Independence Measure (FIM; Uniform Data System for Medical Rehabilitation, 1997)
- Goal Attainment Scaling (GAS; Kiresuk et al., 1994)
- Home and Community Environment Instrument (HCEI; Keysor et al., 2005)
- Independent Living Scales (ILS; Loeb, 1996)
- Index of Activities of Daily Living (Index of ADL; K-ADL; Katz et al., 1963)
- Leisure Assessment Inventory (LAI; Hawkins et al., 2000)
- Leisure Diagnostic Battery (LDB; Ellis et al., 2008)
- Psychosexual Assessment and Treatment Continuum (PATC; Matich-Maroney et al., 2005)
- Scales of Independent Behavior–Revised (SIB-R; Bruininks et al., 1995)
- Supports Intensity Scale (SIS; Thomson et al., 2004)
- Strengths and Difficulties Questionnaire (SDQ; Goodman, 1997)
- Vineland Adaptive Behavior Scales (3rd ed.; Vineland-3; Sparrow et al., 2016)
- Vocational Adaptation Rating Scales–Revised (VARS; Malgady & Barcher, 1982)
- Waisman Activities of Daily Living Scale (WADLS; Maenner et al., 2013)
- Work Adjustment Inventory (WAI; Gilliam, 1994)

Problems/Issues

Activities of Daily Living/Instrumental ADL
- Person may lack knowledge and ability to plan and prepare meals.
- Person may lack knowledge and skills to maintain housekeeping skills (making beds, dusting, cleaning, doing laundry).
- Person may not have knowledge and skills in using public transportation or learning to drive.
- Person may not have knowledge or skills to shop for supplies (groceries, housekeeping supplies, clothing).

Education/Work
- Child/adolescent may have difficulty performing academic tasks (reading, writing, mathematics).
- Child/adolescent may have difficulty performing expected classroom and school behaviors (sitting in seat, sharing materials, waiting in line, asking permission to speak, completing homework as assigned and on time, moving from room to room).
- Person may lack work habits and work skills required for employment (paid or unpaid).

Play/Leisure
- Child/adolescent may not have developed play skills such as cooperative play, following rules, taking turns.
- Person may not have developed or has limited leisure occupations.

Rest/Sleep
- Person may not have developed sleep habits and routines.
- Person may have sleep disturbances in the environment.
- Person may have one or more sleep disorders.

Social Participation
- Person may have limited participation in social activities.

Sensorimotor
- Person may have difficulty with gross motor skills (walking, climbing stairs, stooping, bending, lifting, carrying).
- Person may have difficulty with fine motor skills (grip, grasp, pinch, in-hand manipulation, dexterity).

Cognitive/Perceptual
- Person may have difficulty attending and concentrating attention (easily distracted).
- Person may have difficulty with memory functions, especially working memory.
- Person may have difficulty with executive functions (planning, organizing, problem solving, judgment of safety, time management).

Psychosocial
- Person may be anxious about ability and skills.
- Person may have poor self-concept and self-confidence.
- Person may have difficulty with self-regulation and emotional stability.
- Person may have limited interpersonal skills and social skills.
- Person may have poor quality of life (Dahan-Oliel et al., 2012).

Context/Environment
- Person, family, or caregivers may not be familiar with legislation (state or federal) outlining available services.
- Person, family, or caregivers may not be familiar with community or internet resources.
- Person may need environmental modifications for accessibility or occupational performance.
- Person may experience barriers in physical environment such as a shopping mall (Dahan-Oliel et al., 2016).
- Person may need adapted devices and equipment.
- Family or caregiver may not have self-efficacy beliefs that they can change or improve the child's condition (Bonsall, 2018; Rosenberg et al., 2013).

Intervention/Treatment

Use of "top-down" interventions deliver bigger gains such as behavioral interventions, bimanual training, coaching parents, cognitive interventions, constraint-induced movement therapy, context-focused intervention, early intervention, family-centered care, parent education, goal-directed training, home programs, Kinesio Taping, pain management, pressure care, and weight loss (Novak & Honan, 2019). Models and programs developed by occupational therapy personnel include consultation (Umeda et al., 2017); Documentation of Occupational Therapy Session during Intervention (D.O.T.S.I.; Bart et al., 2011); driving (Unsworth, 2014); facilitating employment (American Occupational Therapy Association, 2015); Play, Leisure, ADLs, and IADLs (Haertl, 2014b); Ross Five-Stage Group Model (Haertl, 2014c); sensory-based approaches (Champagne, 2014); and transitional occupational therapy services (Chou & Duong, 2015). Models and programs developed by other professionals but used by occupational therapy personnel include animal assisted partnerships (Crowe et al., 2019), assistive technology (Hartmann, 2014), Camp Avanti (Erhardt, 2014), cognitive approaches (Herge, 2014), Collaborative Consultation for Participation of Students with IDD (Co-PID; Selanikyo et al., 2016), developmental systems theory (Whitney & Cronin, 2019), early intervention (Dall'Alba et al., 2014), hippotherapy (Weissman-Miller et al., 2017), and Teens making Environment and Activity Modifications (TEAM; Kramer et al., 2018). Team members may include physicians, nursing personnel, psychologists, educators, vocational rehabilitation specialists, social workers, physical therapy personnel, and occupational therapy personnel. Goals include enabling the client to be focused on preparation for community participation, gaining independent living skills, and attaining work skills for employment (Chou & Duong, 2015). The unique contribution of occupational therapy to persons with developmental disabilities is in the profession's ability to "provide professional solutions to the functional limitations" the client "experiences as a result of the intellectual disability" (Yalon-Chamovitz et al., 2010).

Activities of Daily Living/Instrumental ADL
- Participate in transition programs to help clients plan and prepare for community living, including independent living or semi-independent living in housing arrangements such as supported living services, residential care, or group home facilities, and residing with family or relatives.

Education/Work

- Assist in providing recommendations for classroom instruction for clients with developmental disabilities.
- Participate in transition programs for adolescents designed to help clients plan and prepare for postsecondary education and vocational training, including job shadowing and training.
- Assist in providing different types of employment opportunities: supportive, sheltered, at-will (client can quit or be fired or laid off at any time), and competitive.
- Assist client and other professionals to provide opportunities for career exploration, including participation in volunteer and unpaid programs.

Play/Leisure

- Assist in programs for children to develop play skills.
- Assist in helping clients develop leisure occupations both unstructured (individualized) and structured (group).

Rest/Sleep

- Assist client in developing and implementing sleep habits and routines.

Social Participation

- Encourage client to participate in social activities based on ability level.

Sensorimotor

- Create daily exercise programs (record on smartphone app).

Cognitive/Perceptual

- Use chaining techniques to promote learning (backward, errorless, forward).
- Use daily planners or electronic schedules to organize daily schedule.

Context/Environment

- Assist in providing information about legislation, including specific state laws and general federal laws.
- Assist client, family, or caregivers to identify and access community or internet resources that can provide needed services, including referrals to other professionals, access to needed devices and equipment, access to persons who can modify home or work environment, or leisure activities.
- Assist local and state governments through consultation and recommendations to improve services available to persons with developmental disabilities and those who care for them.

Precautions/Safety Considerations

Executive functions such as judgment of safety and ability to anticipate danger may require monitoring.

Prognosis and Outcome

Developmental disability is usually a lifelong, chronic disorder requiring continuous management. Many have complex health conditions and health-care needs not related to the developmental disability that need to be addressed (Majnemer, 2012; Williamson et al., 2017). The degree and type of management depends on the severity of disability, training received by the client, and availability of services. Some clients will be able to live independently and work at productive occupations until retirement age. Other clients will require supervised living conditions and may be limited in their capacity to be productive citizens.

REFERENCES

American Occupational Therapy Association. (2015). *Fact sheet: The role of occupational therapy in facilitating employment of individuals with developmental disabilities.*

Bart, O., Avrech Bar, M., Rosenberg, L., Hamudot, V., & Jarus. T. (2011). Development and validation of the Documentation of Occupational Therapy Session during Intervention (D.O.T.S.I.).

Research in Developmental Disabilities, 32(2), 719–726. https://doi.org/10.1016/j.ridd.2010 .11.008

Bonsall, A. (2018). Narrative transitions in views and behaviors of fathers parenting children with disabilities. *Journal of Family Studies, 24*(2), 95–108. https://doi.org/10.1080/132294 00.2015.1106336

Champagne, T. (2014). Integrating sensory-based approaches for adults with intellectual and developmental disabilities. In K. Haertl (Ed.), *Adults with intellectual and developmental disabilities: Strategies for occupational therapy* (pp. 235–264). AOTA Press.

Chou, W., & Duong M. (2015). Transitional occupational therapy services for youth with neurologic and developmental disabilities. *Career Planning and Adult Development Journal, 31*(4), 179–186.

Crowe, T. K., Deitz, J. C., Winkle, M., Nelson, R. A., & Woolf, J. (2019). Effects of partnerships between adolescents with developmental disabilities and service dogs. *Open Journal of Occupational Therapy, 7*(1), Article 3. https://doi.org/10.15453/2168-6408.1520

Dahan-Oliel, N., Shirkako-Thomas, K., & Majnemer, A. (2012). Quality of life and leisure participation in children with neurodevelopmental disabilities: A thematic analysis of the literature. *Quality of Life Research, 21*, 427–439. https://doi.org/10.1007/s11136-011-0063-9

Dahan-Oliel, N., Shikako-Thomas, K., Mazer, B., & Majnemer, A. (2016). Adolescents with disabilities participate in the shopping mall: Facilitators and barriers framed according to the ICF. *Disability and Rehabilitation, 38*(21), 2102–2113. https://doi.org/10.3109/09739299.2 015.1114033

Dall'Alba, L., Gray, M., Williams, G., & Lowe, S. (2014). Early intervention in children (0–6 years) with a rare developmental disability: The occupational therapy role. *Hong Kong Journal of Occupational Therapy, 24*, 72–80. https://doi.org/10.1016/j.hkjot.2014.12.001

Erhardt, R. P. (2014). Adaptation of a unique pediatric intervention model for adults with intellectual and developmental disabilities. In K. Haertl (Ed.), *Adults with intellectual and developmental disabilities: Strategies for occupational therapy* (pp. 311–335). AOTA Press.

Fisher, A. G., Griswold, L. A., Munkholm, M., & Kottorp, A. (2017). Evaluating domains of everyday functioning in people with developmental disabilities. *Scandinavian Journal of Occupational Therapy, 24*(1), 1–9. https://doi.org/10.3109/11038128.2016.1160147

Haertl, K. (Ed.). (2014a). *Adults with intellectual and developmental disabilities: Strategies for occupational therapy.* AOTA Press.

Haertl, K. (2014b). Play, leisure, ADLs, and IADLs for adults with intellectual and developmental disabilities. In K. Haertl (Ed.), *Adults with intellectual and developmental disabilities: Strategies for occupational therapy* (pp. 265–284). AOTA Press.

Haertl, K. (2014c). Ross's five-stage model for adults with intellectual and developmental disabilities. In K. Haertl (Ed.), *Adults with intellectual and developmental disabilities: Strategies for occupational therapy* (pp. 377–400). AOTA Press.

Hartmann, K. D. (2014). Assistive technology for adults with intellectual and developmental disabilities. In K. Haertl (Ed.), *Adults with intellectual and developmental disabilities: Strategies for occupational therapy* (pp. 337–355). AOTA Press.

Herge, E. A. (2014). Cognitive approaches for adults with intellectual and developmental disabilities. In K. Haertl (Ed.), *Adults with intellectual and developmental disabilities: Strategies for occupational therapy* (pp. 205–234). AOTA Press.

Kramer, J. M., Helfrich, C., Levin, M., Hwang, I.-T., Samuel, P. S. Carrellas, A., Schwartz, A. E., Goeva, A., & Kolaczyk, E. D. (2018). Initial evaluation of the effects of an environmental-focused problem-solving intervention for transition-age young people with developmental disabilities: Project TEAM. *Developmental Medicine & Child Neurology, 60*(8), 801–809. https://doi.org/10.1111/dmcn.13715

Majnemer, A. (2012). Editorial: Vigilance to behavioral problems needed for children with developmental disability. *Physical and Occupational Therapy in Pediatrics, 32*(1), 1–3. https://doi .org/10.3109/01942638.2012.644188

Novak, I., & Honan, I. (2019). Effectiveness of paediatric occupational therapy for children with disabilities: A systematic review. *Australian Occupational Therapy Journal, 66*(3), 258–273. https://doi.org/10.1111/1440-1630.12573

O'Toole, M. T. (Ed.). (2017). *Mosby's dictionary of medicine, nursing & health professions* (10th ed.). Elsevier.

Rosenberg, L., Bart, O., Ratson, N. Z., & Jarus, T. (2013). Personal and environmental factors predict participation of children with and without mild developmental disabilities. *Journal of Child and Family Studies, 22*, 658–671. https://doi.org/10.1007/s10826-012-9619-8

Selanikyo, E., Yalon-Chamovitz, S., & Weintraub, N. (2016). Enhancing classroom participation of students with intellectual and developmental disabilities. *Canadian Journal of Occupational Therapy, 84*(2), 76–86. https://doi.org/10.1177/0008417416661346

Shenai, N. G., & Wadia, D. N. (2014). Development of a self-care skills scale for children with developmental disorders: A pilot study. *Indian Journal of Occupational Therapy, 46*(1), 16–21.

Umeda, C. J., Fogelberg, D. J., Jirikowic, T., Pitonyak, J. S., Mroz, T. M., & Ideishi, R. I. (2017). Expanding the implementation of the Americans With Disabilities Act for populations with intellectual and developmental disabilities: The role of organization-level occupational therapy consultation. *American Journal of Occupational Therapy, 71*(4), Article 7104090010. https://doi.org/10.5014/ajot.2017.714001

Unsworth, C. (2014). Driving for adults with intellectual and developmental disabilities. In K. Haertl (Ed.), *Adults with intellectual and developmental disabilities: Strategies for occupational therapy* (pp. 357–376). AOTA Press.

Weissman-Miller, D., Miller, R. J., & Shotwell, M. P. (2017), Translational research for occupational therapy: Using SPRE in hippotherapy for children with developmental disabilities. *Occupational Therapy International, 2017*, Article 2305402. https://doi.org/10.1155/2017/2305402

Whitney, R., & Cronin, A. (2019). Occupational therapy intervention: Developmental disability, adverse childhood experiences and developmental systems theory. *SIS Quarterly Practice Connections, 4*(3), 2–4.

Williamson, H. J., Contreras, G. M., Rodriguez, E. S., Smith, J. M., & Perkins, E. A. (2017). Health care access for adults with intellectual and developmental disabilities: A scoping review. *OTJR: Occupational Participation and Health, 37*(4), 227–236. https://doi.org/10.1177/15394 49217714148

Yalon-Chamovitz, S., Selanikyo, E., Artzi, N., Prigal, Y., & Fishman, R. (2010). Occupational therapy and intellectual and developmental disability throughout the life cycle: Position paper. *Israeli Journal of Occupational Therapy, 19*(1), E3–E8.

BIBLIOGRAPHY

Davidson, D. A. (2014). Facilitating employment for adults with intellectual and developmental disabilities. In K. Heartl (Ed.), *Adults with intellectual and developmental disabilities: Strategies for occupational therapy* (pp. 285–309). AOTA Press.

Developmental Disabilities Assistance and Bill of Rights Act, 42 U.S.C. § 15002 (2000).

Down Syndrome

Also called trisomy 21, trisomy G, Langdon Down disease.
Obsolete terms: Mongoloidism or Mongolism.
Common misspellings: Downs syndrome, Down's syndrome.
See also Intellectual Disability.

Description

Down syndrome is a congenital disorder caused by one of three anomalies of chromosome 21 in the G group of chromosomes. In about 95% of cases, there is a third chromosome 21, called trisomy 21, which is usually derived from the mother. Such individuals have 47 chromosomes. Most of the remaining 5% of individuals with Down syndrome have a normal count of 46 chromosomes but have an extra chromosome 21 translocated to another chromosome, such as to chromosome 14 called t(14;21) or to chromosome 22 called t(22;21). A few individuals have the mosaic type of Down syndrome, which results from nondisjunction (when chromosomes fail to pass to separate cells) during cell division in the embryo. Individuals with mosaic Down syndrome have two cell lines, one with normal 46 chromosomes and another with 47 chromosomes that includes the extra chromosome 21. Diagnosis is confirmed by cytogenetic (karyotype) analysis (Porter, 2018). Down syndrome is named after an English physician, John Langdon Down (1828–1896).

Individuals with Down syndrome are characterized by intellectual disability, cognitive impairments, motor and language delay, microcephaly, short stature, obesity, and characteristic facies. Infants with Down syndrome are small for their age and hypotonic (have low muscle and postural tone) with laxness of joint ligaments, atlantoaxial and atlanto-occipital instability, poor Moro reflex, and hip dysplasia. The head is small, with a round fattened face (brachycephaly), a flattened occiput and slant to the eyes, depressed nasal bridge, low-set ears, short neck, and a large, protruding tongue that is furrowed, thickened, and lacks a central fissure. The hands are short and broad with a transverse palmar or simian crease; the fingers are stubby and show clinodactyly (lateral or medial bending of the distal phalanx), primarily of the fifth finger. The feet are broad and stubby with a wide space between the first and second toes and a prominent plantar crease. The average intelligence measures from a range of 50 to 75 on standard tests of intelligence, meaning the child is generally trainable and can be reared in home. Other anomalies include bowel defects, congenital heart disease, chronic respiratory infections, hypothyroidism, visual problems (congenital cataracts, glaucoma, strabismus, and nearsightedness), Brushfield spots in the eyes, hearing loss, abnormalities in tooth development, delayed or incomplete sexual development, susceptibility to acute leukemia, and dementia, Alzheimer type (Daunhauer & Fidler, 2011; O'Toole, 2017; Porter, 2018).

Evaluation/Assessment
Areas
- Activities of Daily Living/Instrumental ADL:
  - Infant and Child: eating (chewing and swallowing), dressing and undressing, grooming, bathing or showering, toileting, bed mobility, transfers, weight control
  - Teenager and Adult: meal planning and preparation, homemaking and housekeeping, financial management, shopping, driving, pet care, parenting
- Education/Work: school activities, academic performance, school and work modification, vocational planning, work skills
- Play/Leisure: play skills, leisure interests and occupations
- Rest/Sleep: sleep apnea, sleep disturbances
- Social Participation: social activities
- Sensorimotor: muscle strength, muscle tone, ligament integrity, joint range of motion, coordination, gross motor skills, fine motor and hand functions (grasp, pinch), vision (nearsightedness, strabismus), hearing loss
- Cognitive/Perceptual: attention, memory (working memory), executive functions (planning), visual perception
- Psychosocial: emotional regulation, parent–child bonding
- Context/Environment: health literacy, assistive technology, community integration, independent living, guardianship, life planning
- Development (Infant, Child, Adolescent only): developmental milestones
- Comorbidities: congenital heart disease, respiratory infection, celiac disease, leukemia, repeated ear infections, hypothyroidism, gastrointestinal disorders, dental (missing teeth, faulty bite, and gum diseases), flat feet

Instruments
Instruments Developed by Occupational Therapy Personnel
- Children's Assessment of Participation and Enjoyment and Preferences for Activities of Children (CAPE/PAC; King et al., 2004)
- Leiter International Performance Scale (3rd ed.; Leiter-3; Roid et al., 2013)
- Parent Questionnaire (to sensory experiences; Bruni et al., 2010, in References)
- Pediatric Evaluation of Disability Inventory (PEDI; Haley et al., 1992)
- Revised Knox Preschool Play Scale (RKPPS; Knox, 2008; form in Gokhale et al., 2014, in References)
- School Function Assessment (SFA; Coster et al., 1998)
- Short Sensory Profile (SSP; McIntosh et al., 1999)

Instruments Developed by Other Professionals and Used by Occupational Therapy Personnel
- Bayley Scales of Infant and Toddler Development (4th ed.; Bayley-4; Bayley & Aylward, 2019)
- Behavior Assessment System for Children (3rd ed.; BASC-3; Reynolds & Kamphaus, 2015)
- Behavior Rating Inventory of Executive Function–Preschool Version (BRIEF-P; Gioia et al., 2003)
- Developmental Behavior Checklist (2nd ed.; DBC-2; Gray et al., 2018)
- Gross Motor Function Measure (GMFM; Gémus et al., 2001)
- Oral and Written Language Scales (2nd ed.; OWLS-II; Carrow-Woolfolk, 2011)
- Peabody Developmental Motor Scales (3rd ed.; PDMS-3; Folio & Fewell, 2023)
- Waisman Activities of Daily Living Scale (WADLS; Maenner et al., 2013)

Problems/Issues
Activities of Daily Living/Instrumental ADL
- Infant or child may have difficulty with chewing and swallowing due to low muscle tone and misaligned teeth and gums.
- Child may have difficulty using eating utensils (spoon, fork, knife, cutting knife).
- Child may have difficulty with dressing, undressing, and adjusting clothing items including fasteners (buttons, zippers, lacing, snaps, loops).
- Child may have difficulty brushing teeth, including putting toothpaste on toothbrush, brushing upper and lower teeth, and rinsing out mouth.
- Child may have difficulty washing hands.
- Child may have difficulty with toilet training, including wiping and adjusting clothes.
- Infant or child may demonstrate general delay in developing self-care skills (Frank & Esbensen, 2015).
- Child may need assistance with IADLs, including meal preparation, housekeeping, financial management, transportation (including driving to attain independent living status).

Education/Work
- Child may have difficulty performing activities in the classroom and with academic achievement (Daunhauer, Fidler, & Will, 2014; Will et al., 2017).
- Child may have difficulty performing academic tasks: drawing or coloring within the lines or spaces, printing letters or numbers, completing a jigsaw puzzle, painting, doing math problems.
- Child may have difficulty negotiating school building: cafeteria, auditorium, gymnasium.
- Child may need assistive technology to perform academic tasks.
- Child's school performance may be negatively affected by maladaptive behavior and sensory processing difficulties (Will et al., 2019; Will et al., 2016).

Play/Leisure
- Child may have difficulty playing with toys or playing board games due to hand dysfunction.

- Child may demonstrate limited exploratory play behavior with objects (Fidler, Schworer, Prince, et al., 2019; Fidler et al., 2014).
- Child may engage primarily in solitary and sedentary leisure activities (Oates et al., 2011).

Rest/Sleep
- Not discussed.

Social Participation
- Child may have difficulty participating in group activities (van Jaarsveld et al., 2016).

Sensorimotor
- Child may have difficulty with hand functions such as grasp, pinch, in-hand manipulation and release.
- Child may have difficulty with hand coordination, including catching and throwing, cutting, stacking blocks, snapping pieces together or pulling pieces apart, placing pieces into a puzzle board, pressing and gluing pieces together.
- Child may demonstrate general delay in acquisition of fine motor skills (Frank & Esbensen, 2015).
- Child may have difficulty identifying objects by touch alone (stereognosis).
- Child may be hyper- or hyposensitive to certain sensory stimuli.
- Child may experience difficulties in sensory processing (van Jaarsveld et al., 2016; Will et al., 2019).

Cognitive/Perceptual
- Child may demonstrate difficulty in shifting visual attention (Fidler, Schworer, Will, et al., 2019).
- Child may have difficulty remembering how to perform motor actions (fit shapes in corresponding spaces, match figures with words).
- Child may have difficulty developing executive function skills (Daunhauer, Fidler, Hahn, et al., 2014; Daunhauer et al., 2017; Lee et al., 2011).
- Child may have difficulty with visual-spatial skills.

Psychosocial
- Child may have difficulty with interpersonal relations, especially as skill level does not compare with peers.
- Child or adolescent may demonstrate pattern of depressive and anxiety symptoms (Foley, Bourke, et al., 2015).
- Child or adolescent may demonstrate disruptive and antisocial behavior (Foley, Bourke, et al., 2015).
- Adolescent and family may experience decreased quality of life (Foley, Girdler, et al., 2014).

Context/Environment
- Parents or caregivers may lack knowledge about Down syndrome.
- Child may be restricted to a limited physical environment space thus reducing access to social environments (Foley, Girdler, et al., 2014).
- Child, parents, or caregivers may lack knowledge and instruction on use of assistive technology.
- Child, parents, and caregivers may lack access to community resources.

Intervention/Treatment
Models and programs developed by occupational therapy personnel include the fine motor activities program (Apetrei et al., 2018; Lersilp et al., 2016); "D" Chair (Gawand & Nandagaonkar, 2014); elephant-assisted therapy program (Satiansukpong et al., 2016); friends, fun, and fitness program (Cahill et al., 2015); Handwriting Without Tears (Patton & Hutton, 2016a; Patton &

Hutton, 2017); play-based therapy (Gokhale et al., 2014); and sensory integration dysfunction and vestibular stimulation (Uyanik & Kayihan, 2010). Models and programs developed by other professionals but used by occupational therapy personnel include the Developmental Resource Stimulation Programme (Russell et al., 2016a; Russell et al., 2016b), fine motor activities program (Lersilp et al., 2016), hippotherapy (Champagne & Duguas, 2010), Ludic Model of play (Pelosi et al., 2018), Qigong massage (Silva et al., 2012), neurodevelopmental therapy approach (Uyanik & Kayihan, 2010), retraining approach for eye–hand coordination (Nadkarni et al., 2012), and simultaneous sensory stimulation (Karimi et al., 2010). Team members include physicians, pediatricians, nursing personnel, psychologists, social workers, speech–language pathologists, nutritionists or dieticians, educators, parents and caregivers, physical therapy personnel, and occupational therapy personnel. Goals are to facilitate an individual's acquisition of functional skills, participation in activities of daily living, engagement in significant tasks of life, improvement in educational development and management, and participation in leisure and social activities (Apetrei et al., 2018; Rihtman et al., 2010).

Activities of Daily Living/Instrumental ADL
- Provide practice and guidance to parents and caregivers regarding skills in basic ADLs: eating, dressing and undressing, grooming, bathing or showering, toileting.
- Assist or work with speech–language pathologist to improve chewing and swallowing.
- Provide practice and guidance to parents and caregivers regarding development of independent living skills: meal preparation, housekeeping, money management, shopping, use of transportation.

Education/Work
- Assist educators to develop plans and programs to improve academic skills and participation in school activities (Patton et al., 2015).
- Provide practice in writing readiness (Patton & Hutton, 2016b).
- Provide information and instruction in use of assistive technology in the work setting.

Play/Leisure
- Assist client to develop play skills that are age appropriate.
- Assist client to explore and develop leisure occupations within skill level that are age appropriate.

Rest/Sleep
- See Sleep–Wake Disorders in Section 13: Lifestyle Conditions.

Social Participation
- Encourage client to participate in social activities that are age appropriate.
- Provide suggestions on modifying social activities that permit client to participate.

Sensorimotor
- Provide practice and training in use of hand functions (reach, grasp, manipulate, release).
- Provide practice and training in use of hand skills (throwing, catching, cutting, pinching, pressing).
- Assist client to develop postural control and positioning.
- Assist client to experience different sensory experiences and modify responses if needed.

Cognitive/Perceptual
- Assist client to improve attention, concentration, and memory (especially short-term memory).
- Assist client to develop executive functions (problem solving, planning ahead, goal-directed behavior, judgment of safety).
- Provide instruction to parents and caregivers on approaches to facilitate development of executive functions (Schworer et al., 2019).

Psychosocial

- Assist client in developing emotional regulation (calm down from stress, increase alertness in response to demands).
- Assist client in developing interpersonal skills appropriate to age.
- Provide sense of well-being in relationships, community participation, and independence (Scott et al., 2014).

Context/Environment

- Provide parents and caregivers with information and resources about Down syndrome.
- Assist parents with stress management and coping mechanisms, including use of spirituality and organized religion (Pillay et al., 2012).
- Provide client and parents information and resources for obtaining and caring for assistive technology.
- Provide client and parents with access to available community and internet resources for persons with disabilities.

Precautions/Safety Considerations

Infants and children should be monitored for signs of hypoxia, including skin that turns blue-gray. People with Down syndrome should be monitored closely for signs of infections and respiratory disease, including pneumonia.

Prognosis and Outcome

Down syndrome is a congenital, genetic disorder that is a lifelong condition. The functional level an individual attains depends on a number of person–occupation–environment factors resulting in various outcomes from dependent group living environments to independent living situations. The nature of the disorder changes as development progresses, and dementia may limit potential in individuals who reach age 40 and beyond. Health conditions and lifestyle should be monitored (Pikora et al., 2014; Thomas et al., 2011). Participation in a work setting can reduce behavioral problems (Foley, Jacoby, et al., 2014; Foley et al., 2013).

REFERENCES

Apetrei, L. A., Irsay, L., Borda, M., Ungur, R., Onac, I., & Ciortea, V. (2018). The role of occupational therapy in children with Down's syndrome. *Palestrica of the Third Millennium–Civilization and Sport, 19*(2), 81–85. https://doi.org/10.26659/pm3.2018.19.2.81

Bruni, M., Cameron, D., Dua, S., & Noy, S. (2010). Reported sensory processing of children with Down syndrome. *Physical & Occupational Therapy in Pediatrics, 30*(4), 280–293. https://doi.org/10.3109/01942638.2010.486962

Cahill, S. M., Clone, J., Wilson, K., & Moroni, A. (2015). Friends, fun, and fitness: A 6-week program for adolescents with Down syndrome. *Developmental Disabilities Special Interest Section Quarterly, 39*(2), 1–4.

Champagne, D., & Dugas, C. (2010). Improving gross motor function and postural control with hippotherapy in children with Down syndrome: Case reports. *Physiotherapy Theory and Practice, 26*(8), 564–571. https://doi.org/10.3109/09593981003623659

Daunhauer, L. A., & Fidler, D. J. (2011). The Down syndrome behavioral phenotype: Implications for practice and research in occupational therapy. *Occupational Therapy in Health Care, 25*(1), 7–25. https://doi.org/10.3109/07380577.2010.535601

Daunhauer, L. A., Fidler, D. J., Hahn, L., Will, E., Lee, N. R., & Hepburn, S. (2014). Profiles of everyday executive functioning in young children with Down syndrome. *American Journal on Intellectual and Developmental Disabilities, 119*(4), 303–318. https://doi.org/10.1352/1944-7558-119.4.303

Daunhauer, L. A., Fidler, D. J., & Will, E. (2014). School function in students with Down syndrome. *American Journal of Occupational Therapy, 68*(2), 167–176. https://doi.org/10.5014/ajot.2014.009274

Daunhauer, L. A., Gerlach-McDonald, B., Will, E., & Fidler, D. J. (2017). Performance and ratings based measures of executive function in school-aged children with Down syndrome. *Developmental Neuropsychology, 42*(6), 351–368. https://doi.org/10.1080/87565641.2017.1360303

Fidler, D. J., Schworer, E., Prince, M. A., Will, E. A., Needham, A. W., & Daunhauer, L. A. (2019). Exploratory behavior and developmental skill acquisition in infants with Down syndrome. *Infant Behavior and Development, 54*, 140–150. https://doi.org/10.1016/j.infbeh.2019.02.002

Fidler, D. J., Schworer, E., Will, E. A., Patel, L., & Daunhauer, L. A. (2019). Correlates of early cognition in infants with Down syndrome. *Journal of Intellectual Disability Research, 63*(3), 205–214. https://doi.org/10.1111/jir.12566

Fidler, D. J., Will, E., Daunhauer, L. A., Gerlach-McDonald, B., & Visootsak, J. (2014). Object-related generativity in children with Down syndrome. *Research in Developmental Disabilities, 35*(12), 3379–3385. https://doi.org/10.1016/j.ridd.2014.07.024

Foley, K.-R., Bourke, J., Einfeld, S. L., Tonge, B. J., Jacoby, P., & Leonard, H. (2015). Patterns of depressive symptoms and social relating behaviors differ over time from other behavioral domains for young people with Down syndrome. *Medicine, 94*(19), Article e710. https://doi.org/10.1097/MD.0000000000000710

Foley, K.-R., Girdler, S., Bourke, J., Jacoby, P., Llewellyn, G., Einfeld, S., Tonge, B., Parmenter, T. R., & Leonard, H. (2014). Influence of the environment on participation in social roles for young adults with Down syndrome. *PLOS ONE, 9*(9), Article e108413. https://doi.org/10.1371/journal.pone.0108413

Foley, K.-R., Jacoby, P., Einfeld, S., Girdler, S., Bourke, J., Riches, V., & Leonard, H. (2014). Day occupation is associated with psychopathology for adolescents and young adults with Down syndrome. *BMC Psychiatry, 14*, Article 266. https://doi.org/10.1186/s12888-014-0266-z

Foley, K.-R., Jacoby, P., Girdler, S., Bourke, J., Pikora, T., Lennox, N., Einfeld, S., Llewellyn, G., Parmenter, T. R., & Leonard, H. (2013). Functioning and post-school transition outcomes for young people with Down syndrome. *Child: Care, Health and Development, 39*(6), 789–800. https://doi.org/10.1111/cch.12019

Frank, K., & Esbensen, A. J. (2015). Fine motor and self-care milestones for individuals with Down syndrome using a Retrospective Chart Review. *Journal of Intellectual Disability Research, 59*(8), 719–729. https://doi.org/10.1111/jir.12176

Gawand, N. S., & Nandagaonkar, M. H. (2014). To study the effectiveness of "D" chair on fine motor skills in children with Down's syndrome—A comparative study. *Indian Journal of Occupational Therapy, 46*(3), 77–82.

Gokhale, P., Solanki, P. V., & Agarwal, P. (2014). To study the effectiveness of play based therapy on play behavior of children with Down's syndrome. *Indian Journal of Occupational Therapy, 46*(2), 41–48.

Karimi, H., Nazi, S., Sajedi, F., Akbar Fahimi, N., & Karimloo, M. (2010). Comparison [of] the effect of simultaneous sensory stimulation and current occupational therapy approaches on motor development of the infants with Down syndrome. *Iranian Journal of Child Neurology, 4*(3), 39–44. https://doi.org/10.22037/ijcn.v4i3.2007

Lee, N. R., Fidler, D. J., Blakeley-Smith, A., Daunhauer, L., Robinson, C., & Hepburn, S. L. (2011). Caregiver report of executive functioning in a population-based sample of young children with Down syndrome. *American Journal on Intellectual and Developmental Disabilities, 116*(4), 290–304. https://doi.org/10.1352/1944-7558-116.4.290

Lersilp, S., Putthinoi, S., & Panyo, K. (2016). Fine motor activities program to promote fine motor skills in a case study of Down's syndrome. *Global Journal of Health Science, 8*(12), 60–62. https://doi.org/10.5539/gjhs.v8n12p60

Nadkarni, S., Sumi, S., & Ashok, D. (2012). Enhancing eye-hand coordination with therapy intervention to improve visual spatial abilities using "The Re-training Approach" in children with Down syndrome: Three case studies. *Disability, CBR and Inclusive Development, 23*(2), 107–120. https://doi.org/10.5463/dcid.v23i2.87

Oates, A., Bebbington, A., Bourke, J., Girdler, S., & Leonard, H. (2011). Leisure participation for school-aged children with Down syndrome. *Disability and Rehabilitation, 33*(19-20), 1880–1889. https://doi.org/10.3109/09638288.2011.553701

O'Toole, M. T. (Ed.). (2017). *Mosby's dictionary of medicine, nursing & health professions* (10th ed.). Elsevier.

Patton, S., & Hutton, E. (2016a). Parents' perspectives on a collaborative approach to the application of the Handwriting Without Tears programme with children with Down syndrome. *Australian Occupational Therapy Journal 63*(4), 266–276. https://doi.org/10.1111/1440-1630.12301

Patton, S., & Hutton, E. (2016b). Writing readiness and children with Down syndrome in an Irish context. *Support for Learning, 31*(3), 246–259. https://doi.org/10.1111/1467-9604.12132

Patton, S., & Hutton, E. (2017). Exploring the participation of children with Down syndrome in Handwriting Without Tears. *Journal of Occupational Therapy, Schools, & Early Intervention, 10*(2), 171–184. https://doi.org/10.1080/19411243.2017.1292485

Patton, S., Hutton, E., & MacCobb, S. (2015). Curriculum differentiation for handwriting and occupational therapy/teacher partnership: Collaboration or conflict? *Irish Educational Studies, 34*(2), 107–124. https://doi.org/10.1080/03323315.2015.1032994

Pelosi, M. B., Munaretti, A. S., Nachmento, J. S., & Melo, J. V. (2018). Evolution of the ludic behavior of children with Down syndrome. *Revista de Terapia Ocupacional da Universidade de São Paulo, 29*(2), 170–178. https://doi.org/10.11606/issn.2238-6149.v29i2p170-178

Pikora, T. J., Bourke, J., Bathgate, K., Foley, K. R., Lennox, N., & Leonard, H. (2014). Health conditions and their impact among adolescents and young adults with Down syndrome. *PLOS ONE, 9*(5), Article e96868. https://doi.org/10.1371/journal.pone.0096868

Pillay, D., Girdler, S., Collins, M., & Leonard, H. (2012). "It's not what you were expecting, but it's still a beautiful journey": The experience of mothers of children with Down syndrome. *Disability and Rehabilitation, 34*(18), 1501–1510. https://doi.org/10.3109/09638288.2011.650313

Porter, R. S. (Ed.). (2018). *The Merck manual of diagnosis and therapy* (20th ed.). Merck Sharp & Dohme.

Rihtman, T., Tekuzener, E., Parush, S., Tenenbaum, A., Bachrach, S. J., & Ornoy, A. (2010). Are the cognitive functions of children with Down syndrome related to their participation? *Developmental Medicine & Child Neurology, 52*(1), 72–78. https://doi.org/10.1111/j.1469-8749.2009.03356.x

Russell, D. C., van Heerden, R., van Vuuren, S., Venter, A., & Joubert, G. (2016a). The impact of the "Developmental Resource Stimulation Programme" (DRSP) on children with Down syndrome. *South African Journal of Occupational Therapy, 46*(1), 33–40. http://dx.doi.org/10.17159/2310-3833/2016/v46n1a8

Russell, D. C., van Heerden, R., van Vuuren, S., Venter, A., & Joubert, G. (2016b). Time management guidelines for the intervention of a child with Down syndrome using the Developmental "Resource Stimulation Programme" (DRSP). *South African Journal of Occupational Therapy, 46*(1), 41–44. http://dx.doi.org/10.17159/2310-3833/2016/v46n1a9

Satiansukpong, N., Pongsaksri, M., & Sasat, D. (2016). Thai Elephant-Assisted Therapy Programme in children with Down syndrome. *Occupational Therapy International, 23*(2), 121–131. https://doi.org/10.1002/oti.1417

Schworer, E., Fidler, D. J., Lunkenheimer, E., & Daunhauer, L. A. (2019). Parenting behaviour and executive function in children with Down syndrome. *Journal of Intellectual Disability Research, 63*(4), 298–312. https://doi.org/10.1111/jir.12575

Scott, M., Foley, K.-R., Bourke, J., Leonard, H., & Girdler, S. (2014). "I have a good life": The meaning of well-being from the perspective of young adults with Down syndrome. *Disability and Rehabilitation, 36*(15), 1290–1298. https://doi.org/10.3109/09638288.2013.854843

Silva, L. M. T., Schalock, M., Garberg, J., & Smith, C. L. (2012). Qigong massage for motor skills in young children with cerebral palsy and Down syndrome. *American Journal of Occupational Therapy, 66*(3), 348–355. https://doi.org/10.5014/ajot.2012.003541

Thomas, K., Bourke, J., Girdler, S., Bebbington, A., Jacoby, P., & Leonard, H. (2011). Variation over time in medical conditions and health service utilization of children with Down syndrome. *Journal of Pediatrics, 158*(2), 194–200. https://doi.org/10.1016/j.jpeds.2010.08.045

Uyanik, M., & Kayihan, H. (2010). Down syndrome: Sensory integration, vestibular stimulation and neurodevelopmental therapy approaches for children. In J. H. Stone, & M. Blouin (Eds.), *International encyclopedia of rehabilitation.* Center for International Rehabilitation Research Information Exchange (CIRRIE).

van Jaarsveld, A., van Rooyen, F. C., van Biljon, A.-M., van Rensburg, I. J., James, K., Böning, L., & Haefele, L. (2016). Sensory processing, praxis and related social participation of 5–12 year old children with Down syndrome attending educational facilities in Bloemfontein, South Africa. *South African Journal of Occupational Therapy, 46*(3), 15–20.

Will, E. A., Daunhauer, L. A., Fidler, D. J., Raitano Lee, N., Rosenberg, C. R., & Hepburn, S. L. (2019). Sensory processing and maladaptive behavior: Profiles within the Down syndrome phenotype. *Physical & Occupational Therapy in Pediatrics, 39*(5), 461–476. https://doi.org/10.1080/01942638.2019.1575320

Will, E., Fidler, D. J., Daunhauer, L., & Gerlach-McDonald, B. (2017). Executive function and academic achievement in primary-grade students with Down syndrome. *Journal of Intellectual Disability Research, 61*(2), 181–195. https://doi.org/10.1111/jir.12313

Will, E. A., Gerlach-McDonald, B., Fidler, D. J., & Daunhauer, L. A. (2016). Impact of maladaptive behavior on school function in Down syndrome. *Research in Developmental Disabilities, 59*, 328–337. https://doi.org/10.1016/j.ridd.2016.08.018

BIBLIOGRAPHY

Daunhauer, L. A. (2011). The early development of adaptive behavior and functional performance in young children with Down syndrome: Current knowledge and future directions. *International Review of Research in Developmental Disabilities, 40*(1), 109–137. https://doi.org/10.1016/B978-0-12-374478-4.00005-8

Daunhauer, L. A., & Fidler, D. J. (2013). Executive functioning in individuals with Down syndrome. In K. D. Barrett, N. A. Fox, G. A. Morgan, D. J. Fidler, & L. A. Daunhauer (Eds.), *Handbook of self-regulatory processes in development: New directions and international perspectives* (pp. 453–472). Psychology Press. https://doi.org/10.4324/9780203080719.ch20

Foley, K.-R., Girdler, S., Downs, J., Jacoby, P., Bourke, J., Lennox, N., Einfeld, S., Llewellyn, G., Parmenter, T. R., & Leonard, H. (2014). Relationship between family quality of life and day occupations of young people with Down syndrome. *Social Psychiatry and Psychiatric Epidemiology, 49*(9), 1455–1465. https://doi.org/10.1007/s00127-013-0812-x

Foley, K.-R., Taffe, J., Bourke, J., Einfeld, S. L., Tonge, B. J., Trollor, J., & Leonard, H. (2016). Young people with intellectual disability transitioning to adulthood: Do behavior trajectories differ in those with and without Down syndrome? *PLOS ONE, 11*(7), Article e0157667. https://doi.org/10.1371/journal.pone.0157667

Lee, N. R., Anand, P., Will, E., Adeyemi, E. L., Clasen, L. S., Blumenthal, J. D., Giedd, J. N., Daunhauer, L. A., Fidler, D. J., & Edgin, J. O. (2015). Everyday executive functions in Down syndrome from early childhood to young adulthood: Evidence for both unique and shared characteristics compared to youth with six chromosome trisomy (XXX and XXY). *Frontiers in Behavioral Neuroscience, 9*, Article 264. https://doi.org/10.3389/fnbeh.2015.00264

Leonard, H., Bourke, J., Collins, M.-L., Girdler, S., Bebbington, A., Mulroy, S., Bathgate, K., Foley, K., Povee, K., Thomas, K., Oates, A., Geelhoed, E., Deshpande, A., Knight, O., Pillay, D., & Bower, C. (n.d.). *Understanding Down syndrome: Capturing family experiences through research*. Telethon Institute for Child Health Research. https://www.downsyndrome.org.au/wp-content/uploads/2020/04/understanding_down_syndrome_booklet.pdf

Ornoy, A., Rihtman, T., & Parush, S. (2011). Adaptive and behavioral development in children with Down syndrome at school age with special emphasis on attention deficit hyperactivity disorder (ADHD). In S. Dey (Ed.). *Prenatal diagnosis and screening for Down syndrome* (pp. 17–32). IntechOpen. https://doi.org/10.5772/17455

Thomas, K., Girdler, S., Bourke, J., Deshpande, A., Bathgate, K., Fehr, S., & Leonard, H. (2010). Overview of health issues in school-aged children with Down syndrome. *International Review of Research in Mental Retardation, 39*, 67–106. https://doi.org/10.1016/S0074-7750(10)39003-3

Will, E., Fidler, D. J., & Daunhauer, L. (2014). Executive function and planning in early development in Down syndrome. *International Review of Research in Developmental Disabilities, 47*, 77–98. https://doi.org/10.1016/B978-0-12-800278-0.00003-8

Feeding Disorders in Children

Also called sensory food aversions, food phobia, food neophobia, food avoidance, food selectivity, food refusal, selective food refusal, fear-based food refusal, learning-dependent food refusal.

Description

Pediatric feeding disorder is defined as "impaired oral intake that is not age appropriate, and is associated with medical, nutritional, feeding skills, and/or psychosocial dysfunction" (Goday et al., 2019, p. 125). Impaired oral intake refers to the inability to consume sufficient food and liquids to meet nutritional and hydration requirements. (Note that eating disorders such as anorexia nervosa or bulimia and dysphagia in adults are separate conditions not covered in this chapter.)

Cause

Causes may be medical factors, such as impaired structure/function of the gastrointestinal, cardiorespiratory, and neurological systems; nutritional factors, such as restricted quality, quantity, and variety of foods and beverages consumed; feeding skills factors, such as altered feeding experiences due to illness, injury, or developmental delay; or psychosocial factors, such as mental and behavioral health, social influences or environmental factors in the child, caregiver, or feeding environment that adversely affect feeding (Goday et al., 2019, pp. 126–127).

Definitions

- *Feeding:* Term used to describe process of bringing food to the mouth. Sometimes called self-feeding (American Occupational Therapy Association, 2017).
- *Eating:* Term used to describe keeping and manipulating food or liquid in the mouth and then swallowing it (American Occupational Therapy Association, 2017).
- *Food selectivity:* Term used to describe behaviors such as food refusal, limited food repertoire, and high-frequency single food intake (Bandini et al., 2010).
- *Swallowing:* Term used to describe moving food from the mouth to the stomach (American Occupational Therapy Association, 2017).

Proposed Diagnostic Criteria (Abbreviated; Goday et al., 2019, p. 125)

- A disturbance in oral intake of nutrients, inappropriate for age, lasting at least 2 weeks and associated with one or more of the following:

> Medical dysfunction (cardiorespiratory compromise, gastroesophageal reflux disease, eosinophilic esophagitis, esophageal atresia, chronic lung disease, congenital heart disease, oropharyngeal or laryngeal anomalies). (Note: The medical conditions are not covered in detail because they require medical intervention.)

> Nutritional dysfunction (malnutrition, nutrient deficiency, reliant on enteral feeds or supplements).

> Feeding skill dysfunction (texture modification needed, use of modified feeding position or equipment, use or modified feeding strategies).

> Psychosocial dysfunction (active or passive avoidance behaviors, inappropriate caregiver management, disruption of social functioning with feeding context, disruption of caregiver–child relationship associated with feeding).

- Absence of cognitive processes consistent with eating disorders and pattern of oral intake is not due to lack of food or congruent with cultural norms.

Evaluation/Assessment

Areas

- Activities of Daily Living/Instrumental ADL: dietary diversity, healthy weight, state regulation
- Education/Work: not applicable
- Play/Leisure: interest in playing with food
- Rest/Sleep: sleep disturbances
- Social Participation: feeding as a social activity with caregiver
- Sensorimotor: oral motor skills (lip closure, sip, chew, swallow); hand functions (grip, pinch); hypersensitivity (overresponsivity), especially tactile (oral), taste, temperature, texture, smell, or visual presentation; hyposensitivity to tactile, taste, temperature, texture, or smell
- Cognitive/Perceptual: caregiver beliefs, values, and customs about infant/child feeding and eating
- Psychosocial: anxiety, stress, caregiver–child interaction behaviors
- Context/Environment: adapted devices, adapted positioning, social support, caregiver knowledge of child development, disruptions during feeding and eating time, cultural rituals and expectations, access to nutritious food, dental visits for oral care
- Development (Infant, Child, Adolescent only): age-appropriate foods, liquids, feeding utensils, self-feeding skills, mealtime sitting/positioning, weight
- Comorbidities: neurodevelopmental delay, cerebral palsy, autism spectrum disorder (ASD), attention-deficit/hyperactivity disorder, muscular dystrophy

Instruments

Instruments Developed by Occupational Therapy Personnel

- Eating Profile (EP; Nadon et al., 2011, in References; assessment in French)
- Let's Eat (LE; Little & Wallisch, 2018, in References)
- Sensory Profile (2nd ed.; SP-2; Dunn, 2014)
- Short Sensory Profile (SSP; McIntosh et al., 1999)
- Touch Inventory for Elementary-School-Aged Children (TIE; Royeen & Fortune, 1990)

Instruments Developed by Other Professionals and Used by Occupational Therapy Personnel

- About Your Child's Eating (AYCE; Davies et al., 2007)
- Behavioral Pediatric Feeding Assessment Scale (BPFAS; Crist & Napier-Phillips, 2001)
- Brief Assessment of Motor Function: Oral Motor Deglutition Scale (BAMF-OMD; Sonies et al., 2009)
- Brief Autism Mealtime Behavior Inventory (BAMBI; Lukens & Linscheid, 2008)
- Children's Eating Behavior Inventory (CEBI; Archer et al., 1991)
- Dysphagia Disorder Survey (DDS; Sheppard et al., 2014)
- Eating Checklist (EC; Yack et al., 2002)

- Feeding Demands Questionnaire (FDQ; Faith et al., 2008)
- Fiberoptic Endoscopic Evaluation of Swallowing (FEES; described in Paul & D'Amica, 2013, in References)
- Infant-Toddler Social Emotional Assessment (ITSEA; Briggs-Gowan & Carter, 1998)
- Modified Barium Swallow Study (MBSS; described in Paul & D'Amico, 2013, in References)
- Montreal Children's Hospital Feeding Scale (MCH-FS; Ramsay et al., 2011)
- Multidisciplinary Feeding Profile (MFP; Judd et al., 1989)
- Neonatal Oral-Motor Assessment Scale (NOMAS; Braun & Palmer, 1985)
- Oral Motor Assessment (OMAS; de Oliveira Lira Ortega et al., 2009)
- Parent Mealtime Action Scale (PMAS; Hendy et al., 2009)
- Pediatric Assessment Scale for Severe Feeding Problems (PASSFP; Crist et al., 2004)
- Preterm Infant Breastfeeding Behavior Scale (PIBBS; Nyqvist et al., 1996)
- Schedule of Oral-Motor Assessment (SOMA; Reilly et al., 2000)
- Screening Tool of Eating Problems (STEP; Matson & Kuhn, 2001)
- Video-fluoroscopy: See Modified Barium Swallow Study
- Youth/Adolescent Food Frequency Questionnaire (YAFFQ; Rockett et al., 1997)

Problems/Issues

Activities of Daily Living/Instrumental ADL/Health Maintenance
- Child may experience health risks during feeding, including breathing and swallowing co-ordination, apnea, or bradycardia.
- Child may have an anatomical abnormality such as esophageal atresia (Baird et al., 2015).
- Child may have a gastroesophageal reflux or other gastrointestinal issue (Marcus & Breton, 2013).
- Child may have a swallowing impairment (dysphagia; Marcus & Breton, 2013).
- Child may be underweight or losing weight based on normal weights for age.
- Child is unable to transition to baby food purees by 10 months of age.
- Child is unable to eat food solids by 12 months of age.
- Child is unable to transition from breast or bottle to cup by 16 months based on parent preference.
- Child is unable to be weaned off baby foods by 16 months of age.
- Child eats less than 20 different foods by 24 months (2 years).
- Child may resist brushing teeth due to oral sensitivity or taste of toothpaste.

Education/Work
- Not applicable.

Play/Leisure
- Child may spend more time playing with food than eating.

Rest/Sleep
- Infant or child may have trouble sleeping (not sleeping or sleeping more than expected).
- Infant or child may fall asleep at the beginning of feeding session.
- Infant or child may fall asleep due to fatigue and tiredness related to effort of eating.

Social Participation
- Infant or child and caregiver may not enjoy the social interaction that can occur during feeding time.
- Child may have difficulty conforming to norms expected at social activities involving food and eating behavior.

Sensorimotor
- Infant may have difficulty latching well and consistently to breast or bottle.
- Infant may have more milk coming out of mouth than staying in the mouth.
- Infant or child may frequently spit up, vomit, or have liquid coming from nose.

- Child may lack oral-motor skills due to hypotonia (Crapnell et al., 2013).
- Child may experience fatigue (lack of endurance) during feeding.
- Child may have difficulty using pincher (thumb–fingers) skills to pick up food.
- Child may have difficulty holding and using eating utensils (spoon, fork, knife).
- Child may prefer to walk around while eating and refuse to sit down for more than few seconds.
- Child may be orally defensive (oral hypersensitivity, oral overresponsivity).
- Child may be hypersensitive to certain tastes (salty, bitter, sweet).
- Child may be hypersensitive to certain smells.
- Child may insist that food be presented in a certain shape such as round or square.
- Child may insist that food must be limited to a certain color, such as white.
- Child may insist that food must be of a certain temperature.
- Child may insist that food and liquid be a certain consistency.
- Child has strong preference for certain brands of food and will only eat that brand.
- Child may lack awareness of food in the mouth (hyposensitivity).
- Child may have difficulty forming a bolus and manipulating the bolus in the mouth.
- Child may experience gagging, coughing, or vomiting during feeding.
- Child may require prolonged period of time to finish eating (more than 30 minutes), leading to potential inadequate nutrient intake.
- Child may have tactile sensitivity (tactile defensiveness; Angell, 2010).
- Child may have sensory processing issues (Davis et al., 2013; Nadon et al., 2011; Stein et al., 2012, 2013; Stein et al., 2011; Suarez et al., 2012; Zobel-Lachiusa et al., 2015).

Cognitive/Perceptual
- Eating process and eating "manners" are learned behaviors. Some children with feeding disorders may struggle to master eating manners and behaviors.

Psychosocial
- Infant may refuse to hold the bottle.
- Child may restrict (refuse to eat) food choice.
- Child may not eat any of a certain type of food.
- Child may only eat food from a certain fast-food restaurant.
- Mealtime may be a constant "battle" between caregiver and child.
- Child may be reported to be a "picky" eater.
- Child may be reported to be difficult or hard to feed by all adult caregivers (parents, nanny, grandparents, other relatives or friends).
- Child may not tolerate "new-to-him/her" foods on plate.
- Child cries or arches back when held after feeding (Note: may be sign of medical condition).

Context/Environment
- Child may insist on sitting at the same place and at the same time when eating or refuses to eat.
- Child may only eat if allowed to sit in/on preferred chair or stool.
- Child may need special oral care by a dentist.
- Caregivers may assume the eating is an easy process to perform and comes naturally (actually, eating is a complex process that must be learned and mastered in stages).
- Caregivers may restrict foods to certain meals in the belief that the foods should only be served at those meals (e.g., cereal at breakfast) instead of making the food available at other meal times.
- Caregivers may restrict eating to three meals a day to teach child to eat on the adult's schedule, which may not provide enough food intake for a growing child (five to six small meals may be necessary to obtain sufficient nutrients).
- Caregivers may assume child will eat when hungry and will not starve (child may have medical problems that prevent eating sufficient nutrients to survive).

- Caregivers may assume child should "mind his or her manners" at all meals (food is removed if played with; typically developing children play with their food, so such behavior should be expected of children with feeding problems).

Intervention/Treatment

Models and programs developed by occupational therapy personnel include gastroesophageal reflux (Marcus & Breton, 2013); oral motor dysfunction in cerebral palsy (Siddharth & Gupta, 2016); sensory processing, modulation, and integration (Nadon et al., 2013); and swallowing impairments (Marcus & Breton, 2013). Models and programs developed by other professionals but used by occupational therapy personnel include behavioral approaches (Nadon et al., 2013), cheek and jaw support program (Hwang, Lin, et al., 2010), cognitive approach (Nadon et al., 2013), collaboration (Drobnyk & Rocco, 2011), graduated exposure (Nadon et al., 2013), integrated feeding goals into IEPs (Bruns & Thompson, 2014), neuromuscular electrical stimulation (Song et al., 2015), oral care program (Cermak et al., 2015), premature infant oral motor intervention (Arora et al., 2018; Hwang, Vergara, et al., 2010), selective eating program for ASD (Miyajima et al., 2017), sensorimotor intervention (Fucile et al., 2011; Fucile et al., 2012), and telehealth (Carpenter & Garfinkel, 2019). Team members include general physicians, pediatricians, gastroenterologists, radiologists, psychologists, nursing personnel, dietitians and nutritionists, social workers, speech–language pathologists, dentists, physical therapy personnel, and occupational therapy personnel. Goal is to provide adequate nutritional intake to support growth and development, create a positive caregiver–child interaction process during feeding, provide instruction in best positioning for feeding, provide adapted devices as useful, modify or manage over- or under-responsivity to oral stimulation, and when possible, adapt behavior and food diversity to expected social norms for age and context.

Activities of Daily Living/Instrumental ADL
- Assist caregivers to plan and prepare diversity of food choice.
- Assist caregivers to develop a plan of oral care, including selection of toothbrush and toothpaste at home.

Education/Work
- Not applicable.

Play/Leisure
- Assist caregiver to understand and tolerate that playing with food is normal child behavior.
- Assist caregiver to select foods that can be played with, such a Cheerios and small pretzels.

Rest/Sleep
- Not discussed.

Social Participation
- Assist caregiver to create a positive social activity during feeding time.

Sensorimotor
- Massage: Massage face, lips, and cheeks with various textures and fabrics to gradually decrease sensitivity. Begin with smooth materials (satin, silk) and gradually move to rougher textures.
- Chewing and jaw strengthening: Offer snack foods that require oral muscle activity (heavy chewing: pretzel rods, jerky, Twizzlers; for nonfood items: Chewy Tubes or Theratubing—items can be dipped in juice to add favor).
- Vibration: Use a vibrating (electric) toothbrush or oral massagers on lips, insides of cheeks, palate, tongue, and gums.
- Brushing: Use fingertip massagers, Toothettes, or Brush-Ups (Note: for children 8 years or older).
- Texture: Select several different types of foods that are age appropriate for a "sampling party" or "snack party."

- Temperature: Offer beverages of different temperatures.
- Positioning: Neck flexion with head in midline of body must be maintained (in infants, the rest of the body can be adjusted from horizontal to vertical head up; child should be sitting upright with back extended and feet on a firm surface).

Cognitive/Perceptual
- Not discussed.

Psychosocial
- Behavioral interventions have included use of positive and negative reinforcement, shaping, physical guidance (hand over hand), fading out support, escape extinction, and discrimination between appropriate and inappropriate behavior (Howe & Wang, 2013).

Context/Environment
- Provide education to parents and caregivers on normal development.
- Provide education on facilitating appropriate feeding behaviors.
- Provide education and demonstration of effective caregiver–child interaction.
- Assist parents and caregivers to develop strategies for visits to dentist for oral care.

Precautions/Safety Considerations

- Medical conditions: Aspiration, breathing difficulties such as apnea, cardiac conditions such as bradycardia.
- Nutritional dysfunction: Limit amount of juice and milk before meals because small amounts can decrease appetite.
- Feeding skills: Avoid sharp or pointed edges on eating utensils.
- Psychosocial: Never force-feed a child; never require a child clean or empty a plate.

Prognosis and Outcome

Variable. A number of approaches have been viewed as successful by the researchers, but long-range studies are lacking regarding the management of feeding disorders over the years.

REFERENCES

American Occupational Therapy Association. (2017). The practice of occupational therapy in feeding, eating, and swallowing. *American Journal of Occupational Therapy*, 71(Suppl. 2), Article 7112410015. https://doi.org/10.5014/ajot.2017.716S04

Angell, A. (2010). Selective eaters and tactile sensitivity: A review of classification and treatment methods that address anxiety and support a child's need for a sense of control. *ICAN: Infant, Child & Adolescent Nutrition*, 2(5), 299–303. https://doi.org/10.1177/1941406410382904

Arora, K., Goel, S., Manerkar, S., Konde, N., Panchal, H., Hegde, D., & Mondkar, J. (2018). Prefeeding oromotor stimulation program for improving oromotor function in preterm infants—A randomized controlled trial. *Indian Pediatrics*, 55(8), 675–678. https://doi.org/10.1007/s13312-018-1357-6

Baird, R., Levesque, D., Birnbaum, R., & Ramsay, M. (2015). A pilot investigation of feeding problems in children with esophageal atresia. *Diseases of the Esophagus*, 28(3), 224–228. https://doi.org/10.1111/dote.12178

Bandini, L. G., Anderson, S. E., Curtin, C., Cermak, S., Evans, E. W., Scampini, R. Maslin, M., & Must, A. (2010). Food selectivity in children with autism spectrum disorders and typically developing children. *Journal of Pediatrics*, 157(2), 259–264. https://doi.org/10.1016/j.jpeds.2010.02.013

Bruns, D. A., & Thompson, S. D. (2014). Turning mealtimes into learning opportunities: Integrating feeding goals into IEPs. *Teaching Exceptional Children*, 46(6), 179–186. https://doi.org/10.1177/0040059914534619

Carpenter, K. M., & Garfinkel, M. (2019). Telehealth as a supplemental service to treat pediatric feeding delays and disorders. *SIS Quarterly Practice Connections, 4*(4), 2–4.

Cermak, S. A., Stein Duker, L. I., Williams, M. E., Dawson, M. E., Lane, C. J., & Polido, J. C. (2015). Sensory adapted dental environments to enhance oral care for children with autism spectrum disorders: A randomized controlled pilot study. *Journal of Autism and Developmental Disorders, 45*(9), 2876–2888. https://doi.org/10.1007/s10803-015-2450-5

Crapnell, T. L., Rogers, C. E., Neil, J. J., Inder, T. E., Woodward, L. J., & Pineda, R. G. (2013). Factors associated with feeding difficulties in the very preterm infant. *Acta Paediatrica, 102*(12), e539–e545. https://doi.org/10.1111/apa.12393

Davis, A. M., Bruce, A. S., Khasawneh, R., Schulz, T., Fox, C., & Dunn, W. (2013). Sensory processing issues in young children presenting to an outpatient feeding clinic. *Journal of Pediatric Gastroenterology and Nutrition, 56*(2), 156–160. https://doi.org/10.1097/MPG.0b013e3182736e19

Drobnyk, W., & Rocco, K. (2011). Collaboration between school, family, and occupational therapy coaches to restore oral feeding skills in a young child. *Exceptional Parent Magazine, 41*(2), 10–11.

Fucile, S., Gisel, E. G., McFarland, D. H., & Lau, C. (2011). Oral and non-oral sensorimotor interventions enhance oral feeding performance in preterm infants. *Developmental Medicine & Child Neurology, 53*(9), 829–835. https://doi.org/10.1111/j.1469-8749.2011.04023.x

Fucile, S., McFarland, D. H., Gisel, E. G., & Lau, C. (2012). Oral and nonoral sensorimotor interventions facilitate suck-swallow-respiration functions and their coordination in preterm infants. *Early Human Development, 88*(6), 345–350. https://doi.org/10.1016/j.earlhumdev.2011.09.007

Goday, P. S., Huh, S. Y., Silverman, A., Lukens, C. T., Dodrill, P., Cohen, S. S., Delaney, A. L., Feuling, M. B., Noel, R. J., Gisel, E., Kenzer, A., Kessler, D. B., Kraus de Camargo, O., Browne, J., & Phalen, J. A. (2019). Pediatric feeding disorder: Consensus definition and conceptual framework. *Journal of Pediatric Gastroenterology and Nutrition, 68*, 124–129. https://doi.org/10.1097/MPG.0000000000002188

Howe, T. H., & Wang, T. N. (2013). Systematic review of interventions used in or relevant to occupational therapy for children with feeding difficulties ages birth-5 years. *American Journal of Occupational Therapy, 67*(4), 405–412. https://doi.org/10.5014/ajot.2013.004564

Hwang, Y.-S., Lin, C.-H., Coster, W. J., Bigsby, R., & Vergara, E. (2010). Effectiveness of cheek and jaw support to improve feeding performance of preterm infants. *American Journal of Occupational Therapy, 64*(6), 886–894. https://doi.org/10.5014/ajot.2010.09031

Hwang, Y.-S., Vergara, E., Lin, C.-H., Coster, W. J., Bigsby, R., & Tsai, W.-H. (2010). Effects of prefeeding oral stimulation on feeding performance of preterm infants. *Indian Journal of Pediatrics, 77*(8), 869–873. https://doi.org/10.1007/s12098-010-0001-9

Little, L. M., & Wallisch, A. (2018). Let's Eat: Developmental and reliability of an eating behavior assessment for children with autism spectrum disorders. *Annals of International Occupational Therapy, 1*(1), 24–30. https://doi.org/10.3928/24761222-20180212-03

Marcus, S., & Breton, S. (2013). *Infant and child feeding and swallowing.* AOTA Press.

Miyajima, A., Tateyama, K., Fuji, S., Nakaoka, K., Hirao, K., & Higaki, K. (2017). Development of an intervention programme for selective eating in children with autism spectrum disorder. *Hong Kong Journal of Occupational Therapy, 30*(1), 22–32. https://doi.org/10.1016/j.hkjot.2017.10.001

Nadon, G., Feldman, D., & Gisel. (2013). Feeding issues associated with the autism spectrum disorders. In M. Fitzgerald (Ed.), *Recent advances in autism spectrum disorder* (Vol. 1, pp. 599–632). InTech Open.

Nadon, G., Feldman, D. E.., Dunn, W., & Gisel, E. (2011). Association of sensory processing and eating problems in children with autism spectrum disorders. *Autism Research and Treatment, 2011*, Article 541926. https://doi.org/10.1155/2011/541926

Paul, S., & D'Amico, M. (2013). The role of occupational therapy in the management of feeding and swallowing disorders. *New Zealand Journal of Occupational Therapy, 62*(2), 27–31.

Siddharth, V., & Gupta, A. (2016). Occupational therapy intervention in cerebral palsy children with oral motor dysfunction (OMD) and its impact on occupational goals and quality of life of their mothers. *Indian Journal of Physiotherapy and Occupational Therapy, 10*(4), 159–164.

Song, W. J., Park, J. H., Lee, J. H., & Kim, M. Y. (2015). Effects of neuromuscular electrical stimulation on swallowing functions in children with cerebral palsy: A pilot randomized controlled trial. *Hong Kong Journal of Occupational Therapy, 25*(1), 1–6. https://doi.org/10.1016/j.hkjot.2015.05.001

Stein, L. I., Polido, J. C., & Cermak, S. A. (2012). Oral care and sensory concerns in autism. *American Journal of Occupational Therapy, 66*(5), e73–e76. https://doi.org/10.5014/ajot.2012.004085

Stein, L. I., Polido, J. C., & Cermak, S. A. (2013). Oral care and sensory over-responsivity in children with autism spectrum disorders. *Pediatric Dentistry, 35*(3), 230–235.

Stein, L. I., Polido, J. C., Mailloux, Z., Coleman, G. G., & Cermak, S. A. (2011). Oral care and sensory sensitivities in children with autism spectrum disorders. *Special Care in Dentistry, 31*(3), 102–110. https://doi.org/10.1111/j.1754-4505.2011.00187.x

Suarez, M. A., Nelson, N. W., & Curtis, A. B. (2012). Associations of physiological factors, age, and sensory over-responsivity with food selectivity in children with autism spectrum disorders. *Open Journal of Occupational Therapy, 1*(1). https://doi.org/10.15453/2168-6408.1004

Zobel-Lachiusa, J., Andrianopoulos, M. V., Mailloux, A., & Cermak, S. A. (2015). Sensory differences and mealtime behavior in children with autism. *American Journal of Occupational Therapy, 69*(5), Article 6905185050. https://doi.org/10.5014/ajot.2015.016790

BIBLIOGRAPHY

Cermak, S. A., Curtin, C., & Bandini, L. G. (2010). Food selectivity and sensory sensitivity in children with autism spectrum disorders. *Journal of the American Dietetic Association, 110*(2), 238–246. https://doi.org/10.1016/j.jada.2009.10.032

Cermak, S. A., Curtin, C., & Bandini, L. (2014). Sensory sensitivity and food selectivity in children with autism spectrum disorders. In V. B. Patel, V. R. Preedy, & C. R. Martin (Eds.), *Comprehensive guide to autism* (pp. 2061–2075). Springer. https://doi.org/10.1007/978-1-4614-4788-7_126

Chistol, L. T., Bandini, L. G., Must, A., Phillips, S., Cermak, S. A., & Curtin, C. (2018). Sensory sensitivity and food selectivity in children with autism spectrum disorder. *Journal of Autism and Developmental Disorders, 48*, 583–591. https://doi.org/10.1007/s10803-017-3340-9

Duivestein, J., & Gerlach, A. (2011). Developing clinician expertise in paediatric dysphagia: What is an effective learning model. *International Journal of Therapy and Rehabilitation, 18*(3), 130–138. https://doi.org/10.12968/ijtr.2011.18.3.130

Gal, E., Hardal-Nasser, R., & Engel-Yeger, B. (2011). The relationship between the severity of eating problems and intellectual developmental deficit level. *Research in Developmental Disabilities, 32*(5), 1464–1469. https://doi.org/10.1016/j.ridd.2010.12.003

Korth, K., & Rendell, L. (2015). Feeding intervention. In J. Case-Smith & J. C. O'Brien (Eds.), *Occupational therapy for children and adolescents* (7th ed., pp. 389–415). Elsevier Mosby.

Lane, W. J. (2012). Disorders of eating and feeding and disorders following prenatal substance abuse. In S. J. Lane & A. Bundy (Eds.), *Kids can be kids: A childhood occupations approach* (pp. 417–436). F. A. Davis.

Marshall, J., Ware, R., Ziviani, J., Hill, R. J., & Dodrill, P. (2015). Efficacy of interventions to improve feeding difficulties in children with autism spectrum disorders: A systematic review and meta-analysis. *Child: Care, Health and Development, 41*(2), 278–302. https://doi.org/10.1111/cch.12157

Mazurek, M. O., Vasa, R. A., Kalb, L. G., Kanne, S. M., Rosenberg, D., Keefer, A., Murray, D. S., Freedman, B., & Lowery, L. A. (2013). Anxiety, sensory over-responsivity, and gastrointestinal problems in children with autism spectrum disorders. *Journal of Abnormal Child Psychology, 41*(1), 165–176. https://doi.org/10.1007/s10802-012-9668-x

Nadon, G., Feldman, D. E., Dunn, W., & Gisel, E. (2011). Mealtime problems in children with autism spectrum disorder and their typically developing siblings: A comparison study. *Autism, 15*(1), 98–113. https://doi.org/10.1177/1362361309348943

Snider, L., Majnemer, A., & Darsaklis, V. (2011). Feeding interventions for children with cerebral palsy: A review of the evidence. *Physical & Occupational Therapy in Pediatrics, 31*(1), 58–77. https://doi.org/10.3109/01942638.2010.523397

Speyer, R., Cordier, R., Parsons, L., Denman, D., & Kim, J. H. (2018). Psychometric characteristics of non-instrumental swallowing and feeding assessments in pediatrics: A systematic review using COSMIN. *Dysphagia, 33*, 1–14. https://doi.org/10.1007/s00455-017-9835-x

Stein, L. I., Lane, C. J., Williams, M. E., Dawson, M. E., Polido, J. C., & Cermak, S. A. (2014). Physiological and behavioral stress and anxiety in children with autism spectrum disorders during routine oral care. *BioMed Research International, 2014*, Article 694876. https://doi.org/10.1155/2014/694876

Stein, L. I., Polido, J. C., Najera, S. O., & Cermak, S. A. (2012). Oral care experiences and challenges in children with autism spectrum disorders. *Pediatric Dentistry, 34*(5), 387–391.

Suarez, M. A., Atchison, B. J., & Lagerwey M. (2014). Phenomenological examination of the mealtime experience for mothers of children with autism and food selectivity. *American Journal of Occupational Therapy, 68*(1), 102–107. https://doi.org/10.5014/ajot.2014.008748

Suarez, M. A., Nelson, N. W., & Curtis, A. B. (2014). Longitudinal follow-up of factors associated with food selectivity in children with autism spectrum disorders. *Autism, 18*(81), 924–932. https://doi.org/10.1177/1362361313499457

Fetal Alcohol Spectrum Disorder

Description

Fetal alcohol spectrum disorder (FASD) includes five subcategories of disorders[*]: fetal alcohol syndrome (FAS), partial fetal alcohol syndrome (pFAS), alcohol-related neurodevelopmental disorder (ARND), alcohol-related birth defects (ARBD), and neurobehavioral disorder associated with prenatal alcohol exposure (ND-PAE).

• Fetal alcohol syndrome (FAS) is a diagnosis given to a child or youth who meets the following criteria established by the U.S. Centers for Disease Control and Prevention (n.d.): Facial dysmorphia (smooth philtrum, thin vermillion border, small palpebral fissures), growth problems, central nervous system problems (structural deformities such as small head circumference and functional problems [global cognitive deficit or deficits in three or more domains, including attention and hyperactivity, memory, executive function, motor function, social skills, sensory processing, or language]), and confirmation of maternal alcohol consumption during pregnancy. Set of congenital psychological, behavioral, and physical abnormalities that tend to appear in infants whose mothers consume alcohol during pregnancy. FAS is characterized by typical craniofacial and limb defects, cardiovascular defects, intrauterine growth impairment, delayed development, neurologic dysfunction, and is a leading cause of intellectual disability (O'Toole, 2017; Porter, 2018). FAS can be identified by small stature and typical set of facial traits, including microcephaly, microphthalmia, short palpebral fissures, epicanthal folds, a small or flat midface, a flat elongated philtrum, a thin upper lip, and a small chin. Abnormal palmar creases and joint contracture may also be evident (Porter, 2018).

• Partial fetal alcohol syndrome (pFAS) is described as a diagnosis given to a child or youth who does not meet the full diagnostic criteria for FAS, but has a history of prenatal alcohol exposure and some of the characteristics.

---

[*] These five subtypes are not mutually exclusive. A child or youth may be given a diagnosis of more than one description. In addition, the infant, child, or youth may experience postnatal traumatic experience.

- Alcohol-related neurodevelopment disorder (ARND) is described as a diagnosis given to a child or youth who has a history of prenatal alcohol exposure and has intellectual disabilities as well as problems with cognition, learning, and behavior, such as difficulties with memory, attention, judgment, math, and poor impulse control, but does not have abnormal facial features or growth problems (Centers for Disease Control and Prevention, n.d.).

- Alcohol-related birth defects (ARBD) is described as a diagnosis given to a child or youth who has a history of prenatal alcohol exposure and has problems with how organs were formed and how they function, including the heart, kidneys, bones, vision, or hearing (Centers for Disease Control and Prevention, n.d.).

- Neurobehavioral disorder associated with prenatal alcohol exposure (ND-PAE) is described as a diagnosis given to a child or youth who as problems in three areas: cognition (attention, thinking, memory), behavior (tantrums, irritability, mood shifts), and trouble performing daily activities (bathing, dressing appropriately for the weather, playing with other children). The mother must have consumed more than 13 alcoholic drinks per month of pregnancy or more than two alcoholic drinks in one sitting (Centers for Disease Control and Prevention, n.d.).

Cause

Maternal alcohol consumption leading to alcohol exposure in utero by the fetus. The diagnosis is given to infants, with characteristic findings, born to women who use alcohol during pregnancy (Chung, 2015; Porter, 2018).

Evaluation/Assessment

Areas

- Activities of Daily Living/Instrumental ADL: basic ADLs, mobility, transfers, communication
- Education/Work: academic achievement, academic skills, work skills
- Play/Leisure: play skills, interests, values, frequency, location
- Rest/Sleep: sleep disturbance
- Social Participation: type, frequency, location, with whom
- Sensorimotor: gross motor skills, posture and postural control, fine motor skills, muscle strength, muscle tone, bilateral coordination, range of motion, endurance and activity tolerance, visual motor, sensory processing (seeking, avoidance), sensory modulation
- Cognitive/Perceptual: attention, memory, executive functioning (problem solving, planning, organization), learning, visual field, spatial relations
- Psychosocial: social skills, emotional and self-regulation, irritability, impulsivity, aggression, habituation, anxiety
- Context/Environment: parental knowledge, community or internet resources
- Development (Infant, Child, Adolescent only): developmental delay
- Comorbidities: attention-deficit/hyperactivity disorder, sensory processing disorders

Instruments

Instruments Developed by Occupational Therapy Personnel

- Evaluation Tool of Children's Handwriting (ETCH; Amundson, 1995)
- Infant/Toddler Sensory Profile (ITSP; Dunn, 2002)
- Infant/Toddler Symptom Checklist (ITSC; DeGangi et al., 1995)
- Miller Function and Participation Scales (M-FUN; Miller, 2006)
- Pediatric Clinical Test for Sensory Interaction for Balance (2nd ed.; P-CTSIB-2; Crowe et al., 1991)
- Sensory Processing Measure (SPM) Home Form (SPM-HF; Parham & Ecker, 2007)
- Sensory Processing Measure–Preschool: Home Form (SPM-P-HF; Ecker, & Parham, 2010; see also Hansen & Jirikowic, 2013, in References)

- Sensory Profile (2nd ed.; SP-2; Dunn, 2014; see also Hansen & Jirikowic, 2013, in References)
- Sensory Profile Caregiver Questionnaire (SPCQ; Dunn, 1999)

Instruments Developed by Other Professionals and Used by Occupational Therapy Personnel
- Adaptive Behavior Assessment System (3rd ed.; ABAS-3; Harrison & Oakland, 2015)
- Bayley Scales of Infant and Toddler Development (4th ed.; Bayley-4; Bayley & Aylward, 2019)
- Beery-Buktenica Developmental Test of Visual-Motor Integration (6th ed.; Beery VMI-6; Beery et al., 2010)
- Behavior Rating Inventory of Executive Function (2nd ed.; BRIEF-2; Gioia et al., 2015)
- Child Behavior Checklist (CBCL; Achenbach, 2001)
- Conners' Parent Rating Scale–Revised (CPRS-R; Conners et al., 1998)
- Continuous Performance Test (CPT; Rosvold et al., 1956)
- Developmental Neuropsychological Assessment (2nd ed.; NEPSY-II; Brooks et al., 2009)
- Differential Ability Scales–II (DAS-II; Elliott, 2007)
- Difficult Life Circumstances Scale (2nd ed.; DLC-2; Barnard, 1994)
- Infant Behavior Questionnaire–Revised (IBQ-R; Gartstein & Rothbart, 2003)
- Infant Behavior Questionnaire–Revised, Short Form and Very Short Form (IBQ-R-SF, IBQ-R-VSF; Putnam et al., 2014)
- Kaufman Brief Intelligence Test (2nd ed.; KBIT-2; Kaufman & Kaufman, 2004)
- Movement Assessment Battery for Children (2nd ed.; M-ABC-2; Henderson et al., 2007)
- Multimodal Balance Entrainment Response system (MuMBER; McCoy et al., 2015)
- Peabody Developmental Motor Scales (3rd ed.; PDMS-3; Folio & Fewell, 2023)
- Pediatric Early Elementary Examination (PEEX 2; Levine, 1996)
- Pediatric Examination of Educational Readiness at Middle Childhood (PEERAMID 2; Levine et al., 1988)
- Personality Inventory for Children (2nd ed.; PIC-2; Lachar & Gruber, 2002)
- Process Assessment of the Learner (2nd ed.; PAL-II; Berninger, 2007)
- Quick Neurological Screening Test (3rd ed., revised; QNST-3R; Mutti et al., 2017)
- Roberts Apperception Test for Children (2nd ed.; Roberts-2; Roberts, 2005)
- Scales of Independent Behavior–Revised (SIB-R; Bruininks et al., 1995)
- Sensory Organization Test (SOT; Nashner et al., 1982)
- Social Skills Rating System–Parent Version (SSRS-PV; Hess et al., 2014)
- Test of Nonverbal Intelligence (4th ed.; TONI-4; Brown et al., 2010)
- Wechsler Intelligence Scale for Children (5th ed.; WISC-V; Wechsler, 2014)
- Wechsler Preschool and Primary Scale of Intelligence (4th ed.; WPPSI-IV; Wechsler, 2012)

Problems/Issues

Activities of Daily Living/Instrumental ADL
- Child may have difficulty performing self-care skills.
- Child/youth may have difficulty learning and performing independent living skills.

Education/Work
- Child may have difficulty with handwriting because of use of a cross-thumb grasp, apply heavy writing pressure, and show poor word legibility (Doney et al., 2017).

Play/Leisure
- Child may lack play skills.
- Child may engage in few leisure occupations.

Rest/Sleep
- Child may have sleep disturbances such as a sleep routine.
- Child may need modification of the sleep environment.

Social Participation
- Child may not participate in social activities.

Sensorimotor
- Child may exhibit an array of soft neurological signs (Lucas et al., 2016).
- Child may be delayed in development of gross motor skills.
- Child may have difficulty with maintaining balance and postural control (Jirikowic et al., 2013).
- Child may have difficulty with fine motor skills (dexterity, speed, accuracy).
- Child may have poor hand functions (grasp, pinch, manipulate, position, release).
- Child may have visual impairments.
- Child may have hearing impairments.
- Child may have sensory processing disorders (seeking, avoiding; Carr et al., 2010).
- Child may have sensory registration dysfunction (hyper- or overresponsive, hyporesponsive) especially to auditory sounds (Abele-Webster et al., 2012).

Cognitive/Perceptual
- Child may have difficulty paying attention and concentrating on tasks.
- Child may have difficulty with working memory.
- Child may have difficulty with executive functions (planning, organizing, judgment of safety).

Psychosocial
- Child may demonstrate poor behavior/emotional self-regulation (irritability, mood swings; Gill & Thompson-Hodgetts, 2018; Jirikowic, Chen, et al., 2016).
- Child may have limited social skills.
- Child may be depressed or anxious or fearful.
- Child may have deficits in adaptive behavior skills (Carr et al., 2010).

Context/Environment
- Family and caregivers may lack information about FASD and its management.
- Family and caregivers may lack knowledge about available resources locally, statewide, nationally.
- Family and caregivers may lack information about adaptive devices, their use, and availability.
- Parents may experience stress in coping with a child with FASD (Jirikowic et al., 2012).

Intervention/Treatment

Models and programs developed by occupational therapy personnel include the Alert Program (Wagner et al., 2017; Wells et al., 2012), Kid's Club (Sparks-Keeney et al., 2011), and sample goals and interventions (Chung, 2015). Models and programs developed by other professionals but used by occupational therapy personnel include balance training (Jirikowic, Westcott McCoy, et al., 2016; McCoy et al., 2015); community-based intervention (Quan et al., 2019); intervention recommendations (Jirikowic et al., 2010); Sensorimotor Training to Affect Balance, Engagement and Learning (STABEL; McCoy et al., 2015); and Snoezelen Multisensory Room (Bergstrom et al., 2019). Team members include physicians, nursing personnel, psychologists, educators, and occupational therapy personnel. Goal is to facilitate performance of daily occupations.

Activities of Daily Living/Instrumental ADL
- Improve basic ADL skills (feeding, bathing/showering, toileting, dressing).
- Improve independent living skills through client education and practice (meal preparation, shopping, housekeeping, laundry, finances).

Education/Work
- Improve academic and classroom performance through adapting classroom environment to remove distracting auditory and visual stimuli, rearranging seating, working in small groups, breaking down tasks into smaller units, using visual aids, and providing reminders.
- Provide opportunity to explore work skills and job opportunities through volunteering.

Play/Leisure
- Develop play skills.
- Provide opportunity to explore leisure occupations.

Rest/Sleep
- See Sleep–Wake Disorders in Section 13: Lifestyle Conditions.

Social Participation
- Encourage participation in social activities.

Sensorimotor
- Improve fine motor skills through practice manipulating play items and practicing handwriting.
- Improve sensory processing by altering environment, providing self-regulation strategies, reducing stimuli, using a sensory diet plan, providing proprioceptive (heavy work) and vestibular activities, tactile input (deep pressure, massage, hand fidgets).

Cognitive/Perceptual
- Improve safety awareness through client education, using computer games to simulate safety situations.

Psychosocial
- Improve social skills using social skill-building groups, parent-assisted social skills programs emphasizing roles of social behavior, modeling, rehearsal, performance feedback, and coaching.
- Assist client to improve self-regulation to engage in deliberative and thoughtful actions while remaining attentive, inhibited, and emotionally appropriate for the situation or context (Gill & Thompson-Hodgetts, 2018).

Context/Environment
- Provide family with information about FASD.
- Provide family and caregivers with take-home or take-away instructions to augment practice sessions.
- Assist family and caregivers to identify and use community and internet resources.

Precautions/Safety Considerations

Child/youth may have seizures.

Prognosis and Outcome

There is no cure for FASD. Some persons can lead productive lives depending on characteristics inherited and social and environmental support received, including family, medical, rehabilitation, education and training, and community resources. Risk factors for negative outcomes include delinquency, school failure, alcohol and drug abuse problems, in addition to the type and severity of the FASD (Chung, 2015).

REFERENCES

Abele-Webster, L. A., Magill-Evans, J. E., & Pei, J. R. (2012). Sensory processing and ADHD in children with fetal alcohol spectrum disorder. *Canadian Journal of Occupational Therapy*, 79(1), 60–63. https://doi.org/10.2182/cjot.2012.79.1.8

Bergstrom, V. N. Z., O'Brien-Langer, A., & Marsh, R. (2019). Supporting children with fetal alcohol spectrum disorder: Potential applications of a Snoezelen multisensory room. *Journal of Occupational Therapy, Schools, & Early Intervention*, 12(1), 98–114. https://doi.org/10.1080/19411243.2018.1496869

Carr, J. L., Agnihotri, S., & Keightley, M. (2010). Sensory processing and adaptive behavior deficits of children across the fetal alcohol spectrum disorder continuum. *Alcoholism, Clinical and Experimental Research*, 34(6), 1022–1032. https://doi.org/10.1111/j.1530-0277.2010.01177.x

Centers for Disease Control and Prevention. (n.d.). *Fetal alcohol spectrum disorders (FASDs)*. Retrieved March 20, 2022, from https://www.cdc.gov/ncbddd/fasd/

Chung, A. (2015). *Fetal alcohol syndrome: Occupational therapy*. CINAHL Information Systems.

Doney, R., Lucas, B. R., Jirikowic, T., Tsang, T. W., Watkins, R. E., Sauer, K., Howat, P., Latimer, J., Fitzpatrick, J. P., Oscar, J., Carter, M., & Elliott, E. J. (2017). Graphomotor skills in children with prenatal alcohol exposure and fetal alcohol spectrum disorder: A population-based study in remote Australia. *Australian Occupational Therapy Journal, 64*(1), 68–78. https://doi.org/10.1111/1440-1630.12326

Gill, K., & Thompson-Hodgetts, S. (2018). Self-regulation in fetal alcohol spectrum disorder: A concept analysis. *Journal of Occupational Therapy, Schools, & Early Intervention, 11*(3), 329–345. https://doi.org/10.1080/19411243.2018.1455550

Hansen, K. D., & Jirikowic, T. (2013). A comparison of the Sensory Profile and Sensory Processing Measure Home Form for children with fetal alcohol spectrum disorders. *Physical & Occupational Therapy in Pediatrics, 33*(4), 440–452. https://doi.org/10.3109/01942638.2013.791914

Jirikowic, T., Chen, M., Nash, J., Gendler, B., & Olson, H. C. (2016). Regulatory behaviors and stress reactivity among infants at high risk for fetal alcohol spectrum disorders: An exploratory study. *Journal of Mental Health Research in Intellectual Disabilities, 9*(3), 171–188. https://doi.org/10.1080/19315864.2016.1183246

Jirikowic, T., Gelo, J., & Astley, S. (2010). Children and youth with fetal alcohol spectrum disorders: Summary of intervention recommendations after clinical diagnosis. *Intellectual and Developmental Disabilities, 48*(5), 330–344. https://doi.org/10.1352/1934-9556-48.5.330

Jirikowic, T. L., McCoy, S. W., Lubetzky-Vilnai, A., Price, R., Ciol, M. A., Kartin, D., Hsu, L.-Y., Gendler, B., & Astley, S. J. (2013). Sensory control of balance: A comparison of children with fetal alcohol spectrum disorders to children with typical development. *Journal of Population Therapeutics and Clinical Pharmacology, 20*(3), e212–e228.

Jirikowic, T., Olson, H. C., & Astley, S. (2012). Parenting stress and sensory processing: Children with fetal alcohol spectrum disorders. *OTJR: Occupation, Participation and Health, 32*(4), 160–168. https://doi.org/10.3928/15394492-20120203-01

Jirikowic, T., Westcott McCoy, S., Price, R., Ciol, M. A., Hsu, L.-Y., & Kartin, D. (2016). Virtual sensorimotor training for balance: Pilot study results for children with fetal alcohol spectrum disorders. *Pediatric Physical Therapy, 28*(4), 460–468. https://doi.org/10.1097/PEP.0000000000000300

Lucas, B. R., Latimer, J., Fitzpatrick, J. P., Doney, R., Watkins, R. E., Tsang, T. W., Jirikowic, T., Olson, H. C., Oscar, J., Carter, M., & Elliott, E. J. (2016). Soft neurological signs and prenatal alcohol exposure: A population-based study in remote Australia. *Developmental Medicine & Child Neurology, 58*(8), 861–867. https://doi.org/10.1111/dmcn.13071

McCoy, S. W., Jirikowic, T., Price, R., Ciol, M. A., Hsu, L.-Y., Dellon, B., & Kartin, D. (2015). Virtual sensorimotor balance training for children with fetal alcohol spectrum disorders: Feasibility study. *Physical Therapy, 95*(11), 1569–1581. https://doi.org/10.2522/ptj.20150124

O'Toole, M. T. (Ed.). (2017). *Mosby's dictionary of medicine, nursing & health professions* (10th ed.). Elsevier.

Porter, R. S. (Ed.). (2018). *The Merck manual of diagnosis and therapy* (20th ed.). Merck Sharp & Dohme.

Quan, R., Brintnell, E. S., & Leung, A. W. S. (2019). Elements for developing community-based interventions for adults with fetal alcohol spectrum disorder: A scoping review. *British Journal of Occupational Therapy, 82*(4), 201–212. https://doi.org/10.1177/0308022618790206

Sparks-Keeney, T., Jirikowic, T., & Deitz, J. (2011). The kid's club: A friendship group for school-age children with fetal alcohol spectrum disorders. *Developmental Disabilities Special Interest Section Quarterly, 34*(2), 1–4.

Wagner, B., Fitzpatrick, J., Symons, M., Jirikowic, T., Cross, D., & Latimer, J. (2017). The development of a culturally appropriate school based intervention for Australian Aboriginal children living in remote communities: A formative evaluation of the Alert Program intervention.

Australian Occupational Therapy Journal, 64(3), 243–252. https://doi.org/10.1111/1440-1630
.12352

Wells, A. M., Chasnoff, I. J., Schmidt, C. A., Telford, E., & Schwartz, L. D. (2012). Neurocognitive
habilitation therapy for children with fetal alcohol spectrum disorders: An adaptation of the
Alert Program. *American Journal of Occupational Therapy, 66*(1), 24–34. ttps://doi.org/10.5014/
ajot.2012.002691

BIBLIOGRAPHY

Adebiyi, B., Mukumbang, F. C., Cloete, L. G., & Beytell, A.-M. (2018). Exploring service providers'
perspectives on the prevention and management of fetal alcohol spectrum disorders in South
Africa: A qualitative study. *BMC Public Health, 18,* Article 1238. https://doi.org/10.1186/
s12889-018-6126-x

Ahmed-Landeryou, M. J. (2012). Fetal central nervous system development and alcohol—The
evidence so far. *Fetal and Pediatric Pathology, 31*(6), 349–359. https://doi.org/10.3109/155
13815.2012.659398

Birch, S. M., Carpenter, H. A., Marsh, A. M., McClung, K. A., & Doll, J. D. (2016). The knowledge
of rehabilitation professionals concerning fetal alcohol spectrum disorders. *Occupational
Therapy in Health Care, 30*(1), 69–79. https://doi.org/10.3109/07380577.2015.1053163

Duval-White, C. J., Jirikowic, T., Rios, D., Deitz, J., & Olson, H. C. (2013). Functional handwriting performance in school-age children with fetal alcohol spectrum disorders. *American
Journal of Occupational Therapy, 67*(5), 534–542. https://doi.org/10.5014/ajot.2013.008243

High- or At-Risk Infant or Child

*See also Developmental Delay, Feeding Disorders, Low Birth Weights,
Premature Infant, and specific disorders including Autism Spectrum Disorder,
Congenital Heart Disease, Fetal Alcohol Spectrum Disorder,
Sensory Processing Disorders.*

Description

As used in this handbook, the term *high- or at-risk infant or child* means an "infant who has increasing risk for disability, but the exact disability is not actualized yet" (Pekçetin & Günal, 2017,
p. 1). Risk factors include biological factors such as intracranial hemorrhage, intraventricular
hemorrhage, brachial plexus injury, apnea, asphyxia, sepsis, or diabetic retinopathy. Environmental risk factors include conditions such as mental health problems of parents, substance
abuse of parent, low socioeconomic status, lack of family caregiving skills, and adolescent pregnancy. Medical risk factors include conditions such as genetic disorders, hypertension in the
mother, congenital heart disorders, prematurity, low birth weight, complications during labor
and delivery, and sexually transmitted diseases (Pekçetin & Günal, 2017).

Cause

Causes include demographic social factors, past medical history of the mother, previous pregnan-
cies, factors related to the present pregnancy, issues in labor and delivery, and factors related to
the neonate. Exposure to toxic substances in utero is another risk factor (Rihtman et al., 2012).

Evaluation/Assessment

Areas

- Activities of Daily Living/Instrumental ADL: feeding (sucking, swallowing, tasting), nonnutritive sucking, bathing, diapering, dressing, communication skills, functional mobility, food
preparation for infants and toddlers

- Education/Work: academic skills
- Play/Leisure: play skills
- Rest/Sleep: sleep habits and routines
- Social Participation: social interactions
- Sensorimotor: primitive reflexes (sucking, grasp, Moro, asymmetrical tonic reflex), head control, midline orientation, gross and fine motor skills, positioning (tolerance in prone, prone extension), balance, weight bearing, joint approximation, range of motion, auditory acuity, visual acuity, proprioception, deep pressure, touch, vestibular stimulation
- Cognitive/Perceptual: attention, memory, auditory, perception, tactile perception, visual perception, visual motor perception
- Psychosocial: infant–parent bonding/attachment, stress management, emotional regulation, neurobehavioral organization, parental confidence
- Context/Environment: parenting and caregiver skills (holding, handling), orthotic and adapted devices, environmental home modification
- Development (Infant, Child, Adolescent only): developmental milestones, motor delays, cognitive deficits, regulatory state delays, sensory processing difficulties, social emotional challenges
- Comorbidities: genetic disorders, congenital disorders, maternal substance abuse (smoking, alcoholism, recreational drugs)

Instruments
Instruments Developed by Occupational Therapy Personnel
- Functional Emotional Assessment Scale (FEAS; Greenspan et al., 2001)
- Infant/Toddler Sensory Profile (ITSP; Dunn, 2002)
- Infant/Toddler Symptom Checklist (ITSC; DeGangi et al., 1995)
- Miller Assessment for Preschoolers (MAP; Miller, 1988)
- Miller Function and Participation Scales (M-FUN; Miller, 2006)
- Sensory Profile (2nd ed.; SP-2; Dunn, 2014)
- Sensory Processing Scale Inventory (SPSI; Schoen et al., 2017)
- Structured Preschool Observation (SPO; Golos et al., 2011, in References)
- Toddler and Infant Motor Evaluation (T.I.M.E.; Miller & Roid, 1994)

Instruments Developed by Other Professionals and Used by Occupational Therapy Personnel
- Alberta Infant Motor Scale (AIMS; Piper & Darrah, 1992)
- Autism Detection in Early Childhood (ADEC; Young, 2007)
- Bayley Scales of Infant and Toddler Development (4th ed.; Bayley-4; Bayley & Aylward, 2019)
- Beery-Buktenica Developmental Test of Visual-Motor Integration (6th ed.; Beery VMI-6; Beery et al., 2010)
- Bruininks-Oseretsky Test of Motor Proficiency (2nd ed.; BOT-2; Bruininks & Bruininks, 2005)
- Center for Epidemiological Studies Depression Scale (CES-D; Radloff, 1977)
- Communication and Symbolic Behavior Scales Developmental Profile (CSBS DP) Infant-Toddler Checklist (Wetherby & Prizant, 2002)
- Difficult Life Circumstances Scale (2nd ed.; DLC-2; Barnard, 1994)
- Infant Behavior Questionnaire–Revised (IBQ-R; Gartstein & Rothbart, 2003)
- Infant Neurological International Battery (INFANIB; Ellison et al., 1985)
- Modified Checklist of Autism in Toddlers (M-CHAT; Robins et al., 2001)
- Movement Assessment Battery for Children (2nd ed.; M-ABC-2; Henderson et al., 2007)

Problems/Issues
Activities of Daily Living/Instrumental ADL
- Infant may have difficulty with feeding due to weak sucking or alternating breathing with swallowing.
- Caregivers including first-time parents may not know how to change diapers and bathe an infant due to lack of experience or physical limitations.

Education/Work:
- Child may demonstrate difficulty with handwriting or using scissors in classroom.

Play/Leisure
- Caregivers may not know how to provide appropriate play activities.
- Child may not develop or demonstrate delayed development of play skills, especially cooperative and symbolic.

Rest/Sleep
- Infant may experience sleep disruption for medical procedures.

Social Participation
- Infant may lack social interaction skills with adults.

Sensorimotor
- Infant may lack flexion behaviors if infant was born premature and did experience flexion in utero.
- Child may demonstrate difficulty with fine motor skills, manual dexterity, cutting.
- Child may demonstrate developmental delay and difficulty with gross motor skills including midline functions, balance, jumping, hopping, throwing, and catching (Heathcock et al., 2015).
- Child may demonstrate difficulty with planning and executing purposeful movements and behaviors.
- Infant may lack sensory exposure to facilitate brain development (auditory, gustatory, kinesthetic, olfactory, tactile, vestibular, visual; Philpott-Robinson et al., 2016).
- Child may demonstrate delayed or difficulty with sensory processing skills (Flanagan et al., 2019).

Cognitive/Perceptual
- Infant needs to increase attention skills to facilitate cognitive development.
- Infant needs experience with perceptual activities (visual, auditory).
- Child may demonstrate delays or difficulty with arousal (hypo or hyper).
- Child may have difficulty with maintaining attention or dividing attention.

Psychosocial
- Infant usually has limited coping skills.
- Infant needs interaction with parents to facilitate infant–parent bonding.
- Child may have difficulty with regulatory behavior and stress reactivity (Jirikowic et al., 2016).
- Adolescent or adult may experience decreased quality of life (Dahan-Oliel et al., 2011).

Context/Environment
- Parents and caregivers may lack information on managing an at-risk or high-risk infant.
- Parents and caregivers may lack information about available resources in the community and on the internet.

Intervention/Treatment

Models and programs developed by occupational therapy personnel include auditory stimulation (Sawant, 2011), development support program (Shaikh & Vaidya, 2013), individualized touch and massage (Ehrhard-Wingard et al., 2011), and supplemental sensory stimulation (Shenai & Bijlani, 2013). Models and programs developed by other professionals but used by occupational therapy personnel include the developmental support program (Shaikh & Vaidya, 2013; Shenai & Bijlani, 2013), early intervention program (Golos et al., 2011), ecological model of child development (Golos et al., 2011), and Supporting and Enhancing NICU Sensory Experiences (SENSE; Pineda et al., 2019; Ross et al., 2017). Team members include physicians, neonatologists, nursing personnel, psychologists, physical therapy personnel, dieticians, speech–language pathologists, and occupational therapy personnel. Goals include helping to engage parents in consistently providing positive, developmentally appropriate sensory exposure to high-risk infants (Pineda et al., 2019). When working with high-risk infants, the goal of occupational therapy is to promote optimal development of the child and work with families to support them to engage and participate in their roles as parents and caregivers (Royal College of Occupational Therapists, 2017).

Activities of Daily Living/Instrumental ADL
- Infant may need assistance in learning to suck and swallow.

Education/Work
- Not applicable.

Play/Leisure
- Assist parents to learn to facilitate infant play toys and skills that are age appropriate.

Rest/Sleep
- Assist parents to provide age-appropriate sleep habits and routine.

Social Participation
- Assist parents to provide social and culture activities that are age appropriate and consistent with cultural values and beliefs.

Sensorimotor
- Assist parents to provide activities to promote gross and fine motor development that is consistent with the child's level of occupational performance.
- Assist parents to provide sensory experiences to promote sensory awareness, registration, acuity, and discrimination (Pineda et al., 2019).
  - *Auditory:* Types—quiet conversation, live or recorded music, material voice recording, reading aloud, singing, speaking directly to infant. Dosage—No sound players until 32 weeks postmenstrual age (PMA). One hour/day beginning at 23 weeks to 3 hours/day at 40 weeks PMA.
  - *Gustatory:* Types—milk, water, fluids (may be delayed until suck and swallow reflexes are established). Dosage—depends on whether direct gastrointestinal feedings are also being used.
  - *Kinesthetic:* Types—passive range of motion exercises, joint compression, movement of extremities or body, therapeutic facilitation of muscles. Dosage—Limited to transfers and diaper changes at 23 weeks PMA for total of about 2 minutes, begin intervention at 27 weeks PMA, up to 16 minutes/day at 40 weeks PMA.
  - *Olfactory:* Types—different scents using scent cloths, close contact with parents. Dosage—Daily, no specific time limits.
  - *Tactile:* Types—kangaroo (skin-to-skin care), massage, acupressure, facilitated touch, holding. Dosage—1 hour/day beginning at 23 weeks PMA to 3 hours/day for 40 weeks PMA.
  - *Vestibular:* Types—rocking, bouncing, swinging, unrestricted movement in bassinette/bed. Dosage—2 minutes/day beginning at 23 weeks primarily limited to transfers and diaper changes up to 16 minutes/day for infants 40 weeks PMA.
  - *Vision:* Types—cycled light, color or black and white patterns, eye contact. Dosage—Dim light only until 32 weeks PMA. Cycled light starting at 32 weeks PMA using low level lift (25–100 watts). Always avoid direct and bright lights. Encourage visual attention through human interaction to follow parent or caregiver face. No specific time limits.

Cognitive/Perceptual
- Assist parents to learn child development and what to expect of the child at any specific age and stage of development.
- Assist parents to encourage and support cognitive development of attention, memory, and early executive functions.
- Assist parents to encourage and support development of perceptual skills, especially auditory and visual.

Psychosocial

- Assist parents to feel confident in their ability to parent through training and practice.
- Assist parents to identify family strengths and vulnerabilities.
- Assist parents to recognize signs of stress in infants.
  - ▶ Autonomic cues (breathing, skin color, visceral reactions): irregular or rapid breathing, pale or blotchy colored skin, hiccupping, and gagging.
  - ▶ Motor cues (muscle tone, posture, movement): aching head and trunk, extending arms and legs, squirming or jerky movements, tremors.
  - ▶ Regulation state: high state behaviors (irritable, fussy, crying), low state behaviors (drowsy, sleepy).
- Assist parents to recognize signs of calmness in infants.
  - ▶ Autonomic cues: regular relaxed breathing, pink even color skin, sighing.
  - ▶ Motor cues: body flexion or tucking position, sucking behavior, holding on with fingers, smooth movement of arms and legs.
  - ▶ Regulation state: steady eyes that look alert, smooth transitions from sleep to alertness.

Context/Environment

- Work with other professionals to provide services to at-risk or high-risk infant.
- Provide parent education on managing the needs of an at-risk or high-risk infant (types of food, bedding, clothing, bathing equipment, toys, transportation).
- Provide information on available community and internet resources.
- Provide information on home and environmental modification needed to accommodate an infant for first-time parents (sleeping quarters, feeding and eating space, storage space, play space).
- Provide developmental testing to assist in identifying infants and toddlers at risk or high risk for developing neurological, cognitive, or sensory disorders.
- Assist parents to provide social and culture activities that are age appropriate and consistent with cultural values, beliefs, and traditions regarding child-rearing practices.

Precautions/Safety Considerations

Intervention by therapists is based on the assumption that the infant is medically stable. Adjustments must be made, including discontinuing therapy if infant becomes medically unstable. Always watch for signs of distress.

Prognosis and Outcome

Variable. Some at-risk or high-risk infants progress normally with minimal residual problems. Others begin to demonstrate through developmental testing signs of neurological and cognitive dysfunction, which is characteristic of cerebral palsy, autism spectrum disorder, fetal alcohol spectrum disorder, intellectual disability, sensory processing dysfunction, and other disorders.

REFERENCES

Dahan-Oliel, N., Majnemer, A., & Mazer, B. (2011). Quality of life of adolescents and young adults born at high risk. *Physical & Occupational Therapy in Pediatrics, 31*(4), 362–389. https://doi.org/10.3109/01942638.2011.572151

Ehrhard-Wingard, D., Lowe, J., & Burtner, P. (2011). Individualized touch and massage options: A neurobehavioral, family-centered approach for high risk infants. *Developmental Disabilities Special Interest Section Quarterly, 34*(1), 1–4.

Flanagan, J. E., Schoen, S., & Miller, L. J. (2019). Early identification of sensory processing difficulties in high-risk infants. *American Journal of Occupational Therapy, 73*(2), Article 7302205 130. https://doi.org/10.5014/ajot.2018.028449

Golos, A., Sarid, M., Weill, M., & Weintraub, N. (2011). Efficacy of an early intervention program for at-risk preschool boys: A two-group control study. *American Journal of Occupational Therapy, 65(4)*, 400–408. https://doi.org/10.5014/ajot.2011.000455

Heathcock, J. C., Tanner, K., Robson, D., Young, R., & Lane, A. E. (2015). Retrospective analysis of motor development in infants at high and low risk for autism spectrum disorder. *American Journal of Occupational Therapy, 69(5)*, Article 6905185070. https://doi.org/10.5014/ajot.2015.017525

Jirikowic, T., Chen, M., Nash, J., Gendler, B., & Carmichael Olson, H. (2016). Regulatory behaviors and stress reactivity among infants at high risk for fetal alcohol spectrum disorders: An exploratory study. *Journal of Mental Health Research in Intellectual Disabilities, 9(3)*, 171–188. https://doi.org/10.1080/19315864.2016.1183246

Pekçetin, S., & Günal, A. (2017). Early intervention in pediatric occupational therapy. In M. Huri (Ed.), *Occupational therapy: Occupation focused holistic practice in rehabilitation.* IntechOpen. https://doi.org/10.5772/intechopen.68316

Philpott-Robinson, K., Lane, A. E., & Harpster, K. (2016). Sensory features of toddlers at risk for autism spectrum disorders. *American Journal of Occupational Therapy, 70(4)*, Article 7004220010. https://doi.org/10.5014/ajot.2016.019497

Pineda, R., Raney, M., & Smith, J. (2019). Supporting and enhancing NICU sensory experiences (SENSE): Defining developmentally-appropriate sensory exposures for high-risk infants. *Early Human Development, 133*, 29–35. https://doi.org/10.1016/j.earlhumdev.2019.04.012

Rihtman, T., Parush, S., & Ornoy, A. (2012). Preliminary findings of the developmental effects of *in utero* exposure to topiramate. *Reproductive Toxicology, 34(3)*, 308–311. https://doi.org/10.1016/j.reprotox.2012.05.038

Ross, K., Heiny, E., Conner, S., Spener, P., & Pineda, R. (2017). Occupational therapy, physical therapy and speech–language pathology in the neonatal intensive care unit: Patterns of therapy usage in a level IV NICU. *Research in Developmental Disabilities, 64*, 108–117. https://doi.org/10.1016/j.ridd.2017.03.009

Royal College of Occupational Therapists. (2017). *Occupational therapy in neonatal service and early intervention: Practice guideline.*

Sawant, P. D. (2011). To study the effect of non-linguistic and linguistic auditory stimulation as an adjunct to developmental support program in high-risk infants on their prelinguistic behavior and linguistic performance. *Indian Journal of Occupational Therapy, 43(1)*, 16–21.

Shaikh, S. P., & Vaidya, P. M. (2013). The effect of development support program (DSP) and play through feet on infants at risk for developmental delay. *Indian Journal of Occupational Therapy, 45(3)*, 3–7.

Shenai, N. G., & Bijlani, J. N. (2013). Effect of supplemental sensory stimulation program as an adjunct to developmental support program in high risk infants. *Indian Journal of Occupational Therapy, 45(2)*, 21–27.

BIBLIOGRAPHY

Bigsby, R., LaGasse, L. L., Lester, B. Shankaran, S., Bada, H., Bauer, C., & Liu, J. (2011). Prenatal cocaine exposure and motor performance at 4 months. *American Journal of Occupational Therapy, 65(5)*, e60–e68. https://doi.org/10.5014/ajot.2011.001263

Case-Smith, J. (2013). Systematic review of interventions to promote social-emotional development in young children with or at risk for disability. *American Journal of Occupational Therapy, 67(4)*, 395–404. https://doi.org/10.5014/ajot.2013.004713

Hunter, J., Lee, A., & Altimer, L. (2015). Neonatal intensive care unit. In J. Case-Smith & J. Clifford O'Brien (Eds.), *Occupational therapy for children and adolescents* (7th ed., pp. 595–635). Elsevier.

Intellectual Disability

Also called learning disabilities in most European countries.

See also Autism Spectrum Disorder, Attention-Deficit/Hyperactivity Disorder, Cerebral Palsy, Down Syndrome, Spina Bifida, Traumatic Brain Injury.

Outdated terms: mental retardation, mentally retarded, mental deficiency.

Alternate terms: disorder of intellectual development, global developmental delay, early developmental impairment, mental disability.

Description

Intellectual disability is a term that describes a cluster of conditions characterized by below-average intellectual function and adaptive skills (Suman, 2019). Intellectual disability is characterized by significantly subaverage intellectual functioning (often expressed as an intelligence quotient less than 70 to 75) combined with limitations of more than two of the following: communication, self-direction, social skills, self-care, use of community resources, and maintenance of personal safety (Porter, 2018). The term *learning disabilities* is used in European countries instead of intellectual disability. Disabilities related to specific academic subjects (reading, writing, and mathematics) are covered under the term *specific learning disorders*.

Intellectual disability (intellectual developmental disorder) is a disorder with onset during the developmental period that includes both intellectual and adaptive functioning deficits in conceptual, social, and practical domains. The three criteria that must be met for a diagnosis of intellectual disability are listed in the *Diagnostic and Statistical Manual of Mental Disorders* (5th ed.; *DSM-5*; American Psychiatric Association, 2013).

Cause

Most often, a specific cause cannot be identified. A cause is most likely to be identified in severe cases. Both genetics and environmental situation are involved, including chromosomal abnormalities, genetic metabolic disorders, genetic neurologic disorders, congenital infections, prenatal drug and toxin exposure, severe undernutrition during pregnancy, complications related to prematurity, undernutrition, and environmental deprivation (Porter, 2018).

Evaluation/Assessment

Areas

- Activities of Daily Living/Instrumental ADL: basic ADLs (eating, dressing, grooming, toileting, transfers), independent living skills (meal planning and preparation, housekeeping, shopping, driving, using public transportation), parenting and child care, pet care, sexuality
- Education/Work: academic achievement, vocational planning, workplace modification, work skill training, employer acceptance
- Play/Leisure: interests, type, location, frequency
- Rest/Sleep: sleep habits
- Social Participation: type, location, frequency, with whom
- Sensorimotor: gross motor skills (walking, running, jumping, hopping, skipping, throwing catching, riding a tricycle or bicycle), fine motor skills (holding crayons and writing devices, cutting, gluing and pasting, painting, keyboarding), sensory processing (auditory, gustatory, interoception, olfactory, proprioception, tactile, vestibular, vision)
- Cognitive/Perceptual: attention, memory, executive functions (problem solving, decision making, judgment, time management), time perception, visual perception, auditory perception, tactile perception, including stereognosis
- Psychosocial: social isolation, emotional regulation, quality of life
- Context/Environment: social support, accessibility, social acceptance, adapted devices, community resources, government laws, regulations and policies

- Development (Infant, Child, Adolescent only): developmental delay, developmental milestones
- Comorbidities: anxiety disorder, autism spectrum disorder, attention-deficit/hyperactivity disorder, cerebral palsy, Down syndrome, other congenital disorders, sensory processing disorders, spina bifida, traumatic brain injury

Instruments

Instruments Developed by Occupational Therapy Personnel

- Adolescent/Adults Sensory Profile (AASP; Brown & Dunn, 2002)
- Assessment of Motor and Process Skills (8th ed.; AMPS-8; Fisher & Bray Jones, 2016)
- Assessment of Time Management Skills (ATMS; White et al., 2013)
- Canadian Occupational Performance Measure (5th ed.; COPM-5; Law et al., 2014)
- Children's Assessment of Participation and Enjoyment and Preferences for Activities of Children (CAPE/PAC; King et al., 2004)
- Goal-Oriented Assessment of Lifeskills (GOAL; Miller & Oakland, 2013)
- Jacobs Inventory of Functional Skills (JIFS; Jacobs, 1999)
- KaTid–Child (kit for assessment time processing ability; Janeslätt et al., 2008)
- Model of Human Occupation Screening Tool (Version 2.0; MOHOST 2.0; Parkinson et al., 2006; see also Hawes & Houlder, 2010, in References)
- Occupational Self-Assessment (Version 2.2; OSA 2.2; Baron et al., 2006)
- Revised Knox Preschool Play Scale (RKPPS; Knox, 2008)
- Sensory Profile (2nd ed.; SP-2; Dunn, 2014)
- Time Organisation and Participation Scale (TOPS; Rosenblum, 2012)
- Time-Parent Scale (TPS; Janeslätt et al., 2009)
- Time-Self-Rating Scale (Time-S; Janeslätt et al., 2015; Sköld & Janeslätt, 2017, in References)
- Volitional Questionnaire (Version 4.1; VQ 4.1; de las Heras et al., 2007)
- Work Environment Impact Scale (WEIS; Moore-Corner et al., 1998)

Instruments Developed by Other Professionals and Used by Occupational Therapy Personnel

- Ages and Stages Questionnaire (3rd ed.; ASQ-3; Squires et al., 2009)
- Autonomy Scale (AS; Sigafoos et al., 1988)
- Behavioral Rating Inventory of Executive Function–Adult Version (BRIEF-A; Roth et al., 2005)
- Bruininks-Oseretsky Test of Motor Proficiency (2nd ed., BOT-2; Bruininks & Bruininks, 2005; see also Wuang et al., 2012, in References)
- Goal Attainment Scaling (GAS; Kiresuk et al., 1994)
- Matson Evaluation of Social Skills for Individuals With Severe Retardation (MESSIER; Matson, 1995)
- Movement Assessment Battery for Children (2nd ed., M-ABC-2; Henderson et al.; see also Wuang et al., 2012, in References)
- Patients' Evaluation of Developmental Status (PEDS; Glascoe, 1998)
- Peabody Developmental Motor Scales (3rd ed., PDMS-3; Folio & Fewell, 2023; see also Wuang et al., 2012, in References)
- Screening Tool of Eating Problems (STEP; Matson & Kuhn, 2001)
- World Health Organization Quality of Life–BREF (WHOQOL-BREF) questionnaire (The WHOQOL Group, 1998)

Problems/Issues

Activities of Daily Living/Instrumental ADL

- Toddler or child may have difficulty performing basic ADL tasks, especially if physical limitations are also present.
- Infant or child may have eating or feeding problems including lack of oral-motor skills, hand-to-mouth skills, and risk of aspiration (Gal et al., 2011).
- Child or adolescent may have difficulty learning and performing independent living skills.

Education/Work

- Child or adolescent may have limited ability to perform academic skills (reading, writing, math, science, civics, geography) and require special education services.
- Child or adolescent may have limited ability and opportunity to explore vocational choices and develop work skills and require a transitional training program.
- Adult may face barriers to employment (Berry & Kymar, 2013).
  - ▶ Need for workplace modification.
  - ▶ Inadequate education, training, and experience for the work demands.
  - ▶ Nonacceptance by employers and coworkers.
  - ▶ Difficulty in work–life balance.
  - ▶ Difficulty with accessibility in community transportation.

Play/Leisure

- Toddler or child may have limited play skills (exploratory, symbolic, interactive, cooperative; Fallon & MacCobb, 2013).
- Child or adolescent may engage in few or no leisure occupations.

Rest/Sleep

- Toddler, child, or adolescent may have sleep disturbances.

Social Participation

- Child or adolescent may not participate in or have limited participation in social activities and cultural events.

Sensorimotor

- Child or adolescent may experience developmental delay in acquiring gross motor skills.
- Child or adolescent may have difficulty performing fine motor tasks.
- Child or adolescent may have sensory processing dysfunction in one or more sensory systems (Engel-Yeger et al., 2011, 2016; Joosten & Bundy, 2010).

Cognitive/Perceptual

- Child or adolescent may have difficulty maintaining attention and concentration.
- Child or adolescent may have difficulty with working memory and prospective memory.
- Child or adolescent usually has difficulty with executive functions, including problem solving, planning ahead, decision making, time management and scheduling, organization, judgment of safety (Sharfi & Rosenblum, 2016).

Psychosocial

- Child or adolescent may have limited social interaction skills.
- Child or adolescent may have limited ability to perform social roles.
- Child, adolescent, or adult may have restricted and reduced quality of life.

Context/Environment

- Family or caregivers may lack information about managing persons with intellectual disability.
- Family and friends may not provide social support.
- Adolescents may experience difficult transitioning from school to postschool due environmental factors including family dynamics, communication skills, postschool services and access to transportation (Foley et al., 2012; Foley et al., 2016).
- Individuals with intellectual disability may experience negative attitudes from neighbors toward living in the community independently or in group living homes.
- Community may have limited resources including programs to develop and implement self-determination and independent living.
- Government laws, regulations, and policies may act as barriers as well as facilitators in providing services to person with intellectual disabilities.

Intervention/Treatment

Models and programs developed by occupational therapy personnel include adapting recipes (Delaney, 2014), adaptive play and sensory stimulation (Wilkinson & Chapparo, 1997), Camp Avanti Model (Erhardt, 2014), Cognitive Orientation to daily Occupational Performance (CO-OP; Karunakaran et al., 2018), Collaborative Consultation for Participation of Students with Intellectual Disability (CO-PID; Selanikyo et al., 2018; Selanikyo et al., 2017), community living skills (Sachdeva & Rao, 2012), melotherapy (music therapy; Osiceanu & Zaharescu, 2017), occupational therapy home program (Wuang et al., 2013), occupational therapy intervention process model (OTIPM; Coakley & Bryze, 2018), parenting (Janeslätt, Larsson, et al., 2019), Ross Five-Stage Model (Haertl & Ross, 2014), sensory diet (Shepherd, 2017), and time-processing ability (Janeslätt, Ahlström, & Granlund, 2019; Janeslätt et al., 2010). Models and programs developed by other professionals but used by occupational therapy personnel include electronic planning devices and time aides (Janeslätt et al., 2014; Janeslätt, Lindstedt, et al., 2015; Wennberg & Kjellberg, 2010), intensive interaction (Haythorne, 2019), parenting toolkit (Janeslätt, Larsson, et al., 2019), and supplemental employment (Coakley & Bryze, 2018; Hynes & Harb, 2017). Team members include physicians, pediatricians, orthopedists, neurologists, surgeons, psychologists, physical therapy personnel, speech–language pathologists, audiologists, social workers, educators, nutritionists, and occupational therapy personnel. Goals include consideration of the child or adolescent's current and future needs for occupational performance and adaptive behavior in personal care, social interaction, community engagement, school participation, work settings, and leisure occupations (Suman, 2019).

Activities of Daily Living/Instrumental ADL

- Child:
  - ▶ Provide opportunity to practice basic ADL skills using adaptive techniques and devices if needed.
  - ▶ Dressing: Consider garments without fasteners when possible or adapted with use of Velcro or ring type zipper pull.
- Adolescent and adult:
  - ▶ Provide opportunity to practice independent living skills in a controlled (supervised) environment and then in less restrictive environment if skills are satisfactory.
  - ▶ College experience may be useful for person to learn community skills (Anderson & DaLomba, 2019).

Education/Work

- Child and adolescent: Provide training in use of assistive technology in classroom.
- Adolescent and adult:
  - ▶ Facilitate career exploration.
  - ▶ Provide career training and development of work skills.

Play/Leisure

- Child: Promote development of play skills (symbolic, interactive, cooperative).
- Adolescent and adult: Assist in exploring interests and developing leisure occupations.

Rest/Sleep

- Child: Assist in promoting sleep habits and routines.
- All ages: Monitor for sleep disturbances, which may require referral to sleep specialists (obstructive sleep apnea, central sleep apnea, insomnia).

Social Participation

- Assist in developing skills to participate in social activities and cultural events (attending local community activities, assisting in planning and participating in social events).
- Promote schedule of participation in social activities and cultural events.

Sensorimotor
- Provide program to promote physical fitness tailored to individual needs and abilities.
- Provide sensory awareness and registration (sensory room, sensory experiences).
- Address sensory processing disorders, if present (see Sensory Processing Disorders in Section 2: Sensory Disorders).

Cognitive/Perceptual
- Promote development of arousal, alertness, attending behavior, and concentration.
- Provide practice in memory tasks including use of memory aids (lists, checklist, calendars, timers, smartphone apps, phone calls from family or friends).
- Promote development of functional cognition and executive functions within client's ability, especially autonomy, safety, and problem solving.
- Focus decision making, choices, and control on time and routines, privacy, and use of space and objects (Kåhlin et al., 2016).

Psychosocial
- Provide opportunity to express feelings of anxiety.
- Provide opportunity to practice social skills.

Context/Environment
- Provide information to families and caregivers regarding government financial support such as Supplemental Security Income (SSI) and Medicaid.
- Assist clients to be educated in the least restrictive environment as required under the IDEA (Individuals with Disabilities Education Act).
- Assist clients to take advantage of state vocational education programs.
- Increase and enhance opportunities for clients to participate in a diversity of active use of time and space (Crowe et al., 2015).

Precautions/Safety Considerations

Person may require monitoring for seizures or asthma attacks. Person is at risk for early dementia.

Prognosis and Outcome

Intellectual disability is a lifelong condition. Needs and solutions change as the person ages. The amount of environment support needed by a given individual depends on the severity of the cognitive disability and the skills the individual has mastered over time. Greater ability to perform ADL and IADL skills increased possibility of living in independent or community group home settings (King et al., 2017). Individuals with mild to moderate intellectual disability can support themselves, live independent lives, and be employed at jobs that require basic intellectual skills. Life expectancy may be shortened, depending on the etiology of the disability. Individuals with severe intellectual disability will require lifelong support (Porter, 2018).

Cost Benefit

The College of Occupational Therapists (2014) suggests there are cost benefits to teaching and maintaining skills in independent living that reduce support and care costs: Promoting healthier lifestyles and access to timely primary health care reduces health-care costs, and advice and support on equipment and behavior intervention reduces burden on caregivers.

REFERENCES

American Psychiatric Association. (2013). *Diagnostic and statistical manual of mental disorders* (5th ed.). https://doi.org/10.1176/appi.books.9780890425596

Anderson, M., & DaLomba, E. (2019). A college experience for adults with intellectual and developmental disabilities: Meeting community needs. *SIS Quarterly Practice Connections, 4*(4), 15–18.

Berry, B. S., & Kymar, K. R. (2013). Human resource professionals' perception on disability related barriers to employment of persons with intellectual disability. *Indian Journal of Occupational Therapy, 45*(1), 21–29.

Coakley, K. A., & Bryze, K. (2018). The distinct value of occupational therapy in supported employment of adults with intellectual disabilities. *Open Journal of Occupational Therapy, 6*(2), Article 9. https://doi.org/10.15453/2168-6408.1424

College of Occupational Therapists. (2014). *Fact sheet: The importance of occupational therapy to people with learning disabilities.*

Crowe, T. K., Salazar Sedillo, J., Kertcher, E. F., & LaSalle, J. H. (2015). Time and space use of adults with intellectual disabilities. *Open Journal of Occupational Therapy, 3*(2). https://doi.org/10.15453/2168-6408.1124

Delaney, K. (2014). Adapting recipes for people with learning disabilities. *OT News, 22*(7), 38–39.

Engel-Yeger, B., Hardal-Nasser, R., & Gal, E. (2011). Sensory processing dysfunctions as expressed among children with different severities of intellectual developmental disabilities. *Research in Developmental Disabilities, 32*(5), 1770–1775. https://doi.org/10.1016/j.ridd.2011.03.005

Engel-Yeger, B., Hardal-Nasser, R., & Gal, E. (2016). The relationship between sensory processing disorders and eating problems among children with intellectual developmental deficits. *British Journal of Occupational Therapy, 79*(1), 17–25. https://doi.org/10.1177/0308022615586418

Erhardt, R. P. (2014). Adaptation of a unique pediatric intervention model of r adults with intellectual and developmental disabilities. In K. Haertl (Ed.), *Adults with intellectual and developmental disabilities: Strategies for occupational therapy* (pp. 311–335). AOTA Press.

Fallon, J., & MacCobb, S. (2013). Free play time of children with learning disabilities in a non-inclusive preschool setting: An analysis of play and nonplay behaviours. *British Journal of Learning Disabilities, 41*(3), 212–219. https://doi.org/10.1111/bld.12052

Foley, K. R., Dyke, P., Girdler, S., Bourke, J., & Leonard, H. (2012). Young adults with intellectual disability transitioning from school to post-school: A literature review framed within the ICF. *Disability and Rehabilitation, 20*(34), 1747–1764. https://doi.org/10.3109/09638288.2012.660603

Foley, K. R., Taffe, J., Bourke, J., Einfeld, S. L., Tonge, B. J., Trollor, J., & Leonard, H. (2016). Young people with intellectual disability transitioning to adulthood: Do behavior trajectories differ in those with and without Down syndrome? *PLOS ONE, 11*(7), Article e017667. https://doi.org/10.1371/journal.pone.0157667

Gal, E., Hardal-Nasser, R., & Engel-Yeger, B. (2011). The relationship between the severity of eating problems and intellectual developmental deficit level. *Research in Developmental Disabilities, 32*(5), 1464–1469. https://doi.org/10.1016/j.ridd.2010.12.003

Haertl, K., & Ross, M. (2014). Ross's five-stage model for adults with intellectual and developmental disabilities. In K. Haertl (Ed.), *Adults with intellectual and developmental disabilities: Strategies for occupational therapy* (pp. 377–400). AOTA Press.

Hawes, D., & Houlder, D. (2010). Reflections on using the Model of Human Occupation Screening Tool in a joint learning disability team. *British Journal of Occupational Therapy, 73*(11), 564–567. https://doi.org/10.4276/030802210X12892992239431

Haythorne, R. (2019). A tool for communication. *OT News, 27*(5), 50–52.

Hynes, P. J., & Harb, A. (2017). Practices and roles of Irish occupational therapists' with adults with intellectual disabilities who access supported employment services. *Irish Journal of Occupational Therapy, 45*(2), 78–91. https://doi.org/10.1108/IJOT-06-2017-0016

Janeslätt, G., Ahlström, S. W., & Granlund, M. (2019). Intervention in time-processing ability, daily time management and autonomy in children with intellectual disabilities aged 10-17 years—A cluster randomised trial. *Australian Occupational Therapy Journal, 66*(1), 110–120. https://doi.org/10.1111/1440-1630.12547

Janeslätt, G. K., Granlund, M., Kottorp, A., & Almqvist, L. (2010). Patterns of time processing ability in children with and without developmental disabilities. *Journal of Applied Research in Intellectual Disabilities, 23*(3), 250–262. https://doi.org/10.1111/j.1468-3148.2009.00528.x

Janeslätt, G., Kottorp, A., & Granlund, M. (2014). Evaluating intervention using time aids in children with disabilities. *Scandinavian Journal of Occupational Therapy, 21*(3), 181–190. https://doi.org/10.3109/11038128.2013.870225

Janeslätt, G., Larsson, M., Wickström, M., Springer, L., & Höglund, B. (2019). An intervention using the parenting toolkit "Children—What does it involve?" and the Real-Care-Baby simulator among students with intellectual disability—A feasibility study. *Journal of Applied Research in Intellectual Disabilities, 32*(2), 380–389. https://doi.org/10.1111/jar.12535

Janeslätt, G., Lindstedt, H., & Adolfsson, P. (2015). Daily time management and influence of environmental factors on use of electronic planning devices in adults with mental disability. *Disability and Rehabilitation: Assistive Technology, 10*(5), 371–377. https://doi.org/10.3109/17483107.2014.917124

Joosten, A. V., & Bundy, A. C. (2010). Sensory processing and stereotypical and repetitive behaviour in children with autism and intellectual disability. *Australian Occupational Therapy Journal, 57*(6), 366–372. https://doi.org/10.1111/j.1440-1630.2009.00835.x

Kåhlin, I., Kjellberg, A., & Hagberg, J. E. (2016). Choice and control for people ageing with intellectual disability in group homes. *Scandinavian Journal of Occupational Therapy, 23*(2), 127–137. https://doi.org/10.3109/11038128.2015.1095235

Karunakaran, M., Sugi, S., & Rajendran, K. (2018). Effectiveness of cognitive orientation to daily occupational performance to improve shopping skills in children with learning disability. *Indian Journal of Occupational Therapy, 50*(3), 92–97. https://doi.org/10.4103/0445-7706.244551

King, E., Okodogbe, T., Burke, E., McCarron, M., McCallion, P., & O'Donovan, M. A. (2017). Activities of daily living and transition to community living for adults with intellectual disabilities. *Scandinavian Journal of Occupational Therapy, 24*(5), 357–365. https://doi.org/10.1080/11038128.2016.1227369

Osiceanu, M. E., & Zaharescu, S. (2017). Occupational therapy's role in recovery of children with mental disabilities. *Clinical and Experimental Psychology, 3*(3), Article 1000167. https://doi.org/10.4172/2471-2701.1000167

Porter, R. S. (Ed.). (2018). *Merck manual of diagnosis and therapy* (20th ed.). Merck Sharp & Dohme.

Sachdeva, R., & Rao, C. S. (2012). Community participation activities involving money handling skills of children with learning disabilities as compared to children with typical development aged 10 to 14 years. *Indian Journal of Occupational Therapy, 44*(2), 25–31.

Selanikyo, E., Weintraub, N., & Yalon-Chamovitz, S. (2018). Effectiveness of the Co-PID for students with moderate intellectual disability. *American Journal of Occupational Therapy, 72*(2), Article 7202205090. https://doi.org/10.5014/ajot.2018.024109

Selanikyo, E., Yalon-Chamovitz, S., & Weintraub, N. (2017). Enhancing classroom participation of students with intellectual and developmental disabilities. *Canadian Journal of Occupational Therapy, 84*(2), 76–86. https://doi.org/10.1177/0008417416661346

Sharfi, K., & Rosenblum, S. (2016). Executive functions, time organization and quality of life among adults with learning disabilities. *PLOS ONE, 11*(12), Article e0166939. https://doi.org/10.1371/journal.pone.0166939

Shepherd, K. (2017). Narrative reasoning for a mystery condition: Sensory diet for an adult with intellectual disability. *OT Practice, 22*(20), 22–23.

Sköld, A., & Janeslätt, G. K. (2017). Self-rating of daily time management in children: Psychometric properties of the Time-S. *Scandinavian Journal of Occupational Therapy, 24*(3), 178–186. https://doi.org/10.1080/11038128.2016.1185465

Suman, M. (2019). Best practices in supporting students with intellectual disability. In G. Frolek Clark, J. E. Rioux, & B. E. Chandler (Eds.), *Best practices for occupational therapy in schools* (2nd ed., pp. 271–278). AOTA Press.

Wennberg, B., & Kjellberg, A. (2010). Participation when using cognitive assistive devices—From the perspective of people with intellectual disabilities. *Occupational Therapy International, 17,* 168–176. https://doi.org/10.1002/oti.296

Wilkinson, K., & Chapparo, C. (1997). The immediate effects of three occupational therapy interventions on specific play behaviours of three children with developmental disability. In C. Chapparo and J. Ranka (Eds.), *Occupational Performance Model (Australia): Monograph 1* (pp. 66–82). Occupational Performance Network. http://www.occupationalperformance. com/the-immediate-effects-of-three-occupational-therapy-interventions-on-specific-play-behaviours-of-three-children-with-developmental-disability/

Wuang, Y.-P., Ho, G.-S., & Su, C.-Y. (2013). Occupational therapy home program for children with intellectual disabilities: A randomized, controlled trial. *Research in Developmental Disabilities, 34*(1), 528–537. https://doi.org/10.1016/j.ridd.2012.09.008

Wuang, Y.-P., Su, C.-Y., & Huang, M.-H. (2012). Psychometric comparisons of three measures for assessing motor functions in preschoolers with intellectual disabilities. *Journal of Intellectual Disability Research, 56*(6), 567–578. https://doi.org/10.1111/j.1365-2788.2011 .01491.x

BIBLIOGRAPHY

Association of Occupational Therapists of Ireland. (2010). *Best practice guidelines for occupational therapists: Restrictive practices and people with intellectual disabilities.*

Ball, J., & Fazil, Q. (2013). Does engagement in meaningful occupation reduce challenging behaviour in people with intellectual disabilities? A systematic review of the literature. *Journal of Intellectual Disabilities, 17*(1), 64–77. https://doi.org/10.1177/1744629512473557

Gappmayer, G. (2019). Exploring neoliberalism in care for people with intellectual disabilities: A practice theory approach. *Journal of Occupational Science, 26*(2), 258–274. https://doi.org/ 10.1080/14427591.2019.1596830

Haertl, K. (Ed.). (2014). *Adults with intellectual and developmental disabilities: Strategies for occupational therapy.* AOTA Press.

Janeslätt, G. K., Holmqvist, K. L., White, S., & Holmefur, M. (2018). Assessment of time management skills: Psychometric properties of the Swedish version. *Scandinavian Journal of Occupational Therapy, 25*(3), 153–161. https://doi.org/10.1080/11038128.2017.1375009

Kåhlin, I., Kjellberg, A., Nord, C., & Hagberg, J. E. (2015). Lived experiences of ageing and later life in older people with intellectual disabilities. *Ageing & Society, 35*(3), 602–628. https:// doi.org/10.1017/S0144686X13000949

Leonard, H., Foley, K. R., Pikora, T., Bourke, J., Wong, K., McPherson, L., Lennox, N., & Downs, J. (2016). Transition to adulthood for young people with intellectual disability: The experiences of their families. *European Child & Adolescent Psychiatry, 25*(12), 1369–1381. https:// doi.org/10.1007/s00787-016-0853-2

Lillywhite, A., & Haines, D. (2010). *Occupational therapy and people with learning disabilities: Findings from a research study.* College of Occupational Therapists.

Mahoney, W. J., Roberts, E., Bryze, K., & Parker Kent, J. A. (2016). Occupational engagement and adults with intellectual disabilities. *American Journal of Occupational Therapy, 70*(1), Article 7001350030. https://doi.org/10.5014/ajot.2016.016576

Royal College of Occupational Therapists. (2019). *Leading fulfilled lives: Occupational therapy supporting people with learning disabilities.*

Tinkler, J. (2010). Working with people with learning disabilities—Everyone's job. *Mental Health Occupational Therapy, 15*(2), Article 4546.

Yalon-Chamovitz, S., Selanikyo, E., Artzi, N., Prigal, Y., & Fishman, R. (2010). Occupational therapy and intellectual and developmental disability throughout the life cycle: Position paper. *IJOT: The Israeli Journal of Occupational Therapy, 19*(1), E3–E7.

Low Birth Weights

See also Feeding Disorders, High- or At-Risk Infant or Child, Premature Infant,
and specific disorders such as Developmental Coordination Disorder.

Description

The Centers for Disease Control and Prevention (2020) states that normal birth weight is considered to be 2,500–4,200 grams (5 lb, 8 oz to 9 lb, 4 oz). Low birth weight is less than 2,500 grams (5 lb, 8 oz). Very low birth weight is less than 1,500 grams (3 lb, 4 oz). Extremely low birth weight is less than 1,000 grams (2 lb, 3 oz). Persons born with low birth weights may be more vulnerable to motor and cognitive impairments than those born weighing within normal limits (Oliveira et al., 2011).

Cause

Major causes of low birth weight are premature birth and intrauterine growth restrictions. Other causes are previous history of low birth baby or premature birth; multiple fetuses (twins, triplets, etc.); abnormalities of the cervix or uterus; maternal chronic health problems, including high blood pressure and diabetes; substance abuse; infections in the mother or fetus; inadequate maternal weight gain; African American women; or women under the age of 17 (Centers for Disease Control and Prevention, 2020).

Evaluation/Assessment

Areas
- Activities of Daily Living/Instrumental ADL: feeding, bathing
- Education/Work: school readiness
- Play/Leisure: play games and toys
- Rest/Sleep: sleep routine
- Social Participation: smiling, laughing
- Sensorimotor: primitive reflexes, motor function, postural control, hand functions (grasp, manipulate, release)
- Cognitive/Perceptual: visual tracking
- Psychosocial: social interaction, state regulation, state organization, habituation (conformity to stimuli, consistency of response)
- Context/Environment: parent education, information resources, social support
- Development (Infant, Child, Adolescent only): developmental delay, developmental milestones
- Comorbidities: hypoxia, ischemia, intraventricular hemorrhage, sensorineural injury, respiratory failure, respiratory distress syndrome, cholestatic liver disease, nutrient deficiency, stress
- Sequelae: intellectual deficiency, spastic diplegic cerebral palsy, microcephaly, seizures, hydrocephalus, hearing or visual impairment, retinopathy of prematurity, strabismus, myopia, bronchopulmonary dysplasia, bronchospasm, osteopenia, fractures, failure to thrive, developmental coordination disorder, ventilator dependence

Instruments

Instruments Developed by Occupational Therapy Personnel
- Developmental Coordination Disorder Questionnaire '07 (DCDQ '07; Wilson et al., 2007)

Instruments Developed by Other Professionals and Used by Occupational Therapy Personnel
- Alberta Infant Motor Scale (AIMS; Piper & Darrah, 1992)
- Bruininks-Oseretsky Test of Motor Proficiency (2nd ed.; BOT-2; Bruininks & Bruininks, 2005)
- Early Screening Inventory 3 (ESI-3; Meisels et al., 2019)
- Home Observation for Measurement of the Environment (HOME; Caldwell & Bradley, 2003)

- Infant Neurological International Battery (INFANIB; Ellison, 1994)
- Minnesota Child Development Inventory (MCDI; Kopparthi et al., 1991)
- Movement Assessment Battery for Children (2nd ed.; M-ABC-2; Henderson et al., 2007)
- Neonatal Behavioral Assessment Scale (4th ed.; NBAS-4; Brazelton & Nugent, 2011)
- Neonatal Medical Index (NMI; Korner et al., 1993)
- Peabody Developmental Motor Scales (3rd ed.; PDMS-3; Folio & Fewell, 2023)
- Swanson, Nolan, and Pelham Teacher and Parent Rating Scale (SNAP-IV; Swanson, 2007)
- Test of Infant Motor Performance (3rd ed.; TIMP-3; Campbell et al., 2012)
- Vineland Adaptive Behavior Scales (3rd ed.; Vineland-3; Sparrow et al., 2016)
- Wechsler Intelligence Scale for Children (5th ed.; WISC-V; Wechsler, 2014)
- Wechsler Preschool and Primary Scale of Intelligence (4th ed.; WPPSI-IV; Wechsler, 2012)

Problems/Issues

Activities of Daily Living/Instrumental ADL
- Infant and child may be delayed in acquiring basic ADL skills (feeding, dressing, grooming, bathing, toileting, mobility, communication).[*]

Education/Work
- Child may be delayed in acquiring school readiness and academic achievement (Maitra et al., 2014).

Play/Leisure
- Infant and child may be delayed in acquiring play skills with toys or play simple games.

Rest/Sleep
- Infant and child may have sleep disturbances.

Social Participation
- Child may be delayed in ability to participate in social activities.

Sensorimotor
- Infant and child may demonstrate primitive reflexes beyond time or age normally displayed.
- Infant and child may be delayed in acquiring gross motor skills such as rolling over, sitting up, creeping, and crawling.
- Infant and child may be delayed in acquiring postural control needed for head up in prone, assuming all-four position, weight shifting, standing, walking.
- Infant and child may be delayed in demonstrating hand functions (reach, grasp, manipulate, release, pinch; Wang et al., 2014).
- Infant and child requiring mechanical ventilation may demonstrate delay in gross motor skills (Nazi & Aliabadi, 2015; Tsai et al., 2014).

Cognitive/Perceptual
- Child may be delayed in use of working memory and ability to follow two- or three-step commands/instructions.
- Child may demonstrate delayed (take more) time to make decisions and make more errors.
- Child may be delayed in use of perceptual skills, such as spatial relations.

Psychosocial
- Infant and parent may be delayed in developing infant–parent bonding.
- Child may be delayed in developing social relations skills, such as taking turns or sharing material.
- Child may be delayed in developing habituation (Amini et al., 2016).
- Child at age 5 may demonstrate delayed adaptive behavior (Howe et al., 2016).

---

[*] Pineda (2011) did not find that infants with low birth weight had increased difficulty with breastfeeding.

Context/Environment
- Parents may lack information on managing a low weight infant and what to expect in the future (Dür et al., 2018).
- Parents may lack knowledge and access to community and internet resources.

Intervention/Treatment

Models and programs developed by occupational therapy personnel: None identified. Models and programs developed by other professionals but used by occupational therapy personnel include early intervention (Park et al., 2014), and physical and occupational therapy services (Watkins et al., 2014). Team members include physicians, neonatologists, nursing personnel, psychologists, geneticists, physical therapists, and occupational therapy personnel. Goal is to promote normal growth and development and prevent development delay when possible.

Activities of Daily Living/Instrumental ADL
- Support breastfeeding, but be aware of which maternal groups are at risk for failure (Pineda, 2011).
- Assist in weaning infant off ventilator.
- Monitor development of basic ADL skills.
- Promote early intervention to support development of basic ADL skills.

Education/Work
- Monitor development of school readiness skills.
- Promote early intervention if delays are evident.

Play/Leisure
- Monitor development of play skills (use of toys and engagement in games).
- Promote early intervention if delays are evident.

Rest/Sleep
- Monitor sleep routine.
- Provide assistance to parents to improve sleep behavior.

Social Participation
- Monitor participation in social activities.
- Promote early intervention if delays are noted.

Sensorimotor
- Monitor development of motor skills (rolling over, sitting up, creeping, crawling, standing, walking; Edwards et al., 2011; Zwicker et al., 2013).
- Monitor development of hand skills, especially visual motor integration (Wang et al., 2014).
- Promote early intervention when delay is detected.

Cognitive/Perceptual
- Monitor development of cognitive and perceptual skills.
- Promote early intervention when delay is noted.

Psychosocial
- Assist parents to feel empowered to care for their infant.
- Monitor development of social interaction skills.
- Promote early intervention when delay is reported.

Context/Environment
- Provide information and opportunity to practice skills to parents on caring for low-birth-weight infants.
- Assist parents to make use of available resources such as support groups and online resources.

Precautions/Safety Considerations

Prolonged use of ventilator assistance interferes with neurological development.

Prognosis and Outcome

Variable. Some infants born with low weight values appear to "catch up" with typically developing children by early childhood. Others show varying degrees of delay that are measureable into school age and beyond (Poole et al., 2017; Poole et al., 2018; Poole et al, 2015a, 2015b). Still others develop specific disorders outlined under Sequelae (see above).

REFERENCES

Amini, M., Aliabadi, F., Alizade, M., Kalani, M., & Qorbani, M. (2016). The relationship between motor function and behavioral function in infants with low birth weight. *Iranian Journal of Child Neurology, 10*(4), 49–55.

Centers for Disease Control and Prevention. (2020). *Birthweight and gestation.* https://www.cdc.gov/nchs/factats/birthweight.htm

Dür, M., Brückner, V., Oberleitner-Leeb, C., Fuiko, R., Matter, B., & Berger, A. (2018). Clinical relevance of activities meaningful to parents of preterm infants with very low birth weight: A focus group study. *PLOS ONE, 13*(8), Article e0202189. https://doi.org/10.1371/journal.pone.0202189

Edwards, J., Berube, M., Erlandson, K., Haug, S., Johnstone, H., Meagher, M., Sarkodee-Adoo, S., & Zwicker, J. G. (2011). Developmental coordination disorder in school-aged children born very preterm and/or at very low birth weight: A systematic review. *Journal of Developmental and Behavioral Pediatrics, 32*(9), 678–687. https://doi.org/10.1097/DBP.0b013e31822a396a

Howe, T.-H., Sheu, C.-F., Hsu, Y.-W., Wang, T.-N., & Wang, L.-W. (2016). Predicting neurodevelopmental outcomes at preschool age for children with very low birth weight. *Research in Developmental Disabilities, 48*, 231–241. https://doi.org/10.1016/j.ridd.2015.11.003

Maitra, K., Park, H. Y., Eggenberger, J., Matthiessen, A., Knight, E., & Ng, B. (2014). Difficulty in mental, neuromusculoskeletal, and movement-related school functions associated with low birthweight or preterm birth: A meta-analysis. *American Journal of Occupational Therapy, 68*(2), 140–148. https://doi.org/10.5014/ajot.2014.009985

Nazi, S., & Aliabadi, F. (2015). Comparison of motor development of low birth weight (LBW) infants with and without using mechanical ventilation and normal birth weight infants. *Medical Journal of the Islamic Republic of Iran, 29*, Article 301.

Oliveira, G. E., Magalhães, L. C., & Salmela, L. F. T. (2011). Relationship between very low birth weight, environmental factors, and motor and cognitive development of children of 5 and 6 years old. *Brazilian Journal of Physical Therapy, 15*(2), 138–145. https://doi.org/10.1590/s1413-35552011000200009

Park, H. Y., Maitra, K., Achon, J., Loyola, E., & Rincón, M. (2014). Effects of early intervention on mental or neuromusculoskeletal and movement-related functions in children born low birthweight or preterm: A meta-analysis. *American Journal of Occupational Therapy, 68*(3), 268–276. https://doi.org/10.5014/ajot.2014.010371

Pineda, R. G. (2011). Predictors of breastfeeding and breastmilk feeding among very low birth weight infants. *Breastfeeding Medicine 6*(1), 15–19. https://doi.org/10.1089/bfm.2010.0010

Poole, K. L., Islam, U. A., Schmidt, L., Missiuna, C., Saigal, S., Boyle, M. H., & Van Lieshout, R. J. (2017). Childhood motor function, health related quality of life and social functioning among emerging adults born at term or extremely low birth weight. *Journal of Developmental and Physical Disabilities, 29*, 369–383. https://doi.org/10.1007/s10882-016-9530-0

Poole, K. L., Schmidt, L. A., Ferro, M. A., Missiuna, C., Saigal, S., Boyle, M. H., & Van Lieshout, R. J. (2018). Early developmental influences on self-esteem trajectories from adolescence through adulthood: Impact of birth weight and motor skills. *Development and Psychopathology, 30*(1), 113–123. https://doi.org/10.1017/S0954579417000505

Poole, K. L., Schmidt, L. A., Missiuna, C., Saigal, S., Boyle, M. H., & Van Lieshout, R. J. (2015a). Motor coordination difficulties in extremely low birth weight survivors across four decades. *Journal of Developmental and Behavioral Pediatrics, 36*(7), 521–528. https://doi.org/10.1097/DBP.0000000000000199

Poole, K. L., Schmidt, L. A., Missiuna, C., Saigal, S., Boyle, M. H., & Van Lieshout, R. J. (2015b). Motor coordination and mental health in extremely low birth weight survivors during the first four decades of life. *Research in Developmental Disabilities, 43–44,* 87–96. https://doi.org/10.1016/j.ridd.2015.06.004

Tsai, W.-H., Hwang, Y.-S., Hung, T.-Y., Weng, S.-F., Lin, S.-J., & Chang, W.-T. (2014). Association between mechanical ventilation and neurodevelopmental disorders in a nationwide cohort of extremely low birth weight infants. *Research in Developmental Disabilities, 35*(7), 1544–1550. https://doi.org/10.1016/j.ridd.2014.03.048

Wang, T.-N., Howe, T.-H., Lin, K.-C., & Hsu, Y.-W. (2014). Hand function and its prognostic factors of very low birth weight preterm children up to a corrected age of 24 months. *Research in Developmental Disabilities, 35*(2), 322–329. https://doi.org/10.1016/j.ridd.2013.11.023

Watkins, S., Jonsson-Funk, M., Brookhart, M. A., Rosenberg, S. A., O'Shea, T. M., & Daniels, J. (2014). Preschool motor skills following physical and occupational therapy services among non-disabled very low birth weight children. *Maternal and Child Health Journal 18,* 821–828. https://doi.org/10.1007/s10995-013-1306-x

Zwicker, J. G., Yoon, S. W., MacKay, M., Petrie-Thomas, J., Rogers, M., & Synnes, A. R. (2013). Perinatal and neonatal predictors of developmental coordination disorder in very low birthweight children. *Archives of Disease in Childhood, 98*(2), 118–122. https://doi.org/10.1136/archdischild-2012-302268

Osteogenesis Imperfecta

Also called Adair-Dighton syndrome, brittle bones disorder, osteopsathyrosis, fragilitas ossium.

Description

Osteogenesis imperfecta is a genetic disorder of the collagen (connective) tissue. The disorder is inherited as an autosomal-dominant trait and is characterized by diffuse abnormal brittle and fragile bones that may be fractured by very slight trauma. Other manifestations of the disorder include blue sclera (eye membrane), translucent skin, hyperextensibility (laxity) of ligaments, hypoplasia (underdevelopment) of the teeth, recurrent nose bleeds (epistaxis), excessive sweating (diaphoresis), mild hyperpyrexia (elevated temperature), and a tendency to bruise easily and develop otosclerosis (hardening of bones in the middle ear), resulting in hearing loss (O'Toole, 2017). There are eight types of osteogenesis imperfecta (OI):

- *Type I (autosomal dominant).* Mildest form. Most common and mildest type with few obvious clinical signs. Person is of normal or near normal height when compared with peers and unaffected family members.
- *Type II (autosomal dominant).* Most severe. Infants may die within weeks from respiratory or heart complications. Numerous fractures and bone deformity evident at birth. Person is short in stature with underdeveloped lungs and low birth weight.
- *Type III (autosomal recessive).* Severe. Progressive bone deformity, especially in long bones. Fractures are present at birth. Person has short stature, a barrel-shaped rib cage, spinal curvature, compression fractures of vertebrae, and triangular face.
- *Type IV (autosomal dominant).* Moderate. Between Type I and Type III in severity and height (obtained). Mild to moderate bone deformities, spinal curvature, compression fracture of vertebrae, and barrel-shaped rib cage.

- *Type V (autosomal dominant)*. Moderate. Similar to Type IV in appearance and symptoms. Has large hypertrophic calluses form at fracture or surgical procedure sites. Has calcification of membrane between radius and ulna, restricting forearm rotation.
- *Type VI (autosomal dominant)*. Moderate. Extremely rare. Similar to Type IV in appearance. Distinguished by characteristic mineralization defect seen in biopsied bone.
- *Type VII (autosomal recessive)*. Severe. Phenotype is moderate to severe. Rhizomelia (disproportional, usually shortened proximal bones in the hips and shoulders).
- *Type VIII (autosomal recessive)*. Very severe. Similar to Type II, but with recess inheritance. Severe growth deficiency and undermineralization of the skeleton (Osteogenesis Imperfecta Foundation, n.d.).

Cause

Ninety percent of people who have one of the major types of osteogenesis imperfecta have mutations in the genes encoding the pro-alpha chains of Type I procollagen (a structural component of bones, ligaments, and tendons), *COLIA1* or *COLIA 2* (Porter, 2018).

Evaluation/Assessment

Areas

- Activities of Daily Living/Instrumental ADL: self-maintenance skills are age appropriate (eating, dressing, grooming, bathing/showering, toileting, mobility, transfers), independent living skills are age appropriate (choices, meal planning and preparation, light housekeeping, shopping, driving, pet care)
- Education/Work: school or workplace modification, assistive technology
- Play/Leisure: play skills, types of leisure occupations, location, frequency
- Rest/Sleep: sleep habits
- Social Participation: type, location, frequency, with whom
- Sensorimotor: muscle strength, joint range of motion, endurance, visual impairment, hearing loss
- Cognitive/Perceptual: usually cognition is within normal range
- Psychosocial: interpersonal relations, self-efficacy
- Context/Environment: information and resources, accessibility, adapted devices, assistive technology
- Development (Infant, Child, Adolescent only): developmental milestones
- Comorbidities: respiratory disorders including asthma, short stature, rib cage deformities, scoliosis, hearing loss, brittle teeth, visual impairment, joint and ligament laxity, cardiac defects

Instruments

Instruments Developed by Occupational Therapy Personnel

- Children's Assessment of Participation and Enjoyment and Preferences for Activities of Children (CAPE/PAC; King et al., 2004)
- Impact of OI/Experiences, Challenges and Expectations (I-OI/ECE; Dogba et al., 2016, in References)
- Pediatric Evaluation of Disability Inventory (PEDI; Haley et al., 1992)
- Sample Questionnaire (for activities and participation; see Montpetit et al., 2011, in References)

Instruments Developed by Other Professionals and Used by Occupational Therapy Personnel

- 6-Minute Walk Test (and shorter timed/distance walk tests; American Thoracic Society, 2002)
- Alberta Infant Motor Scale (AIMS; Piper & Darrah, 1992)
- Barthel Index (BI; Mahoney & Barthel, 1965)
- Bayley Scales of Infant and Toddler Development (4th ed.; Bayley-4; Bayley & Aylward, 2019)
- Beighton Score of Hypermobility (Beighton Score; Smits-Engelsman et al., 2011)
- Berg Balance Scale (BBS; Berg et al., 1989)

- Brief Assessment of Motor Function: Oral Motor Deglutition Scale (BAMF-OMD; Sonies et al., 2009)
- Bruininks-Oseretsky Test of Motor Proficiency (2nd ed.; BOT-2; Bruininks & Bruininks, 2005)
- Checklist Individual Strength (CIS; Vercoulen et al., 1994)
- Childhood Health Assessment Questionnaire (CHAQ; Singh et al., 1994)
- Disabilities of the Arm, Shoulder, and Hand (3rd ed.; DASH-3; Kennedy et al., 2011)
- Functional Mobility Test (FMT; Cohen et al., 2012)
- Gillette Functional Assessment Questionnaire (GFAQ; Novacheck et al., 2000)
- Grip strength (dynamometer; Jamar Dynamometer; Wang et al., 2018)
- Joint range of motion (goniometry; Shurtleff & Kaskutuas, 2018)
- Manual Muscle Test (MMT; Kaskutas, 2018)
- Movement Assessment Battery for Children (2nd ed.; M-ABC-2; Henderson et al., 2007)
- Peabody Developmental Motor Scales (3rd ed.; PDMS-3; Folio & Fewell, 2023)
- Pediatric Berg Balance Scale (PBBS; Franjoine et al., 2003)
- Pediatric Outcomes Data Collection Instrument (PODCI; Lerman et al., 2005)
- Timed Up and Go test (TUG; Podsiadlo & Richardson, 1991)
- Tinetti Balance Scale (TBS; Tinnetti et al., 1990)
- Visual Analogue Scale (VAS) Numeric Pain Rating Scale (NPRS) pain scale (scored: 0 = *no pain*, 10 = *worst pain ever*)
- Wong-Baker FACES Pain Rating Scale (FACES; Wong & Baker, 1998)

Problems/Issues

Activities of Daily Living/Instrumental ADL
- Person may lack self-maintenance skills that are age appropriate.
- Person may lack independent living skills that are age appropriate.
- Person may have fragile skin that bruises easily.
- Person may have soft, discolored teeth.

Education/Work
- Person may need assistance with accessibility to school or work (paid or unpaid).
- Person may need assistive technology to help with academic or work assignments.
- Person may need assistance in vocational exploration and choice.

Play/Leisure
- Person may need to develop play skills that are age appropriate.
- Person may need to explore and try out different leisure occupations.

Rest/Sleep
- Person may have breathing problems that interfere with sleep.
- Person may complain of being overheated or excessive sweating at night.

Social Participation
- Person may lack opportunity to participate in social activities that are age appropriate.

Sensorimotor
- Infant/child: all bones, but especially arms and legs, break easily; vertebrae may have compression fractures.
- Person usually has "loose" hyperextensibility, laxity in joints.
- Person may have muscle weakness.
- Person may have bone deformities such as bowing of the legs.
- Person may have a barrel-shaped chest, which may result in breathing restrictions.
- Person may have a curved spine or scoliosis.
- Person may develop joint contractures.
- Person may experience pain (Nghiem et al., 2018).
- Person may experience lack of stamina and fatigue.

- Person may have hearing loss in early adulthood.
- Person may sweat excessively.

Cognitive/Perceptual
- No specific problems due to OI.

Psychosocial (Tsimicalis et al., 2016)
- Person's family or caregivers may be overprotective.
- Person may experience anxiety and depression about future.
- Person may lack self-confidence and a sense of self-efficacy.
- Person may experience decreased quality of life (Dahan-Oliel, Oliel, et al., 2016).
- Person may experience stigma due to physical appearance and decreased ability to "keep up" with others physically.
  - Person may have a triangle-shaped face that is noticeable to others.
  - Person may have an unusual appearance, such as discoloration of the whites of the eye (sclera), which may be blue, purple, or gray, which is noticeable to others.

Context/Environment
- Parents may lack information about OI, including care to reduce fractures.
- Parents and person may lack information about available community and internet resources.
- Parents and person may lack information about adapted devices and assistive technology, including training in use and care for devices and equipment.
- Person may lack social support from family.
- Person may lack access to community resources (Dahan-Oliel, Shikako-Thomas, et al., 2016).

Intervention/Treatment

Models and programs developed by occupational therapy personnel include occupational therapy intervention (de Paiva et al., 2018). Models and programs developed by other professionals but used by occupational therapy personnel include Botox injection (Fortin et al., 2018), consensus statement (Mueller et al., 2018), Fassier-Duval femoral rodding (Ruck et al., 2011), knee surgery (Yang et al., 2010), and multidisciplinary approach (Marr et al., 2017). Team members include physicians, orthopedic surgeons, neurosurgeons, geneticists, psychologists, nursing personnel, physical therapy personnel, speech hearing and language personnel, social workers, dentists, and occupational therapy personnel. Goals are to assist each person to reach maximum in developmental milestones and achieve level of independence while minimizing fractures and deformities (Mueller et al., 2018).

Problems/Issues

Activities of Daily Living/Instrumental ADL
- Infancy
  - Bathing is recommended using a thick towel or foam support in the bath basin and enough water to provide buoyancy to encourage movement and kicking of lower limbs.
  - Clothing should be lightweight cotton to absorb sweating.
- Assist client to learn to perform independently with or without assistive devices; basic ADLs, including eating, dressing, grooming, toileting, bathing, and transfers.
- Assist client to develop and practice independent living skills including meal preparation (cooking, baking), home management, shopping, and managing transportation needs.

Education/Work
- Assist client to explore and participate in paid and unpaid work activities.

Play/Leisure
- Assist child to develop and engage in age-appropriate play activities.
- Assist client to explore and engage in leisure occupations within client's abilities.

Rest/Sleep
- Assist client to review sleep habits, routines, and environment to maximize quality of sleep and decrease sense of being "overheated."
- Consider use of cotton bedding and clothing to absorb sweat.

Social Participation
- Assist client to explore and participate in social activities within client's ability level.

Sensorimotor
- Promote attainment of developmental milestones within client's physical abilities using specialized, adapted equipment such as a crawler designed to fit child's body.
- Assist client to develop and adjust exercise program to maintain range of motion within joint mobility.
- Provide instruction on pain management.
- Provide instruction and practice in energy conservation and work simplification.

Cognitive/Perceptual
- Person may need practice in using executive functions such as planning, problem solving, using judgment of safety, evaluating results.
- Person may need practice in directing others to provide safe transfers.
- Provide instruction in time management including activity pacing.

Psychosocial
- Provide opportunity to discuss with client what roles he or she is able to perform and which roles may be assumed by other household members including family members, partners, or personal care attendants.
- Provide opportunity to discuss with client concerns about others providing too much over-protection and restrictions.
- Provide stress reducing and coping strategies to address anxiety and depression such as meditation, deep-breathing exercises, and mindfulness.
- Provide opportunity to discuss feelings of stigmatization.
- Assist client to achieve and maintain a satisfactory quality of life.

Context/Environment
- Provide instruction to family and caregivers in safe handling techniques to minimize fracture risk.
- Provide instruction to family and caregivers promote good body alignment to decrease potential for deformities. Supine position is suggested for the first 2 years (Marr et al., 2017).
- Assist client in selection, use, and maintenance of assistive devices and technology.
- Support client in learning to promote accessibility to venues and environments.
- Encourage discussion between client and family or caregivers about overprotection versus reality of safety concerns to minimize injury.

Precautions/Safety Considerations

Supine position in infancy may increase risk of brachycephaly and plagiocephaly. Frequent head turning may be important. Prone lying, use of fabric rolls, and wedges can facilitate positioning. Transport using car seats that allow the infant or child to lay flat or with maximum recline are recommended.

Prognosis and Outcome

OI is a chronic, lifelong disorder. Problems and issues change as the person develops and need to be addressed to manage overall health and quality of life to permit maximum performance and participation in everyday occupations.

REFERENCES

Dahan-Oliel, N., Oliel, S., Tsimicalis, A., Montpetit, K., Rauch, F., & Dogba, M. J. (2016). Quality of life in osteogenesis imperfecta: A mixed-methods systematic review. *American Journal of Medical Genetics Part A, 170A*(1), 62–76. https://doi.org/10.1002/ajmg.a.37377

Dahan-Oliel, N., Shikako-Thomas, K., Mazer, B., & Majnemer, A. (2016). Adolescents with disabilities participate in the shopping mall: Facilitators and barriers framed according to the ICF. *Disability & Rehabilitation, 38*(21), 2101–2113. https://doi.org/10.3109/09638288.2015.1114033

de Paiva, D. F., de Oliveira, M. L., & Almohalha, L. (2018). Perceptions of people with osteogenesis imperfecta about the interventions of the occupational therapy and its possibilities of care. *Cadernos Brasileiros de Terapia Ocupacional, 26*(2), 390–407. https://doi.org/10.4322/2526-8910.ctoA01135

Dogba, M. J., Dahan-Oliel, N., Snider, L., Glorieux, F. H., Durigova, M., Palomo, T., Cordey, M., Bédard, M.-H., Bedos, C., & Rauch, F. (2016). Involving families with osteogenesis imperfecta in health service research: Joint development of the OI/ECE Questionnaire. *PLOS ONE, 11*(1), Article e0147654. https://doi.org/10.1371/journal.pone.0147654

Fortin, M., Dahan-Oliel, N., Montpetit, K., Narayanan, U., Saint-Martin, C., & Hamdy, R. C. (2018). Radiological and clinical findings following distraction osteogenesis of the lower limb in children with or without Botox injection: A preliminary report. *Journal of Limb Lengthening & Reconstruction, 4*(1), 41–48. https://doi.org/10.4103/jllr.jllr_16_17

Marr, C., Seasman, A., & Bishop, N. (2017). Managing the patient with osteogenesis imperfecta: A multidisciplinary approach. *Journal of Multidisciplinary Healthcare, 10*, 145–155. https://doi.org/10.2147/JMDH.S113483

Montpetit, K., Dahan-Oliel, N., Ruck-Gibis, J., Fassier, F., Rauch, F., & Glorieux, F. (2011). Activities and participation in young adults with osteogenesis imperfecta. *Journal of Pediatric Rehabilitation Medicine, 4*, 13–22. https://doi.org/10.3233/PRM-2011-0149

Mueller, B., Engelbert, R., Baratta-Ziska, F., Bartels, B., Blanc, N., Brizola, E., Fraschini, P., Hill, C., Marr, C., Mills, L., Montpetit, K., Pacey, V., Rodriguez Molina, M., Schuuring, M., Verhille, C., de Vries, O., Yeung, E. H. K., & Semler, O. (2018). Consensus statement on physical rehabilitation in children and adolescents with osteogenesis imperfecta. *Orphanet Journal of Rare Diseases, 13*, Article 158. https://doi.org/10.1186/s13023-018-0905-4

Nghiem, T., Chougui, K., Michalovic, A., Lalloo, C., Stinson, J., Lafrance, M.-E., Palomo, T., Dahan-Oliel, N., & Tsimicalis, A. (2018). Pain experiences of adults with osteogenesis imperfecta: An integrative review. *Canadian Journal of Pain, 2*(1), 9–20. https://doi.org/10.1080/24740527.2017.1422115

Osteogenesis Imperfecta Foundation. (n.d.). *Physical and occupational therapists guide to treating osteogenesis imperfect.* https://oif.org/wp-content/uploads/2019/08/PT_guide_final.pdf

O'Toole, M. T. (Ed.). (2017). *Mosby's dictionary of medicine, nursing & health professions* (10th ed.). Elsevier.

Porter, R. S. (Ed.). (2018). *The Merck manual of diagnosis and therapy* (20th ed.). Merck Sharp & Dohme.

Ruck, J., Dahan-Oliel, N., Montpetit, K., Rauch, F., & Fassier, F. (2011). Fassier–Duval femoral rodding in children with osteogenesis imperfecta receiving bisphosphonates: Functional outcomes at one year. *Journal of Children's Orthopaedics, 5*(3), 217–224. https://doi.org/10.1007/s11832-011-0341-7

Tsimicalis, A., Denis-Larocque, G., Michalovic, A., Lepage, C., Williams, K., Yao, T. R., Palomo, T., Dahan-Oliel, N., Le May, S., & Rauch, F. (2016). The psychosocial experience of individuals living with osteogenesis imperfecta: A mixed-methods systematic review. *Quality of Life Research 25*, 1877–1896. https://doi.org/10.1007/s11136-016-1247-0

Yang, S. S., Dahan-Oliel, N., Montpetit, K., & Hamdy, R. C. (2010). Ambulation gains after knee surgery in children with arthrogryposis. *Journal of Pediatric Orthopaedics, 30*(8), 863–869. https://doi.org/10.1097/BPO.0b013e3181f5a0c8

PANS and PANDAS

Also called PITAND (pediatric infection-triggered autoimmune neuropsychiatric disorder).

Description

PANS is short for Pediatric Acute-Onset Neuropsychiatric Syndrome. PANDAS stands for Pediatric Autoimmune Neuropsychiatric Disorder Syndrome. Both are considered sequelae to strep (streptococcal) infection. The major symptoms are sudden, dramatic, "overnight" episodes of obsessive-compulsive disorder (OCD), and tics. Periods of symptom exacerbation (relapsing) and remission (remitting) are common. Typical age range is 3–12 years (National Institute of Mental Health, 2019). The diagnosis and existence of the disease are new in the past 25 years. Universal acceptance has not been achieved.

Cause

PANS is associated with streptococcal infection unspecified. PANDAS is associated with group A beta-hemolytic streptococcus infection. Behavioral issues may be related to attacks to the basal ganglia.

Evaluation/Assessment

Areas
- Activities of Daily Living/Instrumental ADL: self-maintenance, including eating patterns (anorexia), urinary frequency, enuresis
- Education/Work: academic performance, especially math, handwriting
- Play/Leisure: age-appropriate play skills
- Rest/Sleep: sleep disturbance, bed-wetting, daytime sleepiness
- Social Participation: age-appropriate social skills
- Sensorimotor: choreiform movements, tics, fine motor skills, joint pain, joint stiffness, sensory processing
- Cognitive/Perceptual: attention, processing speed, visual-spatial relations
- Psychosocial: obsessions, compulsions, hyperactivity, impulsivity, separation anxiety, irritability, rage, mood changes, oppositional behavior, personality changes
- Context/Environment: adapted devices, environmental modifications, family quality of life
- Development (Infant, Child, Adolescent only): age-inappropriate behaviors
- Comorbidities and Misdiagnoses: attention-deficit/hyperactivity disorder, autism spectrum disorder, obsessive compulsive disorder, Tourette's syndrome

Instruments
Instruments Developed by Occupational Therapy Personnel
- Dynamic Loewenstein Occupational Therapy Cognitive Assessment for Children (DLOTCA-Ch; Katz et al., 2012)
- Pediatric Activity Card Sort (PACS; Mandick et al., 2004)
- Short Child Occupational Profile (Version 2.2; SCOPE; Bowyer et al., 2008)

Instruments Developed by Other Professionals and Used by Occupational Therapy Personnel
- Conduct Disorder Scale (CDS; Gilliam, 2002)

Problems/Issues

Activities of Daily Living/Instrumental ADL
- Child may suddenly only eat certain foods.
- Child may be fearful of choking.
- Child's handwriting may become illegible.

Education/Work
- Child's academic performance may decrease, especially in math.

Play/Leisure
- Child may have difficulty playing appropriately with others.
- Child may have restricted areas of interest.

Rest/Sleep
- Child may bed-wet after several months or years of being dry all night.
- Child may have difficulty going to sleep.
- Child may experience daytime sleepiness.

Social Participation
- Child may have difficulty participating in social activities such as sports, parties, or school functions.

Sensorimotor
- Child often develops tics or jerky movements.
- Child may have difficulty with control of fine motor skills.
- Child may complain of pain in the joints.
- Child may have stiffness in the joints.
- Child usually has sensory changes, especially tactile defensiveness.
- Child may develop sensory sensitivities; usually hypersensitive to auditory or visual input.

Cognitive/Perceptual
- Child usually presents cognitive/mental inflexibility.
- Child often has difficulty with functional cognition.
- Child may have difficulty paying attention.
- Child may have difficulty with memory tasks.
- Child may have difficulty with executive functions such as organizing, sequencing, problem solving.
- Child may exhibit slow processing speed.
- Child may exhibit sensory defensive behavior, especially related to clothing.
- Child may seek more and more sensory input.
- Child may have visual or auditory perceptual disorders.

Psychosocial
- Child usually exhibits obsessive compulsive behavior(s).
- Child may exhibit hyperactivity behavior.
- Child may exhibit fidgety behavior.
- Child may exhibit separation anxiety (not wanting to be left alone).
- Child may exhibit mood changes (sadness, irritability, emotional labile).
- Child may exhibit oppositional or argumentative behavior.
- Child may try to injure self.

Context/Environment
- Family, caregivers, and school personnel need information about PANS and PANDAS.

Intervention/Treatment

During exacerbations, adaptation and compensation techniques can be used to address problems. During remission, remedial techniques can be used to address problems. Models and programs developed by occupational therapy personnel include the Montessori classroom (Luborsky, 2017). Models and programs developed by other professionals but used by occupational therapy personnel: No assessments identified. Team members may include speech–language pathologists, special education teachers, school psychologists, social workers, and school nurses. Additional suggested interventions are listed in Tona and Posner (2011). Other articles discuss etiology and early signs of the disease (Demchick & Eglseder, 2019; Demchick et al., 2019; Tona et al., 2017).

Activities of Daily Living/Instrumental ADL
- Food sensitivities: Provide oral desensitization such as deep pressure to hard palate with thumb, modify textures and flavors to increase variety in diet.
- Choking: Modify texture of foods, include moist foods.
- Language: Give extra time to talk (expression) and listen (reception), use augmentative communication approaches such as cue cards or picture cards if needed.

Education/Work
- Handwriting for school work
  - ▶ Paper: Use built-up writing devices, use horizontal lined paper for writing, vertical lined paper for math, raised lined paper may be helpful, graft paper with "boxes" for each letter, use of a template, red line down left margin to maintain alignment.
  - ▶ Computer: Word processing programs, voice recognition.
  - ▶ Assignments: Audio recording to track assignments, suggest some assignments could be completed using audio rather than print format.
- Math: Provide extended time for tests, use calculator if allowed.

Play/Leisure
- No information identified.

Rest/Sleep
- Deep pressure using a weighted blanket.
- Warm bath with Epsom salts before bedtime.
- White noise, calming music, or calming audio books.
- Monitor bedtime/wake time routines.

Social Participation
- No information identified.

Sensorimotor
- Fatigue (muscle weakness/low tone)
  - ▶ During exacerbation: Modify activities to accommodate for deficits, use sensory approaches to increase arousal, encourage activity to maintain strength and endurance.
  - ▶ During remission: Promote strengthening and endurance activities.
- Joint pain: Instruct and promote use of energy conservation (motion economy) techniques, warm baths with Epsom salts may help ease pain, plan activities after pain medication is taken.
- Tics: Use assistive technology if function is compromised, such as weighted or built-up writing devices, use of computer voice-activated programs.
- Somatosensory: Use deep pressure, neutral warmth.
- Sensory seeking: Provide opportunity for tactile input including vibration, different textures, different textures, figure paints.
- Sensory defensive: Decrease extraneous stimulation, avoid light touch.
- Visual perception: Use visual exercises during remission, avoid during exacerbation.
- Auditor perception: Use therapeutic listening programs during remission.

Cognitive/Perceptual
- Attention: Redirect attention as needed, have child sit in front row closest to teacher, use school website to track schedule if available or use smartphone and computer.
- Memory: Checklists, dry/white boards, electronic devices (smartphone, computer).

- Processing speed: Provide visual handouts, have child use gestures (act out responses), use multisensory approaches such as giving information verbally.

Psychosocial

- Mood changes: Teach child to use "safe" places to "get away" to increase self-control, teach child calming techniques such as deep breathing, use of a weighted blanket, petting a dog or toy dog.
- Anxiety: Teach child progressive relaxation exercises, imagery, yoga, relaxation tapes.
- Obsessive-compulsive behavior: Cognitive-behavior therapy, exposure and response prevention therapy, positive behavior support plans, redirection.
- Behavioral disruption: Assist in identifying trigger events (antecedent situation) and recommend modifications to reduce behavioral reactions.

Context/Environment

- Suggest family and caregivers learn stress-reducing techniques such as use of calming music, yoga, progressive relaxation exercises, and deep breathing.
- Assist family and caregivers to modify schedules, activities, and locations as exacerbations and remissions occur (problem solving). Example: homework may need to be completed after medication is taken (reduce pain), in shorter time periods (attention), and with family members present (separation anxiety).
- Work with family to maintain as normal a routine as possible during period of illness and to reestablish normal routine as illness period subsides.

Precautions/Safety Considerations

Child is at risk for suicidal behavior. Child is at risk for infection: Use infection control techniques (avoid use of items such as ball pits, bins of dried beans or rice, and Play-Doh unless the items have been cleaned or are new). Symptoms will come (exacerbate) and go (remission). Generally, symptoms disappear by puberty. Approaches should be considered temporary, not permanent.

Prognosis and Outcome

Disorder is considered to be self-limiting, but the timetable is highly variable lasting weeks or months.

REFERENCES

Demchick, B. B., & Eglseder, K. (2019). PANDAS: What occupational therapy practitioners should know. *OT Practice, 24*(7), 16–21.

Demchick, B. B., Ehler, J., Marramar, S., Mills, A., & Nuneviller, A. (2019). Family quality of life when raising a child with pediatric autoimmune neuropsychiatric disorder associated with streptococcal infection (PANDAS). *Journal of Occupational Therapy, Schools, & Early Intervention, 12*(2), 182–199. https://doi.org/10.1080/19411243.2019.1592052

Luborsky, B. (2017). Helping children with attentional challenges in a Montessori classroom: The role of the occupational therapist. *NAMTA Journal, 42*(2), 287–352.

National Institute of Mental Health. (2019). *PANDAS–Questions and answers*. https://www.nimh.nih.gov/health/publications/pandas/index.shtml

Tona, J. T., Bhattacharjya, S., & Calaprice, D. (2017). Impact of PANS and PANDAS exacerbations on occupational performance: A mixed-methods study. *American Journal of Occupational Therapy, 71*(3), Article 7103220020. https://doi.org/10.5014/ajot.2017.022285

Tona, J., & Posner, T. (2011). Pediatric autoimmune neuropsychiatric disorders. *OT Practice, 16*(20), 14–19.

Premature Infant

*See also Low Birth Weights, High- or At-Risk Infant or Child,
Feeding Disorders in Children, and list of comorbidities below.*

*Also called preterm infant, prematurity, moderate premature, moderate preterm,
very premature, very preterm, extremely premature, extremely preterm.*

Description

Infants born before 37 weeks' gestation are defined as preterm and have an increased incidence of complications and mortality roughly proportional to the degree of prematurity. Infants born less than 34 weeks' gestation are considered moderately premature. Infants born before 32 weeks' gestation are considered very premature, and those born before 28 weeks are considered extremely premature (Porter, 2018).

Cause

The specific cause of an individual case may be unknown. However, there are five groups of identifiable causes in general (O'Toole, 2017; Porter, 2018): (1) fetal (fetal distress, multiple gestation, erythroblastosis, nonimmune hydrops); (2) placental (placental dysfunction, placenta previa, abruption placentae); (3) uterine (bicornuate uterus, incompetent cervix, or premature dilation); (4) maternal (preeclampsia; chronic medical illness, such as cyanotic heart disease or renal disease; infection; drug abuse, such as cocaine, morphine, or fentanyl); and (5) other (premature rupture of membranes, polyhydramnios, iatrogenic, trauma).

Evaluation/Assessment

Areas

- Activities of Daily Living/Instrumental ADL: feeding
- Education/Work (Infant): not applicable; (Child/Adolescent): academic performance, work skills, accessibility
- Play/Leisure: play skills, leisure interests and activities
- Rest/Sleep: sleep disturbance
- Social Participation (Child/Adolescent): type, frequency, location, with whom
- Sensorimotor: primitive reflexes, positioning, muscle tone, bilateral motor patterns, reciprocal motor patterns, pain, visual tracking
- Cognitive/Perceptual: attention, concentration
- Psychosocial (Infant): parent–child bonding, state regulation; (Child/Adolescent): roles, social interaction
- Context/Environment: information resources, health literacy, cultural beliefs and traditions
- Development (Infant, Child, Adolescent only): milestones

Comorbidities

Dysfunctions are associated with respiratory, cardiovascular, hematologic, gastrointestinal, metabolic-endocrine, neurologic, immunologic, and renal systems. Named disorders include Developmental Coordination Disorder (Edwards et al., 2011; Kwok et al., 2019; Zwicker, Yoon, et al., 2013); allergies, asthma, attention-deficit/hyperactivity disorder, autism spectrum disorder, cerebral palsy, epilepsy, hearing impairment, in-utero exposure (McPherson, Haslam, et al., 2015; Zwicker et al., 2016), psychiatric conditions, specific learning disability, speech–language impairment, visual impairment (with or without glasses; Majnemer et al., 2017). Sensory processing disorder (Ryckman et al., 2017).

Instruments

Instruments Developed by Occupational Therapy Personnel

- Behavior-Based Feeding Questionnaire (BFQ; Howe & Ho, 2009)

- Children's Assessment of Participation and Enjoyment and Preferences for Activities of Children (CAPE/PAC; King et al., 2004)
- Head Turn Preference Scale (HTPS; Dunsirn et al., 2016, in References)
- Infant/Toddler Sensory Profile (ITSP; Dunn, 2002)
- Leiter International Performance Scale (3rd ed.; Leiter-3; Roid et al., 2013)
- Pediatric Evaluation of Disability Inventory (PEDI; Haley et al., 1992)
- Short Sensory Profile (SSP; McIntosh et al., 1999)
- Test of Sensory Functions in Infants (TSFI; DeGangi & Greenspan, 1989)

Instruments Developed by Other Professionals and Used by Occupational Therapy Personnel
- Alberta Infant Motor Scale (AIMS; Piper et al., 1991; see also de Albuquerque et al., 2018, in References)
- Assessment of General Movements (GMs; Einspieler & Prechtl, 2005)
- Assessment of Preterm Infants' Behavior (APIB; Als et al., 2005)
- Bayley Scales of Infant Development (4th ed.; Bayley-4; Bayley & Aylward, 2019; see also de Albuquerque et al., 2018, in References)
- Columbia Mental Maturity Scale (3rd ed.; CMS-3; Burgemeister et al., 1972)
- Denver Developmental Screening Test (2nd ed.; Denver II; Frankenburg et al., 1992)
- Dubowitz Neurological Assessment of the Preterm and Full-Term Infant (Dubowitz et al., 1999)
- Infant-Toddler Social Emotional Assessment (ITSEA; Carter & Briggs-Gowan, 2005)
- Movement Assessment Battery for Children (2nd ed.; M-ABC-2; Henderson et al., 2007)
- Neonatal Behavioral Assessment Scale (4th ed.; NBAS; Brazelton & Nugent, 2011)
- Neonatal Intensive Care Unit (NICU) Network Neurobehavioral Scale (NNNS; Lester et al., 2004)
- Neonatal Medical Index (NMI; Korner et al., 1993)
- Neonatal Oral-Motor Assessment Scale (NOMAS; Braun & Palmer, 1985)
- Neurobehavioral Assessment of the Preterm Infant (2nd ed.; NAPI-2; Korner et al., 2000)
- Neuromotor Behavioral Assessment (NMBA; Carmichael et al., 1997)
- Parenting Stress Index (4th ed.; PSI-4; Abidin, 2012)
- Peabody Developmental Motor Scales (3rd ed.; PDMS-3; Folio & Fewell, 2023)
- Prechtl's Assessment of General Movements (GMs; Einspieler & Prechtl, 2005)
- Score for Neonatal Acute Physiology-II (SNAP-II; Richardson, 1993; see also Zwicker, Grunau, et al., 2013, in References)
- Test of Infant Motor Performance (3rd ed.; TIMP-3; Campbell et al., 2012)

Problems/Issues

Activities of Daily Living/Instrumental ADL
- Infant may have inadequate or poor sucking reflex and delayed oral motor skills, among other feeding difficulties (Crapnell et al., 2013).

Education/Work
- Not applicable.

Play/Leisure
- Adolescents may demonstrate lower scores on leisure assessment in areas of hobbies and sport (Dahan-Oliel et al., 2012; Dahan-Oliel, Mazer, Maltais, et al., 2014; Dahan-Oliel, Mazer, Riley, et al., 2014).

Rest/Sleep
- Infant may have difficulty sleeping.

Social Participation
- Adolescents may demonstrate lower scores on participation in social activities (Dahan-Oliel et al., 2012).

Sensorimotor

- Infant may lack primitive reflex reactions (Moro, asymmetrical tonic neck reflex [ATNR], symmetrical tonic neck reflex [STNR]). Infant may demonstrate poor midline orientation.
- Infant may display hyper- or hypotonicity.
- Infant/child may display postural insecurity (Tam et al., 2019).
- Infant may have a severe head turn preference (right is most common), which is a marker for adverse developmental outcome (Dunsirn et al., 2016).
- Infant may display head lag. (Note: may not be a useful predictor of subsequent motor impairment as a single indicator; Pineda et al., 2016.)
- Infant may be hyperresponsive or hyporesponsive to stimuli (auditory, gustatory, olfactory, pressure, taste, touch, vestibular, vision).
- Infant may have retinopathy of prematurity (Glass et al., 2017).
- Child may demonstrate motor impairments. (Note: Interpretations of motor impairment may score differently on the PDMS-2 and the Bayley-III; Gill et al., 2019.)
- Infant or child may demonstrate atypical sensory processing patterns (Crozier et al., 2016; Lecuona et al., 2016).

Cognitive/Perceptual

- Infant may fail to arouse, orient, or attend to stimuli such as an adult's face or maintain only brief contact.

Psychosocial

- Infant may not cuddle or stop crying if held by another person.
- Infant may arch back or squirm in an attempt to get away from another person and avoid handling.
- Infant may not exhibit self-regulatory behaviors (sucking).
- Parents may become stressed caring for a preterm infant.
- Parents may become overprotective of their "fragile" child or adolescent.

Context/Environment

- Parents may experience stress in coping with preterm infant (Howe et al., 2014).
- Parents may lack information about care and development of a preterm infant.
- Parents may be aware of resources (community or internet).

Intervention/Treatment

Models and programs developed by occupational therapy personnel include the Cheek and Jaw Support program (Hwang, Lin, et al., 2010), Early Intervention (Park et al., 2014), Home-Based Occupational Therapy (Chiu et al., 2012), Prefeeding Oral Stimulation (Hwang, Vergara, et al., 2010), Sensorimotor Intervention (Fucile & Gisel, 2010), and Sensory Integration (Pekçetin et al., 2016). Models and programs developed by other professionals but used by occupational therapy personnel include Calmer Robot (Williams et al., 2019), Nonnutritive Oral Motor Stimulation & Infant Massage Therapy (Lau et al., 2012), Oral and Non-Oral Sensorimotor Interventions (Fucile et al., 2011; Fucile et al., 2012), Parental Presence & Holding (Reynolds et al., 2013), Physical Activity Programs (Valizadeh et al., 2017), Positioning (Madlinger-Lewis et al., 2014; Zarem et al., 2013), Prefeeding Oromotor Stimulation Program (Arora et al., 2018), and Therapy Services (Ross et al., 2017; Sturdivant, 2013). Team members include neonatologists, nursing personnel, respiratory and inhalation therapists, dieticians and nutritionists, physical therapy personnel, and occupational therapy personnel. Goals are to address developmental issues related to prematurity such as facilitating oral motor and feeding skills, motor and neurodevelopment, positioning, behavioral regulation, sensory processing skills, and parent education (Ross et al., 2017).

Activities of Daily Living/Instrumental ADL
- Infant: Support coordination of sucking, swallowing, and breathing usually established at about 34 weeks' gestation.
- Child/adolescent: Encourage client to engage in age-appropriate and safe physical activity.

Education/Work
- Child/adolescent: Assist in determining if assistive technology is needed in the classroom.

Play/Leisure
- Infant/Child: Assist client to develop age-appropriate play skills.
- Child/adolescent: Assist client to explore and develop leisure occupations that are age appropriate.

Rest/Sleep
- Not discussed.

Social Participation
- Child/adolescent: Assist client to participate in age-appropriate social activities.

Sensorimotor
- Infant: Stress proper positioning in the NICU to support posture and movement focused on flexed midline-oriented position.
- Infant: Provide passive range of motion of the head and neck to facilitate midline orientation.
- Infant: Provide controlled exposure to varied proprioceptive, tactile, and visual stimuli.
- Infant: Support skin-to-skin contact between infant and mother (kangaroo care).
- Infant: Observe for signs of retinopathy of prematurity (ROP), myopia, and strabismus (crossed eyes).
- Adolescent: Physical activity interventions should be encouraged, especially for females with health problems and movement difficulties (Proulx et al., 2017).

Cognitive/Perceptual
- Not discussed.

Psychosocial
- Infant: Promote a calm, regulated behavior state.
- Infant: Encourage parents to visit and interact with infant.
- Child/adolescent: Assist client to plan and perform activities that will improve the individual's quality of life.

Context/Environment
- Assist in interpreting medical information to parents and caregivers regarding risks to health (activity restrictions and reduced participation) of any conditions associated with prematurity.
- Provide information, training, and care of assistive technology, if needed.

Precautions/Safety Considerations
- Monitor for decreased body temperature (hypothermia) during feedings.
- Monitor for signs of apnea and hypoxia.
- Monitor for signs of aspiration during feeding.
- Seizures are possible and should be considered in any intervention program.
- Cribs should be kept free of fluffy materials, including blankets, quilts, pillows, and stuffed toys, which have been associated with an increased risk of sudden infant death syndrome (SIDS; Porter, 2018).

- Before discharge from the hospital, premature infants should be checked out in a car seat using pulse oximetry to determine whether the infant can maintain patent airway and good oxygen saturation while positioned in the car seat (Porter, 2018).
- High doses of caffeine as an intervention are not recommended (McPherson, Neil, et al., 2015).
- Exposure to stressors in the NICU can decrease brain development (Smith et al., 2011).

Prognosis and Outcome

Prognosis varies depending on the presence and severity of complications. Mortality and likelihood of complications increases with decreased gestational age and birth weight. Infants and young children should be screened regularly for metabolic, central nervous system, and ocular complications (Porter, 2018). Impairment in motor, cognitive, functional, and neurobehavioral performance have been documented (Maggi et al., 2014; Morgan-Feir et al., 2019; Pineda et al., 2013). The relationship between sensory processing and motor, cognition, and language remains controversial (Beltrame et al., 2018; Cabral et al., 2015; Celik et al., 2018).

REFERENCES

Arora, K., Goel, S., Manerkar, S., Konde, N., Panchal, H., Hegde, D., & Mondkar, J. (2018). Prefeeding oromotor stimulation program for improving oromotor function in preterm infants—A randomized controlled trial. *Indian Pediatrics, 55*(8), 675–678. https://doi.org/10.1007s13312-018-1357-6

Beltrame, V. H., de Moraes, A. B., & de Souza, A. P. R. (2018). Sensory profile and its relationship with psychic risk, prematurity and motor and language development in 12-month-old babies. *Revista de Terapia Ocupacional da Universidade de São Paula, 29*(1), 8–18. https://doi.org/10.11606/issn.2238-6149.v29i1p8-18

Cabral, T. I., Pereira da Silva, L. G., Tudella, E., & Simões Martinez, C. M. (2015). Motor development and sensory processing: A comparative study between preterm and term infants. *Research in Developmental Disabilities, 36C*, 102–107. https://doi.org/10.1016/j.ridd.2014.09.018

Celik, H. I., Elbasan, B., Gucuyener, K., Kayihan, H., & Huri, M. (2018). Investigation of the relationship between sensory processing and motor development in preterm infants. *American Journal of Occupational Therapy, 72*(1), Article 7201195020. https://doi.org/10.5014/ajot.2018.026260

Chiu, T. M. L., Wehrmann, S., Reid, D., & Sinclair, G. (2012). Transforming mother–infant interaction within cultural and caregiving contexts: Home-based occupational therapy for preterm infants. *Hong Kong Journal of Occupational Therapy, 22*(1), 17–24. https://doi.org/10.1016/j.hkjot.2012.04.003

Crapnell, T. L., Rogers, C. E., Neil, J. J., Inder, T. E., Woodward, L. J., & Pineda, R. G. (2013). Factors associated with feeding difficulties in the very preterm infant. *Acta Paediatrica, 102*(12), e539–e545. https://doi.org/10.1111/apa.12393

Crozier, S. C., Goodson, J. Z., Mackay, M. L., Synnes, A. R., Grunau, R. E., Miller, S. P., & Zwicker, J. G. (2016). Sensory processing patterns in children born very preterm. *American Journal of Occupational Therapy, 70*(1), Article 7001220050. https://doi.org/10.5014/ajot.2016.018747

Dahan-Oliel, N., Mazer, B., & Majnemer, A. (2012). Preterm birth and leisure participation: A synthesis of the literature. *Research in Developmental Disabilities, 33*(4), 1211–1220. https://doi.org/10.1016/j.ridd.2012.02.011

Dahan-Oliel, N., Mazer, B., Maltais, D. B., Riley, P., Nadeau, L., & Majnemer, A. (2014). Child and environmental factors associated with leisure participation in adolescents born extremely preterm. *Early Human Development, 90*(10), 665–672. https://doi.org/10.1016/j.earlhumdev.2014.08.005

Dahan-Oliel, N., Mazer, B., Riley, P., Maltais, D. B., Nadeau, L., & Majnemer, A. (2014). Participation and enjoyment of leisure activities in adolescents born at ≤ 29 week gestation. *Early Human Development, 90*(6), 307–314. https://doi.org/10.1016/j.earlhumdev.2014.02.010

de Albuquerque, P. L., de Farias Guerra, M. Q., de Carvalho Lima, M., & Eickmann, S. H. (2018). Concurrent validity of the Alberta Infant Motor Scale to detect delayed gross motor development in preterm infants: A comparative study with the Bayley III. *Developmental Neurorehabilitation, 21*(6), 408–414. https://doi.org/10.1080/17518423.2017.1323974

Dunsirn, S., Smyser, C., Liao, S., Inder, T., & Pineda, R. (2016). Defining the nature and implications of head turn preference in the preterm infant. *Early Human Development, 96*, 53–60. https://doi.org/10.1016/j.earlhumdev.2016.02.002

Edwards, J., Berube, M., Erlandson, K., Haug, S., Johnstone, H., Meagher, M. Sarkodee-Adoo, S., & Zwicker, J. G. (2011). Developmental coordination disorder in school-aged children born very preterm and/or at very low birth weight: A systematic review. *Journal of Developmental and Behavioral Pediatrics, 32*(9), 678–687. https://doi.org/10.1097/DBP.0b013e31822a396a

Fucile, S., & Gisel, E. (2010). Sensorimotor interventions improve growth and motor function in preterm infants. *Neonatal Network, 29*(6), 359–366. https://doi.org/10.1891/0730-0832.29 .6.359

Fucile, S., Gisel, E. G., McFarland, D. H., & Lau, C. (2011). Oral and non-oral sensorimotor interventions enhance oral feeding performance in preterm infants. *Developmental Medicine & Child Neurology, 53*(9), 829–835. https://doi.org/10.1111/j.1469-8749.2011.04023.x

Fucile, S., McFarland, D. H., Gisel, E. G., & Lau, C. (2012). Oral and nonoral sensorimotor interventions facilitate suck–swallow–respiration functions and their coordination in preterm infants. *Early Human Development, 88*(6), 345–350. https://doi.org/10.1016/j.earl humdev.2011.09.007

Gill, K., Osiovich, A., Synnes, A., Agnew, J. A., Grunau, R. E., Miller, S. P., & Zwicker, J. G. (2019). Concurrent validity of the Bayley-III and the Peabody Developmental Motor Scales-2 at 18 months. *Physical and Occupational Therapy in Pediatrics 39*(5), 514–524. https://doi.org/10.10 80/01942638.2018.1546255

Glass, T. J. A., Chau, V., Gardiner, J., Foong, J., Vinall, J., Zwicker, J. G., Grunau, R. E., Synnes, A., Poskitt, K. J., & Miller, S. P. (2017). Severe retinopathy of prematurity predicts delayed white matter maturation and poorer neurodevelopment. *Archives of Disease in Childhood: Fetal and Neonatal Edition, 102*(6), F532–F537. https://doi.org/10.1136/archdischild-2016-312533

Howe, T.-H., Sheu, C.-F., Wang, T.-N., & Hsu, Y.-W. (2014). Parenting stress in families with very low birth weight preterm infants in early infancy. *Research in Developmental Disabilities, 35*(7), 1748–1756. https://doi.org/10.1016/j.ridd.2014.02.015

Hwang, Y.-S., Lin, C.-H., Coster, W. J., Bigsby, R., & Vergara, E. (2010). Effectiveness of cheek and jaw support to improve feeding performance of preterm infants. *American Journal of Occupational Therapy, 64*(6), 886–894. https://doi.org/10.5014/ajot.2010.09031

Hwang, Y.-S., Vergara, E., Lin, C.-H., Coster, W. J., Bigsby, R., & Tsai, W.-H. (2010). Effects of prefeeding oral stimulation on feeding performance of preterm infants. *Indian Journal of Pediatrics, 77*(8), 869–873. https://doi.org/10.1007/s12098-010-0001-9

Kwok, C., Mackay, M., Agnew, J. A. Synnes, A., & Zwicker, J. G. (2019). Does the Movement Assessment Battery for Children–2 at 3 years of age predict developmental coordination disorder at 4.5 years of age in children born very preterm? *Research in Developmental Disabilities, 84*, 36–42. https://doi.org/10.1016/j.ridd.2018.04.003

Lau, C., Fucile, S., & Gisel, E. G. (2012). Impact of nonnutritive oral motor stimulation and infant massage therapy on oral feeding skills of preterm infants. *Journal of Neonatal-Perinatal Medicine, 5*(4), 311–317. https://doi.org/10.3233/NPM-1262612

Lecuona, E. P., van Jaarsveld, A., van Heerden, R., & Raubenheimer, J. (2016). The developmental status and prevalence of sensory integration difficulties in premature infants in a tertiary hospital in Bloemfontein, South Africa. *South African Journal of Occupational Therapy, 46*(1), 15–19. http://dx.doi.org/10.17159/23110-3833/2016/v46n1a5

Madlinger-Lewis, L., Reynolds, L., Zarem, C., Crapnell, T., Inder, T., & Pineda, R. (2014). The effects of alternative positioning on preterm infants in the neonatal intensive care unit: A randomized clinical trial. *Research in Developmental Disabilities, 35*(2), 490–497. https://doi.org/10.1016/j.ridd.2013.11.019

Maggi, E. F., Magalhães, L. C., Campos, A. F., & Bouzada, M. C. F. (2014). Preterm children have unfavorable motor, cognitive, and functional performance when compared to term children of preschool age. *Jornal de Pediatria, 90*(4), 377–383. https://doi.org/10.1016/j.jped.2013.10.005

Majnemer, A., Dahan-Oliel, N., Rohlicek, C., Hatzigeorgiou, S., Mazer, B., Maltais, D. B., & Schmitz, N. (2017). Educational and rehabilitation service utilization in adolescents born preterm or with a congenital heart defect and at high risk for disability. *Developmental Medicine & Child Neurology, 59*(10), 1056–1062. https://doi.org/10.1111/dmcn.13520

McPherson, C., Haslam, M., Pineda, R., Rogers, C., Neil, J. J., & Inder, T. E. (2015). Brain injury and development in preterm infants exposed to fentanyl. *Annals of Pharmacotherapy, 49*(12), 1291–1297. https://doi.org/10.1177/1060028015606732

McPherson, C., Neil, J., Tjoeng, T. H., Pineda, R., & Inder, T. E. (2015). A pilot randomized trial of high-dose caffeine therapy in preterm infants. *Pediatric Research, 78*(2), 198–204. https://doi.org/10.1038/pr.2015.72

Morgan-Feir, M., Abbott, A., Synnes, A., Creighton, D., Pillay, T., Zwicker, J. G., & Canadian Neonatal Follow-Up Network. (2019). Comparing standardized and parent-reported motor outcomes of extremely preterm infants. *Children, 6*(8), Article 90. https://doi.org/10.3390/children6080090

O'Toole, M. T. (Ed.). (2017). *Mosby's dictionary of medicine, nursing & health professions* (10th ed.). Elsevier.

Park, H. Y., Maitra, K., Achon, J., Loyola, E., & Rincón, M. (2014). Effects of early intervention on mental or neuromusculoskeletal and movement-related functions in children born low birthweight or preterm: A meta-analysis. *America Journal of Occupational Therapy, 68*(3), 268–276. https://doi.org/10.5014/ajot.2014.010371

Pekçetin, S., Akı, E., Üstünyurt, Z., & Kayıhan, H. (2016). The efficiency of sensory integration interventions in preterm infants. *Perceptual and Motor Skills, 123*(2), 411–423. https://doi.org/10.1177/0031512516662895

Pineda, R. G., Reynolds, L. C., Seefeldt, K., Hilton, C. L., Rogers, C. E., & Inder, T. E. (2016). Head lag in infancy: What is it telling use? *American Journal of Occupational Therapy, 70*(1), Article 7001220010. https://doi.org/10.5014/ajot.2016.017558

Pineda, R. G., Tjoeng, T. H., Vavasseur, C., Kidokoro, H., Neil, J., & Inder, T. (2013). Patterns of altered neurobehavior in preterm infants within the Neonatal Intensive Care Unit. *Journal of Pediatrics, 162*(3), 470–476. https://doi.org/10.1016/j.jpeds.2012.08.011

Porter, R. S. (Ed.). (2018). *The Merck manual of diagnosis and therapy* (20th ed.). Merck Sharp & Dohme.

Proulx, K., Majnemer, A., Dahan-Oliel, N., Mazer, B., Nadeau, L., Vanier, K., & Maltais, D. B. (2017). Factors associated with moderate to vigorous physical activity in adolescents born preterm. *Pediatric Exercise Science, 29*(2), 260–267. https://doi.org/10.1123/pes.2016-0164

Ross, K., Heiny, E., Conner, S., Spener, P., & Pineda, R. (2017). Occupational therapy, physical therapy and speech-language pathology in the neonatal intensive care unit: Patterns of therapy usage in a level IV NICU. *Research in Developmental Disabilities, 64*, 108–117. https://doi.org/10.1016/j.ridd.2017.03.009

Ryckman, J., Hilton, C., Rogers, C., & Pineda, R. (2017). Sensory processing disorder in preterm infants during early childhood and relationships to early neurobehavior. *Early Human Development, 113*, 18–22. https://doi.org/10.1016/j.earlhumdev.2017.07.012

Smith, G. C., Gutovich, J., Smyser, C., Pineda, R., Newnham, C., Tjoeng, T. H., Vavasseur, C., Wallendorf, M., Neil, J., & Inder, T. (2011). Neonatal intensive care unit stress is associated with brain development in preterm infants. *Annals of Neurology, 70*(4), 541–549. https://doi.org/10.1002/ana.22545

Sturdivant, C. (2013). A collaborative approach to defining neonatal therapy. *Newborn and Infant Nursing Reviews, 13*(1), 23–26. https://doi.org/10.1053/j.nainr.2012.12.010

Tam, E. W. Y., Chau, V., Lavoie, R., Chakravarty, M. M., Guo, T., Synnes, A., Zwicker, J., Grunau, R., & Miller, S. P. (2019). Neurologic examination findings associated with small cerebellar volumes after prematurity. *Journal of Child Neurology, 34*(10), 586–592. https://doi.org/10.1177/0883073819847925

Valizadeh, L., Sanaeefar, M., Hosseini, M. B., Jafarabadi, M. A., & Shamili, A. (2017). Effect of early physical activity programs on motor performance and neuromuscular development in infants born preterm: A randomized clinical trial. *Journal of Caring Sciences, 6*(1), 67–79. https://doi.org/10.15171/jcs.2017.008

Williams, N., MacLean, K., Guan, L., Collet, J. P., & Holsti, L. (2019). Pilot testing a robot for reducing pain in hospitalized preterm infants. *OTJR: Occupation, Participation & Health, 39*(2), 108–115. https://doi.org/10.1177/1539449218825436

Zarem, C., Crapnell, T., Tiltges, L., Madlinger, L., Reynolds, L., Lukas, K., & Pineda, R. (2013). Neonatal nurses' and therapists' perceptions of positioning for preterm infants in the neonatal intensive care unit. *Neonatal Network, 32*(2), 110–116. https://doi.org/10.1891/0730-08 32.32.2.110

Zwicker, J. G., Grunau, R. E., Adams, E., Chau, V., Brant, R., Poskitt, K. J., Synnes, A., & Miller, S. P. (2013). SNAP-II predicts corticospinal tract development in premature newborns. *Pediatric Neurology, 45*(2), 123–129.e1. https://doi.org/10.1016/j.pediatrneurol.2012.10.016

Zwicker, J. G., Miller, S. P., Grunau, R. E., Chau, V., Brant, R., Studholme, C., Liu, M., Synnes, A., Poskitt, K. J., Stiver, M. L., & Tam, E. W. (2016). Smaller cerebellar growth and poorer neurodevelopmental outcomes in very preterm infants exposed to neonatal morphine. *Journal of Pediatrics, 172*, 81–87.e2. https://doi.org/10.1016/j.jpeds.2015.12.024

Zwicker, J. G., Yoon, S. W., MacKay, M., Petrie-Thomas, J., Rogers, M., & Synnes, A. R. (2013). Perinatal and neonatal predictors of developmental coordination disorder in very low birthweight children. *Archives of Disease in Childhood, 98*(2), 118–122. https://doi.org/10.1136/archdischild-2012-302268

BIBLIOGRAPHY

Coker-Bolt, P., Woodbury, M. L., Perkel, J., Moreau, N. G., Hope, K., Brown, T., Ramakrishnan, V., Mulvihill, D., & Jenkins, D. (2014). Identifying premature infants at high and low risk for motor delays using motor performance testing and MRS. *Journal of Pediatric Rehabilitation Medicine, 7*(3), 219–232. https://doi.org/10.3233/PRM-140291

Duerden, E. G., Foong, J., Chau, V., Branson, H., Poskitt, K. J., Grunau, R. E., Synnes, A., Zwicker, J. G., & Miller, S. P. (2015). Tract-based spatial statistics in preterm-born neonates predicts cognitive and motor outcomes at 18 months. *AJNR American Journal of Neuroradiology, 36*(8), 1565–1571. https://doi.org/10.3174/ajnr.A4312

Easson, K., Dahan-Oliel, N., Rohlicek, C., Sahakian, S., Brossard-Racine, M., Mazer, B., Riley, P., Maltais, D., Nadeau, L., Hatzigeorgiou, S., Schmitz, N., & Majnemer, A. (2019). A comparison of developmental outcomes of adolescent neonatal intensive care unit survivors born with a congenital heart defect or born preterm. *Journal of Pediatrics, 207*, 34–41.e2. https://doi.org/10.1016/j.jpeds.2018.11.002

Pineda, R., Dewey, K., Jacobsen, A., & Smith, J. (2019). Non-nutritive sucking in the preterm infant. *American Journal of Perinatology, 36*(3), 268–276. https://doi.org/10.1055/s-0038-16 67289

Pineda, R. G., Neil, J., Dierker, D., Smyser, C. D., Wallendorf, M., Kidokoro, H., Reynolds, L. C., Walker, S., Rogers, C., Mathur, A. M., Van Essen, D. C., & Inder, T. (2014). Alterations in brain structure and neurodevelopmental outcome in preterm infants hospitalized in different neonatal intensive care unit environments. *Journal of Pediatrics, 164*(1), 52–60.e2. https://doi.org/10.1016/j.jpeds.2013.08.047

Ranger, M., Zwicker, J. G., Chau, C. M. Y., Park, M. T. M., Chakravarthy, M. M., Poskitt, K., Miller, S. P., Bjornson, B. H., Tam, E. W. Y., Chau, V., Synnes, A. R., & Grunau, R. E. (2015). Neonatal pain and infection related to smaller cerebellum in very preterm children at school age. *Journal of Pediatrics, 167*(2), 292.e.1–298.e.1. https://doi.org/10.1016/j.jpeds.2015.04.055

Reynolds, L. C., Duncan, M. M., Smith, G. C., Mathur, A., Neil, J., Inder, T., & Pineda, R. G. (2013). Parental presence and holding in the neonatal intensive care unit and associations with early neurobehavior. *Journal of Perinatology, 33*(8), 636–641. https://doi.org/10.1038/jp.2013.4

Reynolds, L. C., Inder, T. E., Neil, J. J., Pineda, R. G., & Rogers, C. E. (2014). Maternal obesity and increased risk for autism and developmental delay among very preterm infants. *Journal of Perinatology, 34*(9), 688–692. https://doi.org/10.1038/jp.2014.80

Rett Syndrome

Also called cerebroatrophic hyperammonemia.

Description

Rett syndrome is a pervasive neurodevelopmental disorder affecting the gray matter of the brain. It occurs mostly in females, affecting development after an initial 6-month period of normal development (O'Toole, 2017; Porter, 2018). Most cases are random, spontaneous mutation; less than 1% are inherited or passed from one generation to the next (Porter, 2018). The course, age of onset, and severity of symptoms vary. Four stages are used to describe symptoms:

- *Stage 1 (early onset stage)* usually begins when the child is between 6 and 18 months old, with subtle slowing of development. Symptoms may include less eye contact, decreased interest in toys, delays in sitting or crawling, decreases in head growth, and hand-wringing.
- *Stage 2 (developmental regression or rapid destructive stage)* usually begins between ages 1 and 4 years. Onset may be rapid or gradual, with loss of purposeful hand skills and spoken language. Characteristic hand movement may include wringing, clapping, washing, tapping, and repeatedly bringing hands to mouth. Breathing irregularities such as episodes of apnea and hyperventilation may occur. Walking may be unsteady, and initiating motor movements may be difficult. Impaired social interaction and communication may be present, similar to autism spectrum disorders.
- *Stage 3 (pseudostationary stage)* usually begins between ages 2 and 10 years and can last for years. Seizures, motor deficits, and apraxia are common. Symptoms such as crying, irritability, and autism-like symptoms may decline. Alertness, attention span, communication skills, and interest in surroundings may increase.
- *Stage 4 (late motor deterioration stage)* can last for years or decades. Common characteristics may include decreased mobility, muscle weakness, spasticity, rigidity, or scoliosis. Eye gaze for communication becomes prominent as spoken language is usually absent. Walking may stop, and repetitive hand movements may decrease. Cardiac abnormalities are often present. Person may have difficulty maintaining weight (Porter, 2018).

Cause

The primary cause is the *MECP2* (methyl-CpG-binding protein 2) gene mutation on the child's X chromosome (Xq28). Other known causes include partial gene deletions, and mutation to other genes such as *CDKL5* and *FOXG1* genes that affect brain development in atypical Rett syndrome (Porter, 2018). Eight different mutations have been identified to date (Pidcock et al., 2016). Functional performance is related to the type of mutation the individual has in the genetic profile.

Evaluation/Assessment

Areas

- Activities of Daily Living/Instrumental ADL: feeding, chewing, dressing, grooming, bathing, toileting, mobility, communication skills (including eye contact)
- Education/Work: school readiness, academic performance
- Play/Leisure: play skills (use of toys, tools, and objects)
- Rest/Sleep: sleep habits and routines
- Social Participation: type, location, frequency, with whom
- Sensorimotor: gross motor skills, fine motor skills and hand function (grasp, hold, pinch, manipulate, release), dyspraxia, ataxia, gait abnormalities, muscle tone, contractures, seizures, proprioception, sensory awareness and processing
- Cognitive/Perceptual: intellectual disability, attention, memory, executive function, perceptual skills
- Psychosocial: autistic behavior, lability, and mood swings
- Context/Environment: parent knowledge, social support, community resources, adapted devices (splints)
- Development (Infant, Child, Adolescent only): developmental milestones, developmental delay

Instruments

Instruments Developed by Occupational Therapy Personnel

- Children's Assessment of Participation and Enjoyment and Preferences for Activities of Children (CAPE/PAC; King et al., 2004)
- Kennedy Krieger Institute (KKI) Upper Extremity Measurement Scale (UEMS; Dunkleberger et al., 2006)

Instruments Developed by Other Professionals and Used by Occupational Therapy Personnel

- Communication and Symbolic Behavior Scales Developmental Profile (CSBS DP) Infant-Toddler Checklist; Wetherby & Prizant, 2002)
- Family Resource Scale (FRS; Dunst & Lee, 1987)
- Family Support Scale (FSS; Dunst et al., 1984)
- Functional Ability Checklist (FAC; video-based evaluation; Fyfe et al., 2007)
- Functional Independence Measure for Children (WeeFIM; Uniform Data System for Medical Rehabilitation, 1998)
- Kennedy Krieger Institute (KKI) Physical Abilities and Mobility Scale (PAMS; Suskauer et al., 2006)
- Rett Syndrome Behavior Questionnaire (RSBQ; Mount et al., 2002)
- Rett Syndrome Motor-Behavioral Assessment (RSMBA; Fitzgerald et al., 1990)
- Short Form Health Survey (SF-12; Ware et al., 1996)
- Stem and Leaf Questions (to assess stereotypical hand functions; Downs et al., 2014)

Problems/Issues

Activities of Daily Living/Instrumental ADL

- Child usually loses spoken language but maintains eye communication.
- Child's ability to use speech–language abilities depends on type of *MECP2* mutation (Urbanowicz et al., 2015).
- Adolescent female course of development varies in terms of age at which adrenarche (pubic hair), thelarche (breast development), and menarche (menstruation) occur (Knight et al., 2013).

Education/Work

- Child usually is unable to perform or has difficulty performing classroom skills: holding a book, coloring with a crayon, writing with a pencil, cutting with scissors, picking up and placing puzzle pieces, applying glue to paper, carrying a plastic chair to circle time, imitating hand gestures.

Play/Leisure
- Child may experience difficulty developing play skills involving toys, tools, and objects due to restricted hand use.
- Child/adult may not develop leisure occupations due to restricted hand use.

Rest/Sleep
- Child may have an abnormal sleep pattern.
- Child may grind teeth when asleep (and sometimes when awake).

Social Participation
- Child/adult may be limited in participation in social activities due to lack of communication and/or hand skills.

Sensorimotor
- Child usually loses purposeful hand skills (reach, grasp, hold, pick up, in-hand manipulation, transfer from hand to hand, release).
- Child usually exhibits repetitive hand movements such as wringing, washing, squeezing, clapping, twirling, mouthing, tapping, biting, chewing, or rubbing. Hands may be used together or single.
- Child/adult may have difficulty walking, exhibiting gait abnormalities (such as toe-walking, unsteady, side-based, or stiff-legged walk).
- Child/adult may have difficulty with timing sequencing motor actions (usually slower than average).
- Child/adult may have difficulty sequencing motor actions in correct order.
- Child/adult may perseverate or repeat some action over and over again.
- Child/adult may develop scoliosis.
- Child/adult may have abnormal muscle tone.
- Child/adult may have cold hands and feet, regardless of room temperature or outside temperature.
- Child/adult may develop contractures and skin injuries, especially after age 10 (Hirano & Taniguchi, 2018).
- Child/adult may gaze or fixate on hands.

Cognitive/Perceptual
- Child usually has intellectual disability.
- Child/adult may exhibit ideational dyspraxia (e.g., difficulty understanding how to use objects such as eating utensils or a toothbrush).
- Child/adult may exhibit ideomotor dyspraxia (such as difficulty imitating gestures or performing motor task on command).

Psychosocial
- Child may laugh or scream without relation to situation.

Context/Environment
- Parents usually have limited knowledge of the disorder since it is rare.
- Child/adult may lack social support.
- Parents may have limited access to resources.

Intervention/Treatment

Models and programs developed by occupational therapy personnel: None. Models and programs developed by other professionals but used by occupational therapy personnel include early intervention (Dall'Alba et al., 2014) and management of hand function (Downs et al.,

2014). Team members include physicians, nursing personnel, psychologists, geneticists, physical therapy personnel, speech–language pathologists, and occupational therapy personnel. Goal is to maintain and maximize functional performance for as long as possible by using adaptive and compensatory strategies.

Activities of Daily Living/Instrumental ADL
- Assist in teaching self-feeding, including use of "finger food" and use of eating utensils (modification of eating utensils may be needed).
- Assist in improving oral motor control.
- Assist speech–language pathologist with adapted communication devices (paper, notebooks, electronics, eye gaze).
- Use eye gaze as primary means of communication in therapy (Urbanowicz et al., 2016).
- Assist client in meal preparation, cooking, or baking.
- Assist client in pet care activities.

Education/Work
- No discussion of education or classroom activities.

Play/Leisure
- Encourage recreational and community-based activities, such as visiting the zoo or museum, attending a game or play (Andrews et al., 2014).
- Encourage exploration of toys and objects.

Rest/Sleep
- See Sleep–Wake Disorders in Section 13: Lifestyle Conditions.

Social Participation
- Encourage participation in social and community activities such as shopping with peers or going to movies, concerts, parties, sporting events, or plays, or playing music at home with friends and family.

Sensorimotor
- Encourage physical activities such as swimming, horseback riding, dancing, riding a three- or four-wheeled cycle (Sernheim et al., 2018).
- Optimize motor control, including focus on regulating or directing movement such as generation and coordination of actions of multiple joints and muscles that produce functional movement. Focus can be verbal instructions or nonverbal using environment and prepared setup to facilitate response.

Cognitive/Perceptual
- Optimize motor learning: opportunity to practice; time for intrinsic feedback from the performance and achievement of a task to occur; extrinsic feedback from encouragement and practice; throughout and following completion of task, judicious use of rest periods to avoid fatigue; performance of task in novel conditions; and performance in the actual environment in which the task normally occurs.
- Encourage eye contact on verbal command.

Psychosocial
- Encourage self-expression, such as painting.
- Encourage choice-making by allowing adequate time for a response (Urbanowicz et al., 2018).

Context/Environment
- Provide information to family and caregivers about Rett syndrome and its management.
- Process and facilitate access to community and internet resources.
- Consider use of hand splints to improve self-feeding, elbow splints to reduce hand stereotypy (materials should be soft and comfortable, and worn only for part of the day).

Precautions/Safety Considerations

Child may have seizures. Some repetitive behaviors may result in injury (11 different mutations have been identified, such as excessive rubbing of the skin, biting, chewing the hand, or head banging). Note if a cardiac condition exists. Sudden death has been reported.

Prognosis and Outcome

There is no cure. Rett Syndrome is a chronic, lifelong disorder. Symptoms may change somewhat over the years, but a focus on self-care activities should remain a primary objective. Teenagers and women with the ability to walk maintained greater stability of skills over time than those unable to walk (Foley et al., 2011). Clients with *R133C* and *R294X* mutations are most likely to have hand use; those with *R133C, R295X, R306C*, or small deletions are most likely to be ambulatory; and those with *R133C* are most likely to be verbal (Pidcock et al., 2016).

REFERENCES

Andrews, J., Leonard, H., Hammond, G. C., Girdler, S., Rajapaksa, R., Bathgate, K., & Downs, J. (2014). Community participation for girls and women living with Rett syndrome. *Disability and Rehabilitation, 36*(11), 894–899. https://doi.org/10.3109/09638288.2013.813083

Dall'Alba, L., Gray, M., Williams, G., & Lowe, S. (2014). Early intervention in children (0–6 years) with a rare developmental disability: The occupational therapy role. *Hong Kong Journal of Occupational Therapy, 24*(2), 72–80. https://doi.org/10.1016/j.hkjot.2014.12.001

Downs, J., Parkinson, S., Ranelli, S., Leonard, H., Diener, P., & Lotan, M. (2014). Perspectives on hand function in girls and women with Rett syndrome. *Developmental Neurorehabilitation, 17*(3), 210–217. https://doi.org/10.3109/17518423.2012.758183

Foley, K.-R., Downs, J., Bebbington, A., Jacoby, P., Girdler, S., Kaufmann, W. E., & Leonard, H. (2011). Change in gross motor abilities of girls and women with Rett syndrome over a 3- to 4-year period. *Journal of Child Neurology, 26*(10), 1237–1245. https://doi.org/10.1177/0883 073811402688

Hirano, D., & Taniguchi, T. (2018). Skin injuries and joint contractures of the upper extremities in Rett syndrome. *Journal of Intellectual Disability Research, 62*(1), 53–59. https://doi.org/10.1111/jir.12452

Knight, O., Bebbington, A., Siafarikas, A., Woodhead, H., Girdler, S., & Leonard, H. (2013). Pubertal trajectory in females with Rett syndrome: A population-based study. *Brain & Development, 35*(10), 912–920. https://doi.org/10.1016/j.braindev.2012.11.007

O'Toole, M. T. (Ed.). (2017). *Mosby's dictionary of medicine, nursing & health professions* (10th ed.). Elsevier.

Pidcock, F. S., Salorio, C., Bibat, G., Swain, J., Scheller, J., Shore, W., & Naidu, S. (2016). Functional outcomes in Rett syndrome. *Brain & Development, 38*(1), 76–81. https://doi.org/10.10 16/j.braindev.2015.06.005

Porter, R. S. (Ed.). (2018). *The Merck manual of diagnosis and therapy* (20th ed.). Merck Sharp & Dohme.

Sernheim, A.-S., Hemmingsson, H., Engerström, I. W., & Liedberg, G. (2018). Activities that girls and women with Rett syndrome liked or did not like to do. *Scandinavian Journal of Occupational Therapy, 25*(4), 267–277. https://doi.org/10.1080/11038128.2016.1250812

Urbanowicz, A., Ciccone, N., Girdler S., Leonard, H., & Downs, J. (2018). Choice making in Rett syndrome: A descriptive study using video data. *Disability and Rehabilitation, 40*(7), 813–819. https://doi.org/10.1080/09638288.2016.1277392

Urbanowicz, A., Downs, J., Girdler, S., Ciccone, N., & Leonard, H. (2015). Aspects of speech–language abilities are influenced by *MECP2* mutation type in girls with Rett syndrome. *American Journal of Medical Genetics: Part A, 167A*(2), 354–362. https://doi.org/10.1002/aj mg.a.36871

Urbanowicz, A., Downs, J., Girdler, S., Ciccone, N., & Leonard, H. (2016). An exploration of the use of eye gaze and gestures in females with Rett syndrome. *Journal of Speech, Language, and Hearing Research, 59*(6), 1373–1383. https://doi.org/10.1044/2015_JSLHR-L-14-0185

BIBLIOGRAPHY

Urbanowicz, A., Downs, J., Bebbington, A., Jacoby, P., Girdler, S., & Leonard, H. (2011). Use of equipment and respite services and caregiver health among Australian families living with Rett syndrome. *Research in Autism Spectrum Disorders, 5*(2), 722–732. https://doi.org/10.1016/j.rasd.2010.08.006

Urbanowicz, A., Leonard, H., Girdler, S., Ciccone, N., & Downs, J. (2016). Parental perspectives on the communication abilities of their daughters with Rett syndrome. *Developmental Neurorehabilitation, 19*(1), 17–25. https://doi.org/10.3109/17518423.2013.879940

Specific Learning Disorders

See also Visual Impairment in Children and Adolescents.

Description

Specific learning disorders are difficulties learning and using academic skills that have persisted for at least 6 months, despite the provision of interventions that target those difficulties. The affected academic skills are substantially and quantifiably below those expected for a person's chronological age and cause significant interference with academic or occupational performance, or with activities of daily living. The academic areas affected are impairment in reading (dyslexia), written expression (dysgraphia), and mathematics (dyscalculia). Difficulty may be classified as mild, moderate, or severe (American Psychiatric Association, 2013). In addition, some children have impairment in more than one area, such as dyslexia and dysgraphia, or all three: dyslexia, dysgraphia, and dyscalculia. The learning disability does not pervade all areas of learning but rather is limited to particular scholastic or academic skills (VandenBos, 2015). Affected children typically demonstrate poor school performance, anxiety, social maladaptation, and their problems result in significant parental stress (Karande et al., 2019). Special learning disability is an example of an invisible disability—that is, the disability cannot be seen by casual observation, but only becomes apparent during performance of certain tasks, such as reading, writing, and mathematics (Karande et al., 2019).

Cause

Unknown.

Evaluation/Assessment

Areas

- Activities of Daily Living/Instrumental ADL: basic, independent living
- Education/Work: academic performance and skills (reading, writing, mathematics, handwriting, keyboarding)
- Play/Leisure: play skills (symbolic, cooperative, collaborative)
- Rest/Sleep: not discussed
- Social Participation: type, location, frequency, with whom
- Sensorimotor: manual dexterity, functional mobility especially balance reactions
- Cognitive/Perceptual: attention, memory, learning style, executive function, metacognition

- Psychosocial: hyperactivity, anxiety, depression, oppositional behavior, depression, motivation, quality of life, life roles
- Context/Environment: family and educator knowledge
- Comorbidities: attention-deficit/hyperactivity disorder (ADHD-inattention type, ADHD-hyperactive type, ADHD-mixed type), generalized anxiety disorder, oppositional defiant disorder, tics, social phobia, separation anxiety disorder, convulsions, enuresis, encopresis, obsession, conduct disorder

Instruments
Instruments Developed by Occupational Therapy Personnel
- Child Occupational Self-Assessment (Version 2.2; COSA; Kramer et al., 2014)
- Parent Assessment of Child Occupation (PACO; Yazdani & Nobakht, 2016)
- Pediatric Evaluation of Disability Inventory–Computer Adaptive Test (PEDI-CAT; Kramer et al., 2016)
- Pediatric Volitional Questionnaire (Version 2.1; PVQ; Basu et al., 2008)
- Play History (PH; Takata, 1969)

Instruments Developed by Other Professionals and Used by Occupational Therapy Personnel
- Behavior Rating Inventory of Executive Function (2nd ed.; BRIEF-2; Gioia et al., 2015)
- Child Symptom Inventory–4: Parent Checklist (CSI-4; Sprafkin et al., 2002)
- Motor-Free Visual Perception Test (4th ed.; MVPT-4; Colarusso & Hammill, 2015; see also Köse et al., 2021, in References)
- Movement Assessment Battery for Children (2nd ed.; M-ABC-2; Henderson et al., 2007)

Problems/Issues
Activities of Daily Living/Instrumental ADL
- Child may be delayed in learning to perform some ADL tasks, such as functional mobility (Suhaili et al., 2019).
- Child or adolescent may experience difficulty learning to perform some independent living skills.

Education/Work
- Child with difficulty in reading may demonstrate
  - impairment in word-reading accuracy (mispronunciation, mixing up letter names and sounds, or leaving words out during oral reading);
  - impairment in reading rate or fluency, such as slow or effortful word reading;
  - impairment of reading comprehension, such as reading single words aloud incorrectly or slowly and hesitantly;
  - a frequency of guessing at words;
  - difficulty sounding out words; and
  - difficulty understanding the meaning of what is read.
- Child with difficulties in written expression may include
  - spelling inaccuracy;
  - inaccurate grammar and punctuation, such as making multiple grammatical or punctuation errors with sentences;
  - lack of clarity and organization of written expression;
  - employing poor paragraph organization or expression of ideas that lack clarity; and
  - illegible handwriting.
- Child with difficulty in mathematics may include
  - impairment of number sense;
  - lack of memorization of arithmetic facts (addition, subtraction, multiplication, and division);
  - inaccurate or incorrect calculation;

- ▶ difficulty counting;
- ▶ difficulty recognizing written numbers;
- ▶ inaccuracy of mathematical reasoning;
- ▶ getting lost in the midst of arithmetic computation; and
- ▶ switching procedures during computation.
- Child with difficulty in handwriting may demonstrate problems in speed, accuracy, and legibility.
- Child or adolescent with difficulty in keyboarding may demonstrate problems in speed and accuracy (Weigelt-Marom & Weintraub, 2018).

Play/Leisure
- Child may have difficulty engaging in play activities requiring collaborative and cooperative skills.

Rest/Sleep
- Not discussed.

Social Participation
- Child may have difficulty participating in social activities that require sharing and following rules.

Sensorimotor
- Child may demonstrate poor manual dexterity.
- Child may demonstrate poor balance reactions.

Cognitive/Perceptual
- Child may have difficulty shifting attention.
- Child may have difficulty with activities requiring working memory.
- Child may have difficulty with planning and organizing academic tasks and other life activities.
- Child may have difficulty monitoring activity.
- Child may have visual perceptual problems (Mona et al., 2015).
  - ▶ Dyscalculia: visual discrimination, visual memory, and visual closure.
  - ▶ Dysgraphia: visual memory and spatial relationships.
  - ▶ Dyslexia: visual memory, visual spatial relations, and sequential memory.

Psychosocial (Esmaili et al., 2016)
- Child may have difficulty with emotional control and inhibition.
- Child may demonstrate symptoms consistent with attention-deficit/hyperactivity disorder (inattentive, impulsive, hyperactive).
- Child may demonstrate symptoms consistent with generalized anxiety disorder (fear, inaction).
- Child may demonstrate symptoms consistent with oppositional defiant disorder (stubborn, refusal to act, refusal to follow instructions).

Context/Environment
- Family or caregivers may lack information about specific learning disabilities and management.
- Family or caregivers may be unfamiliar with legal rights to education.
- Family or caregivers may lack information about available community or internet resources.

Intervention/Treatment

Models and programs developed by occupational therapy personnel include information processing strategy training (Juntorn et al., 2017), model of human occupation (MOHO; Esmaili et al., 2019), and technology (Batorowicz et al., 2012). Models and programs developed by other professionals but used by occupational therapy personnel include play-based therapy (Esmaili et al., 2017). Team members include physicians, psychologists, educators, speech–language pathologists and therapists, and occupational therapy personnel. Goals include using both adaptive and compensatory strategies to assist child to participate successfully in school and community.

Activities of Daily Living/Instrumental ADL
- Not addressed.

Education/Work
- Dyscalculia
  - ▸ Use objects (manipulatives) to provide a multisensory approach to learning concrete mathematics facts.
  - ▸ Color code columns of math problems (e.g., write "ones" column in red, and "tens" in blue).
  - ▸ Use mnemonics, such as rhyming, to memorize math concepts.
  - ▸ Use graph paper to assist with lining up numbers for math assignments.
- Dysgraphia
  - ▸ Have child try various pencils and pens to identify which are most comfortable (tri-edge, large diameter, mechanical).
  - ▸ Try out adding a wedge or using a splint to hold a pencil or pen.
  - ▸ Use a multisensory approach to teach writing letters and numbers, such as Handwriting Without Tears program.
  - ▸ Use raised line paper to provide sensory feedback and encourage writing within the lines.
  - ▸ Use fade-out lettering paper, where provided letter formation decreases as practice writing progresses.
- Dyslexia
  - ▸ Use multisensory approach in which sight, sound, and touch are added to reading material.
  - ▸ Use auditory instruction (adult reading out loud or prerecorded book) while following the words on the pages of the book.

Play/Leisure
- Provide opportunity for cooperative play in which materials are shared for individual projects.
- Provide opportunity for collaborative play in which adherence to responsibility and rules are necessary to complete joint projects.

Rest/Sleep
- Not discussed.

Social Participation
- Encourage social participation through play occupations.

Sensorimotor
- Provide training and opportunity to practice manual dexterity tasks.
- Provide opportunity in play activities to practice balance reactions.

Cognitive/Perceptual
- Use of fading techniques in which therapist participates in a leadership role and then slowly withdraws (fades out) participation.

Psychosocial
- See Attention-Deficit/Hyperactivity Disorder (in Section 1: Development Disorders) and Anxiety (in Section 12: Mental and Behavioral Disorders).

Context/Environment
- Provide access to information on specific learning disorders.
- Provide access to community and internet resources.

Precautions/Safety Considerations
- Not discussed.

Prognosis and Outcome

Variable. No consistent findings regarding prognosis or outcome.

Cost

Occupational therapy services (direct therapy costs, indirect such as travel to appointment) constituted 12.63% of total costs in a study conducted in India (Karande et al., 2019). Note that the cost is not divided between public funding versus private family funds, but is a total cost.

REFERENCES

American Psychiatric Association. (2013). *Diagnostic and statistical manual of mental disorders* (5th ed.).

Batorowicz, B., Missiuna, C. A., & Pollock, N. A. (2012). Technology supporting written productivity in children with learning disabilities: A critical review. *Canadian Journal of Occupational Therapy, 79*(4), 211–224. https://doi.org/10.2182/cjot.2012.79.4.3

Esmaili, S. K., Mehraban, A. H., Shafaroodi, N., Yazdani, F., Masoumi, T., & Zarei, M. (2019). Participation in peer-play activities among children with specific learning disability: A randomized controlled trial. *American Journal of Occupational Therapy, 73*(2), Article 7302205110. https://doi.org/10.5014/ajot.2018.028613

Esmaili, S. K., Shafaroodi, N., Mehraban, A. H., Parand, A., Qorbani, M., Yazdani, F., & Mahmoudpour, A. (2016). Prevalence of psychiatric symptoms and mental health services in students with specific learning disabilities in Tehran, Iran. *International Journal of Mental Health and Addiction, 14*, 438–448. https://doi.org/10.1007/s11469-015-9617-3

Esmaili, S. K., Shafaroodi, N., Mehraban, A. H., Parand, A., Zarei, M., & Akbari-Zardkhaneh, S. (2017). Effect of play-based therapy on metacognitive and behavioral aspects of executive function: A randomized, controlled, clinical trial on the students with learning disabilities. *Basic & Clinical Neuroscience, 8*(3), 203–212. https://doi.org/10.18869/nirp.bcn.8.3.203

Juntorn, S., Sriphetcharawut, S., & Munkhetvit, P. (2017). Effectiveness of information processing strategy training on academic task performance in children with learning disabilities: A pilot study. *Occupational Therapy International, 2017*, Article 6237689. https://doi.org/10.1155/2017/6237689

Karande, S., D'souza, S., Gogtay, N., Shiledar, M., & Sholapurwala, R. (2019). Economic burden of specific learning disability: A prevalence-based cost of illness study of its direct, indirect, and intangible costs. *Journal of Postgraduate Medicine, 65*(3), 152–159. https://doi.org/10.4103/jpgm.JPGM_413_18

Köse, B., Karabulut, E., & Aki, E. (2021). Investigating the interchangeability and clinical utility of MVP-3 and MVPT-4 for 7–10 year children with and without specific learning disabilities. *Applied Neuropsychology: Child, 10*(3), 258–265. https://doi.org/10.1080/21622965.2019.1681270

Mona, G., Dhadwad, V., Yeradkar, R., Adhikari, A., & Setia, M. (2015). Study of visual perceptual problems in children with learning disability. *Indian Journal of Basic and Applied Medical Research, 4*(3), 492–497.

Suhaili, I., Harun, D., Kadar, M., Hanif Farhan, M. R., Nur Sakinah, B., & Evelyn Jong, T. H. (2019). Motor performance and functional mobility in children with specific learning disabilities. *Medical Journal of Malaysia, 74*(1), 34–39.

VandenBos, G. R. (Ed.). (2015). *APA dictionary of psychology* (2nd ed.). American Psychological Association. https://doi.org/10.1037/14646-000

Weigelt-Marom, H., & Weintraub, N. (2018). Keyboarding versus handwriting speed of higher education students with and without learning disabilities: Does touch-typing assist in narrowing the gap? *Computers & Education, 117*, 132–140. https://doi.org/10.1016/j.compedu.2017.10.008

Spina Bifida

Description

Spina bifida is defective closure of the vertebral column. Spina bifida, a congenital disorder, is the result of an embryologic failure to fuse one or more neural arches that becomes the vertebral arches (*Stedman's*, 2011). In occult spinal dysraphism (spina bifida occulta), vertebrae do not form normally, and the spinal cord and meninges may also be affected. In spina bifida cystica, the protruding sac can contain meninges (meningocele), spinal cord (myelocele), or both (meningomyelocele, myelomeningocele; Porter, 2018).

Cause

Cause is not known. Low folate levels during pregnancy increase risk, and there seems to be a genetic component. Other risk factors include material use of certain drugs (e.g., valproate) and maternal diabetes (Porter, 2018).

Evaluation/Assessment

Areas

- Activities of Daily Living/Instrumental ADL: self-maintenance activities, catheterization, bowel and bladder management, functional mobility, independent living (adolescent, adult)
- Education/Work: school readiness, handwriting
- Play/Leisure: play skills, leisure interests
- Rest/Sleep: position, nighttime urination
- Social Participation: socialization skills
- Sensorimotor: mobility, hand skills, upper body strength, manipulating toys and objects, contractures (knee, hip)
- Cognitive/Perceptual: attention, memory, executive functions, including problem solving, time management, decision making, planning, visual spatial relationships
- Psychosocial: autonomy, depression (adults)
- Context/Environment: wheelchair access and seating, positioning equipment, home adaptation, including width of entrances to the house, width of bathroom door, access in and out of vehicle, community and environmental exploration
- Development (Infant, Child, Adolescent only): achieving milestones in motor, sensory, cognitive, emotional, and social areas

Instruments

Instruments Developed by Occupational Therapy Personnel

- Assessment of Motor and Process Skills (8th ed.; AMPS-8; Fisher & Bray Jones, 2016)
- Canadian Occupational Performance Measure (5th ed.; COPM-5; Law et al., 2014)
- KaTid–Youth (Janeslätt, 2012)
- School Function Assessment (SFA; Coster et al., 1998)
- Time-Parent Scale (Time-P, TPS; Janeslätt et al., 2009)
- Time Self-Rating Scale (Time-S; Janeslätt et al., 2015)

Instruments Developed by Other Professionals and Used by Occupational Therapy Personnel

- Arc's Self-Determination Scale (ASDS; Wehmeyer, 1995)
- Availability and Participation Scale (APS; Simeonsson et al., 2001)
- Beck Depression Inventory (2nd ed.; BDI-II; Beck et al., 1996)
- Craig Handicap Assessment and Reporting Technique–Short Form (CHART-SF; Walker et al., 2003)
- Goal Attainment Scaling (GAS; Kiresuk & Sherman, 1968)
- Pediatric Quality of Life Inventory–Generic Form, 4.0 (PedsQL-4; Varni et al., 2001)
- Spina Bifida Health Related Quality of Life Questionnaire (SBHRQoLQ; Parkin et al., 1997)

Problems/Issues

Activities of Daily Living/Instrumental ADL
- Child may be delayed in completing toileting training (Gribble et al., 2013).
- Person usually must learn a bowel and bladder management program that may require catheterization.
- Person may experience urinary tract infections.
- Person may experience pressure sores (decubitus ulcers).
- Person may have difficulty with functional mobility (walking versus use of assistive mobility options).
- Person may not learn or be taught independent living skills.
- Person may have health problems that limit the potential for independent living.
- Person may have altered sensation in genital regions during sex or be impotent.

Education/Work
- Person may have difficulty with accessibility and mobility at school.
- Person may lack opportunity to learn work skills suitable for his or her abilities and limitations.
- Person may experience discrimination in job opportunities.

Play/Leisure
- Person may have not developed expected play skills.

Rest/Sleep
- Person may have difficulty with positioning for sleep.

Social Participation
- Person may have limited opportunity to participate in social activities due to health problems or lack of community access.
- Person may experience exclusion and isolation from participation in social activities.

Sensorimotor
- Person usually has difficulty with gross motor skills.
- Person may have difficulty with fine motor skills.
- Person may have muscle weakness and wasting.
- Person may have difficulty with balance and coordination.
- Person may have difficulty with visuomotor skills.
- Person may experience pain, including headaches.
- Person may have spinal deformities (curved spine).
- Person may have foot deformities.
- Person may have a shunt to reduce effect of hydrocephalus.
- Person may have sensory deficits in the lower extremities.
- Person may have tethered cord syndrome.
- Person may have Chiari malformation.

Cognitive/Perceptual
- Person may have reduced attention skills including concentration, shifting from one task to another.
- Person may have reduced memory functions, especially prospective memory.
- Person may have difficulty learning executive functions such as problem solving, planning ahead, initiating a plan, setting goals, making decisions, mental flexibility, time management (managing daily routines, time processing ability).
- Person may experience difficulty with visual perception.

Psychosocial
- Person may experience difficulty achieving autonomy and self-sufficiency due to learned dependency and failure to learn independence living skills (Peny-Dahlstrand et al., 2012).

- Person may have decreased sense of self-esteem.
- Person may experience decreased quality of life and life satisfaction.
- Person may experience symptoms of depression (adult; Dicianno et al., 2015).
- Person may experience discrimination and stigma due to disability.

Context/Environment
- Person, family, and caregivers may lack information about the condition and its management.
- Person and family may lack information about community or national resources.
- Person and family may lack information about available adaptive devices and equipment.
- Person, especially adults, may have no identified health-care management team.
- Person and family may have different perspectives on determining level of or need for autonomy and independence.
- Person may encounter environmental constraints, including no private place to catheterize.
- Person may find that the medical model aimed at protecting the urinary tract dominates over the social model of achieving continence.

Intervention/Treatment
Models and programs developed by occupational therapy personnel include time processing ability (Persson et al., 2017). Models and programs developed by other professionals but used by occupational therapy personnel include self-management catheterization program (Donlau et al., 2013), serial casting (Al-Oraibi et al., 2013), skin-care self-management program (Parmanto et al., 2015), and transition model (Lindsay et al., 2016). Team members include physicians (urologists, neurologists, neurosurgeons, orthopedists), nursing personnel, physical therapists, psychologists, educators, parents and caregivers, and occupational therapy personnel. The goal is to enable the child to achieve the maximum level of function and to facilitate engagement and participation in everyday activities at home, at school, and in the community.

Activities of Daily Living/Instrumental ADL
- Assist in instructing person to use self-management bowel and bladder program, including skin care (Smith et al., 2016).
- Assist in developing or participating in a program designed to promote independent living skills.

Education/Work
- Assist in facilitating participation in school activities including academic and social (Peny-Dahlstrand et al., 2013).
- Assist in developing work-related skills.

Play/Leisure
- Provide opportunity and access to play activities.
- Assist in facilitating engagement in leisure activities, with peers or groups, offered at the school or in the community, such as arts (painting, drawing), crafts, music, computer play, sports and games, home economics, club councils, field trips.

Rest/Sleep
- Assist in providing supported sleep system.

Social Participation
- Assist in providing opportunity to participate in all school activities.

Sensorimotor
- Assist in providing correct seating and positioning support (wheelchair, static seating).
- Develop hand–eye coordination.
- Develop upper body strength.
- Consider whether serial casting would be appropriate if contractures are present in lower extremity (ankle, knee).

Cognitive/Perceptual
- Assist in developing cognitive skills, including attention, memory, and executive functions.
- Assist in developing time-management skills starting with time perception, then time orientation, and finally time planning.

Psychosocial
- No information identified.

Context/Environment
- Person with a shunt should learn the warning signs of shunt dysfunction including headaches, vomiting, vision problems, unusually tired, easily upset or moody, not feeling right, passing out or collapsing, memory problems greater than usual, changes in balance, head and neck pain, numbness in upper extremities, gagging or swallowing problems (West et al., 2011).
- Provide information and training in use of adaptive equipment (wheelchair, seating, stroller).
- Provide information about community resources, especially for adults (West et al., 2011).

Precautions/Safety Considerations

Person is at risk for pressure sores (decubitus ulcers). Person is at risk for renal failure, especially as an adult. Person is at risk for sepsis (infection) associated with catheterization. Person may be at risk for burns due to sensory deficits, especially in the lower extremities. Person may be at risk for fractures, especially in lower extremities. Person may be at risk for shunt dysfunction.

Prognosis and Outcome

Spina bifida is a chronic, lifelong condition. Issues and concerns change as the individual ages.

REFERENCES

Al-Oraibi, S., Tariah, H. A., & Alanazi, A. (2013). Serial casting versus stretching technique to treat knee flexion contracture in children with spina bifida: A comparative study. *Journal of Pediatric Rehabilitation Medicine, 6*(3), 147–153. https://doi.org/10.3233/PRM-130247

Dicianno, B. E., Kinback, N., Bellin, M. H., Chaikind, L., Buhari, A. M., Holmbeck, G. N., Zabel, T. A., Donlan, R. M., & Collins, D. M. (2015). Depressive symptoms in adults with spina bifida. *Rehabilitation Psychology, 60*(3), 246–253. https://doi.org/10.1037/rep0000044

Donlau, M., Mattsson, S., & Glad-Mattsson, G. (2013). Children with myelomeningocele and independence in the toilet activity: A pilot study. *Scandinavian Journal of Occupational Therapy, 20*(1), 64–70. https://doi.org/10.3109/11038128.2012.700729

Gribble, N., Parsons, R., Donlau, M., & Falkmer, T. (2013). Predictors of time to complete toileting for children with spina bifida. *Australian Occupational Therapy Journal, 60*(5), 343–349. https://doi.org/10.1111/1440-1630.12052

Lindsay, S., Cruickshank, H., McPherson, A. C., & Maxwell, J. (2016). Implementation of an inter-agency transition model for youth with spina bifida. *Child: Care, Health and Development, 42*(2), 203–212. https://doi.org/10.1111/cch.12303

Parmanto, B., Pramana, G., Yu, D. X., Fairman, A. D., & Dicianno, B. E. (2015). Development of mHealth system for supporting self-management and remote consultation of skincare. *BMC Medical Informatics and Decision Making, 15*, Article 114. https://doi.org/10.1186/s12911-015-0237-4

Peny-Dahlstrand, M., Krumlinde-Sundholm, L., & Gosman-Hedström, G. (2012). Is autonomy related to the quality of performance of everyday activities in children with spina bifida? *Disability and Rehabilitation, 34*(6), 514–521. https://doi.org/10.3109/09638288.2011.610495

Peny-Dahlstrand, M., Krumlinde-Sundholm, L., & Gosman-Hedström, G. (2013). Patterns of participation in school-related activities and settings in children with spina bifida. *Disability and Rehabilitation, 35*(21), 1821–1827. https://doi.org/10.3109/09638288.2012.758319

Persson, M., Janeslätt, G., & Peny-Dahlstrand, M. (2017). Daily time management in children with spina bifida. *Journal of Pediatric Rehabilitation Medicine, 10*(3-4), 295–302. https://doi.org/10.3233/PRM-170459

Porter, R. S. (Ed.). (2018). *The Merck manual of diagnosis and therapy* (20th ed.). Merck Sharp & Dohme.

Smith, K., Neville-Jan, A., Freeman, K. A., Adams, E., Mizokawa, S., Dudgeon, B. J., Merkens, M. J., & Walker, W. O. (2016). The effectiveness of bowel and bladder interventions in children with spina bifida. *Developmental Medicine & Child Neurology, 58*(9), 979–988. https://doi.org/10.1111/dmcn.13095

Stedman's medical dictionary for the health professions and nursing (7th ed). (2011). Wolters Kluwer.

West, C., Brodie, L., Dicker, J., & Steinbeck, K. (2011). Development of health support services for adults with spina bifida. *Disability and Rehabilitation, 33*(23-24), 2381–2388. https://doi.org/10.3109/09638288.2011.568664

Sensory Disorders

Ayres Sensory Integration Approach

Also called ASI, sensory integration, sensory integration therapy, sensory integrative theory.

See also Sensory Modulation Disorders, Sensory Integration Dysfunction, Sensory Processing Disorders, Sensory-Based Problems in Adults, Sensory Over-Responsiveness.

Description

"Sensory integration is the process by which people register, modulate, and discriminate sensations received through the sensory systems to produce purposeful, adaptive behaviors in response to the environment" (Watling & Mori, 2017, p. 1). Ayres Sensory Integration (ASI) intervention addresses the processing of sensation through active participation in activities that are individually customized, sensory rich and occupation centered, are aimed to support the child's adaptive responses and occupational performance, and are meaningful to the child. ASI theory recognized that there are underlying neurological mechanisms involved in processing sensory information and outlines the relationships between sensation (vestibular, proprioceptive, and tactile), nervous system functions, social and emotional behavior, and occupational performance (Kilroy et al., 2019; Lane et al., 2019; Watling & Mori, 2017). The interventions focus on purposeful activity that requires an adaptive response and active participation by the child and are provided in the context of play (Schaaf & Davies, 2010).[*]

Cause

Multiple factors may cause sensory integrative disorders, including genetic heredity, prenatal and birth complications, and environmental factors.

Terminology: Patterns of Dysfunction (Schaaf & Mailloux, 2015)

- *Poor sensory perception:* Characterized by difficulty in identifying, discriminating, and interpreting sensation in more than one sensory system that interferes with a child's ability to interpret and use sensation to perform tasks such as buttoning clothes or tying shoelaces. The Ayres Sensory Integration Assessment recognizes four problems in sensory perception: Vestibular Processing, Proprioception, Tactile Perception, and Visual Perception.
- *Somatodyspraxia:* Characterized by difficulty with motor planning. The main identifying feature is poor tactile perception and difficulty in imitating, planning, or sequencing actions.
- *Vestibular and bilateral integration deficit:* Characterized by inefficient vestibular processing associated with poor postural, ocular, and bilateral function as shown by delays and difficulties in posture, balance, ocular motor control, bilateral integration, and sequencing skills as observed in riding a bicycle.
- *Visuodyspraxia:* Characterized by difficulty with both visual perception and visual-motor planning. Visuodyspraxia has some similarity to earlier descriptions of perceptual-motor difficulties.

Evaluation/Assessment

Areas

- Activities of Daily Living/Instrumental ADL: oral praxis (feeding, eating), dressing, tying shoelaces
- Education/Work: academic performance, handwriting, classroom behavior
- Play/Leisure: play skills, leisure interests
- Rest/Sleep: sleep disturbances
- Social Participation: type, frequency, location, with whom
- Sensorimotor: bilateral motor control, constructional praxis, design copying, motor accuracy, postural praxis, postrotary nystagmus, sequencing praxis, standing and walking balance

---

[*] Although sensory processing theory is now accepted into ASI, this chapter will focus on the original concepts proposed by Ayres. Sensory processing is covered in a separate chapter.

- Cognitive/Perceptual: concentration, memory, problem solving, organizing, figure ground, finger identification, graphesthesia, kinesthesia, localization of tactile stimulus, manual form perception, praxis on verbal command, spatial (space) visualization
- Psychosocial: emotional regulation, self-esteem, self-control, self-confidence
- Context/Environment: environment modification
- Development (Infant, Child, Adolescent only): no information identified
- Comorbidities: attention-deficit/hyperactivity disorder, autism spectrum disorder, developmental coordination disorder, developmental delay, nonverbal learning disability, regulatory disorders, specific learning disorders (for autism, see Schoen et al., 2019; Watling & Hauer, 2015)

Instruments
Instruments Developed by Occupational Therapy Personnel
- Ayres Sensory Integration Assessment and Interpretation Tool (ASIAIT; Schaaf & Mailloux, 2015, in References)
- Ayres Sensory Integration Fidelity Measure (Fidelity Measure; Parham et al., 2011; see also May-Benson et al., 2014)
- Evaluation in Ayres Sensory Integration (EASI; Mailloux et al., 2018, in References)
- Pediatric Evaluation of Disability Inventory (PEDI; Haley et al., 1992)
- Sensory Integration and Praxis Tests (SIPT; Ayres, 1989)

Instruments Developed by Other Professionals and Used by Occupational Therapy Personnel
- Goal Attainment Scaling (GAS; Kiresuk et al., 1994)

Problems/Issues
Activities of Daily Living/Instrumental ADL
- Child may have difficulty performing self-maintenance skills such as eating and dressing.

Education/Work
- Child may have difficulty managing classroom demands (organizing, executing, interacting).

Play/Leisure
- Child may have difficulty developing play skills (using and manipulating toys, sharing).
- Child may have difficulty engaging in play and leisure activities that are age appropriate.

Rest/Sleep
- Child may have difficulty falling asleep or staying asleep.

Social Participation
- Child may have difficulty participating in family and social activities.

Sensorimotor
- Child may have difficulty performing coordinated motor actions.
- Child may have difficulty registering sensory information.
- Child may have difficulty discriminating among different degrees or amounts of sensory information.
- Child may have difficulty modulating response or responses to sensory information.

Cognitive/Perceptual
- Child may have difficulty attending to tasks.
- Child may have difficulty planning and sequencing motor actions.

Psychosocial
- Child may have difficulty developing social relations.

Context/Environment
- Child may have difficulty dealing with tasks required by home, school, and community.

Intervention/Treatment

Focus is on using knowledge of the dynamic interactions among all sensory systems to provide an understanding of the underlying reasons why a child might be struggling with attaining and using the skills to support occupational engagement. Models and programs developed by occupational therapy personnel include case report (Bellefeuille et al., 2013), data-driven decision making (Faller et al., 2016), and manualization (Hunt et al., 2017). Team members include physicians, psychologists, speech–language pathologists, educators and administrators, parents and caregivers, child care workers, physical therapy personnel, and occupational therapy personnel. Goal is the integration and organization of sensory information into a person's response to adapt to and interact with the environment, and to increase the person's ability to participate in everyday activities and routines, including self-care, school, work, play, and leisure (Schaaf & Mailloux, 2015).

Activities of Daily Living/Instrumental ADL
- No information identified.

Education/Work
- No information identified.

Play/Leisure
- All therapeutic play activities should be child directed and therapist supported.

Rest/Sleep
- Use activities that calm the child before bedtime.
- Modify the sensory environment such as using flannel (cotton based) sheets instead of linen, which may feel scratchy.

Social Participation
- No information identified.

Sensorimotor
- Therapeutic activities should focus on tactile, proprioceptive, and vestibular opportunities.
- Use of activities based in the sensory systems of vestibular and proprioception can contribute to ability to develop adequate posture, balance, muscle tone, gravitational security, and movement of the eyes in coordination with head and body movements.
- Use of activities based in the tactile system can provide a foundation for body awareness, coordination of the two sides of the body, and praxis.
- Therapeutic activities should promote postural control and balance using such equipment as suspended apparatus, scooters, and large therapy balls.

Cognitive/Perceptual
- Therapeutic activities should be designed to challenge the child to develop ideas about what to do.
- Therapeutic activities should allow child to plan out ideas and then successfully carry out plan.

Psychosocial
- No information identified.

Context/Environment
- Therapeutic environment should be physically and emotional safe for the child.
- Therapeutic environment should facilitate adaptive behavior and responses. Examples of equipment include ball pit or ball bag containing variety of sized balls, barrels for rolling, bolster swing, bouncing equipment (trampoline), climbing equipment (steps, ladders, stacking

tires), crash pillow or pad, flexion disc swing, frog swing, incline ramps, inner tubes, gilder swing, large therapy balls, materials for practicing daily living skills (pencils, pens, school supplies, clothing, grooming products), mats, oral toys, pillows made with a variety of materials and textures, platform swing, props for pretend play activities (dress-up clothes, balls and bats, stuffed animals, dolls, puppets, sports equipment, bikes), rubber strips or ropes for pulling, scooter and ramp, stretchy fabric, tire swing, variety of tactile materials (textured fabrics, brushes, carpet squares), vibrating toys, visual targets (balloons, hook-and-loop dartboard, hanging objects), weighted garments, weighted objects (balls, bean bags in a variety of sizes), weighted garments (Schaaf & Mailloux, 2015).

Precautions/Safety Considerations

Mats, cushions, and pillows must always be available to pad the floor underneath any suspended equipment. Therapist should always place hands near the child in anticipation of assisting with difficult maneuvers or movements and to be ready to move or stabilize the child on equipment if needed. Therapist should consider using self to block unsafe situations, such as jumping off a bolster onto a hard surface. Equipment should be checked for wear and tear frequently for safety, especially chains or ropes used for hanging swings. Equipment and supplies should be washed regularly. Equipment not needed for a particular intervention program should be stored out of the way (Schaaf & Mailloux, 2015). Therapists need to follow established guidelines (Mori et al., 2017).

Prognosis and Outcome

Variable. Studies have been criticized for weak methodology and failure to clarify and consistently label concepts. The American Academy of Pediatrics does not recognize sensory integration dysfunction or sensory processing disorder as a diagnosis and there is limited coverage through insurance (American Academy of Pediatrics, 2012). Better outcomes measures have been addressed by May-Benson et al. (2018).

REFERENCES

American Academy of Pediatrics. (2012). Sensory integration therapies for children with developmental and behavioral disorders [Policy statement]. *Pediatrics, 129*(6), 1186–1189. https://doi.org/10.1542/peds.2012-0876

Bellefeuille, I. B., Schaaf, R. C., & Polo, E. R. (2013). Occupational therapy based on Ayres Sensory Integration in the treatment of retentive fecal incontinence in a 3-year-old boy. *American Journal of Occupational Therapy, 67,* 601–606. https://doi.org/10.5014/ajot.2013.008086

Faller, P., Hunt, J., van Hooydonk, E., Mailloux, Z., & Schaaf, R. (2016). Application of data-driven decision making using Ayres Sensory Integration with a child with autism. *American Journal of Occupational Therapy, 70,* Article 7001220020. https://doi.org/10.5014/ajot.2016.016881

Hunt, J., van Hooydonk, E., Faller, P., Mailloux, Z., & Schaaf, R. (2017). Manualization of occupational therapy using Ayres Sensory Integration for autism. *OTJR: Occupation, Participation and Health, 37*(3), 141–149. https://doi.org/10.1177/1539449217697044

Kilroy, E., Aziz Zadeh, L., & Cermak, S. (2019). Ayres theories of autism and sensory integration revisited: What contemporary neuroscience has to say. *Brain Sciences, 9,* Article 68. https://doi.org/10.3390/brainsci9030068

Lane, S. J., Mailloux, Z., Schoen, S., Bundy, A., May-Benson, T. A., Parham, L. D., Smith Roley, S., & Schaaf, R. C. (2019). Neural foundations of Ayres Sensory Integration. *Brain Sciences, 9,* Article 153. https://doi.org/10.3390/brainsci9070153

Mailloux, Z., Parham, L. D., Roley, S. S., Ruzzano, L., & Schaaf, R. C. (2018). Introduction to the evaluation in Ayres Sensory Integration (EASI). *American Journal of Occupational Therapy, 72,* Article 7201195030. https://doi.org/10.5014/ajot.2018.028241

May-Benson, T. A., Roley, S. S., Mailloux, Z., Parham, L. D., Koomar, J., Schaaf, R. C., Van Jaars-veld, A., & Cohn, E. (2014). Interrater reliability and discriminative validity of the structural elements of the Ayres Sensory Integration Fidelity Measure. *American Journal of Occupational Therapy, 68*, 506–513. https://doi.org/10.5014/ajot.2014.010652

May-Benson, T. A., Schaaf, R. C., Clippard, H. L., & Mori, A. B. (2018). Identifying and measuring outcomes in Ayres Sensory Integration. *OT Practice, 23*(3), Article CEA0218.

Mori, A. B., Koester, A. C., Holland, D., Fernandes, P., Rogers, R. G., Roley, S. S., Soechting, E., & VanJaarsveld, A. (2017). Building competency in SI: Evidence-based guidelines for occupational therapy using Ayres Sensory Integration. *OT Practice, 22*(12), 8–13.

Parham, L. D., Roley, S. S., May-Benson, T. A., Koomar, J., Brett-Green, B., Burke, J. P., Cohn, E. S., Mailloux, Z., Miller, L. J., & Schaaf, R. C. (2011). Development of a fidelity measure for research on the effectiveness of the Ayres Sensory Integration intervention. *American Journal of Occupational Therapy, 65*, 133–142. https://doi.org/10.5014/ajot.2011.000745

Schaaf, R. C., & Davies, P. (2010). From the desk of the guest editors: Evolution of the sensory integration frame of reference. *American Journal of Occupational Therapy, 64*(3), 363–367.

Schaaf, R. C., & Mailloux, Z. (2015). *Clinician's guide for implementing Ayres Sensory Integration: Promoting participation for children with autism.* AOTA Press.

Schoen, S. A., Lane, S. J., Mailloux, Z., May-Benson, T., Parham, L. D., Roley, S. S., & Schaaf, R. C. (2019). A systematic review of Ayres Sensory Integration intervention for children with autism. *Autism Research, 12*, 6–19. https://doi.org/10.1002/aur.2046

Watling, R., & Hauer, S. (2015). Effectiveness of Ayres Sensory Integration and sensory-based interventions for people with autism spectrum disorder: A systematic review. *American Journal of Occupational Therapy, 69*, Article 6905180030. https://doi.org/10.5014/ajot.2015.018051

Watling, R., & Mori, A. B. (2017). *Frequently asked questions (FAQ) about: Ayres Sensory Integration.* American Occupational Therapy Association.

BIBLIOGRAPHY

American Occupational Therapy Association. (2015). Occupational therapy for children and youth using sensory integration theory and methods in school-based practice. *American Journal of Occupational Therapy, 69*(Suppl. 3), Article 6913410040. https://doi.org/10.5014/ajot.2015.696S04

Gorman, M. E., & Kashani, N. H. (2017). A. Jean Ayres and the development of sensory integration: A case study in the development and fragmentation of a scientific therapy network. *Social Epistemology, 31*(2), 107–129. https://doi.org/10.1080/02691728.2016.1241322

Mailloux, Z., & Miller-Kuhaneck, H. (2014). Evolution of a theory: How measurement has shaped Ayres Sensory Integration. *American Journal of Occupational Therapy, 68*, 495–499. https://doi.org/10.5014/ajot.2014.013656

Mailloux, Z., Mulligan, S., Roley, S. S., Blanche, E., Cermak, S., Coleman, G. G., Bodison, S., & Lane, C. J. (2011). Verification and clarification of patterns of sensory integrative dysfunction. *American Journal of Occupational Therapy, 65*, 143–151. https://doi.org/10.5014/ajot.2011.000752

May-Benson, T. A., & Schaaf, R. (2015). Ayres Sensory Integration intervention. In I. Söderback (Ed.), *International handbook of occupational therapy interventions* (2nd ed., pp. 633–646). Springer.

Miller-Kuhaneck, H. (2010). The importance of mentoring for the professional involvement of therapists specializing in Ayres Sensory Integration. *Sensory Integration Special Interest Section Quarterly, 33*(2), 1–4.

Parham, L. D., & Mailloux, Z. (2015). Sensory integration. In J. Case-Smith & J. C. O'Brien (Eds.), *Occupational therapy for children and adolescents* (7th ed., pp. 258–303). Elsevier.

Schaaf, R. C., Dumont, R. L., Arbesman, M., & May-Benson, T. A. (2018). Efficacy of occupational therapy using Ayres Sensory Integration: A systematic review. *American Journal of Occupational Therapy, 72*(1), Article 7201190010. https://doi.org/10.5014/ajot.2018.028431

Back Pain and Low Back Pain

Description

Back pain may be acute or chronic. The lower back is a frequent location for chronic back pain and may be related to issues of the lumbar spine such as bony, disk, or ligamentous problems, but pain can also occur in the upper back, often related to poor posture (Hale, 2016). Risk factors include a prior history of back pain; physical and mechanical strains, such as repetitive bending or poor sitting posture; whole body vibration, as experienced in cars or other modes of transportation; and lack of lumbar extension (Mayo & Weissman, 2011). Multiple obstacles and facilitators affect return-to-work status (Dionne et al., 2013).

Cause

Common causes are muscle strain, ligament sprain, spasm, poor posture, decreased strength of stabilizing muscles, or decreased flexibility (Porter, 2018). Specific structural lesions account for only about 15% of symptoms and may be the result of disk herniation, compression fracture, lumbar spinal stenosis, osteoarthritis, or spondylolisthesis (Porter, 2018). Back pain may be related to a past injury or surgery, to another chronic condition such as arthritis or cancer, or may be unrelated to any specific injury or illness (Hale, 2016).

Evaluation/Assessment

Areas

- Activities of Daily Living/Instrumental ADL: change in amount or degree of performance, increased difficulty performing normal ADLs or IADLs
- Education/Work: change in attendance frequency at school or work, ability to perform academic or work tasks
- Play/Leisure: change in interests, frequency, location
- Rest/Sleep: change in sleep habits and routines
- Social Participation: change in type, frequency, location, other participants
- Sensorimotor: description of type of pain (shooting, stabbing, burning, aching, "electrical"), complaints of being sore, feeling "tight" or "stiff," fatigue
- Cognitive/Perceptual: not directly involved, but consider whether comorbidity factors may increase risk of cognitive impairment such as an illness or disorder such as substance abuse
- Psychosocial: changes in mood (anxiety, catastrophizing, depression, feelings of hopelessness, irritability, sense of self-efficacy, stress, worry)
- Context/Environment: overall change in health status (weakened immune system, recent illness, unexplained fever)
- Comorbidities: recent surgery, recent illness, obesity, substance abuse, gastrointestinal or urinary conditions, gynecologic problems, new motor or sensory deficit

Instruments

Instruments Developed by Occupational Therapy Personnel
- Activity Card Sort (2nd ed.; ACS-2; Baum & Edwards, 2008)
- Canadian Occupational Performance Measure (5th ed.; COPM-5; Law et al., 2014)

Instruments Developed by Other Professionals and Used by Occupational Therapy Personnel
- Beck Depression Inventory (2nd ed.; BDI-II; Beck et al., 1996)
- Brief Pain Inventory (BPI; Cleeland & Ryan, 1994)
- Face, Legs, Activity, Cry, and Consolability Pain Scale (FLACC; Merkel et al., 1997)
- Functional Independence Measure (FIM; Uniform Data System for Medical Rehabilitation, 1997)
- Oswestry Disability Index (ODI; Fairbank & Pynsent, 2000)
- Pain Self-Efficacy Questionnaire (PSEQ; Nicholas, 2007)

- Roland-Morris Disability Questionnaire (RMDQ; Roland & Morris, 1983)
- Short-Form 36 Health Survey (SF-36; Ware et al., 1993)
- Visual analogue scale for pain (numeric rating: 0 = *no pain* to 10 = *worst pain ever*)
- Wong-Baker FACES Pain Rating Scale (FACES; Wong & Baker, 1998)

Problems/Issues

Activities of Daily Living/Instrumental ADL
- Person may experience back pain while performing basic ADLs such as dressing, bathing/showering, toileting, mobility in the home.
- Person may experience back pain while performing IADLs such as meal preparation, home making, driving, shopping.
- Person may experience a change in financial status due to reduced income and change in work status (loss of income, increased debt).
- Person may experience difficulty with medication management (following directions, reporting need for medication adjustment).

Education/Work
- Person may experience back pain from prolonged static positions such as use of computer.
- Person may experience back pain while performing work-related movements (lifting, carrying, bending, stopping, walking, climbing).
- Person may miss classes or days of work due to back pain (increased number of days absent from work setting).
- Person may take sick leave due to back pain.

Play/Leisure
- Person may limit or stop engagement in favorite leisure occupations because of back pain.

Rest/Sleep
- Person may report difficulty sleeping due to back pain.

Social Participation
- Person may have limited or stopped participation in certain social activities due to back pain, such as events that require long periods of sitting or require physical activity such as a round of golf.

Sensorimotor
- Person reports or experiences back pain while engaged in everyday activities.
- Person may report decreased muscle strength.
- Person may report decreased endurance.
- Person may be kinesphobic (fearful of movement).
- Person may report increased fatigue and feelings of tiredness.

Cognitive/Perceptual
- See note under Evaluation/Assessment.

Psychosocial
- Person may experience changes such as decreased role performance related directly or indirectly to back pain.
- Person may experience depression, anxiety, fear of reinjury, distress, sense of hopelessness.
- Person may experience reduced sense of self-efficacy, worthlessness, loss of sense of self-control (Richard et al., 2011), and experience a sense of helplessness.
- Person may become more easily irritated, become aggressive, be quick-tempered and in a "bad mood."
- Person may be less tolerant of others and feel that others "just don't understand."
- Person may feel health-care workers do not take pain and complaints seriously.

Context/Environment
- Person and family may lack knowledge and information about available resources.
- Person and family may lack access to information or support groups.
- Person may report decreased social support from family, friends, and colleagues.
- Person may experience lack of environmental accessibility.
- Employer may lack knowledge and information about managing employees with back pain, including policies and procedures that reduce opportunity for person to return to work successfully.
- Employer may be unwilling to manage employees with back pain.

Intervention/Treatment

Models and programs developed by occupational therapy personnel include client-centered occupational therapy analysis (Simon, 2018). Models and programs developed by other professionals but used by occupational therapy personnel include the adapted stress process model (Truchon et al., 2010), biopsychosocial approach (Snodgrass, 2011), myofascial release (Saratchandran & Desai, 2013), return to work in good health program (Richard et al., 2011), yoga (Wattamwar & Nadkami, 2012), and therapeutic modalities (Kennedy-Spaien et al., 2013). Team members include physicians, psychologists, physical therapy personnel, and occupational therapy personnel. Goals are to allow client to complete everyday tasks of living (ADLs, IADLs, work, play, rest, and sleep) and to reengage in social activity, using proper body mechanics, pain management, and coping techniques (Hale, 2016).

Activities of Daily Living/Instrumental ADL
- Medication management: Focused on taking and tapering off pain meds.
- ADLs: See Simon (2018) for examples of dressing, shaving, sex positions.
- IADLs: See Simon (2018) for examples, reaching into a refrigerator, loading/unloading washing machine, child care.

Education/Work
- Stress sense of self-efficacy and locus of control as major elements of a return-to-work program.

Play/Leisure
- Discuss with client interests in existing leisure occupations to determine which are feasible, which can be modified, or which should be discontinued.
- Assist client to explore and develop new leisure occupations that may be added to or replace existing interests.

Rest/Sleep
- See Sleep–Wake Disorders in Section 13: Lifestyle Conditions.

Social Participation
- Assist client to continue participation in social activities with modifications, if needed, such as shorter time periods with more rest breaks, less physically demanding, less distance from home, with people who are educated about back pain, fewer people.

Sensorimotor
- Activity pacing: Instruct client to organize daily activities to permit work and rest cycles.
- Body mechanics: Instruct client in good posture and joint protection.
- Energy conservation: Instruct client in use of energy saving strategies.
- Pain management: No information identified.
- Physical agent modalities: Ice massage, TENS, ultrasound (work with physical therapist or take courses to use modalities).

- Physical conditioning: Instruct client in use of physical exercise within pain tolerance.
- Self-massage: Use tennis ball as massage tool.
- Work simplification: Review with client steps in daily or work tasks to determine whether some steps could be eliminated or combined.

Cognitive/Perceptual
- Assist client and family to problem solve issues related to role performance and responsibilities.

Psychosocial
- Self-management program: Encourage client to take responsibility for pain management, educating self about resources, medication schedule, self-massage, activity pacing.
- Cognitive behavior management: Focus on increasing performance of daily life activities.
- Provide training in stress management techniques including relaxation, yoga, mindfulness, deep-breathing exercises.

Context/Environment
- Ergonomics: Suggest equipment that may reduce stress on back.
- Assistive technology: Suggest technology that may reduce stress and improve performance.

Precautions/Safety Considerations

Most precautions and safety concerns are related to the specific type of back pain, its management, and the environment in which the client lives and functions.

Prognosis and Outcome

Back pain often becomes a chronic condition which may be constant or intermittent. Client needs to function as well as possible within the limits of the back pain, including physical, psychological, and environment factors.

REFERENCES

Dionne, C. E., Bourbonnais, R., Frémont, P., Rossignol, M., Stock, S. R., & Laperrière, È. (2013). Obstacles to and facilitators of return to work after work-disabling back pain: The workers' perspective. *Journal of Occupational Rehabilitation, 23*, 280–289. https://doi.org/10.1007/s10926-012-9399-4

Hale, L. (2016). *Clinical review: Back pain, chronic: Occupational therapy.* Cinahl Information Systems.

Kennedy-Spaien, E., Kohlhofer, D., & Brehm, R. (2013). The challenge of chronic low back pain. *Rehabilitation Management, 26*(6), 46–51.

Mayo, T. P., & Weissman, L. (2011). The noninvasive path to chronic back pain management. *Rehabilitation Management, 24*(8), 18, 20–21.

Porter, R. S. (Ed.). (2018). *The Merck manual of diagnosis and therapy* (20th ed.). Merck Sharp & Dohme.

Richard, S., Dionne, C. E., & Nouwen, A. (2011). Self-efficacy and health locus of control: Relationship to occupational disability among workers with back pain. *Journal of Occupational Rehabilitation, 21*, 421–430. https://doi.org/10.1007/s10926-011-9285-5

Saratchandran, R., & Desai, S. (2013). Myofascial release as an adjunct to conventional occupational therapy in mechanical low back pain. *Indian Journal of Occupational Therapy, 45*(2), 3–7.

Simon, A. U. (2018). Low back pain. In H. M. Pendleton & W. Schulz-Krohn (Eds.), *Pedretti's occupational therapy* (8th ed., pp. 1029–1047). Mosby-Elsevier.

Snodgrass, J. (2011). Effective occupational therapy interventions in the rehabilitation of individuals with work-related low back injuries and illnesses: A systematic review. *American Journal of Occupational Therapy, 65*(1), 37–43. https://doi.org/10.5014/ajot.2011.09187

Truchon, M., Côté, D., Schmouth, M-È., Leblond, J., Fillion, L., & Dionne, C. (2010). Validation of an adaptation of the stress process model for predicting low back pain related long-term disability outcomes: A cohort study. *Spine, 35*(13), 1307–1315.

Wattamwar, R. B., & Nadkami, K. (2012). Effect of conventional occupational therapy and yoga in chronic low back pain. *Indian Journal of Occupational Therapy, 45*(3), 13–20.

BIBLIOGRAPHY

Davies, C., & Howell, D. (2012). A qualitative study: Clinical decision making in low back pain. *Physiotherapy Theory and Practice, 28*(2), 95–107. https://doi.org/10.3109/09593985 .2011.571752[*]

Grangaard, L. (2013). Low back pain. In H. M. Pendleton & W. Schulz-Krohn (Eds.), *Pedretti's occupational therapy* (7th ed., pp. 1091–1109). Mosby-Elsevier.

Gupta, S. (2015). Examining clinimetric and psychometric properties of disability assessment scales for low-back pain: Exploring possibilities for adaptation to Indian context. *Indian Journal of Physiotherapy and Occupational Therapy, 47*(2), 38–45.

Benign Paroxysmal Positional Vertigo

Also called benign positional vertigo, BPPV.
See also Vestibular Disorders.

Description

In benign paroxysmal positional vertigo (BPPV), short (<60 seconds) episodes of vertigo occur when the head is turned in certain positions, such as rolling over in bed or bending over to pick up something. Vertigo occurs due to displacement of otoconial crystals into the semicircular canal. Nausea, vomiting, and nystagmus (rapid movements of the eyes) may develop (Porter, 2018). Tinnitus (ringing in the ear) or hearing loss do not occur. BPPV affects people more frequently as they age and can severely affect balance in the elderly, leading to potential falls (Porter, 2018).

Cause

The etiology is thought to be displacement of the otoconial crystals normally embedded in the saccule and utricle. The displaced material stimulates hair cells most commonly in the posterior semicircular canal, creating the illusion of motion. A few individuals have displaced material in both the posterior and lateral canals. Possible etiologic factors include spontaneous degeneration of the utricular otolithic membranes, labyrinthine concussion, otitis media, ear surgery, viral infection, head trauma, prolonged anesthesia or bed rest, previous vestibular disorders, or occlusion of the anterior vestibular artery (Porter, 2018). Two mechanisms or subtypes have been described: One is *cupulolithiasis,* the presence of otoconial material of the cupula of the semicircular canal. The second is *canalithiasis,* the presence of otoconial material in the semicircular canal. A mix of both may be possible (Cohen & Sangi-Haghpeykar, 2010b).

Evaluation/Assessment

Areas
- Activities of Daily Living/Instrumental ADL: dressing, bathing or showering, meal preparation, household chores (dusting, vacuuming), child care, driving, transportation
- Education/Work: academic setting, work station
- Play/Leisure: types, location, frequency

---

[*] Article is about physical therapy management, even though there is an occupational therapist as author.

- Rest/Sleep: no information identified
- Social Participation: no information identified
- Sensorimotor: balance, moving from one position to another, postural control, postural sway, walking in open spaces, reaching, climbing/descending stairs, using moving equipment (escalator, elevator), nystagmus (rotary, vertical, horizontal), dizziness
- Cognitive/Perceptual: spatial orientation, vertical body orientation
- Psychosocial: role performance, quality of life
- Context/Environment: adaptive devices, health literacy, resources
- Development (Infant, Child, Adolescent only): no information identified
- Comorbidities: sinus or rhinosinusitis disease (Cohen et al., 2010)

Instruments

Instruments Developed by Occupational Therapy Personnel

- Vestibular Disorders Activities of Daily Living Scale (VADL; Cohen & Kimball, 2000)

Instruments Developed by Other Professionals and Used by Occupational Therapy Personnel

- Caloric stimulation (cold and warm water; see Porter, 2018, in References)
  - ▶ Client is supine with head elevated 30°.
  - ▶ Each ear is irrigated sequentially with 3 milliliters of ice water. Alternate approach, 240 milliliters of warm water (40° to 44°C) may be used.
  - ▶ Cold water causes nystagmus to opposite side of stimulation; warm water causes nystagmus to same side (COWS: cold opposite; warm same).
- Clinical Test of Sensory Integration and Balance (CTSIB; Shumway-Cook & Horak, 1986; see also Mulavara et al., 2013, in References)
- Dix-Hallpike Maneuver (Nystagmus Response Test, Barany Test; Porter, 2018)
  - ▶ Client sits on a table with legs extended and eyes open looking straight ahead.
  - ▶ Client's head is turned 45° toward the side to be tested.
  - ▶ Client is rapidly laid down on the table with the nose pitched upward (neck hyperextended) approximately 30° while being supported by the clinician for 30–60 seconds.
  - ▶ Record nystagmus response for up to 3 seconds.
  - ▶ Positive response to test is nystagmus beating toward the test side (Cohen et al., 2014, in References).
- Dizziness Handicap Inventory (DHI; Jacobson & Newman, 1990)
- Mental Rotation Test (MRT; Shepard & Metzler, 1971)
- Persistence of vision (animations; see Holly et al., 2019, in References)
- Rod-and-Frame Test (RFT; Nyborg, 1974; see also Nair et al., 2017, in References)
- Sensory Organization Test (SOT; Nashner et al., 1982; see also Mulavara et al., 2013, in References)
- UCLA Dizziness Questionnaire (UCLA-DQ; Honrubia et al., 1996)
- Vestibular Rehabilitation Benefit Questionnaire (VRBQ; Morris et al., 2008)

Problems/Issues

Activities of Daily Living/Instrumental ADL

- Person may experience difficulty with upper and lower body dressing tasks, especially those requiring balance and postural control.
- Person may have difficulty with bathing or showering due to demand for changes in body position that may exacerbate vertigo or balance disturbance.
- Person may experience difficulty maintaining balance while performing basic mobility tasks, including getting up from lying in bed or sitting in a chair, walking on an uneven surface, walking in wide open or very narrow spaces, walking in crowds, climbing up or descending stairs, walking or climbing while carrying objects (packages, bags).
- Person may experience vertigo or balance disorder while riding in an elevator, using an escalator, or riding in a vehicle (car, train, plane, bus).

- Person may experience vertigo or balance disorder while preparing meals due to demand for reaching, stooping, and standing.
- Person may have difficulty with household chores due to demand for balance, reaching, and climbing if stairs are present.
- Person may experience difficulty driving due to demands for moving the head quickly.
- Person may experience difficulty performing child care activities, including lifting, carrying, bending, and reaching.
- Person may experience difficulty participating in intimate activities (foreplay or sexual activity).
- Person may experience nausea and/or vomiting.
- Person may experience increased perspiration.
- Person may experience increased salivation.
- Person may experience general malaise.

Education/Work
- Person may have difficulty moving about the academic environment, especially if their setting involves a large campus.
- Person may have difficulty completing work tasks that involve frequent changes of position, including lifting, reaching, carrying, bending, and stooping.

Play/Leisure
- Person may have difficulty engaging in favorite leisure occupations that require a lot of movement (golf) and/or many changes in position (gardening).

Rest/Sleep
- No information identified.

Social Participation
- No information identified.

Sensorimotor
- Person may have difficulty with dynamic balance.
- Person may have difficulty with sudden changes in movement demands.
- Person may demonstrate nystagmus (rapid alternating eye movements: getting up, down, in, out, over, under).
- Person may have difficulty moving in different types of spaces, such as narrow aisles, open spaces, uneven ground.

Cognitive/Perceptual
- Person may experience difficulty with spatial orientation.

Psychosocial
- Person may have difficulty performing some role activities that involve movement.
- Person may experience decreased quality of life.

Context/Environment
- Person may need adaptive devices to facilitate safe movement.
- Person may need information about BPPV and its management.
- Person may need social support.
- Person may need access to resources.

Intervention/Treatment

Models and programs developed by occupational therapy personnel: None. Models and programs developed by other professionals but used by occupational therapy personnel include canalith repositioning variations (Cohen & Sangi-Haghpeykar, 2010a), vestibular rehabilitation (Kus & Timmons, 2018), and vestibular therapy (Cronin & Steenerson, 2011). Team members include physicians, psychologists, physical therapy personnel, and occupational therapy personnel. Goals are to reposition the displaced otoconial matter through exercises and passive maneuvers to relieve the sense of vertigo and balance disturbances (Cohen & Sangi-Haghpeykar, 2010a).

Activities of Daily Living/Instrumental ADL
- No information identified.

Education/Work
- No information identified.

Play/Leisure
- No information identified.

Rest/Sleep
- No information identified.

Social Participation
- No information identified.

Sensorimotor
- Assist client to achieve "sensory reweighting" for postural control, the ability to regulate and integrate sensory information dynamically to adapt to changing environments or sensory inputs (Nair et al., 2017). For example, postural control during daylight vision can assist proprioception. At night, without the aid of light to permit vision to function, proprioception becomes the primary sensory system to facilitate postural control. If light is added at night, the two sensory systems can again work together to facilitate postural control.
- Epley maneuver (canalith repositioning maneuver; CRP; Porter, 2018, p. 821)
  - Begin with client sitting upright, facing forward, in the middle of a table.
  - The therapist grasps the head with both hands and rotates the client's head toward the affected ear.
  - The therapist then lowers the client backward to the supine position, with head hanging over the table's edge.
  - The head is then turned to the other side.
  - The head is turned farther, so that the ear is parallel to the floor.
  - The head may be rapidly turned even further, almost facing the floor.
  - The client is returned to the upright position.
  - The head is rotated back to normal position (Porter, 2018).
- Self-CRP exercises: Instruct clients on how to do the Epley maneuver by themselves.
- Semont maneuver (liberatory maneuver; Porter, 2018, p. 820)
  - The client is seated upright, in the middle of a table.
  - The client's head is rotated toward the unaffected ear, and this ration is maintained throughout the maneuver.
  - The torso is lowered laterally onto the table so that the client is lying on the side of the affected ear with the nose pointed up.
  - After 3 minutes in this position, the client is quickly moved through the upright position, without straightening the head, and is lowered laterally to the other side, now with the nose pointed down.
  - After 3 minutes in this position, the client is slowly returned to the upright position, and head is rotated back to normal (Porter, 2018).
- Brandt-Daroff exercise
  - The client sits upright, then lies on side, with the nose pointed up at a 45° angle.
  - The client remains in this position for about 30 seconds, or until the vertigo subsides, and then moves back to the seated position.
  - The same motion is repeated on the opposite side.
  - The cycle is repeated 5 times in a row, 3 times/day, for about 2 weeks, or until vertigo stops (Porter, 2018).

Cognitive/Perceptual
- Self-management: Teach client to perform repositioning maneuver on self.

Psychosocial
- No information identified.

Context/Environment
- No information identified.

Precautions/Safety Considerations

Drugs rarely help and may worsen symptoms. After performing the Epley or Semont maneuvers, the client should remain erect or semi-erect for 1 to 2 days, and avoid neck flexion or extension. Be sure client understands and practices home exercises with therapist present to ensure the exercises are performed correctly. Check client for potential fall risk and provide preventative measures as warranted.

Prognosis and Outcome

Maneuvers often reduce the symptoms immediately. However, the symptoms may return. Certain exercises and self-administered maneuvers can be learned to self-manage symptoms.

REFERENCES

American Occupational Therapy Association (2017) Vestibular impairment, vestibular rehabilitation, and occupational performance. *American Journal of Occupational Therapy, 71*(Suppl. 2) Article 7112410055 https://doi.org/10.5014/ajot.2017.716S09

Cohen, H. S., Mulavara, A. P., Sangi-Haghpeykar, H., Peters, B. T., Bloomberg, J. J., & Pavlik, V. N. (2014). Screening people in the waiting room for vestibular impairments. *Southern Medical Journal, 107*(9), 549–553. https://doi.org/10.14423/SMJ.000000000000017

Cohen, H. S., & Sangi-Haghpeykar, H. (2010a). Canalith repositioning variations for benign paroxysmal positional vertigo. *Otolaryngology–Head and Neck Surgery, 143*(3), 405–412. https://doi.org/10.1016/j.otohns.2010.05.022

Cohen, H. S., & Sangi-Haghpeykar, H. (2010b). Nystagmus parameters and subtypes of benign paroxysmal positional vertigo. *Acta Oto-Laryngologica, 130,* 1019–1023. https://doi.org/10.3109/00016481003664777

Cohen, H. S., Stewart, M. G., Brissett, A. E., Olson, K. L., Takashima, M., & Sangi-Haghpeykar, H. (2010). Frequency of sinus disease in normal subjects and patients with benign paroxysmal positional vertigo. *ORL, 72,* 63–67. https://doi.org/10.1159/000296304

Cronin, G. W., & Steenerson, R. L. (2011). Disequilibrium of aging: Response to a 3-month program of vestibular therapy. *Physical & Occupational Therapy in Geriatrics, 29*(2), 148–155. https://doi.org/10.3109/02703181.2010.544845

Holly, J. E., Cohen, H. S., & Masood, M. A. (2019). Assessing misperception of rotation in benign paroxysmal positional vertigo with static and dynamic visual images. *Journal of Vestibular Research, 29*(5), Article 271279. https://doi.org/10.3233/VES-190676

Kus, E., & Timmons, A. (2018). Vestibular rehabilitation—An emerging role for occupational therapists? *OT News, 26*(9), 28–30.

Mulavara, A. P., Cohen, H. S., Peters, B. T., Sangi-Haghpeykar, H., & Bloomberg, J. J. (2013). New analysis of the Sensory Organization Test compared to the Clinical Test of Sensory Integration and Balance in patients with benign paroxysmal positional vertigo. *The Laryngoscope, 123*(9), 2276–2280. https://doi.org/10.1002/lary.24075

Nair, M. A., Mulavara, A. P., Bloomberg, J. J., Sangi-Haghpeykar, H., & Cohen, H. S. (2017). Visual dependence and spatial orientation in benign paroxysmal positional vertigo. *Journal of Vestibular Research, 27*(5/6), 279–286. https://doi.org/10.3233/VES-170623

Porter, R. S. (Ed.). (2018). *The Merck manual of diagnosis and therapy* (20th ed.). Merck Sharp & Dohme.

Complex Regional Pain Syndrome

Also called RSD, reflex sympathetic dystrophy syndrome, reflex dystrophy, neurovascular dystrophy, neuralgia, causalgia, shoulder-hand syndrome.

Description

Complex regional pain syndrome (CRPS) is a chronic neuropathic pain that follows soft-tissue or bone injury (Type I) or nerve injury (Type II) and lasts longer and is more severe than expected when compared with the original tissue injury or damage (Porter, 2018). Other manifestations may include autonomic changes, such as sweating, or vasomotor abnormalities; motor changes, such as weakness, dystonia; and trophic changes, such as skin or bone atrophy, hair loss, or joint contractures.

Cause

CRPS is thought to be caused by a disturbance to the sympathetic nervous system. CRPS Type I typically follows an injury to the hand or foot, most commonly after crush injuries but also may follow amputation, acute myocardial infarction, stroke, or cancer. CRPS Type II has similar etiology, but involves damage to a peripheral nerve (Porter, 2018).

Evaluation/Assessment

Areas

- Activities of Daily Living/Instrumental ADL: self-care
- Education/Work: ability to work, work status
- Play/Leisure: leisure interests and values, frequency, location
- Rest/Sleep: sleep disturbance
- Social Participation: type, frequency, location, with whom
- Cognition/Perception: report of perceived pain
- Sensorimotor: pain, edema, sensibility, grip and pinch strength, joint range of motion
- Psychosocial: role performance, depression, anxiety
- Context/Environment: social support, environmental modification
- Comorbidity or precipitating event: amputation, cancer, fracture, ligament injury, myocardial infarction, strain injury, surgery

Instruments

Instruments Developed by Occupational Therapy Personnel

- Allodynography (Packham et al., 2020, in References)
- Hamilton Inventory for Complex Regional Pain Syndrome (HI-CRPS; Packham, MacDermid, et al., 2012, in References)
- Patient-Reported Hamilton Inventory for Complex Regional Pain Syndrome (PR-HI-CRPS; Packham, MacDermid, et al., 2012, in References)
- Radboud Evaluation of Sensitivity (RES; Packham, MacDermid, Michlovitz, Cup, et al., 2018, in References)
- Sensory Responsiveness Questionnaire–Intensity Scale (SRQ-IS; Bar-Shalita, Selzer, Vatine, & Yochman, 2009)

Instruments Developed by Other Professionals and Used by Occupational Therapy Personnel

- Beck Depression Inventory (2nd ed.; BDI-II; Beck et al., 1996)
- Budapest Clinical Diagnostic Criteria for CRPS (Budapest Criteria; Harden et al., 2010)
- Disabilities of the Arm, Shoulder, and Hand (3rd ed.; DASH-3; Kennedy et al., 2011)
- Grip strength (JAMAR dynamometer, Lafayette Instrument)
- Joint range of motion (goniometery; Shurtleff & Kaskutuas, 2018)
- McGill Pain Questionnaire (MPQ; Melzack, 1975)
- Pinch meter (pinch strength; B&E Engineering; Mathiowetz et al., 1985)

- Pin (hyperpathia; Abrams & Ivy, 2018, p. 587)
- Rainbow Pain Scale (RPS). Used with Semmes-Weinstein monofilaments (Quintal et al., 2018, in References)
- Semmes-Weinstein Monofilaments (sensory testing; Abrams & Ivy, 2018, p. 588)
- Sensory testing/discrimination (Disk-Criminator; Abrams & Ivy, 2018)
- Short-Form McGill Pain Questionnaire–2 (SF-MPQ-2; Dworkin et al., 2009; see also Packham, Bean, et al., 2019, in References)
- Skin thermometer (skin temperature; Abrams & Ivy, 2018; see also Packham, Fok, et al., 2012, in References)
- State Trait Anxiety Inventory (STAI; Spielberger, 2010)
- Visual analogue scale (VAS; pain scale: 0 = *no pain*, 10 = *severe pain/worst ever*)
- Volumeter or circumference (tape) measure (edema; Stern, 1991)

Problems/Issues
Activities of Daily Living/Instrumental ADL
- Person may be unable to perform self-care activities independently because of pain and inability to move the extremity to perform the task(s). Note that the specifics vary with the person. There is no usual or standard list.
- Person may be unable to perform certain IADLs because of pain and inability to move the extremity to facilitate/accomplish performance of the task(s).

Education/Work
- Person is often unable to continue work activities or perform work tasks.
- Person may be on medical leave or have been terminated because of absenteeism.

Play/Leisure
- Person usually has quit engaging in favorite leisure activities because of pain and loss of movement(s) needed to complete tasks.

Rest/Sleep
- Person may have sleep disturbances due to pain or limited movement.

Social Participation
- Person may have reduced or limited participation with family and friends due to pain and reduced movement or mobility.

Sensorimotor
- Pain
  - ► Person may have allodynia.
  - ► Person may experience cold intolerance (vasomotor change).
  - ► Person may experience hyperpathia to repeated action.
  - ► Person may guard painful extremity to avoid having the painful area touched.
- Autonomic
  - ► Person may have elevated skin temperature over painful area.
  - ► Person may have mottling of skin.
  - ► Person may have sudomotor changes, such as hyperhidrosis (excessive sweating).
  - ► Person may have edema (swelling).
- Trophic
  - ► Person may have excessive or reduced hair growth.
  - ► Person's skin may have abnormal coloring (too red or too white).
  - ► Person's nails may become curled or ridged.
- Motor
  - ► Person may have low or reduced muscle tone.
  - ► Person may have reduced or limited movement of the affected extremity.

- ▶ Person may be uncoordinated (bilateral, dexterity).
- ▶ Person may have greater loss of movement than would be expected given the damage or impact of the original injury on the motor system.
- Sensory
  - ▶ Person may have sensory modulation dysfunction (Bar-Shalita et al, 2018).
  - ▶ Person may be under-responsive to sensory stimulation (sensory under-responsiveness).

Cognitive/Perceptual
- Person may have little or limited understanding of CRPS.

Psychosocial
- Person may become depressed, with a sense of hopelessness about condition.
- Person may express anxiety about the future, given current status of condition.
- Person may not be filling roles (e.g., worker, parent, spouse, friend).

Context/Environment
- Person may have limited support system.
- Person's family, friends, employer, or supervisor may have little knowledge or understanding of CRPS.

Intervention/Treatment

Intervention must be carefully planned to address the condition and situation of the individual client. Standard protocols or guidelines are of limited use. Generally, remedial and compensatory approaches must be used together. Compensatory approaches (adapted techniques, adapted devices) may be started to achieve some pain reduction and increase movement followed by remedial approaches to address range of motion and strength. No practice model in occupational therapy was mentioned in the references. Five models created by other professions are discussed: functional rehabilitation and graded motor imagery (Katholi et al., 2014); somatosensory rehabilitation (SMA; Packham, Spicher, et al., 2018); stress loading program (SLP); mirror visual feedback (MVF); and guided motor imagery (GMI; Harden et al., 2013; Packham & Holly, 2018; Quintal et al., 2018). Team members may include physicians, nursing personnel, physical therapy personnel, recreational therapy personnel, and occupational therapy personnel. Goals are to maximize independence and participation in self-care, school, and leisure activities, while promoting normalized use of the affected limbs (Logan et al., 2012).

Activities of Daily Living/Instrumental ADL
- Encourage client to use involved extremity in daily activities as much as possible. Compensatory approaches (techniques, devices, splints) may be helpful to initiate performance.

Education/Work
- Encourage client to engage in work tasks, if possible, using compensatory approaches as needed to initiate performance. Switch to remedial approaches as client improves.
- Job-specific reconditioning, work hardening, work capacity evaluation, transferable skills analysis, and a functional capacities evaluation program may be helpful.
- Functions to be considered are lifting pushing, pulling, crouching, walking, using stairs, bending at the waist, awkward and/or sustained postures, tolerance for sitting or standing, hot and cold tasks, sustained grip, tool usage, and vibration factors (Harden et al., 2013).

Play/Leisure
- Same as above.

Rest/Sleep
- A pain management program may be useful (see Pain and Chronic Pain in Section 2: Sensory Disorders).
- Review of sleep habits may be useful (see Sleep–Wake Disorders in Section 13: Lifestyle Conditions).

Social Participation
- No information identified.

Sensorimotor
- Somatosensory rehabilitation
  - ▶ Skin is evaluated using a 15-g monofilament to define the territory or zone that is painful to touch.
  - ▶ An anatomical hypothesis is made of the peripheral nerve branch(es) underlying the painful territory/zone and contributing to the aberrant afferent pain signaling and perception.
  - ▶ The painful territory is avoided by minimizing evocation of pain by temporarily limiting touch (and consequently functional use) of the painful zone.
  - ▶ "Counter simulation" (tactile and/or vibratory) is used on an anatomically related cutaneous branch proximal to the zone or arising from the same cord of the brachial plexus (Packham, Spicher, et al., 2018).
- Stress loading program
  - ▶ Program is based on two principles: scrubbing and carrying.
  - ▶ Scrubbing consists of moving the affected extremity in a back-and-forth motion, with weight-bearing through the extremity. A scrub brush may be used to facilitate the action.
  - ▶ Carrying is achieved by weight-loading a small object that is carried in the hand, which can progress to a bag with a handle as heavier weights are added. The weight is carried throughout the day when the client is standing or walking (Harden et al., 2013).
- Mirror visual feedback
  - ▶ Client is asked to close the eyes and describe both the affected and unaffected limb (such as size, location, and perceived differences.
  - ▶ Next, person is asked to imagine movements of both extremities.
  - ▶ Movements are then focused on painful joints and those that are just proximal and distal to the joint.
  - ▶ Client is then asked to look at the mirrored limb without movement in order to try to achieve ownership (Harden et al., 2013).
- Guided motor imagery
  - ▶ Program has three parts:
    - ○ Left/right discrimination using a set of 50 cards showing the hand in different positions. The client is to state which hand (left or right) is shown in each picture as quickly as possible.
    - ○ Explicit motor imagery: Client is asked to close the eyes and visualize the affected hand in a static position.
    - ○ Mirror therapy: Client is asked to move the limb while looking at the mirror (Harden et al., 2013).

Cognitive/Perceptual
- No information identified.

Psychosocial
- No information identified.

Context/Environment
- Provide information to family, friends, employer/supervisor about the condition.

Precautions/Safety Considerations
- Note if condition spreads beyond the original zone or territory of involvement.
- Clients with high pain intensity after distal radius fracture have higher risk of developing CRPS Type I (Farzad et al., 2018).

Prognosis and Outcome

Recovery is possible with effective intervention, but condition may also become chronic or continue to progress to a worse situation. Prognosis varies and is difficult to predict. Condition may remain stable for many years, but may also progress and spread to other areas of the body (Porter, 2018). Outcome should be measured using the following seven concepts: pain, disease severity, participation and physical function, emotional and psychological function, self-efficacy, catastrophizing, and patient's global impression of change (Grieve et al., 2017).

REFERENCES

Bar-Shalita, T., Livshitz, A., Levin-Meltz, Y., Rand, D., Deutsch, L., & Vatine, J.-J. (2018). Sensory modulation dysfunction is associated with complex regional pain syndrome. *PLOS ONE, 13*(8), Article e0201354. https://doi.org/10.1371/journal.pone.0201354

Farzad, M., Layeghi, F., Hosseini, A., Dianat, A., Ahrari, N., Rassafiani, M., & Mirzaei, H. (2018). Investigate the effect of psychological factors in development of complex regional pain syndrome Type I in patients with fracture of the distal radius: A prospective study. *Journal of Hand Surgery (Asian-Pacific Volume), 23*(4), 554–561. https://doi.org/10.1142/S2424835518500571

Grieve, S., Perez, R. S. G. M., Birklein, F., Brunner, F., Bruehl, S., Harden, R. N., Packham, T., Gobeil, F., Haigh, R., Holly, J., Terkelsen, A., Davies, L., Lewis, J., Thomassen, I., Connett, R., Worth, T., Vatine, J.-J., & McCabe, C. S. (2017). Recommendations for a first Core Outcome Measurement set for Complex regional PAin syndrome Clinical sTudies (COMPACT). *Pain, 158*(6), 1083–1090. https://doi.org/10.1097/j.pain.0000000000000866

Harden, R. N., Oaklander, A. L., Burton, A. W., Perez, R. S. G. M., Richardson, K., Swan, M., Barthel, J., Costa, B., Graciosa, J. R., & Bruehl, S. (2013). Complex regional pain syndrome: Practical diagnostic and treatment guidelines, 4th ed. *Pain Medicine, 14*, 180–229. https://doi.org/10.1111/pme.12033

Katholi, B. R., Daghstani, S. S., Banez, G. A., & Brady, K. K. (2014). Noninvasive treatments for pediatric complex regional pain syndrome: A focused review. *PM&R, 6*(10), 926–933. https://doi.org/10.1016/j.pmrj.2014.04.007

Logan, D. E., Carpino, E. A., Chiang, G., Condon, M., Firn, E., Gaughan, V. J., Hogan, M., Leslie, D. S., Olson, K., Sager, S., Sethna, N., Simons, L. E., Zurakowski, D., & Berde, C. B. (2012). A day-hospital approach to treatment of pediatric complex regional pain syndrome: Initial functional outcomes. *Clinical Journal of Pain, 28*(9), 766–774. https://doi.org/10.1097/AJP.0b013e3182457619

Packham, T. L., Bean, D., Johnson, M. H., MacDermid, J. C., Grieve, S., McCabe, C. S., & Harden, R. N. (2019). Measurement properties of the SF-MPQ-2 Neuropathic Qualities subscale in persons with CRPS: Validity, responsiveness, and Rasch analysis. *Pain Medicine, 20*(4), 799–809. https://doi.org/10.1093/pm/pny202

Packham, T. L., Fok, D., Frederiksen, K., Thabane, L., & Buckley, N. (2012). Reliability of infrared thermometric measurements of skin temperature in the hand. *Journal of Hand Therapy, 25*(4), 356–361. https://doi.org/10.1016/j.jht.2012.06.003

Packham, T., & Holly, J. (2018). Mechanism-specific rehabilitation management of complex regional pain syndrome: Proposed recommendations from evidence synthesis. *Journal of Hand Therapy, 31*, 238–249. https://doi.org/10.1016/j.jht.2018.01.007

Packham, T., MacDermid, J. C., Henry, J., & Bain, J. (2012). The Hamilton Inventory for Complex Regional Pain Syndrome: A cognitive debriefing study of the clinician-based component. *Journal of Hand Therapy, 25*(1), 97–111. https://doi.org/10.1016/j.jht.2011.09.007

Packham T. L., MacDermid, J. C., Michlovtiz, S. L., & Buckley, N. (2018). Content validation of the Patient-Reported Hamilton Inventory for complex regional pain syndrome. *Canadian Journal of Occupational Therapy, 85*(2), 99–105. https://doi.org/10.1177/0008417417734562

Packham, T. L., MacDermid, J. C., Michlovitz, S., Cup, E., & Van de Ven-Stevens, L. (2018). Cross cultural adaptation and refinement of the English version of a Dutch patient-reported questionnaire for hand sensitivity: The Radboud Evaluation of Sensitivity. *Journal of Hand Therapy, 31*(3), 371–380. https://doi.org/10.1016/j.jht.2017.03.003

Packham, T. L., Spicher, C. J., MacDermid, J. C., & Buckley, D. N. (2020). Allodynography: Reliability of a new procedure for object clinical examination of static mechanical allodynia. *Pain Medicine, 21*(1), 101–108. https://doi.org/10.1093/pm/pnz045

Packham, T. L., Spicher, C. J., MacDermid, J. C., Michlovitz, S., & Buckley, D. N. (2018). Somatosensory rehabilitation for allodynia in complex regional pain syndrome of the upper limb: A retrospective cohort study. *Journal of Hand Therapy, 31*(1), 10–19. https://doi.org/10.1016/j.jht.2017.02.007

Porter, R. S. (Ed.). (2018). *Merck manual of diagnosis and therapy* (20th ed.). Merck Sharp & Dohme.

Quintal, I., Poiré-Hamel, L., Bourbonnais, D., & Dyer, J.-O. (2018). Management of long-term complex regional pain syndrome with allodynia: A case report. *Journal of Hand Therapy, 31*(2), 255–264. https://doi.org/10.1016/j.jht.2018.01.012

BIBLIOGRAPHY

Cowdry, J. (2014). Perspectives on pain. In C. Cooper (Ed.). *Fundamentals of hand therapy* (2nd ed., pp. 145–150). Mosby/Elsevier.

Ho, E. S., Ponnuthurai, J., & Clarke, H. M. (2014). The incidence of idiopathic musculoskeletal pain in children with upper extremity injuries. *Journal of Hand Therapy, 27*(1), 38–43. https://doi.org/10.1016/j.jht.2013.10.002

Packham, T., MacDermid, J. C., Henry, J., & Bain, J. (2012). A systematic review of psychometric evaluations of outcome assessments for complex regional pain syndrome. *Disability and Rehabilitation, 34*(13), 1059–1069. https://doi.org/10.3109/09638288.2011.626835

Wei, K., Feldmann, R. E., Jr., Brascher, A.-K., & Benrath, J. (2014). Ultrasound-guided stellate ganglion blocks combined with pharmacological and occupational therapy in complex regional pain syndrome (CRPS): A pilot case series. *Pain Medicine, 15*, 2120–2127. https://doi.org/10.1111/pme.12473

Deafness and Hearing Loss

Description

Loss of hearing can be congenital or acquired, progressive or sudden, temporary or permanent, unilateral (affecting one ear) or bilateral, and mild to profound (Porter, 2018). Some terminology includes the following:

- *American Sign Language (ASL):* A visual language that uses hand motions and consists of a distinct vocabulary, grammar, and syntax separate from the English language (Fain, 2019)
- *Cochlear implant:* An electronic device that is surgically implanted into the cochlea of a person with a severe to profound bilateral hearing loss (O'Toole, 2017)
- *Deaf:* Having minimal or no hearing (Fain, 2019)
- *Deaf culture:* A distinct cultural community with its own language, values, and social mores (Fain, 2019)
- *Deaf gain:* Alternate ways of thinking and perceiving sensory information, creative problem-solving, and cultural gains by intensifying observation of the environment, including body language and increasing visual and tactile perceptual skills (Fain, 2019)
- *Deafness:* A condition characterized by loss of hearing in which the person cannot understand speech through hearing alone (O'Toole, 2017)

- *Degree of hearing loss* (in decibels [dB]; Fain, 2019):
  ▶ Normal: –10 to 15 dB (sound level of rustling of leaves and birds chirping)
  ▶ Slight: 16–25 dB (sound level of water dripping, whispering)
  ▶ Mild: 26–40 dB (sound of letters *z, p, h, g, k, f, s, th* and most talking)
  ▶ Moderate: 41–55 dB (sound of letters *j, d, b, n, ng, ee, l, u, a, r, ch, sh*)
  ▶ Moderate severe: 56–70 dB (crying, vacuuming)
  ▶ Severe: 71–90 dB (dog barking, piano playing)
  ▶ Profound: 91+ dB (truck, lawn mower, chain saw, motorcycle, jack hammer, firecracker, playing drums, airplane taking off, siren)
- *Fragmented hearing:* Consists of missing pieces or words in the story or education topic being presented (Fain, 2019)
- *Hard of hearing:* Having some level of hearing loss, but no profound hearing loss (Fain, 2019)
- *Hearing impairment:* Loss of hearing that adversely affects an individual's ability to communicate (O'Toole, 2017)
- *Hearing loss* (Fain, 2019):
  ▶ *Acquired hearing loss:* Occurs after birth
  ▶ *Congenital hearing loss:* Present at birth
  ▶ *Postlingual hearing loss:* Occurs after the acquisition of spoken language
  ▶ *Prelingual hearing loss:* Occurs before or during the acquisition of spoken language
  ▶ *Progressive hearing loss:* Occurs over time
- *Presbycusis:* Sensorineural hearing loss that appears to result from a combination of age, noise exposure, and genetic factors (Porter, 2018)
- *Speech sounds:* Normal speech sounds occur between 20 to 50 decibels (intensity of sound) and 250 to 4,000 frequency (cycles per second; Fain, 2019)
- Types of hearing loss (Fain, 2019):
  ▶ *Conductive hearing loss:* Sound waves are obstructed from traveling to the inner ear by ossified bones or malformed auditory canals
  ▶ *Sensorineural hearing loss:* Damage to the inner ear or auditory nerve prevents the sound message from being sent to the brain for processing
  ▶ *Mixed hearing loss:* Having both a conductive hearing loss and a sensorineural hearing loss
  ▶ *Central auditory processing disorder:* The ear is not damaged, but the neural system involved with processing or understanding language is damaged

Cause

The most common causes are cerumen (ear wax) accumulation, noise, aging, and infections such as otitis media. Other causes include drug toxicity (ototoxicity), genetic disorders, trauma, tumors (benign or malignant), autoimmune disorders, idiopathic malformation, anoxia, and otosclerosis (Porter, 2018).

Evaluation/Assessment
Areas
- Activities of Daily Living/Instrumental ADL: communication skills, verbal apraxia, independent living skills
- Education/Work: academic performance, classroom and school behavior, workplace accommodation
- Play/Leisure: play skills, interests, types, frequency, location
- Rest/Sleep: no information identified
- Social Participation: type, frequency, location, with whom
- Sensorimotor: gross motor skills, fine motor skills, fatigue, balance, coordination, postural stability (static and dynamic), vestibular dysfunction, auditory discrimination, visual motor integration, bilateral integration disorder

- Cognitive/Perceptual: attention, visual memory, auditory memory, executive functions, self-management, time processing and management, visual perceptual skills
- Psychosocial: anxiety, self-esteem, resilience, quality of life
- Context/Environment: adapted devices, assistive technology, environmental modification, social support, resources, advocacy
- Development: developmental delay, developmental milestones
- Comorbidities: attention-deficit/hyperactivity disorder, sensory integration disorder, visual impairment

Instruments

Instruments* Developed by Occupational Therapy Personnel
- None

Instruments Developed by Other Professionals and Used by Occupational Therapy Personnel
- Beery-Buktenica Test of Visual-Motor Integration (6th ed.; VMI-6; Beery et al., 2010)
- Bruininks-Oseretsky Test of Motor Proficiency (2nd ed.; BOT-2; Bruininks & Bruininks, 2005)
- Connor-Davidson Resilience Scale (CD-RISC; Connor & Davidson, 2003)
- Functional Listening Evaluation (FLE; Johnson & VonAlmen, 1997)
- Hearing Handicap Inventory for the Elderly–Screening Version (HHIE-SV; Porter, 2018, pp. 816–817)
- Movement Assessment Battery for Children (2nd ed.; M-ABC-2; Henderson et al., 2007)
- Peabody Developmental Motor Scales (3rd ed.; PDMS-3; Folio & Fewell, 2023)
- Sensory Organization Test (SOT; Nashner et al., 1982)
- Synapsys Posturography System (Marseille, France; see Ebrahimi et al., 2017, in References)
- Test of Auditory Processing Skills (4th ed.; TAPS-4; Martin et al., 2018)

Problems/Issues

Activities of Daily Living/Instrumental ADL
- Child may have tactile sensitivity to certain clothing due to sensory processing disorder.
- Person may not be able to communicate (listen or talk) sufficiently to understand commands and ideas or express needs and follow instructions.
- Person may hear certain sounds well, but not hear other sounds at all (mixed hearing loss).
- Other persons may have difficulty understanding speech of a person with a hearing loss that is caused by congenital conditions or occurred during early childhood.
- Person may have difficulty mastering independent living skills, especially if hearing loss is profound.

Education/Work
- Child may have difficulty following directions in a classroom, especially if the teacher is talking while writing on a chalkboard or whiteboard (facing away from the child).
- Child may not be seated in the classroom where he or she can easily see the teacher or instructor or follow the conversation.
- Person may have difficulty listening to (hearing) conversation in a noisy work environment.

Play/Leisure
- Person may reduce or limit engagement in leisure occupations that occur in a noisy environment.

Rest/Sleep
- No information identified.

---

* Audiologic tests are not included (except for word recognition) because most occupational therapy personnel are not qualified to administer and do not have the necessary soundproof room or equipment.

Social Participation

- Child may have difficulty participating in games and activities in noisy environments or when instructions are not given face-to-face.
- Person may reduce or limit participation in social activities that may occur in a noisy environment, such as indoor sporting events (basketball, hockey) or eating at restaurants that play loud music.

Sensorimotor

- Child may demonstrate balance and vestibular dysfunction.
- Child may be viewed by others as clumsy or uncoordinated.
- Child may have difficulty maintaining postural stability due to difficulty integrating visual, vestibular, and somatosensory information to produce motor responses that maintain balance.
- Child may be developmentally delayed in gross motor skills due to issues with vestibular and proprioceptive systems.
- Child may be developmentally delayed in fine motor skills.
- Child with cochlear implant may be at risk for motor and balance deficits (Ebrahimi et al., 2016; Gronski, 2013).
- Child/person usually experiences greater fatigue due to increased effort needed to compensate for hearing loss.
- Child may have sensory processing disorders, including somatosensory (tactile, proprioception, vestibular) and visual motor integration disorder (Scwpersad, 2014)
- Child may demonstrate difficulty with bilateral integration and sequence due to sensory integration dysfunction.

Cognitive/Perceptual

- Person may have difficulty with maintaining sustained attention and avoiding distractions.
- Person may have difficulty with auditory discrimination, especially of different speech sounds.

Psychosocial

- Person may be anxious about ability to perform expected roles.
- Person is at risk for social isolation.
- Person may experience a decreased quality of life.
- Person may be less resilient, especially if female (Ahmadi et al., 2015).

Context/Environment

- Person and family may lack knowledge about hearing loss and its consequences in daily life.
- Person and family may lack knowledge about laws (federal and state) designed to assist people with hearing loss with participation in society, including accessibility.
- Person and family may lack information about available community or internet resources.
- Person and family may lack information about available adapted devices and augmented communication equipment.
- Person may need environmental modifications in the home, school, or workplace to facilitate participation.

Intervention/Treatment

Models and programs developed by occupational therapy personnel include the Comfortable Cafeteria Program (Prusnek et al., 2019), maximizing independence (Nastasi, 2018), and sensory integration (Koester et al., 2014). Models and programs developed by other professionals but used by occupational therapy personnel include mobile phones (Chiu et al., 2010; Liu et al., 2010), reading improvement (Ghorbani, 2016), and telepractice (Cohn & Cason, 2012). Team members include physicians, audiologists, psychologists, speech–language pathologists, educators and special educators, physical therapy personnel, and occupational therapy personnel. Goals are improving communication and ability to participate in self-care, productive, and leisure occupations.

Activities of Daily Living/Instrumental ADL

- In communicating, use a combination of gestures, facial expressions, body language, and written and pictorial communication techniques.
- Be aware that persons with hearing loss or who are deaf use their eyes and cannot look at an object at the same time a person is talking to them; use combined techniques.
- Be aware that communication modes are unique and shaped by factors such as educational experience, cultural or linguistic identity of the family, and peer influences; check for unique aspects associated with individual child, adolescent, or adult.
- Assist team members to develop and use lipreading methods if selected as a communication method.
- Assist team members to help a child effectively use the cochlear implant as a communication method.
- Assist team members in developing independent living skills (meal planning and preparation, housekeeping, shopping).

Education/Work

- Assist adolescents to participate in transitional school programs designed to teach independent living and work-related skills.
- Make recommendations to employers regarding environment modifications to facilitate worker participation such as added signage, handrails, and written instructions with pictures and illustrations.
- Assist person to optimize work performance including self-accommodation, self-advocacy, self-management, and lobbying (Shaw et al., 2013).

Play/Leisure

- Assist child to develop play skills, especially cooperative and shared activities and games and activities with rules or instructions.
- Assist person to develop leisure occupations.

Rest/Sleep

- No information identified.

Social Participation

- Assist person to participate in social activities that are age appropriate and adapted to account for degree of hearing loss.

Sensorimotor

- Provide practice in gross motor skills, especially those associated with balance, postural stability, and vestibular function (hopping, jumping, skipping, walking on a balance beam).
- Provide practice to increase use of observational and visual perceptual skills.

Cognitive/Perceptual

- Provide practice to increase visual memory.
- Provide practice to improve observation and visual perceptual skills.

Psychosocial

- Discuss with client ways to reduce anxiety.
- Discuss with client what approaches would improve sense of self-efficacy.
- Discuss with client what actions would increase quality of life.

Context/Environment

- Optimize the fit between the person, occupation, and environment using adapted devices and assistive technology if needed.
- Refer child or person to an audiologist if hearing loss is detected and is causing problems identified by the client.

- Refer child to a speech–language pathologist or school-based speech therapist if speech problems are detected.
- Assist client and family to become knowledgeable about federal and state legislation regarding access to services in schools and work environments, such as the Individuals with Disabilities Education Improvement Act (IDEA; 2004).
- Assist client and family to access state, community, and internet resources.

Precautions/Safety Considerations

Monitor for safety.

Prognosis and Outcome

Hearing deficits in early childhood can result in chronic disability throughout life in both receptive and expressive language (Porter, 2018). Children with other disorders (sensory, linguistic, or cognitive deficits) are more severely affected (Porter, 2018).

REFERENCES

Ahmadi, N., Afshari, T., Nikoo, M. R., Rajati, F., Tahmacbi, B., Kamali, M., & Farahani, F. (2015). Does deafness affect resilience? *Middle East Journal of Rehabilitation and Health, 2*(4), Article e32392. https://doi.org/10.17795/mejrh-32392

Chiu, H.-P., Liu, C.-H., Hsieh, C.-L., & Li, R.-K. (2010). Essential needs and requirements of mobile phones for the deaf. *Assistive Technology, 22*(3), 172–195. https://doi.org/10.1080/10400435.2010.483652

Cohn, E. R., & Cason, J. (2012). Telepractice: A wide-angle view for persons with hearing loss. *Volta Review, 112*(3), 207–226. https://doi.org/10.17955/tvr.112.3.m.706

Ebrahimi, A.-A., Movallali, G., Jamshidi, A.-A., Haghgoo, H. A., & Rahgozar, M. (2016). Balance performance of deaf children with and without cochlear implants. *Acta Medica Iranica, 54*(11), 737–742.

Ebrahimi, A.-A., Movallali, G., Jamshidi, A.-A., Rahgozar, M., & Haghgoo, H. A. (2017). Postural control in deaf children. *Acta Medica Iranica, 55*(2), 115–122.

Fain, E. A. (2019). Best practices in supporting students with hearing impairments or deafness. In G. F. Clark, J. E. Rioux, & B. E. Chandler (Eds.), *Best practices for occupational therapy in schools* (2nd ed., pp. 263–270). AOTA Press.

Ghorbani, A. (2016). The impact of multidisciplinary occupational therapy on reading improvement of children with hearing impairment (case study). *Journal of Exceptional Education, 5*(142), 59–63.

Gronski, M. (2013). Balance and motor deficits and the role of occupational therapy in children who are deaf and hard of hearing: A critical appraisal of the topic. *Journal of Occupational Therapy, Schools & Early Intervention, 6*(4), 356–371. https://doi.org/10.1080/19411243.2013.860767

Individuals with Disabilities Education Improvement Act of 2004, 20 U.S.C. § 1400 *et seq.* (2004).

Koester, A. C., Mailloux, Z., Coleman, G. G., Mori, A. B., Paul, S. M., Blanche, E., Muhs, J. A., Lim, D., & Cermak, S. A. (2014). Sensory integration functions of children with cochlear implants. *American Journal of Occupational Therapy, 68*, 562–569. https://doi.org/10.5014/ajot.2014.012187

Liu, C.-H., Chiu, H.-P., & Hsieh, C.-L. (2010). Optimizing the usability of mobile phones for individuals who are deaf. *Assistive Technology, 22*(2), 115–127. https://doi.org/10.1080/10400435.2010.483649

Nastasi, J. A. (2018). Maximizing independence in older adults with visual impairment and hearing loss. *SIS Quarterly Practice Connections, 3*(3), 20–22.

O'Toole, M. T. (Ed.). (2017). *Mosby's dictionary of medicine, nursing & health professions* (10th ed.). Elsevier.

Porter, R. S. (Ed.). (2018). *The Merck manual of diagnosis and therapy* (20th ed.). Merck Sharp & Dohme.

Prusnek, L. L., Griffiths, T., & Provident, I. (2019). Implementing the Comfortable Cafeteria program to foster social participation of students with and without hearing impairments: A look at the outcomes. *Journal of Occupational Therapy, Schools, and Early Intervention, 12*(2), 239–252. https://doi.org/10.1080/19411243.2019.1592055

Sewpersad, V. (2014). Co-morbidities of hearing loss and occupational therapy in preschool children. *South African Journal of Occupational Therapy, 44*(2), 28–32.

Shaw, L., Jennings, M. B., & Southall, K. E. (2013). The standpoint of persons with hearing loss on work disparities and workplace accommodations. *Work, 46*(2), 193–204. https://doi.org/10.3233/WOR-131741

BIBLIOGRAPHY

American Occupational Therapy Association. (2017). Vestibular impairment, vestibular rehabilitation, and occupational performance. *American Journal of Occupational Therapy, 71*(Suppl. 2), Article 7112410055. https://doi.org/10.5014/ajot.2017.716S09

Ebrahimi, A.-A., Jamshidi, A.-A., Movallali, G., Rahgozar, M., & Haghgoo, H. A. (2017). The effect of vestibular rehabilitation therapy program on sensory organization of deaf children with bilateral vestibular dysfunction. *Acta Medica Iranica, 55*(11), 683–689.

Reynolds, S., Kuhaneck, H. M., & Pfeiffer, B. (2016). Systematic review of the effectiveness of frequency modulation devices in improving academic outcomes in children with auditory processing difficulties. *American Journal of Occupational Therapy, 70*(1). https://doi.org/10.5014/ajot.2016.016832

Dyspraxia and Developmental Dyspraxia

Also called somatodyspraxia.

See also Developmental Coordination Disorder and Specific Learning Disorders.

Description

"Praxis is the ability to conceptualize, plan, and successfully complete motor actions in novel situations" (Bodison, 2015, para. 1). Praxis "requires basic motor skills, knowledge or presentation of the movement, and subsequent transcoding of the representation into movement plans" (Abelenda et al., 2015, p. 2). Dyspraxia is defined as "difficulty or inability to perform a planned motor activity when the muscles used in the activity are not paralyzed" (Jacobs & Simon, 2015, p. 89). Dyspraxia is described as "a developmental condition in which the ability to plan unfamiliar motor tasks is impaired" (Bundy et al., 2002, as cited in Abelenda et al., 2015, p. 1). Developmental dyspraxia is characterized by an impairment in the ability to plan and carry out sensory and motor tasks (National Institute of Neurological Disorders and Stroke, 2019). Developmental dyspraxia is a "failure to have acquired the ability to perform appropriate complex motor actions" (Bodison, 2015, para. 2). Types of dyspraxia include visodyspraxia, somatodyspraxia, bilateral integration and sequencing deficits, and dyspraxia on verbal command (Buitendag & Aronstam, 2010).

Cause

May be related to deficits in the central nervous system "related to abnormal connectivity between parietal, premotor, and motor cortices" (Abelenda et al., 2015, p. 2). Also considered to be equivalent to development coordination disorder in some countries.

Evaluation/Assessment
Areas
- Activities of Daily Living/Instrumental ADL: self-care activities such as dressing, eating, functional communication skills
- Education/Work: academics, school activities
- Play/Leisure: types of play activities, play skills
- Rest/Sleep: sleep disturbance
- Social Participation: social activities, type, frequency, location, with whom
- Sensorimotor: motor planning, oral praxis, bilateral integration, praxis on demand, somatodyspraxia, vestibular processing, tactile discrimination, graphesthesia, visual processing (may be a strength)
- Cognitive/Perceptual: gestures (transitive actions, intransitive actions, imitative actions)
- Psychosocial: social skills, such as reciprocal interactions with peers
- Context/Environment: family, community
- Development (Infant, Child, Adolescent only): milestones
- Comorbidities: Autism Spectrum Disorder, Developmental Coordination Disorder, Somatosensory Dysfunction

Instruments
Instruments Developed by Occupational Therapy Personnel
- Comprehensive Praxis Assessment for Children (CPAC; Chang & Yu, 2018, in References)
- Motor Praxis Ability Test (MPAT; Ruttanathantong et al., 2013, in References)
- Sensory Integration and Praxis Tests (SIPT; Ayres, 1989; including the subtests of Imitation of Postures [renamed Postural Praxis], Oral Praxis, Sequencing Praxis, Constructional Praxis, and Praxis on Verbal Command)
- Sensory Profile (2nd ed.; SP-2; Dunn, 2014)
- Sensory Profile School Companion (Dunn, 2006)
- Test of Ideational Praxis (TIP; Lane et al., 2014, in References)

Instruments Developed by Other Professionals and Used by Occupational Therapy Personnel
- Florida Praxis Imagery Test (FPIT; Ochipa et al., 1997)
- Vineland Adaptive Behavior Scales (3rd ed.; Vineland-3; Sparrow et al., 2016)

Problems/Issues
Activities of Daily Living/Instrumental ADL
- Person may have difficulty performing learned skills such as dressing, eating with utensils.
- Person may have difficulty using functional communication effectively to express wants.

Education/Work
- Person may have difficulty with handwriting.

Play/Leisure
- Person may prefer solitary play with stereotypical and repetitive actions.
- Person may have difficulty with imitative or make-believe play activities.
- Person may perform poorly (appears uncoordinated or clumsy) at sports activities, such as kicking a ball.
- Person may have difficulty with interactive or cooperative play.

Rest/Sleep
- Person may have sleep disturbance.

Social Participation
- Person may have difficulty participating in social activities, such as parties.

Sensorimotor

- Person has difficulty with praxis tasks: posture praxis, imitation of postures, oral praxis, sequencing praxis, constructional praxis, praxis on verbal command.
- Person may have poor discrimination of sensory inputs such as tactile, vestibular, or proprioceptive.
- Person may have difficulty with sensory processing including registering, orientating, and responding to sensory input.
- Person may have a sensory modulation disorder characterized by an inability to appropriately adapt one's response to sensory stimulation from one's body or external environment.

Cognitive/Perceptual

- Person may have difficulty generalizing skills learned in one situation or environment to another.
- Person may have difficulty with attending behaviors, including
  - orienting attention to a stimulus, person, or event;
  - sustained attention to maintain the regard of an object or event;
  - shifting attention by disengaging attention to one stimulus and reorienting/engaging to another;
  - social attention to voices and faces of others; and
  - joint attention with others in an educational or social environment.
- Person may have difficulty understanding and responding to transitive gestures (verbal command, pantomimed tool use, make-believe actions—e.g., show me how you brush your teeth with a toothbrush, show me how you hit a nail with a hammer).
- Person may have difficulty understanding and responding to intransitive/nontransitive actions (waving good-bye, saluting, blowing a kiss).
- Person may have difficulty understanding and responding to imitative actions that may be meaningless or nonsymbolic (e.g., lift your index finger from the table, put your right hand on your left shoulder).
- Person may have difficulty copying a model related to perceptual dysfunction.
- Person may have difficulty conceptualizing novel ways to interact with objects (ideation praxis).

Psychosocial

- Person may have difficulty with reciprocal social interactions.

Context/Environment

- Person may be viewed by others as clumsy.

Intervention/Treatment

Intervention is based on the Motor Learning Framework (Buitendag & Aronstam, 2010, 2012), Ayres Sensory Integration (Abelenda et al., 2015), environmental modification (Kinnealey et al., 2012), and compensatory strategies (National Institute of Neurological Disorders and Stroke, 2019). Patten (2013) briefly described six interventions: sensory integrative treatment, perceptual motor approach, sensorimotor approach, cognitive goal-directed approach, compensatory skills development, and consultation. Few details were provided (see Autism Spectrum Disorder and Developmental Coordination Disorder in Section 1: Developmental Disorders, for additional intervention techniques). Focus of intervention is to increase the person's ability to plan, initiate, and carry out an effective motor plan of action in various settings and situations. Team members include physicians, psychologists, educators, physical therapy personnel, and occupational therapy personnel. Goal is to improve the child's participation in self-care, educational, play, leisure, and social activities.

Activities of Daily Living/Instrumental ADL

- Practice eating, dressing, and other tasks in real time with real objects.

Education/Work
- Consider environmental modifications to reduce extraneous sensory stimulation permitting better focus of attention on learning tasks.

Play/Leisure
- Provide opportunity to play with others using different types of play interaction.

Rest/Sleep
- See Sleep–Wake Disorders in Section 13: Lifestyle Conditions.

Social Participation
- Provide opportunity for self-directed participation in meaningful activities in social situations.

Sensorimotor
- Reducing visual and auditory "background" noise may improve attending behavior.

Cognitive/Perceptual
- Encourage novel or creative use of materials and objects.

Psychosocial
- Develop social skills in settings rich in sensory motor experiences (Abelenda et al., 2015).

Context/Environment
- No information identified.

Precautions/Safety Considerations

Person may not generalize learned behavior to new or novel situations.

Prognosis and Outcome

Condition is usually chronic, although performance may be satisfactory in a familiar environment with established routines and tasks. Developmental dyspraxia is a lifelong disorder (National Institute of Neurological Disorders and Stroke, 2019).

REFERENCES

Abelenda, J., Mailloux, Z., & Roley, S. S. (2015). Dyspraxia in autism spectrum disorders: Evidence and implications. *Sensory Integration Special Interest Section Quarterly, 38*(3), 1–3.

Bodison, S. C. (2015). Developmental dyspraxia and the play skills of children with autism. *American Journal of Occupational Therapy, 69*, Article 6905185060. https://doi.org/10.5014/ajot.2015.017954

Buitendag, K., & Aronstam, M. C. (2010). The relationship between developmental dyspraxia and sensory responsivity in children aged four years through eight years: Part 1. *South African Journal of Occupational Therapy, 40*(3), 16–20.

Buitendag, K., & Aronstam, M. C. (2012). The relationship between developmental dyspraxia and sensory responsivity in children aged four to eight years: Part II. *South African Journal of Occupational Therapy, 42*(2), 2–7.

Chang, S.-H., & Yu, N.-Y. (2018). Development and validation of the comprehensive praxis assessment for children aged 6–8. *Human Movement Science, 57*, 332–341. https://doi.org/10.1016/j.humov.2017.09.011

Jacobs, K., & Simon, L. (Eds.). (2015). *Quick reference dictionary to occupational therapy.* Slack.

Kinnealey, M., Pfeiffer, B., Miller, J., Roan, C., Shoener, R., & Ellner, M. L. (2012). Effect of classroom modification on attention and engagement of students with autism or dyspraxia. *American Journal of Occupational Therapy, 66*, 511–519. https://doi.org/10.5014/ajot.2012.004010

Lane, S. J., Ivey, C. K., & May-Benson, T. A. (2014). Test of Ideational Praxis (TIP): Preliminary findings and interrater and test-retest reliability with preschoolers. *American Journal of Occupational Therapy, 68*, 555–561. https://doi.org/10.5014/ajot.2014.012542

National Institute of Neurological Disorders and Stroke. (2019). *Developmental dyspraxia information page.* https://www.ninds.nih.gov/Disorders/All-Disorders/Developmental-Dyspraxia -Information-Page

Patten, N. (2013). *Dyspraxia from an occupational therapy perspective.* Dyspraxia Foundation. https://dyspraxiafoundation.org.uk/wp-content/uploads/2013/10/dyspraxia_and_Occupational_Therapy.pdf

Ruttanathantong, K., Sriphetcharawut, S., Emasithi, A., Saengsuwan, J., Saengsuwan, J., & Sirita-ratiwat, W. (2013). Development of an assessment tool for motor praxis ability in children aged 5–8 years. *Developmental Neurorehabilitation, 16*(3), 172–179. https://doi.org/10.3109 /17518423.2013.769129

Low Vision and Visual Loss

Also called visual impairment, loss of vision, impaired vision, visual dysfunction.

See also Unilateral Spatial Neglect, Visual Impairment in Children and Adolescents, Visual Impairment Due to Neurologic Conditions.

Description

Low vision is defined as best corrected visual acuity between 20/70 and 20/200 and an inability to engage in purposeful activity using one's vision despite the use of corrective lenses, medication, or surgery (National Eye Institute, 2016). Low vision primarily involves reduction in visual acuity or restriction in visual field. Loss of or reduced central (focal, macular) visual acuity decreases ability to read, identify, and locate people, information, and items in the environment. Loss of peripheral vision, such as loss of visual field, decreases ability to move safely within the environment and to identify the location or movement of other people and objects in the environment. Low vision is sometimes referred to as a hidden disability because the problem is not always evident, but it may hinder rehabilitation for another condition, such as a hip fracture (Sternberg, 2013).

Cause

A variety of eye conditions may cause low vision, including age-related macular degeneration (Deemer et al., 2017; Hedlich et al., 2018; Hindman, 2017; Hong et al., 2014), cataracts, glaucoma (Park et al., 2015), retinitis pigmentosa, retinal detachment, corneal injury, or diabetic retinopathy (Sokol-McKay, 2010).

Evaluation/Assessment

Areas

- Activities of Daily Living/Instrumental ADL: dressing, grooming, bathing, toileting, meal preparation, medication management, financial management, shopping, driving (and other transportation needs), functional communication (including reading)
- Education/Work: job performance, retirement planning
- Play/Leisure: type, frequency
- Rest/Sleep: Not mentioned in relation to low vision
- Social Participation: type, frequency, location
- Sensorimotor: energy conservation
- Cognitive/Perceptual: problem solving
- Psychosocial: quality of life, sense of well-being, depression, self-confidence, self-esteem and self-worth, grief and loss (unable to perform previously enjoyed occupations), coping skills, role performance

- Context/Environment: home and community safety, adapted equipment, social support
- Development (Infant, Child, Adolescent only): no information identified
- Comorbidities: diabetes, cardiovascular disease, arthritis, hearing impairment, depression, stroke, neurological problems, cancer, dementia, hypertension, pain

Instruments

Instruments Developed by Occupational Therapy Personnel

- Activity Card Sort (2nd ed.; ACS-2; Baum & Edwards, 2008)
- Brain Injury Visual Assessment Battery for Adult (biVABA; Warren, 1998)
- Canadian Occupational Performance Measure (5th ed.; COPM-5; Law et al., 2014)
- Cognitive Assessment of Minnesota (CAM; Rustad et al., 1993)
- Dynamic Loewenstein Occupational Therapy Cognitive Assessment (DLOTCA; Katz et al., 2012)
- Home Environment Lighting Assessment (HELA; Perlmutter et al., 2013, in References)
- Low Vision Assessment (LVA; Dahlin-Ivanoff et al., 2001)
- Low Vision Independence Measure (LVIM; Smith, 2013, in References)
- Revised Self-Report Assessment of Functional Visual Performance (R-SRAFVP; see Snow et al., 2017, and Zemina et al., 2018, in References)
- Role Checklist (RC; Oakley et al., 1986)
- Self-Report Assessment of Functional Visual Performance (SRAFVP; Gilbert & Baker, 2011)

Instruments Developed by Other Professionals and Used by Occupational Therapy Personnel

- Activities of Daily Vision Scale (ADVS; Mangione et al., 1992)
- Feinbloom Chart Book (measures distance acuity; Feinbloom, 2012)
- Functional Independence Measure for Blind Adults (FIMBA; Long et al., 2000)
- Functional Vision Screening Questionnaire (FVSQ; Horowitz et al., 1991)
- Impact of Vision Impairment (IVI; Lamoureux et al., 2004)
- LEA Numbers Chart for Vision Rehabilitation (Good-Lite; https://www.good-lite.com/products/272100)
- LEA Numbers Low Contrast Test, 10M (Good-Lite; https://www.good-lite.com/products/270400)
- Leisure Interest Measure (LIM; Ragheb & Beard, 1991)
- Low Vision Writing Assessment (LVWA; Watson et al., 2004)
- Manchester Low Vision Questionnaire (MLVQ; Harper et al., 1999)
- Melbourne Low-Vision ADL Index (MLVAI; Haymes et al., 2001)
- Mini-Mental State Examination (MMSE; Folstein et al., 1975)
- MNREAD Acuity Chart (measures near acuity; University of Minnesota, 1994)
- Montreal Cognitive Assessment (MoCA; Nasreddine et al., 2005)
- Morgan Low Vision Reading Comprehension Assessment (MLVRCA; Watson et al., 1996)
- Patient Health Questionnaire-9 (PHQ-9; Löwe et al., 2004)
- Pepper Visual Skills for Reading Test (PVSRT; Watson et al., 1995)
- Short Portable Mental Status questionnaire (SPMSQ; Pfeiffer, 1975)
- Visual Disability Assessment (VDA; Pesudovs & Coster, 1998)
- Visual Function Index (VF-14; Steinberg et al., 1994)
- Visual Functioning Questionnaire-25 (VFQ-25; National Eye Institute, 2000)

Problems/Issues

Activities of Daily Living/Instrumental ADL

- Person with decreased visual acuity may benefit less from rehabilitation services (Cimarolli et al., 2012).
- Person may have difficulty locating clothing by color or type.
- Person may have difficulty with meal preparation because of difficulty locating cooking utensils and food items, and reading instructions or labels.

- Person may experience reduced mobility in the community (Mac Cobb, 2013).
- Person may be unable to continue driving because of decreased vision or be limited to driving in local community during the day.
- Person may have difficulty with paying bills because of limited vision in reading the bill statement and writing a check.

Education/Work

- Person may be unable to complete certain work tasks because of visual limitations, including reading instructions, memos, and emails.
- Person may have difficulty moving about the work environment safely due to poor lighting or frequent changes in the location of equipment or supplies.

Play/Leisure

- Person may decrease participation in community or outdoor leisure occupations because of difficulty managing perceived or real environment risks in which vision is a vital element (Berger, 2012).
- Leisure occupations may differ depending on when in life cycle low vision or visual loss occurred (Khanna & Aikat, 2015).

Rest/Sleep

- No information identified.

Social Participation

- Person may decrease participation in social activities due to concerns of managing social relationships with low vision.
- Person may feel uncomfortable in large group settings because of difficulty following the visual aspects of the event.
- Person may reduce participation due to lack of family support, lack of meaning, or lack of motivation (Nastasi, 2019).

Sensorimotor

- Person may experience increased energy expenditure to deal with the increased demands of planning for dealing with visual loss.
- Person may find that certain visual patterns (busy, multiple stripes, floral, multicolored, low contrast) are difficulty to manage, especially when differentiating important elements in the environment.
- Person may find that certain auditory cues do not substitute for visual loss when the auditory information is given in situations with mixed auditory background and foreground.

Cognitive/Perceptual

- Person may lack problem-solving skills related to figuring out options for low vision issues.
- Person may be unaware of how low vision is restricting participation, attributing the restrictions instead to other factors, such as old age or changes in the environment (e.g., stores closing or moving to another location, lack of sidewalks).
- Person may lack knowledge of self-management skills to manage low vision, especially if comorbidities exist, such as diabetes.
- Person may experience visual hallucination (seeing things that are not there), called Charles Bonnet syndrome.

Psychosocial

- Person may feel vulnerable outside the home, where locations of objects are not predictable.
- Person may feel that use of the white cane makes the individual more vulnerable to attack.
- Person may be depressed about loss of vision and the independence the vision represented.
- Person may resist asking for help, such as driving to a leisure-type event.
- Person may avoid outside activities because of fear of being attacked.

- Person may express feelings of isolation due to decreased interaction with others.
- Person may lack motivation to overcome or meet the challenges of low vision.
- Person may experience changes in role performance and expectations.
- Person may complain that family members or caregivers are overprotective and get in the way of the person doing things for himself or herself.

Context/Environment
- Person may be unable to read a menu or see location of food because of low lighting and poor contrast between food and table setting.
- Person may experience barriers in the environment, including those built into the environment that focus on sighted persons without regard for low vision users (e.g., low-hanging signs and large, open-spaced rooms; extreme visual [busy] or auditory [loud and mixed] sensory background; uneven ground surfaces and objects; inconsistent lighting; Jenkins et al., 2015; McGrath et al., 2017).
- Person may lack social support (Mohler et al., 2015).

Intervention/Treatment

Models and programs developed by occupational therapy personnel include a caregiver training program using the ecology of human performance model (Weisser-Pike, 2013), Computer-Based Training Module (Nipp et al., 2014), Living Life With Vision Loss (Perlmutter & Hussey, 2017), occupational science (Rudman et al., 2010), participation model (Schoessow, 2010), person–environment–occupation model (Mac Cobb, 2013), support group (Digsby-Schoellig, 2010), and visual perception training (Uysal & Düger, 2012). Models and programs developed by other professionals but used by occupational therapy personnel include the Asset-Based Community Development (ABCD; Gagne & Peirce, 2017), assistive technology (Fok et al., 2011; McGrath, 2011), behavioral activation program (Deemer et al., 2017), font characteristics for readability (Hedlich et al., 2018), grounded theory (Rudman et al., 2016), eccentric viewing training (Hong et al., 2014), home-based occupations (Liu et al., 2013), home modification (Young, 2012), Lions Club (Brown, 2019), multidisciplinary rehabilitation (Markowitz et al., 2011), new view (Farrow et al., 2018), self-management program (Girdler et al., 2010), and visual perception training (Uysal & Düger, 2012). Team members include ophthalmologists, optometrists, opticians, vision rehabilitation therapists and teachers, orientation and mobility specialists, certified low vision therapists, nursing personnel, and occupational therapy personnel. Goals include preventing accidents and injury, teaching new (compensatory) skills, modifying tasks and environment, and promoting a healthy and satisfying lifestyle toward maximizing safety and independence with ADLS, IADLs, education, work, play, leisure, and social participation. The focus is on helping clients to use their remaining vision to participate in desired occupations that support healthy and productive living (American Occupational Therapy Association, 2013, 2014; Brown, 2019).

Activities of Daily Living/Instrumental ADL
- Dressing: Organize clothes by color in closets and drawers (put similar colors such as black and navy at opposite ends of the clothes rack or drawer).
- Grocery shopping: Make a list of what is needed according to the aisles, ask for help if needed to retrieve items, or shop online with a store that delivers.
- Meal preparation:
  - Hang frequently used kitchen tools on a wall-mounted pegboard or hooks.
  - Put colored dots or marks on dials for frequently used settings.
  - A microwave may be substituted for a stove.
  - Use good contrast, such a white mug for black coffee or black measuring cups for flour, sugar, or salt.
  - Use oversized timers, dials, or buttons.
  - Make sure countertops and cooking surfaces are well lit.

- Medication management: Mark each pill bottle in a distinctive way (color, label, size, rubber band, button). Use large-print pill boxes. Take pills with meals or use talking medication reminders (American Occupational Therapy Association, 2017).
- Finances: Organize bills and important papers in different-colored trays or folders with large labels. Pay bills and track accounts online where the font can be enlarged or use automatic pay with bank. Use adaptive equipment such as large-print checks, signature guides, or magnifiers.
- Communication: Consider whether magnification (manual or electronic) and better illumination (task lighting, reduce or eliminate fluorescent lights), changing font type and size, increasing contrast might improve readability (alternative: use auditory approaches).
- Driving: Bioptics or prisms, driving simulator training, driver education programs, and orientation and mobility training may be useful (see Driving Fitness in Section 13: Lifestyle Conditions).

Education/Work
- Assistive devices may assist client with reading and writing tasks.
- Organization of the work station can facilitate work performance.
- Review of work setting and conditions (getting to and from work station, location of restroom or breakroom) may facilitate client's ability to continue to work (Markowitz et al., 2011).

Play/Leisure
- Explore and adapt leisure activities, such as using large-faced card decks, playing games on a computer monitor.
- Explore and facilitate ways to help clients participate in leisure activities in the community.

Rest/Sleep
- No information identified.

Social Participation
- Use group activities to engage people in leisure activities that they would not do alone and build a sense of competence.

Sensorimotor
- Glare reduction: use shades or blinds on windows, glare screens for computers and television, wear hats and sunglasses outside.
- Filters: optometrist or physician can prescribe glasses with filters built in.
- Magnification: magnifiers, telescopes, microscopes, and electronic magnifiers.
- Technology: apps on smartphones, computer tablet settings that make reading easier to change to auditory, large monitor, large-screen TV, DVD player.
- Sensory substitution: tactile and auditory cues may be added (e.g., raised dots at selected temperature points on oven, talking watch, home monitors).
- Energy conservation: pacing, time management.
- Eccentric viewing training: useful for some clients.

Cognitive/Perceptual
- Provide opportunity to identify individual problems and problem-solve solutions (Nastasi, 2018; Smallfield et al., 2017).
- Assist person to develop self-management skills to promote healthy living behaviors (Barstow, 2018).

Psychosocial
- Group discussion in a support group about coping behavior and skills.

Context/Environment

- Home safety
  - ▶ Remove clutter, appliance cords, and throw rugs.
  - ▶ Provide good contrast color between furniture, floors, and walls.
  - ▶ Use contrast to distinguish items such as dark bathmat on a light-colored floor, a light-colored cutting board on a dark-colored counter, colored tape on the edge of stair risers, and white sheets with a dark comforter; organize clothes by color in closets and drawers (put similar colors such as black and navy at opposite ends; avoid floral or busy patterns).
  - ▶ Provide good lighting in hallways, stairwells, and outside walkways. Use nightlights, flashlights, or hall lights to illuminate at night.
  - ▶ Label drawers, cabinets, closets, pantries, hampers, and trays.
  - ▶ Use trays and dividers to separate items in drawers.
  - ▶ Organize rooms to keep commonly used items in the same easy-to-locate place.
- Provide instruction to family, friends, coworkers, colleagues, and caregivers about low vision, its effect on everyday living, and how to facilitate the client to participate in everyday life.
  - ▶ Contrast enhancement: Use contrasting colors, black on white, easy-to-read font.
  - ▶ Corrective lenses: Use glasses, goggles, prisms, or magnifiers designed for the task.
  - ▶ Ergonomics: Use proper height for the activity and good posture.
  - ▶ Lighting: Use task-specific lighting for reading, writing, doing handwork activities. Ambient light for walking (see Young, 2012, in References).
  - ▶ Organize: Use organizational strategies to order items by color, number, alphabet, left-to-right, days of the week.
  - ▶ Psychosocial consideration: Try to accommodate person's preferences.
  - ▶ Referral: Refer to vision specialists if vision continues to be a problem.
  - ▶ Resize: Enlarge print for central vision loss, label items with large-print labels, larger screen or monitor.
  - ▶ Restructure routines: Reschedule activities to take place when vision is best.
  - ▶ Safety: Use fall prevention techniques (see Falls in Section 13: Lifestyle Conditions).
  - ▶ Sensory substitution: Use tactile or auditory cues in place of vision.
  - ▶ Simplification: Reduce visual clutter, use solid-colored objects, reduce number of objects in a particular environment (less furniture, fewer clothes, fewer items on tables).
  - ▶ Visual skills: Eccentric viewing, steady strategy, or scrolling.
- Facilitate participation in organized groups, such as those offered by state commission for the blind.
- Provide instruction in the use of low vision devices.

Precautions/Safety Considerations

Person is at high risk for falling, resulting in injury including hip fractures. Environmental modification and adapted devices are critical (Blaylock & Vogtle, 2017; Leland et al., 2012). Person is at risk of harming others inadvertently because of accidents related to low vision. Person is at risk for becoming increasingly dependent on others and losing independence status. Person may progress more slowly than average during rehabilitation.

Prognosis and Outcome

Low vision problems can be managed, but comorbidity issues limit effectiveness.

REFERENCES

American Occupational Therapy Association. (2013). *Tips for living life to its fullest: Living with low vision.* www.aota.org
American Occupational Therapy Association. (2014). *Low vision FAQ.*

American Occupational Therapy Association. (2017). Occupational therapy's role in medication management. *American Journal of Occupational Therapy, 71*(Suppl. 2), Article 7112410025. https://doi.org/10.5014/ajot.2017.716S02

Barstow, B. (2018). Occupational therapy and low vision rehabilitation: Future directions. *British Journal of Occupational Therapy, 81*(1), 3–4. https://doi.org/10.1177/0308022617738158

Berger, S. (2012). Is my world getting smaller? The challenges of living with vision loss. *Journal of Visual Impairment & Blindness, 106*(1), 5–16. https://doi.org/10.1177/0145482X1210600102

Blaylock, S. E., & Vogtle, L. K. (2017). Falls prevention interventions for older adults with low vision: A scoping review. *Canadian Journal of Occupational Therapy, 84*(3), 139–147. https://doi.org/10.1177/0008417417711460

Brown, C. (2018). The Lions Club and occupational therapy: Working together to address low vision. *OT Practice, 23*(12), 26–28.

Deemer, A. D., Massof, R. W., Rovner, B. W., Casten, R. J., & Piersol, C. V. (2017). Functional outcomes of the Low Vision Depression Prevention Trial in Age-Related Macular Degeneration. *Investigative Ophthalmology & Visual Science, 58*, 1514–1520. https://doi.org/10.1167/iovs.16-20001

Digsby-Schoellig, S. (2010). Sharing in the journey: Low vision support groups. *OT Practice, 15*(2), 17–19.

Farrow, K., Holden, C., Lecher, E., & Larges, L. (2018). Increasing access to vision rehabilitation services for seniors through collaboration with occupational therapists. *Journal of Visual Impairment & Blindness, 112*(3), 301–306. https://doi.org/10.1177/0145482X1811200309

Fok, D., Polgar, J. M., Shaw, L., & Jutai, J. W. (2011). Low vision assistive technology device usage and importance in daily occupations. *Work, 39*(1), 37–48. https://doi.org/10.3233/WOR-2011-1149

Gagne, K., & Peirce, C. (2017). Geriatric low vision. *OT Practice, 22*(21), 8–13.

Girdler, S. J., Boldy, D. P., Dhaliwal, S. S., Crowley, M., & Packer, T. L. (2010). Vision self-management for older adults: A randomised controlled trial. *British Journal of Ophthalmology, 94*(2), 223–228. https://doi.org/10.1136/bjo.2008.147538

Hedlich, C., Barstow, E., & Vogtle, L. K. (2018). Age-related macular degeneration and reading performance: Does font style make a difference? *Journal of Visual Impairment & Blindness, 112*(4), 398–403.

Hindman, J. (2017). Adding life to your days through occupational therapy. *OT Practice, 22*(4), 33.

Hong, S. P., Park, H., Kwon, J.-S., & Yoo, E. (2014). Effectiveness of eccentric viewing training for daily visual activities for individuals with age-related macular degeneration: A systematic review and meta-analysis. *NeuroRehabilitation, 34*(3), 587–595. https://doi.org/10.3233/NRE-141055

Jenkins, G. R., Yuen, H. K., & Vogtle, L. K. (2015). Experience of multisensory environments in public space among people with visual impairment. *International Journal of Environmental Research and Public Health, 12*(8), 8644–8657. https://doi.org/10.3390/ijerph120808644

Khanna, A., & Aikat, R. (2015). Correlation between leisure interests and visual function in people with partial and complete (acquired) visual impairment. *Indian Journal of Occupational Therapy, 47*(1), 9–13. http://aiota.org/temp/ijotpdf/ibat15i1p9.pdf

Leland, N. E., Kaldenberg, J., & Lee, I. (2012). Watching their steps: Integrating vision intervention into daily practice to limit fall risk at skilled nursing facilities. *OT Practice, 17*(11), 7–16.

Liu, C.-J., Brost, M. A., Horton, V. E., Kenyon, S. B., & Mears, K. E. (2013). Occupational therapy interventions to improve performance of daily activities at home for older adults with low vision: A systematic review. *American Journal of Occupational Therapy, 67*(3), 279–287. https://doi.org/10.5014/ajot.2013.005512

Mac Cobb, S. (2013). Mobility restriction and comorbidity in vision-impaired individuals living in the community. *British Journal of Community Nursing, 28*(18), 608–613. https://doi.org/10.12968/bjcn.2013.18.12.608

Markowitz, M., Markowitz, R. E., & Markowitz, S. N. (2011). The multi-disciplinary nature of low vision rehabilitation—A case report. *Work, 39*(1), 63–66. https://doi.org/10.3233/WOR-2011-1151

McGrath, C. (2011). Low vision and older adults: The role of occupational therapy. *Occupational Therapy Now, 13*(3), 26–28.

McGrath, C., Rudman, D. L., Spafford, M., Trentham, B., & Polgar, J. (2017). The environmental production of disability for seniors with age-related vision loss. *Canadian Journal on Aging, 36*(1), 55–66. https://doi.org/10.1017/S0714980816000623

Mohler, A. J., Neufeld, P., & Perlmutter, M. S. (2015). Factors affecting readiness for low vision interventions in older adults. *American Journal of Occupational Therapy, 69*(4), Article 6904270020. https://doi.org/10.5014/ajot.2015.014241

Nastasi, J. A. (2018). The everyday lives of older adults with visual impairment: An occupational perspective. *British Journal of Occupational Therapy, 81*(5), 266–275. https://doi.org/10.1177/0308022617752093

Nastasi, J. (2019). The social participation of older adults living with a visual impairment. *Physical & Occupational Therapy in Geriatrics, 37*(4), 282–297. https://doi.org/10.1080/02703181.2019.1648625

National Eye Institute. (2016). *Living with low vision: What you should know.* http://nei.nih.gov/sites/default/files/health-pdfs/LivingWithLowVisionBooklet.pdf

Nipp, C. M., Vogtle, L. K., & Warren, M. (2014). Clinical application of low vision rehabilitation strategies after completion of a computer-based training module. *Occupational Therapy in Health Care, 28*(3), 296–305. https://doi.org/10.3109/07380577.2014.908335

Park, S., Kho, Y. L., Kim, H. J., Kim, J., & Lee, E. H. (2015). Impact of glaucoma on quality of life and activities of daily living. *Hong Kong Journal of Occupational Therapy, 25*(1), 39–44. https://doi.org/10.1016/j.hkjot.2015.04.002

Perlmutter, M. S., Bhorade, A., Gordon, M., Hollingsworth, H., Engsberg, J. E., & Baum, M. C. (2013). Home lighting assessment for clients with low vision, *American Journal of Occupational Therapy, 67*(6), 674–682. https://doi.org/10.5014/ajot.2013.006692

Perlmutter, M. S., & Hussey, G. (2017). Living life with vision loss: A community-based self-management program for people with low vision. *SIS Quarterly Practice Connections, 2*(2), 24–26.

Rudman, D. L., Gold, D., McGrath, C., Zuvela, B., Spafford, M. M., & Renwick, R. (2016). "Why would I want to go out?": Age-related vision loss and social participation. *Canadian Journal on Aging, 33*(4), 465–478. https://doi.org/10.1017/S0714980816000490

Rudman, D. L., Huot, S., Klinger, L., Leipert, B. D., & Spafford, M. M. (2010). Struggling to maintain occupation while dealing with risk: The experiences of older adults with low vision. *OTJR: Occupation, Participation and Health, 30*(2), 87–96. https://doi.org/10.3928/15394492-20100325-04

Schoessow, K. (2010). Shifting from compensation to participation: A model for occupational therapy in low vision. *British Journal of Occupational Therapy, 73*(4), 160–169. https://doi.org/10.4276/030802210X12706313443947

Smallfield, S., Berger, S., Hillman, B., Saltzgaber, P., Giger, J., & Kaldenberg, J. (2017). Living with low vision: Strategies supporting daily activity. *Occupational Therapy in Health Care, 31*(4), 312–328. https://doi.org/10.1080/07380577.2017.1384969

Smith, T. M. (2013). Refinement of the Low Vision Independence Measure: A qualitative study. *Physical & Occupational Therapy in Geriatrics, 31*(3), 182–196. https://doi.org/10.3109/02703181.2013.813619

Snow, M., Warren, M., & Yuen, H. K. (2018). Revised Self-Report Assessment of Functional Visual Performance (R-SRAFVP)–Part II: Construct validation. *American Journal of Occupational Therapy, 72*(5), Article 7205205020. https://doi.org/10.5014/ajot.2018.030205

Sokol-McKay, D. (2010). Vision rehabilitation and the person with diabetes. *Topics in Geriatric Rehabilitation, 26*(3), 241–249. https://doi.org/10.1097/TGR.0b013e3181ef30e4

Sternberg, K. (2013). Low vision strategies for the non-low-vision specialist. *Physical Disabilities Special Interest Section Quarterly, 36*(2), 1–4.

Uysal, S. A., & Düger, T. (2012). Visual perception training on social skills and activity performance in low-vision children. *Scandinavian Journal of Occupational Therapy, 19*(1), 33–41. https://doi.org/10.3109/11038128.2011.582512

Weisser-Pike, O. (2013). Eye witnesses: Keeping low vision caregivers' needs in sight through occupational therapy. *OT Practice, 18*(22), 14–18.

Young, D. (2012). Light the way: Providing effective home modifications for clients with low vision. *OT Practice, 17*(16), 7–12.

Zemina, C. L., Warren, M., & Yuen, H. K. (2018). Revised Self-Report Assessment of Functional Visual Performance (R-SRAFVP)—Part I: Content validation. *American Journal of Occupational Therapy, 72*(5), Article 7205205010. https://doi.org/10.5014/ajot.2018.030197

BIBLIOGRAPHY

American Occupational Therapy Association. (2016). *Fact sheet: Occupational therapy services for persons with visual impairment.*

Barstow, B. A., Warren, M., Thaker, S., Hallman, A., & Batts, P. (2015). Client and therapist perspectives on the influence of low vision and chronic conditions on performance and occupational therapy intervention. *American Journal of Occupational Therapy, 69*(3), Article 6903270010. https://doi.org/10.5014/ajot.2015.014605

Berger, S., McAteer, J., Schreier, K., & Kaldenberg, J. (2013). Occupational therapy interventions to improve leisure and social participation for older adults with low vision: A systematic review. *America Journal of Occupational Therapy, 67*(3), 303–311. https://doi.org/10.5014/ajot.2013.005447

Butler, M. (2016). The role of occupational therapy in visual impairment in Aotearoa/New Zealand. *New Zealand Journal of Occupational Therapy, 64*(1), 31–33.

Cimarolli, V. R., Morse, A. R., Horowitz, A., & Reinhardt, J. P. (2012). Impact of vision impairment on intensity of occupational therapy utilization and outcomes in subacute rehabilitation. *American Journal of Occupational Therapy, 66*(2), 215–223. https://doi.org/10.5014/ajot.2012.003244

Cole, R., Hsu, Y., & Rovins, G. (2014). *Low vision: Modules 1–4.* AOTA Press.

Cole, R. G., Hsu, Y., & Rovins, G. (2013). *Low vision in older adults: Foundations for rehabilitation* (2nd ed.). AOTA Press.

Dirette, D. K. (2012). Low vision disorders. In B. Atchison & D. K. Dirette (Eds.), *Conditions in occupational therapy: Effect on occupational performance* (4th ed., pp. 301–310). Wolter Kluwer.

Golembiewski, D., & Charlton, J. (2011). Living with vision loss. In C. H. Christiansen & K. M. Matuska (Eds.), *Ways of living: Intervention strategies to enable participation* (4th ed., pp. 431–455). AOTA Press.

Hamby, J. R. (2011). Low vision: Strategies for successful intervention. In H. Smith-Gabai (Ed.), *Occupational therapy in acute care* (pp. 605–624). AOTA Press.

Hamby, J. R. (2017). Low vision: Strategies for successful intervention. In H. Smith-Gabai & S. E. Holm (Eds.), *Occupational therapy in acute care* (2nd ed., pp. 627–637). AOTA Press.

Justiss, M. D. (2013). Occupational therapy interventions to promote driving and community mobility for older adults with low vision: A systematic review. *American Journal of Occupational Therapy, 67*(3), 296–302. https://doi.org/10.5014/ajot.2013.005660

Kaldenberg, J. (2014). Optimizing vision and visual processing. In M. V. Radomski & C. A. Trombly Latham (Eds.), *Occupational therapy for physical dysfunction* (7th ed., pp. 699–724). Wolters Kluwer.

Kaldenberg, J. (2019). Low vision rehabilitation services: Perceived barriers and facilitators to access for older adults with visual impairment. *British Journal of Occupational Therapy, 82*(8), 466–474. https://doi.org/10.1177/0308022618821591

Kaldenberg, J., & Smallfield, S. (2013). *Occupational therapy practice guidelines for older adults with low vision*. AOTA Press.

Livengood, H. M., & Baker, N. A. (2015). The role of occupational therapy in vision rehabilitation of individuals with glaucoma. *Disability and Rehabilitation, 37*(13), 1202–1208. https://doi.org/10.3109/09638288.2014.961651

Matti, A. I., Pesudovs, K., Daly, A., Brown, M., & Chen, C. S. (2011). Access to low-vision rehabilitation services: Barriers and enablers. *Clinical & Experimental Optometry, 94*(2), 181–186. https://doi.org/10.1111/j.1444-0938.2010.00556.x

McGrath, C. E., & Rudman, D. L. (2013). Factors that influence the occupational engagement of older adults with low vision: A scoping review. *British Journal of Occupational Therapy, 76*(5), 234–241. https://doi.org/10.4276/030802213X13679275042762

Nastasi, J. A. (2016). Addressing low vision in hospitals and other settings. *OT Practice, 21*(3), 17–18.

Rosenfeld, S. (2011). Vision and occupational therapy: Terminology, tips and trends. *OT Practice, 16*(15), 7–11.

Rudman, D. L., Egan, M. Y., McGrath, C. E., Kessler, D., Gardner, P., King, J., & Ceci, C. (2016). Low vision rehabilitation, age-related vision loss, and risk: A critical interpretive synthesis. *The Gerontologist, 56*(3), e32–e45. https://doi.org/10.1093/geront/gnv685

Smallfield, S., Clem, K., & Myers, A. (2013). Occupational therapy interventions to improve the reading ability of older adults with low vision: A systematic review. *American Journal of Occupational Therapy, 67*(3), 288–295. https://doi.org/10.5014/ajot.2013.004929

Smith, T. M., Krishnan, S., Hong, I., & Reistetter, T. A. (2019). Measurement validity of the Low Vision Independence Measure (LVIM). *American Journal of Occupational Therapy, 73*(3), Article 7303205070. https://doi.org/10.5014/ajot.2019.031070

Velozo, C. A., Warren, M., Hicks, E., & Berger, K. A. (2013). *Generating clinical outputs for self-reports of visual functioning. Optometry and Vision Science, 90*(8), 765–775. https://doi.org/10.1097/OPX.0000000000000007

Warren, M., & Barstow, E. A. (2011). *Occupational therapy interventions for adults with low vision*. AOTA Press.

Warren, M., & Bayeri, D. (2014). *Self-Report Assessment of Functional Visual Performance (SRAFVP) Toolkit*. University of Alabama at Birmingham.

Warren, M., DeCarlo, D. K., & Dreer, L. E. (2016). Health literacy in older adults with and without low vision. *American Journal of Occupational Therapy, 70*(3), Article 7003270010. https://doi.org/10.5014/ajot.2016.017400

Weisser-Pike, O. (2018). A survey of caregivers of people with low vision: A pilot study. *Annuals of International Occupational Therapy, 1*(2), 74–83. https://doi.org/10.3928/24761222-20180409-03

Weisser-Pike, O., & Kaldenberg, J. (2010). Occupational therapy approaches to facilitate productive aging for individuals with low vision. *OT Practice, 15*(3), CE1–CE8.

Pain and Chronic Pain

See also Complex Regional Pain Syndrome.

Description

Pain is an unpleasant sensation caused by noxious stimulation of the sensory nerve endings (O'Toole, 2017). The factors considered to decrease tolerance to pain include anger, anxiety, boredom, depression, fatigue, persistent pain, and stress (O'Toole, 2017). Acute pain usually occurs in response to tissue injury and is the result of activation of peripheral pain receptors and the specific A delta and C sensory nerve fibers. Chronic pain is pain that persists or reoccurs for more than 3 months or persists for more than 1 month after resolution of an acute tissue injury or accompanies a nonhealing lesion (Porter, 2018). Pain may be described as mild, severe, lancinating, burning, dull, sharp, precisely or poorly localized, or referred. Pain intensity is the magnitude of experienced pain and pain interference is the functional consequence of pain intensity (Cook et al., 2013). Hyperalgesia is increased sensitivity to pain (Porter, 2018). Hypoalgesia is decreased sensitivity to pain (Porter, 2018). Allodynia is pain from stimuli that do not normally cause pain. Paraesthesia (or paresthesia) is a subjective feeling of pain (Porter, 2018).

Cause

Causes of acute pain are surgery, trauma (fracture, dislocation), injury (burn, sunburn, cut, abrasion, crushing, penetrating), infection, or inflammation (swelling, edema). Causes of chronic pain include chronic disorders (cancer, arthritis, or diabetes), injuries (herniated disk, torn ligament), and primary pain disorders (fibromyalgia, chronic headache; Porter, 2018). Other examples are arthritis (Kennedy-Spaien & Kohlhofer, 2014), osteoarthritis (Aebischer et al., 2016), cerebral palsy (Hirsh et al., 2011), chronic obstructive pulmonary disease (HajGhanbari et al., 2012), premature infants (Holsti et al., 2011; Meesters et al., 2019; Valeri et al., 2015; Williams et al., 2019), and hand and upper extremity disorders (Hamasaki et al., 2018; Ho et al., 2018; Pelletier, Higgins, & Bourbonnais, 2018; Smith-Forbes et al., 2015).

Evaluation/Assessment

Areas

- Activities of Daily Living/Instrumental ADL: performance of basic ADL tasks, activities or occupations; performance of IADL tasks, activities, or occupations
- Education/Work: performance of academic tasks, performance of classroom or school tasks, activities, or occupations; performance of work-related (paid or unpaid) tasks, activities, or occupations; work interest surveys, work space (office or home) assessment
- Play/Leisure: performance of play or leisure tasks, activities, or occupations, leisure interest survey, type, frequency
- Rest/Sleep: sleep disturbance, sleep habits and routines
- Social Participation: performance of social activities, location, type, frequency, with whom
- Sensorimotor: muscle strength, joint range of motion, endurance and activity tolerance, postural alignment, body mechanics, inflammation (swelling and edema), fatigue and tiredness, sensitivity to touch, vision, hearing, proprioception (joint movement), temperature
- Cognitive/Perceptual: attention and concentration, memory, executive function
- Psychosocial: depressions, anxiety, stress, emotional regulation, quality of life, self-efficacy, pain tolerance, social isolation
- Context/Environment: social support, adaptive devices, resources, health literacy
- Development (Infant, Child, Adolescent only): no information identified
- Comorbidities: existing trauma, injury, infection, disease, disorders, conditions, phantom, imagined

Instruments

(Note that assessments for premature infants and young infants are not well developed.)

Instruments Developed by Occupational Therapy Personnel

- Assessment of Motor and Process Skills (8th ed.; AMPS-8; Fisher & Bray Jones, 2016; see also Amris et al., 2011, in References)
- Effect of Pain Scale (EOP; Hunt et al., 2010, in References)
- Evaluation of Daily Activity Questionnaire (EDAQ; Hammond et al., 2018, in References)

- Left Right Judgement Task (LRJT; Pelletier, Bourbonnais, et al., 2018, in References)
- Pediatric Survey of Pain Attitudes (Peds-SOPA; Engel et al., 2012, in References)
- Rainbow Pain Scale (RPS; Mahon et al., 2015, in References)

Instruments Developed by Other Professionals and Used by Occupational Therapy Personnel
- Adolescent Pediatric Pain Tool (APPT; Jacob et al., 2014)
- Brief Pain Inventory (BPI; Cleeland & Ryan, 1994)
- Checklist of Primary Shoulder Functional Limitations (CPSFL; Smith-Forbes et al., 2015, in References)
- Child Activity Limitations Interview–21 (CALI-21; Palermo et al., 2008)
- Child Health Questionnaire–Parent Form (CHQ-PF50; Landgraf et al., 1996)
- Functional Disability Inventory (FDI; Walker & Greene, 1991)
- McGill Pain Questionnaire (MPQ; Melzack, 1975)
- Numerical rating scale (NRS-11; pain is scored from 0 to 10)
- Pain Catastrophizing Scale (PCS; Sullivan et al., 1995)
- Pain Impact Questionnaire (PIQ-6; Becker et al., 2007)
- Patient Reported Outcome Measurement Information System (PROMIS; Food and Drug Administration, 2009)
- Patient-Specific Functional Scale (PSFS; Stratford et al., 1995)
- PROMIS Pediatric Pain Interference Scale (PPPIS; Varni et al., 2010)
- Purdue Pegboard Test (PPT; Tiffin, 1948)
- QuickDASH (Kennedy et al., 2011; see also Jerosch-Herold et al., 2017, in References)
- Shoulder Pain and Disability Index (SPADI; Roach et al., 1991; see also Jerosch-Herold et al., 2018, in References)
- Verbal rating scale (VRS-6; scoring is based on pain intensity using words or phrases such as *none, mild, moderate, severe*)
- Weinstein enhanced sensory test (WEST; Commercial test instruments, available from several sources)
- West Haven–Yale Multidimensional Pain Inventory (WHYMPI; Kerns et al., 1985)
- Wong-Baker FACES Pain Rating Scale (FACES; Wong & Baker, 1998)

Problems/Issues

Activities of Daily Living/Instrumental ADL
- Any performance task may cause pain.
- Person may have difficulty getting dressed due to pain.
- Person may experience pain while bathing or showering.
- Person may have difficulty with meal preparation due to pain.
- Person may have difficulty completing housekeeping tasks due to pain.
- Person may have difficulty shopping for needed supplies (groceries, cleaning products) due to pain.
- Person may experience pain while driving.

Education/Work
- Child may experience difficulty completing school assignments due to pain.
- Child may have difficulty sitting in class or moving about the school building due to pain.
- Person may have difficulty performing work tasks due to pain.

Play/Leisure
- Child may avoid or restrict play activities due to pain.
- Adolescent or adult may avoid engaging in certain leisure occupations due to pain.

Rest/Sleep
- Person may experience pain that makes falling asleep difficult.

- Person may be awakened by pain and have difficulty falling asleep again.
- Person may report that sleeping in certain positions is painful.

Social Participation

- Person may avoid or restrict participation in certain social activities due to pain (e.g., having to sit or stand for long periods of time; having to walk long distances, such as to a sporting event or playing a round of golf with friends; using certain movements that are repetitive, such as swinging a tennis racket or throwing a ball).

Sensorimotor

- Person may experience pain in specific muscle or muscle groups.
- Person may experience pain in specific joints, such as shoulder, wrist, or knee.
- Person may experience pain after a certain length of time (activity tolerance).
- Person may complain of fatigue (tiredness) in addition to pain.
- Person may experience pain if touched on a certain part of the body.

Cognitive/Perceptual

- Person may experience reduced ability to attend or concentrate due to pain.
- Person may experience difficulty with memory, especially working memory.
- Person may have difficulty with executive functions (problem solving, organizing, time management).

Psychosocial

- Pain may act as a trigger for depression and anxiety.
- Person may report or experience decreased quality of life.
- Person may report decreased sense of self-efficacy, self-confidence, self-competence.
- Person may not be able to perform roles and role tasks previously held and performed.

Context/Environment

- Person may lack knowledge about pain and pain management.
- Person may lack social support from family, friends, supervisors, employers.
- Person may lack knowledge of community and internet resources.
- Person may lack information about adapted devices that may facilitate performance of certain tasks or activities.

Intervention/Treatment

Models and programs developed by occupational therapy personnel include activity pacing (Andrews et al., 2018), biopsychosocial approach (Bridge & Anand, 2017), isometric elastic resistance training (Patil & Sams, 2011), Lifestyle Redesign and lifestyle-based treatment (Lieb, 2019; Simon & Collins, 2017), medication management (American Occupational Therapy Association, 2017; Rowe & Breeden, 2018), nonlinear dynamic systems (Sinclair et al., 2018), and pacing (Guy et al., 2019). Models and programs developed by other professionals but used by occupational therapy personnel include Calmer robot (Holsti et al., 2019), pain and functional restoration program (Kennedy-Spaien & Kohlhofer, 2014), pain spiral (Yee et al., 2016), self-management (Kennedy-Spaien & Maneii, 2015), sucrose to reduce procedural pain (Holsti & Grunau, 2010), and virtual reality (Benham et al., 2019). Team members include physicians, nursing personnel, psychologists, physical therapy personnel, and occupational therapy personnel. Goals are to help clients manage their pain in adaptive ways by reducing physical and emotional demands so they can engage in the occupations they want and need to do every day, and to work toward less reliance on pain medications, such as opioids (American Occupational Therapy Association, 2014; Bridge & Anand, 2017).

Activities of Daily Living/Instrumental ADL

- Review with client whether performing daily self-care activities could be accomplished with less pain by eliminating steps in some tasks, using adapted devices, or modifying how the task is completed.

- Assist client to determine best access to transportation that is within pain tolerance (driving self, private transport with someone else driving, using public transport).
- Assist client to manage medication schedule, especially if opioids are involved, to use as prescribed by physician.
- Assist client to communicate clearly to others when pain interferes with performing daily activities to reduce conflict and frustration with family and friends. Suggest alternative approaches, such as changing some role responsibilities.

Education/Work
- Assist person to return to or continue participation in educational activities.
- Assist person to gain or maintain employment (paid or unpaid).
- Make recommendations for workplace modification or accommodation to improve work station or work conditions.

Play/Leisure
- Assist child to develop play skills within pain tolerance level.
- Assist person to modify or adapt existing leisure occupations within pain tolerance.
- Assist person to identify and explore new leisure occupations, such as journaling or inside gardening.

Rest/Sleep
- Assist client to identify sleep disturbances and alleviate them to facilitate sleep.
- Assist client to review sleep habits and routines to identify problems such as distractions.

Social Participation
- Assist person to modify or adapt participation in social activities within pain tolerance level.

Sensorimotor
- Therapeutic exercises, such as stretching, range of motion, flexibility, strengthening: Assist team members and client to develop an individualized program of therapeutic exercises to maintain general fitness and prevent contractures and deformities.
- Graded functional activity program: Assist team members and client to plan and implement an activity program that is graded to start at the client's level of function and gradually increase activity tolerance level.
- Fatigue management: Avoid overstimulation and "overdoing it" while maximizing rest, relaxation, and sleep.
- Energy conservation: Provide instruction on energy conservation and motion economy to reduce the stress on joints.
- Work simplification: Provide instruction on strategies designed to eliminate some steps or amount of effort required to perform routine tasks (e.g., switching to wrinkle-free clothing to avoid ironing, using automatic cleaning devices for showers and toilet bowls, using robotic vacuum cleaners, buying prechopped vegetables for cooking).
- Fatigue management/activity tolerance: Provide instruction on activity pacing.
- Joint protection: Provide instruction on joint protection strategies.
- Proper body mechanics: Provide practice in using correct body mechanics for lifting, carrying, reaching, climbing, bending, and stooping.
- Mirror therapy: Use of mirror or mirror box that gives the visual illusion of the affected limb. The illusion can help reconcile sensory input and motor output.
- Ice or cold packs: Can be used for localized areas for no more than 10 minutes (note that clients with pain usually are averse to cold temperatures because muscles tend to tighten).
- Heat: Heating pads can be used for localized areas for about 10 minutes. Paraffin wax warmer can be used for hands. Warm water bag heated to more than 100 °F (monitor heat carefully to avoid burns).
- Contrast baths: Start with ice water, submerge hand or foot for 30 seconds, and then switch immediately to warm water for 2 minutes (Jacques, 2011).

Cognitive/Perceptual

- Cognitive dissonance: Encourage client to reflect on pleasant experiences and describe them in verbal form, writing, drawing, painting, photographs, or scrapbooking.
- Assist client to identify and set goals, and means to achieve the goals (action plan) in areas of occupation (ADL/IADL, school/work, play/leisure, rest/sleep, social participation).
- Assist client to develop a self-management program to control pain symptoms by identifying type of pain and how to manage it; identifying when pain most frequently occurs and how to manage it.
- Assist client to create and follow a planned time schedule of daily occupations, habits, and routines.
- Assist client to develop proactive problem-solving strategies to anticipate potential problems and plan for challenges ahead of time.

Psychosocial

- Stress management: Use coping strategies such as mindfulness mediation, deep-breathing exercises, yoga, imagery.
- Distraction: Have client identify a list of distractors and when to employ them.
- Alleviate boredom: Have client identify occupations that reduce boredom and when to employ them.
- Provide occupations that have a sense of meaning (are meaningful): Have client identify occupations that are meaningful and methods to engage or participate in those occupations.
- Improve sense of self-efficacy, self-confidence, and self-competence by enabling client to take more control of responses to pain including self-management strategies.

Context/Environment

- Client education about pain neurophysiology and pain management.
- Environment modification: Provide information and recommendations on ways to reduce motions that cause pain, such as arranging meal preparation items so they are within easy reach.
- Provision of splints: Provide splints and training in use and care that reduce, control, or prevent pain and prevent contractures and deformity. Example: a splint to maintain neutral wrist position (immobilizes) while allowing for functional use of the hand.
- Provision of adapted devices: Provide information and opportunity to practice using adapted devices.
- Refer client to other professionals for additional services as appropriate.

Precautions/Safety Considerations

Client should be regularly reassessed using a pain assessment. Reaction to pain medicines should be monitored and changes reported to prescribing physician or pain management team, including analgesia (insensitivity to pain), activity level, adverse reactions, aberrant behavior, and signs of addiction.

Prognosis and Outcome

Response to pain is influenced by many factors, including physical, mental, biochemical, psychological, physiological, social, cultural, and emotional.

REFERENCES

Aebischer, B., Elsig, S., & Taeymans, J. (2016). Effectiveness of physical and occupational therapy on pain, function and quality of life in patients with trapeziometacarpal osteoarthritis—A systematic review and meta-analysis. *Hand Therapy, 21*(1), 5–15. https://doi.org/10.1177/1758998315614037

Amris, K., Wæhrens, E., Jespersen, A., Bliddal, H., & Danneskiold-Samsøe, B. (2011). Observation-based assessment of functional ability in patients with chronic widespread pain: A cross-sectional study. *Pain, 152*(11), 2470–2476. https://doi.org/10.1016/j.pain.2011.05.027

American Occupational Therapy Association. (2014). *Fact sheet: Occupational therapy and pain rehabilitation.*

American Occupational Therapy Association. (2017). Occupational therapy's role in medication management. *American Journal of Occupational Therapy, 71*(Suppl. 2), Article 7112410025. https://doi.org/10.5014/ajot.2017.716S02

Andrews, N., Strong, J., Meredith, P., & Branjerdporn, G. (2018). Approach to activity engagement and differences in activity participation in chronic pain: A five-day observational study. *Australian Occupational Therapy Journal, 65*(6), 575–585. https://doi.org/10.1111/1440-1630.12516

Benham, S., Kang, M., & Grampurohit, N. (2019). Immersive virtual reality for the management of pain in community-dwelling older adults. *OTJR: Occupation, Participation and Health, 39*(2), 90–96. https://doi.org/10.1177/1539449218817291

Bridge, K., & Anand, H. (2017). Occupational therapy interventions for pain management: CAOT's submission to the Coalition for Safe and Effective Pain Management. *Occupational Therapy Now, 19*(6), 5–7.

Cook, K. F., Dunn, W., Griffith, J. W., Morrison, M. T., Tanquary, J., Sabata, D., Victorson, D., Carey, L. M., Macdermid, J. C., Dudgeon, B. J., & Gershon, R. C. (2013). Pain assessment using the NIH toolbox. *Neurology, 80*(Suppl. 3), S49–S53. https://doi.org/10.1212/WNL.0b013e3182872e80

Engel, J. M., Jensen, M. P., Ciol, M. A., & Bolen, G. M. (2012). The development and preliminary validation of the Pediatric Survey of Pain Attitudes. *American Journal of Physical Medicine & Rehabilitation, 91*(2), 114–121. https://doi.org/10.1097/PHM.0b013e318238a074

Guy, L., McKinstry, C., & Bruce, C. (2019). Effectiveness of pacing as a learned strategy for people with chronic pain: A systematic review. *American Journal of Occupational Therapy, 73*(3), Article 7303205060. https://doi.org/10.5014/ajot.2019.028555

HajGhanbari, B., Holsti, L., Road, J. D., & Darlene Reid, W. (2012). Pain in people with chronic obstructive pulmonary disease (COPD). *Respiratory Medicine, 106*(7), 998–1005. https://doi.org/10.1016/j.rmed.2012.03.004

Hamasaki, T., Pelletier, R., Bourbonnais, D., Harris, P., & Choinière, M. (2018). Pain-related psychological issues in hand therapy. *Journal of Hand Therapy, 31*(2), 215–226. https://doi.org/10.1016/j.jht.2017.12.009

Hammond, A., Prior, Y., Horton, M. C., Tennant, A., & Tyson, S. (2018). The psychometric properties of the Evaluation of Daily Activity Questionnaire in seven musculoskeletal conditions. *Disability and Rehabilitation, 40*(17), 2070–2080. https://doi.org/10.1080/09638288.2017.1323027

Hirsh, A., Kratz, A. L., Engel, J., & Jensen, M. P. (2011). Survey results of pain treatments in adults with cerebral palsy. *American Journal of Physical Medicine & Rehabilitation, 90*(3), 207–216. https://doi.org/10.1097/PHM.0b013e3182063bc9

Ho, E. S., Campos, A. A., Klar, K., & Davidge, K. (2018). Evaluation of pain in pediatric upper extremity conditions. *Journal of Hand Therapy, 31*(2), 206–214. https://doi.org/10.1016/j.jht.2018.02.004

Holsti, L., & Grunau, R. E. (2010). Considerations for using sucrose to reduce procedural pain in preterm infants. *Pediatrics, 125*(5), 1042–1047. https://doi.org/10.1542/peds.2009-2445

Holsti, L., Grunau, R. E., & Shany, E. (2011). Assessing pain in preterm infants in the neonatal intensive care unit: Moving to a "brain-oriented" approach. *Pain Management 1*(2), 171–179. https://doi.org/10.2217/pmt.10.19

Holsti, L., MacLean, K., Oberlander, T., Synnes, A., & Brant, R. (2019). Calmer: A robot for managing acute pain effectively in preterm infants in the neonatal intensive care unit. *PAIN Reports, 4*(2), Article e727. https://doi.org/10.1097/PR9.0000000000000727

Hunt, J., Kassam, L., Kerr, G., Percy, T., & Waithman, L. (2010). The Effect of Pain Scale: A tool to assist in evaluation of client reports of pain and disability. *Occupational Therapy Now, 12*(2), 6–8.

Jacques, E. K. (2011). Controlling neuropathic pain: Tips from an occupational therapist. *Diabetes Self-Management, 28*(5), 41–42, 44.

Jerosch-Herold, C., Chester, R., & Shepstone, L. (2017). Rasch model analysis gives new insights into the structural validity of the QuickDASH in patients with musculoskeletal shoulder pain. *Journal of Orthopaedic and Sports Physical Therapy, 47*(9), 664–672. https://doi.org/10.2519/jospt.2017.7288

Jerosch-Herold, C., Chester R., Shepstone, L., Vincent, J. I., & MacDermid, J. C. (2018). An evaluation of the structural validity of the Shoulder Pain and Disability Index (SPADI) using the Rasch model. *Quality of Life Research, 27*(2), 389–400. https://doi.org/10.1007/s11136-017-1746-7

Kennedy-Spaien, E., & Kohlhofer, D. (2014). Living life to the fullest with arthritis—Tools and treatments. *Rehab Management, 27*(5), 16, 18–19. https://rehabpub.com/resource-center/living-life-fullest-arthritis-tools-treatments/

Kennedy-Spaien, E., & Maneii, F. (2015). Self-managing chronic pain. *Rehab Management, 28*(1), 25–26.

Lieb, L. C. (2019). Occupational therapy, chronic pain, and lifestyle-based treatment. *OT Practice, 24*(11), 20–22.

Mahon, P., Holsti, L., Siden, H., Strahlendorf, C., Turnham, L., & Giaschi, D. (2015). Using colors to assess pain in toddlers: Validation of "The Rainbow Pain Scale"—A proof-of-principle study. *Journal of Pediatric Oncology Nursing, 32*(1), 40–46. https://doi.org/10.1177/1043454214555197

Meesters, N. J., Simons, S. H. P., van Rosmalen, J., Holsti, L., Reiss, I. K. M., & van Dijk, M. (2019). Acute pain assessment in prematurely born infants below 29 weeks: A long way to go. *Clinical Journal of Pain, 35*(12), 975–982. https://doi.org/10.1097/AJP.0000000000000762

O'Toole, M. T. (Ed.). (2017). *Mosby's dictionary of medicine, nursing & health professions* (10th ed.). Elsevier.

Patil, A. S., & Sams, S. B. A. (2011). Effects of isometric elastic resistance training on chronic neck pain. *Indian Journal of Occupational Therapy, 43*(1), 22–31.

Pelletier, R., Bourbonnais, D., Higgins, J., Mireault, M., Danino, M. A., & Harris, P. G. (2018). Left right judgement task and sensory, motor, and cognitive assessment in participants with wrist/hand pain. *Rehabilitation Research and Practice, 2018*, Article 1530245. https://doi.org/10.1155/2018/1530245

Pelletier, R., Higgins, J., & Bourbonnais, D. (2018). Laterality recognition of images, motor performance, and aspects related to pain in participants with and without wrist/hand disorders: An observational cross-sectional study. *Musculoskeletal Science and Practice, 35*, 18–24. https://doi.org/10.1016/j.msksp.2018.01.010

Porter, R. S. (Ed.). (2018). *The Merck manual of diagnosis and therapy* (20th ed.). Merck Sharp & Dohme.

Rowe, N. C., & Breeden, K. L. (2018). Opioid guidelines and their implications for occupational therapy. *OT Practice, 23*(15), CE-1–CE-8.

Simon, A. U., & Collins, C. E. R. (2017). Lifestyle Redesign for chronic pain management: A retrospective clinical efficacy study. *American Journal of Occupational Therapy, 71*(4), Article 7104190040. https://doi.org/10.5014/ajot.2017.025502

Sinclair, C., Meredith, P., & Strong, J. (2018). Case formulation in persistent pain in children and adolescents: The application of the nonlinear dynamic systems perspective. *British Journal of Occupational Therapy, 81*(12), 727–732. https://doi.org/10.1177/0308022618802722

Smith-Forbes, E. V., Moore-Reed, S. D., Westgate, P. M., Kibler, W. B., & Uhl, T. L. (2015). Descriptive analysis of common functional limitations identified by patients with shoulder pain. *Journal of Sport Rehabilitation, 24*(2), 179–188. http://dx.doi.org/10.1123/jsr.2013-0147

Valeri, B. O., Holsti, L., & Linhares, M. B. (2015). Neonatal pain and developmental outcomes in children born preterm: A systematic review. *Clinical Journal of Pain, 31*(4), 355–362. https://doi.org/10.1097/AJP.0000000000000114

Williams, N., MacLean, K., Guan, L., Collet, J. P., & Holsti, L. (2019). Pilot testing a robot for reducing pain in hospitalized preterm infants. *OTJR: Occupation, Participation and Health, 39*(2), 108–115. https://doi.org/10.1177/1539449218825436

Yee, S., Wellum, K., & Wilson, K. (2016). Chronic pain: Finding solutions with clients as partners. *Occupational Therapy Now, 18*(2), 23–25.

BIBLIOGRAPHY

Brown, C. (2012). Pain and occupational therapy: The time is now. *Occupational Therapy Now, 14*(5), 3–4.

Dahl-Popolizio, S., Rogers, O., Muir, S., Carroll, J. K., & Manson, L. (2017). Interprofessional primary care: The value of occupational therapy. *Open Journal of Occupational Therapy, 5*(3), Article 11. https://doi.org/10.15453/2168-6408.1363

Devan, D. (2014). A review of current therapeutic practice for the management of chronic pain. *South African Journal of Occupational Therapy, 44*(1), 48–50.

DiLorenzo, M., Pillai Riddell, P., & Holsti, L. (2016). Beyond acute pain: Understanding chronic pain in infancy. *Children, 3*(4), Article 26. https://doi.org/10.3390/children3040026

Engel, J. M. (2018). Pain management. In H. M. Pendleton & W. Scultz-Krohn (Eds.), *Pedretti's occupational therapy* (8th ed., pp. 701–709). Elsevier.

Engel, J. M., Jensen, M. P., Ciol, M. A., & Bolen, G. M. (2012). The development and preliminary validation of the Pediatric Survey of Pain Attitudes. *American Journal of Physical Medicine & Rehabilitation, 91*(2), 114–121. https://doi.org/10.1097/PHM.0b013e318238a074

Griffiths, K. (2019). The management of analgesia. *OT News, 27*(5), 40–41.

Hesselstrand, M., Samuelsson, K., & Liedberg, G. (2015). Occupational therapy interventions in chronic pain—A systematic review. *Occupational Therapy International, 22*(4), 183–194. https://doi.org/10.1002/oti.1396

Hill, W. (2016). The role of occupational therapy in pain management. *Anaesthesia and Intensive Care Medicine, 17*(9), 451–453. https://doi.org/10.1016/j.mpaic.2016.06.008

Holm, S. E. (2017). Pain management. In H. Smith-Gabai & S. E. Holm (Eds.), *Occupational therapy in acute care* (2nd ed., pp. 673–683). AOTA Press.

Holsti, L., Backman, C. L., & Engel, J. M. (2013). Occupational therapy. In P. J. McGrath, B. J. Stevens, S. M. Walker, & W. T. Zampsky (Eds.), *Oxford textbook of paediatric pain* (pp. 590–599). Oxford University Press. https://doi.org/10.1093/med/9780199642656.003.0057

Holsti, L., Oberlander, T. F., & Brant, R. (2011). Does breastfeeding reduce acute procedural pain in preterm infants in the neonatal intensive care unit? A randomized clinical trial. *Pain, 152*(11), 2575–2581. https://doi.org/10.1016/j.pain.2011.07.022

Jensen, M. P., Moore, M. R., Bockow, T. B., Ehde, D. M., & Engel, J. M. (2011). Psychosocial factors and adjustment to chronic pain in persons with physical disabilities: A systematic review. *Archives of Physical Medicine and Rehabilitation, 92*(1), 146–160. https://doi.org/10.1016/j.apmr.2010.09.021

Klinger, L., & Klassen, B. (2012). What does an occupational therapist do for someone living with chronic pain? *Occupational Therapy Now, 14*(5), 6–7.

Miró, J., Castarlenas, E., de la Vega, R., Solé, E., Tomé-Pires, C., Jensen, M. P., Engel, J. M., & Racine, M. (2016). Validity of three rating scales for measuring pain intensity in youths with physical disabilities. *European Journal of Pain, 20*(1), 130–137. https://doi.org/10.1002/ejp.704

Miró, J., de la Vega, R., Gertz, K. J., Jensen, M. P., & Engel, J. M. (2019). The role of perceived family social support and parental solicitous responses in adjustment to bothersome pain in young people with physical disabilities. *Disability and Rehabilitation, 41*(6), 641–648. https://doi.org/10.1080/09638288.2017.1400594

Miró, J., de la Vega, R., Solé, E., Racine, M., Jensen, M. P., Gálan, S., & Engel, J. M. (2017). Defining mild, moderate, and severe pain in young people with physical disabilities. *Disability and Rehabilitation, 39*(11), 1131–1135. https://doi.org/10.1080/09638288.2016.1185469

Miró, J., de la Vega, R., Tomé-Pires, C., Sánchez-Rodríguez, E., Castarlenas, E., Jensen, M. P., & Engel, J. M. (2017). Pain extent and function in youth with physical disabilities. *Journal of Pain Research, 10*, 113–120. https://doi.org/10.2147/JPR.S121590

Miró, J., Solé, E., Gertz, K., Jensen, M. P., & Engel, J. M. (2017). Pain beliefs and quality of life in young people with disabilities and bothersome pain. *Clinical Journal of Pain, 33*(11), 998–1005. https://doi.org/10.1097/AJP.0000000000000482

Moon, M., McDonald, R., & Van den Dolder, J. (2012). Occupational therapy for pain management in the compensation setting: Context and principles. *Occupational Therapy Now, 14*(5), 16–18.

Robinson, K., Kennedy, N., & Harmon, D. (2011). Review of occupational therapy for people with chronic pain. *Australian Occupational Therapy Journal, 58*(2), 74–81. https://doi.org/10.1111/j.1440-1630.2010.00889.x

Schmid, A., Van Puymbroeck, M., Fruhauf, C., Bair, M., & Portz, J. (2019). Yoga improves occupational performance, depression, and daily activities for people with chronic pain. *Work, 63*(2), 181–189. https://doi.org/10.3233/WOR-192919

van Huet, H., Innes, E., & Stancliffe, R. (2013). Occupational therapists perspectives of factors influencing chronic pain management. *Australian Occupational Therapy Journal, 60*(1), 56–63. https://doi.org/10.1111/1440-1630.12011

Sensory Integrative Dysfunction

Also called sensory integration disorder, SID, DSI.

See also Ayres Sensory Integration Approach, Dyspraxia and Developmental Dyspraxia, Sensory Modulation Disorders, Sensory Processing Disorders, Sensory-Based Problems in Adults, Sensory Over-Responsivity, Somatosensory Dysfunction.

Description

Sensory integration is the ability of the central nervous system to process sensory information to make an adaptive response. Sensory integrative dysfunction is a disorder or irregularity in brain function that makes sensory integration difficult (Jacobs & Simon, 2015). The term *sensory integration* is used to describe many uses of sensory theory and intervention. Strict use of sensory integrative techniques described by Ayres is discussed in the chapter on Ayres Sensory Integration. Description and analysis of articles and books in this chapter may or may not follow the theory and concepts proposed by Ayres. Disorders include autism spectrum disorder (Abelenda et al., 2015; Ashburner et al., 2014; Dunbar et al., 2012; Iwanaga et al., 2014; Kashefimehr et al., 2018; Parham et al., 2019; Pfeiffer et al., 2011; Schaaf, 2010; Schaaf, Benevides, et al., 2012; Schaaf et al., 2014; Schaaf & Case-Smith, 2014; Schaaf, Hunt, et al., 2012), developmental disabilities (Kim et al., 2012; Leong et al., 2015), and premature infant (Lecuona et al., 2017; Pekçetin et al., 2016).

Cause

The cause or causes of sensory integrative dysfunction are not known. Both genetic and environmental factors may be involved.

Terminology

Note: Inconsistent use of terminology is a major issue in sensory integrative dysfunction. The categories below are general and do not necessarily follow any outline provided by various authors.

- *Sensory defensiveness/sensory over-sensitivity:* May demonstrate aversion, anxiety, or negative reaction to sensory input (Schaaf & Lane, 2015).
  - *Auditory defensiveness/sensitivity:* Increased sensitivity (oversensitivity) to sounds such as fire alarms or vacuum cleaners (Jacobs & Simon, 2015).
  - *Oral defensiveness/sensitivity:* Avoidance of certain texture of food and irritation with activities using the mouth (Jacobs & Simon, 2015).
  - *Tactile defensiveness/sensitivity:* Adverse reaction or anxiety to touch or textures (Mailloux et al., 2011; Schaaf & Lane, 2015; Spies & van Rensberg, 2012).
  - *Vestibular sensitivity:* Intolerance to movement.
  - *Visual defensiveness/sensitivity:* Increased reaction to light with feelings of discomfort or pain (Schaaf & Lane, 2015).
- *Sensory (perceptual) discrimination deficits:* Difficulty with accurate perception and interpretation of sensory information (Northrop, 2018).
  - *Tactile–proprioceptive discrimination deficit:* Difficulty discriminating among objects by the sense of touch or feel (Jacobs & Simon, 2015; Northrop, 2018).
  - *Visual–spatial perceptual deficit:* Includes deficits in any of the areas of visual perception (figure–ground, form constancy, or discrimination of size, shape, distance and form of objects; Jacobs & Simon, 2015; Northrop, 2018).
  - *Vestibular discrimination deficit:* Difficulty with bilateral coordination and postural ocular control (Northrop, 2018).
- *Sensory under-sensitivity:* Diminished awareness of sensory input; does not respond to sensory input or takes a lengthened amount of time to respond (Schaaf & Lane, 2015).
  - *Postural disorder:* Demonstrates poor core strength, decreased endurance, poor body awareness, poor postural stability, and poor postural control (Collins & Miller, 2012). Poor postural movement may result in difficulty using antigravity postures needed for stabilization of the neck, trunk, upper extremities through muscle co-contractions in the neck and upper extremities and balance (Lin et al., 2012). Gravitation insecurity (Potegal et al., 2018).
  - *Somatodyspraxia, developmental dyspraxia:* Difficulty perceiving somatosensory information and planning unfamiliar actions (Buitendag & Aronstam, 2010; Lane et al., 2015; Mailloux et al., 2011).
  - *Under-responsive to vestibular input:* May present as overly lethargic (Northrop, 2018).
  - *Vestibular bilateral integration deficits (vestibular bilateral disorder):* Difficulty processing vestibular information and developing postural and bilateral motor control (Lane et al., 2015; Mailloux et al., 2011).
  - *Visuodyspraxia:* Difficulty perceiving visual-spatial information and planning and constructing based on visual data (Lane et al., 2015; Mailloux et al., 2011).

Evaluation/Assessment
Areas
- Activities of Daily Living/Instrumental ADL: basic ADLs (eating, dressing, bathing/showering, grooming, toileting, transfers), driving
- Education/Work: classroom arrangement, academic performance, school activities
- Play/Leisure: type, location, frequency, interests
- Rest/Sleep: sleep disturbance
- Social Participation: type, location, frequency, with whom
- Sensorimotor: gross motor skills, fine motor skills, hand functions, responses to auditory, gustatory, olfactory, pain, proprioception, vestibular, and visual stimuli
- Cognitive/Perceptual: attention, memory, time management and scheduling, self-management
- Psychosocial: anxiety, stress, interaction skills, role performance, quality of life, self-esteem, self-regulation and emotional control
- Context/Environment: environment modification, parent and teacher education, resources

- Development (Infant, Child, Adolescent only): developmental milestones
- Comorbidities: anxiety, autism spectrum disorder, attention-deficit/hyperactivity disorder, cochlear implants, cerebral palsy, developmental coordination disorder, feeding disorders, fetal alcohol spectrum disorder, intellectual disability, prematurity

Instruments

Instruments Developed by Occupational Therapy Personnel

- Comprehensive Observation of Proprioception (COP; Blanche et al., 2012)
- DeGangi-Berk Test of Sensory Integration (DBTSI; DeGangi & Berk, 1983)
- Infant/Toddler Sensory Profile (ITSP; Dunn, 2002)
- Sensory Experience Questionnaire 3.0 (SEQ-3; Baranek et al., 2006)
- Sensory Integration and Praxis Tests (SIPT; Ayres, 1989; see also van Jaarsveld et al., 2012, in References)
- Sensory Processing Measure (SPM) Home Form (SPM-HF; Parham & Ecker, 2007)
- Sensory Processing Measure (SPM) Main Classroom and School Environments Forms (Miller Kuhaneck et al., 2010)
- Sensory Processing Measure–Preschool: Home Form (SPM-P-HF; Ecker & Parham, 2010)
- Sensory Processing Measure (SPM) Main Classroom and School Environments Forms (Miller Kuhaneck et al., 2010)
- Sensory Processing Scales Inventory (SPSI; Schoen et al., 2017)
- Sensory Profile (2nd ed.; SP-2; Dunn, 2014)
- Short Child Occupational Profile (SCOPE; Bowyer et al., 2008)
- Short Sensory Profile (SSP; McIntosh et al., 1999)
- Southern California Postrotary Nystagmus Test (SCPNT; Ayres, 1975)
- Test of Sensory Function in Infants (TSFI; DeGangi & Greenspan, 1989)

Instruments Developed by Other Professionals and Used by Occupational Therapy Personnel

- Bayley Scales of Infant and Toddler Development (4th ed.; Bayley-4; Bayley & Aylward, 2019)
- Beery-Buktenica Developmental Test of Visual-Motor Integration (6th ed.; Beery VMI-6; Beery et al., 2010)
- Goal Attainment Scaling (GAS; Kiresuk & Sherman, 1968)

Problems/Issues

Activities of Daily Living/Instrumental ADL

- Child may demonstrate decreased ability to manage mealtime activities (tactile proprioceptive discrimination).
- Child may avoid finger foods of certain textures (sticky, gooey, messy; tactile defensiveness/sensitivity).
- Child may refuse to wear or avoid wearing clothes that "scratch," "itch," or "feel tight" (tactile defensiveness/sensitivity).
- Child may demonstrate decreased skill in manipulating clothing, such as zipping, buttoning, snapping, tying (tactile-proprioceptive discrimination).
- Child may demonstrate decreased skill in maintaining clean face and hands (tactile-proprioceptive discrimination).
- Child may report feeling sick or nauseated after riding school bus or long car ride (vestibular sensitivity).
- Teenager may have difficulty learning to drive and pass driver's education course (poor bilateral coordination and postural ocular control).

Education/Work

- Child may have decreased handwriting legibility and speed of output (visual-spatial perception).

- Child may lack endurance for handwriting or have decreased handwriting legibility (tactile-proprioceptive discrimination).
- Child may experience decreased keyboard or handwriting speed and accuracy (tactile proprioceptive discrimination).
- Child may have difficulty keeping pace with note-taking and test completion (visual-spatial perception).
- Child may avoid certain classroom activities, such as using glue, paint, clay, Play-Doh, shaving cream, or craft project supplies (tactile defensiveness/sensitivity).

Play/Leisure

- Child may prefer solitary activities and avoid group activities with peers.
- Child may avoid certain play activities, such as sand, gardening, water play (tactile defensiveness/sensitivity).
- Child may become nauseated during play time or recess if activities involve swinging, stretching, doing sit-ups (vestibular oversensitivity).

Rest/Sleep

- Child may have sleep disturbance.

Social Participation

- Child may have difficulty interacting with others because others report roughhousing, being pushed or hit that does not stop (under-responsive vestibular responsivity).
- Child may avoid activities that include loud noises, such as large assembly, pep rallies, cafeteria, or music classes (orchestra, band; auditory sensitivity).
- Child may become anxious and uncomfortable during safety drills for fire, earthquake, or tornado (auditory sensitivity).

Sensorimotor

- Child may try to avoid recess games, physical education, and sport activities (tactile-proprioceptive discrimination and or decreased bilateral coordination and postural ocular control).
- Child may avoid exercises that require movement such as jumping, hopping, skipping, climbing, or running (vestibular sensitivity) or the opposite pattern in which child is in constant motion, including rocking and fidgeting (under-responsivity to vestibular input).

Cognitive/Perceptual

- Child may have difficulty paying attention or take a long time to respond when called upon (under-responsivity).
- Child may have difficulty with visual memory for shapes, size, and orientation recall.
- Child may have difficulty remembering to complete assignments.
- Child may have challenges navigating school building safely and independently.
- Child may have difficulty recognizing faces or reading social cues of peers and teachers.

Psychosocial

- Child may appear to lack motivation and have low frustration tolerance (consider oversensitivity).
- Child appears to have little regard for others feelings or safety (consider undersensitivity).
- Child may experience loss of self-esteem because behavior is not accepted in the classroom or daycare center (consider under-responsivity).
- Child may have difficulty with self-regulation due to low registration.

Context/Environment

- Child may have difficulty opening locks and locker doors (tactile proprioceptive discrimination).

Intervention/Treatment

Models and programs developed by occupational therapy personnel include adaptive response (Stackhouse, 2014), Alert Program (Williams & Shellenberger, n.d.), comprehensive framework (Bodison, 2018), motion-sensing game (Chuang & Kuo, 2016), and weighted garments (Mishra et al., 2011). Models and programs developed by other professionals but used by occupational therapy personnel include interactive metronome training (Kim et al., 2012). Team members include parents and caregivers, child care workers, educators, school administrators, physicians, nurses and nursing personnel, school psychologists and counselors, physical therapy personnel, speech–language pathologists, social workers, and occupational therapy personnel. Goals are to enable the child to participate in everyday activities associated with home, school, and community. The following are examples, but not exhaustive lists, of possible solutions to problems in sensory integrative dysfunction. They are presented separately, but may be used in combination, such as smelling a lavender lotion applied to calm tactile defensiveness.

Activities of Daily Living/Instrumental ADL
- Eating (see Feeding Disorders in Children in Section 1: Development Disorders)
- Clothing
  - ► Defensive: cotton clothing, loose fitting (a size larger than needed), reduce amount of fasteners, avoid tight-fitting collars, wear sandals or slip-on shoes.
  - ► Craving: tight-fitting clothing, belted jeans or slacks, tops with collars, laced shoes.
- Brushing teeth
  - ► Defensive: deep pressure oral massage starting at top of head and working toward mouth, small head brush with soft bristles, plain/no-flavor toothpaste.
  - ► Craving: light touch around mouth, large surface brush, mint or other flavored toothpaste.

Education/Work
- Classroom
  - ► Defensive: have student enter before everyone else and get settled, provide quiet space away from door and traffic pattern in room, reduce visual distractions, talk in soft steady voice, provide a daily printed schedule of classes and special events; headphones to dampen sound may be useful.
  - ► Craving: offer various seating options, allow student to pass out items or collect items to provide opportunity to move about room or take items from classroom to school office; fidget gadgets may be useful.
- School
  - ► Defensive: allow student to move between classes or eat in cafeteria before others, try to schedule classes near each other, have a buddy assigned to assist student during change of class.
  - ► Craving: student may need assistance to learn appropriate behavior for walking in hallways without bumping into or pushing others out of way, not racing up or down the stairs two or three steps at a time, waiting quietly in cafeteria line.

Play/Leisure
- Alerting: action and sports games, interaction and active engagement with others.
- Calming: solitary or parallel activities in a quiet space.

Rest/Sleep
- Calming: smooth silk sheets, soft cotton or flannel blankets, dark room, minimum noise, weighted blanket.

Social Participation
- Alerting: activities that are fast paced, require motor responses, and active participation with several people, such as sports games, attending a "rock star" concert.
- Calming: activities that can be done at a more leisurely pace, such as shuffleboard, doing puzzles together, going to a museum, or orchestra concert.

Sensorimotor
- Auditory
  - ▶ Alerting: fast tempo such as marching music, drum beat.
  - ▶ Calming: slow tempo such as waltz music.
- Gustatory
  - ▶ Alerting: sour, bitter, chewy, irregular texture.
  - ▶ Calming: sweet, uniform smooth texture.
- Olfactory
  - ▶ Alerting scents: cinnamon, citrus, coffee, ginger, jasmine, mint, peppermint, rosemary.
  - ▶ Calming scents: basil, bergamot orange, frankincense, geranium, jasmine, lavender, lemon balm, oregano, rose.
- Proprioception
  - ▶ Alerting: games such as Simon Says, Twister, rock or wall climbing, aiming and throwing at a target.
  - ▶ Calming: weighted vest or blanket, joint compression, rolled tightly in a blanket, "heavy work," such as carrying a heavy load, pushing a loaded grocery cart or wheelbarrow.
- Tactile
  - ▶ Alerting: light touch, "surprise" touch, tickles, searching for objects in rice or sand.
  - ▶ Calming: firm pressure; pressure applied on top of head or shoulders; bear hug; clothing that covers arms, legs, and head; self-brushing; body lotions.
- Vestibular
  - ▶ Alerting: rapid bouncing on a trampoline or therapy ball, swinging in a hammock or on a swing; spinning on swivel chair, scooter board, or sit and spin; rocking in a rocking chair or rocking horse; climbing on a ladder, climbing wall, series of large foam blocks; hanging upside down on a trapeze or monkey bars; sliding on ramp or slide; doing jumping jacks, running, playing hopscotch, swimming, marching, playing sports.
  - ▶ Calming: slow rhythmic, linear swinging, rocking, or bouncing; slow dancing; gentle slow spinning in one direction.
- Vision
  - ▶ Alerting: "bright" colors (red, orange, yellow); flashing lights; rapidly changing pictures on television, videos, movies; florescent lights, "high beam" lights, sunlight.
  - ▶ Calming: "dark" colors (green, blue, purple), soft, steady light, dark or low light conditions, sunglasses.

Cognitive/Perceptual
- Attention: use sensory alerting techniques to increase attention and concentration.
- Memory: matching tasks full view, matching tasks hidden view.
- Executive functions: making daily schedule, organizing study space.

Psychosocial
- Anxiety/fear: step-by-step instructions, errorless learning, scaffolding, reassurance.
- Self-esteem/self-confidence: create "small" successes, use errorless learning.

Context/Environment
- Provide education to parents and caregivers about managing sensory integrative dysfunction in the home, school, and community.
- Provide education and consultation to technicians and professionals about sensory integrative dysfunction and its effect on everyday life in school and community.
- Provide information about available resources.

Precautions/Safety Considerations
Child should always be able to say "stop" and expect immediate compliance. Watch for signs of overstimulation: pale skin, teeth clenching, staring eyes.

Prognosis and Outcome

Positive outcome should be connected to a change in behavior or occupational performance as defined by a specific goal (e.g., child will participate in a structured playground activity, such as T-ball, with one other child without leaving the activity or arguing with the child for 10 minutes during recess or lunch break, two of three opportunities).

REFERENCES

Abelenda, J., Mailloux, A., & Roley, S. S. (2015). Dyspraxia in autism spectrum disorders: Evidence and implications. *Sensory Integration Special Interest Section Quarterly, 38*(3), 1–3.

Ashburner, J. K., Rodger, S. A., Ziviani, J. M., & Hinder, E. A. (2014). Comment on: "An intervention for sensory difficulties in children with autism: A randomized trial" by Schaaf et al. (2013). *Journal of Autism and Developmental Disorders, 44*, 1486–1488. https://doi.org/10.10 07/s10803-014-2083-0

Bodison, S. C. (2018). A comprehensive framework to embed sensory interventions within occupational therapy practice. *SIS Quarterly Practice Connections, 3*(2), 14–16.

Buitendag, K., & Aronstam, M. C. (2010). The relationship between developmental dyspraxia and sensory responsivity in children aged four years through eight years, Part 1. *South African Journal of Occupational Therapy, 40*(3), 16–20.

Chuang, T.-Y., & Kuo, M.-S. (2016). A motion-sensing game-based therapy to foster the learning of children with sensory integration dysfunction. *Educational Technology & Society, 19*(1), 4–16.

Collins, B., & Miller, L. J. (2012, July–August). Sensory-based motor disorders: Postural disorder. *Autism Asperger's Digest*, 46–47. https://www.spdstar.org/sites/default/files/publications/3.%20Jul.-Aug.%202012%20-%20SBMD%2C%20PD_0.pdf

Dunbar, S. B., Carr-Hertel, J., Lieberman, H. A., Perez, B., & Ricks, K. (2012, July 1). A pilot study comparison of sensory integration treatment and integrated preschool activities for children with autism. *Internet Journal of Allied Health Sciences and Practice, 10*(3), Article 6.

Iwanaga, R., Honda, S., Nakane, H., Tanaka, K., Toeda, H., & Tanaka, G. (2014). Pilot study: Efficacy of sensory integration therapy for Japanese children with high-functioning autism spectrum disorder. *Occupational Therapy International, 21*(1), 4–11. https://doi.org/10.1002/oti.1357

Jacobs, K., & Simon, L. (2015). *Quick reference dictionary for occupational therapy* (6th ed.). Slack.

Kashefimehr, B., Kayihan, H., & Huri, M. (2018). The effect of sensory integration therapy on occupational performance in children with autism. *OTJR: Occupation, Participation and Health, 38*(2), 75–83. https://doi.org/10.1177/1539449217743456

Kim, H. H., Bo, G. H., & Yoo, B. K. (2012). The effects of a sensory integration programme with applied interactive metronome training for children with developmental disabilities: A pilot study. *Hong Kong Journal of Occupational Therapy, 22*(1), 25–30. https://doi.org/10.1016/j.hkjot.2012.05.001

Lane, S., Mailloux, Z., Reynolds, S., & Smith Roley, S. (2015). Patterns of sensory integration dysfunction in specific populations: Evidence-based identification. *OT Practice, 20*(17), CE-1–CE-8.

Lecuona, E., van Jaarsveld, A., Raubenheimer, J., & van Heerden, R. (2017). Sensory integration intervention and the development of the premature infant: A controlled trial. *South African Medical Journal, 107*(11), 976–982. https://doi.org/10.7196/SAMJ.2017.v107i11.12393

Leong, H. M., Carter, M., & Stephenson, J. R. (2015). Meta-analysis of research on sensory integration therapy for individuals with developmental and learning disabilities. *Journal of Developmental and Physical Disabilities, 27*, 187–206. https://doi.org/10.1007/s10882-014-9408-y

Lin, C.-K., Lin, C.-H., Wu, P.-F., Wu, H.-M., Wu, Y.-Y., Kuo, B.-C., & Yeung, K.-T. (2012). A small sample test of the factor structure of postural movement and bilateral motor integration using structural equation modeling. *Perceptual and Motor Skills, 115*(2), 544–557. https://doi.org/10.2466/25.03.10.PMS.115.5.544-557

Mailloux, Z., Mulligan, S., Smith Roley, S., Blanche, E., Cermak, S., Coleman, G. G., Bodison, S., & Lane, C. J. (2011). Verification and clarification of patterns of sensory integrative dysfunction. *American Journal of Occupational Therapy, 65*, 143–151. https://doi.org/10.5014/ajot.2011.000752

Mishra, N., Desai, O. P., & Nagar, R. (2011). To study the effectiveness of a specially designed therapy garment in children with sensory integrative dysfunction. *Indian Journal of Occupational Therapy, 43*(1), 32–37.

Northrop, T. (2018). Occupational therapy's critical role in addressing sensory integration to increase academic progress and participation in schools. *SIS Quarterly Practice Connections, 3*(4), 8–10.

Parham, L. D., Clark, G. F., Watling, R., & Schaaf, R. (2019). Occupational therapy interventions for children and youth with challenges in sensory integration and sensory processing: A clinic-based practice case example. *American Journal of Occupational Therapy, 73*(1), Article 7301395010. https://doi.org/10.5014/ajot.2019.731002

Pekçetin, S., Akı, E., Üstünyurt, Z., & Kayıhan, H. (2016). The efficiency of sensory integration interventions in preterm infants. *Perceptual and Motor Skills, 123*(2), 411–423. https://doi.org/10.1177/0031512516662895

Pfeiffer, B. A., Koenig, K., Kinnealey, M., Sheppard, M., & Henderson, L. (2011). Effectiveness of sensory integration interventions in children with autism spectrum disorders: A pilot study. *American Journal of Occupational Therapy, 65*(1), 76–85. https://doi.org/10.5014/ajot.2011.09205

Potegal, M., Pfaff, W. O., & Kroker, E. (2018). Gravitation insecurity in children: A survey of occupational therapists' observations. *Indian Journal of Physiotherapy and Occupational Therapy, 12*(2), 30–37.

Schaaf, R. C. (2010). Interventions that address sensory dysfunction for individuals with autism spectrum disorders: Preliminary evidence for the superiority of sensory integration compared to other sensory approached. In B. Reichow, P. Doehring, D. V. Cichetti, & F. R. Volkmar (Eds.), *Evidence-based practices and treatments for children with autism* (pp. 245–273). Springer Nature.

Schaaf, R. C., Benevides, T. W., Kelly, D., & Mailloux-Maggio, Z. (2012). Occupational therapy and sensory integration for children with autism: A feasibility, safety, acceptability and fidelity study. *Autism, 16*(3), 321–327. https://doi.org/10.1177/1362361311435157

Schaaf, R. C., Benevides, T., Mailloux, Z., Faller, P., Hunt, J., van Hooydonk, E., Freeman, R., Leiby, B., Sendecki, J., & Kelly, D. (2014). An intervention for sensory difficulties in children with autism: A randomized trial. *Journal of Autism and Developmental Disorders, 44*, 1493–1506. https://doi.org/10.1007/s10803-013-1983-8

Schaaf, R. C., & Case-Smith, J. (2014). Sensory interventions for children with autism. *Journal of Comparative Effectiveness Research, 3*(3), 225–227. https://doi.org/10.2217/CER.14.18

Schaaf, R. C., Hunt, J., & Benevides, T. (2012). Occupational therapy using sensory integration to improve participation of a child with autism: A case report. *American Journal of Occupational Therapy, 66*(5), 547–555. https://doi.org/10.5014/ajot.2012.004473

Schaaf, R. C., & Lane, A. E. (2015). Toward a best-practice protocol for assessment of sensory features in ASD. *Journal of Autism and Developmental Disorders, 45*, 1380–1395. https://doi.org/10.1007/s10803-014-2299-z

Spies, R., & van Rensberg, E. (2012). The experience of parents with tactile defensive children. *South African Journal of Occupational Therapy, 43*(3), 1–11.

Stackhouse, T. M. (2014). The adaptive response to the just-right challenge: Essential components of sensory integration intervention. *Sensory Integration Special Interest Section Quarterly, 37*(2), 1–4.

van Jaarsveld, A., Mailloux, Z., & Herzberg, D. S. (2012). The use of the Sensory Integration and Praxis tests with South African children. *South African Journal of Occupational Therapy, 42*(3), 12–18.

Williams, M. S., & Shellenberger, S. (n.d.). *Alert program: Self-regulation made easy.* https://www.alertprogram.com

BIBLIOGRAPHY

American Academy of Pediatrics. (2012). Sensory integration therapies for children with developmental and behavioral disorders. *Pediatrics, 129*(6), 1186–1189. https://doi.org/10.1542/peds.2012-0876 (Note: No OT authors. Reference document.)

American Occupational Therapy Association. (2015). Occupational therapy for children and youth using sensory integration theory and methods in school-based practice. *American Journal of Occupational Therapy, 69*(Suppl. 3), Article 6913410040. https://doi.org/10.5014/ajot.2015.696S04

Brown, C., Filion, D. L., & Wiss, S. J. (2011). Measurement of tactile response and tactile perception. In M. J. Hertenstein & S. J. Weiss (Eds.), *The handbook of touch: Neuroscience, behavioral and health perspectives* (pp. 219–244). Springer.

Kimball, J. G., & May-Benson, T. A. (2013). Complementary sensory-based interventions in occupational therapy using a sensory integration approach. *OT Practice, 18*(22), CE-1– CE-8.

Koziol, L. F., Budding, D. E., & Chidekel, D. (2011). Sensory integration, sensory processing, and sensory modulation disorders: Putative functional neuroanatomic underpinnings. *Cerebellum, 10*, 770–792. https://doi.org/10.1007/s12311-011-0288-8 (Note: No OT authors. Supportive background material.)

Lane, S. J., Smith Roley, S., & Champagne, T. (2014). Sensory integration and processing: Theory and application in occupational performance. In B. A. Boyd Schell, G. Gillen, & M. E. Scaffa (Eds.), *Willard & Spackman's occupational therapy* (12th ed., pp. 816–868). Wolters Kluwer.

McGinnis, A. A., Blakely, E. Q., Harvey, A. C., Hodges, A. C., & Rickards, J. B. (2013). The behavioral effects of a procedure used by pediatric occupational therapists. *Behavioral Interventions, 28*(1), 48–57. https://doi.org/10.1002/bin.1355

Moore, K. M., Cividini-Motta, C., Clark, K. M., & Ahearn, W. H. (2015). Sensory integration as a treatment for automatically maintained stereotypy. *Behavioral Interventions, 30*(2), 95–111. https://doi.org/10.1002/bin.1405

Parham, L. D., & Mailloux, Z. (2010). Sensory integration. In J. Case-Smith & J. C. O'Brien (Eds.), *Occupational therapy for children* (6th ed., pp. 324–372). Mosby.

Parham, L. D., & Mailloux, Z. (2015). Sensory integration. In J. Case-Smith & J. C. O'Brien (Eds.), *Occupational therapy for children* (7th ed., pp. 258–303). Elsevier.

Pfeiffer, B., May-Benson, T. A., & Bodison, S. C. (2018). State of the science of sensory integration research with children and youth. *American Journal of Occupational Therapy, 72*(1), Article 7201170010. https://doi.org/10.5014/ajot.2018.721003

Rodger, S., Ashburner, J., & Hinder, E. (2012). Sensory interventions for children: Where does our profession stand? *Australian Occupational Therapy Journal, 59*(5), 337–338. https://doi.org/10.1111/j.1440-1630.2012.01032.x

Schoen, S. A., Miller, L. J., & Nielsen, D. M. (2014). Sensory integrative theory and treatment: Occupational therapy with a sensory integrative approach. In C. Murray-Slutsky & B. Paris (Eds.), *Autism interventions: Exploring the spectrum of autism* (pp. 27–51). Hammill Institute on Disabilities.

Uyanik, M., & Kayihan, H. (2010). Down syndrome: Sensory integration, vestibular stimulation and neurodevelopmental therapy approaches for children. In *International encyclopedia of rehabilitation* (pp. 1–22). Center for International Rehabilitation Research Information Exchange.

van Jaarsveld, A., Mailloux, Z., Roley, S. S., & Raubenheimer, J. (2014). Patterns of sensory integration dysfunction in children from South Africa. *South African Journal of Occupational Therapy, 44*(2), 2–6.

Watling, R., Koenig, K. P., Davies, P. L., & Schaaf, R. C. (2011). *Occupational therapy practice guidelines for children and adolescents with challenges in sensory processing and sensory integration.* AOTA Press.

Sensory Modulation Disorders

See also Ayres Sensory Integration Approach, Sensory Integration Dysfunction, Sensory Processing Disorders, Sensory Over-Responsivity, Sensory-Based Problems in Adults.

Description

Sensory modulation is the ability to regulate and grade responses to the sensory environment so that responses to sensory input are appropriate to the demands of daily life (Schoen et al., 2014). Sensory modulation is a twofold process. Sensory modulation originates in the central nervous system as the neurological ability to regulate and process incoming sensory stimuli; this process subsequently provides the individual with an opportunity to respond behaviorally to the stimulus in the environment (Brown et al., 2019).

Sensory modulation disorder/dysfunction (SMD) is characterized by difficulty in responding to sensory input in a graded and adaptive manner relative to the degree, nature, or intensity of the sensory input. Individuals with SMD routinely respond to benign sensory input with exaggerated avoidant and defensive behaviors that are inappropriate to the environmental demands (Ostrove & Hartman, 2013; Yochman et al., 2013). "Individuals with SMD demonstrate abnormal responses to naturally occurring stimuli in a manner that interferes with daily life activities" (Bar-Shalita et al., 2012, p. 943). Disorders in which sensory modulation has been identified include autism spectrum disorder (Fernández-Andrés et al., 2018; Hilton et al., 2010; Lane & Reynolds, 2014; Murray-Slutsky & Paris, 2014), dementia (Champagne, 2018), eating disorders (Brand-Gothelf et al., 2016), and juvenile Huntington's disease (Brown & Fisher, 2015).

Cause

Exact cause is unknown. Sensory modulation dysfunction is attributed to a disturbance in the neurophysiological process within the central nervous system to regulate and process sensory stimuli. Genetic and environment factors are likely involved (Ostrove & Hartman, 2013; Román-Oyola, 2011).

Subtypes (Lai et al., 2019; Lane et al., 2010)
- *Sensory over-responsivity* (OR): Person reacts more quickly, more intensely, or for longer than typical durations (see Sensory Over-Responsivity in Section 2: Sensory Disorders).
- *Sensory under-responsivity* (UR): Person disregards or fails to respond to environmental sensory input and does not appear to detect incoming sensory information.
- *Sensory seeking* (SS): Person tends to crave unusual amounts or types of sensory input and appears to have an insatiable desire for sensation.

Evaluation/Assessment

Areas
- Activities of Daily Living/Instrumental ADL: eating and digestion, dressing/clothing, brushing teeth, grooming, toileting
- Education/Work: lighting conditions, types of noises or noisy environments, types of seating, study and workspace arrangement, various educational materials available, consistency of daily schedule, number and type of instructional personnel, cafeteria arrangements, auditorium conditions, playground, busing
- Play/Leisure: type, frequency, interests
- Rest/Sleep: sleep environment (darkness, noise, fabrics in sheets, pillows, pajamas)
- Social Participation: type, frequency, location, number of people

- Sensorimotor: responsiveness to sensory stimuli (auditory, gustatory, olfactory, pain, proprioception, tactile, temperature, vestibular, vision)
- Cognitive/Perceptual: awareness, knowledge, memory, executive functions
- Psychosocial: anxiety, depression, anger, aggression, tantrums (meltdowns), self-efficacy, role performance, quality of life
- Context/Environment: social support, environmental factors, family and community resources
- Development (Infant, Child, Adolescent only): developmental delay, abnormal developmental pattern
- Comorbidities: anxiety, autism spectrum disorder, depression, eating disorders, schizophrenia, Tourette's syndrome.
- Differential diagnosis: SMD have more sensory issues, somatic complaints, anxiety and depression and difficulty adapting that attention-deficit/hyperactivity disorder (Miller et al., 2012; Yochman et al., 2013)

Instruments
Instruments Developed by Occupational Therapy Personnel
- Adolescent/Adult Sensory Profile (AASP; Brown & Dunn, 2002)
- Fabric Prickliness Test (FPT; Bar-Shalita et al., 2012, in References)
- Leiter International Performance Scale (3rd ed.; Leiter-3; Roid et al., 2013)
- Participation in Childhood Occupations Questionnaire (PICO-Q; Bar-Shalita et al., 2009)
- Participation in Physical Activity and Sedentary Behavior Questionnaire (PQ; Cermak, 2007)
- Sensory Processing and Self-Regulation Checklist (SPSRC; Lai et al., 2019, in References)
- Sensory Processing Measure (SPM) Home Form (SPM-HF; Parham & Ecker, 2007)
- Sensory Processing Scale Inventory (SPSI; Schoen et al., 2017, in References)
- Sensory Responsiveness Questionnaire (SRQ; Bar-Shalita et al., 2009)
- Short Sensory Profile (SSP; McIntosh et al., 1999)

Instruments Developed by Other Professionals and Used by Occupational Therapy Personnel
- ACTeRS Teacher & Parent Forms (ACTeRS; Ullman et al., 2000)
- ADD-H Comprehensive Teacher's Rating Scale (see ACTeRS Teacher & Parent Forms)
- Beck Anxiety Inventory (BAI; Beck & Steer, 1993)
- Beck Depression Inventory (2nd ed.; BDI-II; Beck et al., 1996)
- Child Behavior Checklist (CBCL; Achenbach, 2001)
- Raven's Progressive Matrices and Vocabulary Scales (RPMVS; Raven et al., 1998)
- Vibratory Sensory Analyzer (VSA; Medoc)
- Visual analogue scales (mood, level of anxiety, ability to concentrate; Ostrove & Hartman, 2013, in References)
- Von Frey filaments (Smith & Nephew Rolyan, Inc.)

Problems/Issues
Activities of Daily Living/Instrumental ADL
- Person may be a picky eater (OR).
- Person may resist or refuse to wear clothing with tags, seams, or certain fabrics (OR).
- Person may express dislike of hair care, nail trimming, face washing (OR).
- Person may dislike water activities, including bathing or showering (OR).
- Person may not notice he or she is drooling (UR).
- Person may be known to be a messy eater and not seem to care (UR).
- Person may crave salty, spicy foods (UR).
- Person may crave extra chewy and crunchy foods (SS).
- Person may tend to stuff too much food in the mouth at one time without noticing (UR).
- Person may not notice when clothing is soiled, on backwards, or twisted (UR).

Education/Work
- Person may "fall" or frequently slip out of a chair (UR).
- Person has difficulty staying still when seated and is constantly fidgeting (SS).

Play/Leisure
- Person may engage in less play and leisure activities than typically developing peers (OR).
- Person may avoid certain play or leisure activities due to sensory sensitivities, such as "mess" play with finger paints or Play-Doh (OR).
- Person plays rough with others but is aware of hurting others (SS).

Rest/Sleep
- Person has difficulty falling and staying asleep.

Social Participation
- Person may participate in fewer social activities than typically developing peers.

Sensorimotor
- Person may have low muscle tone, slump, slouch, or lean in chair or desk (UR).
- Person may toe walk or have an awkward gait (UR).
- Person may be considered clumsy (UR).
- Person may have poor fine motor skills (UR).
- Person may crave movement and roughhousing (SS).
- Person may be viewed as constantly in motion, "crashing" into walls, or falling down on purpose (SS).
- Person tends to run, jump, or skip everywhere rather than walk (SS).
- Person may dislike and avoid light touch or react with aggression (OR).
- Person with atypical response to oral/olfactory and touch is at risk for social impairment (Hilton et al., 2010).
- Person touches everything in the environment (SS).
- Person may be slow to respond to sights and sounds (UR).
- Person may have a high pain tolerance and not seem to notice cuts and bruises (UR).

Cognitive/Perceptual
- Person may be hyperalert to changes (OR).
- Person may appear to be daydreaming or unfocused on what is going on (UR).
- Person has a short attention span (SS).

Psychosocial
- Person may have a low frustration tolerance, be moody, irritable, or fussy (OR).
- Person may have frequent meltdowns that are out of proportion to the situation (OR).

Context/Environment
- Person may be easily overwhelmed by noisy, busy environment such as birthday parties or crowded shopping malls and stores (OR).

Intervention/Treatment

Models and programs developed by occupational therapy personnel include intervention (Kinnealey et al., 2015), sensory group (Ostrove & Hartman, 2013), and staff training (Machingura & Lloyd, 2017). Models and programs developed by other professionals but used by occupational therapy personnel include the Cutchins program on touch (Caldwell & Champagne, 2018), sensory modulation intervention strategies (SMIS; Brown & Fisher, 2015), SMART therapy room (Warner et al., 2013), and Te Pau Project (Sutton & Nicholson, 2011). Team members include parents and caregivers, educators, psychologists, social workers, speech–language pathologists, physical therapy personnel, and occupational therapy personnel. Goals are to enable the person to participate successfully in the home, school, and community environments.

Activities of Daily Living/Instrumental ADL
- Add condiments to food that is culturally appropriate (UR).
- Use chewy or crunchy foods as snacks (jerky, taffy, pretzels; OR).
- Recommend shopping be done during less busy (quieter) times (OR).
- Recommend driving be done during times when there is less traffic (OR).

Education/Work
- Organize education or work environment with needed items only (OR).
- Reduce background noise, such as radio or TV, during study or work time (OR).
- Provide a quiet place or space with soft light for study or work time (e.g., carrel, a tent, a small room, a corner of a classroom; OR).

Play/Leisure
- Playing sensory-motor games with Nintendo Switch (UR).
- Gardening may be a useful leisure activity (UR).
- Encourage engagement in physical activities during play and leisure activities (all).

Rest/Sleep
- Use of weighted blanket positioned from shoulder to hip applied while lying prone in bed (UR).

Social Participation
- Encourage participation social activities (all).

Sensorimotor
- Use of a vibrating massager held by the person on whatever part of body sensory input is desired (UR).
- Proprioceptive activities: wearing a weighted blanket when walking around home, weight lifting, active prone extension activities on a therapy ball, bouncing a therapy ball (OR).
- Deep pressure TheraBand, weighted objects, rolling prone and supine over a therapy ball (OR).
- Smell: scents of lavender, lemon, mint, rose and pine, flowers.
- Sounds: music, rain sticks, small musical instruments, bells, rattles.
- Taste: sweet and sour candies, lemonade, fruit-flavored ice pops.
- Touch: fidget gadgets including those that are soft, gooey, prickly, or that vibrate.
- Vestibular activities: bouncing, rocking and movement that challenges balance, biking, hiking, tossing a beach ball, playing balloon volleyball, or playing badminton (UR).
- Visual: glasses with different colored lenses; look at photographs of people, place, and food; ooze tubes; magic wands; clear rain sticks.
- Aerobic activities that require constant movement: bike riding, brisk walking, hiking, playing tennis (SS).

Cognitive/Perceptual
- Use of sensory modulation groups can improve focused concentration (Ostrove & Hartman, 2013).

Psychosocial
- A fidget gadget may reduce stress reactions (OR).

Context/Environment
- Reduce clutter or unneeded items in living environment (OR).
- Reduce lighting and noise in living environment (OR).

Precautions/Safety Considerations
- None listed.

Prognosis and Outcome

Experiential groups experiences may provide better outcomes than discussion groups (Ostrove & Hartman, 2013).

REFERENCES

Bar-Shalita, T., Vatine, J. J., Parush, S., Deutsch, L., & Seltzer, Z. (2012). Psychophysical correlates in adults with sensory modulation disorder. *Disability and Rehabilitation, 34*(11), 943–950. https://doi.org/10.3109/09638288.2011.629711

Brand-Gothelf, A., Parush, S., Eitan, Y., Admoni, S., Gur, E., & Stein, D. (2016). Sensory modulation disorder symptoms in anorexia nervosa and bulimia nervosa: A pilot study. *International Journal of Eating Disorders, 49*(1), 59–68. https://doi.org/10.1002/eat.22460

Brown, A., & Fisher, C. A. (2015). Optimizing occupational performance through sensory modulation interventions: Case reports of two young adults diagnosed with juvenile Huntington's disease. *British Journal of Occupational Therapy, 78*(12), 767–771. https://doi.org/10.1177/0308022615569249

Brown, A., Tse, T., & Fortune, T. (2019). Defining sensory modulation: A review of the concept and a contemporary definition for application by occupational therapists. *Scandinavian Journal of Occupational Therapy, 26*(7), 515–523. https://doi.org/10.1080/11038128.2018.1509370

Caldwell, B., & Champagne, T. (2018). Touch In Massachusetts Department of Mental Health (Ed.), *Creating positive cultures of care resource guide* (4th ed., pp. 1–25). https://www.mass.gov/doc/section-one-touch/download

Champagne, T. (2018). *Sensory modulation: Applications for working with people with dementia.* Jessica Kingsley.

Fernández-Andrés, M. I., Sanz-Cerverza, P., Salgado-Burgos, C., Tárraga-Mínguez, R., & Pastor-Cerezuela, G. (2018). Comparative study of sensory modulation vulnerabilities in children with and without ASD in family and school contexts. *Journal of Occupational Therapy, Schools, & Early Intervention, 11*(3), 318–328. https://doi.org/10.1080/19411243.2018.1432448

Hilton, C. L., Harper, J. D., Kueker, R. H., Lang, A. R., Abbacchi, A. M., Todorov, A., & LaVesser, P. D. (2010). Sensory responsiveness as a predictor of social severity in children with high functioning autism spectrum disorders. *Journal of Autism and Developmental Disorders, 40*(8), 937–945. https://doi.org/10.1007/s10803-010-0944-8

Kinnealey, M., Riuli, V., & Smith, S. (2015). Case study of an adult with sensory modulation disorder. *Sensory Integration Special Interest Section Quarterly, 38*(1), 1–4.

Lai, C. Y. Y., Yung, T. W. K., Gomez, I. N. B., & Siu, A. M. H. (2019). Psychometric properties of Sensory Processing and Self-Regulation Checklist (SPSR). *Occupational Therapy International, 2019*, Article 8796402. https://doi.org/10.1155/2019/8796042

Lane, S. J., Lynn, J., & Reynolds, S. (2010). Sensory modulation: A neuroscience and behavioral overview. *OT Practice, 15*(21), CE-1–CE-8.

Lane, S. J., & Reynolds, S. (2014). Sensory modulation. In C. Murray-Slutsky & B. Paris (Eds.), *Autism interventions: Exploring the spectrum of autism* (pp. 57–88). Hammill Institute on Disabilities.

Machingura, T., & Lloyd, C. (2017). A reflection on success factors in implementing sensory modulation in an acute mental health setting. *International Journal of Therapy and Rehabilitation, 24*(1), 35–39. https://doi.org/10.12968/ijtr.2017.24.1.35

Miller, L. J., Nielsen, D. M., & Schoen, S. A. (2012). Attention deficit hyperactivity disorder and sensory modulation disorder: A comparison of behavior and physiology. *Research in Developmental Disabilities, 33*(3), 804–818. https://doi.org/10.1016/j.ridd.2011.12.005

Murray-Slutsky, C., & Paris, B. A. (2014). Intervention strategies for sensory modulation disorders. In C. Murray-Slutsky & B. Paris (Eds.), *Autism interventions: Exploring the spectrum of autism* (pp. 89–150). Hammill Institute on Disabilities.

Ostrove, B., & Hartman, R. (2013). Sound minds: Establishing a sensory modulation education group at a mental health hospital. *OT Practice, 18*(18), 14–18.

Román-Oyola, R. (2011). Risk factors associated with sensory modulation disorder: Applications of a vulnerability model. *Sensory Integration Special Interest Section Quarterly, 34*(2), 1–4.

Schoen, S. A., Miller, L. J., & Sullivan, J. C. (2017). The development and psychometric properties of the Sensory Processing Scale Inventory: A report measure of sensory modulation. *Journal of Intellectual & Developmental Disability, 42*(1), 12–21. https://doi.org/10.3109/136 68250.2016.1195490

Schoen, S. A., Miller, L. J., & Sullivan, J. C. (2014). Measurement in sensory modulation: The Sensory Processing Scale Assessment. *American Journal of Occupational Therapy, 68*(5), 522–530. https://doi.org/10.5014/ajot.2014.012377

Sutton, D., & Nicholson, E. (2011). *Sensory modulation in acute mental health wards: A qualitative study of staff and service user perspectives.* Te Pou o Te Whakaaro Nui. https://www.tepou.co.nz/resources/sensory-modulation-in-acute-mental-health-wards-a-qualitative-study-of-staff-and-service-user-perspectives

Warner, E., Koomar, J., Lary, B., & Cook, A. (2013). Can the body change the score? Application of sensory modulation principles in the treatment of traumatized adolescents in residential settings. *Journal of Family Violence, 28*(7), 729–738. https://doi.org/10.1007/s10896-013-9535-8

Yochman, A., Alon-Beery, O., Sribman, A., & Parush, S. (2013). Differential diagnosis of sensory modulation disorder (SMD) and attention deficit hyperactivity disorder (ADHD): Participation, sensation, and attention. *Frontiers in Human Neuroscience, 7*, Article 862. https://doi.org/10.3389/fnhum.2013.00862

BIBLIOGRAPHY

Champagne, T. (2018). The importance of physical environment. In Massachusetts Department of Mental Health (Ed.), *Creating positive cultures of care resource guide* (4th ed., pp. 1–16). https://www.mass.gov/doc/section-two-the-importance-of-physical-environment/download

Champagne, T. (2010). *Sensory modulation & environment: Essential elements of occupations* (3rd ed., Rev). Pearson.

Hertzog, D., Cermak, S., & Bar-Shalita, T. (2019). Sensory modulation, physical activity and participation in daily occupations in young children. *Canadian Journal of Occupational Therapy, 86*(2), 106–113. https://doi.org/10.1177/0008417419831403

James, K., Miller, L. J., Schaaf, R., Nielsen, D. M., & Schoen, S. A. (2011). Phenotypes within sensory modulation dysfunction. *Comprehensive Psychiatry, 52*(6), 715–724. https://doi.org/10.1016/j.comppsych.2010.11.010

Kinnealey, M., Koenig, K. P., & Smith, S. (2011). Relationships between sensory modulation and social supports and health-related quality of life. *American Journal of Occupational Therapy, 65*(3), 320–327. https://doi.org/10.5014/ajot.2011.001370

Stocks, G. (2019). Training school paraprofessionals in sensory dysfunction. *OT Practice, 24*(6), 16–19.

Sensory Over-Responsivity

Also called hypersensitive, hypersensitivity, hypervigilance, hypervigilant, overvigilance, sensory over-responsiveness, SOR, sensory defensive, sensory defensiveness.

See also Sensory Modulation Disorders, Sensory Integrative Dysfunction, Sensory Processing Disorders, Sensory-Based Problems in Adults.

Description

Sensory over-responsivity is characterized by heightened and unusual reactions to everyday sensory stimuli, such as the sound of a blender or the feel of a shirt tag (Carpenter et al., 2019).

Cause

The hypothesis is that the condition reflects atypical neural integration of sensory input (Brett-Green et al., 2010). Sensory over-responsivity has been reported in disorders such as attention-deficit/hyperactivity disorder (Ben-Sasson, Soto, et al., 2017; Lane et al., 2010; Lane & Reynold, 2019; Lane et al., 2012), autism spectrum disorder (Ben-Sasson et al., 2013; Gee et al., 2013; Green Ben-Sasson, 2010; Green et al., 2012; Mazurek et al., 2013; Syu & Lin, 2018; Tavassoli et al., 2018; Tavassoli et al., 2014), and obsessive-compulsive symptoms (Ben-Sasson, Dickstein, et al., 2017; Ben-Sasson & Podoly, 2017).

Evaluation/Assessment

Areas

- Activities of Daily Living/Instrumental ADL: food selectivity, stomachache, clothing selectivity
- Education/Work: academic performance
- Play/Leisure: play skills, interests, types, location
- Rest/Sleep: sleep disturbance
- Social Participation: types, location, frequency, with whom
- Sensorimotor: sensitivities (heightened or unusual reactions) to visual, tactile, auditory, taste, and olfactory stimuli); pain
- Cognitive/Perceptual: visual perception
- Psychosocial: social interactions, tantrum (meltdown) behavior, anxiety, irritability, quality of life
- Context/Environment: parental stress, community resources
- Development (Infant, Child, Adolescent only): no information identified
- Comorbidities: autism spectrum disorder, attention-deficit/hyperactivity disorder, anxiety disorder, obsessive-compulsive disorder, gastrointestinal disorders (constipation, stool withholding, dysfunctional elimination syndrome), retentive fecal incontinence disorders

Instruments

Instruments Developed by Occupational Therapy Personnel

- Adolescent/Adult Sensory Profile (AASP; Brown & Dunn, 2002)
- Infant/Toddler Sensory Profile (ITSP; Dunn, 2002)
- Sensory Experiences Questionnaire 3.0 (SEQ-3; Baranek et al., 2006)
- Sensory Over-Responsivity (SensOR) Scales (Schoen et al., 2008)
- Sensory Processing Measure (SPM) Home Form (SPM-HF; Parham & Ecker, 2007)
- Sensory Processing Measure (SPM) Main Classroom and School Environments Forms (Miller Kuhaneck et al., 2010)
- Sensory Processing Scale (SP Scale; see Sensory Processing 3-Dimensions Scale [SP-3D])
- Sensory Processing 3-Dimensions Scale (SP-3D; Mulligan et al., 2019)
- Short Sensory Profile (SSP; McIntosh et al., 1999)
- SOR Scale (Suarez et al., 2012, in References)
- Toileting Habit Profile Questionnaire (THPQ; see Beaudry-Bellefeuille & Lane, 2017; and Beaudry-Bellefeuille et al., 2016, in References)

Instruments Developed by Other Professionals and Used by Occupational Therapy Personnel

- Autism Diagnostic Interview–Revised (ADI-R; Rutter et al., 2003)
- Autism Diagnostic Observation Schedule (2nd ed.; ADOS-2; Lord et al., 2012)
- Autism Spectrum Quotient (AQ; Allison et al., 2012)
- Beck Anxiety Inventory (BAI; Beck & Steer, 1993)
- Center for Epidemiologic Studies Depression Scale (CES-D; Radloff, 1977)
- Child Behavior Checklist (CBCL; Achenbach, 2001)
- Empathy Quotient–Child (EQ-C; Auyeung et al., 2009)
- Family Life Impairment Scale (FLIS; Mian et al., 2018)

- Infant-Toddler Social Emotional Assessment (ITSEA; Briggs-Gowan & Carter, 1998)
- Mullen Scales of Early Learning (MSEL; Mullen, 1995)
- Obsessive-Compulsive Inventory (OCI; Foa et al., 1998)
- Parenting Stress Index (4th ed.; PSI-4; Abidin, 2012)
- Preschool Age Psychiatric Assessment (PAPA; Egger et al., 2006)
- Raven's Progressive Matrices and Vocabulary Scales (RPMVS; Raven et al., 1998)
- Revised Childhood Manifest Anxiety Scale (2nd ed.; RCMAS-2; Reynolds & Richmond, 2008)
- Social Communication Questionnaire (SCQ; Rutter et al., 2003)
- Systematizing Quotient–Child (SQ-C; Auyeung et al., 2009)
- UCLA Loneliness Scale (Russell et al., 1978)
- Visual Analogue Scale for Anxiety (VAS-A; Hornblow & Kidson, 1976)

Problems/Issues

Activities of Daily Living/Instrumental ADL

- Child may eat only certain foods based on texture or taste (Suarez et al., 2012).
- Child may only wear certain clothing, such as soft cotton with no tags at the neck.
- Child may refuse to wear "dress up" clothes because they are "scratchy" and "too tight."
- Child may avoid having hair combed or brushed.
- Child may have oral sensitivity to brushing teeth or teeth cleaning (Stein et al., 2013).
- Child may have gastrointestinal problems.
- Child may have language and communication skills below age or norm level.

Education/Work

- Child may present behavior problems in classroom due to oversensitivity.

Play/Leisure

- Child may avoid any play activity that is viewed as "messy" or potentially overstimulating (in view of child).

Rest/Sleep

- Child may have difficulty falling asleep and staying asleep.

Social Participation

- Child may feel discomfort with touching others or being touched by others, affecting interpersonal behavior.
- Child may avoid social events and activities because there are "too many people."

Sensorimotor

- Auditory overresponsiveness (dislikes, avoids, afraid of)
  - ▶ Sudden loud noises.
  - ▶ Electric lights, especially fluorescent lights that emit a sound.
  - ▶ Running water, water falls.
  - ▶ Heater or air conditioning unit starting up.
- Gustatory overresponsiveness (dislikes, avoids, afraid of)
  - ▶ Sticky foods.
  - ▶ Slimy foods.
  - ▶ Greasy foods.
  - ▶ Combination foods.
  - ▶ Having teeth cleaned.
- Olfactory (dislikes, avoids, afraid of)
  - ▶ Strong odors.
  - ▶ Scented candles.
  - ▶ Air fresheners.
- Proprioception (dislikes, avoids, afraid of)

- ► Sudden changes in movement.
- ► Sudden starts and stops.
- Tactile (dislikes, avoids, afraid of)
  - ► Avoids clothes that feel itchy or scratchy.
  - ► Dislikes clothes with tags at neckline.
  - ► May prefer to wear long sleeves.
  - ► Dislikes clothing that hits the back of the legs.
  - ► Dislikes socks with seams.
  - ► Dislikes showers, prefers baths.
  - ► Dislikes skin care, makeup, or hair-care products (lotions, lip balms, lipstick).
  - ► Dislikes wind on bare skin, such as open windows in the car.
  - ► May have high sensitivity to being touched on the neck, back, or face.
  - ► Dislikes touching such as shaking hands, social hugging, holding hands.
  - ► Dislikes certain fabrics on chairs or furniture.
  - ► Dislikes walking barefoot on rugs, grass, or sand.
  - ► May be aversive to touching food during food preparation and cooking.
- Vestibular (dislikes, avoids, afraid of)
  - ► Riding in a car may cause vomiting.
  - ► Avoids walking down a steep flight of steps.
  - ► Demonstrates poor balance (cannot walk on a curb without stepping off).
  - ► Dislikes entertainment parks with rides.
  - ► Dislikes playgrounds with jungle gyms, merry-go-rounds, seesaws, slides.
  - ► Dislikes bounce houses.
- Vision (dislikes, avoids, afraid of)
  - ► Sensitive to visual stimuli that are very bright or have high contrast.
  - ► Avoids looking at moving objects.

Cognitive/Perceptual

- Child may demonstrate hyperarousal, especially toward perceived threatening stimuli.
- Child may be a "neat freak," orderly, organizing.
- Child may prefer set routines and schedules avoiding any deviation.

Psychosocial

- Child may be hypervigilant.
- Child may express general anxiety, tension, and worry.
- Child may expressive feelings of insecurity.
- Child may be fearful or apprehensive, especially of new or different activities.
- Child may express negativity (negative moods) and refuse to participate or do certain activities.
- Child may have limited coping skills and stress reducing strategies.
- Child may refuse to comply with parental demands.
- Child may have "triggers" that set off negative behavior, including crying, screaming, or aggressive behaviors (biting, kicking).

Context/Environment

- Child may have limited family and social support.
- Child may feel discomfort in crowded places such as elevators, buses, subways, restaurants, parties, shopping malls, stores with narrow aisles.

Intervention/Treatment

Models and programs developed by occupational therapists include the Wilbarger Therapressure Protocol (Bhopti & Brown, 2013; Lancaster et al., 2016; Weeks et al., 2012; Wilbarger & Wilbarger, 2014). Models and programs developed by others but used by occupational therapists include the Listening Program. Team members include physicians (psychiatrists), psychologists, social workers, educators, and occupational therapy personnel. Goal is to identify "triggers" and develop compensatory strategies to cope with everyday events and situations.

Education/Work

- Adaptive seating: sitting on therapy ball, use of an air cushion.
- Person may need accommodation during examinations and tests (Lewis & Nolan, 2013).

Play/Leisure

- Plan play activities including type of play items and equipment.

Rest/Sleep

- Maintain consistent bedtime schedule.
- Use cotton bedding.
- Weighted blanket.

Social Participation

- Plan social activities such as playdates in advance.

Sensorimotor

- Auditory
  - Headphones or ear plugs to reduce noise.
  - Use of calming music.
- Gustatory
  - Serve food in a tray with compartments to separate foods or use separate bowls/cups for each food.
  - Avoid mixed fruits or vegetables.
  - Serve dressings or topping separately.
- Olfactory
  - Use calming scents, such as lavender.
- Proprioception
  - Activities such as chair push-ups, bunny hops up several stairs, wheelbarrow walking, jumping jacks.
- Tactile
  - Wear cotton clothing.
  - Remove or buy clothing and socks without seams.
- Vestibular
  - Activities such as rocking, rolling, swinging, sliding that are slow with consistent motion and movement.
- Vision
  - Sunglasses.
  - Tinted glasses (color selected by client).
  - Soft lights.
  - Less overhead lighting; more direct or spot lighting.
  - Reduce computer screen time, especially close to bedtime.

Cognitive/Perceptual

- Self-management: Help client to increase knowledge about overresponsivity and develop management techniques that are most successful for the individual.
- Sensory diet: Help client to identify types of sensory input and control exposure to both positive/pleasant input as well as negative/unpleasant input.
- Time scheduling: Planning and organizing a daily schedule.

Psychosocial

- Instruct in stress-reducing techniques: deep breathing, yoga, mindfulness, meditation, use of calming places and spaces.

Context/Environment
- Create calming and stress-reducing environments: "safe space" such as blanket or pillow tent, small room, protected corner using a wall divider.
- Instruct family, caregivers, educators, and community members about sensory overresponsivity and its management in daily life.
- Provide access to resources for clothing, bedding, and furniture that reduce stress reactions.

Precautions/Safety Considerations
Monitor client for signs of overload and potential meltdown.

Prognosis and Outcome
Variable. Sensory sensitivity is usually a chronic condition but compensatory and learned strategies can increase coping skills and decrease stress reactions.

REFERENCES

Beaudry-Bellefeuille, I., & Lane, S. J. (2017). Examining sensory overresponsivness in preschool children with retentive fecal incontinence. *American Journal of Occupational Therapy, 71*(5), Article 7105220020. https://dol.org/10.5014/ajot.2017.022707

Beaudry-Bellefeuille, I., Lane, S. J., & Ramos-Polo, E. (2016). The Toileting Habit Profile Questionnaire: Screening for sensory based toileting difficulties in young children with constipation and retentive fecal incontinence. *Journal of Occupational Therapy, Schools & Early Intervention, 9*(2), 163–175. https://doi.org/10.1080/19411243.2016.1141081

Ben-Sasson, A., Dickstein, N., Lazarovich, L., & Ayalon, N. (2017). Not just right experiences: Association with obsessive compulsive symptoms and sensory over-responsivity. *Occupational Therapy in Mental Health, 33*(3), 217–234. https://doi.org/10.1080/0164212X.2017.1303418

Ben-Sasson, A., & Podoly, T. Y. (2017). Sensory over responsivity and obsessive compulsive symptoms: A cluster analysis. *Comprehensive Psychiatry, 73*, 151–159. https://doi.org/10.1016/j.comppsych.2016.10.013

Ben-Sasson, A., Soto, T. W., Heberle, A. E., Carter, A. S., & Briggs-Gowan, M. J. (2017). Early and concurrent features of ADHD and sensory over-responsivity symptom clusters. *Journal of Attention Disorders, 21*(10), 835–845. https://doi.org/10.1177/1087054714543495

Ben-Sasson, A., Soto, T. W., Martinez-Pedraza, F., & Carter, A. S. (2013). Early sensory over-responsivity in toddlers with autism spectrum disorders as a predictor of family impairment and parenting stress. *Journal of Child Psychology and Psychiatry, 54*(8), 846–853. https://doi.org/10.1111/jcpp.12035

Bhopti, A., & Brown, T. (2013). Examining the Wilbargers' deep pressure and proprioceptive technique for treating children with sensory defensiveness using a multiple-single-case study approach. *Journal of Occupational Therapy, Schools, & Early Intervention, 6*(2), 108–130. https://doi.org/10.1080/19411243.2013.810944

Brett-Green, B. A., Miller, L. J., Schoen, S. A., & Nielsen, D. M. (2010). An exploratory event-related potential study of multisensory integration in sensory over-responsive children. *Brain Research, 1321*, 67–77. https://doi.org/10.1016/j.brainres.2010.01.043

Carpenter, K. L. H., Baranek, G. T., Copeland, W. E., Compton, S., Zucker, N. Dawson, G., & Egger, H. L. (2019). Sensory over-responsivity: An early risk factor for anxiety and behavioral challenges in young children. *Journal of Abnormal Child Psychology, 47*, 1075–1088. https://doi.org/10.1007/s10802-018-0502-y

Gee, B. M., Thompson, K., & St. John, H. (2013). Efficacy of a sound-based intervention with a child with an autism spectrum disorder and auditory sensory over-responsivity. *Occupational Therapy International, 21*(1), 12–20. https://doi.org/10.1002/oti.1359

Green, S. A., & Ben-Sasson, A. (2010). Anxiety disorders and sensory over-responsivity in children with autism spectrum disorders: Is there a causal relationship? *Journal of Autism and Developmental Disorders, 40*(12), 1495–1504. https://doi.org/10.1007/s10803-010-1007-x

Green, S. A., Ben-Sasson, A., Soto, T. W., & Carter, A. S. (2012). Anxiety and sensory over-responsivity in toddlers with autism spectrum disorders: Bidirectional effects across time. *Journal of Autism and Developmental Disorders, 42*(6), 1112–1119. https://doi.org/10.1007/s10803-011-1361-3

Lancaster, S., Zachry, A., Duck, A., Harris, A., Page, E., & Sanders, J. (2016). Delivery of the Wilbarger Protocol: A survey of pediatric occupational therapy practitioners. *Journal of Occupational Therapy, Schools & Early Intervention, 9*(3), 281–289. https://doi.org/10.1080/19411243.2016.1169243

Lane, S. J., Reynolds, S., & Thacker, L. (2010). Sensory over-responsivity and ADHD: Differentiating using electrodermal responses, cortisol, and anxiety. *Frontiers in Integrative Neuroscience, 4*, Article 8. https://doi.org/10.3389/fnint.2010.00008

Lane, S. J., & Reynolds, S. (2019). Sensory over-responsivity as an added dimension in ADHD. *Frontiers in Integrative Neuroscience, 13*, Article 40. https://doi.org/10.3389/fnint.2019.00040

Lane, S. J., Reynolds, S., & Dumenci, L. (2012). Sensory overresponsivity and anxiety in typically developing children and children with autism and attention deficit hyperactivity disorder: Cause or coexistence? *American Journal of Occupational Therapy, 66*(5), 595–603. https://doi.org/10.5014/ajot.2012.004523

Lewis, K., & Nolan, C. (2013). Practice Brief: Examination accommodations for students with sensory defensiveness. *Journal of Postsecondary Education and Disability, 26*(2), 163–181.

Mazurek, M. O., Vasa, R. A., Kalb, L. G., Kanne, S. M., Rosenberg, D., Keefer, A., Murray, D. S., Freedman, B., & Lowery, L. A. (2013). Anxiety, sensory over-responsivity, and gastrointestinal problems in children with autism spectrum disorders. *Journal of Abnormal Child Psychology, 41*(1), 165–176. https://doi.org/10.1007/s10802-012-9668-x

Stein, L. I., Polido, J. C., & Cermak, S. A. (2013). Oral care and sensory over-responsivity in children with autism spectrum disorders. *Pediatric Dentistry, 35*(3), 230–235.

Suarez, M. A., Nelson, N. W., & Curtis, A. B. (2012). Associations of physiological factors, age, and sensory over-responsivity with food selectivity in children with autism spectrum disorders. *Open Journal of Occupational Therapy, 1*(1), Article 2. https://doi.org/10.15453/2168-6408.1004

Syu, Y.-C., & Lin, L.-Y. (2018). Sensory overresponsivity, loneliness, and anxiety in Taiwanese adults with autism spectrum disorder. *Occupational Therapy International, 2018*, Article 9165978. https://doi.org/10.1155/2018/9165978

Tavassoli, T., Miller, L. J., Schoen, S. A., Brout, J. J., Sullivan, J., & Baron-Cohen, S. (2018). Sensory reactivity, empathizing and systemizing in autism spectrum conditions and sensory processing disorder. *Developmental Cognitive Neuroscience, 29*, 72–77. https://doi.org/10.1016/j.dcn.2017.05.005

Tavassoli, T., Miller, L. J., Schoen, S. A., Nielsen, D. M., & Baron-Cohen, S. (2014). Sensory over-responsivity in adults with autism spectrum conditions. *Autism, 18*(4), 428–432. https://doi.org/10.1177/1362361313477246

Weeks, S., Boshoff, K., & Stewart, H. (2012). Systematic review of the effectiveness of the Wilbarger protocol with children. *Pediatric Health, Medicine and Therapeutics, 3*, 79–89. https://doi.org/10.2147/PHMT.S37173

Wilbarger, P., & Wilbarger, J. (2014). *Sensory defensiveness: A comprehensive treatment approach.* Avanti Educational Programs.

BIBLIOGRAPHY

Ben-Sasson, A., Carter, A. S., & Briggs-Gowan, M. J. (2010). The development of sensory over-responsivity from infancy to elementary school. *Journal of Abnormal Child Psychology, 38*(8), 1193–1202. https://doi.org/10.1007/s10802-010-9435-9

Carter, A. S., Ben-Sasson, A., & Briggs-Gowan, M. J. (2011). Sensory over-responsivity, psychopathology and family impairment in school-aged children. *Journal of the American Academy of Child and Adolescent Psychiatry, 50*(12), 1210–1219. https://doi.org/10.1016/j.jaac.2011.09.010

Tavassoli, T., Brandes-Aitken, A., Chu, R., Porter, L., Schoen, S., Miller, L. J., Gerdes, M. R., Owen, J., Mukherjee, P., & Marco, E. J. (2019). Sensory over-responsivity: Parent report, direct assessment measures, and neural architecture. *Molecular Autism, 10*, Article 4. https://doi.org/10.1186/s13229-019-0255-7

Thomas, S., Bundy, A. C., Black, D., & Lane, S. J. (2015). Toward early identification of sensory over-responsivity (SOR): A construct for predicting difficulties with sleep and feeding in infants. *OTJR: Occupation, Participation and Health, 35*(3), 178–186. https://doi.org/10.1177/1539449215579855

Sensory Processing Disorders: Child

Also called sensory processing dysfunction, sensory processing difficulties.

See also Ayres Sensory Integration Approach, Sensory Modulation Disorders, Sensory Integrative Dysfunction, Sensory-Based Problems in Adults, Sensory Over-Responsivity.

Description

Sensory processing is the interpreting and organizing of varied stimuli, including those acquired by the auditory, gustatory, olfactory, proprioceptive, tactile, vestibular, and visual senses (*Stedman's*, 2011). Sensory processing is the means by which the brain receives, detects, and integrates incoming sensory information for use in producing adaptive responses to one's environment (O'Toole, 2017). Sensory processing is the ability to make meaning out of sensory input (Dunn, 2019). Sensory processing includes physiological and behavior components. *Sensory processing disorders* (SPD) involve difficulty with detecting, integrating, and responding to sensory stimuli (Dunn, 1997). *Sensory processing challenges* are neurologically based problems stemming from the brain's inability to integrate sensory input received from the sensory systems and turn the input into effective responses (Critz et al., 2015).

Cause

The cause of sensory processing disorders is unknown. SPD is associated with several neurodevelopmental disorders such as attention-deficit/hyperactivity disorder and autism spectrum disorder. SPD is also associated with congenital disorders such as Down syndrome. In addition, SPD has been identified in children born prematurely and persons with developmental and intellectual disability.

Terminology

- *Hyperresponsiveness:* An exaggerated behavioral response to sensory stimuli such as aversion to lights, covering ears to sounds, avoidance of touch (Baranek et al., 2013).
- *Hyporesponsiveness:* Refers to lack of a behavioral response, or insufficient intensity of response to sensory stimuli (e.g., lack of orientation to novel sounds, diminished response to pain; Baranek et al., 2013).
- *Sensory avoider/avoiders:* Child responds to ordinary sensory input as though it were aversive and actively avoids input when possible (Dunn, 2014, p. 8).
- *Sensory discrimination:* Refers to interpreting and giving meaning to sensory information (Bodison et al., 2019).
- *Sensory regulation:* Linked to sensory strategies to control the level of alertness and arousal (Blanche et al., 2019).

- *Sensory seeker/seekers:* Child's response to stimuli is characterized by a strong drive to obtain increased intensity, frequency, or duration of the sensory input (Dunn, 2014).
- *Sensory threshold:* Point at which the nervous system has enough information to react (Dunn, 2019).

Evaluation/Assessment

Areas

- Activities of Daily Living/Instrumental ADL: basic ADLs—eating (certain types of foods, with other family members present), dressing (putting on socks, shoes, coat), brushing teeth, bathing, brushing hair, washing hair, cutting fingernails and toenails, changing diapers, toileting, verbal communication (expressive, receptive); IADLs—appointments (doctor, dentist, barber), driving in a vehicle, using public transportation
- Education/Work: classroom activities (cutting, pasting, singing, story time), school behavior (cafeteria, library, bus, gym, playground)
- Play/Leisure: play with toys and objects, play with siblings or other children, symbolic or imaginative play, playing by self, play on a playground
- Rest/Sleep: falling asleep, staying asleep
- Social Participation: eating away from home (at a friend's house, at a restaurant), attending a party, going to a cultural or social event (library, movie theater, concert, sports stadium, museum, parade), going to a community center (swimming pool, water park, amusement park, public park, city or state fair)
- Sensorimotor: level of physical activity (hyper or hypo), balance, posture, primitive reflexes, muscle tone bilateral integration, coordination of the two sides of body, thermoregulation, tactile registration, muscle force and control (proprioception), visual acuity, auditory acuity, smell registration (detection), taste registration (detection)
- Cognitive/Perceptual: visual perception (visual figure ground, spatial perception, depth perception), auditory perception (auditory figure ground, localization of sound, recognition of phonemes and other speech sounds), tactile discrimination (light, deep, textures [rough, smooth, soft, hard], vibration, stereognosis), olfactory discrimination (fruity, fragrant, woody/resinous, chemical, minty, sweet, citrus), taste discrimination (salty, sweet, bitter)
- Psychosocial: interactions (family, peers, teachers, adults in community), depression, anxiety, fear, self-image, self-confidence, coping skills (meltdowns, tantrums)
- Context/Environment: social support, school and community resources, cultural beliefs and values about child rearing and discipline, traveling away from home and community
- Development (Infant, Child, Adolescent only): developmental milestones, developmental delay, uneven developmental
- Comorbidities: attention-deficit/hyperactivity disorder, autism spectrum disorder, developmental delay, intellectual disability, prematurity

Instruments

Instruments Developed by Occupational Therapy Personnel

- Indicators of Developmental Risk Signals (INDIPCD-R; Bolaños et al., 2016, in References)
- Miller Function and Participation Scales (M-FUN; Miller, 2006)
- Parent Effort Scale (PES; Pfeiffer, 2017)
- Participation and Sensory Environment Questionnaire (PSEQ; Pfeiffer et al., 2018)
- Participation and Sensory Environment Questionnaire–Teacher Version (PSEQ-TV; Piller et al., 2017, in References)
- Sensory Experiences Questionnaire (SEQ; Baranek, 1999; Baranek et al., 2006)
- Sensory Integration and Praxis Tests (SIPT; Ayres, 1989)
- Sensory Processing 3-Dimensions Scale (SP-3D; see Mulligan, Schoen, Miller, Valdez, & Magalhaes, 2019; and Mulligan, Schoen, Miller, Valdez, Wiggins, et al., 2019, in References)

- Sensory Processing 3-Dimensions (SP-3D) Parent Inventory (SP-3D-PI; Schoen et al., 2018, in References)
- Sensory Processing Assessment (SPA; Baranek, 1999)
- Sensory Processing Disorder Checklist (SPDC; Sensory Therapies and Research [STAR] Center, 2006)
- Sensory Processing Measure (SPM; Parham et al., 2007; see Parham et al., 2021, in References)
- Sensory Processing Measure (SPM) Home Form (SPM-HF; Parham & Ecker, 2007; see Parham et al., 2021, in References)
- Sensory Processing Measure–Preschool (SPM-P; Miller Kuhaneck et al., 2010; see also Henry & McClary, 2011, and Parham et al., 2021, in References)
- Sensory Processing Measure (SPM) Main Classroom and School Environments Forms (Miller Kuhaneck et al., 2010; see Parham et al., 2021, in References)
- Sensory Processing Measure–Preschool Quick Tips (SPM-P QT; Henry, 2014; see Parham et al., 2021, in References)
- Sensory Processing Scale Inventory (SPSI; Schoen et al., 2014, 2017, in References)
- Sensory Profile (2nd ed.; SP-2; Dunn, 2014; see also van der Linde et al., 2013, in References)
- Sensory Profile School Companion (SPSC; Dunn, 2006)
- Touch Inventory for Elementary-School-Aged Children (TIE; Royeen & Fortune, 1990)

Instruments Developed by Other Professionals and Used by Occupational Therapy Personnel
- Adaptive Behavior Assessment System (3rd ed.; ABAS-3; Harrison & Oakland, 2015)
- Behavior Assessment System for Children (3rd ed.; BASC-3; Reynolds & Kamphaus, 2015)
- Bruininks-Oseretsky Test of Motor Proficiency (2nd ed.; BOT-2; Bruininks & Bruininks, 2005)
- Goal Attainment Scaling (GAS; Kiresuk & Sherman, 1968)
- Mullen Scales of Early Learning (MSEL; Mullen, 1995)
- Preschool Language Scales (5th ed.; PLS-5; Zimmerman et al., 2012)
- Sensory Balance Test (SBT; Nashner, 1993; see also Hu et al., 2010, in References)
- Weiss Functional Impairment Rating Scale (WFIRS; Weiss, 2000)

Problems/Issues
Activities of Daily Living/Instrumental ADL
- Child may be bothered by clothing: certain types of fabrics, tags, seams, ties, belts, turtleneck, or having to wear a certain category of clothing (shorts, skirts, pants, pajamas; tactile defensive).
- Child may state clothing scratches, rubs, presses, is too tight, is uncomfortable (tactile defensive).
- Child dislikes and avoids wearing new or starched clothing that has not been washed with a fabric softener (tactile defensive).
- Child dislikes the feeling of splashing water or shower spray during bathing (tactile defensive).
- Child prefers foods with very strong tastes, spicy flavors, crunchy (such as popcorn, carrots, chips, nuts, pretzels, hard candy; oral hyporesponsive).
- Child has difficulty eating foods with certain textures (lumpy, chewy, crunchy) or mixed textures (oral hyperresponsive).

Education/Work
- Child may have difficulty sitting still in a chair, at a desk, or staying in one place on the floor (vestibular hyporesponsive).
- Child may avoid using classroom materials that involve "getting dirty" (finger paints, modeling clay, playing in a sandbox; tactile defensiveness).
- Child may be covered from head to toe with finger paint, water colors, modeling clay, glue and glitter, sand (tactile hyporesponsive).

Play/Leisure

- Child may avoid playing with certain materials (clay, paint, sand, glitter and glue; tactile defensiveness).
- Child may play "rough" with toys and not seeming to be able to monitor the amount of pressure applied to avoid breaking or damaging the toy (proprioception).
- Child may play "rough" with other children not to be able to differentiate degrees of punches and tackles (proprioception).

Rest/Sleep

- Child has difficulty going to sleep.
- Child has difficulty staying awake during the day.
- Child has difficulty staying asleep or frequently wakes up in the middle of the night.
- Child has difficulty sleeping unless room is completely dark.
- Child is sensitive to bedding materials (tactile defensiveness).

Social Participation

- Child avoids social situations when possible (easily overstimulated).
- Child may not be invited to certain social events or outings because he or she is viewed as clumsy, uncoordinated, or an accident waiting to happen.

Sensorimotor

- Child may have difficulty with gross motor coordination.
  - ► Child may have difficulty learning to ride a bike, scooter, skateboard.
  - ► Child may have difficulty learning to skip, jump, hop, stand on one foot.
  - ► Child may confuse right and left sides of body.
  - ► Child may avoid sports or physical activities.
  - ► Child may have difficulty walking on uneven surfaces.
  - ► Child may bump into people and things.
- Child may have difficulty with fine motor coordination.
  - ► Child may have difficulty with buttoning, zipping, typing, knitting, sewing, closing Ziploc bags, playing games with small parts, keyboarding.
- Child may be high energy and highly active (hyperactivity).
  - ► Child appears to be in motion all the time.
- Child may be low energy and minimally active (hypoactivity).
  - ► Child appears to be contented to stay in one place for long periods of time.
- Child may be easily overstimulated (low threshold of response to stimuli).
  - ► Child is overstimulated and overaroused when people come to the house or child is in a crowded place (mall, restaurant, playground).
  - ► Child becomes overly excited and aroused in group settings.
- Child may be resistant to stimuli (high threshold of response to stimuli).
  - ► Child prefers to avoid crowds and may hide or disappear when people come to the home.
- Child may be hypersensitive to touch (tactile defensiveness, tactile overresponsiveness).
  - ► Child may be bothered by "light touch" such as someone lightly touching, rubbing, or brushing against any part of the body but especially the hand, face, leg, or back.
  - ► Child may be excessively ticklish.
  - ► Child may dislike getting sand on the feet, having sand placed on the body, "digging" in the sand with hands, or getting sand blown on the body.
  - ► Child does not like to go barefoot, but frequently removes socks and shoes.
  - ► Child does not like to be hugged or snuggled.
- Child may be hyposensitive to touch (underresponsiveness/registration).
  - ► Child tries to touch "everything" in sight and reach.

- Child may be hypersensitive to sounds (auditory defensiveness, auditory overresponsiveness).
  - Child often covers ears when "loud" or sudden sounds are present (police or fire siren, vehicle horns, garbage truck, loud speakers, dogs barking, vacuum cleaners, blenders).
  - Child notices sounds that others do not seem to notice or habituate to (clocks, refrigerators, fans, outdoor construction, dishwasher, food disposal, heating system or air conditioner coming on).
  - Child turns down the volume on the speakers (TV, radio, music player).
  - Child dislikes going to places with loud sounds (music concert, indoor sports arena, movie theater).
- Child may be hyposensitive to sounds (under-responsiveness, under-registration).
  - Child seeks loud sounds (turns up the volume all the way on the TV, radio, music player, cell phone; sits as close as possible to the stage at a concert, sits up front at the movie theater or close to the speaker).
- Child may be hypersensitive to oral input (oral defensiveness, oral overresponsiveness).
  - Child resists putting anything in the mouth.
- Child may be hyposensitive to oral input (under-responsiveness/registration).
  - Child constantly chews on the ends of pens or pencils.
- Child may be hypersensitive to smell (olfactory defensiveness, overresponsiveness).
  - Child dislikes, becomes nauseated, or gasps from smells emitted by cooking certain foods, cleaning products, perfume, chlorine, or body odors.
- Child may be hyposensitive to smell (olfactory under-responsiveness).
  - Child enjoys air fresheners, scented candles, strong perfumes, chlorine, foods with strong odors, cleaning products.
- Child may be hypersensitive to moving the body (muscles, joints, tendons) against resistance (proprioceptive overresponsiveness).
  - Child dislikes "rough and tumble" games, wrestling, tug of war, boxing.
- Child may be hyposensitive to moving the body (muscles, joints, tendons) against resistance (proprioceptive under-responsiveness).
  - Child cannot get enough roughhousing, wrestling, pushing, and shoving.
- Child may be hypersensitive to movement of the body in space (vestibular overresponsiveness).
  - Child may frequently become car sick, air sick, motion sick.
  - Child may avoid or have difficulty riding in elevators, on escalators, or standing on a moving sidewalk.
  - Child may avoid playground equipment, carnival rides, or amusement park rides that involve spinning or going upside down.
- Child may be hyposensitive to movement of the body in space (vestibular under-responsiveness).
  - Child may seek fast and sometimes dangerous motion (amusement rides, carnival rides, car racing, action sports).
  - Child often rocks or sways body back and forth while seated or standing still.
  - Child may tip chair back on two hind legs.
  - Child may fidget or "fiddle" with anything available within reach (change in the pocket, keys, pen, pencil, paper clip, rubber band).
  - Child is restless when sitting through a presentation, movie, religious service.
- Child may be hypersensitive to visual stimuli (overresponsiveness).
  - Child prefers spaces and places with dim lights and lighting, shades and blinds closed.
  - Child wants to wear sunglasses outside or avoids going out when sun is brightest, or only plays in shaded areas.
- Child may be hyposensitive to visual stimuli (under-responsiveness).
  - Child prefers bright lights, shades and blinds open, all the lights on.
  - Child avoids wearing sunglasses, and enjoys playing in the sunlight areas.

- Child may be hypersensitive to pain (overresponsiveness).
  - ► Child is very sensitive to any pain (shots, bruises, bumps, scraps, cuts) as compared with others.
- Child may be hyposensitive to pain (under-responsiveness).
  - ► Child does not seem to notice pain (shorts, bruises, bumps, scraps, cuts).
  - ► Child rarely reports feeling anything that hurts, including bites or stings.
- Child may be hypersensitive to changes in ambient temperature.
  - ► Child is sensitive to changes in temperature and wants clothing adapted or removed quickly, including taking off sweaters, jackets, or coats when warm.
- Child may be hyposensitive to changes in ambient temperature.
  - ► Child seems to be insensitive to changes in temperature, especially cold and may be outside in temperatures most people would report as cold, requiring a sweater, jacket, or coat.

Cognitive/Perceptual

- Child may have poor tactile perception and discrimination.
  - ► Child may be unable to identify objects by touch or feel alone (eyes closed); astereognosis.
- Child may have difficulty with visual perception.
  - ► Child may have difficulty locating items in a cupboard, drawer, closet, or grocery shelf.
- Child may have difficulty with visual spatial relations.
  - ► Child may be fearful of heights.
- Child may have difficulty with auditory perception.
  - ► Child has difficulty concentrating on a task or listening if there is a background noise.
- Child may have difficulty with gustatory perception.
- Child may have difficulty with olfactory perception.

Psychosocial

- Child may experience difficulty with social relations due to difficulty establishing or maintaining boundaries (spatial relations).
- Child may have poor self-esteem and self-confidence.

Context/Environment

- Parents and caregivers may be unaware of the condition and its impact on development and participation in everyday activities.
- Educators and other professionals may lack knowledge and management strategies to deal with children with SPD in school or community settings.
- Communities may lack resources to provide families, educators, or others.

Intervention/Treatment

Models and programs developed by occupational therapy personnel include case example (Parham et al., 2019), deep pressure touch (McGinnis et al., 2013), multiple-single-case study (Bhopti & Brown, 2013), retrospective pre–post treatment (Schoen et al., 2018), sensory diet (Pingale et al., 2019; Sahoo & Senapati, 2014), Sensory Processing Measure–Preschool Quick Tips (Olson et al., 2016), and weighted vest (Buckle et al., 2011). Models and programs developed by other professionals but used by occupational therapy personnel include sound therapy/ listening systems (Carley, 2013; May-Benson et al., 2013; Schoen et al., 2014; Villasenor et al., 2018; Wink et al., 2017). Team members include physicians, nursing personnel, psychologists, social workers, physical therapists, and occupational therapy personnel. Goal is to improve a child's adaptive responses to sensory experiences and increase participation in daily activities (Case-Smith et al., 2015; Engel-Yeger et al., 2011).

Activities of Daily Living/Instrumental ADL

- Dressing: for tactile defensiveness, select cotton clothing (wash new clothes before use), remove labels before wearing or buy items without labels, buy socks and underwear without seams, use clip-on ties.

- Dressing: avoid tight-fitting clothing, tight elastic waistbands, turtleneck sweaters, tying ties too tightly.
- Eating: for oral defensiveness, use oral desensitizing approaches.

Education/Work
- Academic: hyperactive or overly sensitive to light and sound; consider reducing stimuli (visual, auditory), arranging work space in a corner away from door(s) or window(s), using a carrel type desk, using portal room divider.
- Lunch: have child eat before others, have lunch in a classroom rather than noisy cafeteria, have parent or caregiver pack lunch with foods child is able to eat.

Play/Leisure
- Increase engagement in different types of play: symbolic, imaginative, manipulative with different types of objects, interactive with others, cooperative in sharing resources.
- Increase engagement in different leisure occupations that are developmentally appropriate.

Rest/Sleep
- Tactile defensive: bedding (sheets, pillow cases) made of smooth cotton or silk, pajamas made of cotton.
- Auditory defensive
  - ▶ Identify ambient and cycled noises: clocks, alarm clocks, radios on timers, refrigerators, coffeemakers on timers, heaters, furnace, air conditioning, car noises from nightshift workers or patrol cars, neon signs, barking dogs, garbage trucks, birds chirping or singing, noisy neighbors with late-night parties.
  - ▶ Minimize: turn off items, remove items from room, close door to bedroom, close windows, add curtains to absorb noise, change location of sleeping quarters, add a white noise to mask cycled noises.
- Visually defensive
  - ▶ Identify ambient and cycled lights: ambient lights on clocks, radios, television sets, computer screens, internet modems, routers, plug-in night-lights, street lights, store signs, traffic lights, outside lights on timers, vehicle headlights.
  - ▶ Minimize: turn off items, cover items with ambient lights, turn the item to the wall, place the item on the floor, remove item from room, place blackout curtains over windows or cardboard insert, change location of sleeping quarters.

Social Participation
- Use play and leisure activities to promote participation in social events and activities with family members and peers.
- Adjust selected activities to ability and developmental level of child.

Sensorimotor
- Gross motor
  - ▶ Provide play and leisure activities and games that require gross motor skills: running, jumping, hopping, skipping, riding tricycle or bicycle, throwing, catching, target practice, batting.
  - ▶ Adjust activity to ability and developmental level of child.
- Fine motor
  - ▶ Provide play and leisure activities and games that require thumb and index fingers (fingertip or lateral pinch) or tripod grasp (cutting, pasting, stringing beads, painting, molding clay, dressing/undressing dolls, Legos, tinker toys, erector sets, building blocks, pick-up sticks, puzzles.
  - ▶ Adjust activity to ability and developmental level of child.
- Hyperactive
  - ▶ Use play and leisure activities that require thought before action: Simon Says, stating before performance if task will be easy or hard, stating in advance consequences of success or failure.

- Hypoactive: Use play and leisure activities that involve more body action, such as gross motor activities with peers, as opposed to solitary or fine motor skills.
- Auditory overresponsive
  - ▶ Use play or leisure activities in an environment with less noise (background and foreground) or use sounds that are calming, such as waltz melodies, easy-listening music, smooth consistent tempo, low volume, low voice tones.
- Auditory under-responsive
  - ▶ Use play or leisure activities with various sounds (bells, whistles, drums, musical instruments, types of music such as marches, jazz, up tempo, high volume, high/loud voice tones).
- Gustatory overresponsive (orally defensive)
  - ▶ Start with bland, soft foods (pudding, soft-cooked eggs, gelatin, grits, oatmeal, no-crust bread, soda crackers, tomato soup, chicken noodle soup, soft cheese, most baby foods, sticky rice, rice cookies, oatmeal cookies).
  - ▶ Use Wilbarger oral desensitizing program.
  - ▶ Slowly introduce new or different foods the family usually eats.
- Gustatory under-responsive
  - ▶ Use different tastes, textures, foods, and objects.
  - ▶ Use crunchy foods (nuts, crackers, pretzels, hard candy, crunchy cereal).
- Olfactory overresponsive
  - ▶ Use scented oils, starting with mild scents (such as lavender and vanilla) to help establish the ability to differentiate between scents and increase awareness (smoke and gas detection).
- Olfactory under-responsive
  - ▶ Use scented oils and food scents with more robust scents to help establish ability to differentiate between scents and increase safety awareness (smoke, gas).
- Proprioceptive overresponsive
  - ▶ Use play or leisure activities that require movement against resistance or gravity push/pull, weight bearing, weight lifting, isometric exercises starting with low-level resistance applied slowly, using a regular tempo, for short periods of time.
- Proprioceptive under-responsive
  - ▶ Same activities as for overresponsiveness, but start with higher level resistance, applied with faster or more irregular tempo for longer periods of time.
- Tactile overresponsive (tactile defensive)
  - ▶ Use play and leisure activities with smooth or dull surfaces (washed cotton, plush toys, smooth plastic) and slowly move to more variety.
- Tactile under-responsive
  - ▶ Use play and leisure activities with various textures and types of input (rough, smooth, dull, sharp [avoid cutting], stereognosis, vibration, fingertip size, full hand size).
- Vestibular overresponsive
  - ▶ Use activities or modalities that requirement movement of the head in one or more planes (yaw, pitch, and roll) to change level of alertness and increase self-perturbation regulation such as rockers, bolster or platform swings, scooter boards, vestibular boards, trampoline, large therapy balls, balance beam, walking heel to toe (tandem walking, Romberg test), yoga. Small excursions (body displacement from center of gravity) or concentrate on maintaining balance, postural control, and equilibrium tasks with slow (controlled) acceleration and deceleration.
- Vestibular under-responsive
  - ▶ Same activities as for overresponsiveness but start with greater excursions (displacements, perturbations) focusing on destabilizing balance and equilibrium with more rapid acceleration and deceleration.

Cognitive/Perceptual
- Plan activities to ensure success (errorless learning).

- Auditory perception: use various sounds, volume of sound, and location of sounds (near, far, under, over); types of sounds (human, animal, equipment manually operated, wind, or water power, electrical); musical instruments (alone, in a band or symphony); and objects (glass, metal, wood, plastic).
- Oral perception (differentiate characteristics between salty, bitter, sweet, smooth texture, lumpy, crunchy).
- Visual perception (figure-ground, spatial perception, depth perception; see Section 2: Visual Impairment in Children and Adolescents).

Psychosocial
- Assist child to improve self-esteem and self-confidence through successful completion of task performance.
- Assist child to improve self-regulation of response to sensory input.

Context/Environment
- Provide information to family and caregivers about management of sensory processing disorders.
- Provide instruction to educators and other professionals about assessment and management of sensory processing disorders.
- Identify community and internet resources.
- Advocate for better coverage of sensory processing disorders in reimbursement systems (private, state, federal).

Precautions/Safety Considerations

All equipment should be checked regularly for safety. All supplies and equipment should be washed and disinfected regularly for infection control.

Prognosis and Outcome

Variable, in part depending on severity of the dysfunction and ability of the child and family/caregivers to self-regulate and self-monitor.

REFERENCES

Baranek, G. T., Watson, L. R., Boyd, B. A., Poe, M. D., David, F. J., & McGuire, L. (2013). Hyporesponsiveness to social and nonsocial sensory stimuli in children with autism, children with developmental delays, and typically developing children. *Development and Psychopathology*, 25(2), 307–320. https://doi.org/10.1017/S0954579412001071

Bhopti, A., & Brown, T. (2013). Examining the Wilbargers' deep pressure and proprioceptive technique for treating children with sensory defensiveness using a multiple-single case study approach. *Journal of Occupational Therapy, Schools, & Early Intervention*, 6(2), 108–130. https://doi.org/10.1080/19411243.2013.810944

Blanche, E. I., Bodison, S. C., Stein Duker, L. I., & Cermak, S. A. (2019). An examination of sensory-related terminology across disciplines: Part two. *SIS Quarterly Practice Connections*, 4(2), 5–7.

Bodison, S. C., Stein Duker, L. I., Cermak, S. A., & Blanche, E. I. (2019). An examination of sensory-related terminology across disciplines: Part one. *SIS Quarterly Practice Connections*, 4(2), 5–7.

Bolaños, C., Gomez, M. M., Ramos, G., & Rios del Rio, J. (2016). Developmental risk signals as a screening tool for early identification of sensory processing disorders. *Occupational Therapy International*, 23(2), 154–164. https://doi.org/10.1002/oti.1420

Buckle, F., Franzsen, D., & Bester, J. (2011). The effect of the wearing of weighted vests on the sensory behavior of learners diagnosed with attention deficit hyperactivity disorder within a school context. *South African Journal of Occupational Therapy*, 41(3), 36–42.

Carley, K. (2013). Sound therapy: A complementary intervention for individuals with sensory integration and processing disorders. Part 1. *Sensory Integration Special Interest Section Quarterly, 36*(1), 1–4.

Case-Smith, J., Weaver, L. L. & Fristad, M. A. (2015). A systematic review of sensory processing interventions for children with autism spectrum disorders. *Autism, 19*(2), 133–148. https://doi.org/10.1177/1362361313517762

Critz, C., Blake, K., & Nogueira, E. (2015). Sensory processing challenges in children. *Journal for Nurse Practitioners, 11*(7), 710–716. https://doi.org/10.1016/j.nurpra.2015.04.016

Dunn, W. (1997). The impact of sensory processing abilities on the daily lives of young children and their families: A conceptual model. *Infants and Young Children, 9*(4), 23–35. https://doi.org/10.1097/00001163-199704000-00005

Dunn, W. (2014). *Sensory Profile* (2nd ed.). Pearson.

Dunn, W. (2019). Best practices in sensory processing to enhance participations. In G. F. Clark, J. E. Rioux, & B. E. Chandler (Eds.), *Best practices for occupational therapy in schools* (pp. 481–488). AOTA Press.

Engel-Yeger, B., Hardal-Nasser, R., & Gal, E. (2011). Sensory processing dysfunctions as expressed among children with different severities of intellectual developmental disabilities. *Research in Developmental Disabilities, 32*(5), 1770–1775. https://doi.org/10.1016/j.ridd.2011.03.005

Henry, D. A., & McClary, M. (2011). The Sensory processing measure–Preschool (SPMP)—Part two: Test–retest and collective collaborative empowerment, including a father's perspective. *Journal of Occupational Therapy, Schools, & Early Intervention, 4*(1), 53–70. https://doi.org/10.1080/19411243.2011.576891

Hu, S. Y., Hinojosa, J., Chiang, P. Y., & Leu, C. S. (2010). Validity of the Sensory Balance Test to screen children for sensory processing impairments. *Journal of Occupational Therapy, Schools, & Early Intervention, 3*(2), 139–153. https://doi.org/10.1080/19411243.2010.491014

May-Benson, T. A., Carley, K., Szklut, S., & Schoen, S. (2013). Sound therapy: A complementary intervention for individuals with sensory integration and processing disorders, Part II. *Sensory Integration Special Interest Section Quarterly, 36*(2), 1–4.

McGinnis, A. A., Blakely, E. Q., Harvey, A. C., Hodges, A. C., & Rickards, J. B. (2013). The behavioral effects of a procedure used by pediatric occupational therapists. *Behavioral Interventions, 28*(1), 48–57. https://doi.org/10.1002/bin.1355

Mulligan, S., Schoen, S. A., Miller, L. J., Valdez, A., & Magalhaes, D. (2019). The Sensory Processing 3-Dimensions Scale: Initial studies of reliability and item analyses. *Open Journal of Occupational Therapy, 7*(1), Article 4. https://doi.org/10.15453/2168-6408.1505

Mulligan, S., Schoen, S., Miller, L., Valdez, A., Wiggins, A., Hartford, B., & Rixon, A. (2019). Initial studies of validity of the Sensory Processing 3-Dimensions Scale. *Physical & Occupational Therapy in Pediatrics, 39*(1), 94–106. https://doi.org/10.1080/01942638.2018.1434717

O'Toole, M. T. (Ed.). (2017). *Mosby's Dictionary of medicine, nursing & health professions* (10th ed.). Elsevier.

Olson, C. H., Henry, D. A., Kliner, A. P., Kyllo, A., Richter, C. M., Charley, J., Whitcher, M. C., Reinke, K. R., Tysver, C. H., Wagner, L., & Walworth, J. (2016). Effectiveness and usability of the Sensory Processing Measure-Preschool Quick Tips: Data-driven intervention following the use of the SPM-Preschool in an early childhood, multiple-case study. *Journal of Occupational Therapy, Schools & Early Intervention, 9*(2), 142–162. https://doi.org/10.1080/19411243.2016.1152933

Parham, L. D., Clark, G. F., Watling, R., & Schaaf, R. (2019). Occupational therapy interventions for children and youth with challenges in sensory integration and sensory processing: A clinic-based practice case example. *American Journal of Occupational Therapy, 73*(1), Article 730139501. https://doi.org/10.5014/ajot.2019.731002

Parham, L. D., Ecker, C. L., Kuhaneck, H., Henry, D. A., & Glennon, T. J. (2021). *Sensory Processing Measure* (2nd ed.). Western Psychological Services. https://www.wpspublish.com/spm-2

Piller, A., Fletcher, T., Pfeiffer, B., Dunlap, K., & Pickens, N. (2017). Reliability of the Participation and Sensory Environment Questionnaire: Teacher Version. *Journal of Autism and Developmental Disorders, 47*(11), 3541–3549. https://doi.org/10.1007/s10803-017-3273-3

Pingale, V., Fletcher, T., & Candler, C. (2019). The effects of sensory diets on children's classroom behaviors. *Journal of Occupational Therapy, Schools & Early Intervention, 12*(2), 225–238. https://doi.org/10.1080/19411243.2019.1592054

Sahoo, S. K., & Senapati, A. (2014). Effect of sensory diet through outdoor play on functional behavior in children with ADHD. *Indian Journal of Occupational Therapy, 44*(2), 49–54.

Schoen, S. A., Miller, L. J., & Flanagan, J. (2018). A retrospective pre-post treatment study of occupational therapy intervention for children with sensory processing challenges. *Open Journal of Occupational Therapy, 6*(1), Article 4. https://doi.org/10.15453/2168-6408.1367

Schoen, S. A., Miller, L. J., & Sullivan, J. C. (2014). Measurement in sensory modulation: The Sensory Processing Scale Assessment. *American Journal of Occupational Therapy, 68*(5), 522–530. https://doi.org/10.5014/ajot.2014.012377

Schoen, S. A., Miller, L. J., & Sullivan, J. C. (2017). The development and psychometric properties of the Sensory Processing Scale Inventory: A report measure of sensory modulation. *Journal of Intellectual & Developmental Disability, 42*(1), 12–21. https://doi.org/10.3109/136 68250.2016.1195490

Stedman's medical dictionary for the health professions and nursing (7th ed.). (2011). Wolters Kluwer.

van der Linde, J., Franzsen, D., & Barnard Ashton, P. (2013). The sensory profile: Comparative analysis of children with specific language impairment, ADHD and autism. *South African Journal of Occupational Therapy, 43*(3), 34–40.

Villasenor, R. F., Smith, S. L., & Jewell, V. D. (2018). A systematic review of sound-based intervention programs to improve participation in education for children with sensory processing and integration challenges. *Journal of Occupational Therapy, Schools, & Early Intervention, 11*(2), 172–191. https://doi.org/10.1080/19411243.2018.1432444

Wink, S., McKeown, L., & Casey, J. (2017). Parents' perspectives of using a therapeutic listening program with their children with sensory processing difficulties: A qualitative study. *Journal of Occupational Therapy, Schools, & Early Intervention, 10*(2), 147–170. https://doi.org/10.1080 /19411243.2017.1304839

BIBLIOGRAPHY

Anzalone, M. E., & Lane, S. J. (2014). Sensory processing disorders. In S. J. Lane & A. C. Bundy (Eds.), *Kids can be kids: A childhood occupations approach* (pp. 437–459). F.A. Davis.

Bialer, D. S., & Miller, L. J. (2011). *No longer a secret.* Future Horizons.

Borkowska, A. R. (2017). Sensory processing disorders—Diagnostic and therapeutic controversies. *Current Issues in Personality Psychology, 5*(3), 196–205. https://doi.org/10.5114/cipp.20 17.70140

Brown, C., Steffen-Sanchez, P., & Nicholson, R. (2019). Sensory processing. In C. Brown, V. Stoffel, & J. Nuñoz (Eds.), *Occupational therapy in mental health* (2nd ed., pp. 323–341). F.A. Davis.

Brown, N. B., & Dunn, W. (2010). Relationship between context and sensory processing in children with autism. *American Journal of Occupational Therapy, 64*(3), 474–483. https://doi .org/10.5014/ajot.2010.09077

Celik, H. I., Elbasan, B., Gucuyener, K., Kayihan, H., & Huri, M. (2018). Investigation of the relationship between sensory processing and motor development in preterm infants. *American Journal of Occupational Therapy, 72*(1), Article 7201195020. https://doi.org/10.5014/ajot.2018.026260

Chiang, W. C., Tseng, M. H., Fu, C. P., Chuang, I. C., Lu, L., & Shieh, J. Y. (2019). Exploring sensory processing dysfunction, parenting stress, and problem behaviors in children with autism spectrum disorder. *American Journal of Occupational Therapy, 73*(1), Article 7301205130. https://doi.org/10.5014/ajot.2019.027607

Cosbey, J., Johnston, S. S., & Dunn, M. L. (2010). Sensory processing disorders and social participation. *American Journal of Occupational Therapy, 64*(3), 462–473. https://doi.org/10.5014/ajot.2010.09076

Cosbey, J., Johnston, S. S., Dunn, M. L., & Bauman, M. (2012). Playground behaviors of children with and without sensory processing disorders. *OTJR: Occupation, Participation and Health, 32*(2), 39–47. https://doi.org/10.3928/15394492-20110930-01

Davies, P. L., & Tucker, R. (2010). Evidence review to investigate the support for subtypes of children with difficulty processing and integrating sensory information. *American Journal of Occupational Therapy, 64*(3), 391–402. https://doi.org/10.5014/ajot.2010.09070

Davis, A. M., Bruce, A. S., Khasawneh, R., Schulz, T., Fox, C., & Dunn, W. (2013). Sensory processing issues in young children presenting to an outpatient feeding clinic. *Journal of Pediatric Gastroenterology and Nutrition, 56*(2), 156–160. https://doi.org/10.1097/MPG.0b013e3182736e19

Dean, E. E., Little, L. M., Wallisch, A., & Dunn, W. (2019). Sensory processing in everyday life. In B. A. B. Schell & G. Gillen (Eds.), *Willard and Spackman's occupational therapy* (13th ed., pp. 942–964). Wolters Kluwer.

Gal, E., Dyck, M. J., & Passmore, A. (2010). Relationships between stereotyped movements and sensory processing disorders in children with and without developmental or sensory disorders. *American Journal of Occupational Therapy, 64*(3), 453–461. https://doi.org/10.5014/ajot.2010.09075

Ghanavati, E., Zarbakhsh, M., & Haghgoo, H. (2013). Effects of vestibular and tactile stimulation on behavioral disorders due to sensory processing deficiency in 3–13 years old Iranian autistic children (Special issue). *Iranian Rehabilitation Journal, 11*(1), 52–57.

Hilton, C. L. (2011). Sensory processing and motor issues. In J. L. Matson & P. Sturmey (Eds.), *International handbook of autism and pervasive developmental disorders* (pp. 175–193). Springer.

Hilton, C. L., Harper, J. D., Kueker, R. H., Lang, A. R., Abbacchi, A. M., Todorov, A., & LaVesser, P. D. (2010). Sensory responsiveness as a predictor of social severity in children with high functioning autism spectrum disorders. *Journal of Autism and Developmental Disorders, 40*(8), 937–945. https://doi.org/10.1007/s10803-010-0944-8

Hochhauser, M., & Engel-Yeger, B. (2010). Sensory processing abilities and their relation to participation in leisure activities among children with high-functioning autism spectrum disorder (HFASD). *Research in Autism Spectrum Disorders, 4*(4), 746–754. https://doi.org/10.1016/j.rasd.2010.01.015

Joosten, A., & Bundy, A. C. (2010). Sensory processing and stereotypical and repetitive behaviour in children with autism and intellectual disability. *Australian Occupational Therapy Journal, 57*(6), 366–372. https://doi.org/10.1111/j.1440-1630.2009.00835.x

Jorquera-Cabrera, S., Romero-Ayuso, D., Rodriguez-Gil, G., & Triviño-Juárez, J. M. (2017). Assessment of sensory processing characteristics in children between 3 and 11 years old: A systematic review. *Frontiers in Pediatrics, 5,* Article 57. https://doi.org/10.3389/fped.2017.00057

Kirby, A. V., Little, L. M., Schultz, B., & Baranek, G. T. (2015). Observational characterization of sensory interests, repetitions, and seeking behaviors. *American Journal of Occupational Therapy, 69*(3), Article 6903220010. https://doi.org/10.5014/ajot.2015.015081

Koenig, K. P., & Rudney, S. G. (2010). Performance challenges for children and adolescents with difficulty processing and integrating sensory information: A systematic review. *American Journal of Occupational Therapy, 64*(3), 430–442.

Koshy, N. M., Sugi, S., & Rajendran, K. (2018). A study to identify prevalence and effectiveness of sensory integration on toilet skill problems among sensory processing disorder. *Indian Journal of Occupational Therapy, 50*(3), 86–91. https://doi.org/10.4103/0445-7706.244548

Kurtz, L. A. (2014). *Simple low-cost games and activities for sensorimotor learning.* Jessica Kingsley.

Lane, A. E., Young, R. L., Baker, A. E. Z., & Angley, M. T. (2010). Sensory processing subtypes in autism: Association with adaptive behavior. *Journal of Autism and Developmental Disorders, 40,* 112–122. https://doi.org/10.1007/s10803-009-0840-2

Little, L. M., Dean, E., Tomchek, S. D., & Dunn, W. (2017). Classifying sensory profiles of children in the general population. *Child: Care, Health and Development, 43*(1), 81–88. https://doi.org/10.1111/cch.12391

Little, L. M., Dean, E., Tomchek, S., & Dunn, W. (2018). Sensory processing patterns in autism, attention deficit hyperactivity disorder, and typical development. *Physical & Occupational Therapy in Pediatrics, 38*(3), 243–254. https://doi.org/10.1080/01942638.2017.1390809

Little, L. M., & Dunn, W. (2019). Adaptation from a sensory processing perspective. In L. C. Grajo & A. K. Boisselle (Eds.), *Adaptation through occupation: Multidimensional perspectives.* Slack.

Matsushima, K., & Kato, T. (2013). Social interaction and atypical sensory processing in children with autism spectrum disorders. *Hong Kong Journal of Occupational Therapy, 23*(2), 89–96. https://doi.org/10.1016/j.hkjot.2013.11.003

Middletown Centre for Autism. (2018, July). Sensory processing (Vol. 2). *Research Bulletin, 26.* https://www.middletownautism.com/files/uploads/da4f1cca803fd337a926bf55fd152bd8.pdf

Miller, L. J., Schoen, S. A., Mulligan, S., & Sullivan, J. (2017). Identification of sensory processing and integration symptom clusters: A preliminary study. *Occupational Therapy International, 2017,* Article ID 2876080. https://doi.org/10.1155/2017/2876080

Miller, L. J., Schoen, S. A., & Nielsen, D. M. (2012). Sensory processing disorder: Implications for multisensory function. In B. E. Stein (Ed.), *The new handbook of multisensory processing* (pp. 707–724). MIT Press.

Moeeni, Z. S., Arshadi, F. K., & Behrouzmanesh, P. (2015). Study of relationship between behavioral and emotional aspects of working memory and symptoms of sensory processing disorder, behavioral disorders and social skills. *Journal of Applied Environmental and Biological Sciences, 4*(12S), 134–141.

Nadon, G., Feldman, D. E., Dunn, W., & Gisel, E. (2011). Association of sensory processing and eating problems in children with autism spectrum disorders. *Autism Research and Treatment, 2011,* Article 541926. https://doi.org/10.1155/2011/541926

Nesayan, A., Gandomani, R. A., Movallali, G., & Dunn, W. (2018). The relationship between sensory processing patterns and behavioral patterns in children. *Journal of Occupational Therapy, Schools, & Early Intervention 11*(2), 124–132. https://doi.org/10.1080/19411243.2018.1432447

O'Donnell, S., Deitz, J., Kartin, D., Nalty, T., & Dawson, G. (2012). Sensory processing, problem behavior, adaptive behavior, and cognition in preschool children with autism spectrum disorders. *American Journal of Occupational Therapy, 66*(5), 586–594. https://doi.org/10.5014/ajot.2012.004168

Pfeiffer, B., Clark, G. F., & Arbesman, M. (2018). Effectiveness of cognitive and occupation-based interventions for children with challenges in sensory processing and integration: A systematic review. *American Journal of Occupational Therapy, 72*(1), Article 7201190020. https://doi.org/10.5014/ajot.2018.028233

Pfeiffer, B., Daly, B. P., Nicholls, E. G., & Gullo, D. F. (2015). Assessing sensory processing problems in children with and without attention deficit hyperactivity disorder. *Physical & Occupational Therapy in Pediatrics, 35,* 1–12. https://doi.org/10.3109/01942638.2014.904471

Pollock, M. R., Metz, A. E., & Barabash, T. (2014). Association between dysfunctional elimination syndrome and sensory processing disorder. *American Journal of Occupational Therapy, 68*(4), 472–477. https://doi.org/10.5014/ajot.2014.011411

Ranford, J., Perez, D. L., & MacLean, J. (2018). Additional occupational therapy considerations for functional neurological disorders: A potential role for sensory processing. *CNS Spectrums, 23*(3), 194–195. https://doi.org/10.1017/S1092852918000950

Reynolds, S., Bendixen, R. M., Lawrence, T., & Lane, S. J. (2011). A pilot study examining activity participation, sensory responsiveness, and competence in children with high functioning autism spectrum disorder. *Journal of Autism and Developmental Disorders, 41*(11), 1496–1506. https://doi.org/10.1007/s10803-010-1173-x

Reynolds, S., Glennon, T. J., Ausderau, K., Bendixen, R. M., Kuhaneck, H. M., Pfeiffer, B., Watling, R., Wilkinson, K., & Bodison, S. C. (2017). Using a multifaceted approach to working with children who have differences in sensory processing and integration. *American Journal of Occupational Therapy, 71*(2), Article 7102360010. https://doi.org/10.5014/ajot.2017.019281

Reynolds S., Miller Kuhaneck, H., & Pfeiffer, B. (2016). Systematic review of the effectiveness of frequency modulation devices in improving academic outcomes in children with auditory processing difficulties. *American Journal of Occupational Therapy, 70*(1), Article 7001220030. https://doi.org/10.5014/ajot.2016.016832

Ribeiro Cavalcanti Buffone, F. R., Eickman, S. H., & de Carvalho, Lima, M. (2016). Sensory processing and cognitive development of preterm and full term infants. *Cadernos de Terapia Ocupacional da UFSCar, 24*(4), 695–701. https://doi.org/10.4322/0104-4931.ctoAO0731

Rybski, D., & Israel, H. (2019). Social skills and sensory processing in preschool children who are homeless or poor housed. *Journal of Occupational Therapy, Schools, & Early Intervention, 12*(2), 170–181. https://doi.org/10.1080/19411243.2018.1523768

Ryckman, J., Hilton, C., Rogers, C., & Pineda, R. (2017). Sensory processing disorder in preterm infants during early childhood and relationships to early neurobehavior. *Early Human Development, 113*, 18–22. https://doi.org/10.1016/j.earlhumdev.2017.07.012

Schaaf, R. C., Benevides, T., Blanche, E. I., Brett-Green, B. A., Burke, J. P., Cohn, E. S., Koomar, J., Lane, S. J., Miller, L. J., May-Benson, T. A., Parham, D., Reynolds, S., & Schoen, S. A. (2010). Parasympathetic functions in children with sensory processing disorder. *Frontiers in Integrative Neuroscience, 4*, Article 4. https://doi.org/10.3389/fnint.2010.00004

Schaaf, R. C., Toth-Cohen, S., Johnson, S. L., Outten, G., & Benevides, T. W. (2011). The everyday routines of families of children with autism: Examining the impact of sensory processing difficulties on the family. *Autism, 15*(3), 373–389. https://doi.org/10.1177/1362361310386505

Schoen, S. A., Miller, L. J., & Sullivan, J. C. (2015). A pilot study of integrated listening systems for children with sensory processing problems. *Journal of Occupational Therapy, Schools, & Early Intervention, 8*(3), 256–276. https://doi.org/10.1080/19411243.2015.1055418

Siaperas, P., Ring, H. A., McAllister, C. J., Henderson, S., Barnett, A., Watson, P., & Holland, A. J. (2012). Atypical movement performance and sensory integration in Asperger's syndrome. *Journal of Autism and Developmental Disorders, 42*(5), 718–725. https://doi.org/10.1007/s108 03-011-1301-2

Spies, R., & van Rensburg, E. (2012). The experiences of parents with tactile defensive children. *South African Journal of Occupational Therapy, 42*(3), 7–11.

Stallings-Sahler, S., Reinoso, G., & Frauwirth, S. (2019). *Neurodevelopmental soft signs: Implications for sensory processing and praxis assessment—Part one* [AOTA Continuing education article no. CEA0919]. AOTA.

Stallings-Sahler, S., Reinoso, G., & Frauwirth, S. (2019). *Neurodevelopmental soft signs: Implications for sensory processing and praxis assessment—Part two* [AOTA continuing education article no. CEA1019]. AOTA.

Stocks, G. (2019). Training school paraprofessionals in sensory dysfunction. *OT Practice, 24*(6), 16–19.

Su, W. C., Lin, C. K., & Chang, S. C. (2015). A study of safety and tolerability of rotatory vestibular input for preschool children. *Neuropsychiatric Disease and Treatment, 11*, 41–49. https://doi.org/10.2147/NDT.S76747

Suzuki, K., Takagai, S., Tsujii, M., Ito, H., Nishimura, T., & Tsuchiya, K. J. (2019). Sensory processing in children with autism spectrum disorder and the mental health of primary caregivers. *Brain & Development, 41*(4), 341–351. https://doi.org/10.1016/j.braindev.2018.11.005

Swami, P. R., & Vaidya, P. M. (2015). Correlation of self-injurious behavior, stereotyped movements and aggressive/destructive behavior with sensory processing disorder in children with autism and mental retardation. *Indian Journal of Occupational Therapy 47*(3), 81–88.

Sweet, M. (2010, Spring/Summer). Helping children with sensory processing disorders: The role of occupational therapy. *Odyssey, 11*(1), 20–22.

Tavassoli, T., Miller, L. J., Schoen, S. A., Brout, J. J., Sullivan, J., & Baron-Cohen, S. (2018). Sensory reactivity, empathizing and systemizing in autism spectrum conditions and sensory processing disorder. *Developmental Cognitive Neuroscience, 29,* 72–77. https://doi.org/10.1016/j.dcn.2017.05.005

Tomchek, S. D., Huebner, R. A., & Dunn, W. (2014). Patterns of sensory processing in children with an autism spectrum disorder. *Research in Autism Spectrum Disorders, 8*(9), 1214–1224. https://doi.org/10.1016/j.rasd.2014.06.006

Tomchek, S. D., Little, L. M., & Dunn, W. (2015). Sensory pattern contributions to developmental performance in children with autism spectrum disorder. *American Journal of Occupational Therapy, 69*(5), Article 6905185040. https://doi.org/10.5014/ajot.2015.018044

Tomchek, S. D., Little, L. M., Myers, J., & Dunn, W. (2018). Sensory subtypes in preschool aged children with autism spectrum disorder. *Journal of Autism and Developmental Disorders, 48*(6), 2139–2147. https://doi.org/10.1007/s10803-018-3468-2

Tseng, M. H., Fu, C. P., Cermak, S. A., Lu, L., & Shieh, J. Y. (2011). Emotional behavioral problems in preschool children with autism: Relationship with sensory processing dysfunction. *Research in Autism Spectrum Disorders, 5*(4), 1441–1450. https://doi.org/10.1016/j.rasd.2011.02.004

van Jaarsveld, A., van Rooyen, F. C., van Biljon, A.-M., van Rensburg, I. J., James, K., Böning, L., & Haefele, L. (2016). Sensory processing, praxis and related social participation of 5-12 year old children with Down syndrome attending educational facilities in Bloemfontein, South Africa. *South African Journal of Occupational Therapy, 46*(3), 15–20. https://dx.doi.org/10.17159/2310-3833/2016/v46n3a4

Walbam, K. M. (2014). The relevance of sensory processing disorder to social work practice: An interdisciplinary approach. *Child and Adolescent Social Work Journal, 31,* 61–70. https://doi.org/10.1007/s10560-013-0308-2

Watling, R., Koenig, K. P., Daies, P. L., & Schaaf, R. C. (2011). *Occupational therapy practice guidelines for children and adolescents with challenges in sensory processing and sensory integration.* AOTA Press.

Watson, L. R., Patten, E., Baranek, G. T., Poe, M., Boyd, B. A., Freuler, A., & Lorenzi, J. (2011). Differential associations between sensory response patterns and language, social, and communication measures in children with autism or other developmental disabilities. *Journal of Speech Language and Hearing Research, 54*(6), 1562–1576. https://doi.org/10.1044/1092-4388(2011/10-0029)

Welters-Davis, M., & Lawson, L. M. (2011). The relationship between sensory processing and parent-child play preferences. *Journal of Occupational Therapy, Schools, & Early Intervention, 4*(2), 108–120. https://doi.org/10.1080/19411243.2011.595300

Wigham, S., Rodgers, J., South, M., McConachie, H., & Freeston, M. (2015). The interplay between sensory processing abnormalities, intolerance of uncertainty, anxiety and restricted and repetitive behaviours in autism spectrum disorder. *Journal of Autism and Developmental Disorders, 45*(4), 943–952. https://doi.org/10.1007/s10803-014-2248-x

Wilbarger, J., Gunnar, M., Schneider, M., & Pollak, S. (2010). Sensory processing in internationally adopted, post-institutionalized children. *Journal of Child Psychology and Psychiatry, 51*(10), 110–114. https://doi.org/10.1111/j.1469-7610.2010.02255.x

Sensory-Based Problems in Adults

See also Ayres Sensory Integration Approach, Sensory Integrative Dysfunction, Sensory Modulation Disorders, Sensory Over-Responsivity, Sensory Processing Disorders: Child.

Description

Terminology includes definitions and descriptions of sensory integration, sensory processing, sensory modulation, including overresponsivity and under-responsivity. The problems may "impact self-concept, emotional regulation, attention, problem solving, behavior control, skill performance and the capacity to develop and maintain interpersonal relationships" (Mori et al., 2017, p. 1). The common denominator is a focus on adolescents and adults in addition to or as opposed to children.

Cause

Specific cause or causes is unknown. Genetics and environment may be factors. Sensory problems in adults have been noted in affective disorders (Engel-Yeger et al., 2016), anxiety (Pfeiffer, 2012), autism spectrum disorder (Syu & Lin, 2018), adolescent trauma (Denison et al., 2018; Warner et al., 2013), depression (Serafini et al., 2017), eating disorders (Brand-Gothelf et al., 2016), intellectual disability (Champagne, 2014), multiple sclerosis (Colbeck, 2018), posttraumatic stress disorder (Champagne, 2011), psychotic symptoms (Annandale et al., 2017), and serious mental disorders (Pfeiffer et al., 2014).

Terminology

- *Sensory-based motor disorders:* Refers to the postural and coordination deficits that are common outcomes of poor sensory discrimination of the sense (e.g., tactile, proprioceptive, vestibular awareness; Champagne & Koomar, 2011, p. 1). Sensory-based motor disorders include dyspraxia and poor postural control.
- *Sensory discrimination:* The ability to take in information from the physical environment and gain spatial, temporal, and perceptual awareness (Champagne & Koomar, 2011, p. 1). Sensory discrimination occurs in all the sensory systems: auditory, gustatory, olfactory, proprioception, tactile, vestibular, and vision.
- *Sensory modulation:* "The capacity to regulate and organize the degree, intensity, and nature of responses to sensory input in a graded and adaptive manner . . . which . . . allows an individual to achieve and maintain an optimal range of performance and to adapt to challenges in daily life" (Champagne & Koomar, 2011, p. 1). Sensory modulation dysfunction includes over-responsivity (sensory defensiveness), under-responsivity, and sensory craving/seeking to certain types of sounds, tastes, smells, positions, touch, movement, and sights.
- *Sensory processing:* Relates to the way one detects, regulates, interprets, and responds to sensory stimuli (Ben-Avi et al., 2012).
- *Sensory sensitivity:* The degree to which one is susceptible to perceiving small changes in stimulus intensity (Harrison et al., 2019).

Evaluation/Assessment

Areas

- Activities of Daily Living/Instrumental ADL: sensory and sensory-motor-based responses in relation to performance of everyday tasks
- Education/Work: sensory and sensory-motor-based responses in relation to the performance of education or work tasks
- Play/Leisure: type, frequency, interests, values
- Rest/Sleep: sleep disturbance, sleep habits
- Social Participation: type, location, frequency
- Sensorimotor: responses (responsivity, discrimination, sensory-motor-based responses) to sounds, tastes, smells, positions of the body, touch, movements of the body and sights/light
- Cognitive/Perceptual: attention, memory, executive functions
- Psychosocial: coping skills, quality of life, social interactions, inappropriate behaviors
- Context/Environment: sensory and sensory-motor-based responses to environments in which the individual exists: home, school, work, yard, neighborhood, community
- Comorbidities: autism spectrum disorder, bipolar disorder, chronic fatigue syndrome, intellectual disabilities, personality disorder, posttraumatic stress disorder, schizophrenia, serious mental illness, substance abuse, trauma (present or past)

Instruments
Instruments Developed by Occupational Therapy Personnel
- Adolescent/Adult Sensory Profile (AASP; Brown & Dunn, 2002)
- Adolescent & Adult SPD Checklist (https://www.sensory-processing-disorder.com/sensory-processing-disorder-checklist.html)
- Adult Sensory Interview (ADULT-SI; Kinnealey et al., 1995)
- Adult Sensory Processing Scale (ASPS; Blanche et al., 2014, in References)
- Adult Sensory Questionnaire (ASQ; Kinnealey & Oliver, 2002 [unpublished]; Pfeiffer & Kinnealey, 2003)
- Allen Cognitive Level Screen (5th ed.; ACLS-5; Allen et al., 2007)
- Dynamic Loewenstein Occupational Therapy Cognitive Assessment (DLOTCA; Katz et al., 2012)
- Sensory Preferences (Checklist; Sensory Integration Task Group, 2017, in References)
- Sensory Responsiveness Questionnaire (SRQ; Bar-Shalita et al., 2009)

Instruments Developed by Other Professionals and Used by Occupational Therapy Personnel
- Beck Anxiety Interview (BAI; Beck & Steer, 1993)
- Global Assessment of Functioning (GAF) scale (Hall, 1995)
- IPAT Anxiety Scale (Krug et al., 1976)
- IPAT Depression Scale (Krug & Laughlin, 1976)
- Mini-Mental State Examination (MMSE; Folstein et al., 1975)
- Minnesota Multiphasic Personality Inventory (2nd ed.; MMPI-2; Butcher et al., 1989)
- Pain Apperception Test (PAT; Petrovich, 1957)
- Positive and Negative Syndrome Scale (PANSS; Kay et al., 1987)
- State Trait Anxiety Inventory (STAI; Spielberger, 2010)

Problems/Issues
Activities of Daily Living/Instrumental ADL
- Person may eat or drink only certain foods or liquids.
- Person may wear only certain types of clothes and avoid others such as ties, turtleneck sweaters, pantyhose.
- Person may avoid medical (being touched, getting shots) and dental (scraping, drilling) procedures.
- Person may have difficulty using household appliances, such as a can opener or vacuum machine.
- Person may have difficulty learning to drive safely, parking between the lines, shifting gears, or entering a freeway.
- Person may be more prone to certain health problems: allergies, migraine headaches, chronic pain, and depression.

Education/Work
- Person may avoid or fail to organize work tasks with aversive sensory characteristics thus reducing work effectiveness and performance.

Play/Leisure
- Person may restrict leisure activities due to sensory modulation reactions, especially over-responsivity.
- Person may avoid certain leisure activities related to aversion to specific sensory input.

Rest/Sleep
- No information identified.

Social Participation
- Person may avoid certain social situations.
- Person may refuse to participate in certain social activities.

- Person may experience high social anxiety when participating in social events.
- Person may have difficulty identifying and understanding the meaning of certain visual and auditory cues in social interactions.
- Person may have difficulty with body awareness in space and understanding the meaning of body boundaries and body image in social situations.

Sensorimotor

- Person may be overresponsive (hypersensitive) to stimuli such as odors, noises, tactile sensitivity to specific fabrics (sensory modulation).
- Person may be under-responsive (hyposensitive) to stimuli in the environment (sensory modulation).
  - ▶ Auditory
    - ○ Sensitive to loud noises and sounds.
    - ○ Irritated by sounds not usually bothersome to others, such as the sound of pencil scratching on paper, lights buzzing, candy wrappers rustling, air conditioner or heater turning on and off.
  - ▶ Proprioceptive
    - ○ Dislikes crowds and jostling in public places.
  - ▶ Tactile
    - ○ Sensitive to textures and tight-fitting clothing.
    - ○ Becomes irritated if touched lightly by others or by unexpected touch.
    - ○ Does not like to touch food during preparation.
  - ▶ Vestibular
    - ○ Has difficulty maintaining balance and dislikes walking on uneven surfaces.
    - ○ Dislikes or becomes disoriented in elevators or on escalators.
    - ○ Becomes nauseated when riding in the car (needs to ride in the front seat or be the driver).
    - ○ Fearful of flying.
- Person may seek and crave sensory input (sensory modulation).
- Person may have poor postural control, using righting and equilibrium adjustments to maintain balance during functional activities (sensory-based motor disorder).
- Person may have dyspraxia: difficulty with planning, sequencing, and executive motor skills (sensory-based motor disorder), manifested in performing new or novel motor activities.
- Person may have poor discrimination ability (lack of awareness) in any single sensory system (auditory/sound, gustatory/taste, olfactory/smell, proprioception/position, tactile/touch, vestibular/movement, or visual/sight discrimination disorder).
- Person may demonstrate poor sensory discrimination of tactile and proprioceptive input (somatosensory organization).
- Person may demonstrate poor ability to access information from the physical environment to gain spatial, temporal, and perceptual awareness (sensory discrimination).
- Person may have problems in coordination of the two sides of the body together (bilateral motor coordination). Person may be viewed by others as clumsy or awkward with motor activities.
- Person may be insensitive to pain sensations that would be considered painful by others.

Cognitive/Perceptual

- Person may be unaware that his or her responses are caused by reactions to stimuli in the environment.
- Person may be very aware of his or her responses to certain stimuli and take extra precautions and behaviors to avoid encountering such stimuli.
- Person may be overly neat and organized, or in contrast have difficulty with organization and planning.
- Person may be overly strict about following the same routine.

Psychosocial

- Person may become aggressive in certain situations.
- Person may express anxiety or anxious behavior.
- Person may be hypervigilant or show avoidance behavior.
- Person may express feelings of fear about certain situations.
- Person may have low self-esteem.
- Person may have poor stress management and coping skills.
- Person may engage in self-injurious behavior.
- Person may have difficulty with emotion regulation resulting in frustration, and anger management issues.

Context/Environment

- Family or friends may avoid certain environments known to upset the person.
- Person may avoid certain types of environments (noisy stadiums, crowded rooms, unfamiliar places, destinations viewed as potentially dangerous).
- Person may have difficulty following navigation directions in the community.

Intervention/Treatment

Models of practice and programs developed by occupational therapy personnel include Dunn's model of sensory processing (Ben-Avi et al., 2012), sensory approaches (Champagne, 2018), sensory discrimination model (Champagne & Koomar, 2011; Champagne et al., 2010), sensory defensiveness (Abernathy, 2010), sensory modulation (Bar-Shalita et al., 2012; Brown & Fisher, 2015; Champagne, 2010; Gardner, 2016; Kinnealey et al., 2015; Ostrove & Hartman, 2013; Warner et al., 2013), sensory room (Loukas, 2011; Novak et al., 2012; Shahgholi et al., 2012; West et al., 2017; Wiglesworth & Farnworth, 2016), sensory strategies (Chinnock & Matson, 2013), and weighted blanket (Champagne et al., 2015; Chen et al., 2012). Models of practice and programs developed by other professionals but used by occupational therapy personnel were not identified in the literature listed in the References below. Team members include physicians (psychiatrists, neurologists), nursing personnel, psychologists, social workers, and occupational therapy personnel. Goals are to increase self-regulation and sensory discrimination to decrease or increase responses to acceptable functional level. Other interventions may include medications (pharmacological agents), electroconvulsive therapy (ECT), group and individual psychotherapy, cognitive behavioral therapy (CBT), case management, and psychosocial skills training.

Activities of Daily Living/Instrumental ADL

- Assist client to develop and maintain a healthy lifestyle, include eating and physical exercise.

Education/Work

- Determine whether modifications in the work environment might reduce sensory distress, such as changes in lighting, wearing colored glasses, wearing noise-canceling headphones, listening to calming music, structuring or organizing the routine.

Play/Leisure

- Explore and try out different leisure activities.

Rest/Sleep

- No information identified.

Social Participation

- Explore different social activities that require different levels of participation. Attention to responses to light, sound, and touch may be helpful.

Sensorimotor

- Auditory
  - ▶ SM (sensory modulation): Listen to calming sounds or music (ocean sounds, slow tempo music, slow chants). Wear noise-canceling headphones.
  - ▶ SD (sensory defensiveness): Use a listening therapy program to increase ability to focus on different sounds and increase auditory awareness.
- Gustatory
  - ▶ SM: Use crunchy foods to decrease oral sensitivity.
  - ▶ SD: Use different textures of food, such as pudding versus popcorn, to aid in discrimination.
- Olfactory
  - ▶ SM: Peppermint increases alertness, lavender calms.
  - ▶ SD: Use different scents to increase discrimination, increase sensitivity to dangerous smells (smoke, sour milk, rotting fruit).
- Proprioceptive
  - ▶ SM: Use isometric exercises to increase joint awareness, play Simon Says game.
  - ▶ SD: Use activities that require moving against resistance (push/pull), weight-bearing activities requiring lifting.
- Tactile
  - ▶ SM: Games or activities that require deep pressure touch.
  - ▶ SD: Games or activities that involve a variety of textures and input (vibration, stereognosis, size).
- Vestibular
  - ▶ SM: Use activities that require movement of the head: rhythmic rocking calms, irregular movement alerts.
  - ▶ SD: Use various movements such as exercises that require changing direction or speed.
- Visual
  - ▶ SM: Decrease light for calming, increase to alert.
  - ▶ SD: Increase contrast to enhance visual figure ground, decrease clutter to permit visual focus on a select number of objects.

Cognitive/Perceptual

- Provide a sensory diet that includes a daily routine and menu plan of individualized supportive sensory strategies that address sensory modulation or sensory discrimination issues.

Psychosocial

- Use therapeutic use of self, group, and individual sensorimotor activities based on assessment of client's needs.
- Develop an individual sensory diet based on the individual's emotional and behavioral reactions to stimuli.
- Provide stress management techniques and coping strategies such as deep breathing, relaxation training, swimming, yoga exercises.
- Assist client to develop insight into the nature of his or her sensory responsivity.
- Assist client to increase self-regulation and emotional regulation through increased knowledge and exploration of individual sensory needs.
- Assist client to become his or her own advocate to make modifications in the living environment and to ask for or make recommendations for modifications in the work or community environment.

Context/Environment

- Recommend changes and modifications of the home or living environment based on individual needs.
- Provide information to family, caregivers, and social support members on sensory processing, sensory discrimination, and sensory-based motor responses as applicable to individual issues.

- Provide environmental modifications such as sensory rooms (rocking chair, quiet space, aromatherapy, weighted blanket, stuffed animals), sensory stations, sensory carts or sensory kits (music, stress balls, items for distraction) to increase or decrease sensory stimulation as needed by the individual.

Precautions/Safety Considerations

Person with reduced sensitivity to pain is at risk for injury and for not taking care of an injury that may have occurred but is not noticed by the individual.

Prognosis and Outcome

Sensory sensitivity and responsivity are lifelong patterns. Self-management and self-regulation can assist in reducing the influence and disruptions of the patterns to the individual's life.

REFERENCES

Abernethy, H. (2010). The assessment and treatment of sensory defensiveness in adult mental health: A literature review. *British Journal of Occupational Therapy, 73*(5), 210–218. https://doi.org/10.4276/030802210X12734991664183

Annandale, T., van Jaarsveld, A., van Heerden, R., & Nel, R. (2017). The incidence of sensory integration problems in distinct sample of individuals with disorders characterised by symptoms of psychosis. *South African Journal of Occupational Therapy, 47*(1), 30–35. http://dx.doi.org/10.17159/2310-3833/2016/v46n3a6

Bar-Shalita, T., Vatine, J. J., Parush, S., Deutsch, L., & Seltzer, Z. (2012). Psychophysical correlates in adults with sensory modulation disorder. *Disability and Rehabilitation, 34*(11), 943–950. https://doi.org/10.3109/09638288.2011.629711

Ben-Avi, N., Almagor, M., & Engel-Yeger, B. (2012). Sensory processing difficulties and interpersonal relationships in adults: An exploratory study. *Psychology, 3*(1), 70–77. https://doi.org/10.4236/psych.2012.31012

Blanche, E. I., Parham, D., Chang, M., & Mallinson, T. (2014). Development of an adult sensory processing scale (ASPS). *American Journal of Occupational Therapy, 68*(5), 531–538. https://doi.org/10.5014/ajot.2014.012484

Brand-Gothelf, A., Parush, S., Eitan, Y., Admoni, S., Gur, E., & Stein, D. (2016). Sensory modulation disorder symptoms in anorexia nervosa and bulimia nervosa: A pilot study. *International Journal of Eating Disorders, 49*(1), 59–68. https://doi.org/10.1002/eat.22460

Brown, A., & Fisher, C. A. (2015). Optimizing occupational performance through sensory modulation interventions: Case reports of two young adults diagnosed with juvenile Huntington's disease. *British Journal of Occupational Therapy, 78*(12), 767–771. https://doi.org/10.1177/0308022615569249

Champagne, T. (2010). *Sensory modulation & environment: Essential elements of occupation* (3rd ed., Rev.). Pearson.

Champagne, T. (2011). The influence of posttraumatic stress disorder, depression, and sensory processing patterns on occupational engagement: A case study. *Work, 38*(1), 67–75. https://doi.org/10.3233/WOR-2011-1105

Champagne, T. (2014). Integrating sensory-based approaches for adults with intellectual and developmental disabilities. In K. Haertel (Ed.), *Adults with intellectual and developmental disabilities* (pp. 235–264). AOTA Press.

Champagne, T. (2018). Sensory approaches. In J. Mikula (Ed.), *Creating positive cultures of care: Resource Guide* (4th ed.). Massachusetts Department of Mental Health. https://www.mass.gov/doc/sensory-approaches/download

Champagne, T., & Koomar, J. (2011). Expanding the focus: Addressing sensory discrimination concerns in mental health. *Mental Health Special Interest Section Quarterly, 34*(1), 1–4.

Champagne, T., Koomar, J., & Olson, L. (2010). Sensory processing evaluation and intervention in mental health. *OT Practice, 15*(5), CE-1–CE-8.

Champagne, T., Mullen, B., Dickson, D., & Krishnamurty, S. (2015). Evaluating the safety & effectiveness of weighted blanket with adults during inpatient mental health hospitalization. *Occupational Therapy in Mental Health, 31*(3), 211–233. https://doi.org/10.1080/0164 212X.2015.1066220

Chen, H.-Y., Yang, H., Cli, H.-J., & Chen, H.-M. (2012). Physiological effects of deep touch pressure on anxiety alleviation: The weighted blanket approach. *Journal of Medical and Biological Engineering, 33*(3), 463–470. https://doi.org/10.5405/jmbe.1043

Chinnock, L., & Matson, R. (2013). Sensory strategies. *OT News, 21*(8), 36–37.

Colbeck, M. (2018). Sensory processing, cognitive fatigue, and quality of life in multiple sclerosis. *Canadian Journal of Occupational Therapy, 85*(2), 169–175. https://doi.org/10.1177/00 08417417727298

Denison, M., Gerney, A., Barbuti Van Leuken, J., & Conklin, J. (2018). The attitudes and knowledge of residential treatment center staff members working with adolescents who have experienced trauma. *Residential Treatment for Children & Youth, 35*(2), 114–138. https://doi.org/10 .1080/0886571X.2018.1458689

Engel-Yeger, B., Muzio, C., Rinosi, G., Solano, P., Geoffroy, P. A., Pompili, M, Amore, M., & Serafini, G. (2016). Extreme sensory processing patterns and their relation with clinical conditions among individuals with major affective disorders. *Psychiatry Research, 236*, 112–118. https://doi.org/10.1016/j.psychres.2015.12.022

Gardner, J. (2016). Sensory modulation treatment on a psychiatric inpatient unit: Results of a pilot program. *Journal of Psychosocial Nursing and Mental Health Services, 54*(4), 44–51. https://doi.org/10.3928/02793695-20160318-06

Harrison, L. A., Kats, A., Williams, M. E., & Aziz-Zadeh, L. (2019). The importance of sensory processing in mental health: A proposed addition to the research domain criteria (RDoC) and suggestions for RDoC 2.0. *Frontiers in Psychology, 10*, Article 103. https://doi.org/10.3389/fpsyg.2019.00103

Kinnealey, M., Riuli, V., & Smith, S. (2015). Case study of an adult with sensory modulation disorder. *Sensory Integration Special Interest Section Quarterly, 38*(1), 1–4.

Loukas, K. M. (2011). Occupational placemaking: Facilitating self-organization through use of a sensory room. *Mental Health Special Interest Section Quarterly, 34*(2), 1–4.

Mori, A. B., Champagne, T., & May Benson, T. A. (2017). *Fact sheet: Occupational therapy using a sensory integration-based approach with adult populations.* American Occupational Therapy Association. https://www.aota.org/~/media/Corporate/Files/AboutOT/Professionals/WhatIsOT/PA/Facts/SI-and-Adults-Fact-Sheet.pdf

Novak, T., Scanlan, J., McCaul, D., MacDonald, N., & Clarke, T. (2012). Pilot study of a sensory room in an acute inpatient psychiatric unit. *Australasian Psychiatry, 20*(5), 401–406. https://doi .org/10.1177/1039856212459585

Ostrove, B., & Hartman, R. (2013). Sound minds: Establishing a sensory modulation education group at a mental health hospital. *OT Practice, 18*(18), 14–18.

Pfeiffer, B. A. (2012). Sensory hypersensitivity and anxiety: The chicken or the egg? *Sensory Integration Special Interest Section Quarterly, 35*(2), 1–4.

Pfeiffer, B., Brusilovskiy, E., Bauer, J., & Salzer, M. S. (2014). Sensory processing, participation, and recovery in adults with serious mental illnesses. *Psychiatric Rehabilitation Journal, 37*(4), 289–296. https://doi.org/10.1037/prj0000099

Sensory Integration Task Group. (2017). *Occupational therapy mental health sensory integration and sensory stimulation guidelines.* South Staffordshire and Shropshire Healthcare.

Serafini, G., Gonda, X., Canepa, G., Pompili, M., Rihmer, Z., Amore, M., & Engel-Yeger, B. (2017). Extreme sensory processing patterns show a complex association with depression, and impul-

sivity, alexithymia and hopelessness. *Journal of Affective Disorders, 210,* 249–257. https://doi
.org/10.1016/j.jad.2016.12.019

Shahgholi, A., Noori, A. K., & Hosseini, S. A. (2012). The effect of sensory room intervention
on perceptual-cognitive performance and the psychiatric status of schizophrenics. *Iranian
Rehabilitation Journal, 10*(16), 5–14.

Syu, Y. C., & Lin, L. Y. (2018). Sensory overresponsivity, loneliness, and anxiety in Taiwanese
adults with autism spectrum disorder. *Occupational Therapy International, 2018,* Article 9165978.
https://doi.org/10.1155/2018/9165978

Warner, E., Koomar, J., Lary, B., & Cook, A. (2013). Can the body change the score? Application
of sensory modulation principles in the treatment of traumatized adolescents in residential
settings. *Journal of Family Violence, 28,* 729–738. https://doi.org/10.1007/s10896-013-9535-8

West, M., Melvin, G., McNamara, F., & Gordon, M. (2017). An evaluation of the use and efficacy
of a sensory room within an adolescent psychiatric inpatient unit. *Australian Occupational
Therapy Journal, 64*(3), 253–263. https://doi.org/10.1111/1440-1630.12358

Wiglesworth, S., & Farnworth, L. (2016). An exploration of the use of a sensory room in a forensic mental health setting: Staff and patient perspectives. *Occupational Therapy International,
23,* 255–264. https://doi.org/10.1002/oti.1428

BIBLIOGRAPHY

Chalmers, A., Harrison, S., Mollison, K., Molloy, N., & Gray, K. (2012). Establishing sensory-
based approaches in mental health inpatient care: A multidisciplinary approach. *Australasian
Psychiatry, 20*(1), 35–39. https://doi.org/10.1177/1039856211430146

Champagne, T., & Frederick, D. (2011). Sensory processing research advances in mental health:
Implications for occupational therapy. *OT Practice, 16*(10), 7–8, 10, 12.

Champagne, T., & Koomar, J. (2012). Evaluating sensory processing in mental health occupational therapy practice. *OT Practice, 17*(5), CE-1–CE-9.

Lashbrook, E., Stone, L., Smillie, K., & Taylor, F. (2016). Allowing better outcomes for service
users. *OT News, 24*(11), 28–30.

May-Benson, T. A. (2011). Understanding the occupational therapy needs of adults with sensory processing disorders. *OT Practice, 16*(10), 13–14, 16–18.

Moore, K. (2016). *Following the evidence: Sensory approaches in mental health.* http://www.sensory
connectionprogram.com/pdf/follow_the_evidence.pdf

Sutton, D., & Nicholson, E. (2011). *Sensory modulation in acute mental health wards: A qualitative
study of staff and service user perspectives.* National Centre of Mental Health Research.

van Jaarsveld, A. (2014). Sensory integration in mental health. In R. Crouch, & V. Alers (Eds.),
Occupational therapy in psychiatry and mental health (5th ed., pp. 295–318). Wiley.

Somatosensory Dysfunction
or Impairment or Disorders

Description

Somatosensory dysfunction refers to the detection, discrimination, and recognition of body
sensations. Somatosensation includes responses to touch, pressure, temperature, pain, and proprioception. Somatosensation includes submodalities of touch sensation, such as light touch,
vibration, firm pressure, and texture discrimination; movement related to the skin and joints,
involving location and movement of body parts; temperature sensation; and pain sensation.

The term *kinesthesia* refers to the ability to detect the movement and position of one's limb in space without vision (Dunn et al., 2013).

Cause

- Autism spectrum disorder (Blanche, Reinoso, et al., 2012; Zetler et al., 2019)
- Burns (Nedelec et al., 2016)
- Cerebral palsy (McLean et al., 2019; McLean et al., 2017; Walmsley et al., 2018)
- Development disability (Blanche, Reinoso, et al., 2012)
- Diabetes (Kim et al., 2016)
- Stroke (Ahn et al., 2016; Bannister et al., 2015; Carey, Abbott, et al., 2016; Carey, Lamp, & Turville, 2016; Carey & Matyas, 2011; Carey et al., 2018; Goodin et al., 2018; Hill et al., 2014; In et al., 2019; Pumpa et al., 2015; Rand, 2018; Sakamoto et al., 2019; Turvill, Cahill, et al., 2019; Turville et al., 2017; Turvill et al., 2018; Turville, Walker, et al., 2019; Yilmazer et al., 2019)

Terminology

- *Haptic perception:* Perception by active touch and intentional exploration of objects and surface (VanderBos, 2015).
- *Interoception (interoceptive) sense:* The ability to detect stimuli originating from within the body that are related to the function of the internal organs or the receptors they activate, such as digestion, excretion, and blood pressure (O'Toole, 2017).
- *Pain sense:* The ability to detect unpleasant sensations caused by noxious stimulation of the sensory nerve endings (O'Toole, 2017; see Pain and Chronic Pain in Section 2: Sensory Disorders).
- *Pressure (deep pressure, deep tactile, mechanical) sense:* Ability to detect when force is applied to the deep layers of the skin, muscles, tendons, or joints. Also called deep sensation (O'Toole, 2017).
- *Proprioception (proprioceptive, posture, postural, position) sense:* The ability to detect and discriminate stimuli originating from within the body related to spatial position and muscular activity or to the sensory receptors that they activate. Proprioceptors are located in muscles, tendons, joints, and the vestibular apparatus that respond to stimuli originating from with the body related to movement and spatial position (O'Toole, 2017).
- *Stereognosis (tactile gnosis):* The ability to perceive and understand (identify and discriminate) the form and nature of objects by the sense of touch alone. Astereognosis (tactile agnosia) is the inability to identify objects or shapes by touch alone (O'Toole, 2017). Apperceptive tactile agnosia is disruption of integration of stimuli, associative tactile agnosia is disruption of meaning.
- *Temperature (thermic) sense:* The ability to detect and register different degrees of temperature of objects or liquids when applied to the skin (cold, cool, warm, hot).
- *Touch (tactile) sense:* The ability to feel objects and to distinguish or discriminate among their various characteristics (sharp, dull, light, soft, moving across the skin; O'Toole, 2017).
- *Vibratory sense:* The ability to perceive vibratory stimuli, such as rapid tapping, when applied to the body. Vibration receptors are found in various locations in the body from the skin surface to membranes covering bones (O'Toole, 2017).

Evaluation/Assessment

Areas

- Activities of Daily Living/Instrumental ADL: eating with utensils, dressing
- Education/Work: no information identified
- Play/Leisure: no information identified
- Rest/Sleep: no information identified
- Social Participation: no information identified

- Sensorimotor: grip strength, hand functions (holding objects), touch awareness, pressure awareness, temperature awareness
- Cognitive/Perceptual: no information identified
- Psychosocial: role performance
- Context/Environment: no information identified
- Comorbidities: autism, burns, cerebral palsy, diabetes, stroke

Instruments

Instruments Developed by Occupational Therapy Personnel

- Activity Card Sort (2nd ed.; ACS-2; Baum & Edwards, 2008)
- Assessment of Self-Regulation (ASR; Mahler, 2015, in References)
- Box and Block Test (BBT; Mathiowetz et al., 1985)
- Canadian Occupational Performance Measure (5th ed.; COPM-5; Law et al., 2014)
- Caregiver Questionnaire for Interoceptive Awareness (CQIA; Mahler, 2015, in References)
- Comprehensive Observations of Proprioception (COP; Blanche, Bodison, et al., 2012, in References)
- Fabric Matching Test (FMT; Carey, 1995)
- Finger Position Sense Test (FPST; Carey et al., 1996)
- Functional Tactile Object Recognition Test (fTORT; Carey et al., 2006; see also Taylor, Girdler, et al., 2018, in References)
- Hand Function Survey (HFS; Blennerhassett et al., 2008)
- Interoceptive Awareness Interview (IAI; Mahler, 2015)
- Kinesthesia Test (KT; Ayres, 1989; part of the Sensory Integration and Praxis Tests [SIPT])
- Manual Form Perception Test (MFPT; Ayres, 1989; part of the Sensory Integration and Praxis Tests [SIPT])
- Sensory Integration and Praxis Tests (SIPT; Ayres, 1989)
- Tactile Discrimination Test (TDT; Carey et al., 1997)
- Tactile Object Recognition Test (see Functional Tactile Object Recognition Test)
- Wrist Position Sense Test (WPST; Carey et al., 1996)

Instruments Developed by Other Professionals and Used by Occupational Therapy Personnel

- Action Research Arm Test (ARAT; Lyle, 1981)
- Aesthesiometer (instrument; available from rehabilitation equipment and supply vendors)
- Boley gauge (instrument; available from rehabilitation equipment and supply vendors)
- Disk-Criminator (instrument; available from rehabilitation equipment and supply vendors)
- Functional Independence Measure (FIM; Uniform Data System for Medical Rehabilitation, 1997)
- Functional Reach Test (FRT; Duncan et al., 1990)
- Jebsen-Taylor Hand Function Test (JTHFT; Jebsen et al., 1969)
- Kinaesthetic Sensitivity Test (KST; Laszlo & Baivstow, 1980)
- Manual Function Test (MFT; Michimata et al., 2008)
- Mini-Mental Status Examination (MMSE; Folstein et al., 1975)
- Modified Ashworth Scale (MAS; Bohannon & Smith, 1987)
- Motor Activity Log-28 (MAL-28; Uswatte et al., 2006)
- National Institutes of Health Toolbox: Dimensional Card Sort Test (NIH Toolbox-DCST; Weintraub et al., 2013)
- Nottingham Sensory Assessment–Revised (NSA-R; University of Nottingham, 2007)
- Postural Assessment Scale for Stroke (PASS; Benaim et al., 1999)
- Rivermead Assessment of Somatosensory Performance (2nd ed.; RASP-2; Winward et al., 2002)
- Sequential Occupational Dexterity Assessment (SODA; van Lankveld et al., 1999)
- Shape/Texture Identification Test (STIT; Rosén & Lundborg, 1998)

Problems/Issues

Activities of Daily Living/Instrumental ADL
- Child/Person may grasp objects so tightly that they are difficult to use, such as a spoon, or break, such as a plastic cup.
- Child/Person may pet animals with too much force.

Education/Work
- Child may grasp objects, such as a pencil, so tightly that it is difficult to use the object.
- Child may have difficulty with handwriting (printing, cursive).
- Child may hold a crayon with such force that it breaks.

Play/Leisure
- Child may put too much pressure on a toy or game piece, breaking or bending it.
- Child may "play rough" (pushing, shoving, punching) with other children.

Rest/Sleep
- Person may have continuing problem with enuresis (bed-wetting) because the person does not respond to a signal that bladder is full.

Social Participation
- Person may tend to squeeze another person's hand too tightly (hurts other person) during a handshake.

Sensorimotor
- Interoception
  ▸ Person may have difficulty identifying emotional reactions and responding.
  ▸ Person may have difficulty responding to signals from internal organs such as feeling full, feeling hungry, full bladder, full bowel.
- Pressure (see also Pressure Ulcers in Section 10: Skin Disorders)
  ▸ Person may not recognize pressure on skin, wrinkled socks, or shoes that are too tight due to reduced sensation due to a condition such as diabetes.
- Proprioception
  ▸ Person may have difficulty identifying where body or limbs are in space based on information from joints, muscles, and tendons alone.
  ▸ Person may have decreased muscle tone.
  ▸ Person may have joint hyperactivity.
  ▸ Person may have poor joint alignment and co-contraction.
  ▸ Person may have decreased postural control.
  ▸ Person may have inefficient grading of force.
  ▸ Person may tend to tiptoe when walking.
  ▸ Person may tend to crash into things, fall frequently, push into others, or run everywhere.
  ▸ Person may have difficulty with fluid movement related to excess grasp or grip of object in hand.
- Stereognosis
  ▸ Person may have difficulty discriminating by texture, size, or shape, objects in the hand based on touch alone (astereognosis).
  ▸ Person may have difficulty retrieving wallet from back pocket because he or she cannot see and sense of touch is impaired.
  ▸ Person may have difficulty finding objects in a purse such as a cell phone without looking directly into the purse.
  ▸ Person may have difficulty identifying objects in the dark.
- Tactile
  ▸ Person may have difficulty manipulating objects in the hand based on touch.
  ▸ Person may have difficulty gripping objects with the hand based on touch.

- Vibration
  - ▶ Person may not recognize vibration.

Cognitive/Perceptual
- No information identified.

Psychosocial
- No information identified.

Context/Environment
- Person may not recognize symptoms of somatosensory dysfunction and its management.
- Person may not be aware of potential adaptive devices or compensatory strategies that may reduce the impact of somatosensory dysfunction on everyday life.
- Person may not know about community or internet resources.

Intervention/Treatment

Models and programs developed by occupational therapy personnel: Interception (Mahler, 2015). Models and programs developed by other professionals but used by occupational therapy personnel include cross-modal plasticity (McCormack, 2014), mesh grove and mirror therapy (Lin et al., 2014), SENSe: Study of Effectiveness of Neurorehabilitation on Sensation (Carey et al., 2011; Taylor, McLean, et al., 2018), somatosensory discrimination intervention (McLean et al., 2017), and somatosensory training (Song et al., 2013). Team members include physicians, neurologists, physiologists, psychologists, physical therapy personnel, and occupational therapy personal. Goal is to train or retrain the client's ability to discriminate sensory information for use in everyday living (Carey et al., 2011).

Activities of Daily Living/Instrumental ADL
- Person may need visual reminders or supports such as a "to do" list of morning occupations: go to bathroom, brush teeth, comb hair, get dressed, eat breakfast, take medication, do self-regulation exercises, preview day's schedule, put on coat, go to school bus stop, or drive to work.

Education/Work
- No information identified.

Play/Leisure
- Play a game where therapist passively positions a joint and the child tries to verbally identify the location without vision (blindfold, block vision with a piece of cardboard or blanket; verbal identification).
- Play a game where therapist passively moves a joint and child tries to move the joint back to original position (unilateral limb matching). May start by allowing child to look and then progress to occluding vision.
- Play a game where therapist passively moves joint on one side of body and child tries to match the position on the other side of the body (contralateral limb matching).
- Play a game where therapist touches a digit on one hand and child tries with other hand to touch the same spot with vision occluded (location identification).
- Play a game where therapist positions a limb and child is asked to hold the position without looking (isometric contraction).
- Place weights in each hand and have child identify which hand has the heavier weight. Start with contrast (5 lb vs. 1 lb) and slowly decrease difference. Also include weights that are the same in a random pattern.

Rest/Sleep
- No information identified.

Social Participation
- No information identified.

Sensorimotor
- General
  - Desensitization strategies, such as repeated exposure to sensory stimuli beginning with quick or weak stimuli and gradually increasing time or strength of exposure.
  - Regular retesting of body sensations to monitor progress or need for revision of intervention strategy.
- Interoception
  - Identifying different emotions.
  - Identifying different visceral sensations.
- Pressure/deep pressure
  - Weighted blanket.
  - Squeezing theraputty of different consistencies.
- Proprioception
  - Discrimination of limb positions and movement (see items under Play/Leisure, above).
  - Joint approximation: press one joint into other 3 to 5 times.
- Stereognosis
  - Finding objects in different mediums (sand, rice).
  - Match or identify objects of different textures, shapes, or sizes.
- Tactile
  - Sensory reeducation (touch, tactile): feeling, touching, and handling different types of textures or objects.
  - Light touch stimulation: person identifies whether and where a light touch was applied without vision (cotton ball, pencil tip, rounded end of a paper clip).
  - Two-point discrimination: using an esthesiometer, Boley gauge, or Disk-Criminator, therapist starts with widest distance and moves toward narrow distance. Tips of fingers are most able to detect narrow distance (millimeters). Palm or dorsal surface less so.
- Temperature
  - Repeated exposure to drawing water for different purposes.
  - Repeated exposure to objects that are heated during cooking or baking versus objects that are cooled or frozen (kept in a refrigerator or freezer).
- Vibration
  - Graded exposure to different frequencies.

Cognitive/Perceptual
- Not discussed.

Psychosocial
- Not discussed.

Context/Environment
- Not discussed.

Precautions/Considerations

Person with poor interoception may be at risk for obesity from overeating. Persons who cannot detect temperature differences are at risk for burns.

Prognosis and Outcome

Variable. Original diagnosis, severity of condition, age, and general health are all contributing factors to recovery of sensation and ability to use the information effectively in everyday occupations.

REFERENCES

Ahn, S.-N., Lee, J.-W., & Hwang, S. (2016). Tactile perception for stroke induce changes in electroencephalography. *Hong Kong Journal of Occupational Therapy, 28*(1), 1–6.

Bannister, L. C., Crewther, S. G., Gavrilescu, M., & Carey, L. M. (2015). Improvement in touch sensation after stroke is associated with resting functional connectivity changes. *Frontiers in Neurology, 6*, Article 165. https://doi.org/10.3389/fneur.2015.00165

Blanche, E. I., Bodison, S., Chang, M. C., & Reinoso, G. (2012). Development of the Comprehensive Observations of Proprioception (COP): Validity, reliability, and factor analysis. *American Journal of Occupational Therapy, 66*(6), 691–698. https://doi.org/10.5014/ajot.2012.003608

Blanche, E. I., Reinoso, G., Chang, M. C., & Bodison, S. (2012). Proprioceptive processing difficulties among children with autism spectrum disorders and developmental disabilities. *American Journal of Occupational Therapy, 66*(5), 621–624. https://doi.org/10.5014/ajot.2012.004234

Carey, L. M., Abbott, D. F., Lamp, G., Puce, A., Seitz, R. J., & Donnan, G. A. (2016). Same intervention—Different reorganization: The impact of lesion location on training-facilitated somatosensory recovery after stroke. *Neurorehabilitation and Neural Repair, 30*(10), 988–1000. https://doi.org/10.1177/1545968316653836

Carey, L. M., Lamp, G., & Turville, M. (2016). The state-of-the-science on somatosensory function and its impact on daily life in adults and older adults and following stroke: A scoping review. *OTJR: Occupation, Participation and Health, 36*(Suppl. 2), 27S–41S. https://doi.org/10.1177/1539449216643941

Carey, L., Macdonell, R., & Matyas, T. A. (2011). SENSe: Study of the Effectiveness of Neurorehabilitation on Sensation: A randomized controlled trail. *Neurorehabilitation and Neural Repair, 25*(4) 304–313. https://doi.org/10.1177/1545968310397705

Carey, L. M., & Matyas, T. A. (2011). Frequency of discriminative sensory loss in the hand after stroke in a rehabilitation setting. *Journal of Rehabilitation Medicine, 43*(3), 257–263. https://doi.org/10.2340/16501977-0662

Carey, L. M., Matyas, T. A., & Baum, C. (2018). Effects of somatosensory impairment on participation after stroke. *American Journal of Occupational Therapy, 72*, Article 7203205100. https://doi.org/10.5014/ajot.2018.025114

Dunn, W., Griffith, J. W., Morrison, M. T., Tanquary, J., Sabata, D., Victorson, D., Carey, L. M., & Gershon, R. C. (2013). Somatosensation assessment using the NIH Toolbox. *Neurology, 80*(11, Suppl. 3), S41–S44. https://doi.org/10.1212/WNL.0b013e3182872c54

Goodin, P., Lamp, G., Vidyasagar, R., McArdle, D., Seitz, R. J., & Carey, L. M. (2018). Altered functional connectivity differs in stroke survivors with impaired touch sensation following left and right hemisphere lesions. *NeuroImage: Clinical, 18*, 342–355. https://doi.org/10.1016/j.nicl.2018.02.012

Hill, V. A., Fisher, T., Schmid, A. A., Crabtree, J., & Page, S. J. (2014). Relationship between touch sensation of the affected hand and performance of valued activities in individuals with chronic stroke. *Topics in Stroke Rehabilitation, 21*(4), 339–346. https://doi.org/10.1310/tsr2104-339

In, T.-S., Jung, J.-H., Jang, S.-H., Kim, K.-H., Jung, K.-S., & Cho, H.-Y. (2019). Effects of light touch on balance in patients with stroke. *Open Medicine, 14*(1), 259–263 https://doi.org/10.1515/med-2019-0021

Kim, Y. J., Rogers, J. C., Kwok, G., Dunn, W., & Holm, M. B. (2016). Somatosensation differences in older adults with and without diabetes, and by age group. *Occupational Therapy in Health Care, 30*(3), 231–244. https://doi.org/10.3109/07380577.2015.1136758

Lin, K.-C., Chen, Y.-T., Huang, P.-C., Wu, C.-Y., Huang, W.-L., Yang, H.-W., Lai, H.-T., & Lu, H.-J. (2014). Effect of mirror therapy combined with somatosensory stimulation on motor recovery and daily function in stroke patients: A pilot study. *Journal of the Formosan Medical Association, 113*(7), 422–428. https://doi.org/10.1016/j.jfma.2012.08.008

Mahler, K. (2015). *Interoception: The eighth sensory system: Practical solutions for improving self-regulation, self-awareness and social understanding of individual with autism spectrum and related disorders*. AAPC.

McCormack, G. L. (2014). The significance of somatosensory stimulation to the hand: Implications for occupational therapy practice. *Open Journal of Occupational Therapy, 2*(4), Article 7. https://doi.org/10.15453/2168-6408.1141

McLean, B., Girdler, S., Taylor, S., Valentine, J., Carey, L., & Elliott, C. (2019). Experience of engagement in a somatosensory discrimination intervention for children with hemiplegic cerebral palsy: A qualitative investigation. *Developmental Neurorehabilitation, 22*(5), 348–358. https://doi.org/10.1080/17518423.2018.1503620

McLean, B., Taylor, S., Blair, E., Valentine, J., Carey, L., & Elliott, C. (2017). Somatosensory discrimination intervention improves body position sense ad motor performance in children with hemiplegic cerebral palsy. *American Journal of Occupational Therapy, 71*(3), Article 72013190060. https://doi.org/10.5014/ajot.2016.024968

Nedelec, B., Calva, V., Chouinard, A., Couture, M. A., Godbout, E., de Oliveira, A., & LaSalle, L. (2016). Somatosensory rehabilitation for neuropathic pain in burn survivors: A case series. *Journal of Burn Care & Research, 37*(1), e37–e46. https://doi.org/10.1097/BCR.0000000000000321

O'Toole, M. T. (Ed.). (2017). *Mosby's dictionary of medicine, nursing & health professions* (10th ed.). Elsevier.

Pumpa, L. U., Cahill, L. S., & Carey, L. M. (2015). Somatosensory assessment and treatment after stroke: An evidence-practice gap. *Australian Occupational Therapy Journal, 62*(2), 93–104. https://doi.org/10.1111/1440-1630.12170

Rand, D. (2018). Mobility, balance and balance confidence—Correlations with daily living of individuals with and without mild proprioception deficits post-stroke. *NeuroRehabilitation, 43*(2), 219–226. https://doi.org/10.3233/NRE-172398

Sakamoto, K., Yokoi, K., Hirayama, K., Yamaguchi, J., & Shinoda, A. (2019). A case of somatoparaphrenia characterized by very mild somatosensory disturbance and absence of anosognosia for hemiplegia and personal neglect. *Cortex, 120,* 603–606. https://doi.org/10.1016/j.cortex.2019.03.008

Song, B. K., Chung, S. M., & Hwang, B. Y. (2013). The effects of somatosensory training focused on the hand on hand function, postural control and ADL of stroke patients with unilateral spatial neglect and sensorimotor deficits. *Journal of Physical Therapy Science, 25*(3), 297–300. https://doi.org/10.1589/jpts.25.297

Taylor, S., Girdler, S., Parsons, R., McLean, B., Falkmer, T., Carey, L., Blair, E., & Elliott, C. (2018). Construct validity and responsiveness of the functional Tactile Object Recognition Test for children with cerebral palsy. *Australian Occupational Therapy Journal, 65*(5), 420–430. https://doi.org/10.1111/1440-1630.12508

Taylor, S., McLean, B., Blair, E., Carey, L. M., Valentine, J., Girdler, S., & Elliott, C. (2018). Clinical acceptability of the sense_assess® kids: Children and youth perspectives. *Australian Occupational Therapy Journal, 65*(2), 79–88. https://doi.org/10.1111/1440-1630.12429

Turville, M. L., Cahill, L. S., Matyas, T. A., Blennerhassett, J. M., & Carey, L. M. (2019). The effectiveness of somatosensory retraining for improving sensory function in the arm following stroke: A systematic review. *Clinical Rehabilitation, 33*(5), 834–846. https://doi.org/10.1177/0269215519829795

Turville, M., Carey, L. M., Matyas, T. A., & Blennerhassett, J. (2017). Change in functional arm use is associated with somatosensory skills after sensory retraining poststroke. *American Journal of Occupational Therapy, 71*(3), Article 7103190070. https://doi.org/10.5014/ajot.2017.024950

Turville, M. L., Matyas, T. A., Blennerhassett, J. M., & Carey, L. M. (2018). Initial severity of somatosensory impairment influences response to upper limb sensory retraining post-stroke. *NeuroRehabilitation, 43*(4), 413–423. https://doi.org/10.3233/NRE-182439

Turville, M. L., Walker, J., Blennerhassett, J. M., & Carey, L. M. (2019). Experiences of upper limb somatosensory retraining in persons with stroke: An interpretative phenomenological analysis. *Frontiers in Neuroscience, 13,* Article 756. https://doi.org/10.3389/fnins.2019.00756

VandenBos, G. (Ed.). (2015). *APA dictionary of psychology* (2nd ed.). American Psychological Association. https://doi.org/10.1037/14646-000

Walmsley, C., Taylor, S., Parkins, T., Carey, L., Girdler, S., & Elliott, C. (2018). What is the current practice of therapists in the measurement of somatosensation in children with cerebral palsy and other neurological disorders? *Australian Occupational Therapy Journal, 65*(2), 89–97. https://doi.org/10.1111/1440-1630.12431

Yilmazer, C., Boccuni, L., Thijs, L., & Verheyden, G. (2019). Effectiveness of somatosensory interventions on somatosensory motor and functional outcomes in the upper limb post-stroke: A systematic review and meta-analysis. *NeuroRehabilitation, 44*(4), 459–477. https://doi.org/10.3233/NRE-192687

Zetler, N. K., Cermak, S. A., Engel-Yeger, B., & Gal, E. (2019) Somatosensory discrimination in people with autism spectrum disorder: A scoping review. *American Journal of Occupational Therapy, 73*(5), Article 730520501. https://doi.org/10.5014/ajot.2019.029728

BIBLIOGRAPHY

Abrams, M. R., & Ivy, C. C. (2018). Evaluation of sensation and intervention for sensory dysfunction. In H. M. Pendleton & W. Schultz-Krohn (Eds.), *Pedretti's occupational therapy* (8th ed., pp. 580–593). Elsevier.

Carey, L. M. (2012). Touch and body sensation. In L. M. Carey (Ed.), *Stroke rehabilitation: Insights from neuroscience and imaging* (pp. 157–172). Oxford University Press. 10.1093/med/9780199797882.003.0012

Cheng, C.-H. (2018). Effects of observing normal and abnormal goal-directed hand movements on somatosensory cortical activation. *European Journal of Neuroscience, 47*(1), 48–57. https://doi.org/10.1111/ejn.13783

Cheng, C.-H., Chan, P.-Y. S., Baillet, S., & Lin, Y. Y. (2015). Age-related reduced somatosensory gating is associated with altered alpha frequency desynchronization. *Neural Plasticity, 2015,* Article 302878. https://doi.org/10.1155/2015/302878

Cheng, C.-H., Tseng, Y.-J., Chen, R.-S., & Lin, Y.-Y. (2016). Reduced functional connectivity of somatosensory network in writer's cramp patients. *Brain and Behavior, 6*(3), Article e00433. https://doi.org/10.1002/brb3.433

Chu, V. W. T. (2017). Assessing proprioception in children: A review. *Journal of Motor Behavior, 49*(4), 458–466. https://doi.org/10.1080/00222895.2016.1241744

Dunn, W., Griffith, J. W., Sabata, D., Morrison, M. T., MacDermid, J. C., Darragh, A., Schaaf, R., Dudgeon, B., Connor, L. T., Carey, L., & Tanquary, J. (2015). Measuring change in somatosensation across the lifespan. *American Journal of Occupational Therapy, 69*(3), Article 6903290020. https://doi.org/10.5014/ajot.2015.014845

Lamp, G., Goodin, P., Palmer, S., Low, E., Barutchu, A., & Carey, L. M. (2019). Activation of bilateral secondary somatosensory cortex with right hand touch stimulation: A meta-analysis of functional neuroimaging studies. *Frontiers in Neurology, 9,* Article 1129. https://doi.org/10.3389/fneur.2018.01129

Puce, A., & Carey, L. (2010). Somatosensory function. In I. B. Weiner & W. E. Craighead (Eds.), *The Corsini encyclopedia of psychology* (pp. 1678–1680). Wiley.

Taylor, S., McLean, B., Falkmer, T., Carey, L., Girdler, S., Elliott, C., & Blair, E. (2016). Does somatosensation change with age in children and adolescents? A systematic review. *Child: Care, Health and Development, 42*(6), 809–824. https://doi.org/10.1111/cch.12375

Theis, J. L. (2014). Assessing abilities and capacities: Sensation. In M. V. Radomski & C. A. Thombly Latham (Eds.), *Occupational therapy for physical dysfunction* (7th ed., pp. 276–305). Wolter-Kluwer.

Vestibular Disorders

See also Benign Paroxysmal Positional Vertigo (BPPV).

Description

Vestibular disorders include BPPV (see Benign Paroxysmal Positional Vertigo in Section 2: Sensory Disorders), Ménière's disease, labyrinthitis, vestibular neuritis, vestibular neuronitis, and central vestibular disorders such as an acoustic neuroma, also called vestibular schwannoma; (Porter, 2018). Vestibular rehabilitation is the use of activities and exercises to treat vertigo (sensation of spinning or whirling motion), dizziness, faintness, unsteadiness, imbalance, disequilibrium (poor balance), visual disturbances, functional limitation, and psychosocial complications cause by vestibular dysfunction. Vestibular rehabilitation therapy (VRT) includes use of compensatory, adaptive, substitution, and movement retraining through exercise-based activities (American Occupational Therapy Association, 2017).

Cause

The cause of Ménière's disease and acoustic neuroma are unknown. Labyrinthitis, vestibular neuritis, and vestibular neuronitis may be caused by a viral infection.

Terminology

- *Bilateral peripheral vestibular lesions:* Disorder or symptoms are present on both sides of the body.
- *Central disorders:* Disorders involving vestibular nuclei and their pathways in the brain stem and cerebellum (Porter, 2018).
- *Central vestibular system disorders:* Brain stem hemorrhage, cerebellar hemorrhage, migraine, multiple sclerosis, vertebral artery dissection, vertebrobasilar insufficiency (Porter, 2018).
- *Dizziness:* Includes sensations such as faintness or syncope, lightheadedness, feeling of imbalance or unsteadiness, and spinning sensation (Porter, 2018).
- *Mixed systems disorder:* Conditions or symptoms are present involving both the central vestibular system and the peripheral vestibular system.
- *Oscillopsia:* Illusion of object movement in the environment during head movement (American Occupational Therapy Association, 2017; O'Toole, 2017).
- *Peripheral disorders:* Disorders involving the inner ear and 8th (vestibulocochlear) cranial nerve (Porter, 2018).
- *Peripheral unilateral impairment/weakness:* Disorder or symptoms are present on one side of the body.
- *Peripheral vestibular system disorders:* Benign paroxysmal positional vertigo, Ménière's disease, vestibular neuronitis, labyrinthitis, otitis media, acoustic neuroma, ototoxic drugs, herpes zoster oticus, chronic motion sickness, and trauma such as tympanic membrane rupture, labyrinthine contusion, perilymphatic fistula, temporal bone fracture, post-concussion (Porter, 2018).
- *Sensory weighting:* A cognitive process in which one of several potentially redundant sensory systems (vision, vestibular, and proprioception) is selected and favored over another.
- *Unequal bilateral impairment:* Disorder or symptoms are present on both sides of the body but one side is more involved (shows more symptoms or a more severe symptom) than the other side.
- *Unilateral vestibular hypofunction:* Poor or low vestibular function on one side of the body.
- *Vestibulo-ocular reflex (VOR):* normal reflex in which eye position compensates for movement of the head (O'Toole, 2017).
- *Vertigo:* Illusion or false sense of self-motion or movement such as spinning or falling (American Occupational Therapy Association, 2017; Porter, 2018). Sensations of instability, giddiness, loss of equilibrium, wheeling, or rotation (O'Toole, 2017; Porter, 2018).

- *Visual vertigo:* Syndrome where symptoms are triggered or exacerbated in situations involving rich visual conflict or intense visual stimulation such as a supermarket or city driving. Assumed to be caused by a sensory conflict or mismatch between visual, vestibular, and musculoskeletal systems.

Evaluation/Assessment

Areas
- Activities of Daily Living/Instrumental ADL: dressing, bathing or showering, meal preparation, household chores (dusting, vacuuming), child care, driving, transportation
- Education/Work: academic setting, work task, work history
- Play/Leisure: types, location, frequency
- Rest/Sleep: sleep disturbance
- Social Participation: types, location, frequency, with whom
- Sensorimotor: balance (disequilibrium, poor balance), vertigo (illusion of spinning or falling), changing body positions (standing up, bending down), postural control, postural sway, walking in open spaces, reaching, climbing/descending stairs, using moving equipment (escalator, elevator), nystagmus, dizziness, hearing loss, tinnitus, visual impairment
- Cognitive/Perceptual: attention, memory, executive functions, spatial orientation, vertical body orientation
- Psychosocial: role performance, quality of life, anxiety, stress, panic attack, hyperventilation
- Context/Environment: adaptive devices, health literacy, resources
- Development (Infant, Child, Adolescent only): developmental delay (motor functions)
- Comorbidities: medication toxicity, brain injury, heart disease, deafness, profound hearing loss, attention-deficit/hyperactivity disorder, autism, cerebral palsy, Down syndrome, hydrocephalus, posterior brain tumor, Wallenberg syndrome (stroke in brain stem, vertebral or posterior inferior cerebellar artery)

Instruments

Instruments Developed by Occupational Therapy Personnel
- Canadian Occupational Performance Measure (5th ed.; COPM-5; Law et al., 2014)
- Driving Habits Questionnaire (DHQ; Cohen et al., 2003)
- Miller Function and Participation Scales (M-FUN; Miller, 2006)
- Modified Clinical Test of Sensory Interaction and Balance (MCTSIB; Cohen et al., 2019, in References)
- Reintegration to Normal Living Index (RNLI; Wood-Dauphinee et al., 1988)
- Role Evaluation of Activities of Life (REAL; Roll & Roll, 2013)
- Vestibular Disorders Activities of Daily Living Scale (VADL; Cohen & Kimball, 2000; see also Cohen, 2014; Mehrkian et al., 2018; and Ricci et al., 2014, in References)

Instruments Developed by Other Professionals and Used by Occupational Therapy Personnel
(Note: Oculomotor screening tests did not detect vestibular disorders; Cohen et al., 2018, in References.)

- Activities-Specific Balance Confidence (ABC) Scale (Powell & Myers, 1995)
- Balance perturbation (see Goel et al., 2019, in References)
- Berg Balance Scale (BBS; Berg et al., 1989)
- Bruininks-Oseretsky Test of Motor Proficiency (2nd ed.; BOT-2; Bruininks & Bruininks, 2005)
- "Bucket test" (BT; Zwergal et al., 2009; see also Cohen & Sangi-Haghpeykar, 2012, in References)
- Clinical Test of Sensory Integration and Balance (CTSIB; Shumway-Cook & Horak, 1986)
- Dizziness Handicap Inventory (DHI; Jacobson & Newman, 1990)
- Dynamic Gait Index (DGI; Marchett & Whitney, 2006; see also Dye et al., 2013, in References)
- Dynamic visual acuity (DVA) test (measurement instrument; see Dye et al., 2013, in References)
- Five-Times-Sit-to-Stand Test (FTSST; Whitney et al., 2005)

- Four Square Step Test (FSST; Whitney et al., 2007)
- Fukuda Stepping Test (FST; Fukuda, 1959)
- Functional Mobility Test (FMT; Johnson Space Functional Mobility Test; Cohen, Kimball, et al., 2012, in References)
- Head impulse test (HIT)
  - ▶ Examiner sits in front of subject and instructs subject to stare at examiner's nose.
  - ▶ The examiner briskly or quickly rotates the head approximately 20 degrees leftward or rightward in jaw rotations (side to side) stopping suddenly and approximating a step of velocity.
  - ▶ Response is positive if a saccade (eye movement) contralateral to the head movement is observed.
- Peabody Developmental Motor Scales (3rd ed.; PDMS-3; Folio & Fewell, 2023)
- Pediatric Berg Balance Scale (PBBS; Franjoine et al., 2003)
- Posturography (see Cohen, Kimball, et al., 2012, in References)
- Romberg Balance Test (RBT; and variations of Tandem Walking: 10 steps, arms crossed, eyes open, then eyes closed; Cohen et al., 1993; see also Cohen, Mulavara, et al., 2012; Cohen et al., 2013; and Cohen et al., 2018, in References)
- Standing balance (see Cohen et al., 2014, in References)
- Tandem Walking Test (see Romberg Test)
- Timed Up and Go test (TUG; Podsiadlo & Richardson, 1991)
- Tinetti Balance Scale (TBS; Tinetti et al., 1986)
- UCLA Dizziness Questionnaire (UCLA-DQ; Honrubia et al., 1996)
- Vertical and torsional alignment (see Schubert et al., 2017, in References)
- Vertigo Handicap Questionnaire (VHQ; Yardley & Putman, 1992)
- Vestibular Activities and Participation Measure (VAPM; Alghwiri et al., 2012)
- Vestibular Rehabilitation Benefit Questionnaire (VRBQ; Morris et al., 2008)
- Visual acuity screening (see Peters et al., 2013, and Peters et al., 2012, in References)
- Walking speed (see Cohen & Sangi-Haghpeykar, 2011, in References)

Problems/Issues

Activities of Daily Living/Instrumental ADL
- Person may experience symptoms when bending over to put on socks and shoes.
- Person may experience symptoms while preparing a meal, such as raising the head up to reach for items on a shelf or bending down to retrieve a pan from a lower cabinet.
- Person may experience symptoms while driving, especially during busy traffic times.
- Person may experience symptoms while shopping in a grocery store with many different visual displays that require many head movements.
- Person may decrease engagement in driving or shopping to avoid dizziness (Plutschack & Moore, 2018).

Education/Work
- Person may experience symptoms while performing work tasks that require moving about and changing position, such as stock clerk or delivery driver.
- Person may have quit a job in which symptoms have occurred.

Play/Leisure
- Person may experience symptoms while playing sports games that require rapid and repeated head movements to perform actions (golf swing) or follow the ball (catch a baseball).
- Person may avoid engagement in leisure occupations in which symptoms have occurred.

Rest/Sleep
- Sleep disturbance.

Social Participation
- Person may experience symptoms while participating in social activities that require rapid or repeated head movements, such as following a conversation in a large group of people.
- Person may reduce or limit participation in social activities to avoid symptom flare-up (Plutschack & Moore, 2018).

Sensorimotor
- Person may experience symptoms when bending over or changing the position of head rapidly.
- Person may experience symptoms when the body turns quickly.
- Person may experience difficulty walking while engaged in dual-task performance (Roberts et al., 2011).

Cognitive/Perceptual
- Person may have difficulty understanding and following instructions due to difficulty with attending behavior and memory.
- Person may have difficulty with executive functions that reduce person's ability to use judgment of safety, planning, and problem solving.

Psychosocial
- Person may have difficulty coping with symptoms and experience increased stress.
- Person may have reduced or stopped performing certain roles or role tasks to avoid symptoms.
- Person may have reduced quality of life.

Context/Environment
- Person may lack knowledge about specific vestibular disorder and management.
- Person may lack social support.
- Person may lack information and use of assistive devices that may be helpful in managing symptoms.
- Person may lack knowledge about available resources in the community or on the internet.

Intervention/Treatment

Models and programs developed by occupational therapy personnel: None. Models and programs developed by other professionals but used by occupational therapy personnel include stochastic vestibular stimulation/resonance (Goel et al., 2015; Mulavara et al., 2011), vestibular rehabilitation (Bhovad & Kale, 2015; Bush & Dougherty, 2015; Cohen, 2011, 2016; Cohen et al., 2011), and vestibular therapy (Cronin & Steenerson, 2011). Team members include physicians, neurologists, otolaryngologists, nursing personnel, physical therapy personnel, and occupational therapy personnel. Goals are to decrease symptoms, increase independence, and enhance occupational performance, participation, safety, self-efficacy, and perceived quality of life (American Occupational Therapy Association, 2017; Kannenberg, 2014).

Activities of Daily Living/Instrumental ADL
- Discuss and review with client if any tasks or activities cause symptoms while performing basic ADLs (dressing, bathing/showering, toileting). Assist client to modify, minimize, or eliminate those tasks or activities.
- Discuss and review with client if any tasks or activities cause symptoms while performing IADLs (meal preparation, housekeeping, shopping, driving, child- or pet care). Assist client to modify, minimize, or eliminate those tasks or activities.
- Recommend wearing flat shoes (no heels), or orthotic designed shoes to improve balance and reduce fall risk.

Education/Work
- Discuss with client if any tasks or activities at work cause symptoms. Assist client to modify, minimize, or eliminate those tasks or activities.

Play/Leisure

- Discuss with client if any tasks or activities cause symptoms while engaging in leisure occupations. Assist client to modify, minimize, or eliminate those tasks or activities.
- Assist client to identify leisure occupations that may be enjoyable but also provide vestibular exercise using the eyes while the head and body are in motion, such as golf, bowling, tennis, racquetball, or ping-pong. Dancing, tai chi, and martial arts may also be considered.

Rest/Sleep

- No information identified.

Social Participation

- Discuss with client if any tasks or activities cause symptoms while participating in social activities. Assist client to modify, minimize, or eliminate those tasks or activities.

Sensorimotor

- Balance and gait training: Exercises may involve standing on one foot for 15 seconds, eyes open, eyes closed, and then the other; walking heel to toe on a line; standing on a spongy surface; yoga; tai chi.
- Bilateral vestibular exercises
  - ▶ Place two targets horizontally in front of a client on a wall. Ask client to look at one target for 10 seconds. Next, ask the client to look at the next target with head fixed. Third, ask client to move the head toward the second target. Perform actions for 2–3 minutes. After horizontal exercises, repeat exercises with targets placed vertically. Repeat exercises by doing them faster. The active eye–head movement will facilitate the saccadic or smooth pursuit strategies.
  - ▶ Client looks at different targets with high eye speed with eyes fixed for 30 seconds to facilitate gaze stabilization using saccadic eye movements.
  - ▶ Client stands with open eyes while opening arms in front for 20 seconds. Next, ask client to do the same exercise with eyes closed (simultaneous use of vestibular and somatosensory inputs).
  - ▶ Ask client to repeat previous exercise on a firm surface with eyes opened and closed for 20 seconds (simultaneous use of vestibular and visual inputs).
  - ▶ Ask client to sit in front of a target and look at it. Next, ask client to close the eyes, remembering the location of the target. Ask client to open eyes to check whether client has remembered location of target. Ask client to repeat 10 times. Check for accuracy.
- Cawthorne-Cooksey exercises
  - ▶ In bed or sitting
    - ○ Eye movements: at first slow, then quickly.
      - ▷ Move eyes up and down.
      - ▷ Move eyes side to side.
      - ▷ Focus eyes on finger moving from 3 feet to 1 foot away from face.
    - ○ Head movements.
      - ▷ Bend head forward and backward.
      - ▷ Turn head from side to side.
  - ▶ Sitting
    - ○ Eye movements and head movements as above.
    - ○ Shrug shoulders, do circles with shoulders.
    - ○ Bend forward and pick up objects from the ground or floor.
  - ▶ Standing
    - ○ Eye, head, and shoulder movement, as above.
    - ○ Change from sitting to standing position, eyes open and closed.
    - ○ Throw a small ball from hand to hand above eye level (so person must look up).

○ Throw a small ball from hand to hand behind the knee (so person must bend forward with legs slightly apart and one foot slight forward).

○ From a sitting position, stand up and turn in a complete circle while staying in one place, then sit back down. Alternate direction turned.

▶ Moving (in a large room free of obstacles)

○ Helper stands in the center of a large circle. While person circles the perimeter of the circle, the helper throws a large ball to the client, who then throws the ball back to the helper.

○ Walk across room first with eyes open; when dizziness improves, walk with eyes closed.

○ Walk up and down a slope surface first with eyes open; when dizziness improves, walk with eyes closed.

○ Walk up and down stairs with eyes open and then closed.

○ Play any game that involves stooping, stretching, or aiming, such as bowling, tennis, golf, table tennis, basketball.

● Frenzel goggles/lenses/glasses: Magnification system with a light used to observe client for presence of nystagmus.

● Gaze stabilization exercises: Enhance gaze stability.

▶ Duration of exercises is usually short (1–2 minutes) especially for children. Total time for adults, 30 minutes spaced over the day. Duration adjusted so person feels "dizzy" but stop if person feels "sick."

▶ Number of exercise repetitions: usually 8–10.

▶ Instructions: A small card (business card) is attached to a wall at eye level. Client is positioned at midline in front of the card. Client is instructed to look straight ahead at the card. Then the client is instructed to turn the head 45 degrees toward the right (while maintaining eye contact with the card). Next, the client is instructed to turn the head 45 degrees toward the left (while maintaining eye contact with the card). Speed of turning the head (slow, medium, fast), frequency of exercises during the day/week, target distance (near/far), background (blank, busy, very busy), head position on trunk (midline left, right, up, down), and head position in respect to gravity (upright, supine, prone) can be varied.

● Postural stability: Enhance postural stability.

▶ Ergonomics: Stoop (bend at the knees) rather than bending over to reach objects.

▶ Therapeutic

○ Stand with feet heel to toe, with both arms extended for 15 seconds.

○ Sway back and forth on heels and toes. Place person behind a chair and before a wall for safety. Repeat 10 times.

○ March in place for 15 seconds with eyes open and then closed.

○ Walk straight 20 steps while turning head. Walking close to a wall is helpful.

○ Walk forward on a hard surface for 10 seconds, and then walk backward. Next, have client walk on foam or uneven surface.

○ Start exercise with feet shoulder-width apart, with eyes open looking at a target on wall for 20 seconds. Then ask client to narrow base of support to semi-heel-to-toe position. Next, ask client to do the same exercise with eyes closed.

● Stochastic vestibular stimulation (SVS): Based on concept of stochastic resonance, which uses a signal too weak to be detected by a sensor but can be boosted by adding white noise to the signal. SVS uses a small amount of electrical noise applied to the vestibular system to improve balance control during standing and walking (see Goel et al., 2015; Goel et al., 2019).

● Unilateral vestibular exercises

▶ Client moves the head horizontally at different speeds while looking at a target in front for 1 minute. Next, the client moves the head vertically while looking at the target.

▶ Client looks at his or her thumb while moving the head and trunk together on a rotating chair for 30 seconds.

- ▶ Client looks at a target on a wall while walking, moving the head horizontally for 15 seconds. Next, the client moves head vertically.
- ▶ Client sits down on a therapy ball and looks at a target in front while moving the body up and down on the ball for 1 minute.
- Vertigo habituation exercises: No information identified.
- Visual desensitization exercises/visual dependence training: Use of a mixture of gaze stabilization and balance exercises with an emphasis on suppressing abnormal visual input in real-life situations.
- Work simplification: Explore with client if certain steps in tasks or activities can be eliminated or reduced in frequency if they cause symptoms. Explore whether certain other steps or group of steps could be substituted for those that cause symptoms.

Cognitive/Perceptual

- Assist client to determine what tasks are being performed that elicit symptoms during self-care, work, driving, shopping, socializing, and other areas of everyday living.
- Assist client to use problem-solving strategies to minimize or eliminate symptoms associated with self-care, work, driving, shopping, socializing, or other areas of everyday living, such as work simplification or use of exercises designed to reduce symptoms.

Psychosocial

- Assist client to identify situations and activities in which symptoms occur.
- Reduce stress through tai chi or yoga exercises.
- Assist client to examine if modifications in task performance would improve role performance.

Context/Environment

- Suggest used of assistive devices (gait aids) such as a cane, walker, walker with wheels.
- Suggest environmental adaptations to promote safety and prevent falls: grab bars, tub benches, night-lights, lighted canes, single long-distance lenses rather than bifocal or trifocal lenses, providing clear and unobstructed pathways in the home, organizing cooking and food items within easy reach.
- Provide education in fall prevention and safety promotion.
- Assist client to identify resources in the community or on the internet.

Precautions/Safety Considerations

Person is at risk for falls regardless of environmental modifications recommended or implemented (Plutschack & Moore, 2018). Pediatric clients should be over age 4 (Lotfi et al., 2016). Stress reactions in children may be observed/heard in crying, blushing, or fear reaction.

Prognosis and Outcome

Prognosis using vestibular rehabilitation for clients with stable peripheral conditions is generally good. Clients with central lesions (migraine vertigo, transient ischemic attacks or TIAs), unstable conditions (Ménière's disease), or mixed central and peripheral lesion may be more limited. Medical management or surgical approaches should be considered (Lotfi et al., 2016).

REFERENCES

American Occupational Therapy Association. (2017). Vestibular impairment, vestibular rehabilitation, and occupational performance. *American Journal of Occupational Therapy, 71*(Suppl. 2), Article 7112410055. https://doi.org/10.5014/ajot.2017.716S09

Bhovad, R. P., & Kale, J. (2015). The effectiveness of early vestibular rehabilitation on balance after acoustic neuroma surgery: A comparative study. *Indian Journal of Occupational Therapy, 47*(2), 31–37.

Bush, M. L., & Dougherty, W. (2015). Assessment of vestibular rehabilitation therapy training and practice patterns. *Journal of Community Health, 40*(4), 802–807. https://doi.org/10.1007/s10900-015-0003-7

Cohen, H. S. (2011). Vestibular rehabilitation and stroke. In G. Gillen (Ed.), *Stroke rehabilitation: A function-based approach* (3rd ed., pp. 210–217). Elsevier Mosby.

Cohen, H. S. (2014). Use of the Vestibular Disorders Activities of Daily Living Scale to describe functional limitations in patients with vestibular disorders. *Journal of Vestibular Research, 24*(1), 33–38. https://doi.org/10.3233/VES-130475

Cohen, H. S. (2016). Vestibular rehabilitation and stroke. In G. Gillen (Ed.), *Stroke rehabilitation: A function-based approach* (4th ed., pp. 416–423). Elsevier Mosby.

Cohen, H. S., Gottshall, K. R., Graziano, M., Malmstrom, E. M., Sharpe, M. H., & Whitney, S. L. (2011). International guidelines for education in vestibular rehabilitation therapy. *Journal of Vestibular Research, 21,* 243–250. https://doi.org/10.3233/VES-2011-0424

Cohen, H. S., Kimball, K. T., Mulavara, A. P., Bloomberg, J. J., & Paloski, W. H. (2012). Posturography and locomotor tests of dynamic balance after long-duration spaceflight. *Journal of Vestibular Research, 22,* 191–196. https://doi.org/10.3233/VES-2012-0456

Cohen, H. S., Mulavara, A. P., Peters, B. T., Sangi-Haghpeykar, H., & Bloomberg, J. (2014). Standing balance tests for screening people with vestibular impairments. *The Laryngoscope, 124*(2), 545–550. https://doi.org/10.1002/lary.24314

Cohen, H. S., Mulavara, A. P., Peters, B. T., Sangi-Haghpeykar, H., & Bloomberg, J. (2012). Tests of walking balance for screening vestibular disorders. *Journal of Vestibular Research: Equilibrium & Orientation, 22*(2-3), 95–104. https://doi.org/10.3233/VES-2012-0443

Cohen, H. S., Mulavara, A. P., Peters, B. T., Sangi-Haghpeykar, H., Kung, D. H., Mosier, D., & Bloomberg, J. J. (2013). Sharpening the tandem walking test for screening peripheral neuropathy. *Southern Medical Journal, 106*(10), 565–569. https://doi.org/10.1097/SMJ.0000000000000009

Cohen, H. S., Mulavara, A. P., Stitz, J., Sangi-Haghpeykar, H., Williams, S. P., Peters, B. T., & Bloomberg, J. J. (2019). Screening for vestibular disorders using the Modified Clinical Test of Sensory Interaction and Balance and tandem walking with eyes closed. *Otology & Neurotology, 40*(5), 658–665. https://doi.org/10.1097/MAO.0000000000002173

Cohen, H. S., & Sangi-Haghpeykar, H. (2011). Walking speed and vestibular disorders in a path integration task. *Gait & Posture, 33*(2), 211–213. https://doi.org/10.1016/j.gaitpost.2010.11.007

Cohen, H. S., & Sangi-Haghpeykar, H. (2012). Subjective visual vertical in vestibular disorders measured with the bucket test. *Acta Oto-Laryngology, 132*(8), 850–854. https://doi.org/10.3109/00016489.2012.668710

Cohen, H. S., Stitz, J., Sangi-Haghpeykar, H., Williams, S. P., Mulavara, A. P., Peters, B. T., & Bloomberg, J. J. (2018). Tandem walking as a quick screening test for vestibular disorders. *The Laryngoscope, 128*(7), 1687–1691. https://doi.org/10.1002/lary.27022

Cronin, G. W., & Steenerson, R. L. (2011). Disequilibrium of gaining: Response to a 3-month program of vestibular therapy. *Physical & Occupational Therapy in Geriatrics, 29*(2), 148–155. https://doi.org/10.3109/02703181.2010.544845

Dye, D. C., Eakman, A. M., & Bolton, K. M. (2013). Assessing the validity of the Dynamic Gait Index in a balance disorders clinic: An application of Rasch analysis. *Physical Therapy, 93*(6), 809–818. https://doi.org/10.2522/ptj.20120163

Goel, R., Kofman, J., Jeevarajan, J., De Dios, Y., Cohen, H. S., Bloomberg, J. J., & Mulavara, A. P. (2015). Using low levels of stochastic vestibular stimulation to improve balance function. *PLOS ONE, 10*(8), Article 30136335. https://doi.org/10.1371/journal.pone.0136335

Goel, R., Rosenberg, M. J., Cohen, H. S., Bloomberg, J. J., & Mulavara, A. P. (2019). Calibrating balance perturbation using electrical stimulation of the vestibular system. *Journal of Neuroscience Methods, 311,* 193–199. https://doi.org/10.1016/j.jneumeth.2018.10.012

Kannenberg, K. (2014). Vestibular rehabilitation in occupational therapy practice. *OT Practice, 19*(1), 8.

Lotfi, Y., Rezazadeh, N., Moossavi, A., Haghgoo, H. A., Moghadam, S. F., Pishyareh, E., Bakhshi, E., Rostami, R., Sadeghi, V., & Khodahandelou, Y. (2016). Review paper: Introduction of pediatric balance therapy in children with vestibular dysfunction: Review of indications, mechanisms, and key exercises. *Iranian Rehabilitation Journal, 14*(1), 4–14. https://doi.org/10.15412/J.IRJ .08140102

Mehrkian, S., Erfanimanesh, Z., & Bakhshi, E. (2018). Validity and reliability of the Persian version of the vestibular disorders activities of daily living scale. *Auditory and Vestibular Research, 27*(1), 25–50.

Mulavara, A. P., Fiedler, M. J., Kofman, I. S., Wood, S. J., Serrador, J. M., Peters, B., Cohen, H., Reschke, M. F., & Bloomberg, J. J. (2011). Improving balance function using vestibular stochastic resonance: Optimizing stimulus characteristics. *Experimental Brain Research, 210*(2), 303–312. https://doi.org/10.1007/s00221-011-2633-z

O'Toole, M. T. (Ed.). (2017). *Mosby's dictionary of medicine, nursing and health professions* (10th ed.). Elsevier.

Peters, B. T., Cohen, H. S., Sangi-Haghpeykar, H., & Bloomberg, J. J. (2013). Effects of distance and duration on vertical dynamic visual acuity in screening healthy adults and people with vestibular disorders. *Journal of Vestibular Research, 23*(6), 285–291. https://doi.org/10.3233/ VES-130502

Peters, B. T., Mulavara, A. P., Cohen, H. S., Sangi-Haghpeykar, H., & Bloomberg, J. J. (2012). Dynamic visual acuity testing for screening patients with vestibular impairments. *Journal of Vestibular Research, 22*(2), 145–151. https://doi.org/10.3233/VES-2012-0440

Plutschack, D., & Moore, S. (2018). Addressing psychosocial needs in the vestibular population. *OT Practice, 23*(11), 22–24.

Porter, R. S. (Ed.). (2018). *The Merck manual of diagnosis and therapy* (20th ed.). Merck Sharp & Dohme.

Ricci, N. A., Aratani, M. C., Caovilla, H. H., Cohen, H. S., & Ganança, F. F. (2014). Evaluation of properties of the Vestibular disorders Activities of Daily Living Scale (Brazilian version) in an elderly population. *Brazilian Journal of Physical Therapy, 18*(2), 174–182. https://doi.org/ 10.1590/S1413-35552012005000144

Roberts, J. C. Cohen, H. S., & Sangi-Haghpeykar, H. (2011). Vestibular disorders and dual task performance: Impairment when walking a straight path. *Journal of Vestibular Research, 21*(3), 167–174. https://doi.org/ 10.3233/VES-2011-0415

Schubert, M. C., Stitz, J., Cohen, H. S., Sangi-Haghpeykar, H., Mulavara, A. P., Peters, B. T., & Bloomberg, J. J. (2017). Prototype tests of vertical and torsional alignment nulling for screening vestibular function. *Journal of Vestibular Rehabilitation, 27*(2-3), 173–176. https:// doi.org/10.3233/VES-170618

BIBLIOGRAPHY

Cohen, H. S. (2011). Assessment of functional outcomes in patients with vestibular disorders after rehabilitation. *NeuroRehabilitation, 29*(2), 173–178. https://doi.org/10.3233/NRE-20 11-0692

Cohen, H. S. (2019). A review on screening tests for vestibular disorders. *Journal of Neurophysiology, 122*(1), 81–92. https://doi.org/ 10.1152/jn.00819.2018

Cohen, H. S., Mulavara, A. P., Sangi-Haghpeykar, H., Peters, B. T., Bloomberg, J. J., & Pavlik, V. N. (2014). Screening people in the waiting room for vestibular impairments. *Southern Medical Journal, 107*(9), 549–553. https://doi.org/10.14423/SMJ.000000000000017

Cohen, H. S., Sangi-Haghpeykar, H., Ricci, N., Kampangkaew, J., & Williamson, R. A. (2014). Utility of stepping, walking, and head impulses for screening patients for vestibular impairments. *Otolaryngology–Head and Neck Surgery, 151*(1), 131–136. https://doi.org/10.1177/01 94599814527724

Cohen, H. S., Stitz, J., Sangi-Haghpeykar, H., Williams, S. P., Mulavara, A. P., Peters, B. T., & Bloomberg, J. J. (2018). Utility of quick oculomotor tests for screening the vestibular system in the subacute and chronic populations. *Acta Oto-Laryngologica, 138*(4), 382–386. https://doi.org/10.1080/00016489.2017.1398838

Li, C.-M., Hoffman, H. J., Ward, B. K., Cohen, H. S., & Rine, R. M. (2016). Epidemiology of dizziness and balance problems in children in the United States: A population-based study. *Journal of Pediatrics, 171*, 240–247. https://doi.org/10.1016/j.jpeds.2015.12.002

Visual Impairment Due to Neurologic Conditions

Also called visual dysfunction, vision dysfunction, vision impairment.
See also Low Vision and Visual Loss, Unilateral Spatial Neglect,
Visual Impairment in Children and Adolescents.

Description

This chapter discusses visual impairment due to neurological conditions such as a stroke, multiple sclerosis, brain injury, or brain tumor. Visual impairment or dysfunction can result in changes to visual acuity, visual fields, color vision, night vision, contrast sensitivity, glare sensitivity, ocular motor (accommodation, alignment, vergence), cranial nerve palsy, visual fixation, visual perception, visual pursuit, or visual motor integration (Chung & Slowman, 2017).

Cause

Most frequent causes are disease, injury, aging, or a combination of the three. Anatomical location of impairment may be the parietal lobe (visual attention, spatial relations), occipital lobe and optic tract (visual field loss), temporal lobe (visual perception, discrimination color), eye structures, or cranial nerves II, III, IV, and VI (oculomotor control; Blanchard et al., 2016; Chung & Slowman, 2017). Norup et al. (2016) reported, in a consecutive sample of stroke clients, that a quarter had visual or visuo-attentional deficits during the initial assessment. Visual concerns continue into the poststroke period (Smith et al., 2018).

Types of Visual Impairment

- *Accommodation deficits:* Difficulty changing the focus from distant to near or near to distant objects. Involves pupil constriction, vergence, and change in convexity of the lens (Chung & Slowman, 2017).
- *Alignment/misalignment (binocular vision):* If the eyes are not aligned and do not work together, diplopia (double vision) occurs, in which the images may be displaced horizontally, vertically, or diagonally in relation to each other (Burgess & Jewell, 2018; Chung & Slowman, 2017).
- *Asthenopia:* Eye strain.
- *Binocular vision deficit:* Difficulty of the visual system to fuse or combine the information from the right and left eyes to form one image (Wagener et al., 2013).
- *Contrast sensitivity deficit:* Difficulty detecting the borders of objects by contrast from their backgrounds (Maskill & Grieve, 2017).
- *Convergence insufficiency:* Inability of the eye muscles to stay focused on one point or object (Chung & Slowman, 2017). (Note: not a synonym for visual neglect or attention deficit.)
- *Cranial nerve palsy:* Paralysis of one or more the cranial nerves controlling eye muscles (C-III, C-IV, or C-VI), which limits eye movements.
- *Depth perception (lack of):* Difficulty determining the distance of objects from the body based on vision alone.

- *Diplopia (double vision):* See Alignment/Misalignment (above).
- *Esophoria:* One or both eyes have a tendency to turn out.
- *Exophoria:* One or both eyes have a tendency to turn in.
- *Fixation deficit:* Difficulty fixing or stopping the gaze on specific visual data.
- *Functional/dysfunctional vision:* Functional vision is the effective use of vision to perform everyday activities such as mobility, learning, communicating, applying knowledge, ADLs, IADLs, interpersonal interactions, leisure activities, work, and relationships. Dysfunction is the degree to which impaired visual function at the organ level interferes with or prevents the person from performing everyday activities (Roberts et al., 2016).
- *Hemispatial inattention:* Refers to the brain's inability to attend to one side of the client's environment as strongly as it does to the opposite side (Lighthill et al., 2013).
- *Hyperphoria:* One eye has a tendency to turn upward.
- *Ocular motor control dysfunction:* Difficulty performing the eye mobility functions that allow the eyes to move in a smooth and coordinated manner. Areas of ocular motor function that can be affected include alignment of the eyes, vergence, accommodation, scanning, and saccades (Chung & Slowman, 2017).
- *Pattern recognition:* Involves identifying the salient features of an object and using these features to distinguish the object from its surroundings (Warren, 2018).
- *Posttrauma vision syndrome (PTVS):* Characterized by exotropia, exophoria, convergence, and accommodative insufficiency, oculomotor dysfunction, and myopia. Client may report systems such as diplopia, blurred near vision eye strain (asthenopia), sensitivity to light (photophobia), and perceived movement of print or stationary objects (Hudac et al., 2012).
- *Saccade deficits:* Difficulty performing rapid eye movements from one point to another that affects tracking and reading (Chung & Slowman, 2017).
- *Scanning, tracking, or pursuit deficits:* Difficulty seeing visual data in an organized manner, usually from left to right but can be top to bottom (Chung & Slowman, 2017).
- *Scotoma:* Dark or blind spot within the visual field.
- *Strabismus:* Deficit of binocularity in which the two eyes do not work together to pursue or track visual data. The result may be that visual data is lost or repeated depending on where one eye leaves off and the other one picks up.
- *Vergence deficits:* Difficulty or inability to focus the eyes on a single point by simultaneous movement of the pupils toward (convergence) or away from (divergence) one another to adjust for different distances between the eyes and the visual target (Chung & Slowman, 2017).
- *Visual acuity deficits:* Difficulty seeing details clearly at all distances from the eyes. Includes nearsightedness and farsightedness. Usually measured using high-contrast letter charts (Hunt & Bassi, 2010; Maskill & Grieve, 2017).
- *Visual agnosia:* The inability to recognize familiar objects by sight in the absence of any other significant visual or intellectual impairment (Maskill & Grieve, 2017).
  - ▸ *Apperceptive agnosia:* Failure to form a stable perceptual representation of objects. Person is unable to match or copy shapes or objects based on visual alone. More common in right hemisphere lesions.
  - ▸ *Associative (sematic) agnosia:* Inability to recognize familiar objects when visual perception is intact. Person can name objects, but cannot describe the function of the object. More common in left hemisphere lesions.
- *Visual attention deficit:* Lack of or difficulty attending to visual objects or information (Warren, 2018).
- *Visual cognition (visuocognition):* Ability to manipulate visual input and integrate vision with other sensory information to gain knowledge, solve problems, formulate plans, and make decision (Warren, 2018).
- *Visual field deficits:* The visual field is the area of view of the external world seen by the two eyes without movement of the head (Blaylock et al., 2016; Faieta & Page, 2016; Grider et al.,

2014, Maskill & Grieve, 2017). Deficits are blind segments in one or more areas of the field of vision.

- ► *Homonymous hemianopsia:* Blind areas in the right visual field of both eyes or left visual field of both eyes.
- ► *Homonymous quadrantanopia:* Blind areas in right or left visual field that affect superior or inferior quadrants of both eyes (Chung & Slowman, 2017).
- *Visual memory deficit:* Difficulty creating, retaining, and recalling memories of visual images to use for comparison during visual analysis (Warren, 2018).
- *Visual midline shift syndrome (VMSS):* Causes an altered sense of midline orientation. When standing or walking, client may lean excessively to their nonaffected side, attempting to compensate for the altered sense of midline (Lighthill et al., 2013). Client may report that the walls appear to be moving and floor tilted (Hudac et al., 2012).
- *Visual motor deficits:* Impairment in the ability to integrate visual data with motor planning and action.
- *Visual perception deficits:* Impairment in the ability to integrate visual data taken in through the eyes with the sensory system for higher cognitive function (Chung & Slowman, 2017). Includes deficits in figure–ground, form constancy, and size discrimination.
- *Visual scanning:* see Scanning (above).
- *Visual stress:* Term used to describe visual discomfort and perceptual distortions in print text.

Evaluation/Assessment

Areas

- Activities of Daily Living/Instrumental ADL: reading directions and labels, writing checks, functional mobility, medication management, driving, shopping
- Education/Work: academic performance, reading comprehension
- Play/Leisure: type, frequency, location, level of satisfaction
- Rest/Sleep: sleep disturbances such as headache or pain
- Social Participation: type, frequency, location, with whom
- Sensorimotor: balance with eyes open versus closed, navigation in space, ocular motor function, visual motor integration
- Cognitive/Perceptual: visual attention and concentration, visual memory, visual perception skills, visual agnosia
- Psychosocial: depression, anxiety, role performance, self-efficacy, quality of life
- Context/Environment: lighting, home and community safety, resources
- Comorbidities: stroke, traumatic brain injury, tumor, Parkinson's disease, multiple sclerosis, cerebral palsy, other neurological condition affecting the brain and visual system, diabetes, diabetic retinopathy, macular degeneration, cataracts, glaucoma, presbyopia

Instruments

Instruments Developed by Occupational Therapy Personnel

- Assessment of Motor and Process Skills (8th ed.; AMPS-8; Fisher & Bray Jones, 2016)
- Brain Injury Visual Assessment Battery for Adults (biVABA; Warren, 1998; see also Wagener et al., 2013, in References)
- Occupational Therapy Vision Screening (OTVS; Herron, 2016, in References)
- Self-Report Assessment of Functional Visual Performance (SRAFVP; Gilbert & Baker, 2011; see also Mennem et al., 2012, in References)

Instruments Developed by Other Professionals and Used by Occupational Therapy Personnel

- Adult Developmental Eye Movement Test (A-DEM; Sampedro et al., 2005)
- Amsler grid (assessment chart): Person looks at a dot matrix on a grid with each eye separately to detect visual field losses or damage to the macula (if the person perceives wavy lines or missing squares on the grid)

- Behavioral Inattention Test (BIT; Wilson et al., 1987)
- Biometrics E-LINK evaluation (computerized dynamometer; https://www.biometricsltd.com/rehab.htm)
- Chronister Pocket Acuity Chart (CPAC; Gulden Ophthalmics; https://guldenophthalmics.com/)
- College of Optometrists in Vision Development Quality of Life Assessment (COVD-QOL; Mozlin, 1995; see also Wagener et al., 2013, in References)
- Convergence test: Move a penlight toward the bridge of the nose until it reaches point of convergence, usually about 3 inches from bridge of nose, to observe the eye's ability to converge
- Cover test: Focus on a central target, with one eye covered, to determine whether uncovered eye can fixate
- Developmental Test of Visual Perception–Adolescent and Adult (2nd ed.; DTVP-A:2; Reynolds et al., 2021)
- Dynamic Functional Task Observation Checklist (DFTOC; Sister Kenny Rehabilitation Institute; see Wagener et al., 2013, in References)
- Functional Vision Performance Test (FVPT; McCabe et al., 2000)
- Gulden Fixation Stick (Gulden Ophthalmics; https://guldenophthalmics.com)
- Hirschberg technique: Fixate on a penlight and observe light reflection in eyes to see where the light is reflected on the cornea to detect ocular misalignment
- LEA Numbers Chart for Vision Rehabilitation (Good-Lite: https://www.good-lite.com)
- LEA Numbers Low-Contrast Test, 10M (Good-Lite; https://www.good-lite.com)
- Lea Symbols Test (Good-Lite; https://www.good-lite.com)
- MNREAD Acuity Chart (Regents of the University of Minnesota, 1994)
- Morgan Low Vision Reading Comprehension Assessment (MLVRCA; Watson et al., 1996)
- Motor-Free Visual Perceptual Test (4th ed.; MVPT-4; Colarusso & Hammill, 2015)
- National Eye Institute Visual Function Questionnaire (NEIVFQ; Mangione et al., 1998)
- Northeastern State College of Optometry (NSUCO) Oculomotor Test (Pursuits and Saccades; Maples et al., 1992; see also Wagener et al., 2013, in References)
- Pepper Visual Skills Reading Test (PVSRT; Watson et al., 1995)
- Posturography (see Taylor et al., 2012, in References)
- Saccades test: Alternate fixating between two objects at 6 inches apart and 16 inches from bridge of nose to observe eye's ability to rapidly and smoothly move between objects
- Sister Kenny Dynamic Visual Task Observation Checklist (SKDVTOC; see Dynamic Visual Task Observation Checklist)
- Snellen chart: Eye acuity chart test
- Stereo Randot Test (Bernell VTP; https://www.bernell.com; see also Wagener et al., 2013, in References)
- Stereo Randot Test (SRT; Lombart Instrument; https://lombartinstrument.com/store/stereo-randot-test)
- Target and fixation test: Have person visually locate and fixate on a target
- Test of Visual Perceptual Skills (nonmotor; 4th ed.; TVPS-4; Martin, 2017)
- Visual Functioning Questionnaire 25 (VFQ-25; National Eye Institute, 2000)

Problems/Issues

Activities of Daily Living/Instrumental ADL

- Person may experience difficulty reading recipes or labels to prepare meals or use an object.
- Person may have difficulty seeing the correct amount of financial statements, such as bills, and write checks or enter amounts online incorrectly.
- Person may have difficulty reading instructions to take medications correctly or lose track of location of medication due to visual field loss.
- Person may have difficulty putting on makeup or shaving mustache.

- Person may have difficulty locating items and getting the correct items when shopping due to slow scanning or failure to see items in the visual field.
- Person may be unable to drive (see Driving Fitness in Section 13: Lifestyle Conditions).

Education/Work
- Person may experience difficulty reading and following instructions for classroom or work assignments.
- Person may be unable to continue working or engaging in a specific occupation if work tasks involve certain visual skills, such as rapid saccades, sustained visual attention/concentration, or excellent eye–hand coordination.

Play/Leisure
- Person may avoid leisure activities that require visual skills, such as reading, or sports that rely on visuomotor integration, such as batting or kicking a ball.

Rest/Sleep
- Not discussed.

Social Participation
- Person may be unable to participate in social activities that require visual skills, such as rapid saccades, or good visual perception, such as playing a card game.
- Person may discontinue participation because of perceived inability to "keep up" with others in processing visual information.

Sensorimotor
- Person may have impaired mobility or get lost due to visual dysfunction.
- Person may have poor eye–hand coordination (visual motor integration).
- Person may have decreased saccadic eye movements affecting ability of the eyes to move rapidly to look from one place to another, impacting reading, walking, and driving.
- Person may have decreased vertical eye movements affecting the ability to look up and down, as may be needed to read a large menu or a list of names and locations in an office building.
- Person may experience diplopia or double vision, which may interfere with walking, driving, reading, watching TV, or engaging in leisure activities.
- Person may experience convergent insufficiency, which may make focusing the eyes on a single object or target difficult.
- Person may lack visual accommodation, which interferes with the ability to quickly change focus from far to near or vice versa, making changing focus while driving difficult.
- Person may lack eye alignment (binocularity), resulting in double vision.
- Person may have difficulty scanning or visually searching the environment.
- Person may complain of headaches or tired eyes after performing visual tasks.
- Person may experience nausea or dizziness after performing visual tasks.
- Person may complain the visual images are blurry or the straight horizontal and vertical lines are wavy or squiggly.
- Person may squint to avoid light or reduce glare.
- Person may tilt or cock the head to one side.
- Person may use fingers or hands as guides along a wall when walking or touch furniture while navigating a room.
- Person may have difficulty judging distances due to lack of depth perception.
- Person may be unable to fixate eye gaze if head is turned (isolating head/eye movement).

Cognitive/Perceptual
- Person may experience visual neglect (see Unilateral Spatial Neglect in Section 11: Cognitive-Perceptual Disorders).
- Person may experience light sensitivity (glare).

- Person may experience decreased visual attention and concentration.
- Person may have visual agnosia, resulting in difficulty recognizing objects.
- Person may have difficulty with form discrimination, making differentiation and recognition of shapes and forms difficult.
- Person may be unable to recognize and identify pictures.

Psychosocial
- Person may lose self-confidence and sense of self-efficacy related to loss of visual skills.
- Person may experience fear and frustration due to visual impairment.
- Person may experience increasing social isolation because of visual impairment.
- Person may have difficulty recognizing family and friends (prosopagnosia).
- Person may experience decreased quality of life.

Context/Environment
- Person may have difficulty navigating home and community safely and securely.
- Family and friends may not understand the problem is related to visual impairment, not dementia or motor impairment.

Intervention/Treatment

Models and programs developed by occupational therapy personnel include the hierarchy of visual perceptual processing model (Warren, 2018), and person-environment-occupation model (Perea & Anise, 2019). Models and programs developed by other professionals but used by occupational therapy personnel include computer-based compensatory therapy (Mödden et al., 2012), constraint-induced therapy with eye patching (Wu et al., 2013), Dynavision (Anderson et al., 2011; Wagener et al., 2013), independence matters (Sant, 2017), scanning training (Hazelton et al., 2019), treating homonymous hemianopia (Perea & Anise, 2019), visual scanning training (Turton, 2014; Turton et al., 2015; Turton et al., 2018), and yoked prism lenses (Lighthill et al., 2013). Team members may include neuro-ophthalmologists, optometrists/neuro-optometrists, vision rehabilitation specialists, other types of physicians, nursing personnel, physical therapists, speech–language pathologists, neuropsychologists, psychologists, social workers, therapeutic recreation specialists, and occupational therapy personnel. Most intervention goals are based on compensatory and adaptive approaches since many remedial approaches have little evidence of reversing or repairing visual dysfunction. The focus is to enable the client to use current visual abilities to participate in valued and meaningful activities and occupations (Warren, 2018).

Activities of Daily Living/Instrumental ADL
- Reading a recipe, preparing a meal, setting the table.
- Washing, drying, sorting clothes, ironing, putting clothes away, organizing closet/drawers.
- Organizing pantry, spice rack, freezer, clothes closet, drawers.
- Dusting, vacuuming, cleaning up.
- Walking outdoors, including crossing roads.
- Shopping: groceries, clothing.
- Riding bicycle in a park or in limited traffic area.
- Visiting a park, searching for wildlife.

Education/Work
- Organizing work tools and space (a place for everything and everything in its place).
- Simplify/declutter work environment so essential tools are within easy reach.

Play/Leisure
- Card games: use cards with enlarged pips (numbers, symbols).
- Table/board games: use large pieces with unique colors or markings.
- Computer games: enlarge symbols on screen, add sound if available.

- Games on smartphone: add sound.
- Ball games (throwing and catching): use large balls with unique colors or markings and/or sounds.

Rest/Sleep
- Not discussed (see Sleep–Wake Disorders in Section 13: Lifestyle Conditions).

Social Participation
- Participate in social activities with family and friends.

Sensorimotor
- Auditory stimulation (AVT) may be useful to encourage visual field exploration. A visual stimulus is presented such as a light-emitting diode accompanied by a white noise auditory stimulus. When the client presses a button or flips a switch to turn off the light, the auditory stimulus is also shut off.
- Vision restorative therapy uses lights, letters, or objects randomly outside the intact field of view and asks the client to locate the items. Minimum evidence of effectiveness (Berger et al., 2016).
- Prisms: Partial occlusion: used for binocular diplopia.

Cognitive/Perceptual
- Visual perception training/retraining should begin with training/retraining the three basic elements of the visual hierarchy: oculomotor control, visual fields, and visual acuity, followed by attention, scanning, pattern recognition, visual memory, visuo-cognition leading to adaptation through vision.
- Visual acuity: Compensatory strategies
  - ▶ Lighting: Determine best lighting/illumination for the task that also minimizes glare, place light below client's glasses or optical device if possible, use task lamps for reading (near vision tasks).
  - ▶ Increase contrast: Use black on white, dark on light, contrasting colored tape to mark edge of the stairs or door.
  - ▶ Increase/enlarge: Enlarge print, use think markers, enlarge computer font, use magnification: handheld, stand, or lobe magnifiers.
  - ▶ Decrease background pattern or clutter: Use solid-colored bedspreads, use plain dishes and solid-colored placemats, reduce number of different items stored together.
  - ▶ Organize the environment: Put objects/items/things away, organize storge places, label drawers.
  - ▶ Visual markers: For reading, a ruler under the line being read; for dials, put tape or stickers on most commonly used settings.
  - ▶ Provide sensory substitution using assistive devices or tactile cues.
- Saccade exercises
  - ▶ Have client scan the table to match labeled lids to appropriate can or jars.
  - ▶ Have client move eyes from one target (thumb, pencil) to another starting with short distance and increasing distance as quickly as possible.
- Convergence
  - ▶ Have client copy information from a wall chart or white board to paper on table.
  - ▶ Have client hold out both index fingers, one at arm's length away and the other about 3 inches from the nose. Client alternates looking at distant finger the then close finger and back again.
- Pursuits
  - ▶ In a darkened room have client use a flashlight to search for a list of items.
  - ▶ Have client follow a pencil top or finger in all directions in a smooth and consistent motion while keeping head still.

- Gaze stabilization/Focused attention
  - ▶ Client fixes gaze on a target at midline and eye level. Client then turns head side to side wile maintain eyes forward and fixed on the target.
- Visual memory: Clients are asked to recall words, letters, or numbers, and touch them on a screen or white board in a certain order.
- Grade tasks from simple to more complex.
  - ▶ Begin setting up tasks in organized manner and move to more disorganized visual array.
  - ▶ Start with easy to discriminate objects and more to those that are harder to discriminate in shape, size, or function.
  - ▶ Begin without timing the task and then add timing component.
  - ▶ Change body position from seated, to standing, or to ambulatory.
  - ▶ Start with high contrast and move to less contrast.
  - ▶ Start with large, widely spaced print and move to smaller, less separated print.
  - ▶ Start with structured items in evenly spaced rows or columns, using the same sized font and move to unevenly spaced rows or columns, using a mixed of fonts and sizes.
  - ▶ Start with low-density visual stimuli (object and background are clearly differentiated and the number of stimuli are limited) and move to high-density visual stimuli (object and background are not clearly differentiated and the number of stimuli are unlimited; e.g., high-density shelves in a grocery store or pharmacy section shelf).

Psychosocial

- Social skills training
  - ▶ If client has not previously worn glasses, discuss with client advantages and disadvantages of wearing glasses in public places and social activities.
  - ▶ Practice with client asking for help when visual assistance is needed, such as in a dark movie theater.
  - ▶ Practice placing hand on person's arm near the elbow so sighted person is moving slightly ahead.

Context/Environment

- Educate family and caregivers about proper use of glasses. Proper glasses for tasks such as distance, reading, or computer monitor. Progressive or trifocal glasses; upper portion is for distance, middle portion for immediate (reading computer monitor/screen), and lower for reading.
- Educate family and caregivers about proper use of monovision contacts: One eye is used for distance and other for near vision.
- Educate family and caregivers about visual impairment and how to manage the client in the home and community.
- Consider use of talking/audio devices to assist vision.
- Modifications in lighting, contrast, pattern, and size can facilitate (or impede) person's ability to engage and function better within the environment. Principles are as follows:
  - ▶ Increase contrast of key components of a task and environment: increase contrast between background and object such as black or white.
  - ▶ Reduce or eliminate background patterns: use solid colors, not patterns, and reduce clutter and unneeded objects.
  - ▶ Enlarge critical features of objects and environments (magnifiers, font size).
  - ▶ Provide adequate, good-quality illumination.
  - ▶ Provide clear pathways for navigating environment.
  - ▶ Educate staff to check that glasses or other visual aids are available during performance of ADLs and rehabilitation sessions.

Precautions/Safety Considerations

Person with visual impairments is at risk for falls. Person with homonymous hemianopsia is at increased risk for bumping into objects, causing bruising or cuts. Medications may cause visual impairment. Person with blast injuries is at risk for visual dysfunction. Older persons with any neurological disorder should be screened for visual impairment (Roche et al., 2014; Siong et al., 2014).

Prognosis and Outcome

Variable. Many people can adjust to limited or impaired vision. Numerous devices are available to assist and compensate for visual deficits. Attitude, ability, and willingness to learn and adapt are key elements to a successful outcome

REFERENCES

Anderson, L., Cross, A., Wynthein, D., Schmidt, L., & Grutz, K. (2011). Effects of Dynavision training as a preparatory intervention status postcerebrovascular accident: A case report. *Occupational Therapy in Health Care, 25*(4), 270–282. https://doi.org/10.3109/07380577.2011.589888

Berger, S., Kaldenberg, J., Selmane, R., & Carlo, S. (2016). Effectiveness of interventions to address visual and visual-perceptual impairments to improve occupational performance in adults with traumatic brain injury: A systematic review. *American Journal of Occupational Therapy, 70*(3), Article 7003180010. https://doi.org/10.5014/ajot.2016.020875

Blanchard, S., Change, W. P., Heronema, A. M., Rancharan, D. D., Stanton, K. L., & Stollberg, J. E. (2016). Common occupational therapy vision rehabilitation interventions for impaired and low vision associated with brain injury. *Optometry & Performance, 4*(5), 265–274.

Blaylock, S. E., Warren, M., Yuen, H. K., & DeCarlo, D. K. (2016). Validation of a reading assessment for persons with homonymous hemianopia or quadrantanopia. *Archives of Physical Medicine and Rehabilitation, 97*(9), 1515–1519. https://doi.org/10.1016/j.apmr.2016.02.022

Burgess, G., & Jewell, V. D. (2018). Occupational therapists' perspectives on binocular diplopia in neurorehabilitation: A national survey. *NeuroRehabilitation, 42*(2), 223–233. https://doi.org/10.3233/NRE-172263

Chung, A., & Slowman, L. S. (2017). *Clinical review: Visual dysfunction: Occupational therapy.* EBSCO Information Services.

Faieta, J., & Page, S. (2016). Visual impairment after a stroke. *Archives of Physical Medicine and Rehabilitation, 97*(11), 2021–2022. https://doi.org/10.1016/j.apmr.2016.06.002

Grider, S. L., Yuen, H. K., Vogtle, L. K., & Warren, M. (2014). Visual concerns that interfere with daily activities in patients on rehabilitation units: A descriptive study. *Occupational Therapy in Health Care, 28*(4), 362–370. https://doi.org/10.3109/07380577.2014.933946

Hazelton, C., Pollock, A., Walsh, G., & Brady, M. C. (2019). Scanning training for rehabilitation of visual field loss due to stroke: Identifying and exploring training tools in use. *British Journal of Occupational Therapy, 82*(8), 502–511. https://doi.org/10.1177/0308022618809900

Herron, S. (2016). Review of experience with a collaborative eye care clinic in inpatient stroke rehabilitation. *Topics in Stroke Rehabilitation, 23*(1), 67–75. https://doi.org/10.1179/1074935715Z.00000000065

Hudac, C. M., Kota, S., Nedrow, J. L., & Molfese, D. L. (2012). Neural mechanisms underlying neurooptometric rehabilitation following traumatic brain injury. *Eye and Brain, 2012*(4), 1–12. https://doi.org/10.2147/EB.S27290

Hunt, L. A., & Bassi, C. J. (2010). Near-vision acuity levels and performance on neuropsychological assessments used in occupational therapy. *American Journal of Occupational Therapy, 64*(1), 105–113. https://doi.org/10.5014/ajot.64.1.105

Lighthill, C. R., Perez, E. E., & McWilliams, K. B. (2013). Coming into focus: Brain injury and vision therapy. *Rehab Management, 26*(9), 20–23.

Maskill, L., & Grieve, J. (2017). Visual perception, recognition and agnosia. In L. Maskill & S. Tempest (Eds.), *Neuropsychology for occupational therapists* (4th ed., pp. 89–111). Wiley Blackwell.

Mennem, T. A., Warren, M., & Yuen, H. K. (2012). Preliminary validation of a vision-dependent activities of daily living instrument on adults with homonymous hemianopia. *American Journal of Occupational Therapy, 66*(4), 478–482. https://doi.org/10.5014/ajot.2012.004762

Mödden, C., Behrens, M., Damke, I., Eilers, N., Kastrup, A., & Hildebrandt, H. (2012). A randomized controlled trial comparing 2 interventions for visual field loss with standard occupational therapy during inpatient stroke rehabilitation. *Neurorehabilitation and Neural Repair*, 26(5), 463–469. https://doi.org/10.1177/1545968311425927

Norup, A., Guldberg, A. M., Friis, C. R., Deurell, E. M., & Forchhammer, H. B. (2016). An interdisciplinary visual team in an acute and sub-acute stroke unit: Providing assessment and early rehabilitation. *NeuroRehabilitation*, 39(3), 451–461. https://doi.org/10.3233/NRE-161376

Perea, J. D., & Anise, M. C. (2019). Beyond cueing to the life and a red line: Treatment methods for homonymous hemianopia. *SIS Quarterly Practice Connections*, 4(2), 28–30.

Roberts, P. S., Rizzo, J.-R., Hreha, K., Wertheimer, J., Kaldenberg, J., Hironaka, D., Riggs, R., & Colenbrander, A. (2016). A conceptual model for vision rehabilitation. *Journal of Rehabilitation Research and Development*, 53(6), 693–704. https://doi.org/10.1682/JRRD.2015.06.0113

Roche, S., Vogtle, L., Warren, M., & O'Connor, K. A. (2014). Assessment of the visual status of older adults on an orthopedic unit. *American Journal of Occupational Therapy*, 68(4), 465–471. https://doi.org/10.5014/ajot.2014.010231

Sant, C. (2017). Living with sight loss. *OT News*, 25(11), 38–39.

Siong, K. H., Woo, G. C., Chan, D. Y.-L., Chung, K. Y. K., Li, L. S. W., Cheung, H. K. Y., Lai, C. K. Y., & Cheong, A. M. Y. (2014). Prevalence of visual problems among stroke survivors in Hong Kong Chinese. *Clinical and Experimental Optometry*, 97(5), 433–441. https://doi.org/10.1111/cxo.12166

Smith, T. M., Pappadis, M. R., Krishnan, S., & Reistetter, T. A. (2018). Stroke survivor and caregiver perspectives on post-stroke visual concerns and long-term consequences. *Behavioral Neurology*, 2018, Article 1463429. https://doi.org/10.1155/2018/1463429

Taylor, L., Poland, F., & Stephenson, R. (2012). A pilot study exploring head and shoulder movement in visual field deficits following stroke. *International Journal of Therapy and Rehabilitation*, 19(8), 471–477.

Turton, A. (2014). *Final project report: Description and measurement of visual scanning training in occupational therapy for patients with visual search deficits following stroke*. College of Occupational Therapists.

Turton, A. J., Angilley, J., Chapman, M., Daniel, A., Longley, V., Clatworthy, P., & Gilchrist, I. D. (2015). Visual search training occupational therapy—an example of expert practice in community-based stroke rehabilitation. *British Journal of Occupational Therapy*, 78(11), 674–687. https://doi.org/10.1177/0308022615600180

Turton, A. J., Angilley, J., Longley, V., Clatworthy, P., & Gilchrist, I. D. (2018). Search training for people with visual field loss after stroke: A cohort study. *British Journal of Occupational Therapy*, 81(5), 255–265. https://doi.org/10.1177/0308022617743481

Warren, M. (2018). Evaluation and treatment of visual deficits after brain injury. In H. M. Pendleton & W. Schultz-Krohn (Eds.), *Pedretti's occupational therapy: Practice skills for physical dysfunction* (8th ed., pp. 594–630). Elsevier.

Wagener, S. G., Anheluk, M., Arulanantham, C., & Scheiman, M. (2013). Vision assessment and intervention. In M. Weightman, M. V. Radomski, P. A. Mashima, & C. R. Roth (Eds.), *Mild traumatic brain injury rehabilitation toolkit* (pp. 97–146). Borden Institute.

Wu, C.-Y., Wang, T.-N., Chen, Y.-T., Lin, K.-C., Chen, Y.-A., Li, H.-T., & Tsai, P.-L. (2013). Effects of constraint-induced therapy combined with eye patching on functional outcomes and movement kinematics in poststroke neglect. *American Journal of Occupational Therapy*, 67(2), 236–245. https://doi.org/10.5014/ajot.2013.006486

BIBLIOGRAPHY

American Academy of Ophthalmology. (2017). *Vision rehabilitation preferred practice pattern: Appendix 6. Occupational therapy for patients with vision loss*. https://doi.org/10.1016/j.ophtha.2017.09.030

Brown, T., Elliott, S., Bourne, R., Sutton, E., Wigg, S., Morgan, D., Glass, S., & Lalor, A. (2011). The discriminative validity of three visual perception tests. *New Zealand Journal of Occupational Therapy, 58*(2), 14–22.

Butler, M., & Hollestelle, E. (2017). Visual impairment following acquired brain injury: A survey of occupational therapy practice in New Zealand. *New Zealand Journal of Occupational Therapy, 64*(2), 32–38.

Hellerstein, L. F., Scheiman, M., Fishman, B., & Whittaker, S. G. (2011). Visual rehabilitation for patients with brain injury. In M. Scheiman (Ed.), *Understanding and managing vision deficits: A guide for occupational therapists* (3rd ed., pp. 201–232). Slack.

Jarvis, K., Grant, E., Rowe, F., Evans, J., & Cristino-Amenos, M. (2012). Impact of visual impairment assessment of functional recovery in stroke patients: A pilot randomized controlled trial. *International Journal of Therapy and Rehabilitation, 19*(1), 11–20.

Pollock, A., Hazelton, C., & Brady, M. (2011). Visual problems after stroke: A survey of current practice by occupational therapists working in UK stroke inpatient settings. *Topics in Stroke Rehabilitation, 18*(Suppl. 1), 643–651. https://doi.org/10.1310/tsr18s01-643

Scheiman, M. (2011). *Understanding and managing vision deficits: A guide for occupational therapists* (3rd ed.). Slack.

APPENDIX A

The following vision assessments, commonly used, are described in Wagener et al. (2013).

- Distance Visual Acuity Testing, p. 104
- Accommodative Amplitude Test, pp. 105–106
- Near Point Convergence, pp. 107–108
- Binocular Vision: Eye Alignment Test, pp. 108–110
- Saccades: Developmental Eye Movement Test, pp. 110–112
- Confrontation Field Test, pp. 116–118

APPENDIX B

The following vision interventions are described in Wagener et al. (2013).

- Poor Acuity, pp. 123–125
- Impaired Pursuits, pp. 125–127, 129
- Impaired Saccades, pp. 127–128, 129
- Impaired Accommodation, pp. 128, 130
- Impaired Convergence, pp. 131–133
- Diplopia, pp. 133–134
- Visual Field Loss, pp. 135–136
- Visual Neglect and Inattention, pp. 136–139
- Glare/Photophobia Management pp. 139–140

Visual Impairment in Children and Adolescents

See also Low Vision, Visual Impairments Due to Neurologic Conditions.

Description

Visual impairment is defined by the Individuals with Disabilities Education Improvement Act (2004) as "any impairment in vision that even with correction adversely affects a child's educational performance" (Sec. 300.8[c][13]).

Cause

Etiologies may include congenital eye conditions, acquired brain injuries, tumors, diseases or injuries affecting the eye, optic nerve, optic tract, optic chiasm, or optic lobe. Examples include retinopathy of prematurity, ocular malformations, congenital glaucoma, optic atrophy, retinal dystrophies, congenital cataracts, toxoplasmic macular retinochoroiditis, and degenerative disorders of the retina and macula. Additional sources of visual impairment include neurological disorders such as cerebral palsy (Denver et al., 2017).

Terminology

- *Visual agnosia:* Loss or impairment of ability to recognize and understand the nature of visual stimuli (VandenBos, 2015).
- *Visual attention:* Process by which one item (the target) is selected for analysis from among several competing items (the distractors; VandenBos, 2015).
- *Visual closure:* Ability to identify a familiar object from an incomplete visual presentation (VandenBos, 2015).
- *Visual field:* Extent of visual space over which vision is possible with the eyes held in a fixed position (VandenBos, 2015).
- *Visual form discrimination:* Ability to discriminate visually between different shapes (VandenBos, 2015).
- *Visual discrimination:* Ability to distinguish shapes, patterns, hidden figures, or other images from similar objects that differ in subtle ways (VandenBos, 2015).
- *Visual memory:* Capacity to remember what has previously been seen in the form of visual images (VandenBos, 2015).
- *Visual motor coordination:* Ability to coordinate vision with movements of the body or parts of the body (Jacobs & Simon, 2015).
- *Visual motor integration:* Coordinating the interaction of information from the eyes with body movement during activity (Jacobs & Simon, 2015).
- *Visual perception:* Awareness of visual sensation that arises between the physiology of the visual system and internal and external environments of the observer (VandenBos, 2015).
- *Visual pursuit:* Movement of the eyes in an attempt to maintain fixation on a moving target (also called ocular pursuit: visual tracking; VanderBos, 2015).
- *Visual recognition:* Ability to recognize an object visually (VandenBos, 2015).
- *Visual search:* Process of detecting a target visual stimulus among distractor stimuli (VandenBos, 2015).
- *Visual spatial ability (visuospatial):* Ability to comprehend and conceptualize visual representations and spatial relationships in learning and in performance of task such as reading maps, navigating mazes, conceptualizing object in space from different perspectives, and executing various geometric operation (VandenBos, 2015).
- *Visual spatial agnosia:* Inability to analyze spatial relationships or to perform simple construction tasks under visual control (O'Toole, 2017).

Evaluation/Assessment

Areas

- Activities of Daily Living/Instrumental ADL: independent living skills
- Education/Work: academic performance, academic skills
- Play/Leisure: interests, type, frequency, location
- Rest/Sleep: sleep habits
- Social Participation: frequency, location, type, with whom
- Sensorimotor: gross and fine motor skills, visual acuity, visuomotor control, oculomotor control, vergence, visual pursuit, visual scanning, visual discrimination
- Cognitive/Perceptual: visual cognition, visual memory, visual perception, visual figure–ground, visual closure, contrast sensitivity

- Psychosocial: social skills, resilience, social participation, role performance, quality of life
- Context/Environment: adapted devices, social support, community resources
- Development (Infant, Child, Adolescent only): developmental milestone

Instruments

Instruments Developed by Occupational Therapy Personnel

- Canadian Occupational Performance Measure (5th ed.; COPM-5; Law et al., 2014)
- Children's Visual Behaviour Checklist: Age 7–12 (CVBC; Sullivan et al., 2018, in References)
- Erhardt Developmental Visual Assessment (EDVA; Erhardt, 1990)

Instruments Developed by Other Professionals and Used by Occupational Therapy Personnel

- 15 Dimension Questionnaire, Vision scale (15-D; Sintonen & Richardson, 1994)
- Atkinson Battery for Child Development for Examining Functional Vision (ABCDEFV; Atkinson et al., 2002)
- Callier Azusa Scale (CAS; Stillman, 1974)
- Developmental Test of Visual Perception (3rd ed.; DTVP-3; Hammill et al., 2014)
- Functional Vision Screening Questionnaire (FVSQ; Horowitz et al., 1991)
- Health Status Classification System–Preschool, Vision scale (HSCS-PS; Saigal et al., 2005)
- Institutes' Developmental Profile–Visual Competence Scale (IDP-VC; Malkowicz et al., 2006)
- Low Vision Checklist (LVC; Salati et al., 2001)
- Motor-Free Visual Perception (4th ed.; MVPT-4; Colarusso, & Hamill, 2015)
- Perkins-Roman CVI Range (PR-CVI; Perkins School for the Blind)
- Preverbal Visual Assessment (PreViAs; Pueyo et al., 2014)
- Psychological Sense of School Membership (PSSM; Goodenow, 1993)
- Schedule of Growing Skills, Visual Skills Domain (SGS; Bellman & Cash, 1987)
- Social Skills Assessment Tool for Children With Visual Impairments (SSAT-VI; Barclay & Sacks, 2006)
- Test of Visual Perceptual Skills (4th ed.; TVPS-4; Martin, 2017)
- Visual Assessment Procedure–Capacity, Attention, and Processing (VAP-CAP; Blanksby, 1998)
- Visual Skills Inventory (VSI; McCulloch et al., 2007)

Problems/Issues

Activities of Daily Living/Instrumental ADL

- Child may experience difficulty with mobility and be considered clumsy.

Education/Work

- Child may not find academic work challenging due to lack of content for visually impaired students.
- Child/adolescent may not be fully integrated into school schedule and activities.
- Child/adolescent may not be receiving work skills training.

Play/Leisure

- Child may need leisure exploration, especially with peers.
- Child or adolescent may spend much of out of school alone at home (Jessup, Bundy, Broom, & Hancock, 2018).

Rest/Sleep

- No information identified.

Social Participation

- Child may have few friends or social interactions with peers.
- Child may interact primarily with adults (teachers, caregivers, personal assistants).

Sensorimotor

- Child may exhibit a delayed response to visual stimuli.

- Child may have difficulty with accommodation: moving eyes quickly between two items (people, objects) that are near or far.
- Child may have difficulty with saccades, tracking: moving eyes to search the environment.
- Child may have difficulty with pursuits: moving eyes to follow a moving object or persons.
- Child may have difficulty maintaining visual gaze to locate and find an object or person.

Cognitive/Perceptual
- Child may have difficulty maintaining sustained visual contact with objects or persons (inability to keep looking or attending visually).
- Child may have difficulty shifting attention from one object or person to another.
- Child may have difficulty with visual perceptual skills such as form constancy, figure–ground discrimination, position in space, visualization, spatial relations, and visual discrimination.

Psychosocial
- Child may lack social skills with peers.
- Child/adolescent may lack opportunity for self-determination.

Context/Environment
- Child may need additional adapted devices or reassessment of current devices.
- Community resources for visual impaired children/adolescents may be affected by lack of transportation, venues, equipment, information and lack of qualified instructors or people who have positive expectations of them (Jessup et al., 2010).

Intervention/Treatment

Models or programs developed by occupational therapy personnel include the developmental approach for visual perception (Vlok et al., 2011), sensory modulation program (Southwell & Hunt, 2011), and visual perception training (Atasavun Uysal & Düger, 2012). Models or programs developed by other professionals but used by occupational therapy personnel include discrimination training (Tsai et al., 2013), multimedia visual perceptual training (Chen et al., 2013), and online learning (Capili et al., 2019). Team members include ophthalmologists, optometrists, educators (teachers, special education teachers, teacher's aides), psychologists, physical therapists, speech–language pathologists, and occupational therapy personnel. The goal of occupational therapy is to enable the child or adolescent to promote self-help skills and independence, develop motor and perceptual skills in relation to the performance of functional tasks, develop problem solving skills, modify behavior, and provide advice on the purchase of adapted or specialized equipment (Southwell & Hunt, 2011).

Activities of Daily Living/Instrumental ADL
- Assist in instructing client to learn independent living skills such as cooking, cleaning, shopping, using the phone, using public transportation.

Education/Work
- Increase opportunity of students to fully access the curriculum alongside their peers.
- Encourage students to explore, identify, and build on personal strengths.
- Encourage inclusion in school activities (Jessup, Bundy, Broom, & Hancock, 2018).

Play/Leisure
- Increase exploration and development of leisure skills.
- Games can be used to improve visual motor and visual perceptual skills.
- Provide opportunity for play and leisure activities with peers.

Rest/Sleep
- Not discussed.

Social Participation
- Provide opportunities for social activities in a variety of settings.
- Provide opportunities for social interactions with peers.

Sensorimotor
- Practice in visual/tactile discrimination is useful to clients.

Cognitive/Perceptual
- Practice in visual memory is useful in helping clients learn to cope with their environment.

Psychosocial
- Facilitate opportunities to develop friendships with peers.
- Facilitate opportunity to have control (make choices) in situations.
- Facilitate self-determination including sense of autonomy.
- Facilitate self-esteem including sense of confidence and competence.
- Facilitate interpersonal and social skills with peers.
- Facilitate increased sense of resiliency (ability to thrive amid adversity; Jessup et al., 2013; Jessup et al., 2010).
- Facilitate inclusion in social activities (Jessup, Bundy, Hancock, & Broom, 2018).

Context/Environment
- Facilitate learning and practicing moving about safely in the environments including home, school, neighborhood, and frequently visited community buildings (Mashele & Smit, 2011).
- Explore and facilitate use of assistive devices such as talking books, binoculars, image-enlarging video systems, and large-print displays on computers.
- Encourage inclusion in community activities and recreation (Jessup, Bundy, Broom, & Hancock, 2018).

Precautions/Safety Considerations
No information identified.

Prognosis and Outcome
Visual impairment and visual perceptual problems are likely to be lifelong conditions. Compensatory techniques, including adapted orthotic devices, provide useful assistance in managing visual problems.

REFERENCES
Atasavun Uysal, S., & Düger, T. (2012). Visual perception training on social skills and activity performance in low-vision children. *Scandinavian Journal of Occupational Therapy, 19*(1), 33–41. https://doi.org/10.3109/11038128.2011.582512

Capili, T. D., Watson, J. L., & Duffy, J. O. (2019). *Increased accessibility for people with visual impairments in an online learning environment.* American Occupational Therapy Association. https://www.aota.org/-/media/Corporate/Files/Publications/CE-Articles/CE-Article-August-2019.pdf

Chen, Y.-N., Lin, C.-K., Wei, T.-S., Liu, C.-H., & Wuang, Y.-P. (2013). The effectiveness of multimedia visual perceptual training groups for the preschool children with developmental delay. *Research in Developmental Disabilities, 34*(12), 4447–4454. https://doi.org/10.1016/j.ridd.2013.09.023

Denver, B. D., Adolfsson, M., Froude, E., Rosenbaum, P., & Imms, C. (2017). Methods for conceptualising "visual ability" as a measurable construct in children with cerebral palsy. *BMC Medical Research Methodology, 17,* Article 46. https://doi.org/10.1186/s12874-017-0316-6

Individuals with Disabilities Education Improvement Act of 2004, 20 U.S.C. § 1400 *et seq.* (2004). https://sites.ed.gov/idea/regs/b/a/300.8/c/13

Jacobs, K., & Simon, L. (2015). *Quick reference dictionary for occupational therapy.* Slack.

Jessup, G., Bundy, A. C., Broom, A., & Hancock, N. (2018). Fitting in or feeling excluded: The experiences of high school students with visual impairments. *Journal of Visual Impairment & Blindness, 112*(3), 261–273. https://doi.org/10.1177/0145482X1811200305

Jessup, G. M., Bundy, A. C., & Cornell, E. (2013). To be or to refuse to be? Exploring the concept of leisure as resistance for young people who are visually impaired. *Leisure Studies, 32*(2), 191–205. https://doi.org/10.1080/02614367.2012.695388

Jessup, G., Bundy, A. C., Hancock, N., & Broom, A. (2018). Being noticed for the way you are: Social inclusion and high school students with vision impairment. *British Journal of Visual Impairment, 36*(1), 90–103. https://doi.org/10.1177/0264619616686396

Jessup, G., Cornell, E., & Bundy, A. C. (2010). The treasure in leisure activities: Fostering resilience in you people who are blind. *Journal of Visual Impairment & Blindness, 104*(7), 419–430. https://doi.org/10.1177/0145482X1010400705

Mashele, N. P. C., & Smit, N. (2011). Comparing the effect of different living environments on the development of independent living skills in children with visual impairment. *South African Journal of Occupational Therapy, 41*(3), 79–84.

O'Toole, M. T. (Ed). (2017). *Mosby's dictionary of medicine, nursing & health professions* (10th ed.). Elsevier.

Southwell, C., & Hunt, D. (2011). *Visual impairment and occupational therapy: The best of both: Working together to support children with visual impairment and additional complex needs.* RNIB.

Sullivan, C., Lynch, H., & Kirby, A. (2018). Does visual perceptual testing correlate with caregiver and teacher reported functional visual skill difficulties in school-aged children? Considerations for practice. *Irish Journal of Occupational Therapy, 46*(2), 89–105. https://doi.org/10.1108/IJOT-03-2018-0005

Tsai, L.-T., Meng, L.-F., Wu, W.-C. Jang, Y., & Su, Y.-C. (2013). Effects of visual rehabilitation on a child with severe visual impairment. *American Journal of Occupational Therapy, 67*(4), 437–447. https://doi.org/10.5014/ajot.2013.007054

VandenBos, G. R. (Ed.). (2015). *APA dictionary of psychology* (2nd ed.). American Psychological Association.

Vlok, E. D., Smit, N. E., & Bester, J. (2011). A developmental approach: A framework for the development of an integrated visual perception programme. *South African Journal of Occupational Therapy, 41*(3), 25–33. http://www.sajot.co.za/index.php/sajot/article/view/45

BIBLIOGRAPHY

Brown, T. (2012). Are motor-free visual perception skill constructs predictive of visual-motor integration skill constructs? *Hong Kong Journal of Occupational Therapy, 22*(2), 48–59. https://doi.org/10.1016/j.hkjot.2012.06.003

Chaikin, L. R. (2013). Disorders of vision and visual-Perceptual dysfunction. In D. A. Umphred, G. U. Burton, R. T. Lazaro, & M. L. Roller (Eds.), *Umphred's neurological rehabilitation* (6th ed., pp. 863–894). Elsevier.

Dahan-Oliel, N., Shikako-Thomas, K., Mazer, B., & Majnemer, A. (2016). Adolescents with disabilities participate in the shopping mall: Facilitators and barriers framed according to the ICF. *Disability and Rehabilitation, 38*(21), 2102–2113. https://doi.org/10.3109/09638288.2015.1114033

Jessup, G., Bundy, A. C., Broom, A., & Hancock, N. (2013). Sampling social experiences in school: Feasibility of experience sampling methodology on an iPlatform. *Journal of the South Pacific Educators in Vision Impairment, 6*(1), 140–152.

Jessup, G., Bundy, A. C., Broom, A., & Hancock, N. (2017). The social experiences of high school students with visual impairments. *Journal of Visual Impairment & Blindness, 111*(1), 5–19. https://doi.org/10.1177/0145482X1711100102

Lampert, J. (2019). Best practices in supporting students with visual impairments. In G. Frolek Clark, J. E. Rioux, & B. E. Chandler (Eds.), *Best practices for occupational therapy in schools* (2nd ed., pp. 321–330). AOTA Press.

Loukas, K. M., & Nagaishi, P. S. (2015). Intervention for children who are blind or who have visual impairment. In J. Case-Smith & J. C. O'Brien (Eds.), *Occupational therapy for children and adolescents* (7th ed., pp. 747–765). Elsevier-Mosby.

Salminen, A. L., & Karhula, M. E. (2014). Young persons with visual impairment: Challenges of participation. *Scandinavian Journal of Occupational Therapy, 21*(4), 267–276. https://doi.org /10.3109/11038128.2014.899622

Schneck, C. (2019). Best practices in visual perception and visual-motor skills to enhance participation. In G. Frolek Clark, J. E. Rioux, & B. E. Chandler (Eds.), *Best practices for occupational therapy in schools* (2nd ed., pp. 489–498). AOTA Press.

Nervous System Disorders

Amyotrophic Lateral Sclerosis

*Also called ALS, Lou Gehrig's disease, Charcot syndrome,
motor neuron disease, motor degenerative disorder.*

Description

Amyotrophic lateral sclerosis (ALS) is characterized by steady, progressive degeneration of corticospinal tracts, anterior horn cells, bulbar motor nuclei, or a combination. Symptoms vary in severity and usually start with random, asymmetric presentation consisting of cramps, weakness, and muscle atrophy of the hands or feet. Weakness progresses to the forearms, shoulder, and lower limbs. Other symptoms may include fasciculations, spasticity, hyperactive deep tendon reflexes, extensor plantar reflexes, clumsiness, stiffness of movement, weight loss, fatigue, and difficulty controlling facial expression. Client may experience hoarseness, dysphagia, slurred speech, difficulty swallowing, increased salivation, and tendency to choke on liquids (Porter, 2018). There are two types of ALS: sporadic and familial.

Cause

The etiology of sporadic ALS is unknown. The familial form of ALS has a genetic link. Possible causes include gene mutation, metabolic disorders, metal toxicity, autoimmune factors, and viral infection (Foti, 2018). In some clients the disorder may have started with a minor injury in an arm or leg that did not heal properly. People who engage in intense physical activities, such as professional athletes or military personnel, are more likely to be affected. Death is usually caused by respiratory muscle failure (Porter, 2018).

Six stages of the disease are recognized (adapted from Foti, 2018):

- *Phase 1: Stage 1:* Description: ambulatory, no problems with ADLs, but may have mild weakness. Intervention: normal activities, exercises to maintain active joint range of motion, gentle strengthening.
- *Phase 1: Stage 2:* Description: ambulatory, moderate weakness in certain muscle groups. Intervention: lifestyle and environmental modifications, active assisted exercises in joint range of motion, orthotic support.
- *Phase 1: Stage 3:* Description: ambulatory, severe weakness in certain muscle groups. Intervention: joint pain management, continue assisted exercises, deep-breathing exercises, focus on engagement in pleasurable activities.
- *Phase 2: Stage 4:* Description: partially independent, wheelchair user, severe leg weakness, mostly independent in ADLs. Intervention: passive range of motion, arm supports, hand and wrist splints, anti-edema measures.
- *Phase 2: Stage 5:* Description: partially independent, wheelchair dependent, severe leg and arm weakness. Intervention: increasing ADL dependence, passive range of motion, continue pain management, skin inspection.
- *Phase 3: Stage 6:* Description: dependent, bedridden. Intervention: ADL dependent, maximum assistance required, continue pain management and passive range of motion, prevent decubitus ulcers and venous thrombosis.

Evaluation/Assessment

Areas

- Activities of Daily Living/Instrumental ADL: self-care, swallowing, feeding, writing, communication, home management, transfers, transportation, pet care, child care
- Education/Work: work skill loss
- Play/Leisure: quantity, interests
- Rest/Sleep: sleep disturbance
- Social Participation: quantity

- Sensorimotor: fine and gross motor tasks, grip and pinch strength, muscle strength, joint range of motion, hand and wrist positioning, pain, fatigue, skin integrity, activity tolerance
- Cognitive/Perceptual: dementia
- Psychosocial: coping skills, role performance, perceived loss, emotional regulation
- Context/Environment: assistive technology, mobility equipment, environmental modification, caregiver education
- Comorbidity: no information identified

Instruments

Instruments Developed by Occupational Therapy Personnel

- No information identified.

Instruments Developed by Other Professionals and Used by Occupational Therapy Personnel

- Amyotrophic Lateral Sclerosis Functional Rating Scale-R (ALSFRS-R; Cedarbaum et al., 1999)
- Functional Independence Measure (FIM; Uniform Data System for Medical Rehabilitation, 1997)
- Grip strength (dynamometry; JAMAR, Lafayette Instrument; Wang et al., 2018)
- Joint range of motion (goniometry; Shurtleff & Kaskutas, 2018)
- Manual Muscle Test (MMT; muscle strength; Kaskutas, 2018)
- Pinch meter (pinch strength; Mathiowetz et al., 1985)
- Resident Assessment Instrument (RAI 2.0; interRAI Organization; available from https://catalog.interrai.org/)
- Resident Assessment Instrument–Home Care (RAI-HC; interRAI Organization; https://catalog.interrai.org/)

Problems/Issues

Activities of Daily Living/Instrumental ADL

- Person experiences increasing difficulty with self-care activities, such as dressing and using eating utensils, as the disease progresses.
- Person may have dysphagia (difficulty swallowing).
- Person may require gastrostomy feeding.
- Person may lose ability to communicate through oral speech.
- Person may experience body weight loss.
- Person experiences increasing loss of ability of drive independently and increasing difficulty using other forms of transportation.
- Person experiences increasing difficulty with home management tasks and shopping.
- Person, if a pet parent, will experience loss of ability to care for pet or pets.
- Person, if a parent of a young child, will experience loss of ability to perform child care tasks.
- Note: eye function, bowel and bladder function, and sensory function are not involved.

Education/Work

- Person may be unable to continue work activities, especially those related to motor skills and functions.

Play/Leisure

- Person may be unable to continue engagement in favorite leisure activities.

Rest/Sleep

- No information identified.

Social Participation

- Person may be unable to engage in social activities due problems with dysarthria or dysphagia.

Sensorimotor

- Person may experience symmetrical foot drop or weakness in small muscles of the hand as initial symptoms (Dirette, 2017).

- Person always experiences loss of muscle strength.
- Person always experiences loss of range of motion.
- Person always experiences loss of energy and endurance.
- Person usually experiences increased fatigue.
- Person usually experiences pain including in the shoulder (Gicalone et al., 2019).
- Person with corticospinal tract involvement experiences spasticity and hyperreactive reflexes.
- Person with lower motor neuron involvement experiences muscle atrophy (distal to proximal starting with intrinsic muscles of hand and/or tongue), muscle cramping, and muscle twitching.
- Person may have changes in muscle tone.
- Person may have difficulty with postural control.
- Person may require assistance with ventilation.

Cognitive/Perceptual
- Person may experience frontotemporal dementia depending on the type of ALS.
- Person may experience impairment of executive function.
- Person may be aware of the increased burden of care assumed by family members or other carers (Foley et al., 2016).

Psychosocial
- Person always experiences loss of control over everyday life activities (Foley et al., 2014b; Lemoignan & Ells, 2010).
- Person usually experiences loss of role performance.
- Person usually experiences loss of hope for the future.
- Person may have difficulty coping with loss of abilities and occupational performance.
- Person may have loss of self-esteem and self-efficacy.
- Person may experience emotional lability.
- Person may experience guilt and regret regarding increased burden of care experiences by family and caregivers as loss of function increases (Foley et al., 2016).
- Person and caregivers may experience decreased quality of life (Johnson et al., 2017).

Context/Environment
- Provide information to family and caregivers on safe handling during transfers, use and maintenance of assistive devices and equipment.
- Focus on assistive devices and equipment that require little or no hand function such as voice activation, timer control, or other parts of body (head, elbow, shoulder, foot).
- Provide information on community resources, including getting a disabled parking sticker.

Intervention/Treatment

Models and programs developed by occupational therapy personnel include assistive technology clinic (Casey, 2011) and home-based therapy (Schielder, 2016). Models and programs developed by other professionals but used by occupational therapy personnel include home exercise program (Arbesman & Sheard, 2014), multidisciplinary approach (Hogden et al., 2017), power wheelchairs program (Ward et al., 2015; Ward et al., 2010), and resistive exercise (Arbesman & Sheard, 2014). Team members include physicians, nursing personnel, physical therapy personnel, respiratory or inhalation therapists, and occupational therapy personnel. The primary goal is to maintain occupational performance for as long as possible using compensatory strategies, adaptive devices, home and work modification, and community resources to assist or substitute for loss of function (Muscular Dystrophy Association ALS Division, 2010).

Activities of Daily Living/Instrumental ADL
- Maintain independent performance of ADLs for as long as possible using assistive devices or compensatory techniques, such as use of a bidet (Jenkins, 2012).
- Maintain performance of IADLs using assistive devices, compensatory techniques, or shared performance with others.

Education/Work

- Maintain work activities for as long as possible using modified work strategies (shorter hours, change to light duty, work from home) or compensatory techniques.

Play/Leisure

- Maintain engagement in leisure occupations for as long as possible using compensatory techniques.
- Assist client to explore new or different leisure occupations that require less physical actions as physical abilities decline.

Rest/Sleep

- Assist client to review and revise sleep habits and routines to maintain or improve sleep and rest.

Social Participation

- Assist client to continue participation in social activities using modifications such as outings of shorter duration, more home-based activities, use of wheelchair for mobility, outings with more opportunity for passive participation rather than active.

Sensorimotor

- Maintain muscle strength.
- Maintain range of motion.
- Implement education and use of joint protection program.
- Implement education and use of pain management program.
- Provide splints and orthotics devices.
- Implement fatigue management program such as activity pacing (alternate work and rest cycles), organizing most important activities when energy level is highest.
- Implement education and use of energy conservation (motion economy) techniques.

Cognitive/Perceptual

- Assist client to provide instructions to others regarding care, including prepared written or audio instructions.
- Encourage joint decision making between client and family/caregivers (Foley & Hynes, 2017; Foley et al., 2014a, 2014b).

Psychosocial

- Assist client to discuss issues related to decreased ability to perform independently and how to manage and cope with increased dependence on others.
- Assist client to transition role performance to others.
- Assist client to maintain sense of self-efficacy and self-worth.
- Assist caregivers to cope with increased burden of caregiving through discussion and information (Sanguinett de Almeida et al., 2017).
- Focus on improving quality of life (Soofi et al., 2018).

Context/Environment

- Provide caregiver education on proper lifting techniques and body mechanics education.
- Provide information and suggestions for home modification, including environmental controls.
- Provide assistive equipment as needed and train client and caregivers in use and maintenance, such as raised toilet seat or commode chair, bathtub seat or lift, mechanical lifts.
- Provide assistive devices for activities of daily living and include training and maintenance, such as reachers, long-handled sponge for bathing, utensils with enlarged handles, mugs with large handles, doorknob turner, Velcro/elastics to replace buttons or zippers.
- Provide assistance with mobility equipment such as canes, walkers, manual or power wheelchairs, and scooters.

Precautions/Safety Considerations

Person may be at risk for falls, especially as disease progresses. Monitor for respiratory and breathing functions.

Prognosis and Outcome

There is no cure for ALS. The disease is progressive, requiring palliative care until death. Life expectancy from the onset of symptoms is on average 2–4 years. Clients with early bulbar involvement generally have a poorer prognosis. Clients with ALS usually have a number of health issues requiring therapy, medical interventions, and psychotropic drug use (Kehyayan et al., 2014).

REFERENCES

Arbesman, M., & Sheard, K. (2014). Systematic review of the effectiveness of occupational therapy–related interventions for people with amyotrophic lateral sclerosis. *American Journal of Occupational Therapy, 68*(1), 20–26. https://doi.org/10.5014/ajot.2014.008649

Casey, K. S. (2011). Creating an assistive technology clinic: The experience of the Johns Hopkins AT clinic for patients with ALS. *NeuroRehabilitation, 28*(3), 281–293. https://doi.org/10.3233/NRE-2011-0656

Dirette, D. P. (2017). Progressive neurodegenerative disorders: Amyotrophic lateral sclerosis. In B. J. Atchison & D. P. Dirette (Eds.), *Conditions in occupational therapy* (5th ed., pp. 413–416). Wolters-Kluwer.

Foley, G., & Hynes, G. (2018). Decision-making among patients and their family in ALS care: A review. *Amyotrophic Lateral Sclerosis and Frontotemporal Degeneration, 19*(3/4), 173–193. https://doi.org/10.1080/21678421.2017.1353099

Foley, G., Timonen, V., & Hardiman, O. (2014a). Acceptance and decision making in amyotrophic lateral sclerosis from a life-course perspective. *Qualitative Health Research, 24*(1), 67–77. https://doi.org/10.1177/1049732313516545

Foley, G., Timonen, V., & Hardiman, O. (2014b). Exerting control and adapting to loss in amyotrophic lateral sclerosis. *Social Science & Medicine, 101*, 113–119. https://doi.org/10.1016/j.socscimed.2013.11.003

Foley, G., Timonen, V., & Hardiman, O. (2016). "I hate being a burden": The patient perspective on carer burden in amyotrophic lateral sclerosis. *Amyotrophic Lateral Sclerosis and Frontotemporal Degeneration, 17*(5/6), 351–357. https://doi.org/10.3109/21678421.2016.1143512

Foti, D. (2018). Degenerative diseases of the central nervous system: Amyotrophic lateral sclerosis. In H. M. Pendleton & W. Schultz-Krohn (Eds.), *Pedretti's occupational therapy* (8th ed., pp. 873–878). Elsevier.

Gicalone, A. R., Heckman, M. G., Otto, E., & McVeigh, K. H. (2019). Shoulder pain among patients with amyotrophic lateral sclerosis: A case series. *American Journal of Occupational Therapy, 73*(5), Article 7305345020. https://doi.org/10.5014/ajot.2019.031757

Hogden, A., Foley, G., Henderson, R. D., James, N., & Aoun, S. M. (2017). Amyotrophic lateral sclerosis: Improving care with a multidisciplinary approach. *Journal of Multidisciplinary Healthcare, 10*, 205–215. https://doi.org/10.2147/JMDH.S134992

Jenkins, G. (2012). Assisting clients with amyotrophic lateral sclerosis: The bidet. *OT Practice, 17*(5), 18.

Johnson, S., Alonso, B., Faulkner, K., Roberts, H., Monroe, B., Lehman, L., & Kearney, P. (2017). Quality of life perspectives of people with amyotrophic lateral sclerosis and their caregivers. *American Journal of Occupational Therapy, 71*, Article 7103190010. https://doi.org/10.5014/ajot.2017.024828

Kehyayan, V., Korngut, L., Jetté, N., & Hirdes, J. P. (2014). Profile of patients with amyotrophic lateral sclerosis across continuum of care. *Canadian Journal of Neurological Sciences, 41*(2), 246–252. https://doi.org/10.1017/s0317167100016656

Lemoignan, J., & Ells, C. (2010). Amyotrophic lateral sclerosis and assisted ventilation: How patients decide. *Palliative and Supportive Care, 8*(2), 207–213. https://doi.org/10.1017/S1478951510000027

Muscular Dystrophy Association ALS Division. (2010). *Everyday life with ALS: A practical guide.*

Porter, R. S. (Ed.). (2018). *The Merck manual of diagnosis and therapy* (20th ed.). Merck Sharp & Dohme.

Sanguinett de Almeida, L. M., Falcão, I. V., & Carvalho, T. L. (2017). Evaluation of overloading on caregivers of people with amyotrophic lateral sclerosis (ALS). *Cadernos Brasileiros de Terapia Ocupacional Sãn Carlos, 25*(3), 585–593. https://doi.org/10.4322/2526-8910.ctoAO0871

Schielder, B. (2016). Easing the way for life-limiting illnesses: Treating clients with ALS in the home. *OT Practice, 21*(22), 22–24.

Soofi, A. Y., Dal Bello-Haas, V., Kho, M. E., & Letts, L. (2018). The impact of rehabilitative interventions on quality of life: A qualitative evidence synthesis of personal experiences of individuals with amyotrophic lateral sclerosis. *Quality of Life Research, 27,* 845–856. https://doi.org/10.1007/s11136-017-1754-7

Ward, A. L., Hammond, S., Holsten S., Bravver, E., & Brooks, B. R. (2015). Power wheelchair use in persons with amyotrophic lateral sclerosis: Change over time. *Assistive Technology 27,* 238–245. https://doi.org/10.1080/10400435.2015.1040896

Ward, A. L., Sanjak, M., Duffy, K., Bravver, E., Williams, N., Nichols, M., & Brooks, B. R. (2010). Power wheelchair prescriptions, utilization, satisfaction, and cost for patients with amyotrophic lateral sclerosis: Preliminary data for evidence-based guidelines. *Archives of Physical Medicine and Rehabilitation, 91,* 268–272. https://doi.org/10.1016/j.apmr.2009.10.023

BIBLIOGRAPHY

Foley, G., Timonen, V., & Hardiman, O. (2012a). Experience of services as a key outcome in amyotrophic lateral sclerosis (ALS) care: The case for a better understanding of patient experiences. *American Journal of Hospice and Palliative Medicine, 29*(5), 362–367. https://doi.org/10.1177/1049909111423774

Foley, G., Timonen, V., & Hardiman, O. (2012b). Patients' perceptions of services and preferences for care in amyotrophic lateral sclerosis: A review. *Amyotrophic Lateral Sclerosis, 13,* 11–24. https://doi.org/10.3109/17482968.2011.607500

Preissner, K. (2014). *Occupational therapy practice guidelines for adults with neurodegenerative diseases.* AOTA Press.

Ward, A. L. (2013). Occupational therapy for persons with amyotrophic lateral sclerosis. *OT Practice, 18*(17), 10–11.

Ward, A. L., & Brooks, B. R. (2012). Occupational therapy. In R. S. Bedlack & H. Mitsumoto (Eds.), *Amyotrophic lateral sclerosis: A patient care guide for clinicians* (pp. 119–136). Demos Medical.

Ataxia

Description

Ataxia is an impaired ability to coordinate movement (lack of coordination), which is often characterized by a staggering gait and postural imbalance (O'Toole, 2017). Ataxia is a primary sign of cerebral dysfunction (Porter, 2018). Types include congenital malformation, hereditary ataxia (Friedreich ataxia, spinocerebellar ataxia), and acquired condition. Onset for hereditary types may occur between ages 5–15 (Porter, 2018). Median survival time from onset is 21 years (Silva et al., 2010).

Cause

Causes of each type are listed below.

- Congenital: Usually sporadic malformation of the central nervous system (CNS), including the cerebellum such as Dandy-Walker malformation (Porter, 2018)
- Hereditary ataxia
  - ▶ Friedreich ataxia: Autosomal recessive gene mutation causing abnormal repetition of the DNA sequence GAA in the gene coded for mitochondrial protein frataxin leading to iron overload and impaired mitochondrial function. Condition is progressive (Porter, 2018).
  - ▶ Spinocerebellar ataxia (SCA) is autosomal dominant. Many different subtypes have been described leading to various classification systems. SCA Type 3 (Machado-Joseph disease) is considered most common. Condition is progressive (Porter, 2018).
  - ▶ Note: Ataxia-telangiectasia is not specifically covered, although some symptoms and interventions may apply.
- Acquired condition: Conditions such as multiple system atrophy, systemic disorders, multiple sclerosis, cerebellar strokes, traumatic brain injury, toxin exposure, alcoholic cerebellar degeneration, celiac disease, heatstroke, hypothyroidism, and vitamin E deficiency. In children, primary cause is brain tumor, epilepsy, or diffuse cerebellar dysfunction following viral infection (Porter, 2018). Some acquired conditions may be temporary, and ataxic condition may be reversible, but those associated with neurological conditions subject to degeneration often are permanent and may be progressive.

Evaluation/Assessment

Areas

- Activities of Daily Living/Instrumental ADL: eating and swallowing (deglutition), dressing, grooming, toileting and incontinence, dysarthria, meal preparation, home management, communication, mobility and transfers, child care, driving and public transportation
- Education/Work: work requirements, computer use
- Play/Leisure: leisure interests, type, frequency, location, restrictions
- Rest/Sleep: sleep disorder
- Social Participation: location, type, active or passive, frequency, with whom
- Sensorimotor:
  - ▶ Friedreich ataxia: gait unsteadiness, paresis in lower extremities, tremor, reflexes, proprioception, scoliosis, upper extremity ataxia, "claw hand" deformity, club feet
  - ▶ Spinocerebellar ataxia: restless leg syndrome, pyramidal signs, facial twitching, ophthalmoplegia, bulging eyes, Babinski sign
- Cognitive/Perceptual: cognitive impairment, dementia
- Psychosocial: depression, anxiety, quality of life, social roles
- Context/Environment: adapted devices, education and information, fall prevention
- Comorbidities: cardiomyopathy, epilepsy, visual impairment

Instruments

Instruments Developed by Occupational Therapy Personnel

- Assessment of Motor Process Skills (8th ed.; AMPS-5; Fisher & Bray Jones, 2016)
- Canadian Occupational Performance Measure (5th ed.; COPM-5; Law et al., 2014)

Instruments Developed by Other Professionals and Used by Occupational Therapy Personnel

- Barthel Index (BI; Mahoney & Barthel, 1965)
- Berg Balance Scale (BBS; Berg et al., 1989)
- Friedreich Ataxia Rating Scale (FARS; Subramony et al., 2005; see also Tai et al., 2015, in References)

- Fugl-Meyer Assessment (FMA; Fugl-Meyer et al., 1975)
- Functional Independence Measure (FIM; Uniform Data System for Medical Rehabilitation, 1997; see also Tai et al., 2015, in References)
- Functional Independence Measure–Functional Assessment Measure (FIM-FAM; Turner-Stokes et al., 1999)
- Generalized Self-Efficacy Scale (GSES; Kakudate et al., 2010)
- Goal Attainment Scaling (GAS; Kiresuk & Sherman, 1968)
- Hamilton Rating Scale for Depression (HRSD; Hamilton, 1960)
- Hasegawa Dementia Scale Revised (HDS-R; Kim et al., 2005)
- International Cooperative Ataxia Rating Scale (ICARS; Trouillas et al., 1997; see also Tai et al., 2015, in References)
- Modified Ashworth Scale (MAS; Bohannon & Smith, 1987)
- Modified Barthel Index (MBI; Shah et al., 1989; see also Tai et al., 2015, in References)
- Neurological Examination Scale for Spinocerebellar Ataxia (NESSCA; Kieling et al., 2008)
- Scale for Assessment and Rating of Ataxia (SARA; Schmitz-Hübsch et al., 2006)
- World Health Organization Quality of Life–BREF (WHOQOL-BREF; The WHOQOL Group, 1998)

Problems/Issues
Activities of Daily Living/Instrumental ADL
- Person may have difficulty performing certain self-maintenance activities.
- Person may have difficulty with communication (vocal due to dysarthria and written due to decreased hand function).
- Person may have difficulty with mobility (safe walking in home or community).

Education/Work
- Person may be unable to perform or have difficulty performing specific work-related tasks.
- Person may have difficulty getting to place of work (transportation) or to work station (mobility).

Play/Leisure
- Person may have difficulty engaging in favorite leisure activities.

Rest/Sleep
- Person may have sleep disorders.

Social Participation
- Person may have difficulty participating in social activities.
- Person may withdraw from participating in social activities.

Sensorimotor
- Person may have a wide-based gait.
- Person may have extrapyramidal signs (dystonia, rigidity, bradykinesia).
- Person may have lower motor neuron disease (fasciculation and amyotrophy, loss of sensation, eyelid retraction, weight loss).
- Person may have an inability to correctly sequence fine, coordinated acts.
- Person may have dysdiadochokinesia (inability to perform rapid alternating movements).
- Person may have dysmetria (inability to control range of movement).
- Person may have decreased muscle tone (hypotonia).
- Person may have nystagmus (involuntary, rapid oscillation of the eyeballs), in a horizontal, vertical, or rotary direction, with fast component maximal toward the side of cerebellar lesion.

- Person may have tremor (rhythmic, alternating, oscillatory movement of a limb as it approaches a target; intention tremor or proximal).
- Person may have limitation of upward gaze and convergence.

Cognitive/Perceptual
- Person may experience cognitive impairment and dementia.

Psychosocial
- Person may experience depression and anxiety as disease progresses.
- Person may experience decreased quality of life.
- Person may lose ability to perform valued social roles.
- Person may lack sense of self-efficacy.

Context/Environment
- Person may need adapted devices, such as a wheelchair or walker for mobility, splinting for positioning, or hand function.
- Person is at risk for falls due to changes or poor balance reactions.
- Person, family, and others may need information and resources about ataxic disorders.

Intervention/Treatment

Models and programs developed by occupational therapy personnel include functional approach (Sawant & Gokhale, 2015) and self-efficacy intervention (Tohyama & Usuki, 2015). Models and programs developed by other professionals but used by occupational therapy personnel include client-centered care (Swaminathan et al., 2014) and repetitive transcranial magnetic stimulation (Urushidani et al., 2017). Team members include physicians, nursing personnel, physical therapy personnel, speech–language pathologists, and occupational therapy personnel. Goals are focused on assisting the person to maintain independence and quality of life, enabling the person to participate in self-maintenance, work, and leisure activities for as long as possible. In the early stages, rehabilitation and educative approaches can support occupational engagement, but compensatory approaches will likely be needed as the degenerative disease progresses (Bonney et al., 2016). Overall, occupational therapy may improve global function status (Fonteyn et al., 2014).

Activities of Daily Living/Instrumental ADL
- Provide advice on managing activities of daily living.
- Bathing/Showering: Encourage client to sit with a back support.
- Washing: Limit temperature of water, use lever handles/taps rather than round type.
- Dressing: For limited hand function, use zipper pulls or button hooks; consider replacing fastenings with Velcro.
- Toileting: Consider use of adapted toilet seat with hand rails.
- Consult with speech–language pathologist on feeding assessment.
- Eating: Review positioning and use of devices during meals.
  - Postural control: Add lumbar support to back if needed.
  - Use nonslip mat, such as Dycem.
  - Suggest use of plate guard, rocker knife to reduce degree of movement needed.
  - Weighted cutlery may be useful if tremor is present.
  - Use of lidded or insulated cups or cups with straws for drinking may avoid spills.
  - Use of sports bottle, cups with wide bases and narrow tops.
  - Hydraulic feeder may be useful for severely involved client.
- Meal preparation
  - Consider whether microwave oven would be safer to use than conventional oven.
  - Review whether oven or stove are waist-high for safety.

- ▶ Recommend sliding instead of lifting, using a cart to move items, putting small items in an apron front pocket instead of carrying.
- ▶ Use food processor to help with slicing and chopping vegetables or fruits.
- ▶ Use of ergonomically designed grip knives and cooking utensils can improve hand use.
- ▶ Use of a chopping board with attached cutting blade can be safer than using a separate knife.
- Communication
  - ▶ Consider use of voice-activated or autodial numbers on phones.
  - ▶ Handwriting: Thick barreled (fat handles) pens, triangle shaped pens, or weighted pens may be easier to grip; felt-tipped pens may require less pressure.
- Home management
  - ▶ Instruct person to avoid carrying items if possible. If carrying is essential, carry item as close to body as possible and in a pocket or sack over arm to leave hands free. Use a cart to transport items.
  - ▶ Remove throw rugs or scatter rugs in walkway areas. Walkways should be clear of all unnecessary items and clutter.
  - ▶ Remove loose electrical cables or extension cords.
  - ▶ Install good lighting for mobility and task performance areas.
- Transfers
  - ▶ Check bed mobility as well as bed to chair.
  - ▶ Ensure height of bed and chair is correct for person.
  - ▶ Bed should have a firm mattress.
  - ▶ Recommend use of chair with armrests and back.
  - ▶ A hoist may be needed for those with advanced disease. Training will be needed for family or caregivers.
- Assisting in determining driving status and transportation, such as taxi or bus, for persons with mobility limitations.
- Educate person and family on safe entry and exit from a vehicle.
  - ▶ Sit first before moving legs to enter and vice versa to exit.
  - ▶ Be sure vehicle door is fully open in locked position before entering or exiting to avoid door moving and destabilizing person.
  - ▶ Consider if a swivel transfer mat might be useful.

Education/Work

- Assist client to maintain worker role for as long as possible or desired by client.
- Review computer use to determine whether word prediction or voice-activated software may be helpful to reduce need to keyboard (Note: dysarthria may preclude use of voice-activated software).
- Modifications such as use of "sticky keys," using a tracker ball, enlarging font type, or changing background to blue may be useful.
- Determine whether ergonomic setup and seating of computer workstation is desirable, including use of lumbar support.
- Reduce clutter and maximize organization of work station.

Play/Leisure

- Determine whether leisure sites (restaurants, shops, parks, stadiums) are wheelchair accessible.
- Consider modifying participation in sports to roles such as score keeping, event scheduling, or participation on committees.
- For hobbies such as gardening, consider whether raised garden beds, container gardening, or indoor gardening may be a suitable replacement.
- For reading, recommend large-print books or an electronic book reader, which allows print font to be changed to different sizes if vision is a problem, or consider talking books.

- Elastic bands can be used to hold pages and rubber thimbles can be used to turn pages to compensate for grasp and fine motor coordination.
- For outdoor activities, a wheelchair or scooter may be needed for longer mobility situations.

Rest/Sleep
- No information identified.

Social Participation
- No information identified.

Sensorimotor
- Promote normal postural alignment and movement.
- Improve proximal stability and automatic equilibrium reactions.
- Assist in determining best seating system for clients with early and advanced disorder (stable cushions and back supports). Avoid canvas backs, as such material does not provide enough support.
- Provide fatigue-management program, such as rest-activity-rest schedule or grouping important activities at a time when client has the most energy.

Cognitive/Perceptual
- If cognitive impairment is present, instructions may need to be modified to include reminders (verbal, pictures, posted instructions, gestures).

Psychosocial
- Support continued engagement in social roles with modifications acceptable to client.
- Discuss with client ideas and programs to maintain as much quality of life as possible.

Context/Environment
- Determine whether seating evaluation is needed for wheelchair or scooter mobility.
- Provide education on disease and management to client, family, caregivers, or employers.
- Consider enlarging small switches (light switches, on-off switch on appliances) to make on-off devices easier to manage.
- Consider whether repositioning (higher or lower) wall sockets and switches would make access easier and avoid bending, squatting, and reaching.
- Recommend devices to compensate for decreased hand functions, such as built-up and modified handles and cuffs to compensate for loss of hand grip functions.
- Fall prevention.
  - ▶ Recommend well-fitted shoes.
  - ▶ Recommend avoiding long clothing.
  - ▶ Recommend nonslip flooring in home.
  - ▶ Instruct person and family members on how to get up safely from the floor.
  - ▶ Suggest person wear a security care alarm necklace or button.

Precautions/Safety Considerations

Person may have progressive cardiomyopathy including arrhythmia or heart failure (Porter, 2018).

Prognosis and Outcome

Clients usually progress to wheelchair use and later become bedridden if ataxia is due to hereditary disorders (Silva et al., 2010).

REFERENCES

Bonney, H., de Silva, R., Giunti, P., Greenfield, J., & Hunt, B. (2016). *Management of the ataxias: Towards best clinical practice* (3rd ed.). Ataxia UK. Ataxia_UK_2016_Management_of_the_ataxias_towards_best_clinical.pdf

Fonteyn, E. M. R., Keus, S. H. J., Verstappen, C. C. P., Schöls, L., de Groot, I. J. M., & van de Warrenburg, B. P. C. (2014). The effectiveness of allied health care in patients with ataxia: A systematic review. *Journal of Neurology, 261*(2), 251–258. https://doi.org/10.1007/s00415-013-6910-6

O'Toole, M. T. (Ed.). (2017). *Mosby's dictionary of medicine, nursing & health professions* (10th ed.). Elsevier.

Porter, R. S. (Ed.). (2018). *The Merck manual of diagnosis and therapy* (20th ed.). Merck Sharp & Dohme.

Sawant, P., & Gokhale, P. (2015). Functional approach in spino-cerebellar ataxia-occupational therapy perspective. *Indian Journal of Physiotherapy and Occupational Therapy, 9*(4), 223–228.

Silva, R. C. R., Saute, J. A. M., Silva, A. C. F., Coutinho, A. C. O., Saraiva-Pereira, M. L., & Jardim, L. B. (2010). Occupational therapy in spinocerebellar ataxia Type 3: An open-label trial. *Brazilian Journal of Medical and Biological Research, 43*(6), 537–542. https://doi.org/10.1590/s0100-879x2010005000009

Swaminathan, A., Jahagirdar, S., & Kulkarni, C. (2014). Client centred care: Looking through the lens of quantitative and qualitative measures—Case studies. *Indian Journal of Occupational Therapy, 46*(1), 10–15.

Tai, G., Corben, L. A., Gurrin, L., Yiu, E. M., Churchyard, A., Fahey, M., Hoare, B., Downie, S., & Delatycki, M. B. (2015). A study of up to 12 years of follow-up of Friedreich ataxia utilising four measurement tools. *Journal of Neurology, Neurosurgery & Psychiatry, 86*(6), 660–666. https://doi.org/10.1136/jnnp-2014-308022

Tohyama, S., & Usuki, F. (2015). Occupational therapy intervention to inspire self-efficacy in a patient with spinal ataxia and visual disturbance. *BMJ Case Reports, 86*(6), Article bcr2014 208259. https://doi.org/10.1136/bcr-2014-208259

Urushidani, N., Okamoto, T., Kinoshita, S., Yamane, S., Tamashiro, H., Kakuda, W., & Abo, M. (2017). Combination treatment of low-frequency repetitive transcranial magnetic stimulation and intensive occupational therapy for ataxic hemiparesis due to thalamic hemorrhage. *Case Reports in Neurology, 9*(2), 179–187. https://doi.org/10.1159/000478975

Guillain-Barré Syndrome

Also called Landry's syndrome, polyradiculoneuritis,
acute idiopathic neuropathy, infectious polyneuropathy.

Description

Guillain-Barré syndrome (GBS) is an acute, usually rapidly progressive but self-limited inflammatory polyneuropathy characterized by muscular weakness and mild distal sensory loss. In some variants of the syndrome, demyelination predominates; other variants affect the axon. In about two-thirds of patients, the syndrome begins 5 days to 3 weeks after an infectious disorder, surgery, or vaccination (Porter, 2018). Weakness usually begins in the legs, proceeds to the arms, and may affect the respiratory system and facial nerve. GBS is an acquired immune-mediated inflammatory disorder of the peripheral nervous system (GBS/CIDP Foundation International, 2012). Typically, the immune system destroys the myelin sheath (demyelination) that surrounds the axons of the peripheral nerves or the axons themselves, damaging the ability of the nerve to transmit signals effectively to the muscles (George, 2018).

Cause

The cause is thought to be autoimmune. There are several variants, including Miller-Fisher syndrome and the pharyngeal-cervical-brachial motor variant (Hamby, 2017).

Phases of GBS (Hamby, 2017):

Initial or Acute Phase
- Lasts from first conclusive symptoms until there is no further decline in physical status.
- Phase may last up to 4 weeks.

Plateau Phase
- Physical state stabilizes.
- Phase may last for a few weeks, during which the status remains unchanged.

Recovery Phase
- Slow recovery begins as symptoms gradually decrease.
- Physical ability starts to recover.
- Phase may last from 6 months to 2 years.

Evaluation/Assessment

Areas
- Activities of Daily Living/Instrumental ADL: basic ADLs, dysphasia, transfers, mobility, independent living skills
- Education/Work: education level, work history, work skill requirements
- Play/Leisure: interests, type, frequency, location
- Rest/Sleep: sleep disturbance
- Social Participation: type, location, frequency, with whom
- Sensorimotor: muscle strength, muscle tone, muscle belly tenderness, deep tendon reflexes, joint range of motion, endurance, fatigue, pain, sensory awareness, skin inspection
- Cognitive/Perceptual: executive functions
- Psychosocial: depression, anxiety, self-efficacy, quality of life
- Context/Environment: social support system, adapted equipment, environment modification
- Comorbidities: Previous viral infection, pneumonia, upper respiratory infections, pulmonary thrombosis, deep vein thrombosis (DVT), autonomic dysfunction, decubitus ulcers (pressure sores)

Instruments

Instruments Developed by Occupational Therapy Personnel
- Home Safety Self-Assessment Tool (Version 5; HSSAT 5.0; Tomita, 2017)

Instruments Developed by Other Professionals and Used by Occupational Therapy Personnel
- Activities-Specific Balance Confidence Scale (ABC; Powell & Myers, 1995)
- Center for Epidemiology Studies Depression Scale (CES-D; Radloff, 1977)
- Community Integration Questionnaire (CIQ; Willer et al., 1993)
- Dermatome mapping (Abrams & Ivy, 2018)
- Fatigue Severity Scale (FSS; Krupp et al., 1989; Lerdal et al., 2011)
- Functional Independence Measure (FIM; Uniform Data System for Medical Rehabilitation, 1997)
- Joint range of motion (goniometry; Shurtleff & Kaskutas, 2018)
- Manual Muscle Test (MMT; Kaskutas, 2018)
- Modified Barthel Index (MBI; Shah et al., 1989)
- Older Americans Resources and Services (OARS) Program (Fillenbaum, 1988)
- Semmes-Weinstein Monofilaments (SWMs; Patterson Medical Supply)
- Timed Up and Go test (TUG; Podsiadlo & Richardson, 1991)
- World Health Organization Quality of Life–BREF (WHOQOL-BREF; The WHOQOL Group, 1998)

Problems/Issues

Activities of Daily Living/Instrumental ADL

- Person usually is dependent on others for self-care during the plateau phase.
- Person may experience dysphagia if oropharyngeal and facial muscle weakness occurs due to cranial nerve VII involvement.
- Person may experience difficulty speaking because of weakness in respiratory muscles.
- Person may experience dysautonomia, including abnormal heart rate, high or low blood pressure, and breathing changes.
- Person may experience problems such as blood clots or infections related to dysfunctions of the autonomic nervous system.
- Person may require a respirator to breathe if respiratory muscles are affected.

Education/Work

- Person usually is unable to attend school or complete work activities during the course of the disorder until recovery has progressed and motor skills have returned.

Play/Leisure

- Person usually is unable to participate in leisure activities that require motor skills.

Rest/Sleep

- Person may experience sleep disturbance or disruptions.

Social Participation

- Person usually is unable to engage in social activities or events in the community.

Sensorimotor

- Person usually experiences rapidly progressive ascending symmetric weakness or paralysis occurring bilaterally.
- Person usually experiences weakness progressing distal to proximal (feet to trunk, hands to trunk, and possibly upward to the face). Sometimes called "stocking glove" distribution because the loss occurs as if wearing knee-high stocking or long gloves.
- Person usually has flaccid muscle tone.
- Person usually loses both gross and fine motor skills during the acute phase.
- Person usually has loss of endurance and increased sense of fatigue.
- Person may experience loss of deep tendon reflexes or the reflexes may become hyper-reflexive. (Note: Anal reflex and tone, and eye wink reflexes usually are preserved.)
- Person may experience muscle belly tenderness.
- Person may experience sensory loss or disturbances such as inability to feel textures, temperature, and other sensations.
- Person may experience overresponsiveness to certain stimuli, such as light or touch.
- Person may report initial sensations such as tingling, "crawling skin," or painful sensations.
- Person may be at increased risk of falling due to decreased motor skills.
- Person may experience radicular back pain and neuropathic pain.
- Person may require sensory reeducation.

Cognitive/Perceptual

- Not affected directly by the disease. Knowledge of previous status may be helpful in planning intervention.

Psychosocial

- Person and family usually experience difficulty in coping with the symptoms of the disorder.
- Person usually is frightened by the progressive loss of function and increased weakness or paralysis.
- Person may grieve over loss of function and abilities.

- Person may become despondent and depressed at the perceived slow rate of recovery.
- Person may find maintaining motivation difficult as recovery progresses.

Context/Environment
- Person's family and friends are usually frightened by seeing the progression of the disorder and increased weakness or paralysis occurring.
- Person's living environment may need modification to increase safety.

Intervention/Treatment

Models and programs developed by occupational therapy personnel include fatigue management (Sawant & Ferzandi, 2015), model of human occupation (Brooks, 2014), and person-environment-occupation (Brooks, 2014; Tomita et al., 2016). Remedial techniques are needed to regain motor skills, but compensatory techniques are also needed during the plateau and recovery periods. Models and programs developed by other professionals but used by occupational therapy personnel include guidelines (GBS/CIDP Foundation International, 2012), multidisciplinary rehabilitation team (Khanzada & Zameer, 2016), and resistive exercises (Ko et al., 2017). Team members include physicians, nursing personnel, psychologists, pulmonologists and respiratory therapists, physical therapy personnel, and occupational therapy personnel. The goal is to help the person achieve optimal neuromotor function, resume an activity level that is as close to the previous lifestyle as possible, and return to full community integration (Tomita et al., 2016).

Activities of Daily Living/Instrumental ADL
- Schedule self-care activities according to energy expenditure with list of items needed for each activity.
- Encourage client to perform self-care activities as independently as possible. Provide assistive devices as needed, even if only needed for a short time, such as long-handled aids, plate guard, or enlarged handles on eating utensils and grooming items, and use compensatory techniques such as holding a cup or bottle with two hands or use of a universal cuff to hold items instead of fingers.
- Work on transfer skills, such as transfer from bed to chair and back again.
- Provide assistive devices for homemaking activities as needed.

Education/Work
- If a student, discuss plans for return to school and what modifications may be needed, such as taking online courses.
- If employed, discuss plans for return to work and what modifications may be useful, such as working from home, working part time or working flex time. May need to involve employer as well.

Play/Leisure
- Discuss plans for return to leisure activities.
- Explore possibilities for adapting some leisure activities to reduce fatigue or need for muscle strength.
- Explore possibilities for engaging in new leisure activities.

Rest/Sleep
- See Sleep–Wake Disorders in Section 13: Lifestyle Disorders.

Social Participation
- Encourage person to reengage in social activities with family and in the community.

Sensorimotor
- Provide passive range of motion to maintain joint range during acute and plateau phases and active joint range of motion during recovery.

- Provide graded therapeutic exercises, such as by using a TheraBand.
- Increase graded practice in using gross and fine motor skills as reactivation of motor neurons occurs.
- Encourage walking by providing a pedometer or use of an app on the smartphone.
- Use deep-breathing exercises, bridging, and dissociative rolling to build core (trunk) strength.
- Increase mobility skills, including rolling in bed, supine to sit, body weight transfer on both hands, trunk rotation, sit to stand, and reaching for objects.
- Teach energy conservation (motion economy) techniques to manage fatigue.
- Teach activity pacing (rest and work/activity cycles).
- Teach activity grading, based from simple/minimum energy expenditure to complex/energy intense.
- Consider whether a hand splint may improve range of motion of metacarpophalangeal and proximal interphalangeal joint function.
- Provide desensitization program if needed.
- Provide a home program when discharged. Print format or access online program is desirable.

Cognitive/Perceptual
- Communicate instructions clearly and repeat at each therapy session.
- Maintain general level of functional cognition.
- Involve client in decision making and participation in recovery program.

Psychosocial
- Assist client to develop and implement coping behaviors and stress management (relaxation techniques, deep breathing, mindfulness, yoga).
- Respect client's values and spirituality.

Context/Environment
- Provide access to correct information about intervention and prognosis to client, family, and social support group members.
- Anticipate need for and training in use of assistive equipment as needed, such as a walker to aid mobility, transfer (powder) board, or slings.
- Provide information and suggestions for modifying living environment to increase safety, such as grab bars in the bathroom.

Precautions/Safety Considerations

While family members and others can assist in range of motion exercises, they should be cautioned to follow instructions exactly to avoid overstretching or overexerting the muscles. All exercises should be stopped if pain occurs, vital signs (heart rate, blood pressure, respiratory rate) are too low or too high, and should never be performed to the point of exhaustion. Watch for muscle substitutions during exercises such as shoulder movement instead of forearm movement or hip-hiking and circumduction gait pattern to substitute for weak hip flexors. During the acute stage, avoid prolonged hip and knee flexion such as putting a pillow under the knees to reduce possibility of contractures. Change position of the body at least every 2 hours in bed and perform regular pressure reliefs when sitting to avoid pressure sores. Support weak upper extremities with an armrest, a wheelchair tray, or pillows to prevent stretching shoulder muscles and joint. Train caregivers in proper body mechanics for lifting, transferring, or positioning client. Ensure home program fits with client's current activity level. Inform client and caregivers of increased risk of falling and instruct in fall prevention.

Prognosis and Outcome

There is no known cure for GBS. Recovery depends on the extent of involvement and may take weeks to many months. Although technically full recovery is possible, many individuals will experience long-term residual deficits such as distal numbness, fatigue, general weakness, or weakness in specific muscle groups, which interfere with performing daily function. Death can occur from pneumonia adult respiratory distress syndrome, autonomic dysfunction, or pulmonary embolism. A relapse of muscle weakness and tingling sensation occurs in some clients years after the initial attack (George, 2018).

REFERENCES

Brooks, S. A. N. (2014). Commentary: Inside Guillain-Barré syndrome: An occupational therapist's perspective. *South African Journal of Occupational Therapy, 44*(3), 40–43.

GBS/CIDP Foundation International. (2012). *Guidelines for physical and occupational therapy: Guillain-Barré syndrome, CIDP and variants.* https://www.gbs-cidp.org/wp-content/uploads/2014/09/Physical-and-Occupational-Therapy-Guidelines.pdf

George, A. H. (2018). Disorders of the motor unit: Guillain-Barré syndrome. In H. M. Pendleton & W. Schultz-Krohn (Eds). *Pedretti's occupational therapy* (8th ed., pp. 931–934). Elsevier.

Hamby, J. R. (2017). The nervous system: Guillain-Barré Syndrome. In H. Smith-Gabai & S. E. Holm (Eds.), *Occupational therapy in acute care* (2nd ed., pp. 339, 341, 347–348). AOTA Press.

Khanzada, F. J., & Zameer, S. (2016). Effectiveness of occupational therapy in rehabilitation of Guillain Barré syndrome: A case study. *Physical Medicine and Rehabilitation International, 3*(2), Article 1083.

Ko, K.-J., Ha, G.-C., & Kang, S.-J. (2017). Effects of daily living occupational therapy and resistance exercise on the activities of daily living and muscular fitness in Guillain-Barré syndrome: A case study. *Journal of Physical Therapy Science, 29*(5), 950–953. https://doi.org/10.1589/jpts.29.950

Porter, R. S. (Ed.). (2018). *The Merck manual of diagnosis and therapy* (20th ed.). Merck Sharp & Dohme.

Sawant, P., & Ferzandi, Z. (2015). Effect of occupational therapy on fatigue and quality of life in patients with Guillain Barré syndrome. *Indian Journal of Physiotherapy and Occupational Therapy, 9*(4), 209–215.

Tomita, M. R., Buckner, K., Saharan, S., Persons, K., & Liao, S. H. (2016). Extended occupational therapy reintegration strategies for a woman with Guillain-Barré syndrome: Case report. *American Journal of Occupational Therapy, 70*(4), Article 7004210010. https://doi.org/10.5014/ajot.2016.017871

Huntington's Disease

Also called Huntington's chorea.

Description

Huntington's disease (HD) is an autosomal dominant genetic disease that is characterized by movement disorders (voluntary and involuntary), behavioral and neuropsychiatric disturbances, progressive cognitive deterioration, and ultimately dementia. Adult onset typically manifests beginning in middle age. Diagnosis is made by genetic testing (Cook et al., 2012a, 2012b; Porter, 2018). Signs of juvenile onset Huntington's disease differ from adult onset in that voluntary movement abnormalities, rigidity, and spasticity may be manifest early, and myoclonus (brief jerks of muscle groups) may be evident. In addition, seizures are more likely (Cook et al., 2012a, 2012b).

Cause

Huntington's disease is caused by a mutation on chromosome 4, which results in atrophy of the caudate nucleus and putamen (basal ganglia) and degeneration of the corpus striatum. Changes start in the dorsal caudate nucleus and gradually spread throughout the frontostriatal system (Cook et al., 2012a, 2012b; Porter, 2018).

Stages of Huntington's Disease (Cook et al., 2012b; Schultz-Krohn, 2018)

- *Presymptom Stage (UHDRS I):* Decreased speed of finger tapping on the Unified Huntington's Disease Rating Scale (UHDRS) may be an early sign. Initial symptoms vary but may include choreiform (rapid, involuntary, irregular) movements of the hands causing difficulty with manipulation of small objects, alterations in behavior such as irritability or depression, or changes in cognitive function such as forgetfulness or difficulty concentrating.
- *Early Stage (UHDRS II):* Some neurological and psychiatric features are present. Changes may be noticed at work, driving ability may be affected, and some home tasks requiring rapid task switching may be apparent. Person is able to care for self independently.
- *Mid Stage (UHDRS III):* Person has ceased work or changed to less challenging position. Executive function decline is demonstrated. Involuntary movement may be obvious. Person is still able to care for self.
- *Late Stage (UHDRS IV, V):* Employment is not possible due to loss of motor and cognitive functions. Person is unable to live independently. Cognitive decline is obvious. Person may be able to perform some self-care tasks, but movement disorders, both voluntary and involuntary, create increasing difficulties. Communication may be limited, and person needs assistance to participate in social activities.

Evaluation/Assessment

Areas

- Activities of Daily Living/Instrumental ADL: self-care (eating, fastening buttons, holding a phone), swallowing, bowel and bladder control, communication (speech, handwriting), driving
- Education/Work: work task performance, safety
- Play/Leisure: frequency of engagement, type, interests
- Rest/Sleep: no information identified
- Social Participation: frequency, location, type
- Sensorimotor: grip strength, manual dexterity, coordination, postural control
- Cognitive/Perceptual: attention and concentration, memory, executive function, dementia
- Psychosocial: aggression, depression, anxiety, motivation, irritability, antisocial behavior, psychotic symptoms (bipolar or schizophreniform)
- Context/Environment: safety, adapted equipment, environmental modification
- Comorbidities: dementia, psychosis

Instruments

Instruments Developed by Occupational Therapy Personnel

- ADL Taxonomy (Törnquist & Sonn, 2014)
- Adolescent/Adult Sensory Profile (AASP; Brown & Dunn, 2002)
- Assessment of Motor and Process Skills (8th ed.; AMPS-8; Fisher & Bray Jones, 2016)
- Canadian Occupational Performance Measure (5th ed.; COPM-5; Law et al., 2014)
- Model of Human Occupation Screening tool (Version 2.0; MOHOST 2.0; Parkinson et al., 2006)
- Occupational Performance History Interview-II (Version 2.1; OPHI-II; Kielhofner et al., 2004)
- Perceive, Recall, Plan, Perform (PRPP) System of Task Analysis (Chapparo & Ranka, 2014)
- Worker Role Interview (Version 10.0; WRI 10.0; Braveman et al., 2005)

Instruments Developed by Other Professionals and Used by Occupational Therapy Personnel

- Dementia Care Mapping (DCM; Bradford Dementia Group, 1997)
- Posturography (see Fekete et al., 2012, in References)
- Stroop Color and Word Test (SCWT; Golden, & Freshwater, 2002)

- Symbol Digit Modalities Test (SDMT; Smith, 1973)
- Total Functional Capacity Scale (TFCS; part of the Unified Huntington's Disease Rating Scale)
- Unified Huntington's Disease Rating Scale (UHDRS; Huntington Study Group, 1996)
- Verbal Fluency Test (VFT; Benton et al., 1994)

Problems/Issues

Activities of Daily Living/Instrumental ADL
- Person usually experiences dysphagia (difficulty swallowing).
- Person usually loses ability to walk in late stage of disease.
- Person may have difficulty coordinating breathing and chewing while eating.
- Person may experience weight loss as a result of difficulty swallowing and need to increase caloric intake due to increased body movement.
- Person may have dysarthria resulting is loss of voice clarity and decreased intelligibility of speech.
- Person may become incontinent in bowel and bladder.
- Person's handwriting may become enlarged and slanted and shape of letters may become distorted.
- Person may be unable to maintain financial records, including budgeting and bill paying.

Education/Work
- Person may be unable to perform certain work tasks at required level of performance.
- Person may be unable to perform tasks safely, including getting to and from work station as well as performing required work activities.
- Person may be dismissed from work setting due to poor job performance.

Play/Leisure
- Person may discontinue engagement in favorite leisure activities.

Rest/Sleep
- No information identified.

Social Participation
- Person may reduce or stop participation in social activities.

Sensorimotor
- Person usually has chorea, myoclonic jerk, and pseudo-tics, which interfere with maintaining control of limb movements.
- Person usually has a gait disturbance, sometimes called "puppet-like gait."
- Person usually demonstrates a slowing of intentional movement (bradykinesia).
- Person usually demonstrates dystonia in which contracting of specific muscle groups causes balance problems and increasing risk of falls.
- Person may display a wide-based gait to compensate for motor dysfunction.
- Person may have hypertonicity and rigidity in later stages of disease, which may replace the choreatic movements.
- Person may have difficulty walking on uneven surfaces.
- Person may have a "staggering gait" that makes the person appear to be drunk (alcohol substance abuse).
- Person may be unable to sustain a motor act (motor impersistence), such as tongue protrusion or grasping.
- Person may have reduced manual dexterity and coordination, making performance of manual tasks difficult, especially manipulation of small objects.
- Person may have reduced grip strength.
- Person may drop objects from hand frequently (motor impersistence).
- Person may complete voluntary motor tasks slowly (bradykinesia).
- Person may experience fatigue resulting in reduced endurance affecting all tasks.

- Person may have decreased speed of ocular pursuit (difficulty moving the eyes quickly, oculomotor apraxia).
- Person may have difficulty with visual perception or visual motor perception.
- Person may have sensory modulation difficulties including over- and underreactivity.

Cognitive/Perceptual

- Person may experience bradyphrenia (generalized slowing of thinking processes).
- Person may have impaired attention span and ability to concentrate on a task or difficulty switching attention from one task to another (focused attention, divided attention, sustained attention, dual task attention, or switch attention).
- Person may have difficulty with procedural and episodic memory due to basal ganglia deterioration.
- Person may demonstrate impaired executive function, such as difficulty with problem solving and decision making, lack of insight, poor abstract thinking ability, decreased ability to perform mathematical skills, poor temporal sequencing, difficulty multitasking, and distractibility.
- Note: Verbal comprehension is usually maintained until late stages of the disease.

Psychosocial

- Person may demonstrate signs of aggression (Brown et al., 2017; Fisher et al., 2014).
- Person may have reduced motivation, variable motivation, and apathy.
- Person may demonstrate depression and flat or shallow affect.
- Person may demonstrate mood swings from sadness to euphoria.
- Person may confabulate (tell tales and untruths not based on facts).
- Person may become easily confused.
- Person may demonstrate anxiety, including fear and avoidance of certain situations.
- Person may demonstrate lack of concern for others, including a lack of concern for social rules.
- Person may be unable to inhibit certain behavioral responses (disinhibition, impulsivity).
- Person may be restless and unable to stay in one place.
- Person may perseverate.
- Person may demonstrate signs of dementia.
- Person may demonstrate signs of psychosis, especially paranoid ideology.

Context/Environment

- Person is at risk for falls.

Intervention/Treatment

Models and programs developed by occupational therapy personnel include framework for intervention (Cook et al., 2012a), model of human occupation (Brown & Fisher, 2015), and sensory modulation (Brown & Fisher, 2015; Fisher & Brown, 2017). Intervention is supportive. Early intervention may include remedial approaches, but later intervention is primarily compensatory, such as adapting the environment or changing routines. Intervention usually involves a multidisciplinary team including physicians, psychologists, geneticists, nursing personnel, physical therapy personnel, speech–language pathologists, dietitians, dentists, and occupational therapy personnel. Goals in self-care are to enable the individual to survive and to promotor and maintain health. In productivity the goal is to include occupations that make a social or economic contribution, or provide economic sustenance. In leisure, goals are to propose and promote enjoyment in socializing, creative expression, and participation in outdoor activities and sports (Cook et al., 2012b). Overall, the goal is to encourage and support participation in occupational performance throughout the stages of the disease.

Activities of Daily Living/Instrumental ADL

- Consult with dietician to suggest and modify food selection to reduce effect of dysphagia. Person may need to eat smaller meals more frequently (five times per day). Soft food and thickened fluids are recommended rather than chewy foods. In late stage, a feeding tube may be needed.

- Positioning during feeding, especially good trunk support, is important.
- Recommend client sit while performing daily activities or lean against sturdy furniture or walls to compensate for decreased balance.
- Recommend alternations to clothing, such as wearing clothing with no fasteners or changing fasteners to Velcro or elastic closures. When possible, avoid clothing with small buttons, snaps, hooks, and small zippers.
- Suggest use of enlarged or built-up handles on eating and cooking utensils.
- Inform person about mobility equipment and assist person in selection in late stage.
- Consider if alternative forms of communication (language or symbol boards) might be useful if verbal communication is lost or not functional. Consult with a speech pathologist or speech therapist.
- Assist client in determining alternative forms of mobility to assist walking, such as walkers, scooters, or wheelchairs. (Note: Client may be better able to move a wheelchair using feet than hands.)
- Assist client in determining when driving should cease, and considering alternative forms of transportation.

Education/Work
- Consider whether changing work requirements to a position with less demand for motor and cognitive skills may be possible.
- Consider whether work setting modifications may improve safety.

Play/Leisure
- Assist client in determining leisure interests, including developing new ones if previous interests are no longer feasible.
- Assist client in engaging in purposeful and meaningful activities.

Rest/Sleep
- See Sleep–Wake Disorders in Section 13: Lifestyle Conditions.

Social Participation
- Encourage participation in pleasurable social activities.

Sensorimotor
- Provide a fatigue management program to prioritize most important activities.
- Teach client energy conservation (motion economy) techniques, including work simplification tasks.
- Assist client to develop and implement an activity pacing program (alternate work and rest cycles).
- Assist client to determine which activities require the most energy, and schedule those when energy level is greatest.
- Splints may be needed in later stages to prevent contractures.
- Provide sensory modulation strategies (see Brown & Fisher, 2015, for examples).

Cognitive/Perceptual
- Use of lists, notebooks, sticky notes, diary, calendars, or white (wipe) board may be useful to organize tasks and provide prompts and reminders.
- Assist client to establish a consistent daily routine.
- Assist client to label drawers and cupboards.
- Assist client to develop and use prompts to aid retrieval of information.
- Suggest family and caregivers offer choices rather that asking open-ended questions, such as "Do you want coffee or tea?" rather than "What do you want to drink?"
- Break down complex tasks into smaller steps.
- Write instructions in sequential order, such as in a checklist.

- Encourage client to complete one task before starting another to deal with loss of ability to multitask.
- Use short, declarative sentences when giving instructions.
- Eliminate external stimuli whenever possible to assist in focusing attention. Turn off the television or radio when performing tasks.

Psychosocial

- Assist family and caregivers to identify triggers and escalators for aggressive or other undesirable behavior. Examples include monitoring for pain or mild infection, as well as stressors and unintended changes in routine.

Context/Environment

- Provide family and caregivers information and training on safe handling and transfers.
- Recommend assistive devices and environmental modifications and provide opportunity to practice to develop habits while cognition is still relatively intact.
- Provide home safety check. Eliminate throw rugs and clutter, install grab bars and shower chair, use of unbreakable dishes, sturdy chairs with arm rests, railings on stairs.
- Environmental controls may be useful in late stages of the disease.

Precautions/Safety Considerations

Person is at risk for aspiration due to loss of swallowing reflexes. Person is at risk for falling due to decreased motor control. Person may have uncontrolled behavioral changes, such as aggression, which need to be monitored. Person is at risk for self-harm and suicidal behavior in an early stage. Person should avoid use of sharp instruments due to decreased motor control. Person may need additional support and stabilization to perform activities to compensate for poor motor control.

Prognosis and Outcome

There is no cure. Huntington's disease is progressive, degenerative, and fatal. Palliative care may be needed. Death usually occurs 13 to 15 years after symptoms occur (Porter, 2018). A common cause of the death is pneumonia (Schultz-Krohn, 2018).

REFERENCES

Brown, A., & Fisher, C. (2015). Optimising occupational performance through sensory modulation interventions: Case reports of two young adults diagnosed with juvenile Huntington's disease. *British Journal of Occupational Therapy, 78*(12), 767–771. https://doi.org/10.1177/03 08022615569249

Brown, A., Sewell, K., & Fisher, C. A. (2017). Characterisation of aggression in Huntington's disease: Rates, types and antecedents in an inpatient rehabilitation setting. *Journal of Clinical Nursing, 26*(19-20), 2922–2931. https://doi.org/10.1111/jocn.13614

Cook, C., Page, K., Wagstaff, A., Simpson, S. A., & Rae, D. (2012a). Development of guidelines for occupational therapy in Huntington's disease. *Neurodegenerative Disease Management, 2*(1), 79–87. https://doi.org/10.2217/NMT.11.81

Cook, C., Page, K., Wagstaff, A., Simpson, S., & Rae, D. (2012b). *Occupational therapy for people with Huntington's disease: Best practice guidelines.* European Huntington's Disease Network.

Fekete, R., Davidson, A., Ondo, W. G., & Cohen, H. S. (2012). Effect of tetrabenazine on computerized dynamic posturography in Huntington disease patients. *Parkinsonism & Related Disorders, 18*(7), 896–898. https://doi.org/10.1016/j.parkreldis.2012.04.029

Fisher, C. A., & Brown, A. (2017). Sensory modulation intervention and behaviour support modification for the treatment of severe aggression in Huntington's disease: A single case experimental design. *Neuropsychological Rehabilitation, 27*(6), 891–903. https://doi.org/10.1 080/09602011.2015.1091779

Fisher, C. A., Sewell, K., Brown, A., & Churchyard, A. (2014). Aggression in Huntington's disease: A systematic review of rates of aggression and treatment methods. *Journal of Huntington's Disease, 3*(4), 319–332. https://doi.org/10.3233/JHD-140127

Porter, R. S. (Ed.). (2018). *The Merck manual of diagnosis and therapy* (20th ed.). Merck Sharp & Dohme.

Schultz-Krohn, W. (2018). Huntington's disease. In H. M. Pendleton & W. Schultz-Krohn (Eds.), *Pedretti's occupational therapy* (8th ed., pp. 885–889). Elsevier.

Motor Neuron Diseases

Also called motor neurone diseases, MNDs.
See also Amyotrophic Lateral Sclerosis, Post-Polio Syndrome.

Description

Motor neuron diseases (MNDs) are characterized by steady, relentless, progressive degeneration of corticospinal tracts, anterior horn cells, bulbar motor nuclei, or a combination. MNDs are more common among men, most often appearing during their 50s, except for progressive muscular atrophy, which may have an onset in childhood. MNDs can be classified as upper and lower. Upper MNDs affect neurons of the motor cortex, which extend to the brain stem (corticobulbar tracts) or spinal cord (corticospinal tracts). Upper MNDs are distinguished by hyperactive reflexes and increased tone, but atrophy and fasciculations are absent. Lower MNDs affect the anterior horn cells, cranial nerve motor nuclei, or their efferent axons to the skeletal muscles. Lower MNDs are distinguished by presence of atrophy and fasciculations, but reflexes are diminished or absent and tone is decreased or absent. In bulbar type palsies, only the cranial nerve motor nuclei in the brain stem (bulbar nuclei) are affected. Cause of death is usually respiratory failure and/or repeated chest infections (Motor Neurone Disease Association, 2017; Porter, 2018).

Cause

The etiology is often unknown, and most cases are sporadic. An exception is childhood onset of progressive muscular atrophy, which is an inherited autosomal recessive disorder.

Types

- *Primary lateral sclerosis* (PLS; spastic primary paraplegia)
  - ▶ Accounts for approximately 2% of MND cases.
  - ▶ Characterized by spasticity and brisk reflexes, including a positive Babinski sign.
  - ▶ Neurons of the motor cortex are affected, which extend to the brain stem (corticobulbar tracts) or spinal cord (corticospinal tracts).
  - ▶ Balance is often impaired.
  - ▶ Muscle stiffness and signs of distal motor weakness gradually increase, affecting the limbs.
  - ▶ Person may experience bladder involvement in the form of spasms and urinary urgency.
  - ▶ Survival is often more than 10 years from symptom onset (Motor Neurone Disease Association, 2017; Porter, 2018).
- *Progressive bulbar palsy* (PBP; progressive bulbar atrophy)
  - ▶ Accounts for approximately 5% of MND cases.
  - ▶ Muscles innervated by cranial nerves and corticobulbar tracts are predominantly affected.
  - ▶ Characterized by rapidly progressive speech (nasal voice, dysarthria), chewing, and swallowing (dysphagia) problems.
  - ▶ Weak movement of facial muscles and tongue and weak palatal movement may occur.
  - ▶ Aspiration and choking are risk factors.
  - ▶ Bulbar-level symptoms may be present for several months before limbs become involved.

▶ Muscles in upper limbs, neck, and shoulder girdle may become progressively weaker (Motor Neurone Disease Association, 2017; O'Toole, 2017; Porter, 2018).

- *Progressive muscular atrophy* (PLS)
  ▶ Accounts for 5%–10% of MND cases.
  ▶ Anterior horn cell involvement may occur alone or is more prominent than corticospinal involvement.
  ▶ Has limb onset, with muscle wasting and weakness.
  ▶ Twitching or rippling under the skin (fasciculations) may be visible.
  ▶ Disorder is characterized by slowly progressive, symmetrical, proximal upper limb weakness (flail arms). Flail legs may occur.
  ▶ Survival is typically more than 4 years. If only one flail arm or leg is present, survival is 5–10 years from onset (Motor Neurone Disease Association, 2017; Porter, 2018).
- *Progressive pseudobulbar palsy*
  ▶ Muscle stiffness and signs of distal motor weakness gradually increase, affecting the lower cranial nerves.
  ▶ Fasciculations and muscle atrophy may follow.
  ▶ Emotional lability may occur.
  ▶ Disorder usually takes several years to result in total disability (Porter, 2018).

Evaluation/Assessment

Areas

- Activities of Daily Living/Instrumental ADL: basic ADLs: eating (chewing, swallowing, weight loss), dressing, toileting and continence, bathing/showering, transfers, functional mobility, functional communication (dysarthria, voice volume, keyboarding); independent living skills: financial management, medication management, meal preparation, housekeeping, home maintenance, shopping, driving
- Education/Work: work performance, work site modification
- Play/Leisure: interests, types, frequency, locations
- Rest/Sleep: sleep disturbances
- Social Participation: types, frequency, location, with whom
- Sensorimotor: hyper or hypo tendon and muscle reflexes, muscle weakness, muscle atrophy, fatigue, joint range of motion, falls, hand dexterity, grip strength, muscle cramps, fasciculations. (Note: sensory changes to sight, hearing, and touch are not associated with MND, but limitations may be present due to other causes.)
- Cognitive/Perceptual: not affected directly, but dementia is a comorbidity
- Psychosocial: emotional lability, role performance, loss of independence, depression, anxiety, fear, death and dying, quality of life, sense of hopelessness and helplessness, sense of well-being
- Context/Environment: family and caregiver education, social support, referrals to other professionals/agencies, assistive devices, home modification, electronic environmental controls, community and internet resources
- Comorbidities: amyotrophic lateral sclerosis, obesity, frontotemporal dementia

Instruments

Instruments Developed by Occupational Therapy Personnel

- Assessment of Motor and Process Skills (8th ed.; AMPS-8; Fisher & Bray Jones, 2016)
- Pool Activity Level (PAL) Instrument for Occupational Profiling (4th ed.; PAL-4; Pool, 2012)

Instruments Developed by Other Professionals and Used by Occupational Therapy Personnel

- Amyotrophic Lateral Sclerosis Functional Rating Scale-R (ALSFRS-R; Cedarbaum et al., 1999)

Problems/Issues

Activities of Daily Living/Instrumental ADL

- Person may experience difficulty using regular eating utensils due to decreased muscle strength.

- Person may become incontinent or constipated.
- Person may have difficulty bathing or showering due to lack of energy/fatigue.
- Person may have difficulty transferring due to muscle weakness.
- Person may need assistance with managing medications, which may change type and dosage frequently as disease progresses.
- Person may have difficulty shopping related to fatigue and muscle weakness.
- Person may be unable to continue driving due to muscle weakness.

Education/Work
- Person may be unable to continue to perform work tasks.
- Person may need to retire due to loss of functional abilities.

Play/Leisure
- Person may be unable to engage in favorite leisure occupations due to decreased abilities/skills needed for such engagement.
- Person may refuse to consider engaging in new leisure occupations due to loss of hope about living.

Rest/Sleep
- Person may experience sleep disturbances, including decreased ability to turn over in bed due to progressive motor weakness.
- Person may experience insomnia.

Social Participation
- Person may be unable to participate actively in social activities due to decreased communication skills, difficulty with chewing and swallowing, or decreased motor skills.
- Person may avoid or refuse to participate in social activities because of changes in occupational performance abilities/skills.

Sensorimotor
- Person may have increased or decreased reflex responses depending on type of MND.
- Person usually experiences muscle weakness.
- Person may experience muscle atrophy.
- Person may experience stumbles, tripping, or falls.
- Person may experience loss of grip strength.
- Person may experience decreased hand dexterity.
- Person may experience muscle cramps.
- Person may have fasciculations depending on type of MND.

Cognitive/Perceptual
- Person may experience dementia depending on the type of MND.
- Person may experience changes in visuospatial perception.

Psychosocial
- Person usually becomes increasingly dependent on others for care.
- Person may experience depressive thoughts.
- Person may be fearful and anxious about the future.
- Person may experience emotional lability (inappropriate or excessive crying or laughter).
- Person may express feelings of hopelessness, helplessness, and decreased sense of well-being.
- Person may experience loss of ability to perform role-related tasks.
- Person may experience decreased quality of life.
- Caregivers must cope with increasing burden of caregiving role as person's functional ability declines (Foley, 2016).

Context/Environment
- Person may not have access to adaptive devices or equipment to permit/facilitate occupational performance.

- Person, family, and caregivers may not have access to informational resources on the nature and management of MND conditions.
- Person and family may not have access to information and techniques to modify home or living environment to facilitate transfers and mobility.

Intervention/Treatment

Models and programs developed by occupational therapy personnel include Living Well With MND (Dunn, 2019), occupational therapy in hospice care (Stevens, 2017), occupational therapy services (Motor Neurone Disease Association, 2017), and wheelchair services (Rolfe, 2012). Models and programs developed by other professionals but used by occupational therapy personnel include communications technology (Mackenzie et al., 2016). Team members include physicians, neurologists, psychologists, nursing personnel, physical therapy personnel, dieticians or nutritionists, speech–language pathologists, social workers, recreation specialists, and occupational therapy personnel. Goals are to provide information, techniques, equipment and devices to assist person to complete everyday activities for as long as possible as the condition advances (Motor Neurone Disease Association, 2017).

Activities of Daily Living/Instrumental ADL
- Assist client to perform ADL tasks that are important to the individual.
- Assist client to perform IADL tasks that are meaningful to the individual.

Education/Work
- No information identified.

Play/Leisure
- Encourage client to continue engagement in leisure occupations. Use of adaptive devices or technology may be useful.
- Explore with client new interests that might be substituted for those that cannot be continued as activity restrictions and physical limitations increase due to disease progression.

Rest/Sleep
- Bed sheets with satin panels or satin sheets may facilitate turning over in bed.

Social Participation
- Assist client to maintain participation in social activities for as long as possible.
- Recommend adjustments or adaptations to participation, such as use of mobility devices (walkers, scooters, wheelchairs), assistive devices for eating, shorter outings, less physically demanding activities, more passive activities, fewer demands for communication or more use of adaptive or augmentative communication, more use of computer-assisted communication (e.g., Skype, Zoom).

Sensorimotor
- Energy conservation: Educate and provide practice in ways to conserve energy, such as sitting for dressing.
- Fatigue management: Education in activity pacing using alternate rest and activity cycles.
- Posture and positioning: Educate and provide equipment as needed to maintain good posture in sitting or semireclining positions.

Cognitive/Perceptual
- Encourage development of a self-management program.
- Assist client and others to plan ahead for future needs for assistive technology.

Psychosocial
- Provide stress management techniques: relaxation training, deep breathing, mindfulness.
- Explore with client and others what activities will increase quality of life and sense of well-being within individual's capacities, family situation, or community resources.

- Establish rapport with client, family, and caregivers to facilitate discussion involving functional loss and future planning to minimize crisis situations.
- Assist client to maintain sense of control over daily life through active choices (Sakellariou et al., 2013).

Context/Environment

- Provide adaptive devices, such as adaptive cutlery and plates, leg lifters, and large-grip household items.
- Explore with client use of specialized adaptive equipment, such as mobile arm supports, head and neck supports, seating systems, electronic switches (for lights, TV, radio, computer, music player, microwave), electronic feeders, electronic standing aids or electric wheelchair.
- Explore with client different types of communication technology: desktop, laptop, tablets, mobile phone, prediction software, alphabet boards, picture boards, picture notebooks, voice-activated, apps (applications).
- Provide instruction in use and care of any adaptive equipment, devices, or augmentative communication systems.
- Provide family and caregivers with access to information about MND, its management, and its progressive course.
- Recommend home modifications to facilitate mobility and improve safety.
- Provide information about available community and internet resources.

Precautions/Safety Considerations

Aspiration is a risk factor for those with bulbar types. Falls are risk factors for those with lower limb involvement. Frequency reevaluations may be needed because changes in function can occur quickly.

Prognosis and Outcome

There is no cure. MND kills one-third of people affected within 1 year, and more than half within 2 years of diagnosis.

REFERENCES

Dunn, Y. (2019). Living well with MND. *OT News, 27*(4), 41.

Foley, G. (2016). Burden by obligation: Recognising the caring roles of people with motor neurone disease. *Palliative Medicine, 30*(10), 981–982. https://doi.org/10.1177/0269216316661687

Mackenzie, L., Bhuta, P., Rusten, K., Devine, J., Love, A., & Waterson, P. (2016). Communications technology and motor neuron disease: An Australian survey of people with motor neuron disease. *JMIR Rehabilitation and Assistive Technologies, 3*(1), Article e2. https://doi.org/10.2196/rehab.4017

Motor Neurone Disease Association. (2017). *Occupational therapy for motor neurone disease* (Version 1.2).

O'Toole, M. T. (Ed.). (2017). *Mosby's dictionary of medicine, nursing & health professions* (10th ed.). Elsevier.

Porter, R. S. (Ed.). (2018). *The Merck manual of diagnosis and therapy* (20th ed.). Merck Sharp & Dohme.

Rolfe, J. (2012). Planning wheelchair service provision in motor neurone disease: Implications for service delivery and commissioning. *British Journal of Occupational Therapy, 75*(5), 217–222. https://doi.org/10.4276/030802212X13361458480243

Sakellariou, K., Boniface, G., & Brown, P. (2013). Experiences of living with motor neurone disease: A review of qualitative research. *Disability and Rehabilitation, 35*(21), 1765–1773. https://doi.org/10.3109/09638288.2012.753118

Stevens, B. (2017). Supporting people with motor neurone disease. *OT News, 25*(7), 28–30.

Multiple Sclerosis
Also called MS.

Description

Multiple sclerosis is a disorder of demyelination in the brain and spinal cord causing patches of sclerosis (plaques), which occurs primarily in young adults. Symptoms depend on the location and size of the plaques. Typical symptoms include visual loss, diplopia, nystagmus, dysarthria, muscle weakness, gait disturbances, vertigo, clumsiness, spasticity, paresthesia, urinary dysfunction, mood alterations (emotional lability, apathy, euphoria, depression), fatigue, and cognitive dysfunction (inattention, poor judgment). Typically, the symptoms show exacerbations and remissions (Porter, 2018; *Stedman's*, 2011).

Four variations or patterns are recognized:

- *Relapsing-remitting pattern:* Exacerbations alternate with remissions. During remission, partial or full recovery may occur, and symptoms are stable. Remissions may last for months or years. Pattern is the most common.
- *Primary progressive pattern:* The disease progresses with no remissions, although some plateaus may occur in which the disease does not seem to be progressing.
- *Secondary progressive pattern:* The disease begins with relapses alternating with remission, but then progresses without remissions.
- *Progressive relapsing pattern:* The disease progresses slowly, but progression is interrupted by relapses. Pattern is rare (Porter, 2018).

Cause

MS is believed to be an immunologic disorder caused by infection of a latent virus which when activated triggers a secondary autoimmune response. Possible viruses include a human herpes virus such as Epstein-Barr virus. Living in temperate climates, low levels of vitamin D, and cigarette smoking appear to increase risk (Porter, 2018).

Evaluation/Assessment

Areas

- Activities of Daily Living/Instrumental ADL: self-care (dressing, eating, bathing, toileting), dysphagia (difficulty swallowing), dysarthria (difficulty speaking), slurred speech, bowel and bladder function (incontinence), homemaking skills, meal preparation, mobility, handwriting
- Education/Work: education level, work requirements (hand functions, reading), work environment
- Play/Leisure: interests, type and frequency of engagement, location, level of satisfaction
- Rest/Sleep: sleep disturbance, sleep disorders
- Social Participation: type and frequency of participation, location, with whom
- Sensorimotor: muscle strength, balance and postural stability, ataxia and clumsiness, tremor, gait, dizziness, gross and fine motor coordination, spasticity, stiffness, spasms, proprioception, functional motor skills (bending, lifting, carrying, reaching), sensory changes (numbness on one side of the body, tingling, temperature regulation), visual changes (diplopia [double vision], scotoma [spot of vision loss]), decreased vividness of color red, dimming of vision, optic neuritis (pain when moving the eyes), fatigue and lethargy, changes in physical activity
- Cognitive/Perceptual: attending behavior, working memory, processing speed, executive functions, mental flexibility, time management, body image, stereognosis, kinesthesia, visuospatial relationships
- Psychosocial: emotional regulation (euphoria, depression), anxiety, self-efficacy, values and beliefs, role performance and expectation, quality of life, self-concept

- Context/Environment: assistive devices and equipment, home safety, home and community accessibility and barriers, home/living environment modification, social support, cultural values and expectations, costs
- Comorbidity: no information identified

Instruments
Instruments Developed by Occupational Therapy Personnel

- Actual Reality (AR; Goverover & DeLuca, 2018; Goverover, Hass, & DeLuca, 2016; and Goverover et al., 2010, in References)
- Adolescent/Adult Sensory Profile (AASP; Brown & Dunn, 2002)
- Canadian Occupational Performance Measure (5th ed.; COPM-5; Law et al., 2014)
- Community Integration Measure (CIM; McColl et al., 2001)
- Dynamic Loewenstein Occupational Therapy Cognitive Assessment (DLOTCA; Katz et al., 2012)
- Executive Function Performance Test (EFPT; Baum & Wolf, 2013; see also Voelbel et al., 2011, in References)
- Functional Behavior Profile (FBP; Baum et al., 1993)
- Impact on Participation and Autonomy (IPA; Cardol et al., 1999)
- MS Cognitive Impairment Impact on Occupational Profile Questionnaire (MSCIIOPQ; Abraham & Rege, 2012, in References)
- Multidimensional Assessment of Tremor (MAT; Daudrich et al., 2010, in References)
- Nine Hole Peg Test (NHPT; Kellor et al., 1971; Mathiowetz et al., 1985)
- Occupational Performance History Interview (Version 2.1; OPHI-II; Kielhofner et al., 2004)
- Occupational Self Assessment–Daily Living Scales (OSA-DLS; Scott, 2016)
- Reintegration to Normal Living Index (RNLI; Wood-Dauphinee & Willams, 1987; Wood et al., 1988)
- Satisfaction With Daily Occupations (SDO; Eklund, 2004)
- Self-Efficacy for Performing Energy Conservation Strategies Assessment (SEPECSA; Leipold & Mathiowetz, 2005)
- Weekly Calendar Planning Activity (WCPA; Toglia, 2015)
- Western University's On-Road Assessment (WUORA; Classen et al., 2017, in References)

Instruments Developed by Other Professionals and Used by Occupational Therapy Personnel

- Action Research Arm Test (ARAT; Lyle, 1981)
- Behavior Rating Inventory of Executive Function–Adult Version (BRIEF-A; Roth et al., 2005)
- Behavioural Assessment of the Dysexecutive Syndrome (BADS; Wilson et al., 1996)
- Brief International Cognitive Assessment for Multiple Sclerosis (BICAMS; Langdon et al., 2012; see also Goverover, Chiaravalloti, & DeLuca, 2016, in References)
- Brief Visuospatial Memory Test–Revised (BVMT-R; Benedict, 1997)
- California Verbal Learning Test (3rd ed.; CVLT-3; Delis et al., 2017)
- Checklist Individual Strength (CIS; Vercoulen et al., 1994)
- Chicago Multiscale Depression Inventory (CMDI; Nyenhuis & Luchetta, 1998)
- Community Participation Indicators (CPI; Butterfoss, 2006)
- Delis-Kaplan Executive Function System (D-KEFS; Delis et al., 2001)
- Dysexecutive Questionnaire Revised (DEX-R; Simblett et al., 2017)
- Everyday Memory Questionnaire–Revised (EMQ-R; Royle & Lincoln, 2008)
- Expanded Disability Status Scale (EDSS; Kurtzke 1983)
- Fatigue Impact Scale (FIS; Fisk et al., 1994)
- Fatigue Severity Scale (FSS; Krupp et al., 1989; see also Johansson et al., 2014, in References)
- Functional Assessment of Chronic Illness Therapy–Fatigue Scale (FACIT-F; Smith, 2010)
- Functional Assessment of Multiple Sclerosis (FAMS; Cella et al., 1996)
- Functional Independence Measure (FIM; Uniform Data System for Medical Rehabilitation, 1997)

- Grip strength (dynamometer; JAMAR, Lafayette Instrument; Wang et al., 2018)
- Jebsen-Taylor Hand Function Test (JTHFT; Jebsen et al., 1969)
- Leeds Multiple Sclerosis Quality of Life (LMSQoL; Ford et al., 2001)
- Manual Muscle Test (MMT; see Bennett et al., in References, for scoring)
- Minimal Assessment of Cognitive Function in Multiple Sclerosis (MACFIMS; Benedict et al., 2006)
- Modified Fatigue Impact Scale (MFIS; Ritvo et al., 1997; see Bennett et al., 2015, p. 50, in References)
- Montreal Cognitive Assessment (MoCA; Nasreddine et al., 2005)
- Multidimensional Fatigue Inventory (MFI; Smets et al., 1995)
- Multiple Sclerosis Functional Composite (MSFC; Cutter et al., 1999)
- Multiple Sclerosis Neuropsychological Questionnaire (MSNQ; Benedict et al., 2003)
- Multiple Sclerosis Quality of Life-54 (MSQOL-54; National Multiple Sclerosis Society, 1997)
- Multiple Sclerosis Resilience Scale (MSRS; Gromisch et al., 2018)
- Multiple Sclerosis Self-Management Scale (MSSMS; Bishop et al., 2008; see also Ghahari et al., 2014, in References)
- Open-Trial Selective Reminding Test (OTSRT; Chiaravalloti et al., 2009)
- Patient Health Questionnaire (PHQ-9; Löwe et al., 2004)
- Purdue Pegboard Text (PPT; Tiffin, 1948)
- Rivermead Mobility Index (RMI; Collen et al., 1991)
- Short-Form 36 Health Survey (SF-36; Ware et al., 1993)
- Symbol Digit Modalities Test (SDMT; Smith, 1973)
- Tower of London (TOL-DX; Culbertson & Zillmer, 2001)
- Trail Making Tests (TMT; Reitan & Wolfson, 1995)
- Visual Analogue Scale (VAS) Numeric Pain Rating Scale (NPRS; pain scale: 0 = *no pain*, 10 = *worst pain ever*)

Problems/Issues

Activities of Daily Living/Instrumental ADL
- Person may have dysarthria (poor articulation).
- Person may have dysphagia.
- Person may have incontinence in bladder, bowel, or both.
- Person may have erectile dysfunction.
- Person may have difficulty managing money and financial matters.
- Person may have difficulty performing tasks related to child care or pet care.

Education/Work
- Person may be unable to complete assignments that require visual skills, such as reading, due to changes in visual system.
- Person may have difficulty performing work activities that require hand dexterity skills such as keyboarding, handwriting, and other manual tasks.
- Person may be unable to work because of physical barriers or policy restrictions in the work environment (lack of close-by and covered disabled parking, stairs, elevators, height of desk and chair, temperature in work space, accessible toilets).
- Other symptoms that affect education or work activities include fatigue, pain, incontinence, memory loss, decreased ability to concentrate, depression, and anxiety.

Play/Leisure
- Person may report giving up doing favorite leisure activities because of difficulty performing certain tasks or activities.

Rest/Sleep
- Person may experience sleep disturbance due to pain.

Social Participation
- Person may have stopped engaging in social activities because of symptoms.

Sensorimotor
- Person may have incoordination and poor balance.
- Person may have impaired muscle tone.
- Person may experience muscle weakness that may appear in one limb, one side of body, or in multiple limbs on either side of the body.
- Person may experience decreased gross and fine motor skills.
- Person may have tremors.
- Person may be clumsy and ataxic.
- Person may experience exercise intolerance.
- Person may report feeling cold even in rooms that are warm.
- Person may report being hypersensitive to heat.
- Person may have visual impairments including double vision, loss of vision, decreased oculomotor control, nystagmus, color blindness, optic neuritis, sensitivity to light and glare.
- Person may experience fatigue and lethargy.
- Person may experience pain.

Cognitive/Perceptual
- Person may have cognitive impairment in attention, speed of processing information, memory, and executive functions.
- Person may have cognitive impairment in planning and problem solving.
- Person may have impaired self-awareness of and lack of insight into disability.
- Person may experience decreased cognitive functioning due to being in an exacerbation in which symptoms are increased in number, severity, or both; depression, fatigue, taking certain medications, and stress (Buzaid et al., 2013).

Psychosocial
- Person may experience euphoria and depression.
- Person may experience difficulty with behavioral regulation.
- Person may experience emotional lability.
- Person may experience apathy and lack of motivation.
- Person may experience loss of self-confidence and self-efficacy.
- Person may experience loss of self-esteem and self-worth.
- Person may want to hide disability for fear of discrimination.
- Person may experience increased difficulty coping with stress.

Context/Environment
- Person's home/living environment may include safety hazards.
- Person's home and community may present accessibility barriers.
- Person may need a social support system.
- Person may lack information on legal rights for persons with disabilities, including discrimination, disability pay, health-care insurance.

Intervention/Treatment

Models of practice and intervention programs developed by occupational therapists include Being, Belonging and Becoming (Stern & Goverover, 2018), case studies (Athmann & Molitor, 2019; Finlayson, 2011; Preissner et al., 2016), client-centered therapy (Eyssen et al., 2014; Eyssen et al., 2013), cognitive occupation-based program for people with multiple sclerosis (Reilly & Hynes, 2018), early intervention (Sweetland et al., 2014), inpatient energy management education program (Hersche et al., 2019), one-to-one fatigue management course (Van Heest et al., 2017), person-environment-occupation model (Ghahari & Finlayson, 2018), person-environment-occupational performance (Reilly & Hynes, 2018), model of sensory processing

(Colbeck, 2018), and weekly calendar planning activity (WCPA; Goverover et al., 2020). Models developed by other professionals but used by occupational therapy personnel include the cognitive occupation-based program (Hynes & Forwell, 2019), Community Reintegration for Socially Isolated Patients (CRISP; Kalina et al., 2018), fall prevention program (Sosnoff et al., 2015), fatigue management (Asano & Finlayson, 2014), relapse management (Asano, Hawken, et al., 2015), functional electrical stimulation (Esnouf et al., 2010), self-generation learning (Goverover et al., 2013, 2014; Goverover et al., 2018), Nintendo Wii Fit (Plow & Finlayson, 2014), self-management (Ghahari et al., 2019; Kos et al., 2016), speed of processing training (SPT; Chiaravalloti et al., 2018), teleconference-delivered program (Asano, Preissner, et al., 2015; Dunleavy et al., 2013), and vocational rehabilitation intervention (Jellie et al., 2014). Intervention can be based on preventative, educational, compensatory, remedial or consultative approaches. The focus is on enabling clients to participate in occupations that have value and meaning to them by developing and implementing practical solutions to the challenges of everyday living with MS (Ghahari & Finlayson, 2018). Team members include physicians, nurses, physical therapists, psychologists, neuropsychology, speech–language pathologists, and occupational therapists (Conrad et al., 2012). The most common goals are related to self-care activities, instrumental activities of daily living, productive activities, and leisure activities (Asano, Preissner, et al., 2015).

Activities of Daily Living/Instrumental ADL

- Teach one-handed techniques, including use of devices such as a buttonhook, Velcro fasteners, elastic shoelaces, wall-mounted electric can opener, clamp-on peeler, rocker knife.
- Recommend use of assistive devices to facilitate self-care activities such as eating, dressing, or taking a shower.
- Recommend equipment for mobility: scooter, wheelchair (manual, power).
- Assist in training personal care attendant (PCA) by providing clear instructions on duties needed by client (transfers, dressing, bathing, bowel and bladder management, body positioning client in bed or wheelchair, meal preparation, housekeeping, shopping); role-playing with client may assist in developing client's communication skills.
- Consider a safe driving evaluation if person is still driving.

Education/Work

- Assist in modifying work environment through consultation and recommendations to reduce barriers and increase access to work environment (travel, parking, getting to assigned work station, performing tasks in work station, access to other areas in work environment such as toilets, break room, conference room).
- Consult with employers to support accommodations in the work environment.

Play/Leisure

- Encourage engagement in leisure activities with modifications as needed.
- Explore new leisure activities if previous activities are no longer possible.

Rest/Sleep

- See Sleep–Wake Disorders in Section 13: Lifestyle Conditions.

Social Participation

- Engage client to participate in social and community activities. "Dry runs" and practice may be needed to alleviate fears and solve problems.

Sensorimotor

- Educate client and caregivers in fall prevention and safety.
- Suggest and implement modifications to work and home environment to accommodate for visual impairments and sensitivities such as increasing font size, maximizing background–foreground contrast, using antiglare filters on computer monitor.

- Teach energy conservation (motion economy) and work simplification program to reduce energy demand.
- Assist client to develop a fatigue management program.
- Facilitate exercise program by integrating exercises into everyday activities, such as cooking, housekeeping, and shopping.
- Suggest wearing cooling vest or other cooling devices when performing activities that tend to heat the body. Assist client to identify situations and activities that may contribute to over-heating, such as using too much hot water while bathing or showering.
- Management of tremor
  - Hand-over-hand technique: Use nondominant hand to support dominant hand.
  - Weighted wrist: Use a weights wrist band (1/2 to 2 lb) on dominant arm starting with 1/2-lb increment from lightest to heaviest.
  - Weighted tool: Use a weighted object starting with 1/2-lb increments.
  - Weighted tool: Use a soft weighted pen wrap (foam, pipe insulation) for handwriting.
  - Splint: Use a commercial universal wrist splint to provide distal support or fabricated splint.
  - Combine any two approaches.

Cognitive/Perceptual

- Assist client in developing a self-management program including time management, activity schedule, and necessary reminders for appointments and medication renewals.
- Memory tasks may be facilitated by use of apps on a smartphone for medication management, appointments, and shopping lists.
- Memory training may be improved by using mass and spaced practice.
- Providing training to improve processing speed (Chiaravalloti et al., 2018).
- Provide training in time management.
- Provide training in energy conservation (motion economy).

Psychosocial

- Assist client to develop a self-management strategy, including adjusting outlook, managing stress, managing symptoms, heathy lifestyle, effective communication, and setting priorities (Ghahari et al., 2019).

Context/Environment

- Instruct client in maintenance and simple repair of wheelchair and other equipment.
- Assist in training PCA in safe handling (lifting, transferring, carrying), body mechanics to prevent back injuries, energy conservation (motion economy), wheelchair/scooter maintenance and repair.
- Provide information on home and community accessibility to client, family, and caregivers and recommendations for modifications.
- Assist client and family in maintaining a safe living environment to prevent falls and other injuries, such as rearranging furniture, adding lighting to stairs and hallways, tacking down loose floorboards, removing small rugs, installing grab bars in the tub or showers, throwing out worn shoes.
- Encourage client to participate in social support groups.
- Provide information on legal rights and support services.

Precautions/Safety Considerations

Person is at risk for falling. Person should be monitored for cognitive decline.

Prognosis and Outcome

There is no known cure. Disease is degenerative, but course of disease is highly variable. Person may live for many years with the disease, although severe forms do shorten life span (Porter, 2018).

REFERENCES

Abraham, P., & Rege, P. V. (2012). A study of cognitive impairments in multiple sclerosis—Occupational therapy perspective. *Indian Journal of Occupational Therapy, 44*(1), 2–12.

Asano, M., & Finlayson, M. L. (2014). Meta-analysis of three different types of fatigue management interventions for people with multiple sclerosis: Exercise, education, and medication. *Multiple Sclerosis International, 2014*, Article 798285. https://doi.org/10.1155/2014/798285

Asano, M., Hawken, K., Turpin, M., Eitzen, A., & Finlayson, M. (2015). The lived experience of multiple sclerosis relapse: How adults with multiple sclerosis processed their relapse experience and evaluated their need for postrelapse care. *Multiple Sclerosis International, 2015*, Article 351416. https://doi.org/10.1155/2015/351416

Asano, M., Preissner, K., Duffy, R., Meixell, M., & Finlayson, M. (2015). Goals set after completing a teleconference-delivered program for managing multiple sclerosis fatigue. *American Journal of Occupational Therapy, 69*(3), Article 6903290010. https://doi.org/10.5014/ajot.2015.015370

Athmann, A., & Molitor, W. L. (2019). Occupational therapy for multiple sclerosis. *OT Practice, 24*(11), 12–14.

Bennett, S. E., Bednarik, P., Bobryk, P., & Smith C. (2015). *A practical guide to rehabilitation in multiple sclerosis*. Consortium of Multiple Sclerosis Centers and the France Foundation. https://www.cmeaims.org/resources/AIMS-rehab-primer.pdf

Buzaid, A., Dodge, M. P., Handmacher, L., & Kiltz, P. J. (2013). Activities of daily living: Evaluation and treatment in persons with multiple sclerosis. *Physical Medicine and Rehabilitation Clinics of North America, 24*(4), 629–638. https://doi.org/10.1016/j.pmr.2013.06.008

Chiaravalloti, N. D., Goverover, Y., Costa, S. L., & DeLuca, J. (2018). A pilot study examining speed of processing training (SPT) to improve processing speed in persons with multiple sclerosis. *Frontiers in Neurology, 9*, Article 685. https://doi.org/10.3389/fneur.2018.00685

Classen, S., Krasniuk, S., Alvarez, L., Monahan, M., Morrow, S. A., & Danter, T. (2017). Development and validity of Western University's on-road assessment. *OTJR: Occupation, Participation and Health, 37*(1), 14–29. https://doi.org/10.1177/1539449216672859

Colbeck, M. (2018). Sensory processing, cognitive fatigue, and quality of life in multiple sclerosis. *Canadian Journal of Occupational Therapy, 85*(2), 169–175. https://doi.org/10.1177/0008417417727298

Conrad, A., Coenen, M., Schmalz, H., Kesselring, J., & Cieza, A. (2012). Validation of the Comprehensive ICF Core Set for multiple sclerosis from the perspective of occupational therapists. *Scandinavian Journal of Occupational Therapy, 19*(6), 468–487. https://doi.org/10.3109/11038128.2012.665475

Daudrich, B., Hurl, D., & Forwell, S. (2010). Multidimensional assessment of tremor in multiple sclerosis: A useful instrument. *International Journal of MS Care, 12*(1), 23–32. https://doi.org/10.7224/1537-2073-12.1.23

Dunleavy, L., Preissner, K. L., & Finlayson, M. L. (2013). Facilitating a teleconference-delivered fatigue management program: Perspectives of occupational therapists. *Canadian Journal of Occupational Therapy, 80*(5), 304–313. https://doi.org/10.1177/0008417413511787

Esnouf, J. E., Taylor, P. N., Mann, G. E., & Barrett, C. L. (2010). Impact on activities of daily living using a functional electrical stimulation device to improve dropped foot in people with multiple sclerosis, measured by the Canadian Occupational Performance Measure. *Multiple Sclerosis, 16*(9), 1141–1147. https://doi.org/10.1177/1352458510366013

Eyssen, I. C. J. M., Dekker, J., de Groot, V., Steultjens, E. M., Knol, D. L., Polman, C. H., & Steultjens, M. P. (2014). Client-centred therapy in multiple sclerosis: More intensive diagnostic evaluation and less intensive treatment. *Journal of Rehabilitation Medicine, 46*(6), 527–531. https://doi.org/10.2340/16501977-1797

Eyssen, I. C. J. M., Steultjens, M. P. M., de Groot, V., Steultjens, E. M. J., Knol, D. L., Polman, C. H., & Dekker, J. (2013). A cluster randomised controlled trial on the efficacy of client-centred occupational therapy in multiple sclerosis: Good process, poor outcome. *Disability and Rehabilitation, 35*(19), 1636–1646. https://doi.org/10.3109/09638288.2012.748845

Finlayson, M. (2011). *Clinical bulletin information for health professionals: Occupational therapy in multiple sclerosis rehabilitation.* National Multiple Sclerosis Society. https://www.nation almssociety.org/NationalMSSociety/media/MSNationalFiles/Brochures/Clinical-Bulletin -OT.pdf

Ghahari, S., & Finlayson, M. (2018). *A resource for healthcare professionals: Occupational therapy in multiple sclerosis rehabilitation.* National Multiple Sclerosis Society. https://www.nationalms society.org/PRC

Ghahari, S., Forwell, S. J., Suto, M. J., & Morassaei, S. (2019). Multiple sclerosis self-management model: Personal and contextual requirements for successful self-management. *Patient Education and Counseling, 102*(5), 1013–1020. https://doi.org/10.1016/j.pec.2018.12.028

Ghahari, S., Khoshbin, L. S., & Forwell, S. J. (2014). The Multiple Sclerosis Self-Management Scale: Clinicometric testing. *International Journal of MS Care, 16*(2), 61–67. https://doi.org/10 .7224/1537-2073.2013-019

Goverover, Y., Chiaravalloti, N., & DeLuca, J. (2013). The influence of executive functions and memory on self-generation benefit in persons with multiple sclerosis. *Journal of Clinical and Experimental Neuropsychology, 35*(7), 775–783. https://doi.org/10.1080/13803395.2013.824553

Goverover, Y., Chiaravalloti, N. D., & DeLuca, J. (2014). Task meaningfulness and degree of cognitive impairment: Do they affect self-generated learning in persons with multiple sclerosis? *Neuropsychological Rehabilitation, 24*(2), 155–171. https://doi.org/10.1080/09602011 .2013.868815

Goverover, Y., Chiaravalloti, N., & DeLuca, J. (2016). Brief International Cognitive Assessment for Multiple Sclerosis (BICAMS) and performance of everyday life tasks: Actual reality. *Multiple Sclerosis, 22*(4), 544–550. https://doi.org/10.1177/1352458515593637

Goverover, Y., Chiaravalloti, N., Genova, H., & DeLuca, J. (2018). A randomized controlled trial to treat impaired learning and memory in multiple sclerosis: The self-GEN trial. *Multiple Sclerosis, 24*(8), 1096–1104. https://doi.org/10.1177/1352458517709955

Goverover, Y., & DeLuca, J. (2018). Assessing everyday life functional activity using actual reality in persons with MS. *Rehabilitation Psychology, 63*(2), 276–285. https://doi.org/10.1037/ rep0000212

Goverover, Y., Haas, S., & DeLuca, J. (2016). Money management activities in persons with multiple sclerosis. *Archives of Physical Medicine and Rehabilitation, 97*(11), 1901–1907. https://doi .org/10.1016/j.apmr.2016.05.003

Goverover, Y., O'Brien, A. R., Moore, N. B., & DeLuca, J. (2010). Actual reality: A new approach to functional assessment in persons with multiple sclerosis. *Archives of Physical Medicine and Rehabilitation, 91*(2), 252–260. https://doi.org/10.1016/j.apmr.2009.09.022

Goverover, Y., Toglia, J., & DeLuca, J. (2020). The weekly calendar planning activity in multiple sclerosis: A top-down assessment of executive functions. *Neuropsychological Rehabilitation, 30*(7), 1372–1387. https://doi.org/10.1080/09602011.2019.1584573

Hersche, R., Weise, A., Michel, G., Kesselring, J., Barbero, M., & Kool, J. (2019). Development and preliminary evaluation of a 3-week inpatient energy management education program for people with multiple sclerosis-related fatigue. *International Journal of MS Care, 21*(6), 265–274. https://doi.org/10.7224/1537-2073.2018-058

Hynes, S. M., & Forwell, S. (2019). A cognitive occupation-based programme for people with multiple sclerosis: A new occupational therapy cognitive rehabilitation intervention. *Hong Kong Journal of Occupational Therapy, 32*(1), 41–52. https://doi.org/10.1177/1569186119841263

Jellie, B., Sweetland, J., Riazi, A., Cano, S. J., & Playford, E. D. (2014). Staying at work and living with MS: A qualitative study of the impact of a vocational rehabilitation intervention. *Disability and Rehabilitation, 36*(19), 1594–1599. https://doi.org/10.3109/09638288.2013.854842

Johansson, S., Kottorp, A., Lee, K. A., Gay, C. L., & Lerdal, A. (2014). Can the Fatigue Severity Scale 7-item version be used across different patient populations as a generic fatigue measure—A comparative study using a Rasch model approach. *Health and Quality of Life Outcomes, 12*, Article 24. https://doi.org/10.1186/1477-7525-12-24

Kalina, J. T., Hinojosa, J., Strober, L., Bacon, J., Donnelly, S., & Goverover, Y. (2018). Randomized controlled trial to improve self-efficacy in people with multiple sclerosis: The Community Reintegration for Socially Isolated Patients (CRISP) program. *American Journal of Occupational Therapy, 72*(5), Article 7205205030. https://doi.org/10.5014/ajot.2018.026864

Kos, D., Duportail, M., Meirte, J., Meeus, M., D'hooghe, M. B., Nagels, G., Willekens, B., Meurrens, T., Ilsbroukx, S., & Nijs, J. (2016). The effectiveness of a self-management occupational therapy intervention on activity performance in individuals with multiple sclerosis-related fatigue: A randomized-controlled trial. *International Journal of Rehabilitation Research, 39*(3), 255–262. https://doi.org/10.1097/MRR.0000000000000178

Plow, M., & Finlayson, M. (2014). A qualitative study exploring the usability of Nintendo Wii Fit among persons with multiple sclerosis. *Occupational Therapy International, 21*, 21–32. https://doi.org/10.1002/oti.1345

Porter, R. S. (Ed.). (2018). *The Merck manual of diagnosis and therapy* (20th ed.). Merck Sharp & Dohme.

Preissner, K., Arbesman, M., & Lieberman, D. (2016). Occupational therapy interventions for adults with multiple sclerosis. *American Journal of Occupational Therapy, 70*(3), Article 7003 395010. https://doi.org/10.5014/ajot.2016.703001

Reilly, S., & Hynes, S. M. (2018). A cognitive occupation-based programme for people with multiple sclerosis: A study to test feasibility and clinical outcomes. *Occupational Therapy International, 2018*, Article 1614901. https://doi.org/10.1155/2018/1614901

Sosnoff, J. J., Moon, Y., Wajda, D. A., Finlayson, M. L., McAuley, E., Peterson, E. W., Morrison, S., & Motl, R. W. (2015). Fall risk and incidence reduction in high risk individuals with multiple sclerosis: A pilot randomized control trial. *Clinical Rehabilitation, 29*(10), 952–960. https://doi.org/10.1177/0269215514564899

Stedman's medical dictionary for the health professions and nursing (7th ed.). (2011). Wolters Kluwer.

Stern, B. Z., & Goverover, Y. (2018). Everyday technology use for men with multiple sclerosis: An occupational perspective. *British Journal of Occupational Therapy, 81*(12), 709–716. https://doi.org/10.1177/0308022618777985

Sweetland, J., Playford, D. E., & Radford, K. A. (2014). What is "early intervention" for work related difficulties for people with multiple sclerosis: A case study report. *Journal of Neurology & Neurophysiology, 5*(6), Advance online publication. https://doi.org/10.4172/2155-9562.1000252

Van Heest, K. N. L., Mogush, A. R., & Mathiowetz, V. G. (2017). Effects of a one-to-one fatigue management course for people with chronic conditions and fatigue. *American Journal of Occupational Therapy, 71*(4), Article 7104100020. https://doi.org/10.5014/ajot.2017.023440

Voelbel, G. T., Goverover, Y., Gaudino, E. A., Moore, N. B., Chiaravalloti, N., & DeLuca, J. (2011). The relationship between neurocognitive behavior of executive functions and the EFPT in individuals with multiple sclerosis. *OTJR: Occupation, Participation and Health, 31*(Suppl. 1), S30–S37. https://doi.org/10.3928/15394492-20101108-06

BIBLIOGRAPHY

Abdullah, E. J., Badr, H. E., & Manee, F. (2018). MS people's performance and satisfaction with daily occupations: Implications for occupational therapy. *OTJR: Occupation, Participation and Health, 38*(1), 28–37. https://doi.org/10.1177/1539449217719867

Asano, M., Berg, E., Johnson, K., Turpin, M., & Finlayson M. L. (2015). A scoping review of rehabilitation interventions that reduce fatigue among adults with multiple sclerosis. *Disability and Rehabilitation, 37*(9), 729–738. https://doi.org/10.3109/09638288.2014.944996

Classen, S., Krasniuk, S., Morrow, S. A., Alvarez, L., Monahan, M., Danter, T., & Rosehart, H. (2018). Visual correlates of fitness to drive in adults with multiple sclerosis. *OTJR: Occupation, Participation and Health, 38*(1), 15–27. https://doi.org/10.1177/1539449217718841

Dirette, D. P. (2017). Progressive neurodegenerative disorders: Multiple sclerosis. In B. J. Atchison & D. P. Dirette (Eds.), *Conditions in occupational therapy* (5th ed., pp. 403–408). Wolters Kluwer.

Fakolade, A., Bisson, E. J., Pétrin, J., Lamarre, J., & Finlayson, M. (2016). Effect of comorbidities on outcomes of neurorehabilitation interventions in multiple sclerosis: A scoping review. *International Journal of MS Care, 18*(6), 282–290. https://doi.org/10.7224/1537-2073.2016-015

Falk-Kessler, J., Kalina, J. T., & Miller, P. (2012). Influence of occupational therapy on resilience in individuals with multiple sclerosis. *International Journal of MS Care, 14*(3), 160–168. https://doi.org/10.7224/1537-2073-14.3.160

Finlayson, M. (Ed.). (2013). *Multiple sclerosis rehabilitation: From impairment to participation.* CRC Press.

Finlayson, M., Peterson, E., & Matsuda, P. N. (2014). Participation as an outcome in multiple sclerosis falls—Prevention research: Consensus recommendation from the International MS Falls Prevention Research Network. *International Journal of MS Care, 16*(4), 171–177. https://doi.org/10.7224/1537-2073.2014-053

Finlayson, M. L., & Cho, C. C. (2011). A profile of support group use and need among middle-aged and older adults with multiple sclerosis. *Journal of Gerontological Social Work, 54*(5) 475–493. https://doi.org/10.1080/01634372.2011.575446

Fogelberg, D. J., Hughes, A. J., Vitiello, M. V., Hoffman, J. M., & Amtmann, D. (2016). Comparison of sleep problems in individuals with spinal cord injury and multiple sclerosis. *Journal of Clinical Sleep Medicine, 12*(5), 695–701. https://doi.org/10.5664/jcsm.5798

Forwell, S. J., Hugos, L., Copperman, L. F., & Ghahari, S. (2014). Neurodegenerative diseases: Multiple sclerosis. In M. V. Radomski & C. A. T. Latham (Eds.), *Occupational therapy for physical dysfunction* (7th ed., pp. 1079–1088). Wolters Kluwer.

Foti, D. (2018). Multiple sclerosis. In H. M. Pendleton & W. Schultz-Krohn (Eds.), *Pedretti's occupational therapy* (8th ed., pp. 889–893). Elsevier.

Fritz, N. E., Eloyan, A., Baynes, M., Newsome, S. D., Calabresi, P. A., & Zackowski, K. M. (2018). Distinguishing among multiple sclerosis fallers, near-fallers and non-fallers. *Multiple Sclerosis and Related Disorders, 19*, 99–104. https://doi.org/10.1016/j.msard.2017.11.019

Ghahari, S., & Forwell, S. J. (2016). Social media representation of chronic cerebrospinal venous insufficiency intervention for multiple sclerosis. *International Journal of MS Care, 18*(2), 49–57. https://doi.org/10.7224/1537-2073.2014-073

Ghahari, S., Parvaneh, S., & Packer, T. (2013). Fatigue in progressive neurological conditions: A literature review. *Iranian Rehabilitation Journal, 11*, 85–90.

Goverover, Y., Basso, M., Wood, H., Chiaravalloti, N., & DeLuca, J. (2011). Examining the benefits of combining two learning strategies on recall of functional information in persons with multiple sclerosis. *Multiple Sclerosis, 17*(12), 1488–1497. https://doi.org/10.1177/1352458511406310

Goverover, Y., Chiaravalloti, N. D., O'Brien, A. R., & DeLuca, J. (2018). Evidenced-based cognitive rehabilitation for persons with multiple sclerosis: An updated review of the literature from 2007 to 2015. *Archives of Physical Medicine and Rehabilitation, 99*(2), 390–407. https://doi.org/10.1016/j.apmr.2017.07.021

Goverover, Y., Genova, H., Griswold, H., Chiaravalloti, N., & DeLuca, J. (2014). Metacognitive knowledge and online awareness in persons with multiple sclerosis. *NeuroRehabilitation, 35*(2), 315–323. https://doi.org/10.3233/NRE-141113

Goverover, Y., Sandroff, B. M., & DeLuca, J. (2018). Dual task of fine motor skills and problem solving in individuals with multiple sclerosis: A pilot study. *Archives of Physical Medicine and Rehabilitation, 99*(4), 635–640. https://doi.org/10.1016/j.apmr.2017.10.012

Goverover, Y., Strober, L., Chiaravalloti, N., & DeLuca, J. (2015). Factors that moderate activity limitation and participation restriction in people with multiple sclerosis. *American Journal of Occupational Therapy, 69*(2), Article 692260020. https://doi.org/10.5014/ajot.2015.014332

Hamby, J. R. (2017). The nervous system: Multiple sclerosis. In H. Smith-Gabai & S. E. Holm (Eds.), *Occupational therapy in acute care* (2nd ed., pp. 347, 349–351). AOTA Press.

Hawes, F., Billups, C., & Forwell, S. (2010). Interventions for upper-limb intention tremor in multiple sclerosis. *International Journal of MS Care, 12*(3), 122–132. https://doi.org/10.7224/1537-2073-12.3.122

Hwang, J. E., Cvitanovich, D. C., Doroski, E. K., & Vajarakitipongse, J. G. (2011). Correlations between quality of life and adaptation factors among people with multiple sclerosis. *American Journal of Occupational Therapy, 65*(6), 661–669. https://doi.org/10.5014/ajot.2011.001487

Kalb, R., Beier, M., Benedict, R. H. B., Charvet, L., Costello, K., Feinstein, A., Gingold, J., Goverover, Y., Halper, J., Harris, C., Kostich, L., Krupp, L., Lathi, E., LaRocca, N., Thrower, B., & DeLuca, J. (2018). Recommendations for cognitive screening and management in multiple sclerosis care. *Multiple Sclerosis Journal, 24*(13), 1665–1680. https://doi.org/10.1177/1352458518803785

Khan, F., & Amatya, B. (2017). Rehabilitation in multiple sclerosis: A systematic review of systematic reviews. *Archives of Physical Medicine and Rehabilitation, 98*(2), 353–367. https://doi.org/10.1016/j.apmr.2016.04.016

Kraft, G. H., Amtmann, D., Bennett, S. E., Finlayson, M., Sutliff, M. H., Tullman, M., Sidovar, M., & Rabinowicz, A. L. (2014). Assessment of upper extremity function in multiple sclerosis: Review and opinion. *Postgraduate Medicine, 126*(5), 102–108. https://doi.org/10.3810/pgm.2014.09.2803

Krasniuk, S., Classen, S., Morrow, S. A., Tippett, M., Knott, M., & Akinwuntan, A. (2019). Clinical determinants of fitness to drive in persons with multiple sclerosis: Systematic review. *Archives of Physical Medicine and Rehabilitation, 100*(8), 1534–1555. https://doi.org/10.1016/j.apmr.2018.12.029

Lexell, E. M., Flansbjer, U.-B., & Lexell, J. (2014). Self-perceived performance and satisfaction with performance of daily activities in persons with multiple sclerosis following interdisciplinary rehabilitation. *Disability and Rehabilitation, 36*(5), 373–378. https://doi.org/10.3109/09638288.2013.797506

Lexell, E. M., Iwarsson, S., & Lund, M. L. (2011). Occupational adaptation in people with multiple sclerosis. *OTJR: Occupation, Participation and Health, 31*(3), 127–134. https://doi.org/10.3928/15394492-20101025-01

Maitra, K., Hall, C., Kalish, T., Anderson, M., Dugan, E. Rehak, J., Rodríguez, V., Tamas, J., & Zeitlin, D. (2010). Five-year retrospective study of inpatient occupational therapy outcomes for patients with multiple sclerosis. *American Journal of Occupational Therapy, 64*(5), 689–694. https://doi.org/10.5014/ajot.2010.090204

McCreary, J. K., Rogers, J. A., & Forwell, S. J. (2018). Upper limb intention tremor in multiple sclerosis: An evidence-based review of assessment and treatment. *International Journal of MS Care, 20*(5), 211–223. https://doi.org/10.7224/1537-2073.2017-024

Mesa, A., Anderson, K. H., Askey-Jones, S., Gray, R., & Silber, E. (2012). The mental health needs of individuals living with multiple sclerosis: Implications for occupational therapy practice and research. *Mental Health Special Interest Section Quarterly, 35*(2), 1–4.

Morrow, S. A., Classen, S., Monahan, M., Danter, T., Taylor, R., Krasniuk, S., Rosehart, H., & He, W. (2018). On-road assessment of fitness-to-drive in persons with MS with cognitive impairment: A prospective study. *Multiple Sclerosis Journal, 24*(11), 1499–1506. https://doi.org/10.1177/1352458517723991.

Newsome, S. D., von Geldern, G., Shou, H., Baynes, M., Marasigan, R. E. R., Calabresi, P. A., & Zackowski, K. M. (2019). Longitudinal assessment of hand function in individuals with multiple sclerosis. *Multiple Sclerosis and Related Disorders, 32*, 107–113. https://doi.org/10.1016/j.msard.2019.04.035

Newsome, S. D., Wang, J. I., Kang, J. Y., Calabresi, P. A., & Zackowski, K. M. (2011). Quantitative measures detect sensory and motor impairments in multiple sclerosis. *Journal of the Neurological Sciences, 305*(1-2), 103–111. https://doi.org/10.1016/j.jns.2011.03.003

Plow, M. A., Finlayson, M., & Rezac, M. (2011). A scoping review of self-management interventions for adults with multiple sclerosis. *PM&R, 3*(3), 251–262. https://doi.org/10.1016/j.pmrj.2010.11.011

Plow, M. A., Finlayson, M., Gunzler, D., & Heinemann, A. W. (2015). Correlates of participation in meaningful activities among people with multiple sclerosis. *Journal of Rehabilitation Medicine, 47*(6), 538–545. https://doi.org/10.2340/16501977-1948

Preissner, K. (2014). *Adults with neurodegenerative diseases.* AOTA Press.

Preston, J., Haslam, S., & Lamont, L. (2012). What do people with multiple sclerosis want from an occupational therapy service? *British Journal of Occupational Therapy, 75*(6), 264–270. https://doi.org/10.4276/030802212X13383757345102

Preston, J., Hammersley, R., & Gallagher, H. (2013). The executive dysfunctions most commonly associated with multiple sclerosis and their impact on occupational performance. *British Journal of Occupational Therapy, 76*(5), 225–233. https://doi.org/10.4276/030802213X13679275042726

Prodinger, B., Weise, A. P., Shaw, L., & Stamm, T. A. (2010). A Delphi study on environmental factors that impact work and social life participation of individuals with multiple sclerosis in Austria and Switzerland. *Disability and Rehabilitation, 32*(3), 183–195. https://doi.org/10.3109/09638280903071883

Salomè, A., Sasso D'Elia, T., Franchini, G., Santilli, V., & Paolucci, T. (2019). Occupational therapy in fatigue management in multiple sclerosis: An umbrella review. *Multiple Sclerosis International, 2019,* Article 2027947. https://doi.org/10.1155/2019/2027947

Sarsak, H. I. (2018). The effectiveness of energy conservation techniques in reducing fatigue in clients with multiple sclerosis. *Researches in Arthritis & Bone Study, 1*(3), 1–2. https://crimsonpublishers.com/rabs/pdf/RABS.000512.pdf

Schmitt, M. M., Goverover, Y., DeLuca, J., & Chiaravalloti, N. (2014). Self-efficacy as a predictor of self-reported physical, cognitive, and social functioning in multiple sclerosis. *Rehabilitation Psychology, 59*(1), 27–34. https://doi.org/10.1037/a0035288

Souza, A., Kelleher, A., Cooper, R., Cooper, R. A., Iezzoni, L. I., & Collins, D. M. (2010). Multiple sclerosis and mobility-related assistive technology: Systematic review of literature. *Journal of Rehabilitation Research and Development, 47*(3), 213–224. https://doi.org/10.1682/JRRD.2009.07.0096

Squillace, M., Ray, S., & Milazzo, M. (2015). Changes in gross grasp strength and fine motor skills in adolescents with pediatric multiple sclerosis. *Occupational Therapy in Health Care, 29*(1), 77–85. https://doi.org/10.3109/07380577.2014.967441

Stern, B. Z., Strober, L., DeLuca, J., & Goverover, Y. (2018). Subjective well-being differs with age in multiple sclerosis: A brief report. *Rehabilitation Psychology, 63*(3), 474–478. https://doi.org/10.1037/rep0000220

Stout, K., & Finlayson, M. (2011). Management in chronic illness: The role of occupational therapy. *OT Practice, 16*(1), 16–19, 26.

Sweetland, J., Howse, E., & Playford, D. (2012). A systematic review of research undertaken in vocational rehabilitation for people with multiple sclerosis. *Disability and Rehabilitation, 34*(24), 2031–2038. https://doi.org/10.3109/09638288.2012.669019

Tarakci, E., & Uyanik, M. (2012). Comparison of effectiveness of ergothrapy in different types of multiple sclerosis. *Türkiye Klinikleri Journal of Medical Sciences, 32*(2), 316–323. https://doi.org/10.5336/medsci.2011-22633

Turpin, M., Kerr, G., Gullo, H., Bennett, S., Asano, M., & Finlayson, M. (2018). Understanding and living with multiple sclerosis fatigue. *British Journal of Occupational Therapy, 81*(2), 82–89. https://doi.org/10.1177/0308022617728679

Valadbeigi, A., Weisi, F., Rohbakhsh, N., Rezaei, M., Heidari, A., & Rahmani Rasa, A. (2014). Central auditory processing and word discrimination in patients with multiple sclerosis. *European Archives of Oto-Rhino-Laryngology*, *271*, 2891–2896. https://doi.org/10.1007/s00405-013-2776-6

Wendebourg, M. J., Heesen, C., Finlayson, M., Meyer, B., Pöttgen, J., & Köpke, S. (2017). Patient education for people with multiple sclerosis-associated fatigue: A systematic review. *PLOS ONE*, *12*(3), Article e0173025. https://doi.org/10.1371/journal.pone.0173025

Yu, C. H., & Mathiowetz, V. (2014). Systematic review of occupational therapy-related interventions for people with multiple sclerosis: Part 1. Activity and participation. *American Journal of Occupational Therapy*, *68*(1), 27–32. https://doi.org/10.5014/ajot.2014.008672

Yu, C. H., & Mathiowetz, V. (2014). Systematic review of occupational therapy-related interventions for people with multiple sclerosis: Part 2. Impairment. *American Journal of Occupational Therapy*, *68*(1), 33–38. https://doi.org/10.5014/ajot.2014.008680

Zackowski, K. M., Wang, J. I., McGready, J., Calabresi, P. A., & Newsome, S. D. (2015). Quantitative sensory and motor measures detect change over time and correlate with walking speed in individuals with multiple sclerosis. *Multiple Sclerosis and Related Disorders*, *4*(1), 67–74. https://doi.org/10.1016/j.msard.2014.11.001

Parkinson's Disease

Also called Parkinson Disease, Parkinsonism, PD.
See also Executive Dysfunction, Depression, Anxiety, Sleep–Wake Disorders.

Description

Parkinson's disease is a slowly progressive, degenerative disorder of the nervous system characterized by resting muscle tremor, stiffness (rigidity of movement), hypomimia (masklike facies), dysarthria (speech disarticulation), dysphagia (difficulty swallowing), bradykinesia (slow and decreased movement), gait festination (shortened stride length, shuffling), droopy shoulder and back posture, and postural instability (impaired balance reflexes; R. S. Porter, 2018).

Cause

The most common cause is deficiency of the neurotransmitter dopamine as a consequence of degenerative, vascular, or inflammatory changes in the basal ganglia. About 10% of clients have a family history of Parkinson's disease (PD), which is autosomal dominant (R. S. Porter, 2018; Stedman's, 2011).

Stages of Parkinson's Disease (Hoehn and Yahr Scale; Adapted from Dirette, 2017; Jansa & Aragon, 2015; Schultz-Krohn, 2018)

- *Stage 1:* Signs of Parkinson's disease are evident on one side of the body, unilateral tremor, micrographia, poor endurance for previous occupations, and fatigue. Occupational therapy focuses on acquisitional occupation, restorative occupation, and occupation-based education programs.
- *Stage 2:* Signs of bilateral motor disturbance, mild rigidity, difficulties with simultaneous tasks, difficulties with executive function. Occupational therapy focuses on acquisitional occupation, restorative occupation, occupation-based education programs, and adaptive occupation.
- *Stage 3:* Signs of PD are bilateral and balance is impaired, delayed reactions, difficulty with skilled sequential tasks. Occupational therapy focuses on acquisitional occupation, restorative occupation, occupation-based education programs, and adaptive occupation.
- *Stage 4:* PD is functionally disabling, with fine motor control severely compromised and oral motor deficits. Occupational therapy focuses on adaptive occupation, restorative occupation, acquisitional occupation, and occupation-based education programs.

- *Stage 5:* The person is confined to bed or a wheelchair, dependent in performing ADLs. Occupational therapy focuses on adaptive occupation and occupation-based education programs.

Evaluation/Assessment

Areas

- Activities of Daily Living/Instrumental ADL: swallowing (dysphagia), speech disturbances, reduced bowel and bladder function, handwriting
- Education/Work: ability to perform tasks
- Play/Leisure: interests, values, type, frequency, location
- Rest/Sleep: sleep habits, sleep disturbances
- Social Participation: type, frequency, location, with whom
- Sensorimotor: tremor, cogwheel rigidity, bradykinesia, postural changes (stooped, unsteady, instability), balance and gait (falls, shuffling gait, reduced arm swing), postural reflexes (righting, equilibrium), coordination, grip strength, oculomotor control, facial expression (masking), sensory disturbances, seborrhea (oily skin and dandruff), orthotic hypotension, fatigue
- Cognitive/Perceptual: attention, memory, executive functions
- Psychosocial: depression, anxiety, stress, hallucinations, role performance, self-efficacy, self-esteem, self-worth, self-identity, stigma, quality of life
- Context/Environment: home safety check, home modification, community accessibility
- Comorbidities: dementia, psychosis, substance abuse (self-medication)

Instruments

Instruments Developed by Occupational Therapy Personnel

- Assessment of Motor and Process Skills (8th ed.; AMPS-8; Fisher & Bray Jones, 2016)
- Canadian Occupational Performance Measure (5th ed.; COPM-5; Law et al., 2014)
- Complex Task Performance Assessment (CTPA; Wolf et al., 2008; see also Davis et al., 2019, in References)
- Nottingham Extended Activities of Daily Living (NEADL; Nouri & Lincoln, 1987)

Instruments Developed by Other Professionals and Used by Occupational Therapy Personnel

- Berg Balance Scale (BBS; Berg et al., 1989)
- Client Satisfaction Questionnaire-8 (CSQ-8; Larsen et al., 1979)
- Credibility/Expectancy Questionnaire (C/EQ; Devilly & Borkovec, 2000)
- Dot cancellation test, or Bourdon–Wiersma test (tests visual perception and vigilance; original source in Dutch)
- Dynamometer (grip strength; JAMAR, Lafayette Instrument; Wang et al., 2018; see also Villafañe et al., 2016, in References)
- European Quality of Life 5-Dimension Scale (EQ-5D; EuroQol Group, 1990)
- Finger-to-Nose Test (Swaine et al., 2005)
- Functional Independence Measure (FIM; Uniform Data System for Medical Rehabilitation, 1997)
- Functional Reach Test (FRT; Duncan et al., 1990)
- Functioning Disability Evaluation Scale–Adult Version (Chinese version of the WHODAS 2.0)
- Hoehn and Yahr Scale (H&Y Scale; Hoehn & Yahr, 1967; see also Modified Hoehn and Yahr Scale)
- Modified Hoehn and Yahr Scale (Goetz et al., 2004)
- Montreal Cognitive Assessment (MoCA; Nasreddine et al., 2005; see also Stillerova et al., 2016, in References)
- Non-Motor Symptoms Scale (NMSS; Chaudhuri et al., 2007)
- Parkinson's Disease Questionnaire-8 (PDQ-8; Jenkinson et al., 1997)
- Parkinson's Disease Questionnaire-39 (PDQ-39; Jenkinson et al., 1995)

- Rapid pace walk (RPW). Measures time in seconds person takes to walk 10 feet, turn around, and walk back as quickly and safely as possible. Seven seconds is the cutoff point. (Marottoli et al., 1994)
- Rey Complex Figure Test and Recognition Trial (Meyers & Meyers, 1995)
- Trail Making Tests A and B (TMT-A, TMT-B; Bowie & Harvey, 2006)
- Unified Parkinson's Disease Rating Scale (UPDRS; Goetz et al., 2008)
- Useful Field of View (UFOV; Ball & Owsley, 1993)
- Zarit Burden Interview (ZARIT-BI; Zarit et al., 1980)

Problems/Issues

Activities of Daily Living/Instrumental ADL
- Person may have swallowing difficulties.
- Person's handwriting may become very small in size (micrographia).
- Person may have soft, monotone voice, and reduced volume of speech due to poor breath support.
- Person may have difficulty maintaining a medication schedule to take medications on time to avoid "on/off" effects.
- Person may have continence problems, such as urinary urgency, constipation, and incontinence.
- Person may experience erectile dysfunction or reduced libido. (Note: Hypersexuality may develop as a side effect of some anti-Parkinson's medication.)
- Person may have sensorimotor deficits that make driving a vehicle unsafe, such as poor contrast sensitivity, decreased visual processing speed, and psychomotor retardation (see Classen, 2014, and other articles in Appendix: Driving Fitness in Clients With Parkinson's Disease).

Education/Work
- Person may be reluctant to tell employer or work colleagues of diagnosis.
- Person may be at risk for injury in the workplace.
- Person may be unable to perform some work tasks due to motor or cognitive impairments.

Play/Leisure
- Person may stop or reduce engagement in favorite leisure activities because of motor or cognitive impairment.

Rest/Sleep
- Person may have excessive daytime sleepiness.
- Person may have changes in REM (rapid eye movement) sleep called RBD (REM behavior disorder, including verbal and physical disruptive behaviors).
- Person may experience insomnia.
- Person may experience sleep fragments.
- Person may experience vivid or disturbing dreams.

Social Participation
- Person may have withdrawn or reduced social participation in favorite social activities.
- Person may experience social isolation due to lack of understanding by others or personal withdrawal.
- Person may report lower activity participation (Foster & Hershey, 2011).
- Person may experience social rejection related to facial masking (hypomimia; Gunnery et al., 2016).

Sensorimotor
- Person usually has akinesia or dyskinesia (lack of movement or difficulty with movement).
- Person usually has bradykinesia (slowness of movement).
- Person usually has hypokinesia (reduced scaling of movements that may affect balance, coordination, speech, swallowing, handwriting, and facial expression).

- Person may have a shuffling or festinating gait and shortened stride length (short steps).
- Person usually has rigidity (raised and sustained high muscle tone and stiffness).
- Person may have a resting or pill rolling tremor.
- Person may have postural instability related to balance and gait problems.
- Person may have difficulty changing directions or turning.
- Person may have writhing movements (usually a side effect of medication).
- Person may not swing arms while walking.
- Person may have an asymmetric posture when standing.
- Person may have reduced reflexes.
- Person may have numbness, tingling, or burning sensation.
- Person may experience autonomic failure, such as postural hypotension (a sudden fall in blood pressure when rising from lying or sitting).
- Person may report increased level of fatigue (Ghahari et al., 2013).
- Person may experience pain related to muscle rigidity, which may include dystonic muscle cramps.
- Person may experience the "on/off" syndrome (abrupt changes in mobility in some clients taking levodopa medication in which there is an unpredictable shift from relative ability to move to being unable to move, and vice versa).
- Person may experience "start hesitation," in which the person appears to begin an action, and then does not carry through.
- Person may experience "freezing," in which the action stops suddenly without the person intending to actually do so.
- Person may experience visuospatial disturbances including difficulty judging depth and width.
- Person may experience changes in ability to detect contrast sensitivity, color vision, object recognition, and the perception of motion.
- Person may lose sense of smell (anosmia).

Cognitive/Perceptual

- Person may experience reduced ability to concentrate or pay attention, including maintaining a train of thought and difficulty switching from one topic to another.
- Person may have difficulty remembering events.
- Person may have difficulty reading an analogue-faced clock.
- Person may experience dysexecutive problems such as difficulty in planning, decision making, problem solving, and organization.
- Person may exhibit reduced or slowing of thinking processes.
- Person may have difficulty multitasking (doing more than one thing at a time).
- Person may have difficulty with working memory.
- Person is at risk for developing dementia.

Psychosocial

- Person may experience visual hallucinations (seeing objects, persons, or animals that are not actually present).
- Person may have delusional beliefs.
- Person may experience anxiety, depression, and irritability.
- Person may experience apathy and lack of motivation.
- Person may experience mood swings (flat affect to euphoria).
- Person may express feelings of embarrassment, stress, or frustration at being slow or clumsy.
- Person may express feelings of grief and loss of control at being diagnosed with the disease.
- Person may experience stress resulting from coping with daily life and effects of Parkinson's disease.
- Person may experience symptoms of anxiety (Lutz et al., 2016).
- Person may experience discrepancies in role identity and role expectations following diagnosis (Ravenek et al., 2017).

- Person and partner may experience role reversals requiring negotiations with family.
- Person may feel a loss of power and control in everyday activities.
- Person may express feelings of hostility and resentment due to changes in status and role performance.
- Person may experience loss of self-esteem and self-worth related to changes in role and status.
- Person may experience stigma in social interactions.
- Person may experience decreased quality of life.

Context/Environment
- Person may be misunderstood by others who misinterpret changes in behavior.
- Person and family may lack information about Parkinson's disease and its management.
- Person and family may lack knowledge and information about assistive technology and adapted devices.
- Person and family may lack knowledge about available community and internet resources.

Intervention/Treatment

Models and programs developed by occupational therapy personnel include adapted devices and aids (Jackson, 2019); Canadian Practice Process Framework (Jansa & Aragon, 2015); cognitive strategy training (Foster et al., 2018); community-based occupational therapy (Chapman & Nelson, 2014); occupational therapy in Parkinson's disease (OTiP; Saint-Hilaire, 2014; Sturkenboom et al., 2013; Sturkenboom et al., 2014); Parkinson's men's group (S. Porter et al., 2011); Perceive, Recall, Plan and Perform system (Van Keulen-Rouweler et al., 2017); self-management rehabilitation (Tickle-Degnen et al., 2010); and sensory-motor training (Taghizadeh et al., 2018). Models and programs developed by other professionals but used by occupational therapy personnel include adaptive strategies (Sperens et al., 2018), multidisciplinary rehabilitation program (Monticone et al., 2015), and tai chi (Toh, 2013). Team members include physicians, nursing personnel, psychologists and counselors, physical therapy personnel, and occupational therapy personnel. Goal is to provide holistic assessment and intervention for clients living with Parkinson's disease that enable them to engage in meaningful roles and activities and supports self-management (Aragon & Kings, 2018; Radder et al., 2017).

Activities of Daily Living/Instrumental ADL
- Discuss and support maintaining a healthy weight through diet.
- Using a mug to "drink" soup instead of using a spoon may assist when eating.
- Provide opportunity to discuss sexual well-being and discuss available resources (signs of hypersexuality should be referred to the prescribing physician).
- Assist client to determine whether he or she is fit to drive a vehicle, and when driving self should cease.
- Assist client to explore alternative transportation to driving own vehicle.
- Assist client to explore other mobility equipment, such as a walker, scooter, or wheelchair.
- Assist client to explore alternatives to going shopping, such as ordering items online that have delivery service.
- Provide opportunity to practice safe transfers.

Education/Work
- Support continued participation in work activities.
- Discuss with client whether employer should be told of diagnosis, and when.
- Assist client to determine whether individual can safely and feasibly return to work setting including accessibility, workplace modification, work task adaptation, flexible or part-time work.
- Assist client and employer in determining whether alterative work settings, such as home or other location, may be acceptable.
- Continue to evaluate client's physical and cognitive difficulties.
- If client is unable to continue working, assist client with emotional, practical, and financial impact of stopping work.

Play/Leisure
- Assist client to engage in meaningful leisure activities, making adaptations as needed as disease progresses.
- Assist client to explore new interests that are within physical and cognitive limitations.

Rest/Sleep
- Review nighttime routines to reduce sleep disturbances.
- Suggest wearing satin pajamas in bed to ease turning over or moving in bed.

Social Participation
- Encourage client to maintain participation in social activities and pleasurable pastimes with adaptations as needed.
- Assist client to explore new social activities that are congruent with level of physical and cognitive abilities.

Sensorimotor
- Support engagement in physical fitness programs (recalibration training), such as cardiovascular exercise (walking, dancing, cycling, tai chi), as part of client's regular routine.
- Implement a fatigue management program.
- If needed, provide a stop-smoking program and reduced alcohol intake approach.
- Teach work simplification techniques; focus on most important elements of the task.
- Encourage the use of cognitive and sensory cues and triggers to guide motor performance, including internal cues such as mental rehearsal, visualization, or internal dialogue, and external cues such as positioning furniture to simplify visual impact of layout, using floor markers to increase stride length, using a metronome to overcome start hesitation, using music and rhythm to maintain flow of movement (Aragon & Kings, 2018).
- A visual demonstration of movement to be performed may be useful.
- Verbal directions should be brief, clear descriptions of actions and emphasize key words.
- A hands-on approach to physically facilitate movement may be useful.
- Backwards chaining (start with last movement to first movement) may be useful when learning a movement sequence.
- Focus on one task at a time (do not ask client to walk and talk at the same time). Focus on walking: to talk, stop walking, allow client to hold onto a surface, and then talk; stop talking before restarting walking.

Cognitive/Perceptual
- Encourage client to develop and maintain a self-management program for as long as possible.
- Assist client to develop an activity pacing schedule to pursue outdoor activities, such as determining when medication is most effective.
- Develop a time-management schedule, such as determining when shops are likely to be less busy, reducing risk of falling and allowing a more leisurely pace for decision making.
- Encourage planning ahead when leaving the house to determine best route, location of toilets, amount of walking, possible architectural barriers.
- Use recall aids (cue cards, prompt sheets, and short written reminders), but avoid overload.
- Break down sequences into smaller parts, such as Think-Look-Plan-Do.
- Participation in reminiscence sessions may help with memory.

Psychosocial
- Assist client to develop positive stress and coping strategies (mindfulness, relaxation, yoga).
- Assist client to maintain meaningful roles and role performance, making adaptations as disease progresses.

Context/Environment
- Offer client, family, and others education, advice, and information to promote participation.

- Consult with client and family about modifying living arrangements to avoid stairs inside and out, such as installing a ramp, using an elevator, or arranging to live on the ground floor.
- Provide information on local services, including support groups and health and wellness groups such as mindfulness training meditation, relaxation, or yoga training.
- Support caregiver with information and training as needed (Berger et al., 2019).
- Ensure that safety issues are addressed, including grab bars, adequate lighting, indoor and outdoor railings, clear pathways.
- Assist person to get a handicapped (disabled) parking sticker.

Precautions/Safety Considerations

Person is at risk for falls. Safety issues should always be addressed. Family and caregivers should be trained in safe transfer techniques.

Prognosis and Outcome

There is no cure. Disease is progressive and results in increased incapacitation. Person usually needs palliative care (Murdock et al., 2015).

Cost Effectiveness

The two reports found no benefit of occupational therapy and physical therapy versus no therapy long term for clients with Parkinson's disease (Clarke, Patel, Ives, Rick, Dowling, et al., 2016; Clarke, Patel, Ives, Rick, Woolley, et al., 2016). Sturkenboom et al. (2015) found that adding occupational therapy did not significantly impact the total cost of care but the positive effective was significant only for caregivers. Foster et al. (2014) found moderate to strong evidence exists for task-specific management and cognitive-behavior strategies and moderate evidence for use of external supports during functional movement activities. Clients were satisfied with the intervention (Foster et al., 2014; Sturkenboom et al., 2016).

REFERENCES

Aragon, A., & Kings, J. (2018). *Occupational therapy for people with Parkinson's* (2nd ed.). Royal College of Occupational Therapists. https://www.rcot.co.uk/file/2806/download?token=hq e17blb

Berger, S., Chen, T., Eldridge, J., Thomas, C. A., Habermann, B., & Tickle-Degnen, L. (2019). The self-management balancing act of spousal care partners in the case of Parkinson's disease. *Disability and Rehabilitation, 41*(8), 887–895. https://doi.org/10.1080/09638288.2017.1413427

Chapman, L., & Nelson, D. (2014). Person-centered, community-based occupational therapy for a man with Parkinson's disease: A case study. *Activities, Adaptation & Aging, 38*(2), 94–112. https://doi.org/10.1080/01924788.2014.901045

Clarke, C. E., Patel, S., Ives, N., Rick, C. E., Dowling, F., Woolley, R., Wheatley, K., Walker, M. F., Sackley, C. M., & PD REHAB Collaborative Group. (2016). Physiotherapy and occupational therapy vs no therapy in mild to moderate Parkinson Disease: A randomized clinical trial. *JAMA Neurology, 73*(3), 291–299. https://doi.org/10.1001/jamaneurol.2015.4452

Clarke, C. E., Patel, S., Ives, N., Rick, C. E., Woolley, R., Wheatley, K., Walker, M. F., Zhu, S., Kandiyali, R., Yao, G., & Sackley, C. M. (2016). Clinical effectiveness and cost-effectiveness of physiotherapy and occupational therapy versus no therapy in mild to moderate Parkinson's disease: A large pragmatic randomised controlled trial (PD REHAB). *Health Technology Assessment, 20*(63), 1–96. https://doi.org/10.3310/hta20630

Davis, A., Wolf, T. J., & Foster, E. R. (2019). Complex Task Performance Assessment (CTPA) and functional cognition in people with Parkinson's disease. *American Journal of Occupational Therapy, 73*(5), Article 7205205060. https://doi.org/10.5014/ajot.2019.031492

Dirette, D. P. (2017). Progressive neurodegenerative disorders: Parkinson's disease. In B. J. Atchison & D. P. Dirette (Eds.), *Conditions in occupational therapy* (5th ed., pp. 408–413). Wolters-Kluwer.

Foster, E. R., Bedekar, M., & Tickle-Degnen, L. (2014). Systematic review of the effectiveness of occupational therapy-related interventions for people with Parkinson's disease. *American Journal of Occupational Therapy, 68*(1), 39–49. https://doi.org/10.5014/ajot.2014.008706

Foster, E. R., & Hershey, T. (2011). Everyday executive function is associated with activity participation in Parkinson disease without dementia. *Occupational Therapy Journal of Research: Occupation, Participation, and Health, 31*(1, Suppl.), S16–S22. https://doi.org/10.3928/15394492 -20101108-04

Foster, E. R., Spence, D., & Toglia, J. (2018). Feasibility of a cognitive strategy training intervention for people with Parkinson's disease. *Disability and Rehabilitation, 40*(1), 1127–1134. https://doi.org/10.1080/09638288.2017.1288275

Ghahari, S., Parvaneh, S., & Packer, T. L. (2013). Fatigue in progressive neurological conditions: A literature review. *Iranian Rehabilitation Journal, 11*(1), 85–90.

Gunnery, S. D., Habermann, B., Saint-Hilaire, M., Thomas, C. A., & Tickle-Degnen, L. (2016). The relationship between the experience of hypomimia and social wellbeing in people with Parkinson's disease and their care partners. *Journal of Parkinson's Disease, 6*(3), 625–630. https://doi.org/10.3233/JPD-160782

Jackson, A. (2019). Aids for activities of daily living in people with Parkinson's disease. *British Journal of Community Nursing, 24*(5), 229–232. https://doi.org/10.12968/bjcn.2019.24.5.229

Jansa, J., & Aragon, A. (2015). Living with Parkinson's and the emerging role of occupational therapy. *Parkinson's Disease, 2015,* Article 196303. https://doi.org/10.1155/2015/196303

Lutz, S. G., Holmes, J. D., Ready, E. A., Jenkins, M. E., & Johnson, A. M. (2016). Clinical presentation of anxiety in Parkinson's disease: A scoping review. *OTJR: Occupation, Participation and Health, 36*(3), 134–147. https://doi.org/10.1177/1539449216661714

Monticone, M., Ambrosini, E., Laurini, A., Rocca, B., & Foti, C. (2015). In-patient multidisciplinary rehabilitation for Parkinson's disease: A randomized controlled trial. *Movement Disorders, 30*(8), 1050–1058. https://doi.org/10.1002/mds.26256

Murdock, C., Cousins, W., & Kernohan, W. G. (2015). "Running water won't freeze": How people with advanced Parkinson's disease experience occupation. *Palliative & Supportive Care, 13*(5), 1363–1372. https://doi.org/10.1017/S1478951514001357

Porter, R. S. (Ed.). (2018). *The Merck manual of diagnosis and therapy* (20th ed.). Merck Sharp & Dohme.

Porter, S., Mazonson, N., & Tickle-Degnen, L. (2011). Supporting social participation in individuals with Parkinson's disease: A story of the Parkinson's men's group. *OT Practice, 16*(15), 17–18.

Radder, D. L. M., Sturkenboom, I. H., van Nimwegen, M., Keus, S. H., Bloem, B. R., & de Vries, N. M. (2017). Physical therapy and occupational therapy in Parkinson's disease. *International Journal of Neuroscience, 127*(10), 930–943. https://doi.org/10.1080/00207454.2016 .1275617

Ravenek, M., Rudman, D. L., Jenkins, M. E., & Spaulding, S. (2017). Understanding uncertainty in young-onset Parkinson disease. *Chronic Illness, 13*(4), 288–298. https://doi.org/10.1177/ 1742395317694699

Saint-Hilaire, M. (2014). Occupational therapy for Parkinson's disease: Increasing awareness. *Lancet Neurology, 13*(6), 527–529. https://doi.org/10.1016/S1474-4422(14)70074-2

Schultz-Krohn, W. (2018). Parkinson's disease. In H. M. Pendleton & W. Schultz-Krohn (Eds.), *Pedretti's occupational therapy* (8th ed., pp. 893–898). Elsevier.

Sperens, M., Hamberg, K., & Hariz, G. M. (2018). Challenges and strategies among women and men with Parkinson's disease: Striving toward *joie de vivre* in daily life. *British Journal of Occupational Therapy, 81*(12), 700–708. https://doi.org/10.1177/0308022618770142

Stedman's medical dictionary for the health professions and nursing (7th ed). (2011). Wolters Kluwer.

Stillerova, T., Liddle, J., Gustafsson, L., Lamont, R., & Silburn, P. (2016). Could everyday technology improve access to assessments? A pilot study on the feasibility of screening cognition in people with Parkinson's disease using the Montreal Cognitive Assessment via Internet videoconferencing. *Australian Occupational Therapy Journal, 63*(6), 373–380. https://doi.org/10.1111/1440-1630.12288

Sturkenboom, I. H., Graff, M. J., Borm, G. F., Veenhuizen, Y., Bloem, B. R., Munneke, M., & Nijhuis-van der Sanden, M. W. (2013). The impact of occupational therapy in Parkinson's disease: A randomized controlled feasibility study. *Clinical Rehabilitation, 27*(2), 99–112. https://doi.org/10.1177/0269215512448382

Sturkenboom, I. H., Graff, M. J. L., Hendriks, J. C., Veenhuizen, Y., Munneke, M., Bloem, B. R., & Nijhuis-van der Sanden, M. W. (2014). Efficacy of occupational therapy for patients with Parkinson's disease: A randomised controlled trial. *Lancet Neurology, 13*(6), 557–566. https://doi.org/10.1016/S1474-4422(14)70055-9

Sturkenboom, I. H., Hendriks, J. C., Graff, M. J., Adang, E. M., Munneke, M., Nijhuis-van der Sanden, M. W., & Bloem, B. R. (2015). Economic evaluation of occupational therapy in Parkinson's disease: A randomized controlled trial. *Movement Disorders, 30*(8), 1059–1067. https://doi.org/10.1002/mds.26217

Sturkenboom, I. H., Nijhuis-van der Sanden, M. W., & Graff, M. J. (2016). A process evaluation of a home-based occupational therapy intervention for Parkinson's patients and their caregivers performed alongside a randomized controlled trial. *Clinical Rehabilitation, 30*(12), 1186–1199. https://doi.org/10.1177/0269215515622038

Taghizadeh, G., Azad, A., Kashefi, S., Fallah, S., & Daneshjoo, F. (2018). The effect of sensory-motor training on hand and upper extremity sensory and motor function in patients with idiopathic Parkinson disease. *Journal of Hand Therapy, 31*(4), 486–493. https://doi.org/10.1016/j.jht.2017.08.001

Tickle-Degnen, L., Ellis, T., Saint-Hilaire, M. H., Thomas, C. A., & Wagenaar, R. C. (2010). Self-management rehabilitation and health-related quality of life in Parkinson's disease: A randomized controlled trial. *Movement Disorders, 25*(2), 194–204. https://doi.org/10.1002/mds.22940

Toh, S. F. M. (2013). A systematic review of the effectiveness of tai chi exercise in individuals with Parkinson's disease from 2003 to 2013. *Hong Kong Journal of Occupational Therapy, 23*(2), 69–81. https://doi.org/10.1016/j.hkjot.2013.11.001

Van Keulen-Rouweler, B. J., Sturkenboom, I. H., Kottorp, A., Graff, M. J., Nijhuis-van der Sanden, M. W., & Steultjens, E. M. (2017). The Perceive, Recall, Plan and Perform (PRPP) system for persons with Parkinson's disease: A psychometric study. *Scandinavian Journal of Occupational Therapy, 24*(1), 65–73. https://doi.org/10.1080/11038128.2016.1233291

Villafañe, J. H., Valdes, K., Buraschi, R., Martinelli, M., Bissolotti, L., & Negrini, S. (2016). Reliability of the handgrip strength test in elderly subjects with Parkinson disease. *Hand, 11*(1), 54–58. https://doi.org/10.1177/1558944715614852

BIBLIOGRAPHY

Aragon, A., & Kings, J. (2010). *Occupational therapy for people with Parkinson's: Best practice guidelines.* College of Occupational Therapists.

Forwell, S. J., Hugos, L., Copperman, L. F., & Ghahari, S. (2014). Neurodegenerative diseases: Parkinson's disease. In M. V. Radomski & C. A. T. Latham (Eds.), *Occupational therapy for physical dysfunction* (7th ed., pp. 1088–1090). Wolters-Kluwer.

Gunnery, S. D., Naumova, E. N., Saint-Hilaire, M., & Tickle-Degnen, L. (2017). Mapping spontaneous facial expression in people with Parkinson's disease: A multiple case study design. *Cogent Psychology, 2017*(1), Article 1376425. https://doi.org/10.1080/23311908.2017.1376425

Hanby, J. R. (2017). The nervous system: Table 18.14, Parkinson's disease, normal pressure hydrocephalus, and essential tremor. In H. Smith-Gabai & S. E. Holm (Eds.), *Occupational therapy in acute care* (2nd ed., pp. 325–327). AOTA Press.

Hsu, T. H., Liou, T. H., Chou, K. R., Chi, W. C., Yen, C. F., Liao, H. F., & Tseng, I. J. (2018). Large-scale assessment of function and disability in patients with Parkinson's disease using the

Functioning Disability Evaluation Scale–Adult Version. *International Journal of Environmental Research and Public Health, 15*(12), Article 2788. https://doi.org/10.3390/ijerph15122788

Preissner, K. (2014). *Occupational therapy practice guidelines for adults with neurodegenerative diseases.* AOTA Press.

Schenkman, M., Ellis, T., Christiansen, C., Baron, A. E., Tickle-Degnen, L., Hall, D. A., & Wagenaar, R. (2011). Profile of functional limitations and task performance among people with early- and middle-stage Parkinson disease. *Physical Therapy, 91*(9), 1339–1354. https://doi.org/10.2522/ptj.20100236

Takahashi, K., Tickle-Degnen, L., Coster, W. J., & Latham, N. K. (2010). Expressive behavior in Parkinson's disease as a function of interview context. *American Journal of Occupational Therapy, 64*(3), 484–495. https://doi.org/10.5014/ajot.2010.09078

Tickle-Degnen, L., Zebrowitz, L. A., & Ma, H. (2011). Culture, gender and health care stigma: Practitioners' response to facial masking experienced by people with Parkinson's disease. *Social Science & Medicine, 73*(1), 95–102. https://doi.org/ 10.1016/j.socscimed.2011.05.008

Wang, S. M., & Tickle-Degnen, L. (2018). Emotional cues from expressive behavior of women and men with Parkinson's disease. *PLOS ONE, 13*(7), Article e0199886. https://doi.org/10.1371/journal.pone.0199886

APPENDIX: DRIVING FITNESS IN CLIENTS WITH PARKINSON'S DISEASE

Alvarez, L., & Classen, S. (2018). Driving with Parkinson's disease: Cut points for clinical predictors of on-road outcomes. *Canadian Journal of Occupational Therapy, 85*(3), 232–241. https://doi.org/10.1177/0008417418755458

Classen, S. (2014). Consensus statements on driving in people with Parkinson's disease. *Occupational Therapy in Health Care, 28*(2), 140–147. https://doi.org/10.3109/07380577.2014.890307

Classen, S., & Alvarez, L. (2016). Caregivers' impressions predicting fitness to drive in persons with Parkinson's. *OTJR: Occupation, Participation, and Health, 36*(1), 5–13. https://doi.org/10.1177/1539449215601117

Classen, S., Brumback, B., Crawford, K., & Jenniex, S. (2019). Visual attention cut points for driver fitness in Parkinson's disease. *OTJR: Occupation, Participation and Health, 39*(4), 257–265. https://doi.org/10.1177/1539449219836689

Classen, S., Brumback, B., Monahan, M., Malaty, I. I., Rodriguez, R. L., Okun, M. S., & McFarland, N. R. (2014). Driving errors in Parkinson's disease: Moving closer to predicting on-road outcomes. *American Journal of Occupational Therapy, 68*(1), 77–85. https://doi.org/10.5014/ajot.2014.008698

Classen, S., Holmes, J. D., Alvarez, L., Loew, K., Mulvagh, A., Rienas, K., Walton, V., & He, W. (2015). Clinical assessments as predictors of primary on-road outcomes in Parkinson's Disease. *OTJR: Occupation, Participation and Health, 35*(4), 213–220. https://doi.org/10.1177/1539449215601118

Classen, S., Witter, D. P., Lanford, D. N., Okun, M. S., Rodriguez, R. L., Romrell, J., Malaty, I., & Fernandez, H. H. (2011). Usefulness of screening tools for predicting driving performance in people with Parkinson's disease. *American Journal of Occupational Therapy, 65*(5), 579–588. https://doi.org/10.5014/ajot.2011.001073

Crizzle, A. M., Classen, S., Lanford, D. N., Malaty, I. A., Okun, M. S., Wang, Y., Wagle Shukla, A., Rodriguez, R., & McFarland, N. R. (2013). Postural/gait and cognitive function as predictors of driving performance in Parkinson's disease. *Journal of Parkinson's Disease, 3*(2), 153–160. https://doi.org/10.3233/JPD-120152

Crizzle, A. M., Classen, S., Lanford, D., Malaty, I. A., Okun, M. S., Wagle Shukla, A., & McFarland, N. R. (2013). Driving performance and behaviors: A comparison of gender differences in Parkinson's disease. *Traffic Injury Prevention, 14*(4), 340–345. https://doi.org/10.1080/15389588.2012.717730

Crizzle, A. M., Classen, S., & Uc, E. Y. (2012). Parkinson disease and driving: An evidence-based review. *Neurology, 79*(20), 2067–2074. https://doi.org/10.1212/WNL.0b013e3182749e95

Devos, H., Morgan, J. C., Onyeamaechi, A., Bogle, C. A., Holton, K., Kruse, J., Sasser, S., & Akin-wuntan, A. E. (2016). Use of a driving simulator to improve on-road driving performance and cognition in persons with Parkinson's disease: A pilot study. *Australian Occupational Therapy Journal, 63*(6), 408–414. https://doi.org/10.1111/1440-1630.12263

Lee, H. C., Yanting Chee, D., Selander, H., & Falkmer. T. (2012). Is it reliable to assess visual attention of drivers affected by Parkinson's disease from the backseat? A simulator study. *Emerging Health Threats Journal, 5*(1), Article 15343. https://doi.org/10.3402/ehtj.v5i0.15343

Ma, H. I., Saint-Hilaire, M., Thomas, C. A., & Tickle-Degnen, L. (2016). Stigma as a key determinant of health-related quality of life in Parkinson's disease. *Quality of Life Research, 25*(12), 3037–3045. https://doi.org/10.1007/s11136-016-1329-z

Perinatal and Pediatric Stroke

Also called intrauterine infarct, neonatal cerebral infarction.
See also Cerebral Palsy: Infant and Child.

Description

Perinatal stroke is a stroke occurring between the 20th week of fetal life and the 28th postnatal day (Basu, 2014). A pediatric stroke is defined as a stroke occurring before age 18, but usually the age is 10 or younger. Correct diagnosis of a stroke in infants and young children is often difficult to determine because the motor symptoms present in older children or adults may not be apparent until a magnetic resonance imaging (MRI) is ordered or developmental delay is established, such as missing specific developmental milestones or observed unequal bilateral skills of legs, arms, and hands (noticeable hemiplegia). Therefore, the exact age at which the stroke occurred may be uncertain.

Cause

Perinatal stroke is caused by an interrupted blood supply to part of the brain before birth or age less than 28 days (Basu et al., 2017). A pediatric stroke is also caused by an interrupted blood supply to part of the brain, but the age is after 1 month. There are several different causes of strokes depending on the type of interruption or structures involved, including arterial ischemic, hemorrhagic, diffuse brain injury following trauma, hypoxic ischemic encephalopathy, and periventricular leukomalacia. Infarct to the spinal cord have also been reported (Felter et al., 2019).

Evaluation/Assessment

Areas

(Note: Specific areas are age and skill-level dependent. All items must be selected based on age or ability level.)

- Activities of Daily Living/Instrumental ADL: feeding, eating, diapering, bathing, dressing and undressing, toileting, mobility, transfers, communication, self-management or dependent on adults; for older children, some IADL tasks may be included, such as doing chores, helping with meal preparation, doing laundry, dusting, vacuuming
- Education/Work: school activities, academic performance, building modification, assistive technology
- Play/Leisure: play skills
- Rest/Sleep: sleep habits and routines (infant, parents)
- Social Participation: socialization skills

- Sensorimotor: reflexes (primitive, righting, equilibrium), gross motor skills (sit, stand, walk, ride a bike, jump, skip, hop, kick), positioning, balance, fine motor hand functions (grasp, hook, pinch, throw, catch), coordination (bimanual, eye–hand), dexterity, sensory processing, sensory discrimination (auditory, gustatory, olfactory, pressure, proprioception, tactile, vestibular, and visual)
- Cognitive/Perceptual: attention, concentration, memory, executive functions, visual perception skills
- Psychosocial: parent–child interaction, emotional regulation, stress behavior (fussing crying, arching, fisting, tremors, or startles)
- Context/Environment: parent education and health literacy, adapted devices, splinting, community and internet resources
- Development (Infant, Child, Adolescent only): age-stage development, developmental milestones
- Comorbidities: cerebral palsy (unilateral, hemiplegic), seizures, hydrocephalus, lethargy, poor feeding behavior

Instruments
Instruments Developed by Occupational Therapy Personnel
- Assisting Hand Assessment (Kids-AHA 5.0; Holmefur & Krumlinde-Sundholm, 2016)
- Canadian Occupational Performance Measure (5th ed.; COPM-5; Law et al., 2014)
- Pediatric Evaluation of Disability Inventory (PEDI; Haley et al., 1992)
- Pediatric Stroke Quality of Life Measure (PAQLM; Fiume et al., 2018, in References)
- Perceived Efficacy and Goal Setting (PEGS; Missiuna & Pollock, 2000)
- Quality of Upper Extremity Skills Test (QUEST; DeMatteo et al., 1993)
- Rehabilitation Engineering Laboratory Hand Function Test (RELHF; Popovic et al., 2006)
- Simple Test for Evaluating Hand Function (STEF; Kaneko & Muraki, 1990)

Instruments Developed by Other Professionals and Used by Occupational Therapy Personnel
- Alberta Infant Motor Scale (AIMS; Piper & Darrah, 1994)
- Bayley Scales of Infant and Toddler Development (4th ed.; Bayley-4; Bayley & Aylward, 2019)
- Fugl-Meyer Assessment (FMA; Fugel-Meyer et al., 1975)
- Pediatric Quality of Life Inventory (PedsQL 4.0; Varni et al., 2001)
- Pediatric Stroke Outcome Measure (PSOM; deVeber et al., 2000; see also Cooper et al., 2018; Kitchen et al., 2012; and Lo et al., 2014, in References)
- Ten-second test (10-ST; Hatanaka et al., 2007)
- Test of Infant Motor Performance (3rd ed.; TIMP-3; Campbell et al., 2012)
- Toronto Rehabilitation Institute Hand Function Test (see Rehabilitation Engineering Laboratory Hand Function Test in Appendix A)
- Wolf Motor Function Test (WMFT; Taub et al., 2011)

Problems/Issues
Activities of Daily Living/Instrumental ADL
- Infant or child may have difficulty with feeding or independent eating, including use of eating utensils (cutlery).
- Child may have difficulty undressing or dressing, including management of fasteners (buttons, zippers, snaps, loops) involving both upper and lower dressing skills.
- Child may have difficulty mastering bladder and bowel functions.
- Child may have difficulty learning independent washing or bathing skills.

Education/Work
- Child may have difficulty with handwriting.
- Child may need assistance with academic and/or school tasks, such as extra time to complete a task or assistive technology to perform a task.

- Child may need modification to building structure for accessibility.
- Child may need modification to time schedule to change from one classroom to another, or to a cafeteria, gym, auditorium, or to exit building to playground or transportation.

Play/Leisure
- Infant or child may be unable to engage in independent (by self) play.
- Child may be unable to engage in parallel play.
- Child may be unable to engage in cooperative play.
- Child may not have an identified leisure interest (hobby, games, sports).

Rest/Sleep
- Child may have difficulty falling or staying asleep.

Social Participation
- Child may have difficulty participating in social and group activities.
- Child may demonstrate poorer social adjustment (Greenham et al., 2018).

Sensorimotor
- Child may lack gross motor skills or have difficulty performing them with accuracy and speed (Cooper et al., 2019).
- Child may be unable to reach, grasp, manipulate, release toys or objects with one or both hands.
- Child may have hyper- or hypotonicity (spasticity, flaccidity).
- Child may have difficulty maintaining good posture and positioning.
- Child may have limited joint range of motion.
- Child may have limited endurance or activity tolerance (fatigue, tiredness).
- Child may have sensory hypersensitivities or overresponsivities to stimuli.
- Child may have sensory hyposensitivities or underresponsivities to stimuli.

Cognitive/Perceptual
- Overall cognition and executive functions may be reduced (Anderson et al., 2020; Araujo et al., 2017).
- Infant or child may have difficulty focusing and maintaining attention.
- Infant or child may have difficulty with memory functions appropriate to age.
- Child may have difficulty with executive functions.
- Child may have difficulty with visual perception.

Psychosocial
- Child may have difficulty with emotional (state, behavioral) regulation.
- Child may have difficulty bonding with parent or caregiver.
- Child may have difficulty with interpersonal relations.
- Child may have limited or poor quality of life (Friefeld et al., 2011; Neuner et al., 2011).

Context/Environment
- Child may require adapted devices such as a wheelchair for mobility and positioning.
- Child may require environmental modification to school building, playground equipment, or community recreational facility.
- Parents or caregivers may have limited information or knowledge about perinatal or pediatric stroke.
- Parents or caregivers may have limited information or knowledge about assistive devices or technology.
- Parents or caregivers may be unaware of community or internet resources.
- Parents and caregivers may experience increased amount of caregiver burden (Galvin et al., 2011).

Intervention/Treatment

Models and programs developed by occupational therapy personnel include bimanual activities, positioning aids, sensory integration, and splinting (Marcroft et al., 2019). Models and programs developed by other professionals but used by occupational therapy personnel include Constraint-Induced Movement Therapy (CIMT or Modified CIMT; Gillick et al., 2014; Kirton et al., 2016; Marcroft et al., 2019), early therapy in perinatal stroke (eTIPS) program (Basu et al., 2017), functional electrical stimulation (Kapadia et al., 2014), functional taping (Kinesio Taping; Marcroft et al., 2019), high-frequency rTMS (Niimi et al., 2013), low-frequency rTMS (Gillick et al., 2014; Rich et al., 2016), neurodevelopmental therapy (Bobath; Marcroft et al., 2019), synactive theory (Roan & Bell, 2017), and transcranial direct current simulation (Kirton et al., 2017). Team members include physicians, neonatologists, pediatric neurologists, nursing personnel, physical therapists, educators, and occupational therapy personnel. Goals include tasks in the domains of self-care, productivity, and leisure (Galvin et al., 2010; Gordon et al., 2018).

Activities of Daily Living/Instrumental ADL
- Provide age- and skill-appropriate training in basic ADLs.
- If needed, provide age- and skill-appropriate training in IADLs.

Education/Work
- Provide information and training on use of assistive technology.
- Provide advice and recommendations for building or schedule modification.

Play/Leisure
- Provide age- and skill-appropriate play occupations.
- Assist client to explore and develop age- or skill-appropriate leisure occupations.

Rest/Sleep
- Assist parents or caregivers to provide appropriate sleeping routine.
- Assist parents or caregivers to provide appropriate sleepwear and bedding.

Social Participation
- Encourage participation in social activities.

Sensorimotor
- Premature infants might require assistance in promoting physiologic flexion and bilateral movement patterns, including hand-to-mouth movement, side lying position with support to decrease effect of gravity and encourage midline and adducted position.
- Assist in providing opportunity to practice age- and skill-appropriate gross motor skills.
- Provide training in age- and skill-appropriate fine motor and hand skills, including reach, grasp, manipulate, and release.
- Assist in providing positioning for spasticity.
- Assist in increasing endurance and activity tolerance.
- Child may need modification of sensory environment.

Cognitive/Perceptual
- Assist in improving attention, memory, and executive skills to age-appropriate level. Attention may be promoted through tactile, proprioceptive, vestibular, auditory, and sensory stimulation.
- Assist in providing visual perception training if needed.

Psychosocial
- Assist in developing stress reduction (soothing) and emotional regulation, including use of external supports such as dimming lights, reducing noise, and reducing visual distractions, and client supports such as palmar grasp, hand containment, and nonnutritive sucking.

- Assist parents or caregivers to develop parent–child bonding.
- Provide opportunities to practice social interaction skills.

Context/Environment

- Parent education about pediatric stroke and possible health issues such as cerebral palsy and seizures.
- Parent education about facilitating play activities.
- Parent education on parent–infant bonding.
- Parent education on interpreting and responding to infant behavior, including not over-stimulating.
- Provide information and training on use of adapted devices or technology as needed.
- Provide information on community and internet resources.

Precautions/Safety Considerations

Be aware of potential for seizures.

Prognosis and Outcome

Variable. Infant and child response to stroke varies from little or no major residual, to minor disability for which compensatory approaches work well, to severe spastic hemiplegic cerebral palsy as a chronic lifelong disorder. Larger lesion size is associated with poorer gross motor outcomes (Cooper et al., 2017; Greenham, Anderson, Cooper, et al., 2017). Sensorimotor functional outcome is dependent on corticospinal tract integrity (Gordon et al., 2012). Psychosocial outcome is dependent on multiple factors (Greenham, Anderson, Hearps, et al., 2017). Multiple community-based services are needed posthospitalization (McKevitt et al., 2019).

REFERENCES

Anderson, V., Darling, S., Mackay, M., Monagle, P., Greenham, M., Cooper, A., Hunt, R. W., Hearps, S., & Gordon, A. L. (2020). Cognitive resilience following paediatric stroke: Biological and environmental predictors. *European Journal of Paediatric Neurology, 25,* 52–58. https://doi .org/10.1016/j.ejpn.2019.11.011

Araujo, G. C., Antonini, T. N., Anderson, V., Vannatta, K. A., Salley, C. G., Bigler, E. D., Taylor, H. G., Gerhardt, C., Rubin, K., Dennis, M., Lo, W., Mackay, M. T., Gordon, A., Hajek Koterba, C., Gomes, A., Greenham, M., & Yeates, K. O. (2017). Profiles of executive function across children with distinct brain disorders: Traumatic brain injury, stroke, and brain tumor. *Journal of the International Neuropsychological Society, 23*(7), 529–538. https://doi.org/10.1017/S1355617717000364

Basu, A. P. (2014). Early intervention after perinatal stroke: Opportunities and challenges. *Developmental Medicine & Child Neurology, 56*(6), 516–521. https://doi.org/10.1111/dmcn.12407

Basu, A. P., Pearse, J. E., Baggaley, J., Watson, R. M., & Rapley, T. (2017). Participatory design in the development of an early therapy intervention for perinatal stroke. *BMC Pediatrics, 17,* Article 33. https://doi.org/10.1186/s12887-017-0797-9

Cooper, A. N., Anderson, V., Greenham, M., Hearps, S., Hunt, R. W., Mackay, M. T., Ditchfield, M., Coleman, L., Monagle, P., & Gordon, A. L. (2019). Motor function daily living skills 5 years after paediatric arterial ischaemic stroke: A prospective longitudinal study. *Developmental Medicine & Child Neurology, 61*(2), 161–167. https://doi.org/10.1111/dmcn.13915

Cooper, A. N., Anderson, V., Hearps, S., Greenham, M., Ditchfield, M., Coleman, L., Hunt, R. W., Mackay, M. T., Monagle, P., & Gordon, A. L. (2017). Trajectories of motor recovery in the first year after pediatric arterial ischemic stroke. *Pediatrics, 140*(2), Article e2013870. https://doi .org/10.1542/peds.2016-3870

Cooper, A. N., Anderson, V., Hearps, S., Greenham, M., Hunt, R. W., Mackay, M. T., Monagle, P., & Gordon, A. L. (2018). The Pediatric Stroke Outcome Measure: A predictor of outcome following arterial ischemic stroke. *Neurology, 90*(5), e365–e372. https://doi.org/10.1212/WNL.0000000000004906

Felter, C. E., Neuland, E. E., Iuculano, S. C., & Dean, J. (2019). Interdisciplinary, intensive, activity-based treatment for intrauterine spinal cord infarct: A case report. *Topics in Spinal Cord Injury Rehabilitation, 25*(1), 97–103. https://doi.org/10.1310/sci18-00025

Fiume, A., Deveber, G., Jang, S.-H., Fuller, C., Viner, S., & Friefeld, S. (2018). Development and validation of the Pediatric Stroke Quality of Life Measure. *Developmental Medicine & Child Neurology, 60*(6), 587–595. https://doi.org/10.1111/dmcn.13684

Friefeld, S. J., Westmacott, R., MacGregor, D., & deVeber, G. A. (2011). Predictors of quality of life in pediatric survivors of arterial ischemic stroke and cerebral sinovenous thrombosis. *Journal of Child Neurology, 26*(9), 1186–1192. https://doi.org/10.1177/0883073811408609

Galvin, J., Randall, M., Hewish, S., Rice, J., & MacKay, M. T. (2010). Family-centred outcome measurement following paediatric stroke. *Australian Occupational Therapy Journal, 57*(3), 152–158. https://doi.org/10.1111/j.1440-1630.2010.00853.x

Galvin, J., Hewish, S., Rice, J., & Mackay, M. T. (2011). Functional outcome following paediatric stroke. *Developmental Neurorehabilitation, 14*(2), 67–71. https://doi.org/10.3109/17518423.2010.547241

Gillick, B. T., Krach, L. E., Feyma, T., Rich, T. L., Moberg, K., Thomas, W., Cassidy, J. M., Menk, J., & Carey, J. R. (2014). Primed low-frequency repetitive transcranial magnetic stimulation and constraint-induced movement therapy in pediatric hemiparesis: A randomized controlled trial. *Developmental Medicine & Child Neurology, 56*(1), 44–52. https://doi.org/10.1111/dmcn.12243

Gordon, A. L., Nguyen, L., Panton, A., Mallick, A. A., Ganesan, V., Wraige, E., & McKevitt, C. (2018). Self-reported needs after pediatric stroke. *European Journal of Paediatric Neurology, 22*(5), 791–796. https://doi.org/10.1016/j.ejpn.2018.06.003

Gordon, A. L., Wood, A., Tournier, J. D., & Hunt, R. W. (2012). Corticospinal tract integrity and motor function following neonatal stroke: A case study. *BMC Neurology, 12*, Article 53. https://doi.org/10.1186/1471-2377-12-53

Greenham, M., Anderson, V., Cooper, A., Hearps, S., Ditchfield, M., Coleman, L., Hunt, R. W., Mackay, M. T., Monagle, P., & Gordon, A. L. (2017). Early predictors of psychosocial functioning 5 years after paediatric stroke. *Developmental Medicine & Child Neurology, 59*(10), 1034–1041. https://doi.org/10.1111/dmcn.13519

Greenham, M., Anderson, V., Hearps, S., Ditchfield, M., Coleman, L., Mackay, M. T., Monagle, P., & Gordon, A. L. (2017). Psychosocial function in the first year after childhood stroke. *Developmental Medicine & Child Neurology, 59*(10), 1027–1033. https://doi.org/10.1111/dmcn.13387

Greenham, M., Gordon, A. L., Cooper, A., Ditchfield, M., Coleman, L., Hunt, R. W., Mackay, M. T., Monagle, P., & Anderson, V. (2018). Social functioning following pediatric stroke: Contribution of neurobehavioral impairment. *Developmental Neuropsychology, 43*(4), 312–328. https://doi.org/10.1080/87565641.2018.1440557

Kapadia, N. M., Nagai, M. K., Zivanovic, V., Bernstein, J., Woodhouse, J., Rumney, P., & Popovic, M. R. (2014). Functional electrical stimulation therapy for recovery of reaching and grasping in severe chronic pediatric stroke patients. *Journal of Child Neurology, 29*(4), 493–499. https://doi.org/10.1177/0883073813484088

Kirton, A., Andersen, J., Herrero, M. Nettel-Aguirre, A., Carsolio, L., Damji, O., Keess, J., Mineyko, A., Hodge, J., & Hill, M. D. (2016). Brain stimulation and constraint for perinatal stroke hemiparesis: The PLASTIC CHAMPS trial. *Neurology, 86*(18), 1659–1667. https://doi.org/10.1212/WNL.0000000000002646

Kirton, A., Ciechanski, P., Zewdie, E., Andersen, J., Nettel-Aguirre, A., Carlson, H., Carsolio, L., Herrero, M., Quigley, J., Mineyko, A., Hodge, J., & Hill, M. (2017). Transcranial direct current stimulation for children with perinatal stroke and hemiparesis. *Neurology, 88*(3), 259–267. https://doi.org/10.1212/WNL.0000000000003518

Kitchen, L., Westmacott, R., Friefeld, S., MacGregor, D., Curtis, R., Allen, A., Yau, I., Askalan, R., Moharir, M., Domi, T., & deVeber, G. (2012). The Pediatric Stroke Outcome Measure: A validation and reliability study. *Stroke, 43*(6), 1602–1608. https://doi.org/10.1161/STROKEAHA.111.639583

Lo, W., Gordon, A. L., Hajek, C., Gomes, A., Greenham, M., Anderson, V., Yeates, K. O., & Mackay, M. T. (2014). Pediatric Stroke Outcome Measure: Predictor of multiple impairments in childhood stroke. *Journal of Child Neurology, 29*(11), 1524–1530. https://doi.org/10.1177/0883073813503186

Marcroft, C., Tsutsumi, A., Pearse, J., Dulson, P., Embleton, N. D., & Basu, A. P. (2019). Current therapeutic management of perinatal stroke with a focus on the upper limb: A cross-sectional survey of UK physiotherapists and occupational therapists. *Physical & Occupational Therapy in Pediatrics, 39*(2), 151–167. https://doi.org/10.1080/01942638.2018.1503212

McKevitt, C., Topor, M., Panton, A., Mallick, A. A., Ganesan, V., Wraige, E., & Gordon, A. (2019). Seeking normality: Parents' experiences of childhood stroke. *Child: Care, Health and Development, 45*(1), 89–95. https://doi.org/10.1111/cch.12622

Neuner, B., von Mackensen, S., Krümpel, A., Manner, D., Friefeld, S., Nixdorf, S., Frühwald, M., deVeber, G., & Nowak-Göttl, U. (2011). Health-related quality of life in children and adolescents with stroke, self-reports, and parent/proxies reports: Cross-sectional investigation. *Annals of Neurology, 70*(1), 70–78. https://doi.org/10.1002/ana.22381

Niimi, M., Kakuda, W., Takekawa, T., Momosaki, R., Hara, T., Ito, H., Kameda, Y., & Abo, M. (2013). Therapeutic application of high-frequency rTMS combined with intensive occupational therapy for pediatric stroke patients with upper limb hemiparesis: A case series study. *Journal of Behavioral and Brain Science, 3*(2), 188–193. https://doi.org/10.4236/jbbs.2013.32019

Rich, T. L., Menk, J., Krach, L. E., Feyma, T., & Gillick, B. T. (2016). Repetitive transcranial magnetic stimulation/behavioral intervention clinical trial: Long-term follow-up of outcomes in congenital hemiparesis. *Journal of Child and Adolescent Psychopharmacology, 26*(7), 598–605. https://doi.org/10.1089/cap.2015.0157

Roan, C., & Bell, A. (2017). Occupational therapy in the neonatal intensive care unit for a neonate with perinatal stroke: A case report. *Physical & Occupational Therapy in Pediatrics, 37*(3), 283–291. https://doi.org/10.1080/01942638.2016.1185503

BIBLIOGRAPHY

Gordon, A. L. (2014). Functioning and disability after stroke in children: Using the ICF-CY to classify health outcome and inform future clinical research priorities. *Developmental Medicine & Child Neurology, 56*(5), 434–444. https://doi.org/10.1111/dmcn.12336

Gordon, A. L., Anderson, V., Ditchfield, M., Coleman, L., Mackay, M. T., Greenham, M., Hunt, R. W., & Monagle, P. (2015). Factors associated with six-month outcome of pediatric stroke. *International Journal of Stroke, 10*(7), 1068–1073. https://doi.org/10.1111/ijs.12489

Grigoratos, D. N., Mazarakis, N. K., Lumsden, D. E., Kariyawasam, S., Bhangoo, R., Gordon, A., Lin, J. P., & Dlamini, N. (2013). Good outcome following emergency decompressive craniectomy in a case of malignant middle cerebral artery infarction in a 14-month-old infant. *British Journal of Neurosurgery, 27*(5), 694–695. https://doi.org/10.3109/02688697.2013.776668

Post-Polio Syndrome

Also called post-poliomyelitis syndrome, post-poliomyelitis muscular atrophy (PPMA).

Description

Post-polio syndrome is a group of symptoms that reoccurs years or decades after the original illness of acute paralytic poliomyelitis and usually, but not always, affects the same groups of muscles as in the original infectious attack (O'Toole, 2017; Porter, 2018).

Cause

The cause may be related to further loss of anterior horn cells due to aging process in a group of neurons already depleted by the initial polio virus infection (Porter, 2018; Southam et al., 2013).

Evaluation/Assessment

Areas

- Activities of Daily Living/Instrumental ADL: bathing, dressing, meal preparation, medication management, swallowing, functional mobility
- Education/Work: paid and unpaid work skills, work history
- Play/Leisure: interests, types, frequency, location
- Rest/Sleep: sleep quality
- Social Participation: type, frequency, location, family and community participation
- Sensorimotor: endurance, fatigue related to chronic condition, functional range of motion, joint and muscle pain, muscle strength and tone, sensibility (temperature tolerance)
- Cognitive/Perceptual: executive functions
- Psychosocial: coping behavior, adjustment to decreased ability, quality of life
- Context/Environment: environmental modification, lifestyle modification, assistive device and technology

Instruments

Instruments Developed by Occupational Therapy Personnel

- Canadian Occupational Performance Measure (5th ed.; COPM-5; Law et al., 2014)
- Knowledge of Polio Test (KPT; Young, 1991)
- Semistructured Interview (Atwal et al., 2019, in References)

Instruments Developed by Other Professionals and Used by Occupational Therapy Personnel

- Joint range of motion (goniometry; Shurtleff & Kaskutas, 2018)
- Manual Muscle Test (MMT; Kaskutas, 2018)
- Ways of Coping Questionnaire–Revised (WoC-R or WCQ-R; Folkman et al., 1986)

Problems/Issues

Activities of Daily Living/Instrumental ADL

- Person may experience decreased bladder and bowel control.
- Person may experience increased breathing difficulties.
- Person may be obese and have difficulty with diet management.
- Person may have budget and financial concerns.
- Person may have difficulty driving or with other transportation systems.

Education/Work

- Person may have difficulty performing home management tasks.
- Person may have difficulty with employment status (getting/keeping a job).

Play/Leisure

- Person may have abandoned certain hobbies and leisure-time activities.
- Person may experience difficulty performing tasks associated with selected hobbies and leisure-time activities.

Rest/Sleep

- Person may be experiencing sleep disturbance.
- Person may not have an established sleep routine.

Social Participation

- Person may experience difficulty maintaining interpersonal relations.
- Person may have discontinued participation in favorite community activities.

Sensorimotor

- Person may develop contractures.
- Person may experience increased difficulty with mobility (walking and climbing stairs).
- Person may experience increased joint and muscle pain.
- Person may experience new and increased muscle atrophy.
- Person may have progressive muscle weakness.
- Person may experience muscle cramps.
- Person may experience increased muscle weakness and muscular fatigability.
- Person may experience degenerative disk disease due to abnormal biomechanics.
- Person may experience increased fatigue due to chronic condition, making everyday tasks more difficult to perform (Note: fatigue in chronic conditions is defined as "an overwhelming sustained sense of exhaustion and decreased capacity for physical and mental work at usual level"; Ghahari et al., 2013, p. 85).
- Person may develop osteoporosis and be at greater risk for fractures.
- Person may experience changes in posture and postural control.
- Person may develop scoliosis.
- Person may have difficulty with transfers.
- Person may experience increased cold intolerance.

Cognitive/Perceptual

- Person may lack of knowledge about the existence of post-polio syndrome and its effects.

Psychosocial

- Person may experience depression related to increased symptoms.
- Person may experience anxiety about the future as disabling symptoms increase.
- Person may experience stress in coping with daily life demands.
- Person may be angry about life situation.
- Person may deny symptoms are a problem or that "anything has changed" in his or her life situation.
- Person may experience difficulty "fitting in" and with feeling of being accepted.
- Person may experience decreased life satisfaction.
- Person may experience feelings of hopelessness and helplessness.
- Person may feel a of lack of social support and understanding of symptoms.
- Person may feel discriminated against because of disability by society.
- Person may feel a decreased sense of competence as symptoms progress.
- Person may experience decreased quality of life.
- Person may feel he or she is a burden to others or may become a burden.

Context/Environment

- Person may have increased difficulty with finding an accessible environment.
- Family members may have difficulty accepting change in status of person as disability increases.
- Social acquaintances may not understand what has happened to the person as disability status increases.

Intervention/Treatment

Focus is on compensatory and adapted techniques and equipment. Use of remedial techniques is not realistic given the degenerative course of the disorder. Multidisciplinary team should be involved. Models and programs developed by occupational therapy personnel: No information identified. Models and program developed by other professionals but used by occupational therapy personnel: No information identified. Team members include physicians, psychologists, social workers, nursing personnel, physical therapy personnel, and occupational therapy personnel. Goal is to maintain occupational performance and life satisfaction for as long as possible using adaptive and compensatory strategies as needed to enable person to function with a chronic condition. Journal references are from the United Kingdom (Atwal et al., 2019; Atwal et al., 2013; Atwal et al., 2015; Spiliotopoulou et al., 2012), Sweden (Santos-Tavares & Thorén-Jönsson, 2013; Silva & Thorén-Jönsson, 2015), and Israel (Shoseyov et al., 2017). No recent studies were identified from the United States or Canada, possibly reflecting the decreased number of clients receiving occupational therapy services.

Activities of Daily Living/Instrumental ADL

- With dietician or nutritionist help, assist client to develop a diet and nutritional management plan to maintain a healthy weight and nutritional balance.
- Assist client to develop and follow a medication management plan. Work with physician to determine and select best medications available within client's financial resources.
- Assist client to create and follow a plan for shopping for groceries and other items (plan may include using delivery programs).
- Assist client's ability to continue to drive independently. Explore other transportation options.

Education/Work

- Patient education: increase client's understanding of post-polio syndrome.

Play/Leisure

- Assist client to modify or adapt tasks that have restricted client from engaging in hobbies or leisure activities.
- Assist client to develop new leisure activities if previous activities cannot be modified to the client's satisfaction.

Rest/Sleep

- Assist client to modify or adapt sleep routines.
- Assist management team to determine whether breathing-assistance equipment is needed to maintain adequate ventilation.

Social Participation

- Assist client to modify or adapt activities or actions that facilitate social participation activities.

Sensorimotor

- Provide a falls training program based on client's risk factors.
- Develop, with client input, fatigue management based on pacing (alternate cycles of rest and activity, selecting which activities or tasks are most important and performing them when energy level is highest, determining whether other people could assist with some tasks; concept of "Changing the Rhythm of Life" may help client with acceptance).
- Develop, with client input, a joint protection plan that best protects joints from injury and external trauma, including use of external aids.
- Encourage use of good body mechanics and posture.
- Explore, with team management, a pain-management program that includes pharmaceutical and nonpharmaceutical agents (heat compresses, hydrotherapy).
- Explore with client compensatory techniques for performing tasks requiring use of upper extremity, including use of adaptive equipment and splinting.
- With assistance from and consultation with a physician, physical therapist, or exercise physiologist, consider developing an exercise plan with the client. (Note that the benefits of exercise are controversial. Per occupational therapy tradition, exercise can be built into everyday activities that are routinely performed as part of the client's daily routine.)

Cognitive/Perceptual

- Assist client to gain a better understanding of approaches to successfully manage post-polio symptoms.
- Assist client with information to be used in discussion with family, friends, and coworkers as to how they can be helpful without feeling overwhelmed as symptoms progress.

Psychosocial
- Assist client to develop coping skills, including adjustment to life as a post-polio survivor.
- Increase client's self-awareness of strengths and limitation.
- Assist client to deal effectively with emotions such as shyness to admit, shame, or embarrassment about disability.
- Assist client to express feelings appropriately dealing with anger and denial.
- Increase sense of competence and self-esteem, and decrease sense of hopelessness and helplessness.

Context/Environment
- Facilitate lifestyle modification, including home and local community modification.
- Assist client to select and use assistive technology for facilitated occupational performance.
- Provide ergonomic training for client to more effectively and efficiently perform tasks.
- Provide training in work simplification techniques.
- Provide information on ergonomic principles.
- Provide educational information to family, friends, and coworkers about post-polio syndrome and its impact on them.
- Provide staff and professional training about post-polio syndrome and its management.

Precautions/Safety Considerations

Fall prevention should be an important consideration in all activities. Fatigue management may determine if employment is feasible (Ghahari et al., 2013).

Prognosis and Outcome

Condition is chronic. Reliance on compensatory techniques and assistive devices is likely to increase.

REFERENCES

Atwal, A., Duncan, H., Queally, C., & Cedar, S. H. (2019). Polio survivors perceptions of a multi-disciplinary rehabilitation programme. *Disability and Rehabilitation*, *41*(2), 150–157. https://doi.org/10.1080/09638288.2017.1381184

Atwal, A., Giles, A., Spiliotopoulou, G., Plastow, N., & Wilson, L. (2013). Living with polio and postpolio syndrome in the United Kingdom. *Scandinavian Journal of Caring Sciences*, *27*(2), 238–245. https://doi.org/10.1111/j.1471-6712.2012.01029.x

Atwal, A., Spiliotopoulou, G., Coleman, C., Harding, K., Quirke, C., Smith, N., Osseiran, Z., Plastow, N., & Wilson, L. (2015). Polio survivors' perceptions of the meaning of quality of life and strategies used to promote participation in everyday activities. *Health Expectations*, *18*(5), 715–726. https://doi.org/10.1111/hex.12152

Ghahari, S., Parvaneh, S., & Packer, T. L. (2013). Fatigue in progressive neurological conditions: A literature review. *Iranian Rehabilitation Journal*, *11*, 85–90.

O'Toole, M. T. (Ed.). (2017). *Mosby's dictionary of medicine, nursing & health professions* (10th ed.). Elsevier.

Porter, R. S. (Ed.). (2018). *The Merck manual of diagnosis and therapy* (20th ed.). Merck Sharp & Dohme.

Santos-Tavares, I., & Thorén-Jönsson, A.-L. (2013). Confidence in the future and hopelessness: Experiences in daily occupations of immigrants with late effects of polio. *Scandinavian Journal of Occupational Therapy*, *20*(1), 9–20. https://doi.org/10.3109/11038128.2012.660193

Shoseyov, D., Cohen-Kaufman, T., Schwartz, I., & Portnoy, S. (2017). Comparison of activity and fatigue of the respiratory muscles and pulmonary characteristics between post-polio patients and controls: A pilot study. *PLOS ONE*, *12*(7), Article e0182036. https://doi.org/10.1371/journal.pone.0182036

Silva, I. S. T., & Thorén-Jönsson, A.-L. (2015). Struggling to be part of Swedish society: Strategies used by immigrants with late effects of polio. *Scandinavian Journal of Occupational Therapy, 22*(6), 450–461. https://doi.org/10.3109/11038128.2015.1057222

Southam, M., Schmidt, A., & Hewitt George, A. (2013). Disorders of the motor unit: Polio-myelitis and postpolio syndrome. In H. M. Pendleton & W. Schultz-Krohn (Eds.), *Pedretti's occupational therapy* (7th ed., pp. 989–991). Elsevier.

Spiliotopoulou, G., Fowkes, C., & Atwal, A. (2012). Assistive technology and prediction of happiness in people with post-polio syndrome. *Disability and Rehabilitation: Assistive Technology, 7*(3), 199–204. https://doi.org/10.3109/17483107.2011.616921

Stroke: Acute

Also called cerebrovascular accident, CVA, apoplexy, cerebral infarction.

See also Cognitive Impairment, Dementia, Depression and Depressive Disorders, Executive Dysfunction, Falls, Memory Impairment, Sleep–Wake Disorders, Stroke: Chronic, Stroke: Hemiplegia, Swallowing Disorders: Adult, Visual Impairment Due to Neurologic Conditions.

Description

The term *stroke* refers to a heterogeneous group of disorders that involve sudden, focal interruption of cerebral blood flow, leading to various neurologic deficits. An ischemic stroke is the result of a thrombosis or embolism blocking blood flow in the brain. A hemorrhage stroke is the result of vascular rupture, such as a subarachnoid hemorrhage or intracerebral hemorrhage. Transient ischemic attacks (TIAs) are symptoms that typically last less than 1 hour but do not show evidence of infarction on a magnetic resonance imaging (MRI) (Porter, 2018). The term *acute stroke* includes the period of inpatient status in a hospital (typically 5–7 days) or rehabilitation unit and may include the term *subacute stroke*. Poststroke or chronic stroke includes the period after hospitalization or discharge from a rehabilitation unit regardless of whether the person goes home or to a nursing facility (Miller et al., 2010).

Cause

The blockage or hemorrhage usually involves the arteries of the brain—either the anterior circulation (branches of the internal carotid artery) or the posterior circulation (branches of the vertebral and basilar arteries).

Evaluation/Assessment

Areas

(Note: RH = right hemisphere; LH = left hemisphere.)

- Activities of Daily Living/Instrumental ADL: self-maintenance (eating, dressing, bathing/showering, brushing teeth, grooming, shaving, toileting), functional mobility, functional communication (aphasia [LH], anomia). (Note: Most IADL and health management issues are addressed under Stroke: Chronic Stroke or Stroke: Hemiplegia.)
- Education/Work: alexia (LH), agraphia (LH), acalculia (LH), work demands (paid or unpaid), work-site layout
- Play/Leisure: interests, values, frequency, location
- Rest/Sleep: sleep disturbance, sleep habits
- Social Participation: type, frequency, location, with whom
- Sensorimotor: muscle weakness (hemiplegia or hemiparesis), muscle strength, joint range of motion, endurance, posture and postural control (hand functions: grip strength, pinch

strength, grasp and release, two hand coordination, stereognosis), pain, tactile, pressure, proprioception, temperature, visual acuity (near, distance), visual field of vision, visual tracking, visuospatial neglect, visual scanning, ocular (eye) movements, pattern recognition, diplopia (double vision), unilateral motor apraxia (RH), bilateral motor apraxia (LH)

- Cognitive/Perceptual: attention (visual and auditory), memory (visual and auditory), executive function, left unilateral body neglect (RH), left unilateral visual neglect (RH), body image (RH), visuospatial relationships, agnosia (LH)
- Psychosocial: depression, anxiety, self-image, liability, apathy (lack of motivation), perseveration, frustration tolerance (LH), anosognosia (RH, lack of awareness of disability)
- Context/Environment: social support, adapted devices, home environmental modification, family or caregiver education
- Comorbidities: diabetes, hypertension, fractures, osteoporosis, dementia, cognitive impairment, visual impairment

Instruments

Instruments Developed by Occupational Therapy Personnel

- A-ONE (see Arnadottir OT-ADL Neurobehavioral Evaluation)
- Acute Stroke Dysphagia Screen (ASDS; Edmiaston et al., 2010, in References; also called the Barnes-Jewish Hospital-Stroke Dysphagia Screen [BIH-SDS]; Edmiaston et al., 2014, in References)
- Adapted Four-Item Shopping Task (Nir-Hadad et al., 2017, in References)
- Allen Cognitive Level Screen (5th ed.; ACLS-5; Allen et al., 2007; see also Krumlinde-Sundholm et al., 2019, in References)
- Arnadottir OT-ADL Neurobehavioral Evaluation (A-ONE; Arnadottir, 1990)
- Assessment of Motor and Process Skills (8th ed.; AMPS-8; Fisher & Bray Jones, 2016)
- Australian Therapy Outcome Measures (3rd ed.; AusTOMs-3; Unsworth & Duncombe, 2014; see also Chen & Eng, 2015, in References)
- Box and Block Test (BBT; Holser & Fuchs, 1957, 1960; Mathiowetz et al., 1985)
- Brain Injury Visual Assessment Battery for Adults (biVABA; Warren, 1998)
- Canadian Occupational Performance Measure (5th ed.; COPM-5; Law et al., 2014)
- Executive Function Performance Test (EFPT; Baum & Wolf, 2013)
- Kettle Test (KT; Hartman-Maeir et al., 2009)
- Nine Hole Peg Test (9HPT; Kellor et al., 1971; Mathiowetz et al., 1985)
- Nottingham Extended Activities of Daily Living (NEADL; Nouri & Lincoln, 1987)
- Nottingham Stroke Dressing Assessment (NSDA; Fletcher-Smith et al., 2010)
- Occupational Therapy Adult Perceptual Screening Test (OT-APST; Cooke et al., 2005; see also Razemba et al., 2017, in References)
- Stroke Assessment of Fall Risk (SAFR; Breisinger et al., 2014, in References)
- Test of Grocery Shopping Skills (TGSS; Brown et al., 2009)

Instruments Developed by Other Professionals and Used by Occupational Therapy Personnel

- Activity Measure of Post-Acute Care (AM-PAC; Sandel et al., 2013)
- Addenbrooke's Cognitive Examination III (ACE-III; Hsieh et al., 2013)
- Animal Naming (Tombaugh et al., 1999)
- Barthel Index (BI; Mahoney & Barthel, 1965)
- Barthel Index-Based Supplementary Scales (BI-SS; Lee et al., 2014, in References; see also Lee et al., 2017, in References)
- Behavioral Inattention Test (BIT; Wilson et al., 1987)
- Benton Controlled Oral Word Association Test (Ruff et al., 1996)
- Berg Balance Scale (BBS; Berg et al., 1989)
- Chedoke-McMaster Stroke Assessment (CMSA; Barreca et al., 2004)
- European Quality of Life 5-Dimension Scale (EuroQol 5; EuroQol Group, 1990)
- Fall Harm Risk Screen (FHRS; Breisinger et al., 2014, in References)

- Fatigue Severity Scale (FSS; Krupp et al., 1989)
- Five-Digit Test (FDT; Sedo, 2005, in Spanish; see also Lin et al., 2016, in References)
- Functional Independence Measure (FIM; Uniform Data System for Medical Rehabilitation, 1997)
- General Health Questionnaire (GHQ; Goldberg & Williams, 1988)
- Grip strength (dynamometer; JAMAR, Lafayette Instrument; Wang et al., 2018)
- Hopkins Verbal Learning Test–Revised (HVLT-R; Benedict et al., 1998)
- Modified Ashworth Scale (MAS; Bohannon & Smith, 1987)
- Mini-Mental State Examination (MMSE; Folstein et al., 1975; see also Toglia et al., 2011, in References)
- Modified Barthel Index (MBI; Collin et al., 1988)
- Modified Rankin Scale (mRS; van Swieten et al., 1988)
- Montreal Cognitive Assessment (MoCA; Nasreddine et al., 2005; see also Jaywant et al., 2019; Toglia et al., 2017; and Toglia et al., 2011, in References)
- Motor-Free Visual Perception Test (4th ed.; MVPT-4; Colarusso & Hamill, 2015)
- Multiple Errands Test (MET; Shallice & Burgess, 1991)
- National Institute of Neurologic Disorders and Stroke (NINDS)–Canadian Stroke Network (CSN) Battery (NINDS-CSN; Hachinski et al, 2006)
- National Institutes of Health (NIH) Stroke Scale (NIHSS; Brott et al., 1989)
- Pinch strength (pinch meter; B&E Engineering; Mathiowetz et al., 1985)
- Postural Assessment Scale for Stroke (PASS; Benaim et al., 1999)
- Rivermead Behavioural Memory Test (3rd ed.; RBMT-3; Wilson et al., 2008)
- Rivermead Motor Assessment (RMA; Lincoln & Leadbitter, 1979)
- Short Form 36 Health Survey (SF-36; Ware et al., 1993)
- Stroke Aphasia Depression Questionnaire (SADQ; Lincoln et al., 2000)
- Stroke Assessment of Fall Risk (SAFR; Breisinger & Campbell, 2011; see also Breisinger et al., 2014, in References)
- Stroke Impact Scale (Version 2.0; SIS-2; Duncan et al., 1999)
- Stroke Impairment Assessment Set (SIAS; Chino et al., 1996)
- Stroke Rehabilitation Assessment of Movement (STREAM; Daley et al., 1999)
- Sunnybrook Neglect Assessment Procedure (SNAP; Ebert et al., 2001)
- Symbol Digit Modalities Test (SDMT; Smith, 1973; see also NINDS-CSN Battery)
- Trail Making Tests A & B (TMT-A, TMT-B; Bowie & Harvey, 2006)

Problems/Issues

Activities of Daily Living/Instrumental ADL

- Person may be unable or has difficulty performing basic self-maintenance tasks (eating, dressing, toileting, grooming, bathing/showering, functional mobility, functional communication).
- Person may have difficulty performing IADL tasks (probably not necessary to determine during acute stage; meal preparation or laundry may be exceptions).

Education/Work

- Person usually is unable to perform or has difficulty performing work-related tasks (paid or unpaid), such as keyboarding.
- Person may report difficulty negotiating the work environment (accessibility).

Play/Leisure

- Person may be unable to engage or has difficulty engaging in favorite leisure occupations, especially active involvement in sports.
- Person may be unable to engage in some passive or quiet leisure activities because of decreased hand dexterity and coordination, including changing channel on TV remote or holding a magazine or book to read.

Rest/Sleep
- Person may experience sleep disturbance (unable to fall asleep or stay asleep).
- Person may have difficulty maintaining a sleep routine.

Social Participation
- Person may be unable to participate or have difficulty participating in social activities (accessibility).
- Person may withdraw from participation in social activities (psychosocial issues).

Sensorimotor
- Person usually has muscle weakness or paralysis (hemiparesis or hemiplegia).
- Person may have a stereotypical synergy pattern (flexion or extension).
- Person may have reduced joint range of motion.
- Person may experience reduced endurance, fatigue, tiredness, activity tolerance.
- Person may have decreased sensory awareness (tactile, proprioception).
- Person may demonstrate motor apraxia or dyspraxia (difficulty with motor planning).
- Person may experience visual changes (visual acuity, visual field of vision, ocular movement, binocular function such as diplopia, visual scanning, pattern recognition, visual tracking) such as the following:
  - Person has difficulty reading printed materials (hospital menu forms, newspaper, magazine) or says the text is blurry (visual acuity).
  - Person loses place while reading (visual tracking).
  - Person does not read part of text (visual neglect).
  - Person cannot find beginning of next line when reading (visual spatial).
  - Person squints or closes one eye when reading (binocular dysfunction, diplopia).
  - Person looks down while ambulating, even if told to look ahead (decreased visual field of vision).
  - Person runs into walls or trails the wall while ambulating (missing visual field of vision).

Cognitive/Perceptual
- Person may have reduced ability to attend and concentrate on a task or activity.
- Person may have difficulty remembering instructions.
- Person may demonstrate poor judgment of safety, such as trying to walk without support.
- Person may be unable to problem solve or has difficulty problem solving or planning ahead.
- Person may appear to ignore one side (usually the left side) of visual field and environment.
- Person may have difficulty with spatial relationships.

Psychosocial
- Person appears depressed or expresses depressive thoughts.
- Person expresses anxiety or fear.
- Person's mood changes quickly (lability) from anger to smiling to crying.
- Person is apathetic (low motivation).

Context/Environment
- Person, family, and caregivers may lack knowledge about stroke or its management.
- Person, family, and caregivers may lack information about available resources in community or on internet.
- Person may lack social support.
- Person may need adapted devices or mobility aids.

Intervention/Treatment

Models and programs developed by occupational therapy personnel include Aid for Decision-Making in Occupation Choice (ADOC; Tomori et al., 2015); case study (Schriner & Ziegler

Delahunt, 2017); client-centered, self-care intervention (CCSCI; Guidetti & Ytterberg, 2011); Cognitive Orientation to daily Occupational Performance (CO-OP; Skidmore et al., 2011); dressing program (Mew, 2010; Walker et al., 2012); home visits (HOVIS; Drummond et al., 2013); and model of human occupation (Shinohara et al., 2012). Models and programs developed by other professionals but used by occupational therapy personnel include direct skill training (Skidmore et al., 2017), Graded Repetitive Arm Supplementary Program (GRASP; Murdolo et al., 2017; Schneider et al., 2019; University of British Columbia [2011, 2016]), orthotics (SaeboFlex: Andriske et al., 2017), rehabilitation gaming system (Seitz & Carey, 2013), robotic system (Abdullah et al., 2011; Iwamoto et al., 2019), strategy training (Skidmore et al., 2015; Skidmore et al, 2014), taping (Bell & Muller, 2013; Hayner, 2012), virtual reality (Imam & Jarus, 2014), visual field loss (Mödden et al., 2012), wheelchair skills program (Mountain et al., 2010), and Wii Sports (Celinder & Peoples, 2012). Team members include physicians, nursing personnel, psychologists, physical therapists, speech–language pathologists, social workers, neuropsychologists, and occupational therapy personnel. Goals should be relevant to the needs of the client (Langhorne et al., 2011). In acute care, the primary focus is on occupational performance of basic activities of daily living, but other occupational areas may be addressed.

Activities of Daily Living/Instrumental ADL
- Bathing/Showering: transfer bench, tub bench, handheld shower nozzle, grab bar, nonskid surface, extended handle brush to wash back, soft handles on towel to dry back.
- Bed mobility: silk sheets and pajamas, handle on bed, position chair or nightstand near bed for stability, commode chair.
- Dressing: buttonhook, elastic shoelaces or Velcro fasteners, long-handled shoehorn, zipper pull, hook and loop fasteners, reacher or grabber.
- Dysphagia (see Swallowing Disorders: Adult in Section 3: Nervous System Disorders; use of the Acute Stroke Dysphagia Screen is important first step; Edmiaston et al., 2010).
- Eating: universal cuff, built-up handles, rocker knife, plate guard, plates with lips, scoop dish, extended handle utensils, nonslip or nonskid mats, hook and loop fasteners, suction cup, double handle cups.
- Functional mobility: wheelchair, scooter, walker, cane.
- Grooming: built-up handles, extended handles.
- Toileting: raised commode chair, grab bars, hook and loop fasteners on pants or elastic waist pants, pump soap dispenser, toilet safety frame.
- Transfers: equipment—transfer board, transfer bench.
- Home management: laundry and clothes care, vacuuming, dusting, organizing closets.
- Meal planning, preparation and cleanup: simplify meal plan and preparation, use more ready-to-eat or easy-to-prepare products, use microwave.
- Finances: budgeting, check writing, or internet banking.
- Driving: operational skills, tactical skills, strategic planning skills.
- Pet care: walking, feeding, grooming, health care, safety.
- Child care: feeding, dressing, washing/bathing, grooming, play activities, safety.
- Shopping: groceries, sundries, clothes, household goods.

Education/Work
- Physical demands (crouching, bending, stooping, reaching, lifting, carrying, climbing, moving objects; consider whether pertinent to return to work).
- Work-related cognitive demands: attention, memory, executive functions (consider whether pertinent to return to work).
- Work-related social skills: interpersonal skills, supervisee/supervisor relationships (consider whether pertinent to return to work).
- Specific task skills: hand skills, computer skills (consider whether pertinent to return to work).

Play/Leisure

- Active leisure occupations: Assist client to select in which leisure occupations the client wants to continue active engagement.
- Passive leisure occupations: Assist client to select in which leisure occupations the client can engage passively.

Rest/Sleep

- Sleep routines
  - ▶ Joint positioning: Client should be positioned to maximize pain-free degrees of shoulder abduction and external rotation while maintaining shoulder joint alignment. Facility staff and family members should be educated on correct positioning (see Semenko et al., 2015, pp. 30–31, in References, for sample forms).
- Rest routines
  - ▶ Assist client to schedule regular rest routines.
  - ▶ Assist client to determine whether more activities could be shared with others to provide more rest time.

Social Participation

- Active participation: Assist client to determine which social activities involve active participation in order to be of value to the client.
- Passive participation: Assist client to determine which social activities would continue to be valued if the client's role changed from active to a more passive one.
- Community integration: Assist client to maintain participation in community activities (concerts, theater, religious, book club).

Sensorimotor

- Musculoskeletal
  - ▶ Aerobic exercise: Activity must be of sufficient intensity, duration, and frequency to improve oxygen consumption from client's present level of function during an occupation. Client might begin by sitting in bed supported for increased lengths of time, sitting on side of bed without support, walking more steps to toilet, taking a shower using shower bench without assistance, getting dressed without assistance (may require monitoring of heart rate, pulse, and oxygen level).
  - ▶ Edema control
    - ○ Elevation: Place hand above the level of heart. Place hand and forearm on pillows in bed or when sitting.
    - ○ Massage: Apply lotion first. Use fingertips and firm pressure with long, smooth strokes.
    - ○ Active use: Tighten and relax muscle of hand to act as a pump to push fluid out of hand up the arm.
  - ▶ Joint range of motion and mobility: Use active range of motion as much as possible while engaging client in everyday activities such as eating, grooming, dressing, bathing, toileting.
  - ▶ Spasticity management
    - ○ Botulinum toxin (BTX) alone or in combination with therapy significantly decreases spasticity in the upper extremity.
    - ○ Splinting can be used to provide a prolonged stretch to improve muscle length, correct and prevent contractures, and maximize function.
  - ▶ Strengthening activities/exercises: Use progressive resistive exercises.
- Neuromuscular rehabilitation
  - ▶ Balance control and postural awareness.
    - ○ Sitting: Sitting on side of bed using hands for support, sitting on side of bed without hand support, sitting in chair with arms, sitting in chair or bench without arm supports.
    - ○ Standing with equal weight on both feet, shifting weight from one side to the other while standing in one place, standing on one foot while holding onto a support, standing on

one foot without support, stepping forward and backward holding onto a support, stepping forward and backward without support.

▶ Constraint-Induced Movement Therapy (CIMT): Use of repetitions of task-specific training of the affected limb while the unaffected limb is restrained using a glove or sling. May be done for a few hours or all day.

▶ Functional Electrical Stimulation (FES): Used in combination with a task-specific activity. Example: Wrap the involved hand around a cup when the stimulator is off; have client let go of the cup when the muscle stimulator is on to facilitate extension.

▶ Motor learning and coordination: Practice involves repeating either specific movements (reaching, grasping, releasing) or performing functional tasks (washing face, holding and eating a banana, squeezing toothpaste on a toothbrush, putting on a T-shirt).

▶ Neurodevelopmental Therapy (NDT, Bobath): Although popular, NDT approach is not superior to any other type of therapy (Miller et al., 2010).

▶ Repetitive task training: Repeated practice within a single training session of an active motor sequence that is aimed toward a specific functional objective.

- Compensatory
  ▶ Activity pacing
    o Schedule periods of occupation and rest throughout the day.
    o Frequent short rests are usually more beneficial that longer ones.
    o Avoid occupations that cannot be stopped immediately if they become stressful
    o Maintain a balance of work, leisure, and rest.
  ▶ Adapted/self-help devices
    o Built-up handles (easier to grip, such as enlarged handles for eating utensils).
    o Elongated or extended handles and reachers/grabbers (substitute for decreased range of motion or decreased flexibility).
    o Electric powered (substitute for hand functions such as an electric can opener or electric toothbrush).
    o Suction cup or nonskid mounted (substitute for supporting or assisting hand).
    o Flexible "goose" neck (substitute for range of motion or decreased ability to position body).
    o Mounted or shaped hooks (substitute for hand dexterity, such as a buttonhook, or decreased range of motion, such as a dressing hook).
  ▶ Energy conservation: Techniques to minimize muscle fatigue, joint stress, and pain including planning ahead, prioritizing occupation, changing ways in which occupations are done including combining or eliminating specific tasks. Example: sit while dressing upper extremity, organize tasks within easy reach between waist and shoulder height.
  ▶ Fatigue management: Includes activity pacing, energy conservation, and work simplification.
  ▶ Kinesio Taping: Therapeutic taping of joints designed to alleviate pain and facilitate lymphatic drainage by microscopically lifting the skin.
  ▶ Mirror therapy: Use of mirror alongside the unaffected limb so the mirror image seems to be the affected limb.
  ▶ One-handed techniques (see Ryan et al., 2016)
  ▶ Slings: May be used temporarily for decreased tone, acute edema, acute pain, or decreased sensory or less than 10 degrees of active shoulder movement in any plane. Use with caution and never for long-term use.
  ▶ Splints/orthotic devices
    o Static: No information identified.
    o Dynamic: Dynamic wrist hand orthosis that positions the wrist and hand functionally and assists with finger/thumb extension may enable participation in repetitive task-oriented activities. Example: SaeboReach or SaeboFlex orthoses (Andriske et al., 2017).
  ▶ Work simplification: Eliminate or modify method of performing task. Example: Wear loafers or sandals rather than shoes with shoelaces.

- Sensory
  - ▸ Pain management for shoulder (see also Pain and Chronic Pain in Section 2: Sensory Disorders).
    - ○ Sling: Support weight of arm while allowing elbow to straighten; do not use slings that hold elbow and forearm close to body, which promotes stiffness.
    - ○ Mental practice: Rehearse a physical activity by memory without body movement.
    - ○ Practice a given task that requires shoulder movement.
  - ▸ Sensory stimulation (see Stroke: Hemiplegia in Section 3: Nervous System Disorders)
  - ▸ Visual (see Visual Impairments Due to Neurologic Conditions in Section 2: Sensory Disorders)
    - ○ Determine whether client wears glasses and if glasses are being worn during rehabilitation sessions.
    - ○ Consider whether enlarged print or magnifying glass may be useful.
    - ○ If menus are used in facility, check for visual field neglect and have menu read to client or double-checked.

Cognitive/Perceptual

- Cognitive therapy
  - ▸ Backward chaining: The last step in a sequence is taught or retaught first, then the second to last is added, then the third to last is added, and so forth until all steps in sequence are learned; finally, the sequence is started at the beginning.
  - ▸ Cues: Verbal (live or recorded), nonverbal (metronome), gestures (live or pictures), or physical (guided, scaffolding) can be used to assist client to perform a specific activity or task.
- Mental imagery: Approach is usually done immediately before or after practicing actual movements of the affected upper extremity. Client is instructed to imagine all of the steps of a successful function activity. Before starting mental imagery, therapist should be sure affected upper extremity is placed in the correct position for the start of the movement that is to be imagined. Written or recorded instruction describing the activity to be imagined should be included for a home program. Example: Reach for a towel and dry the other arm with it.
- Executive functions (see Executive Dysfunction in Section 11: Cognitive-Perceptual Disorders).
- Perceptual training (see Unilateral Spatial Neglect in Section 11: Cognitive-Perceptual Disorders).

Psychosocial

- Depression management (also see Depression and Depressive Disorders in Section 12: Mental and Behavioral Disorders)
  - ▸ Monitor for signs of depression and continue to assess.
  - ▸ Use occupations, tasks, and activities familiar to and valued by client.
  - ▸ Maintain a routine schedule familiar to the client.
- Impulsive behavior
  - ▸ Monitor environment for personal and caregiver safety to avoid injury.
  - ▸ Encourage client to "take a deep breath" before taking action.
  - ▸ Discuss with client situations that have been shown to result in impulsive actions.
  - ▸ Ignore impulsive behavior unless it is unsafe.
- Aggressive behavior
  - ▸ Remain calm, speak directly to client using soothing words (a gentle touch and playing soft music in background might help).
  - ▸ Avoid arguing with client; listen and try to understand what is triggering the behavior and make adjustments accordingly.
  - ▸ Keep environment orderly and avoid distractions as much as possible.
  - ▸ Try to redirect response to acceptable behavior that involves physical activity (taking deep breaths, going for a walk, taking a bath or shower, doing a routine and familiar task such as sorting or putting objects away).

▸ Back away keeping a safe distance if aggressive behavior is directed toward therapist.

▸ Get help from other staff if client is in danger of harming self or others.

- Frustration tolerance
  ▸ Simplify task into easier-to-do steps or fewer steps if possible.
  ▸ Allow more time; encourage client to take as much time as needed; do not rush.
  ▸ Change to a different occupation (redirect attention) if client becomes too frustrated.
  ▸ Maintain schedule as much as possible and explain in advance if changes are needed.
  ▸ Use occupations the client already knows how to do before engaging in unfamiliar occupations.
  ▸ Explain new occupation each time before starting, do not expect client to remember.

Context/Environment

- Compensatory
  ▸ Environmental adaption (home safety assessment, home and community accessibility).
  ▸ Home and work modification (ergonomics, energy conservation, and work simplification principles).
- Educational
  ▸ Client education (falls prevention, wheelchair maintenance, dysphagia, home safety).
  ▸ Caregiver education (stress management, coping skills).
  ▸ Staff education (safe transfers, visual impairments).
- Equipment
  ▸ Adaptive equipment (self-help devices, household electronics; sources, training in correct use, and maintenance).
  ▸ Mobility management (wheelchair, scooter, walker, cane; sources, training in correct use, and maintenance).

Precautions/Safety Considerations

- Cardiac conditions: Hypertension, coronary artery disease, and congestive heart failure may continue to be factors for consideration in any intervention strategy.
- Dysphagia: Choking is a factor in any eating or drinking activity; working with a speech–language pathologist should be considered (see Swallowing Disorders: Adult in Section 3: Nervous System Disorders).
- Falls: Monitoring for falls is a factor (see Falls in Section 13: Lifestyle Conditions).
- Home safety: Arrange for a home safety check if possible; use of phone video may be useful.
- Joint contractures: Positioning in bed to avoid knee contractures (no pillows under knees).
- Pressure sores: Bed mobility should be facilitated and maintained (see Pressure Ulcers in Section 10: Skin Disorders).
- Slings: Never use for long-term solution; never leave a client with a sling unattended in a bed or sitting position.
- Transfers: Excessive traction should be avoided during assisted movements, such as transfers; protect and support affected arm during wheelchair use by using a hemi-tray or arm trough.

Prognosis and Outcome

Variable. Hospitals with higher use of occupational therapy had lower adjusted readmission rates (Burke et al., 2014). There is no specific recommendation related to therapy intensity during inpatient rehabilitation (Foley et al., 2012).

Cost Effectiveness

- England: Cost effectiveness of predischarge occupational therapy home visits was found to be slightly more effective than a hospital interview (Sampson et al., 2014).

- Japan: In terms of quality adjusted life years (QALYs), the intervention group was significantly higher than the control group (p = .001, difference 95% confidence interval [CI]), and total costs were not statistically different. The probability of an occupation-based approach being cost effective was estimated to be 65.3% (Nagayama et al., 2017).

REFERENCES

Abdullah, H. A., Tarry, C., Lambert, C., Barreca, S., & Allen, B. O. (2011). Results of clinicians using a therapeutic robotic system in an inpatient stroke rehabilitation unit. *Journal of NeuroEngineering and Rehabilitation, 8*, Article 50. https://doi.org/10.1186/1743-0003-8-50

Andriske, L., Verikios, D., & Hitch, D. (2017). Patient and therapist experiences of the Saebo-Flex: A pilot study. *Occupational Therapy International, 2017*, Article 5462078. https://doi.org/10.1155/2017/5462078

Bell, A., & Muller, M. (2013). Effects of Kinesio Tape to reduce hand edema in acute stroke. *Topics in Stroke Rehabilitation, 20*(3), 283–288. https://doi.org/10.1310/tsr2003-283

Breisinger, T. P., Skidmore, E. R., Niyonkuru, C., Terhorst, L., & Campbell, G. B. (2014). The Stroke Assessment of Fall Risk (SAFR): Predictive validity in inpatient stroke rehabilitation. *Clinical Rehabilitation, 28*(12), 1218–1224. https://doi.org/10.1177/0269215514534276

Burke, J. F., Skolarus, L. E., Adelman, E. E., Reeves, M. J., & Brown, D. L. (2014). Influence of hospital-level practices on readmission after ischemic stroke. *Neurology, 82*(24), 2196–2204. https://doi.org/10.1212/WNL.0000000000000514

Celinder, D., & Peoples, H. (2012). Stroke patients' experiences with Wii Sports during inpatient rehabilitation. *Scandinavian Journal of Occupational Therapy, 19*(5), 457–463. https://doi.org/10.3109/11038128.2012.655307

Chen, A., & Eng, J. Y. (2015). Use of the Australian Therapy Outcome Measures for Occupational Therapy (AusTOMs-OT) in an early supported discharge programme for stroke patients in Singapore. *British Journal of Occupational Therapy, 78*(9), 570–575. https://doi.org/10.1177/0308022614562582

Drummond, A. E. R., Whitehead, P., Fellows, K., Sprigg, N. Sampson, C. J., Edwards, C., & Lincoln, N. B. (2013). Occupational therapy predischarge home visits for patients with a stroke (HOVIS): Results of a feasibility randomized controlled trial. *Clinical Rehabilitation, 27*(5), 387–397. https://doi.org/10.1177/0269215512462145

Edmiaston, J., Connor, L. T., Loehr, L., & Nassief, A. (2010). Validation of a dysphagia screening tool in acute stroke patients. *American Journal of Critical Care, 19*(4), 357–364. https://doi.org/10.4037/ajcc2009961

Edmiaston, J., Connor, L. T., Steger-May, K., & Ford, A. L. O. (2014). A simple bedside stroke dysphagia screen, validated against videofluoroscopy, detects dysphagia and aspiration with high sensitivity. *Journal of Stroke and Cerebrovascular Diseases, 23*(4), 712–716. https://doi.org/10.1016/j.jstrokecerebrovasdis.2013.06.030

Foley, N., Pereira, S., Salter, K., Meyer, M., McClure, J. A., & Teasell, R. (2012). Are recommendations regarding inpatient therapy intensity following acute stroke really evidence-based? *Topics in Stroke Rehabilitation, 19*(2), 96–103. https://doi.org/10.1310/tsr1902-96

Guidetti, S., & Ytterberg, C. (2011). A randomised controlled trial of a client-centred self-care intervention after stroke: A longitudinal pilot study. *Disability and Rehabilitation, 33*(6), 494–503. https://doi.org/10.3109/09638288.2010.498553

Hayner, K. A. (2012). Effectiveness of the California tri-pull taping method for shoulder subluxation poststroke: A single-subject ABA design. *American Journal of Occupational Therapy, 66*(6), 727–736. https://doi.org/10.5014/ajot.2012.004663

Imam, B., & Jarus, T. (2014). Virtual reality rehabilitation from social cognitive and motor learning theoretical perspectives in stroke population. *Rehabilitation Research and Practice, 2014*, Article 594540. https://doi.org/10.1155/2014/594540

Iwamoto, Y., Imura, T., Suzukawa, T., Fukuyama, H., Ishii, T., Taki, S., Imada, N., Shibukawa, M., Inagawa, T., Araki, H., & Araki, O. (2019). Combination of exoskeletal upper limb robot and occupational therapy improve activities of daily living function in acute stroke patients. *Journal of Stroke and Cerebrovascular Diseases, 28*(7), 2018–2025. https://doi.org/10.1016/j.jstrokecerebrovasdis.2019.03.006

Jaywant, A., Toglia, J., Gunning, F. M., & O'Dell, M. W. (2019). The diagnostic accuracy of the Montreal Cognitive Assessment in inpatient stroke rehabilitation. *Neuropsychological Rehabilitation, 29*(8), 1163–1176. https://doi.org/10.1080/09602011.2017.1372297

Krumlinde-Sundholm, L., Lindkvist, B., Plantin, J., & Hoare, B. (2019). Development of the assisting hand assessment for adults following stroke: A Rasch-built bimanual performance measure. *Disability and Rehabilitation, 41*(4), 472–480. https://doi.org/10.1080/09638288.2017.1396365

Langhorne, P., Bernhardt, J., & Kwakkel, G. (2011). Stroke rehabilitation. *Lancet, 377*(9778), 1693–1702. https://doi.org/10.1016/S0140-6736(11)60325-5

Lee, Y.-C., Chen, S.-S., Koh, C.-L., Hsueh, I.-P., Yao, K.-P., & Hsieh, C.-L. (2014). Development of two Barthel Index-based supplementary scales for patients with stroke. *PLOS ONE, 9*(10), Article e110494. https://doi.org/10.1371/journal.pone.0110494

Lee, Y.-C. Yu, W.-H., Hsueh, I.-P., Chen, S.-S., & Hsieh, C.-L. (2017). Test-retest reliability and responsiveness of the Barthel Index-based Supplementary Scales in patients with stroke. *European Journal of Physical and Rehabilitation Medicine, 53*(5), 710–718. https://doi.org/10.23736/S1973-9087.17.04454-9

Lin, G.-H., Lu, Y., Wu, C.-T., Chiu, E.-C., Huang, S.-L. Hsueh, I.-P., & Hsieh, C.-L. (2016). Psychometric properties of the Five-Digit Test in patients with stroke. *Disability and Rehabilitation, 38*(1), 97–102. https://doi.org/10.3109/09638288.2015.1031288

Mew, M. (2010). Normal movement and functional approaches to rehabilitate lower limb dressing following stroke: A pilot randomised controlled trial. *British Journal of Occupational Therapy, 73*(2), 64–70. https://doi.org/10.4276/030802210X12658062793807

Miller, E. L., Murray, L., Richards, L., Zorowitz, R. D., Bakas, T., Clark, P., & Billinger, S. A. (2010). Comprehensive overview of nursing and interdisciplinary rehabilitation care of the stroke patient: A scientific statement from the American Heart Association. *Stroke, 41*(10), 2402–2448. https://doi.org/10.1161/STR.0b013e3181e7512b

Mödden, C., Behrens, M., Damke, I., Eilers, N., Kastrup, A., & Hildebrandt, H. (2012). A randomized controlled trial comparing 2 interventions for visual field loss with standard occupational therapy during inpatient stroke rehabilitation. *Neurorehabilitation and Neural Repair, 26*(5), 463–469. https://doi.org/10.1177/1545968311425927

Mountain, A. D., Kirby, R. L., Eskes, G. A., Smith, C., Duncan, H., MacLeod, D. A., & Thompson, K. (2010). Ability of people with stroke to learn powered wheelchair skills: A pilot study. *Archives of Physical Medicine and Rehabilitation, 91*(4), 596–601. https://doi.org/10.1016/j.apmr.2009.12.011

Murdolo, Y., Brown, T., Fielding, L., Elliott, S., & Castles, E. (2017). Stroke survivors' experiences of using the Graded Repetitive Arm Supplementary Program (GRASP) in an Australian acute hospital setting: A mixed-methods pilot study. *Australian Occupational Therapy Journal, 64*(4), 305–313. https://doi.org/10.1111/1440-1630.12363

Nagayama, H., Tomori, K., Ohno, K., Takahashi, K., Nagatani, R., Izumi, R., Moriwaki, K., & Yamauchi, K. (2017). Cost effectiveness of the occupation-based approach for subacute stroke patients: Result of a randomized controlled trial. *Topics in Stroke Rehabilitation, 24*(5), 337–344. https://doi.org/10.1080/10749357.2017.1289686

Nir-Hadad, S. Y., Weiss, P. L., Waizman, A., Schwartz, N., & Kizony, R. (2017). A virtual shopping task for the assessment of executive functions: Validity for people with stroke. *Neuropsychological Rehabilitation, 27*(5), 808–833. https://doi.org/10.1080/09602011.2015.1109523

Porter, R. S. (Ed.). (2018). *The Merck manual of diagnosis and therapy* (20th ed.). Merck Sharp & Dohme.

Razemba, F., Jacobs, L., & Franzsen, D. (2017). Convergent validity of the Occupational Therapy Adult Perceptual Screening Test (OT-APST) with to other cognitive-perceptual tools in a South African context. *South African Journal of Occupational Therapy, 47*(2), 3–10. https://doi.org/10.17159/2310-3833/2017/v47n2a2

Ryan, P. A., Sullivan, J. W., & Gillen, G. (2016). Activities of daily living adaptations: Managing the environment with one-handed techniques. In G. Gillen (Ed.), *Stroke rehabilitation: A function-based approach* (4th ed., pp. 136–154). Mosby.

Sampson, C., James, M., Whitehead, P., & Drummond, A. E. R. (2014). An introduction to economic evaluation in occupational therapy: Cost-effectiveness of pre-discharge home visits after stroke (HOVIS). *British Journal of Occupational Therapy, 77*(7), 330–335. https://doi.org/10.4276/030802214X14044755581664

Schneider, E. J., Ada, L., & Lannin, N. A. (2019). Extra upper limb practice after stroke: A feasibility study. *Pilot and Feasibility Studies, 5*, Article 156. https://doi.org/10.1186/s40814-019-0531-5

Schriner, M., & Zigler Delahunt, J. (2017). Cerebrovascular accident. In B. J. Atchison & D. P. Dirette (Eds.), *Conditions in occupational therapy* (5th ed., pp. 291–327). Wolters Kluwer.

Seitz, R. J., & Carey, L. M. (2013). Neurorehabilitation after stroke. *European Medical Journal Neurology, 1*(1), 38–45. https://www.emjreviews.com/neurology/article/neurorehabilitation-after-stroke/

Semenko, B., Thalman, L., Ewer, E., Delorme, R., Hui, S., Flett, H., & Lavoie, N. (2015). *An evidence based occupational therapy toolkit for assessment and treatment of the upper extremity post stroke.* Winnipeg Regional Health Authority. https://professionals.wrha.mb.ca/old/professionals/occupational-therapy/files/Stroke-UEToolkit.pdf

Shinohara, K., Yamada, T., Kobayashi, N., & Forsyth, K. (2012). The Model of Human Occupation-based intervention for patients with stroke: A randomized trial. *Hong Kong Journal of Occupational Therapy, 22*(2), 60–69. https://doi.org/10.1016/j.hkjot.2012.09.001

Skidmore, E. R., Butters, M., Whyte, E., Grattan, E., Shen, J., & Terhorst, L. (2017). Guided training relative to direct skill training for individuals with cognitive impairments after stroke: A pilot randomized trial. *Archives of Physical Medicine and Rehabilitation, 98*(4), 673–680. https://doi.org/10.1016/j.apmr.2016.10.004

Skidmore, E. R., Dawson, D. R., Butters, M. A., Grattan, E. S., Juengst, S. B., Whyte, E. M., Begley, A., Holm, M. B., & Becker, J. T. (2015). Strategy training shows promise for addressing disability in the first 6 months after stroke. *Neurorehabilitation and Neural Repair, 29*(7), 668–676. https://doi.org/10.1177/1545968314562113

Skidmore, E. R., Dawson, D. R., Whyte, E. M., Butters, M. A., Dew M. A., Grattan, E. S., Becker, J. T., & Holm, M. B. (2014). Developing complex interventions: Lessons learned from a pilot study examining strategy training in acute stroke rehabilitation. *Clinical Rehabilitation, 28*(4), 378–387. https://doi.org/10.1177/0269215513502799

Skidmore, E. R., Holm, M. B., Whyte, E. M., Dew, M. A., Dawson, D., & Becker, J. T. (2011). The feasibility of meta-cognitive strategy training in acute inpatient stroke rehabilitation: Case report. *Neuropsychological Rehabilitation, 21*(2), 208–223. https://doi.org/ 10.1080/09602011.2011.552559

Toglia, J., Askin, G., Gerber, L. M., Taub, M. C. Mastrogiovanni, A. R., & O'Dell, M. W. (2017). Association between 2 measures of cognitive instrumental activities of daily living and their relation to the Montreal Cognitive Assessment in persons with stroke. *Archives of Physical Medicine and Rehabilitation, 98*(11), 2280–2287. https://doi.org/10.1016/j.apmr.2017.04.007

Toglia, J., Fitzgerald, K. A., O'Dell, M. W., Mastrogiovanni, A. R., & Lin, C. D. (2011). The Mini-Mental State Examination and Montreal Cognitive Assessment in persons with mild subacute stroke: Relationship to functional outcome. *Archives of Physical Medicine and Rehabilitation, 92*(5), 792–798. https://doi.org/10.1016/j.apmr.2010.12.034

Tomori, K., Nagayama, H., Ohno, K., Nagatani, R., Saito, Y., Takahashi, K., Sawada, T., & Higashi, T. (2015). Comparison of occupation-based and impairment-based occupational therapy for subacute stroke: A randomized controlled feasibility study. *Clinical Rehabilitation, 29*(8), 752–762. https://doi.org/10.1177/0269215514555876

University of British Columbia. (2011). *GRASP: Graded repetitive arm supplementary program: Exercise manual: Level 1.*

University of British Columbia. (2016). *GRASP: Graded repetitive arm supplementary program: Instructor's manual for Hospital GRASP and Home GRASP version 2.* https://neurorehab.med.ubc.ca/files/2016/08/GRASP-Instructor-Manual-Ver2.pdf

Walker, M. F., Sunderland, A., Fletcher-Smith, J., Drummond, A., Logan, P., Edmans, J. A., Garvey, K., Dineen, R. A., Ince, P., Horne, J., Fisher, R. J., & Taylor, J. L. (2012). The DRESS trial: A feasibility randomized controlled trial of a neuropsychological approach to dressing therapy for stroke inpatients. *Clinical Rehabilitation, 26*(8), 675–685. https://doi.org/10.1177/0269215511431089

BIBLIOGRAPHY

Arya, K. N. (2018). Evolution of motor therapies in stroke rehabilitation: An eternal path. *Neurology India, 66*(5), 1303–1305. https://doi.org/10.4103/0028-3886.241379

Barrett, M., Snow, J. C., Kirkland, M. C., Kelly, L. P., Gehue, M., Downer, M. B., McCarthy, J., & Ploughman, M. (2018). Excessive sedentary time during in-patient stroke rehabilitation. *Topics in Stroke Rehabilitation, 25*(5), 366–374. https://doi.org/10.1080/10749357.2018.1458461

Bartels, M. N., Duffy, C. A., & Beland, H. E. (2016). Pathophysiology, medical management, and acute rehabilitation of stroke survivors. In G. Gillen (Ed.), *Stroke rehabilitation: A function-based approach* (4th ed., pp. 2–45). Elsevier.

Cahill, L. S., Carey, L. M., Lannin, N. A., Turville, M., & O'Connor, D. (2017). Implementation interventions to promote the uptake of evidence-based practices in stroke rehabilitation. *Cochrane Database of Systematic Reviews, 3*, Article CD012575. https://doi.org/10.1002/14651858.CD012575

Fujita, T., Iokawa, K., Sone, T., Yamane, K., Yamamoto, Y., Ohira, Y., & Otsuki, K. (2019). Effects of the interaction among motor functions on self-care in individuals with stroke. *Journal of Stroke and Cerebrovascular Diseases, 28*(11), Article 104387. https://doi.org/10.1016/j.jstrokecerebrovasdis.2019.104387

Gillen, G. (Ed.). (2011). *Stroke rehabilitation: A function-based approach* (3rd ed.). Mosby.

Gillen, G. (Ed.). (2016). *Stroke rehabilitation: A function-based approach* (4th ed.). Mosby.

Gillen, G. (2018). Cerebrovascular accident. In H. M. Pendleton & W. Schultz-Krohn (Eds.), *Pedretti's occupational therapy* (8th ed., pp. 809–840). Elsevier.

Guidetti, S., Andersson, K., Andersson, M., Tham, K., & Von Koch, L. (2010). Client-centred self-care intervention after stroke: A feasibility study. *Scandinavian Journal of Occupational Therapy, 17*(4), 276–285. https://doi.org/10.3109/11038120903281169

Gustafsson, L., & Bootle, K. (2013). Client and carer experience of transition home from inpatient stroke rehabilitation. *Disability and Rehabilitation, 35*(16), 1380–1386. https://doi.org/10.3109/09638288.2012.740134

Hanby, J. R. (2019). The nervous system: Cerebrovascular accident. In H. Smith-Gabai & S. E. Holm (Eds.), *Occupational therapy in acute care* (2nd ed., pp. 309–316). AOTA Press.

Harvey, L. A., Katalinic, O. M., Herbert, R. D., Moseley, A. M., Lannin, N. A., & Schurr, K. (2017). Stretch for the treatment and prevention of contracture: An abridged republication of a Cochrane Systematic Review. *Journal of Physiotherapy, 63*(2), 67–75. https://doi.org/10.1016/j.jphys.2017.02.014

Horn, S. D., Deutscher, D., Smout, R. J., DeJong, G., & Putman, K. (2010). Black–white differences in patient characteristics, treatments, and outcomes in inpatient stroke rehabilitation. *Archives of Physical Medicine and Rehabilitation, 91*(11), 1712–1721. https://doi.org/10.1016/j.apmr.2010.04.013

Hsieh, C. H., Putman, K., Nichols, D., McGinty, M. E., DeJong, G., Smout, R. J., & Horn, S. (2010). Physical and occupational therapy in inpatient stroke rehabilitation: The contribution of therapy extenders. *American Journal of Physical Medicine & Rehabilitation, 89*(11), 887–898. https://doi.org/10.1097/PHM.0b013e3181f70fb1

Jaywant, A., Toglia, J., Gunning, F. M., & O'Dell, M. W. (2018). The clinical utility of a 30-minute neuropsychological assessment battery in inpatient stroke rehabilitation. *Journal of the Neurological Sciences, 390*, 54–62. https://doi.org/10.1016/j.jns.2018.04.012

Levack, W. M. M., Dean, S. G., Siegert, R. J., & McPherson, K. M. (2011). Navigating patient-centered goal setting in inpatient stroke rehabilitation: How clinicians control the process to meet perceived professional responsibilities. *Patient Education and Counseling, 84*(2), 206–213. https://doi.org/10.1016/j.pec.2011.01.011

Miller-Scott, C. (2016). Stroke rehab enriched by technology. *Rehab Management, 29*(2), 20–22.

Morrison, M. T., Edwards, D. F., & Giles, G. M. (2015). Performance-based testing in mild stroke: Identification of unmet opportunity for occupational therapy. *American Journal of Occupational Therapy, 69*(1), Article 6901360010. https://doi.org/10.5014/ajot.2015.011528

O'Toole, M. T. (Ed.). (2017). *Mosby's Dictionary of medicine, nursing & health professions* (10th ed.). Elsevier.

Rapolienè, J., Endzelytè, E., Jasevičienè, I., & Savickas, R. (2018). Stroke patients motivation influence on the effectiveness of occupational therapy. *Rehabilitation Research and Practice, 2018*, Article 9367942. https://doi.org/10.1155/2018/9367942

Sasaki, T., Kitajima, H., Kanaya, K., Sugama, K., & Sengoku, Y. (2010). A preliminary study on the usability of head mount display (HMD) for evaluating attentional behavioral disturbance. *Asian Journal of Occupational Therapy, 8*(1), 21–29. https://doi.org/10.11596/asiajot.8.21

Schiavi, M., Costi, S., Pellegrini, M., Formisano, D., Borghi, S., & Fugazzaro, S. (2018). Occupational therapy for complex inpatients with stroke: Identification of occupational needs in post-acute rehabilitation setting. *Disability and Rehabilitation, 40*(9), 1026–1032. https://doi.org/10.1080/09638288.2017.1283449

Skidmore, E. R., Whyte, E. M., Holm, M. B., Becker, J. T., Butters, M. A., Dew, M. A., Munin, M. C., & Lenze, E. J. (2010). Cognitive and affective predictors of rehabilitation participation after stroke. *Archives of Physical Medicine and Rehabilitation, 91*(2), 203–207. https://doi.org/10.1016/j.apmr.2009.10.026

Skolarus, L. E., Feng, C., & Burke, J. F. (2017). No racial difference in rehabilitation therapy across all post-acute care settings in the year following a stroke. *Stroke, 48*(12), 3329–3335. https://doi.org/10.1161/STROKEAHA.117.017290

Vratsistas-Curto, A., Sherrington, C., & McCluskey, A. (2021). Dosage and predictors of arm practice during inpatient stroke rehabilitation: An inception cohort study. *Disability and Rehabilitation, 43*(5), 640–647. https://doi.org/10.1080/09638288.2019.1635215

Wolf, T. J., Barbee, A. R., & White, D. (2011). Executive dysfunction immediately after mild stroke. *OTJR: Occupation, Participation and Health, 31*(Suppl. 1), S23–S29. https://doi.org/10.3928/15394492-20101108-05

Wolf, T. J., & Birkemeier, R. (2011). Intervention to increase performance and participation following stroke. In C. H. Christiansen & K. M. Matuska (Eds.), *Ways of living* (4th ed., pp. 281–298). AOTA Press.

Woodson, A. M. (2014). Stroke. In M. V. Radomski & C. A. Trombly Latham (Eds.), *Occupational therapy for physical dysfunction* (7th ed., pp. 999–1041). Wolters Kluwer.

Stroke: Chronic

Also called poststroke. Person may be also called a stroke survivor.

Description

The working definition of poststroke varies in the literature from the time period following acute hospital discharge at 5–7 days following the stroke to the period of time at or greater than 6 months since the original stroke occurred. Stroke as a chronic condition causes loss of control over a person's body and may result in motor and cognitive sequelae, changes in functional capacity, and loss of valued activities, meaningful skills, and social roles (Caro & Cruz, 2017; Engel-Yeger et al., 2018; Miller et al., 2010). This chapter includes studies and reports that concentrate on the time period following acute, inpatient, hospitalized care to whenever clients were studied poststroke.

Cause
Residual or long-term effects of the stroke.

Evaluation/Assessment
Areas
- Activities of Daily Living/Instrumental ADL: basic ADLs (eating, dressing, bathing/showering, toileting, grooming, shaving, sexual function); independent living (meal preparation, housekeeping, home and yard maintenance and repair, shopping, driving, public transportation, transfers, finances); health management (medications, nutritional management, physical activity)
- Education/Work: work tasks (paid, unpaid), work accommodations
- Play/Leisure: interests, values, frequency, location
- Rest/Sleep: sleep disturbances
- Social Participation: type, location, frequency, with whom
- Sensorimotor: muscle strength, muscle tone, joint range of motion, joint mobility, posture and postural coordination, endurance, hand functions (grip, grasp, dexterity, two-hand coordination, in-hand manipulation), sensation and sensibility (tactile, stereognosis, touch pressure, temperature), edema, pain, visual impairment
- Cognitive/Perceptual: attention, memory, executive function (especially problem solving), functional cognition, unilateral spatial neglect
- Psychosocial: depression, anxiety, motivation, irritability, aggression, frustration tolerance, role performance, interpersonal relations, quality of life, self-efficacy
- Context/Environment: social support, adapted equipment, community resources
- Comorbidities: diabetes, hypertension, hemiplegia, dementia

Instruments
Instruments Developed by Occupational Therapy Personnel
- Arnadottir OT-ADL Neurobehavioral Evaluation (A-ONE; Arnadottir, 1990)
- Assessment of Motor and Process Skills (8th ed.; AMPS-8; Fisher & Bray Jones, 2016)
- Box and Block Test (BBT; Holser & Fuchs, 1957; norms in Mathiowetz, Volland, et al., 1985)
- Canadian Occupational Performance Measure (5th ed.; COPM-5; Law et al., 2014)
- Catherine Bergego Scale (CBS; see Kessler Foundation Neglect Assessment Process)
- Community Integration Measure (CIM; McColl et al., 2001)
- Functional Tactile Object Recognition Test (fTORT; Carey et al., 2006; see also Carey et al., 2020, in References)
- Kessler Foundation Neglect Assessment Process (KF-NAP; Chen et al., 2015)
- Leisure Interest Checklist (LIC; Gillen, 2016; adapted from Interest Checklist, Matsutsuyu, 1969)
- Nine Hole Peg Test (9HPT; Kellor et al., 1971; norms in Mathiowetz et al., 1985)
- Occupational Questionnaire (OQ; Smith et al., 1986)
- Participation Strategies Self-Efficacy Scale (PS-SES; D. Lee et al., 2018, in References)
- Performance Quality Rating Scale (PQRS; Martini et al., 2015)
- Reintegration to Normal Living Index (RNLI; Wood-Dauphinee et al., 1988)
- Weekly Calendar Planning Activity (WCPA; Toglia, 2015)

Instruments Developed by Other Professionals and Used by Occupational Therapy Personnel
(Note: See Bushnell et al., 2015, in References, for review of instruments.)

- Action Research Arm Test (ARAT; Lyle, 1981)
- Arm Motor Ability Test (AMAT; Kopp et al., 1997)
- Barthel Index (BI; Mahoney & Barthel, 1965)
- Behavioral Inattention Test (BIT; Wilson et al., 1987)
- Berg Balance Scale (BBS; Berg et al., 1989)
- Birmingham Cognitive Screen (BCoS; Bickerton et al., 2012; see Bisiker & Bickerton, 2013, in References)
- Brunnstrom Recovery Stages (BRS; see Stroke: Hemiplegia in Section 3: Nervous System Disorders)
- Chedoke Arm and Hand Activity Inventory (CAHAI; Barreca et al., 2004)
- Chedoke-McMaster Stroke Assessment (CMSA; Gowland et al., 1993)
- Client Satisfaction Questionnaire-8 (CSQ-8; Attkisson & Greenfield, 1994)
- Diadochokinesis: Have client alternate between supination and pronation arm movements (palm up, palm down) while supporting arm on thigh or other hand. Record number of repetitions in 10 seconds.
- Finger-to-Nose Test (FNT; Swaine et al., 2005): Have client move index finger from nose to therapist's index finger (placed an arm's length away from client). Record number of repetitions in 10 seconds.
- Flanker Inhibitory Control & Attention Test (FICA; Slotkin et al., 2012)
- Frenchay Activities Index (FAI; Holbrook & Skilbeck, 1983)
- Fugl-Meyer Assessment (FMA) Upper Extremity (FM-UE) and Lower Extremity (FM-LE) Scales (Fugl-Meyer et al., 1975)
- Functional Ambulation Category (FAC; Martin & Cameron, 1996)
- Functional Independence Measure (FIM; Uniform Data System for Medical Rehabilitation, 1997)
- Functional Reach Test (FRT; Duncan et al., 1990)
- Functional Test Battery (FTB; Sabini et al., 2013, in References)
- General Activity Motivation Measure (GAMM; Caro et al., 2005)
- General Health Questionnaire (GHQ; Goldberg & Williams, 1988)
- Goal Attainment Scaling (GAS; Kiresuk et al., 1968; Kiresuk et al., 1994)
- Grip strength (dynamometer; JAMAR, Lafayette Instrument)
- Intrinsic Motivation Inventory (IMI; Ryan et al., 1990)
- Jebsen-Taylor Hand Function Test (JTHFT; Jebsen et al., 1969)
- Leisure Competence Measure (LCM; Kloseck & Crilly, 1997; Kloseck et al., 1996)
- Leisure Diagnostic Battery (LDB; Ellis et al., 2008)
- Leisure Satisfaction Measure (LSM; Ragheb & Beard, 1991)
- Life Space Questionnaire (LSQ; Stalvey et al., 1999)
- Manual Muscle Test (MMT; Kaskutas, 2018)
- McGill Pain Questionnaire (MPQ; Melzack, 1975)
- Mini-Mental State Examination (MMSE; Folstein et al., 1975)
- Modified Ashworth Scale (MAS; Bohannon & Smith, 1987)
- Modified Barthel Index (MBI; Shah et al., 1989)
- Modified Rivermead Mobility Index (MRMI; Tsang et al., 2014)
- Montreal Cognitive Assessment (MoCA; Nasreddine et al., 2005)
- Motor Activity Log (MAL; Taub, 2011)
- Motor Assessment Scale (MAS; Carr et al., 1985)
- Multidimensional Health Locus of Control (MHLC) Scales (Wallston et al., 1978)
- National Institutes of Health (NIH) Stroke Scale (NIHSS; Brott et al., 1989)

- NeuroFlexor (measure botulinum toxin A; Gäverth et al., 2014; and Gäverth et al., 2013, in References)
- NIH Toolbox Dimensional Card Sort Test (NIH Toolbox; Weintraub et al., 2013)
- Nottingham Sensory Assessment–Revised (NSA-R; Lincoln et al., 1998)
- Patient Health Questionnaire-9 (PHQ-9; Kroenke et al., 2001)
- Patient-Reported Outcomes Measurement Information System (PROMIS; Hahn et al., 2014)
- Pittsburgh Sleep Quality Index (PSQI; Buysse et al., 1989)
- Quality of Life in Neurological Disorders (Version 2.0; Neuro-QoL-2.0; National Institute of Neurological Disorders and Stroke, 2015)
- Rankin Scale, modified (mRS; Bonita & Beaglehole, 1988)
- Rivermead Mobility Index (RMI; Collen et al., 1991)
- Rivermead Visual Gait Assessment (RVGA; Lord et al., 1998)
- Semmes-Weinstein Monofilaments (SWMs; Patterson Medical, commercial test instruments)
- Stroke Adapted Sickness Impact Profile-30 (SA-SIP30; van Straten et al., 1997)
- Stroke Impact Scale (Version 3.0; SIS-3; Duncan et al., 2003)
- Stroke Rehabilitation Assessment of Movement (STREAM; Daley et al., 1999)
- Stroke Specific Quality of Life Scale (SS-QOL; Williams et al., 1999)
- Virtual Peg Insertion Test (VPIT; Fluet et al., 2011; see also Tobler-Ammann et al., 2016, in References)
- Visual Analogue Scale (VAS) Numeric Pain Rating Scale (NPRS; pain scale; 0 = *no pain*, 10 = *worst pain ever*)
- Wolf Motor Function Test (WMFT; Wolf et al., 1989)
- World Health Organization Quality of Life–BREF (WHOQOL-BREF; The WHOQOL Group, 1998)
- World Health Organization Well-Being Index (WHO-5; The WHOQOL Group, 1998)

Problems/Issues

Activities of Daily Living/Instrumental ADL
- Person usually has difficulty performing basic ADLs such as eating, dressing and undressing, bathing/showering, brushing teeth, toileting, grooming, shaving, medication management including side effects, functional communication and mobility, safe transfers.
- Person usually has difficulty performing instrumental ADLs such as meal preparation, housekeeping, doing laundry, home and yard maintenance and repair, money management (paying bills, budgeting, loss of income), shopping for groceries and supplies, driving, using public transportation, sexual functions, child care and pet care.

Education/Work
- Person may limit or retire from paid or unpaid work due to issues related to chronic stroke such as mobility, communication, and hand function.

Play/Leisure
- Person may reduce or quit engaging in favorite leisure occupations due to problems such as difficulty with mobility, communication, and hand function.
- Person may experience loss of interest in favorite leisure occupations.

Rest/Sleep
- Person may experience sleep disturbance due to pain or difficulty with bed mobility.

Social Participation
- Person may stop or limit participation in social activities due to factors related to chronic stroke, such as mobility, communication, or hand function.

Sensorimotor

- Person may have difficulty with shoulder–elbow coordination, such as reaching and retrieving a dish on a shelf or wiping up spilled liquid.
- Person may have difficulty performing movements that require supination and pronation, such picking up a raisin from a dish and putting in the mouth.
- Person may have difficulty with three-finger grasp and object manipulation, such as picking up a pen and writing his or her name.
- Person may have difficulty with visuomotor coordination and proprioception, such as touch nose with finger (eyes open and closed).
- Person may have difficulty with stereognosis, such as identifying coins with eyes closed.
- Person may have difficulty using index finger (digit two) to dial a number on a phone or individually use fingers to touch type on a keyboard.
- Person may have difficulty with bilateral asymmetry, such as putting on a coat or cutting meat.
- Person may have difficulty with bilateral coordination, such as holding a dinner tray with both hands.
- Person may have difficulty with bilateral dexterity, such as tying shoelaces or buttoning a coat.

Cognitive/Perceptual

- Person may have difficulty with attention and concentration.
- Person may have difficulty with memory functions, especially working memory.
- Person may have difficulty with executive functions, such as problem solving, planning ahead, time management, and judgment of safety.
- Person may have difficulty with visuomotor coordination.
- Person may experience unilateral spatial neglect.

Psychosocial

- Person may become depressed or despondent.
- Person may express anxiety, fear, or apprehension about doing certain occupations, such as going up and down stairs or going outdoors for fear of falling.
- Person may become irritable and aggressive.
- Person may experience emotional lability alternating between sad and happy states.
- Person may experience increased stress and decreased coping skills.
- Person may experience loss of motivation or increased sense of apathy.
- Person may express feelings of hopelessness and helplessness.
- Person may experience loss of role performance.
- Person may experience decreased sense of self-efficacy, self-esteem, and self-worth.
- Person may experience decreased quality of life and life satisfaction.
- Person may experience increased thoughts of suicide.

Context/Environment

- Person may need information and training in use of adapted devices and equipment.
- Person may need information and resources about home modification to increase safety and accessibility.
- Person, family, and caregivers may need information about management of poststroke problems and issues.
- Person, family, and caregivers may need information about community and internet resources, such as local support groups.

Intervention/Treatment

Models and programs developed by occupational therapy personnel include activity tips (American Occupational Therapy Association, 2013), client-centered therapy (J.-H. Park, 2018), coaching (Kessler et al., 2017, 2018), Cognitive Orientation to daily Occupational Performance (CO-OP; McEwen et al., 2010), dialogue-based intervention (Hjelle et al., 2019), dressing task-specific practice (Christie et al., 2011), Improving Participation after Stroke Self-Management Program (IPASS; Wolf et al., 2016), interactive metronome (Yu et al., 2017), lifestyle redesign (Ng et al., 2013), lifestyle groups (Lund et al., 2018), neurofunctional treatment program (Rotenberg-Shpigelman et al., 2012), practice guidelines (Wolf & Nilsen, 2015), sensory retraining (Doyle et al., 2013; Pumpa et al., 2015; Turville et al., 2017; Turville et al., 2018), task-oriented approach (Almhdawi et al., 2016; Hsieh et al., 2017; Rowe & Neville, 2019), and time-use intervention (J.-H. Park, 2019b).

Models and programs developed by other professionals but used by occupational therapy personnel include bilateral arm training (Lin et al., 2010; Sethy et al., 2018; Stoykov & Stinear, 2010; Wu et al., 2011); biofeedback functional electrical stimulation (J. H. Kim & Lee, 2015); cognitive behavioral therapy (Kneebone et al., 2010); Community Participation Transition After Stroke (COMPASS; Stark et al., 2018); constraint-induced movement therapy (C.-S. Hung, Hsieh, et al., 2019; C.-S. Hung, Lin, et al., 2019; Sethy et al., 2016; Takebayashi et al., 2015; Wu et al., 2011); dual task training (Mishra, 2015; J.-H. Park, 2019a); electromyogram-triggered neuromuscular stimulation (EGM-stim; S.-H. Kim et al., 2016); fatigue (Eskes et al., 2015; Flinn & Stube, 2010); home exercise program (Kara & Ntsiea, 2015; Simpson et al., 2017); interactive metronome (Hill et al., 2011; Yu et al., 2017); interlimb coupling (Arya et al., 2020); Lee Silverman Voice Treatment (LSVT BIG; Metcalfe et al., 2019; requires certification—originally designed for Parkinson's disease); mental practice (Ali Hosseini et al., 2012; Cha et al., 2012; Nilsen et al., 2010; Page et al., 2011); mirror therapy (Arya & Pandian, 2013; G. K. N. Hung et al., 2015; J. H. Kim & Lee, 2015; Lin et al., 2014; J.-Y. Park et al., 2015; Y. Park et al., 2015; Wu, Huang, et al., 2013); motor training (Pandian et al., 2014); Modified Constraint-Induced Movement Therapy (Baldwin et al., 2018); myoelectric orthosis (Dunaway et al., 2017; McCabe et al., 2019; Nijenhuis et al., 2017); Neuro-15 program (low-frequency repetitive transcranial magnetic stimulation & OT; Yamane et al., 2018); neurofunctional treatment (Rotenberg-Shpigelman et al., 2012); photovoice (Maratos et al., 2016); return to work (Mohapatra & Mokashi, 2010); robotic-assisted therapy (Hsieh et al., 2017; C.-S. Hung, Lin, et al., 2019; Liao et al., 2012; Linder et al., 2013; Wu, Yang, et al., 2013; Wu et al., 2012; Yang et al., 2012); stroke guidelines—mobility (McCluskey et al., 2015); stroke guidelines—mood cognition, fatigue (Lanctôt et al., 2020); stroke guidelines—psychological care (Gillham & Clark, 2011); taping/Kinesio Taping (Hayner, 2012; D.-H. Lee et al., 2015); task-specific training (Birkenmeier et al., 2010; Page et al., 2011); telerehabilitation (Linder et al., 2013); transfer training (Pavol et al., 2018); videogame group intervention (Rand et al., 2018); virtual reality (Boone et al., 2019; Saposnik et al., 2010); and yoga (Atler et al., 2017; Schmid et al., 2012).

Team members include physicians, nursing personnel, neuropsychologists, physical therapists, speech–language pathologists, social workers, vocational rehabilitation counselors, orthotists–prosthetists, recreational therapy personnel, and occupational therapy personnel. Goals are to focus on those occupations that maintain or improve a client's health and well-being (Chae & Chang, 2016). The goal of occupational therapy is to address the physical, cognitive, and emotional challenges brought on by the stroke and to help stroke survivors engage in the occupations they want and need to do (American Occupational Therapy Association, 2013). The goal is to improve the ability to carry out activities of daily living (Legg et al., 2017).

Activities of Daily Living/Instrumental ADL

- Assist person to manage dressing tasks (dressing upper body, lower body), tying a tie, putting on jewelry (consider two hands, one handed, with assistance of someone else).
- Assist person with cutting food (consider two handed or use of adapted device such as a rocker knife).
- Assist person with bathing/showering (consider safely getting in and out, and use of adapted devices such as a tub bench or handheld shower).
- Assist person with meal preparation (consider alternate cooking equipment [microwave, slow cooker], adapted equipment [one-handed cutting board, enlarged handles on cooking utensils,

electric can opener], or rearranging kitchen for safety and ease of retrieving frequently used items).

- Assist client with homemaking chores (making beds, doing laundry, cleaning bathrooms, washing floors; consider scheduling, pacing work and rest breaks, using carts for supplies, hiring a housekeeper, keeping duplicate supplies to prevent having to carry).
- Assist with using telephone or smartphone (consider larger dial for telephone and programming frequently used numbers on smartphone).
- Assist with shopping (consider consolidating trips, organizing list by grocery store aisle, using a delivery service).
- Assist with using computer programs, keyboarding, and internet.
- Assist with check writing (consider a check template or automatic bill paying).
- Assist with watering plants (consider using a long-stemmed watering can or changing water schedule so only a few plants are watered at one time).
- Assist client with outdoor mobility (consider ramps, railings, and outdoor lighting).
- Assist client in renewing driver's license or using alternate transportation.
- Assist client with child care or pet care functions to improve performance, including sharing responsibilities with other family members or caregivers.
- Discuss with client whether sexual dysfunction is an issue and provide resources.

Education/Work

- Discuss with client options for paid or unpaid work, such as shorter schedules, different work tasks, application of energy conservation and work simplification principles, economically designed tools and workstation, alternate transportation arrangements.

Play/Leisure

- Assist client to engage in favorite leisure occupations by reducing barriers and improving access based on physical limitations.
- Games may be used to practice cognitive and motor coordination skills.
- Assist client to explore new leisure occupations if past leisure occupations must be discontinued or are no longer of interest.

Rest/Sleep

- Discuss with client sleep habits and problems with sleeping (see also Sleep–Wake Disorders in Section 13: Lifestyle Conditions).

Social Participation

- Assist client to participate in social activities such as visiting with family and friends (consider whether type of activity needs modification, such as length of time of visit or location at home versus going to someone's home).
- Assist client to participate in social events such as going to movies, concerts, or sporting events (consider transportation needs, both wheeled and walking, stair climbing, sitting for long periods of time).

Sensorimotor (Semenko et al., 2015)

- Constraint-induced movement therapy (CIMT), modified and hybrid.
  - ▶ Objective: Work toward active movement of the involved extremity and hand.
  - ▶ Technique: Restrain unimpaired limb in a glove or mitt for a period of time each day (up to 6 hours) for as long as 2 weeks, forcing use of impaired hand and arm to perform everyday activities with the involved hand and perform specific activities during rehabilitation session. Person must have some active movement in involved hand for the technique to be useful. A signed contract of agreement between client/family and therapist regarding amount of time in glove/mitt and type of activities performed is useful.
- Dual-task training
  - ▶ Objective: Client is engaged in two motor tasks at the same time.

▶ Technique: Client uses upper extremities to engage in a fine motor task requiring eye–hand coordination or coordination plus cognition while sitting on an unstable surface requiring balance reactions. Upper extremities tasks included moving beans with a spoon and opening bottle caps. Cognitive motor task required classifying wooden blocks by color and grouping them together (J.-H. Park, 2019a, 2019b).

- Electromyogram-triggered neuromuscular stimulation (EMG-stim)
  ▶ Objective: Used in conjunction with task-oriented training.
  ▶ Technique: Applied to affected arm muscle(s) for 30 minutes per day, 5 days per week, for 4 weeks. Client must have some voluntary muscle contraction (S.-H. Kim et al., 2016).
- Edema management (see also Lymphedema in Section 9: Immunologic and Infection Diseases)
  ▶ Objective: Control and reduce swelling.
  ▶ Technique: Encourage active, active-assisted, and passive movement. Consider use of retrograde massage, use of compression techniques, and use of custom or prefabricated splint. Educate regarding positioning and elevation.
- Functional dynamic orthoses (SaeboFlex or SaeboReach)
  ▶ Objective: Work toward active and passive movement required for functional activity (positioning wrist and hand for grasp, and especially for use of finger and thumb extension to release objects).
  ▶ Technique: Use orthosis with goal of two 45-minute sessions per day, followed by functional activities without orthosis.
- Functional electrical stimulation (FES)
  ▶ Objective: Increase wrist extension or prevent shoulder subluxation.
  ▶ Technique: Target wrist extensor and forearm muscles while engaged in task specific activities. Example: When muscle stimulation is on, work on straightening wrist and pushing into standing position. Target shoulder girdle while engaged in shoulder shrugs when muscle stimulation is on.
- Interlimb coupling (lower extremity coordination)
  ▶ Objective: Address primary function of lower limbs—coordination as opposed to focusing attention primarily on affected limb only.
  ▶ Technique: Intervention (three sessions of 1 hour each per week) composed of activities requiring coordinated, alternate, and rhythmic use of both lower extremity limbs together.
- Joint positioning
  ▶ Objective: Prevent stretching, dislocation, or subluxation of joint structures causing additional injury or dysfunction by using proper body positioning.
  ▶ Technique: (1) Educate carers (family and staff) regarding handling and joint protection when sitting, lying, mobilizing, or transferring; (2) use splints, taping, or slings to maintain proper body positioning (illustrations and list of positioning devices available in Semenko et al., 2015).
- Mirror therapy
  ▶ Objective: Use of visual feedback about motor performance to improve functional skills.
  ▶ Technique: Client places affected hand and forearm inside the mirror box with the unaffected hand and forearm in front to mirror. Client is directed to perform a movement with the unaffected hand and simultaneously attempt to copy the movement with the hidden affected hand. Client should be looking at the image in the mirror while attempting to move the affected hand. Example: Direct client to "Make a fist and then open your hand fully. Attempt to copy movement with involved hand." Repeat 15 times.
- Motor retraining
  ▶ Objective: Provide equal amounts of retraining to both sides (ipsilateral and contralateral).
  ▶ Technique: Progressive resistive exercises and bimanual activities such as arm cycling, rowing, and postural transition (Pandian et al., 2014).
- Range of motion
  ▶ Objective: Maintain or improve joint movement.

▸ Technique: Use active movement, both bilateral and unilateral, in positions where gravity is reduced to those against gravity. Use passive movement with caution and do not use pulleys, which may result in stretching or injury to joint structures especially in shoulder.

- Sensory stimulation and retraining: tactile perception exploration (Ahn et al., 2016)
  ▸ Objective: Protect from injury, especially skin, and facilitate regaining effective use of sensory system.
  ▸ Technique: Educate client and caregivers about purpose of sensation, safety concerns, and upper extremity protection. Modify environment for safety, such as changing water temperature in bath/shower. Introduce various textures and sensations to involved hand and arm (e.g., washcloth, rice, macaroni, mixed cereals). Use different weights, sizes, and shapes of objects to promote discrimination. Use vision as a compensatory strategy, and then occlude vision relying on stereognosis by hiding objects in rice, macaroni, or sack and asking client to locate and name objects without using vision.

- Spasticity management
  ▸ Objective: Decrease pain and dysfunction due to spasticity.
  ▸ Techniques: Botox injections may be useful when combined with strengthening antagonist muscles postinjection. Serial splinting has been used.

- Strength training
  ▸ Objective: Maintain or improve muscle strength and endurance.
  ▸ Technique: Use strength training (progressive resistive exercises) throughout available range of motion. Focus on use of naturally occurring activities (carrying, lifting, moving, reaching, weight shifting). Mobile arm supports may be useful in early stage. Do not use pulleys during acute recovery, and carefully monitor any use of pulleys in postrecovery or chronic stage to avoid injury.

- Task-specific training
  ▸ Objective: Achieve ability to perform functional, goal-oriented activities.
  ▸ Technique: Select task(s) that are simple but challenging enough for the client to do that encourage problem solving. Increase the number of repetitions of the movement(s), amount of time, and intensity. The optimal number of repetitions is unknown, but Birkenmeier et al. (2010) suggested that within 1 hour, three different tasks can be repeated 100 times each. Examples: eating finger foods, position involved hand from thigh to table and back.

- Transfer training (three-word stand-pivot technique; Pavol et al., 2018)
  ▸ Objective: Safety transfer from or to bed, chair, toilet, or wheelchair.
  ▸ Technique: (1) Position client's feet on floor. (2) Position client's hand(s) on chair arms or rails. (3) Say "STAND"; provide cues (nonverbal) and physical assistance as needed. (4) Say "TURN"; position hands as needed, provide cues (nonverbal) and physical assist as needed, repeat command as needed. (5) Say "SIT"; position hands as needed, provide cues (nonverbal) and physical assistance as needed.

Cognitive/Perceptual

- Mental practice/imagery
  ▸ Objective: Uses mental imagery to practice functional and useful everyday activities.
  ▸ Technique: Used most frequently as homework with written or oral instructions. Start with simple one item instructions and increase complexity as client improves. Examples: Imagine picking up a pen and positioning it in the hand for writing; imagine reaching for a towel with the involved hand and drying the other arm with it; using the involved hand, imagine wiping a counter with a towel; imagine throwing a ball with the involved arm.

- Procedural memory: Use behaviorally (sensorimotor) learned responses that do not rely (or rely less) on language or conscious awareness. Examples: Smelling coffee brewing may move client toward breakfast area; hearing running water may help move client to bathroom for bath or shower.

- Problem-solving situations: Encourage client to participate in solving problems experienced by client in everyday living (functional tasks).
- Unilateral spatial neglect (see Unilateral Spatial Neglect in Section 11: Cognitive-Perceptual Disorders).
- Virtual reality

Psychosocial
- Encourage client to set achievable goals to improve motivation.
- Discuss with client feelings of depression and anxiety.
- Discuss with client and family possible modifications in role performance.

Context/Environment
- Adapted equipment: Provide information, resources, instructions for use and care.
- Community resource: Explore with client community activities and events that may be of interest.
- Personal assistance: Discuss with client if personal attendant may be helpful.

Precautions/Safety Considerations

- Monitor environment to prevent falls (slippery, wet surface; rugs, uneven surface).
- Monitor for tingling in the thumb and fingers if wrist is splinted to avoid median nerve compression.
- Monitor skin integrity whenever splints, slings, or other devices are used against the skin because touch sensation may be compromised due to the stroke.
- Person is at risk for a second stroke within 1 year if lifestyle risks or physiologic risks are present:
  - ▶ Lifestyle: obesity, lack of balanced diet, smoking, substance abuse, lack of exercise.
  - ▶ Physiologic: diabetes, high blood pressure, poor medication compliance.

Prognosis and Outcome

Outcome is variable. Recovery can continue to occur, but compensatory techniques are usually needed. For outcome measures, see Bushnell et al. (2015).

Cost Effectiveness

Sackley et al. (2016) in United Kingdom found no evidence of improvement in functional activity, mobility, mood, or health related quality of life between residents receiving a targeted course of occupational therapy versus those receiving usual care without therapy.

REFERENCES

Ahn, S.-N., Lee, J.-W., & Hwang, S. (2016). Tactile perception for stroke induce changes in electroencephalography. *Hong Kong Journal of Occupational Therapy, 28*(1), 1–6. https://doi.org/10.1016/j.hkjot.2016.10.001

Ali Hosseini, S., Fallahpour, M., Sayadi, M., Gharib, M., & Haghgoo, H. (2012). The impact of mental practice on stroke patients' postural balance. *Journal of the Neurological Sciences, 322*(1-2), 263–267. https://doi.org/10.1016/j.jns.2012.07.030

Almhdawi, K. A., Mathiowetz, V. G., White, M., & delMas, R. C. (2016). Efficacy of occupational therapy task-oriented approach in upper extremity post-stroke rehabilitation. *Occupational Therapy International, 23*, 444–456. https://doi.org/10.1002/oti.1447

American Occupational Therapy Association. (2013). *Tips for living life to its fullest: Recovering from a stroke.* AOTA Press.

Arya, K. N., & Pandian, S. (2013). Effect of task-based mirror therapy on motor recovery of the upper extremity in chronic stroke patients: A pilot study. *Topics in Stroke Rehabilitation, 20*(3), 210–217. https://doi.org/10.1310/tsr2003-210

Arya, K. N., Pandian, S., Sharma, A., Kumar, V., & Kashyap, V. K. (2020). Interlimb coupling in poststroke rehabilitation: A pilot randomized controlled trial. *Topics in Stroke Rehabilitation, 27*(4), 272–289. https://doi.org/10.1080/10749357.2019.1682368

Atler, K. E., Van Puymbroeck, M., Portz, J. D., & Schmid, A. A. (2017). Participant-perceived outcomes of merging yoga and occupational therapy: Self-management intervention for people post stroke. *British Journal of Occupational Therapy, 80*(5), 294–301. https://doi.org/10.1177/0308022617690536

Baldwin, C. R., Harry, A., Power, L. J., Pope, K. L., & Harding, K. E. (2018). Modified constraint-induced movement therapy is a feasible and potentially useful addition to the Community Rehabilitation tool kit after stroke: A pilot randomised control trial. *Australian Occupational Therapy Journal, 65*(6), 503–511. https://doi.org/10.1111/1440-1630.12488

Birkenmeier, R., Prager, E. M., & Lang, C. E. (2010). Translating animal doses of task-specific training to people with chronic stroke in 1-hour therapy sessions: A proof-of-concept study. *Neurorehabilitation and Neural Repair, 24*(7), 620–635. https://doi.org/10.1177/1545968310361957

Bisiker, J., & Bickerton, W. (2013). Using a comprehensive and standardised cognitive screen to guide cognitive rehabilitation to stroke. *British Journal of Occupational Therapy, 76*(3), 151–156. https://doi.org/10.4276/030802213X13627524435261

Boone, A. E., Wolf, T. J., & Engsberg, J. R. (2019). Combining virtual reality motor rehabilitation with cognitive strategy use in chronic stroke. *American Journal of Occupational Therapy, 73*(4), Article 7304345020. https://doi.org/10.5014/ajot.2019.030130

Bushnell, C., Bettger, J. P., Cockroft, K. M., Cramer, S. C., Edelen, M. O., Hanley, D., Katzan, I. L., Mattke, S., Nilsen, D. M., Piquado, T., Skidmore, E. R., Wing, K., & Yenokyan, G. (2015). Chronic stroke outcome measures for motor function intervention trials: Expert panel recommendations. *Circulation: Cardiovascular Quality and Outcomes, 8*(6, Suppl. 3), S163–S169. https://doi.org/10.1161/CIRCOUTCOMES.115.002098

Carey, L. M., Mak-Yuen, Y. Y. K., & Matyas, T. A. (2020). The Functional Tactile Object Recognition Test: A unidimensional measure with excellent internal consistency for haptic sensing of real objects after stroke. *Frontiers in Neuroscience, 14*, Article 542590. https://doi.org/10.3389/fnins.2020.542590

Caro, C. C., & Cruz, D. M. C. (2017). Correlação entre independência funcional e cognição em homens com AVC [Correlation between cognition and functional independence in male stroke patients]. *Revista de Terapia Ocupacional da Universidade de São Paulo, 28*(2), 173–180. https://doi.org/10.11606/issn.2238-6149.v28i2p173-180

Cha, Y.-J., Yoo, E.-Y., Jung, M.-Y., Park, S.-H., & Park, J.-H. (2012). Effects of functional task training with mental practice in stroke: A meta analysis. *NeuroRehabilitation, 30*(3), 239–246. https://doi.org/10.3233/NRE-2012-0751

Chae, G. S., & Chang, M. (2016). The correlation between occupational performance and well-being in stroke patients. *Journal of Physical Therapy Science, 28*(6), 1712–1715. https://doi.org/10.1589/jpts.28.1712

Christie, L., Bedford, R., & McCluskey, A. (2011). Task-specific practice of dressing tasks in a hospital setting improved dressing performance post-stroke: A feasibility study. *Australian Occupational Therapy Journal, 58*(5), 364–369. https://doi.org/10.1111/j.1440-1630.2011.00945.x

Doyle, S., Bennett, S., & Gustafsson, L. (2013). Occupational therapy for upper limb post-stroke sensory impairments: A survey. *British Journal of Occupational Therapy, 76*(10), 434–442. https://doi.org/10.4276/030802213X13807217284143

Dunaway, S., Dezsi, D. B., Perkins, J., Tran, D., & Naft, J. (2017). Case report on the use of a custom myoelectric elbow-wrist-hand orthosis for the remediation of upper extremity paresis and loss of function in chronic stroke. *Military Medicine, 182*(7), e1963–e1968. https://doi.org/10.7205/MILMED-D-16-00399

Engel-Yeger B., Tse, T., Josman, N., Baum, C., & Carey, L. M. (2018). Scoping review: The trajectory of recovery of participation outcomes following stroke. *Behavioural Neurology, 2018*, Article 5472018. https://doi.org/10.1155/2018/5472018

Eskes, G. A., Lanctôt, K. L., Herrmann, N., Lindsay, P., Bayley, M., Bouvier, L., Dawson, D., Egi, S., Gilchrist, E., Green, T., Gubitz, G., Hill, M. D., Hopper, T., Khan, A., King, A., Kirton, A., Moorhouse, P., Smith, E. E., Green, J., Foley, N., Salter, K., & Swartz, R. H. (2015). Canadian stroke best practice recommendations: Mood, cognition and fatigue following stroke practice guidelines, Update 2015. *International Journal of Stroke, 10*(7), 1130–1140. https://doi.org/10.1111/ijs.12557

Flinn, N. A., & Stube, J. E. (2010). Post-stroke fatigue: Qualitative study of three focus groups. *Occupational Therapy International, 17*(2), 81–91. https://doi.org/10.1002/oti.286

Gäverth, J., Eliasson, A. C., Kullander, K., Borg, J., Lindberg, P. G., & Forssberg, H. (2014). Sensitivity of the NeuroFlexor method to measure change in spasticity after treatment with botulinum toxin A in wrist and finger muscles. *Journal of Rehabilitation Medicine, 46*(7), 629–634. https://doi.org/10.2340/16501977-1824

Gäverth, J., Sandgren, M., Lindberg, P. G., Forssberg, H., & Eliasson, A. C. (2013). Test–retest and inter-rater reliability of a method to measure wrist and finger spasticity. *Journal of Rehabilitation Medicine, 45*(7), 630–636. https://doi.org/10.2340/16501977-1160

Gillham, S., & Clark, L. (2011). *Psychological care after stroke: Improving stroke services for people with cognitive and mood disorders*. National Health Services, NHS Improvement. https://www.nice.org.uk/media/default/sharedlearning/531_strokepsychologicalsupportfinal.pdf

Hayner, K. A. (2012). Effectiveness of the California tri-pull taping method for shoulder subluxation poststroke: A single-subject ABA design. *American Journal of Occupational Therapy, 66*(6), 727–736. https://doi.org/10.5014/ajot.2012.004663

Hill, V., Dunn, L., Dunning, K., & Page, S. J. (2011). A pilot study of rhythm and timing training as a supplement to occupational therapy in stroke rehabilitation. *Topics in Stroke Rehabilitation, 18*(6), 728–737. https://doi.org/10.1310/tsr1806-728

Hjelle, E. G., Bragstad, L. K., Kirkevold, M., Zucknick, M., Bronken, B. A., Martinsen, R., Kvigne, K. J., Kitzmüller, G., Mangset, M., Thommessen, B., & Sveen, U. (2019). Effect of a dialogue-based intervention on psychosocial well-being 6 months after stroke in Norway: A randomized controlled trial. *Journal of Rehabilitation Medicine, 51*(8), 557–565. https://doi.org/10.2340/16501977-2585

Hsieh, Y.-W., Wu, C.-Y., Wang, W.-E., Lin, K.-C., Chang, K.-C., Chen, C.-C., & Liu, C.-T. (2017). Bilateral robotic priming before task-oriented approach in subacute stroke rehabilitation: A pilot randomized controlled trial. *Clinical Rehabilitation, 31*(2), 225–233. https://doi.org/10.1177/0269215516633275

Hung, C.-S., Hsieh, Y.-W., Wu, C.-Y., Chen, Y.-J., Lin, K.-C., Chen, C.-L., Yao, K. G., Liu, C.-T., & Horng, Y.-S. (2019). Hybrid rehabilitation therapies on upper-limb function and goal attainment in chronic stroke. *OTJR: Occupation, Participation and Health, 39*(2), 116–123. https://doi.org/10.1177/1539449218825438

Hung, C.-S., Lin, K.-C., Chang, W.-Y., Huang, W.-C., Chang, Y.-J., Chen, C.-L., Yao, K.-G., & Lee, Y.-Y. (2019). Unilateral vs bilateral hybrid approaches for upper limb rehabilitation in chronic stroke: A randomized controlled trial. *Archives of Physical Medicine and Rehabilitation, 100*(12), 2225–2232. https://doi.org/10.1016/j.apmr.2019.06.021

Hung, G. K. N., Li, C. T. L., Yiu, A. M., & Fong, K. N. K. (2015). Systematic review: Effectiveness of mirror therapy for lower extremity post-stroke. *Hong Kong Journal of Occupational Therapy, 26*(1), 51–59. https://doi.org/10.1016/j.hkjot.2015.12.003

Kara, S., & Ntsiea, M. V. (2015). The effect of a written and pictorial home exercise prescription on adherence for people with stroke. *Hong Kong Journal of Occupational Therapy, 26*(1), 33–41. https://doi.org/10.1016/j.hkjot.2015.12.004

Kessler, D., Egan, M., Dubouloz, C. J., McEwen, S., & Graham, F. P. (2017). Occupational performance coaching for stroke survivors: A pilot randomized controlled trial. *American Journal of Occupational Therapy, 71*(3), Article 7103190020. https://doi.org/10.5014/ajot.2017.024216

Kessler, D., Egan, M. Y., Dubouloz, C. J., McEwen, S., & Graham, F. P. (2018). Occupational performance coaching for stroke survivors (OPC-Stroke): Understanding of mechanisms of actions. *British Journal of Occupational Therapy, 81*(6), 326–337. https://doi.org/10.1177/0308022618756001

Kim, J. H., & Lee, B.-H. (2015). Mirror therapy combined with biofeedback functional electrical stimulation for motor recovery of upper extremities after stroke: A pilot randomized controlled trial. *Occupational Therapy International, 22*(2), 51–60. https://doi.org/10.1002/oti.1384

Kim, S.-H., Park, J.-H., Jung, M.-Y., & Yoo, E.-Y. (2016). Effects of task-oriented training as an added treatment to electromyogram triggered neuromuscular stimulation on upper extremity function in chronic stroke patients. *Occupational Therapy International, 23*(2), 165–174. https://doi.org/10.1002/oti.1421

Kneebone, I., Baker, J., & O'Malley, H. (2010). Screening for depression after stroke. Developing protocols for the occupational therapists. *British Journal of Occupational Therapy, 73*(2), 71–76. https://doi.org/10.4276/030802210X12658062793843

Lanctôt, K. L., Lindsay, M. P., Smith, E. E., Sahlas, D. J., Foley, N., Gubitz, G., Austin, M., Ball, K., Bhogal, S., Blake, T., Herrmann, N., Hogan, D., Khan, A., Longman, S., King, A., Leonard, C., Shoniker, T., Taylor, T., Teed, M., de Jong, A., Mountain, A., Casaubon, L. K., Dowlatshahi, D., & Swartz, R. H. (2020). *Canadian Stroke Best Practice Recommendations: Mood, cognition and fatigue following stroke,* 6th edition update 2019. *International Journal of Stroke, 15*(6), 668–688. https://doi.org/10.1177/1747493019847334

Lee, D., Fogg, L., Baum, C. M., Wolf, T. J., & Hammel, J. (2018). Validation of the Participation Strategies Self-Efficacy Scale (PS-SES). *Disability and Rehabilitation, 40*(1), 110–115. https://doi.org/10.1080/09638288.2016.1242172

Lee, D.-H., Kim, W.-J., Oh, J.-S., & Chang, M. (2015). Taping of the elbow extensor muscle in chronic stroke patients: Comparison between before and after three-dimensional motion analysis. *Journal of Physical Therapy Science, 27*(7), 2101–2103. https://doi.org/10.1589/jpts.27.2101

Legg, L. A., Lewis, S. R., Schofield-Robinson, O. J., Drummond, A., & Langhorne, P. (2017). Occupational therapy for adults with problems in activities of daily living after stroke. *Cochrane Database of Systematic Reviews, 7,* Article CD003585. https://doi.org/10.1002/14651858.CD003585.pub3

Liao, W.-W., Wu, C.-Y., Hsieh, Y.-W., Lin, K.-C., & Chang, W.-Y. (2012). Effects of robot-assisted upper limb rehabilitation on daily function and real-world arm activity in patients with chronic stroke: A randomized controlled trial. *Clinical Rehabilitation, 26*(2), 111–120. https://doi.org/10.1177/0269215511416383

Lin, K.-C., Chen, Y.-A., Chen, C.-L., Wu, C.-Y., & Chang, Y.-F. (2010). The effects of bilateral arm training on motor control and functional performance in chronic stroke: A randomized controlled study. *Neurorehabilitation and Neural Repair, 24*(1), 42–51. https://doi.org/10.1177/1545968309345268

Lin, K.-C., Chen, Y.-T., Huang, P.-C., Wu, C.-Y., Huang, W.-L., Yang, H.-W., Lai, H.-T., & Lu, H.-J. (2014). Effect of mirror therapy combined with somatosensory stimulation on motor recovery and daily function in stroke patients: A pilot study. *Journal of the Formosan Medical Association, 113*(7), 422–428. https://doi.org/10.1016/j.jfma.2012.08.008

Linder, S. M., Reiss, A., Buchanan, S., Sahu, K., Rosenfeldt, A. B., Clark, C., Wolf, S. L., & Alberts, J. L. (2013). Incorporating robotic-assisted telerehabilitation in a home program to improve arm function following stroke. *Journal of Neurologic Physical Therapy, 37*(3), 125–132. https://doi.org/10.1097/NPT.0b013e31829fa808

Lund, A., Melhus, M., & Sveen, U. (2018). Enjoyable company in sharing stroke experiences: Lifestyle groups after stroke. *Scandinavian Journal of Occupational Therapy, 25*(2), 127–135. https://doi.org/10.1080/11038128.2017.1341958

Maratos, M., Huynh, L., Tan, J., Lui, J., & Jarus, T. (2016). Picture this: Exploring the lived experience of high-functioning stroke survivors using photovoice. *Qualitative Health Research, 26*(8), 1055–1066. https://doi.org/10.1177/1049732316648114

McCabe, J. P., Henniger, D., Perkins, J., Skelly, M., Tatsuoka, C., & Pundik, S. (2019). Feasibility and clinical experience of implementing a myoelectric upper limb orthosis in the rehabilitation of chronic stroke patients: A clinical case series report. *PLOS ONE, 14*(4), Article e0215311. https://doi.org/10.1371/journal.pone.0215311

McCluskey, A., Ada, L., Kelly, P. J., Middleton, S., Goodall, S., Grimshaw, J. M., Logan, P., Longworth, M., & Karageorge, A. (2015). Compliance with Australian stroke guideline recommendations for outdoor mobility and transport training by post-inpatient rehabilitation services: An observational cohort study. *BMC Health Services Research, 15*, Article 296. https://doi.org/10.1186/s12913-015-0952-7

McEwen, S. E., Polatajko, H., Huijbregts, M. P., & Ryan, J. D. (2010). Inter-task transfer of meaningful, functional skills following a cognitive-based treatment: Results of three multiple baseline design experiments in adults with chronic stroke. *Neuropsychological Rehabilitation, 20*(4), 541–561. https://doi.org/10.1080/09602011003638194

Metcalfe, V., Egan, M., & Sauvé-Schenk, K. (2019). LSVT BIG in late stroke rehabilitation: A single-case experimental design study. *Canadian Journal of Occupational Therapy, 86*(2), 87–94. https://doi.org/10.1177/0008417419832951

Miller, E. L., Murray, L., Richards, L., Zorowitz, R. D., Bakas, T., Clark, P., & Billinger, S. A. (2010). Comprehensive overview of nursing and interdisciplinary rehabilitation care of the stroke patient: A scientific statement from the American Heart Association. *Stroke, 41*(10), 2402–2448. https://doi.org/10.1161/STR.0b013e3181e7512b

Mishra, N. (2015). Comparison of effects of motor imagery, cognitive and motor dual task training methods on gait and balance of stroke survivors. *Indian Journal of Occupational Therapy, 47*(2), 46–57.

Mohapatra, J., & Mokashi, S. P. (2010). Influence of modified therapeutic work program on return to work abilities in individual with CVA. *Indian Journal of Occupational Therapy, 42*(3), 3–8.

Ng, S. S. W., Chan, D. L., Chan, M. K. L., & Chow, K. K. Y. (2013). Long-term efficacy of occupational lifestyle redesign programme for strokes. *Hong Kong Journal of Occupational Therapy, 23*(2), 46–53. https://doi.org/10.1016/j.hkjot.2013.09.001

Nilsen, D. M., Gillen, G., & Gordon, A. M. (2010). Use of mental practice to improve upper-limb recovery after stroke: A systematic review. *American Journal of Occupational Therapy, 64*, 695–708. https://doi.org/10.5014/ajot.2010.09034

Nijenhuis, S. M., Prange-Lasonder, G. B., Stienen, A. H., Rietman, J. S., & Buurke, J. H. (2017). Effects of training with a passive hand orthosis and games at home in chronic stroke: A pilot randomised controlled trial. *Clinical Rehabilitation, 31*(2), 207–216. https://doi.org/10.1177/0269215516629722

Page, S. J., Murray, C., Hermann, V., & Levine, P. (2011). Retention of motor changes in chronic stroke survivors who were administered mental practice. *Archives of Physical Medicine and Rehabilitation, 92*(11), 1741–1745. https://doi.org/10.1016/j.apmr.2011.06.009

Pandian, S., Arya, K. N., & Kumar, D. (2014). Does motor training of the nonparetic side influences[*] balance and function in chronic stroke? A pilot RCT. *Scientific World Journal, 2014*, Article 769726. https://doi.org/10.1155/2014/769726

Park, J.-H. (2018). The influences of client-centered therapy on the level of performance, the level of satisfaction of activity of daily living, and the quality of life of the chronic stroke patients. *Journal of Physical Therapy Science, 30*(2), 347–350. https://doi.org/10.1589/jpts.30.347

Park, J.-H. (2019a). Dual task training effects on upper extremity function and performance of daily activities of chronic stroke patients. *Osong Public Health and Research Perspectives, 10*(1), 2–5. https://doi.org/10.24171/j.phrp.2019.10.1.02

Park, J.-H. (2019b). The effects of time-use intervention on the quality of life of outpatients with chronic stroke. *Journal of Physical Therapy Science, 31*(1), 36–38. https://doi.org/10.1589/jpts.31.36

---

[*] The published article includes this typo.

Park, J.-Y., Chang, M., Kim, K.-M., & Kim, H.-J. (2015). The effect of mirror therapy on upper-extremity function and activities of daily living in stroke patients. *Journal of Physical Therapy Science, 27*(6), 1681–1683. https://doi.org/10.1589/jpts.27.1681

Park, Y., Chang, M., Kim, K.-M., & An, D.-H. (2015). The effects of mirror therapy with tasks on upper extremity function and self-care in stroke patients. *Journal of Physical Therapy Science, 27*(5), 1499–1501. https://doi.org/10.1589/jpts.27.1499

Pavol, M. A., Bassile, C., Lehman, J. R., Harmon, E., Ferreira, N., Shinn, B., St. James, N., Callender, J., & Stein, J. (2018). Modified Approach to Stroke Rehabilitation (MAStR): Feasibility study of a method to apply procedural memory concepts to transfer training. *Topics in Stroke Rehabilitation, 25*(5), 351–358. https://doi.org/10.1080/10749357.2018.1458462

Pumpa, L. U., Cahill, L. S., & Carey, L. M. (2015). Somatosensory assessment and treatment after stroke: An evidence-practice gap. *Australian Occupational Therapy Journal, 62*(2), 93–104. https://doi.org/10.1111/1440-1630.12170

Rand, D., Givon, N., & Avrech Bar, M. (2018). A video-game group intervention: Experiences and perceptions of adults with chronic stroke and their therapists. *Canadian Journal of Occupational Therapy, 85*(2), 158–168. https://doi.org/10.1177/0008417417733274

Rotenberg-Shpigelman, S., Erez, A. B., Nahaloni, I., & Maeir, A. (2012). Neurofunctional treatment targeting participation among chronic stroke survivors: A pilot randomized controlled study. *Neuropsychological Rehabilitation, 22*(4), 532–549. https://doi.org/10.1080/09602011.2012.665610

Rowe, V. T., & Neville, M. (2019). The feasibility of conducting task-oriented training at home for patients with stroke. *Open Journal of Occupational Therapy, 7*(1), Article 6. https://doi.org/10.15453/2168-6408.1514

Sabini, R. C., Dijkers, M. P. J. M., & Raghavan, P. (2013). Stroke survivors talk while doing: Development of a therapeutic framework for continued rehabilitation of hand function post stroke. *Journal of Hand Therapy, 26*(2), 124–131. https://doi.org/10.1016/j.jht.2012.08.002

Sackley, C. M., Walker, M. F., Burton, C. R., Watkins, C. L., Mant, J., Roalfe, A. K., Wheatley, K., Sheehan, B., Sharp, L., Stant, K. E., Fletcher-Smith, J., Steel, K., Barton, G. R., Irvine, L., & Peryer, G. (2016). An occupational therapy intervention for residents with stroke-related disabilities in UK care homes (OTCH): Cluster randomised controlled trial with economic evaluation. *Health Technology Assessment, 20*(15), 1–138. https://doi.org/10.3310/hta20150

Saposnik, G., Teasell, R., Mamdani, M., Hall, J., McIlroy, W., Cheung, D., Thorpe, K. E., Cohen, L. G., Bayley, M., & the Stroke Outcome Research Canada (SORCan) Working Group. (2010). Effectiveness of virtual reality using Wii gaming technology in stroke rehabilitation: A pilot randomized clinical trial and proof of principle. *Stroke, 41*(7), 1477–1484. https://doi.org/10.1161/STROKEAHA.110.584979

Schmid, A. A., Van Puymbroeck, M., Altenburger, P. A., Schalk, N. L., Dierks, T. A., Miller, K. K., Damush, T. M., Bravata, D. M., & Williams, L. S. (2012). Poststroke balance improves with yoga: A pilot study. *Stroke, 43*(9), 2402–2407. https://doi.org/10.1161/STROKEAHA.112.658211

Semenko, B., Thalman, L., Ewert, E., Delorme, R., Hui, S., Flett, H., & Lavoie, N. (2015). *An evidence based occupational therapy toolkit for assessment and treatment of the upper extremity post stroke.* Winnipeg Regional Health Authority. https://professionals.wrha.mb.ca/old/professionals/occupational-therapy/files/Stroke-UEToolkit.pdf

Sethy, D., Bajpai, P., Kujur, E. S., Mohakud, K., & Sahoo, S. (2016). Effectiveness of modified constraint induced movement therapy and bilateral arm training on upper extremity function after chronic stroke: A comparative study. *Open Journal of Therapy and Rehabilitation, 4*(1), 1–9. https://doi.org/10.4236/ojtr.2016.41001

Sethy, D., Sahoo, S., Kujur, E. S., & Bajpai, P. (2018). Stroke upper extremity rehabilitation: Effect of bilateral arm training. *International Journal of Health & Allied Sciences, 7*(4), 217–221.

Simpson, L. A., Eng, J. J., & Chan, M. (2017). H-GRASP: The feasibility of an upper limb home exercise program monitored by phone for individuals post stroke. *Disability and Rehabilitation, 39*(9), 874–882. https://doi.org/10.3109/09638288.2016.1162853

Stark, S., Keglovits, M., Somerville, E., Hu, Y.-L., Conte, J., & Yan, Y. (2018). Feasibility of a novel intervention to improve participation after stroke. *British Journal of Occupational Therapy, 81*(2), 116–124. https://doi.org/10.1177/0308022617736704

Stoykov, M. E., & Stinear, J. W. (2010). Active-passive bilateral therapy as a priming mechanism for individuals in the subacute phase of post-stroke recovery: A feasibility study. *American Journal of Physical Medicine & Rehabilitation, 89*(11) 873–878. https://doi.org/10.1097/PHM.0b013e3181f1c31c

Takebayashi, T., Amano, S., Hanada, K., Umeji, A., Takahashi, K., Marumoto, K., Kodama, N., Koyama, T., & Domen, K. (2015). A one-year follow-up after modified constraint-induced movement therapy for chronic stroke patients with paretic arm: A prospective case series study. *Topics in Stroke Rehabilitation, 22*(1), 18–25. https://doi.org/10.1179/1074935714Z.0000000028

Tobler-Ammann, B. C., de Bruin, E. D., Fluet, M. C., Lambercy, O., de Bie, R. A., & Knols, R. H. (2016). Concurrent validity and test-retest reliability of the Virtual Peg Insertion Test to quantify upper limb function in patients with chronic stroke. *Journal of NeuroEngineering Rehabilitation, 13*, Article 8. https://doi.org/10.1186/s12984-016-0116-y

Turville, M., Carey, L. M., Matyas, T. A., & Blennerhassett, J. (2017). Change in functional arm use is associated with somatosensory skills after sensory retraining poststroke. *American Journal of Occupational Therapy, 71*(3), Article 7103190070. https://doi.org/10.5014/ajot.2017.024950

Turville, M., Matyas, T. A., Blennerhassett, J. M., & Carey, L. M. (2018). Initial severity of somatosensory impairment influences response to upper limb sensory retraining post-stroke. *NeuroRehabilitation, 43*(4), 413–423. https://doi.org/10.3233/NRE-182439

Wolf, T. J., Baum, C. M., Lee, D., & Hammel, J. (2016). The development of the Improving Participation after Stroke Self-Management Program (IPASS): An exploratory randomized clinical study. *Topics in Stroke Rehabilitation, 23*(4), 284–292. https://doi.org/10.1080/10749357.2016.1155278

Wolf, T. J., & Nilsen, D. M. (2015). *Occupational therapy practice guidelines for adults with stroke.* AOTA Press.

Wu, C.-Y., Chuang, L.-L., Lin, K.-C., Chen, H.-C., & Tsay, P.-K. (2011). Randomized trial of distributed constraint-induced therapy versus bilateral arm training for the rehabilitation of upper-limb motor control and function after stroke. *Neurorehabilitation and Neural Repair, 25*(2), 130–139. https://doi.org/10.1177/1545968310380686

Wu, C.-Y., Huang, P.-C., Chen, Y.-T., Lin, K.-C., & Yang, H.-W. (2013). Effects of mirror therapy on motor and sensory recovery in chronic stroke: A randomized controlled trial. *Archives of Physical Medicine and Rehabilitation, 94*(6), 1023–1030. https://doi.org/10.1016/j.apmr.2013.02.007

Wu, C.-Y., Yang, C.-L., Chen, M.-D., Lin, K.-C., & Wu, L.-L. (2013). Unilateral versus bilateral robot-assisted rehabilitation on arm-trunk control and functions post stroke: A randomized controlled trial. *Journal of NeuroEngineering and Rehabilitation, 10*, Article 35. https://doi.org/10.1186/1743-0003-10-35

Wu, C.-Y., Yang, C.-L., Chuang, L.-L., Lin, K.-C., Chen, H.-C., Chen, M.-D., & Huang, W.-C. (2012). Effect of therapist-based versus robot-assisted bilateral arm training on motor control, functional performance and quality of life after chronic stroke: A clinical trial. *Physical Therapy, 92*(8), 1006–1016. https://doi.org/10.2522/ptj.20110282

Yamane, S., Urushidani, N., Tamashiro, H., Kurushima, T., Abo, M., Okamoto, T., & Hanaoka, H. (2018). The impact of NEURO-15 on performance skills and related factors in activities of daily living in patients in the chronic phase of stroke. *Asian Journal of Occupational Therapy, 14*(1), 43–52. https://doi.org/10.11596/asiajot.14.43

Yang, C.-L., Lin, K.-C., Chen, H.-C., Wu, C.-Y., & Chen, C.-L. (2012). Pilot comparative study of unilateral and bilateral robot-assisted training on upper-extremity performance in patients with stroke. *American Journal of Occupational Therapy, 66*(2), 198–206. https://doi.org/10.5014/ajot.2012.003103

Yu, G. H., Lee, J.-S., Kim, S.-K., & Cha, T.-H. (2017). Effects of interactive metronome training on upper extremity function, ADL and QOL in stroke patients. *NeuroRehabilitation, 41*(1), 161–168. https://doi.org/10.3233/NRE-171468

BIBLIOGRAPHY

Barnsley, L., McCluskey, A., & Middleton, S. (2012). What people say about travelling outdoors after their stroke: A qualitative study. *Australian Occupational Therapy Journal, 59*(1), 71–78. https://doi.org/10.1111/j.1440-1630.2011.00935.x

Burke, J. F., Skolarus, L. E., Adelman, E. E. Reeves, M. J., & Brown, D. L. (2014). Influence of hospital-level practices on readmission after ischemic stroke. *Neurology, 82*(24), 2196–2204. https://doi.org/10.1212/WNL.0000000000000514

Carey, L. M., Matyas, T. A., & Baum, C. (2018). Effects of somatosensory impairment on participation after stroke. *American Journal of Occupational Therapy, 72*(3), Article 7203205100. https://doi.org/10.5014/ajot.2018.025114

Carey L. M., Seitz, R. J., Parsons, M., Levi, C., Farquharson, S., Tournier, J. D., Palmer, S., & Connelly, A. (2013). Beyond the lesion: Neuroimaging foundations for post-stroke recover. *Future Neurology, 8*(5), 507–527. https://doi.org/10.2217/FNL.13.39

Cawood, J., & Visagie, S. (2015). Environmental factors influencing participation of stroke survivors in a Western Cape setting. *African Journal of Disability, 4*(1), Article 198. https://doi.org/10.4102/ajod.v4i1.198

Cawood, J., Visagie, S., & Mji, G. (2016). Impact of post-stroke impairments on activities and participation as experienced by stroke survivors in a Western Cape setting. *South African Journal of Occupational Therapy, 46*(2), 10–15. http://dx.doi.org/10.17159/2310-3833/2016/v46n2a3

Derakhshanrad, S. A., Piven, E. F., & Ghoochani, B. Z. (2017). Adaption to stroke: A nonlinear thinking approach in occupational therapy. *Occupational Therapy in Health Care, 31*(3), 255–269. https://doi.org/10.1080/07380577.2017.1335922

Fletcher-Smith, J., Drummond, A., Sackley, C., Moody, A., & Walker, M. (2014). Occupational therapy for care home residents with stroke: What is routine national practice? *British Journal of Occupational Therapy, 77*(5), 265–273. https://doi.org/10.4276/030802214X13990455043601

Fukuzawa, I., Tokumaru, O., Eshima, N., Bacal, K., Kitano, T., & Yokoi, I. (2018). Re-employment of people with chronic stroke: A single-centre retrospective study. *Australian Occupational Therapy Journal, 65*(6), 598–605. https://doi.org/10.1111/1440-1630.12523

Gillen, G. (Ed.). (2011). *Stroke rehabilitation: A function-based approach* (3rd ed.). Mosby.

Gillen, G. (2015). What is the evidence for the effectiveness of interventions to improve occupational performance after stroke? *American Journal of Occupational Therapy, 69*(1), Article 6901170010. https://doi.org/10.5014/ajot.2015.013409

Gillen, G. (2016). Leisure participation after stroke. In G. Gillen (Ed.), *Stroke rehabilitation: A function-based approach* (4th ed., pp. 296–308). Mosby.

Gillen, G. (Ed.). (2016). *Stroke rehabilitation: A function-based approach* (4th ed.). Mosby.

Hassan, S. A. M., Visagie, S., & Mji, G. (2012). The achievement of community integration and productive activity outcomes by CVA survivors in the Western Cape Metro Health District. *South African Journal of Occupational Therapy, 42*(1), 11–16.

Hildebrand, M. W. (2015). Effectiveness of interventions for adults with psychological or emotional impairment after stroke: An evidence-based review. *American Journal of Occupational Therapy, 69*(1), Article 6901180050. https://doi.org/10.5014/ajot.2015.012054

Hjelle, E. G., Bragstad, L. K., Zucknick, M., Kirkevold, M., Thommessen, B., & Sveen, U. (2019). The General Health Questionnaire-28 (GHQ-28) as an outcome measurement in a randomized controlled trial in a Norwegian stroke population. *BMC Psychology, 7*, Article 18. https://doi.org/10.1186/s40359-019-0293-0

Hogan, C., Fleming, J., Cornwell, P., & Shum, D. (2016). Prospective memory after stroke: A scoping review. *Brain Impairment, 17*(2), 123–142. https://doi.org/10.1017/BrImp.2016.12

Hreha, K., Mulry, C., Gross, M., Jedziniak, T., Gramas, N., Ohevshalom, L., Sheridan, A., Szabo, G., Davison, C., & Barrett, A. M. (2017). Assessing chronic stroke survivors with aphasia sheds light on prevalence of spatial neglect. *Topics in Stroke Rehabilitation, 24*(2), 91–98. https://doi.org/10.1080/10749357.2016.1196906

Ilić, N. V., Dubljanin-Raspopović, E., Nedeljković, U., Tomanović-Vujadinović, S., Milanović, S. D., Petronić-Marković, I., & Ilić, T. V. (2016). Effects of anodal tDCS and occupational therapy on fine motor skill deficits in patients with chronic stroke. *Restorative Neurology & Neuroscience, 34*(6), 935–945. https://doi.org/10.3233/RNN-160668

Johansson, S., Kottorp, A., Lee, K. A., Gay, C. L., & Lerdal, A. (2014). Can the Fatigue Severity Scale 7-item version be used across different patient populations as a generic fatigue measure—A comparative study using a Rasch model approach. *Health and Quality of Life Outcomes, 12*, Article 24. https://doi.org/10.1186/1477-7525-12-24

Kitzmüller, G., Mangset, M., Evju, A. S., Angel, S., Aadal, L., Martinsen, R., Bronken, B. A., Kvigne, K., Bragstad, L. K., Hjelle, E. G., Sveen, U., & Kirkevold, M. (2019). Finding the way forward: The lived experience of people with stroke after participation in a complex psychosocial intervention. *Qualitative Health Research, 29*(12), 1711–1724. https://doi.org/10.1177/1049 732319833366

Kneebone, I., Stone, N., Robertson, S., & Walker-Samuel, N. (2013). Screening for depression after stroke: Occupational therapists' performance to protocols. *Occupational Therapy in Mental Health, 29*(2), 106–113. https://doi.org/10.1080/0164212X.2013.788971

Kniepmann, K. (2012). Female family carers for survivors of stroke: Occupational loss and quality of life. *British Journal of Occupational Therapy, 75*(5), 208–216. https://doi.org/10.4276/ 030802212X13361458480207

Kootker, J. A., Rasquin, S. M. C., Smits, P., Geurts, A. C. van Heugten, C. M., & Fasotti, L. (2015). An augmented cognitive behavioural therapy for treating post-stroke depression: Description of a treatment protocol. *Clinical Rehabilitation, 29*(9), 833–843. https://doi.org/10.1177/02 69215514559987

Lin, K. C., Fu, T., Wu, C. Y., & Hsieh, C. J. (2011). Assessing the Stroke-Specific Quality of Life for outcome measurement in stroke rehabilitation: Minimal detectable change and clinically important difference. *Health and Quality of Life Outcomes, 9*, Article 5. https://doi.org/10.1186/ 1477-7525-9-5

Lund, A., Mangset, M., Wyller, T. B., & Sveen, U. (2015). Occupational transaction after stroke constructed as threat and balance. *Journal of Occupational Science, 22*(2), 146–159. https:// doi.org/10.1080/14427591.2013.770363

Lund, A., Michelet, M., Kjeken, I., Wyller, T. B., & Sveen, U. (2012). Development of a person-centred lifestyle intervention for older adults following a stroke or transient ischaemic attack. *Scandinavian Journal of Occupational Therapy, 19*(2), 140–149. https://doi.org/10.3109/110381 28.2011.603353

Lund, A., Michelet, M., Sandvik, L., Wyller, T., & Sveen, U. (2012). A lifestyle intervention as supplement to a physical activity programme in rehabilitation after stroke: A randomized controlled trial. *Clinical Rehabilitation, 26*(6), 502–512. https://doi.org/10.1177/0269215511 429473

Martinsen, R., Kirkevold, M., & Sveen, U. (2012). Younger stroke survivors' experiences of family life in a long-term perspective: A narrative hermeneutic phenomenological study. *Nursing Research and Practice, 2012*, Article 948791. https://doi.org/10.1155/2012/948791

Martinsen, R., Kirkevold, M., & Sveen, U. (2015). Young and midlife stroke survivors' experiences with the health services and long-term follow-up needs. *Journal of Neuroscience Nursing, 47*(1), 27–35. https://doi.org/10.1097/JNN.0000000000000107

Nicholson, C. (2018). Creating music to facilitate recovery after stroke. *OT News, 26*(7), 34–36.

O'Brien, A. N., & Wolf, T. (2010). Determining work outcomes in mild to moderate stroke survivors. *Work, 36*(4), 441–447. https://doi.org/10.3233/WOR-2010-1047

O'Sullivan, C., & Chard, G. (2010). An exploration of participation in leisure activities post-stroke. *Australian Occupational Therapy Journal, 57*(3), 159–166. https://doi.org/10.1111/j.14 40-1630.2009.00833.x

Park, J. (2019). A study on the sleep quality, pain, and instrumental activities of daily living of outpatients with chronic stroke. *Journal of Physical Therapy Science, 31*(2), 149–152. https:// doi.org/10.1589/jpts.31.149

Park, J. (2019). Effects of the sleep quality of chronic stroke outpatients on patterns of activity performance and quality of life. *Sleep and Hypnosis, 21*(3), 228–232. https://doi.org/10.5350/ Sleep.Hypn.2019.21.0190

Pascoe, M. C., Crewther, S. G., Carey, L. M., & Crewther, D. P. (2011). Inflammation and depression: Why poststroke depression may be the norm and not the exception. *International Journal of Stroke, 6*(2), 128–135. https://doi.org/10.1111/j.1747-4949.2010.00565.x

Plante, M., Demers, L., Swaine, B., & Desrosiers, J. (2010). Association between daily activities following stroke rehabilitation and social role functioning upon return to the community. *Topics in Stroke Rehabilitation, 17*(1), 47–57. https://doi.org/10.1310/tsr1701-47

Poulin, V., Korner-Bitensky, N., Bherer, L., Lussier, M., & Dawson, D. R. (2017). Comparison of two cognitive interventions for adults experiencing executive dysfunction post-stroke: A pilot study. *Disability and Rehabilitation, 39*(1), 1–13. https://doi.org/ 10.3109/09638288.20 15.1123303

Sansonetti, D., & Hoffmann, T. (2013). Cognitive assessment across the continuum of care: The importance of occupational performance-based assessment for individuals post-stroke and traumatic brain injury. *Australian Occupational Therapy Journal, 60*(5), 334–342. https:// doi.org/10.1111/1440-1630.12069

Schiavi, M., Costi, S., Pellegrini, M., Formisano, D., Borghi, S., & Fugazzaro, S. (2018). Occupational therapy for complex inpatients with stroke: Identification of occupational needs in post-acute rehabilitation setting. *Disability and Rehabilitation, 40*(9), 1026–1032. https://doi .org/10.1080/09638288.2017.1283449

Schulz, C. H., Hersch, G. I., Foust, J. L., Wyatt, A. L., Godwin, K. M., Virani, S., & Ostwald, S. K. (2012). Identifying occupational performance barriers of stroke survivors: Utilization of a home assessment. *Physical & Occupational Therapy in Geriatrics, 30*(2), 109–123. https://doi .org/10.3109/02703181.2012.687441

Scott, S. L., & Bondoc, S. (2018). Return to work after stroke: A survey of occupational therapy practice patterns. *Occupational Therapy in Health Care, 32*(3), 195–215. https://doi.org/10.10 80/07380577.2018.1491083

Simpson, E. K., Ramirez, N. M., Branstetter, B., Reed, A., & Lines, E. (2018). Occupational therapy practitioners' perspectives of mental health practices with clients in stroke rehabilitation. *OTJR: Occupation, Participation and Health, 38*(3), 181–189. https://doi.org/10.1177/ 1539449218759627

Skolarus, L. E., Feng, C., & Burke, J. F. (2017). No racial difference in rehabilitation therapy across all post-acute care settings in the year following a stroke. *Stroke, 48*(12), 3329–3335. https://doi.org/10.1161/STROKEAHA.117.017290

Spitzer, J., Tse, T., Baum, C. M., & Carey, L. M. (2011). Mild impairment of cognition impacts on activity participation after stroke in a community-dwelling Australian cohort. *OTJR: Occupation, Participation and Health, 31*(1), S8–S15. https://doi.org/10.3928/15394492-20101108-03

Stewart, C., Subbarayan, S., Paton, P., Gemmell, E., Abraha, I, Myint, P. K., O'Mahony, D., Cruz-Jentoft, A. J., Cherubini, A., & Soiza, R. L. (2018). Non-pharmacological interventions for the improvement of post-stroke activities of daily living and disability amongst older stroke survivors: A systematic review. *PLOS ONE, 13*(10), Article e0204774. https://doi.org/10.1371/ journal.pone.0204774

Terrill, A. L., Schwartz, J. K., & Belagaje, S. R. (2018). Best practices for the interdisciplinary rehabilitation team: A review of mental health issues in mild stroke survivors. *Stroke Research and Treatment, 2018,* Article 6187328. https://doi.org/10.1155/2018/6187328

Tse, T., Yusoff, S. Z. B., Churilov, L., Ma, H., Davis, S., Donnan, G. A., Carey, L. M., & the START research team. (2017). Increased work and social engagement is associated with increased stroke specific quality of life in stroke survivors at 3 months and 12 months post-stroke: A longitudinal study of an Australian stroke cohort. *Topics in Stroke Rehabilitation, 24*(6), 405–414. https://doi.org/10.1080/10749357.2017.1318339

Williams, S., & Murray, C. (2013). The lived experience of older adults' occupational adaptation following a stroke. *Australian Occupational Therapy Journal, 60*(1), 39–47. https://doi.org/10.1111/1440-1630.12004

Wolf, T. J., Chuh, A., Floyd, T., McInnis, K., & Williams, E. (2015). Effectiveness of occupation-based interventions to improve areas of occupation and social participation after stroke: An evidence-based review. *American Journal of Occupational Therapy, 69*(1), Article 6902280060. https://doi.org/10.5014/ajot.2015.012195

Stroke: Hemiplegia

See also Stroke: Acute, Stroke: Chronic, Apraxia, Cognitive Impairment, Dementia, Depression and Depressive Disorders, Executive Dysfunction, Driving Fitness, Driving Cessation and Driving Retirement, Swallowing Disorders: Adult, Unilateral Spatial Neglect, Visual Impairment Due to Neurologic Conditions, Sleep Wake Disorders.

Description

Hemiplegia is defined as paralysis of one side of the body. Hemiparesis is defined as muscular weakness of one side of the body (O'Toole, 2017). This chapter focuses on hemiplegia and hemiparesis occurring as result of a stroke or cerebrovascular accident (CVA). Hemiplegia in cerebral palsy or resulting from brain injury is included in the chapters on cerebral palsy in Section 1: Development Disorders or brain injury in Section 6: Injuries.

Cause

Stroke or cerebrovascular accident (CVA), either ischemic (blockage) or hemorrhage (rupture), involving the anterior circulation (branches of the internal carotid artery) or posterior circulation (branches of the vertebral and basilar arteries; Porter, 2018).

Stages of Recovery for Arm (Originally proposed by Signe Brunnstrom, PT; Adapted from Sabari et al., 2014; Schultz-Krohn & Mclaughlin-Gray, 2018)

- Stage I: Flaccidity—No voluntary movement, muscle tone, or reflex responses are present.
- Stage II: Synergy patterns (flexion and extension) may be observed, spasticity is developing. (Note: Actually eliciting synergy patterns is no longer considered good therapy.)
- Stage III: Voluntary movement is beginning but only within synergy patterns, severe spasticity may be present.
- Stage IV: Spasticity begins to decrease; some voluntary movements are mastered separate from synergy patterns.
- Stage V: Control of isolated voluntary movements increases; dominance of synergy patterns decreases.
- Stage VI: Isolated motor control and joint movement is possible; spasticity is minimal.
- Stage VII: Normal speed and coordination of voluntary motor functions.

Stages of Recovery for Hand (Pandian et al., 2012)

- Stage I: Flaccidity.
- Stage II: Little or no active finger flexion.
- Stage III: Mass grasp, use of hook grasp but no release, no voluntary finger extension, reflex extension of fingers possible.

- Stage IV: Lateral prehension possible with release by thumb movement, semivoluntary finger extension of fingers, range of motion varies.
- Stage V: Palmar prehension for cylindrical and spherical gap, voluntary mass extension of fingers, variable range of motion.
- Stage VI: All prehension type under voluntary control, skills improving, full range of voluntary extension of fingers, individual finger movements present but less accurate than on opposite side.

Evaluation/Assessment

Areas

- Activities of Daily Living/Instrumental ADL: basic ADLs—dressing, eating, toileting, grooming, bathing/showering, functional communication, functional mobility, transfers; independent living—homemaking, meal preparation, shopping, driving
- Education/Work: work tasks, work demands, work accommodations, ergonomics
- Play/Leisure: interests, values, types, frequency
- Rest/Sleep: sleep disturbance
- Social Participation: type, location, frequency, with whom
- Sensorimotor: joint range of motion, balance, postural control, grip and pinch strength, hand functions, object manipulation, pain
- Cognitive/Perceptual: attention, memory, executive function, body awareness, tactile perception, proprioception, somatosensory awareness, ideomotor apraxia
- Psychosocial: depression, anxiety, self-confidence, self-efficacy, quality of life
- Context/Environment: adapted equipment, home modification, community resources, social support
- Comorbidities: diabetes, dementia, cognitive impairment

Instruments

Instruments Developed by Occupational Therapy Personnel

- Box and Block Test (BBT; Mathiowetz et al., 1985)
- Canadian Occupational Performance Measure (5th ed.; COPM-5; Law et al., 2014)
- Hand Function Survey (HFS; Blennerhassett et al., 2008; see also Blennerhassett et al., 2010, in References)
- Manual Ability Measure-16 (MAM-16; Chen et al., 2005)
- Manual Ability Measure-36 (MAM-36; Chen & Bode, 2010)
- Rating of Everyday Arm-use in the Community and Home (REACH) scale (Simpson et al., 2013, in References)
- Upper Extremity Performance Test for the Elderly (TEMPA; Desrosiers et al., 1993)

Instruments Developed by Other Professionals and Used by Occupational Therapy Personnel

- ABILHAND Questionnaire (Penta et al., 2001)
- Action Research Arm Test (ARAT; Lyle, 1981)
- Arm Motor Ability Test (AMAT; Kopp et al., 1997)
- Berg Balance Scale (BBS; Berg et al., 1989)
- Brunnstrom recovery stages (BRS; see Stages of Recovery, above; also see Huang et al., 2016; and Pandian et al., 2012, in References)
- Chedoke Arm and Hand Activity Inventory (CAHAI; Barreca et al., 2004)
- Florida Apraxia Battery–Extended and Revised Sydney (FABERS; Power et al., 2010)
- Fugl-Meyer Assessment (FMA; Fugl-Meyer et al., 1975; see also Page et al., 2012, in References)
- Functional Independence Measure (FIM; Uniform Data System for Medical Rehabilitation, 1997)
- Grip strength (dynamometry; JAMAR, Lafayette Instrument; see also Bertrand et al., 2015, in References)
- Joint range of motion (goniometer; Shurtleff & Kaskutas, 2018)

- Jebsen-Taylor Hand Function Test (JTHFT; Jebsen et al, 1969)
- Modified Barthel Index (MBI; Shah et al., 1989)
- Motor-Free Visual Perception Test (4th ed.; MVPT-4; Colarusso & Hammill, 2015)
- Motor Activity Log (MAL; Taub et al., 2011)
- Motricity Index (MI; Demeurisse et al., 1980; Collin & Wade, 1990)
- NeuroFlexor (instrument; Aggero MedTech AB, Sweden; Gäverth et al., 2014; and Gäverth et al., 2013, in References)
- Wolf Motor Function Test (WMFT; Wolf et al., 1989)

Problems/Issues

Activities of Daily Living/Instrumental ADL

- Person may have difficulty holding and drinking from a glass or cup with involved hand.
- Person may have difficulty holding and using eating utensils to scoop, spear, or cut food.
- Person may have difficulty cutting, peeling, pouring, mixing, or stirring foods.
- Person may have difficulty swallowing certain kinds of foods (see Swallowing Disorders: Adult, this section).
- Person may have difficulty putting toothpaste on a toothbrush and brushing teeth.
- Person may have difficulty putting on and taking off clothes on upper (including gloves) and lower extremities (including shoes and boots).
- Person may have difficulty buttoning buttons, zipping zippers, snapping snaps, fastening a belt or necklace, tying a tie, straightening a collar, or lacing and tying shoelaces.
- Person may have difficulty with medication management including removing or unscrewing bottle caps, reading labels on dosage and scheduling correctly, setting up a timetable to take medication, and swallowing large pills.
- Person may have difficulty with housecleaning tasks that require reaching, opening, pouring, holding, squeezing, wringing out (as in a washcloth), towel drying (as in drying dishes or pans), sweeping, dusting, pushing and pulling a vacuum cleaner.
- Person may have difficulty doing laundry tasks such as sorting and folding clothes, reaching into washing machine, turning knobs, selecting wash cycle, opening laundry detergent box or bottle.
- Person may have difficulty with meal preparation, including opening jars, cans, boxes, or containers; opening refrigerator door or cabinets; reaching and retrieving objects; turning knobs on stove or blender to required setting (Poole et al., 2011).
- Person may have difficulty putting in or taking out paper money from a wallet or pocket, or picking up coins and placing them in a coin purse.
- Person may have difficulty dialing a rotary phone or pushing buttons on touch phone.
- Person may have difficulty writing a check or using a keyboard for online banking.
- Person may have difficulty getting in and out of a vehicle (car, truck, bus, van, train).
- Person may have difficulty with mobility, including turning over in bed, getting up from a bed or chair, changing direction while walking, walking outside, walking on uneven surfaces, climbing up and down stairs.
- Person may have difficulty driving a vehicle, including turning the wheel, depressing gas pedal, changing to brake pedal, staying in proper lane, making left-hand turns, gauging the speed of traffic (see Driving Fitness or Driving Cessation and Driving Retirement in Section 13: Lifestyle Conditions).
- Person may have difficulty speaking clearly (dysarthria) and selecting correct words (expressive aphasia).
- Person may experience difficulty taking care of young children including assisting with dressing, bathing, and toileting; meal management; getting ready for school; providing supervision for safety and behavioral management.
- Person may have difficulty taking care of pet, including fixing meals, putting on and taking off collar and leash, going for walks safely.

Education/Work

- Person may have difficulty getting to and from paid or unpaid work site.
- Person may have difficulty performing tasks at workstation, such as keyboarding, answering calls, opening mail, operating a machine.
- Person may have difficulty performing body movements such as reaching up or down, bending, stooping, moving side to side, changing speed of walking, or climbing stairs or a ladder.
- Person may have difficulty with actions that require carrying, holding, lifting, retrieving, grabbing, placing, swiping, stamping, sorting, punching.

Play/Leisure

- Person may have difficulty turning on television knobs or pushing buttons on remote.
- Person may have difficulty manipulating small items such as pieces of a puzzle or moving game pieces such as checkers or chess.
- Person may have difficulty recalling or following rules of a game due to cognitive impairment (see Cognitive Impairment in Section 11: Cognitive-Perceptual Disorders).

Rest/Sleep

- Person may have difficulty with bed mobility, especially turning over.
- Person may have changes in sleep habits if pain is present.
- Person may experience sleep disturbances (see Sleep–Wake Disorders in Section 13: Lifestyle Conditions).

Social Participation

- Person may have difficulty talking with family and friends due to speech problems (dysarthria, aphasia).
- Person may have difficulty walking long distances, such as walking on a golf course.
- Person may not have the motor coordination to participate in sports activities, such as swinging a racket or club or steering a boat.
- Person may not have the eye–hand coordination to participate in sports where accuracy is required, such as throwing darts or playing table tennis.

Sensorimotor

- Person may have muscle weakness on one side of the body that affects both upper and lower extremity.
- Person may have reduced joint range of motion on one side of the body, especially when compared to other side.
- Person may have reduced endurance and experience fatigue and tiredness.
- Person may present with a flexion synergy (scapular retraction and/or elevation, shoulder abduction and external rotation, elbow flexion, forearm pronation, wrist and finger flexion).
- Person may present with an extension synergy (scapular protraction, shoulder horizontal adduction and internal rotation, elbow extension and forearm pronation; wrist and hand position may vary).
- Person may experience loss of or decreased efficiency and effectiveness of hand functions such as grip, grasp, pinch, dexterity (speed, accuracy), two-hand coordination, in-hand manipulation.
- Person may experience pain, especially in shoulder and hand.
- Person may experience edema, especially in the hand.
- Person may experience loss or impairment in sensory modalities in the affected upper extremity, such as light touch, pressure, proprioception, stereognosis, temperature, discrimination of size, shape, or texture.

Cognitive/Perceptual

- Person may have decreased attention span and concentration.
- Person may have memory loss, especially short term or immediate recall.
- Person may experience reduced executive functioning, especially in problem solving, planning ahead, and time management.

- Person may have unilateral spatial neglect, thus not seeing or reacting to persons or objects on one side of the environment (more commonly the left but can occur to the right; see chapter on Unilateral Spatial Neglect in Section 11: Cognitive-Perceptual Disorders).
- Person may have reduced tactile perception, thus having difficulty feeling and identifying objects by size, shape, or texture, especially in the hand.
- Astereognosis may be present (inability to identify objects by touch or feel alone; e.g., person cannot identify correctly the type of coins in pocket without looking).
- Person may have reduced proprioception and body awareness, thus having difficulty knowing where body parts (most often arm, hand, or leg) are located in space without looking.
- Person may have difficulty with spatial orientation (left sleeve versus right sleeve, inside of garment versus outside of garment, back of garment versus front of garment).
- Person may have difficulty with spatial relations, including inability to perceive midline, leading to sitting postures that are misaligned from vertical.
- Person may have ideomotor apraxia, especially after left hemisphere stroke.

Psychosocial

- Person may become depressed (depression may be part of stroke syndrome and/or related to situation of reduced abilities).
- Person may be anxious about situation of reduced ability.
- Person may be fearful of moving, such as fear of falling.
- Person may experience loss of self-confidence and self-efficacy.
- Person may experience reduced quality of life.

Context/Environment

- Person, family members, and caregivers may be unaware or lack knowledge about available community or internet resources.
- Person may need assistance in obtaining adapted equipment or make better use of existing electronic devices.
- Person may need home modification, such as installing grab bars in tub or shower, adding a handheld showerhead, adding a tub transfer board, adding lighting in hallways, providing sturdy bannisters, adding railings on outside stairs, adding ramps, removing small rugs from walking pathway in house, reducing clutter, providing sturdy chairs with armrests.
- Person may need information and instruction on use of adapted devices such as wheelchairs, scooters, transfer chairs, splints, reachers or grabbers, commode chairs, enlarged-handled eating utensils, long-handled brush and comb, electric can opener, "sticky keys" on keyboard, word-predicting software.

Intervention/Treatment

Models and programs developed by occupational therapy personnel include computer-based rhythm and timing training (Beckelhimer et al., 2011), dual-task training (lower extremities; Mishra, 2015), dual-task training (upper extremities; J. H. Park, 2019), dynamic splinting (Hookstadt et al., 2012), Graded Repetitive Arm Supplementary Program (GRASP; Murdolo et al., 2017), hand edema (Giang et al., 2016), in-home intensive therapy (Poole et al., 2019), meaningful task-specific training (Amini, 2014; Arya et al., 2012), multisensory stimulation (Law et al., 2018), Occupational Therapy Stroke Arm & Hand Treatment Record (OT-STAR; Jarvis et al., 2014), orthotics and splints (Andriske et al., 2017; Hookstadt et al., 2012; Royal College of Occupational Therapists, 2015), SENSe (Study of the Effectiveness of Neurorehabilitation on Sensation; Carey et al., 2016; Carey et al., 2011), tactile exploration (Ahn et al., 2016), taping or Kinesio Taping (Hayner, 2012; D.-H. Lee et al., 2015), and task-specific occupational therapy (Hubbard et al., 2015; Prager et al., 2011; Shirahama et al., 2016).

Models and programs developed by other professionals but used by occupational therapy personnel include bilateral arm training (Hung et al., 2019; Jung et al., 2013; M.-J. Lee et al., 2017; Lin et al., 2010; Sethy et al., 2018; Stoykov & Stinear, 2010; C.-Y. Wu et al., 2010), biofeedback (J. H. Kim & Lee, 2015; Rayegani et al., 2014), botulinum toxin (Yamada et al., 2014), Brunnstrom movement therapy (Huang et al., 2016; Pandian & Arya, 2012; Pandian et al., 2012), cognitive sensory motor training therapy (Chanubol et al., 2012), combined task-oriented training and electromyogram-triggered neuromuscular simulation (S.-H. Kim et al., 2016), compression therapy for edema (Gustafsson et al., 2014), computer-based training (Beckelhimer et al., 2011), constraint-induced movement therapy (Amini, 2014; Earley et al., 2010; Jonasson et al., 2012; Tanabe et al., 2011; C.-Y. Wu et al., 2011; C.-Y. Wu et al., 2010), extra practice (Schneider et al., 2019), functional electrical stimulation (Marquez-Chin et al., 2017), handling skills (Davis, 2012), Home-Graded Repetitive Arm Supplementary Program (H-GRASP; Simpson et al., 2017), horticulture (M.-Y. Kim et al., 2010), interactive metronome (Yu et al., 2017), meaning task-specific training (MTST; Arya et al., 2012), mental practice (Cha et al., 2012; Kho et al., 2014; Nilsen et al., 2010; Page et al., 2011; A. I. Wu et al., 2011), mirror therapy (Arya et al., 2015; Birkenmeier et al., 2010; Cantero-Téllez et al., 2019; J. H. Kim & Lee, 2015; Lin et al., 2014; Paik et al., 2014; J.-Y. Park et al., 2015; Y. Park et al., 2015; Pérez-Cruzado et al., 2017; Samuelkamaleshkumar et al., 2014; Toh & Fong, 2012; C.-Y. Wu, Huang, et al., 2013), Modified Constraint-Induced Movement Therapy (Baldwin et al., 2018; Earley et al., 2010; J.-H. Kim & Chang, 2018; McCall et al., 2011; Sethy et al., 2016), motor relearning/training (Hubbard et al., 2015; Pandian et al., 2014), neuromuscular electrical stimulation (Amini, 2014), Nintendo Wii (Kam et al., 2012; Saposnik et al., 2010), orthotics (Andriske et al., 2017; Royal College of Occupational Therapists, 2015), rhythmic auditory stimulation (J.-R. Kim et al., 2014), robotic or robot-assist therapy (Amini, 2014; Ferreira et al., 2018, Hsieh et al., 2017; M.-J. Lee et al., 2018; Liao et al., 2012; Lu et al., 2011; Pila et al., 2018; Takahashi et al., 2016; Villafañe et al., 2018; C.-Y. Wu, Yang, et al., 2013; C.-Y. Wu et al., 2012; Yang et al., 2012), self-management (Bower et al., 2012), sensorimotor stimulation (Go & Lee, 2016), sensory retraining (Turville et al., 2017; Turville et al., 2018; Umeki et al., 2019), taping/Kinesio Taping (Hayner, 2012), task-oriented training (S.-H. Kim et al., 2016), transcranial stimulation (rTMS; Ilić et al., 2016; Kakuda et al., 2010; Kakuda, Abo, Kobayashi, Momosaki, Yokoi, Fukuda, Ito, & Tominaga, 2011; Kakuda, Abo, Kobayashi, Momosaki, Yokoi, Fukuda, Ito, Tominaga, Umemori, & Kameda, 2011; Kakuda et al., 2012; Kinoshita et al., 2016; Yamada, Kakadu, Kondo, et al., 2013; Yamada, Kakuda, Senoo, et al., 2013), upper limb exercises (Connell et al., 2014), video games (Chen et al., 2015; Kam et al., 2012), virtual reality (Adams et al., 2019; Saposnik et al., 2010; Sin & Lee, 2013; Yin et al., 2014), voice and electromyography-driven actuated (VAEDA) glove (Thielbar et al., 2017), Xbox Kinect (Sin & Lee, 2013), and yoga (Schmid et al., 2012).

Team members include physicians, nursing personnel, social workers, psychologists, rehabilitation engineers, physical therapists, and occupational therapy personnel. Goals include improving the functional performance of the upper extremity and hand, and lower extremity in everyday tasks.

Activities of Daily Living/Instrumental ADL

- Eating: Adaptive devices may be needed (see also Swallowing Disorders, this section, if dysphagia is present).
- Dressing: Adaptive devices may be needed; one-handed techniques may be needed.
- General: Client with right hemisphere damage more likely to need more time to perform motor task. Left hemisphere damage more likely to include cognitive impairment affecting understanding, following instructions, and working memory (Ahn, 2016; Gokhale & Kale, 2015; Poole et al., 2011).

Education/Work

- Work tasks: See General comment above.
- Work modification: Consider if modification of work tasks, workstation, or work environment (including transportation and ambulation) may increase ability to return to work or apply for work.

Play/Leisure

- Identify favorite leisure occupations and assist client to modify, if possible (see General comment under ADL/IADL).
- Explore with client new leisure occupations that can be accomplished within client's functional limitations.

Rest/Sleep

- Identify issues in sleeping and assist client to modify, such as changing location of bed in room, using different bedding (such as silk sheets and pajamas to make rolling over easier), providing a bedside commode, getting an electric bed that assists with sitting up, providing an easy-to-reach bedside light.

Social Participation

- See General comment under ADL/IADL.
- Encourage client to participate in social activities (changes can be suggested, such as shorter time periods, less crowded venues, most accessible venues, passive versus active venues, more familiar places).

Sensorimotor

- Compensatory strategies
  - ► Assistive technology
    - ○ Rationale: Assistive devices and equipment can compensate for lost or damaged motor functions and improve occupational performance.
    - ○ Technique: Devices and equipment should be selected or recommended based on individual need; cognitive function should be considered before devices or equipment are issued or purchased.
  - ► Contextual training
    - ○ Rationale: Tasks should be practiced in the environment or context in which they are normally performed to maximize learning and performance.
    - ○ Technique: Training involves practicing a task in the specific environment or context until the task is learned or becomes habitual.
  - ► Neurofunctional approach
    - ○ Rationale: Clients with severe cognitive deficits can be taught habit-based performance with little or no expectation of generalization to novel situations that may occur in everyday life.
    - ○ Technique: Therapist selects habits to be acquired based on the client's living situation and provides practice until each habit is established; usually, person must live in a supervised environment because individual cannot generalize behavior to new or novel situations.
  - ► One-handed techniques
    - ○ Rationale: A person can learn to function using one-handed approach and some environmental adaptations (devices and equipment).
    - ○ Technique: Therapist focuses on helping client to use the nonaffected extremity as the dominant hand and the affected or involved hand as an assist when possible; assistive devices may be added when useful.
  - ► Taping (Kinesio Taping)
    - ○ Rationale: Relieve shoulder pain and subluxation.
    - ○ Technique: Three pieces of tape are applied to the client's shoulder on top of self-adhesive cotton tape. The first (medial) is "applied from 1.5 in. below the deltoid tuberosity running straight up the middle of the arm to 2 in. above the top of the glenoid fossa between the clavicle and the spine of the scapula" (Hayner, 2012, p. 731). Second piece (posterior) is placed "1.5 in. below the deltoid tuberosity to 1.5 in. above the middle of the spine of the scapula" (Hayner, 2012, p. 731). Third piece (anterior) is placed "1.5

in. below the deltoid tuberosity to . . . front of the humeral head and over the coracoid process, up to 1.5 in. above the clavicle" (Hayner, 2012, p. 731). Tape removed and replaced 3 times per week for 3 consecutive weeks (Hayner, 2012).

- Remediation strategies
  - ▶ General theory
    - ○ Rationale: Everyday skills and tasks can be improved or retrained through practices following a neurological event such as stroke.
    - ○ Technique: Strategies focus on improvement or retraining of motor skills used to perform a whole task as much as possible with intent to encourage transfer of skills; feedback should be provided that encourages problem solving (Prager et al., 2011).
  - ▶ Brunnstrom movement therapy[*]
    - ○ Rationale: Motor impairment is caused by synergies.
    - ○ Technique: Movements should focus on reflexive, synergistic, and out-of-synergy movements focusing on inducing voluntary motor control such as sit-to-stand, stooping, reaching, and sideward walking or straight-line walking (Huang et al., 2016; Pandian & Arya 2012).
  - ▶ Constraint-Induced Movement Therapy (CIMT)
    - ○ Rationale: Counter effects of learned nonuse.
    - ○ Technique: Restraining unimpaired limb in a glove or mitten for up to 6 hours each day for as long as 2 weeks, forcing the use of impaired hand and arm to perform everyday activities with the involved hand and perform specific activities during rehabilitation sessions.
  - ▶ Functional (task-oriented, task-specific) approaches
    - ○ Rationale: Focusing on functional tasks that are purposeful and meaningful to the clients increases motivation and orientation to everyday living activities (Arya et al., 2012).
    - ○ Technique: Select tasks that are part of the client's daily life. Use teaching strategies that facilitate performance (forward or backward chaining, visual or auditory supports, simplify task such as starting dressing task with garments that are easy to put on with no fasteners).
  - ▶ Motor learning theory
    - ○ Rationale: Impaired components of a task or skill can be isolated and practiced separately until mastered and then integrated back into the total task or skill.
    - ○ Technique: Functional activity is identified, limited motor components are analyzed, impaired components are practiced in isolation through visual, verbal, and manual guidance and then the component is practiced in context of the total task with intent of integrating the components (Prager et al., 2011).
  - ▶ Motor control theory
    - ○ Rationale: Intervention should emphasize practice of functional skills used in the person's everyday life as a means of organizing motor behavior.
    - ○ Technique: Therapist determines and modifies the tasks and environmental demands to focus on practicing tasks and activities in a natural context).
  - ▶ Neurodevelopmental Treatment (NDT; Bobath Approach)[**]
    - ○ Rationale: Correct abnormal tonicity in muscles and eliminate unwanted muscle activity.
    - ○ Technique: Retrain muscles using normal, functional patterns of movement.
  - ▶ Sensorimotor theory (Rood approach)
    - ○ Rationale: Focus on enhancing the integration of reflexes and emergence of voluntary motor behaviors concerned with posture and locomotion.

---

[*] Note that Brunnstrom movement therapy has not been updated in many years (Gillen, 2015).
[**] Studies have not found NDT to be superior to other approaches (Gillen, 2015).

    ○ Technique: Primitive reflexes are to be integrated so they do not interfere in voluntary movement and righting and equilibrium reflexes are to be promoted to improve postural control and functional ambulation.

Cognitive/Perceptual
- Compensatory approaches
  - ▶ Cognitive Orientation to daily Occupational Performance (CO-OP)
    - ○ Rationale: Model is designed to enable skill acquisition through a process of developing and using specific cognitive linked behavior strategies.
    - ○ Technique: Strategies include use of reinforcement, modeling, shaping, prompting, fading, and chaining techniques and is built on a cognitive approach that assumes learning as an active process of acquiring, remembering, and using knowledge to perform actions and tasks (problem-solving strategy is "Goal, Plan, Do, Check").
  - ▶ Cognitive rehabilitation strategies
    - ○ Rationale: Cognitive rehabilitation focuses on compensating for deficits through the use of internal or external cognitive-based strategies or both.
    - ○ Technique: Examples of internal strategies include mental imagery, self-awareness training, self-cueing strategies, or use of mnemonic cues. Examples of external strategies include cueing devices, developing written plans before performance, or using memory and planning aids. Choice of strategies depends of client's deficits, skills, abilities, and the specific occupation or occupations in which the person is trying to reengage. A combination of internal and external strategies may be used.
  - ▶ Dynamic interactional model of cognition
    - ○ Rationale: Environmental cues or task alterations can be used to compensate for neurological deficits.
    - ○ Technique: Focus is on developing internal strategies that increase the client's awareness of existing deficits and teaching how to compensate by changing the environment or changing the task.
- Self-management (Bower et al., 2012)

Psychosocial
- Assist person to participate in occupations to engage mind and body.

Context/Environment
- Provide commercial or custom-made splints including information on use and care.
  - ▶ Dynamic wrist/hand orthosis to provide wrist and finger positioning and facilitate wrist extension.
- Provide information and contacts for available resources in community or internet.
- Provide information on access to and training on use and care of adapted devices and equipment.
- Provide information and training on living with a chronic disorder such as hemiplegia or hemiparesis.

Precautions/Safety Considerations

Person is at risk for falls. Person may be at risk to burns, cuts, or scrapes on the involved side due to reduced sensation.

Prognosis and Outcome

Person can expect some degree of recovery, although the length of time varies depending on the amount of damage. Peak recovery occurs within the first 6 months but some recovery may occur for up to a year. The amount of rehabilitation services received does impact the amount of recovery.

REFERENCES

Adams, R. J., Ellington, A. L., Armstead, K., Sheffield, K., Patrie, J. T., & Diamond, P. T. (2019). Upper extremity function assessment using a glove orthosis and virtual reality system. *OTJR: Occupation, Participation and Health, 39*(2), 81–89. https://doi.org/10.1177/1539449219829862

Ahn, S. (2016). Association between daily activities, process skills, and motor skills in community dwelling patients after left hemiparetic stroke. *Journal of Physical Therapy Science, 28*(6), 1829–1831. https://doi.org/10.1589/jpts.28.1829

Ahn, S.-N., Lee, J.-W., & Hwang, S. (2016). Tactile perception for stroke induce changes in electroencephalography. *Hong Kong Journal of Occupational Therapy, 28*(1), 1–6. https://doi.org/10.1016/j.hkjot.2016.10.001

Amini, D. (2014). Hand therapy and the neurologically involved hand. *Rehab Management, 27*(3), 10, 12–13. https://rehabpub.com/resource-center/hand-therapy-neurologically-involved-hand/

Andriske, L., Verikios, D., & Hitch, D. (2017). Patient and therapist experiences of the Saebo-Flex: A pilot study. *Occupational Therapy International, 2017*, Article 5462078. https://doi.org/10.1155/2017/5462078

Arya, K. N., Pandian, S., Kumar, D., & Puri, V. (2015). Task-based mirror therapy augmenting motor recovery in poststroke hemiparesis: A randomized controlled trial. *Journal of Stroke and Cerebrovascular Diseases, 24*(8), 1738–1748. https://doi.org/10.1016/j.jstrokecerebrovasdis.2015.03.026

Arya, K. N., Verma, R., Garg, R. K., Sharma, V. P., Agarwal, M., & Aggarwal, G. G. (2012). Meaningful task-specific training (MTST) for stroke rehabilitation: A randomized controlled trial. *Topics in Stroke Rehabilitation, 19*(3), 193–211. https://doi.org/10.1310/tsr1903-193

Baldwin, C. R., Harry, A. J., Power, L. J., Pope, K. L., & Harding, K. E. (2018). Modified Constraint-Induced Movement Therapy is a feasible and potentially useful addition to the community rehabilitation tool kit after stroke: A pilot randomised control trial. *Australian Occupational Therapy Journal, 65*(6), 503–511. https://doi.org/10.1111/1440-1630.12488

Beckelhimer, S. C., Dalton, A. E., Richter, C. A., Hermann, V., & Page, S. J. (2011). Computer-based rhythm and timing training in severe stroke-induced arm hemiparesis. *American Journal of Occupational Therapy, 65*(1), 96–100. https://doi.org/10.5014/ajot.2011.09158

Bertrand, A. M., Fournier, K., Wick Brasey, M. G., Kaiser, M. L., Frischknecht, R., & Diserens, K. (2015). Reliability of maximal grip strength measurements and grip strength recovery following a stroke. *Journal of Hand Therapy, 28*(4), 356–362. https://doi.org/10.1016/j.jht.2015.04.004

Birkenmeier, R. L., Prager, E. M., & Lang, C. E. (2010). Translating animal doses of task-specific training to people with chronic stroke in 1-hour therapy sessions: A proof-of-concept study. *Neurorehabilitation and Neural Repair, 24*(7), 620–635. https://doi.org/10.1177/1545968310361957

Blennerhassett, J. M., Avery, R. M., & Carey, L. M. (2010). The test-retest reliability and responsiveness to change for the Hand Function Survey during stroke rehabilitation. *Australian Occupational Therapy Journal, 57*(6), 431–438. https://doi.org/10.1111/j.1440-1630.2010.00884.x

Bower, K., Gustafsson, L., Hoffmann, T., & Barker, R. (2012). Self-management of upper limb recovery after stroke: How effectively do occupational therapists and physiotherapists train clients and carers? *British Journal of Occupational Therapy, 75*(4), 180–187. https://doi.org/10.4276/030802212X13336366278130

Cantero-Téllez, R., Naughton, N., Algar, L., & Valdes, K. (2019). Outcome measurement of hand function following mirror therapy for stroke rehabilitation: A systematic review. *Journal of Hand Therapy, 32*(2), 277–291. https://doi.org/10.1016/j.jht.2018.01.009

Carey, L. M., Abbott, D. F., Lamp, G., Puce, A., Seitz, R., & Donnan, G. A. (2016). Same intervention-different reorganization: The impact of lesion location on training-facilitated somatosensory recovery after stroke. *Neurorehabilitation and Neural Repair, 30*(10), 988–1000. https://doi.org/ 10.1177/1545968316653836

Carey, L., Macdonell, R., & Matyas T. A. (2011). SENSe: Study of the effectiveness of neurorehabilitation on sensation: A randomized controlled trial. *Neurorehabilitation and Neural Repair, 25*(4), 304–313. https://doi.org/10.1177/1545968310397705

Cha, Y.-J., Yoo, E.-Y, Jung, M.-Y., Park, S.-H., & Park, J.-H. (2012). Effects of functional task training with mental practice in stroke: A meta analysis. *NeuroRehabilitation, 30*(3), 239–246. https:// doi.org/10.3233/NRE-2012-0751

Chanubol, R., Wongphaet, P., Chavanich, N., Werner, C. Hesse, S., Bardeleben, A., & Merholz, J. (2012). A randomized controlled trial of cognitive sensory motor training therapy on the recovery of arm function in acute stroke patients. *Clinical Rehabilitation, 26*(12), 1096–1104. https://doi.org/10.1177/0269215512444631

Chen, M.-H., Huang, L.-L., Lee, C.-F., Hsieh, C.-L., Lin, Y.-C., Liu, H., Chen, M.-I., & Lu, W.-S. (2015). A controlled pilot trial of two commercial video games for rehabilitation of arm function after stroke. *Clinical Rehabilitation, 29*(7), 674–682. https://doi.org/10.1177/0269215514 554115

Connell, L. A., McMahon, N. E., Eng, J. J., & Watkins, C. L. (2014). Prescribing upper limb exercises after stroke: A survey of current UK therapy practice. *Journal of Rehabilitation Medicine, 46*(3), 212–218. https://doi.org/10.2340/16501977-1268

Davis, J. (2012, October 8). Shoulder pain and stroke: Reducing hemiplegic shoulder pain through practical handling skills. *OT Practice*, 9–13. https://www.icelearningcenter.com/s/ OTP-Shoulder-Pain-and-Stroke.pdf

Earley, D., Herlache, E., & Skelton, D. R. (2010). Use of occupations and activities in a modified constraint-induced movement therapy program: A musician's triumphs over chronic hemiparesis from stroke. *American Journal of Occupational Therapy, 64*(5), 735–744. https://doi.org/ 10.5014/ajot.2010.08073

Ferreira, F. M. R. M., Chaves, M. E. A., Oliveira, V. C., Van Petten, A. M. V. N., & Vimieiro, C. B. S. (2018). Effectiveness of robot therapy on body function and structure in people with limited upper limb function: A systematic review and meta-analysis. *PLOS ONE, 13*(7), Article e0200330. https://doi.org/10.1371/journal.pone.0200330

Gäverth, J., Eliasson, A.-C., Kullander, K., Borg, J., Lindberg, P. G., & Forssberg, H. (2014). Sensitivity of the NeuroFlexor method to measure change in spasticity after treatment with botulinum toxin A in wrist and finger muscles. *Journal of Rehabilitation Medicine, 46*(7), 629–634. https://doi.org/10.2340/16501977-1824

Gäverth, J., Sandgren, M., Lindberg, P. G., Forssberg, H., & Eliasson, A.-C. (2013). Test–retest and inter-rater reliability of a method to measure wrist and finger spasticity. *Journal of Rehabilitation Medicine, 45*(7), 630–636. https://doi.org/10.2340/16501977-1160

Giang, T. A., Ong, A. W. G., Krishnamurthy, K., & Fong, K. N. K. (2016). Rehabilitation interventions for poststroke hand oedema: A systematic review. *Hong Kong Journal of Occupational Therapy, 27*(1), 7–17. https://doi.org/10.1016/j.hkjot.2016.03.002

Gillen, G. (2015). What is the evidence for the effectiveness of interventions to improve occupational performance after stroke? *American Journal of Occupational Therapy, 69*(1), Article 6901170010. https://doi.org/10.5014/ajot.2015.013409

Go, E.-J., & Lee, S.-H. (2016). Effect of sensorimotor stimulation on chronic stroke patients' upper extremity function: A preliminary study. *Journal of Physical Therapy Science, 28*(12), 3350–3353. https://doi.org/10.1589/jpts.28.3350

Gokhale, P. S., & Kale, J. (2015). To study the effect of occupational therapy on balance and its impact on activities of daily living in patients with right and left cerebral infarct: A comparative study. *Indian Journal of Physiotherapy and Occupational Therapy, 9*(4), 216–222. https:// doi.org/10.5958/0973-5674.2015.00175.6

Gustafsson, L., Walter, A., Bower, K., Slaughter, A., & Hoyle, M. (2014). Single-case design evaluation of compression therapy for edema of the stroke affected hand. *American Journal of Occupational Therapy, 68*(2), 203–211. https://doi.org/10.5014/ajot.2014.009423

Hayner, K. A. (2012). Effectiveness of the California tri-pull taping method for shoulder subluxation poststroke: A single-subject ABA design. *American Journal of Occupational Therapy, 66*(6), 727–736. https://doi.org/10.5014/ajot.2012.004663

Hookstadt, K., Filarowicz, M., & Rieks, J. (2012). Raising the bar for upper extremity goals. *Rehab Management, 25*(3), 9–13. https://rehabpub.com/conditions/neurological/stroke-neurological/raising-the-bar-for-upper-extremity-goals/

Hsieh, Y.-W., Wu, C.-Y., Wang, W.-E., Lin, K.-C., Chang, K.-C., Chen, C.-C., & Liu, C.-T. (2017). Bilateral robotic priming before task-oriented approach in subacute stroke rehabilitation: A pilot randomized controlled trial. *Clinical Rehabilitation, 31*(2), 225–233. https://doi.org/10.1177/0269215516633275

Huang, C.-Y., Lin, G.-H., Huang, Y.-J., Song, C.-Y., Lee, Y.-C., How, M.-J., Chen, Y.-M., Hsueh, I.-P., Chen, M.-H., & Hsieh, C.-L. (2016). Improving the utility of the Brunnstrom recovery stages in patients with stroke: Validation and quantification. *Medicine, 95*(31), Article e4508. https://doi.org/10.1097/MD.0000000000004508

Hubbard, I. J., Carey, L. M., Budd, T. W., Levi, C., McElduff, P., Hudson, S., Bateman, G., & Parsons, M. W. (2015). A randomized controlled trial of the effect of early upper-limb training on stroke recovery and brain activation. *Neurorehabilitation and Neural Repair, 29*(8), 703–713. https://doi.org/10.1177/1545968314562647

Hung, C.-S., Lin, K.-C., Chang, W.-Y., Huang, W.-C., Chang, Y. J., Chen, C.-L., Yao, K. G., & Lee, Y.-Y. (2019). Unilateral vs bilateral hybrid approaches for upper limb rehabilitation in chronic stroke: A randomized controlled trial. *Archives of Physical Medicine and Rehabilitation, 100*(12), 2225–2232. https://doi.org/10.1016/j.apmr.2019.06.021

Ilić, N. V., Dubljanin-Raspopović, E., Nedeljković, U., Tomanović-Vujadinović, S., Milanović, S. D., Petronić-Marković, I., & Ilić, T. V. (2016). Effects of anodal tDCS and occupational therapy on fine motor skill deficits in patients with chronic stroke. *Restorative Neurology and Neuroscience, 34*(6), 935–945. https://doi.org/10.3233/RNN-160668

Jarvis, K., Reid, G., Edelstyn, N., & Hunter, S. (2014). *Occupational therapy stroke arm and hand treatment record (OT-STAR) booklet.* Keele University & University of Liverpool. http://pcwww.liv.ac.uk/ehls/health-sciences/ot-star/treatment-schedule-instructions.pdf

Jonasson, I., Baigi, A., Marklund, B., & Månsson, J. (2012). A new primary care model for the rehabilitation of stroke patients with impaired arm and hand function—A pilot study. *Nordic Journal of Nursing Research, 32*(2), 15–20. https://doi.org/10.1177/010740831203200204

Jung, N.-H., Kim, K.-M., Oh, J.-S., & Chang, M. (2013). The effects of bilateral arm training on reaching performance and activities of daily living of stroke patients. *Journal of Physical Therapy Science, 25*(4), 449–452. https://doi.org/10.1589/jpts.25.449

Kakuda, W., Abo, M., Kaito, N., Ishikawa, A., Taguchi, K., & Yokoi, A. (2010). Six-day course of repetitive transcranial magnetic stimulation plus occupational therapy for post-stroke patients with upper limb hemiparesis: A case series study. *Disability and Rehabilitation, 32*(10), 801–807. https://doi.org/10.3109/09638280903295474

Kakuda, W., Abo, M., Kobayashi, K., Momosaki, R., Yokoi, A., Fukuda, A., Ito, H., & Tominaga, A. (2011). Combination treatment of low frequency rTMS and occupational therapy with levodopa administration: An intensive neurorehabilitative approach for upper limb hemiparesis after stroke. *International Journal of Neuroscience, 121*(7), 373–378. https://doi.org/10.3109/00207454.2011.560314

Kakuda, W., Abo, M., Kobayashi, K., Momosaki, R., Yokoi, A., Fukuda, A., Ito, H., Tominaga, A., Umemori, T., & Kameda, Y. (2011). Anti-spastic effect of low-frequency rTMS applied with occupational therapy in post-stroke patients with upper limb hemiparesis. *Brain Injury, 25*(5), 496–502. https://doi.org/10.3109/02699052.2011.559610

Kakuda, W., Abo, M., Shimizu, M., Sasanuma, J., Okamoto, T., Yokoi, A., Taguchi, K., Mitani, S., Harashima, H., Urushidani, N., Urashima, M., & NEURO Investigators. (2012). A multi-center study on low-frequency rTMS combined with intensive occupational therapy for upper limb hemiparesis in post-stroke patients. *Journal of NeuroEngineering and Rehabilitation, 9*, Article 4. https://doi.org/10.1186/1743-0003-9-4

Kam, N., Struzik, J., Jarus, T., & Rand, D. (2012). Is the Nintendo Wii suitable for stroke rehabilitation? A pilot feasibility and usability study. *Israeli Journal of Occupational Therapy, 21*(1), e3–e25.

Kho, A. Y., Liu, K. P. Y., & Chung, R. C. K. (2014). Meta-analysis on the effect of mental imagery on motor recovery of the hemiplegic upper extremity function. *Australian Occupational Therapy Journal, 61*(2), 38–48. https://doi.org/10.1111/1440-1630.12084

Kim, J.-H., & Chang, M.-Y. (2018). Effects of modified constraint-induced movement therapy on upper extremity function and occupational performance of stroke patients. *Journal of Physical Therapy Science, 30*(8), 1092–1094. https://doi.org/10.1589/jpts.30.1092

Kim, J. H., & Lee, B.-H. (2015). Mirror therapy combined with biofeedback functional electrical stimulation for motor recovery of upper extremities after stroke: A pilot randomized controlled trial. *Occupational Therapy International, 22*, 51–60. https://doi.org/10.1002/oti.1384

Kim, J.-R., Jung, M.-Y., Yoo, E.-Y., Park, J.-H., Kim, S.-H., & Lee, J. (2014). Effects of rhythmic auditory stimulation during hemiplegic arm reaching in individuals with stroke: An exploratory study. *Hong Kong Journal of Occupational Therapy, 24*(2), 64–71. https://doi.org/10.1016/j.hkjot.2014.11.002

Kim, M.-Y., Kim, G.-S., Matson, N.-S., & Kim, W.-S. (2010). Effects of horticultural occupational therapy on the physical and psychological rehabilitation of patients with hemiplegia after stroke. *Horticultural Science & Technology, 28*(5), 884–890.

Kim, S.-H., Park, J.-H., Jung, M.-Y., & Yoo, E.-Y. (2016). Effects of task-oriented training as an added treatment to electromyogram-triggered neuromuscular stimulation on upper extremity function in chronic stroke patients. *Occupational Therapy International, 23*(2), 165–174. https://doi.org/10.1002/oti.1421

Kinoshita, S., Kakuda, W., Yamada, N., Momosaki, R., Okuma, R. Watanabe, S., & Abo, M. (2016). Therapeutic administration of atomoxetine combined with rTMS and occupational therapy for upper limb hemiparesis after stroke: A case series study of three patients. *Acta Neurologica Belgica, 116*(1), 31–37. https://doi.org/10.1007/s13760-015-0503-3

Law, L. L. F., Fong, K. N. K., & Li, R. K. F. (2018). Multisensory stimulation to promote upper extremity motor recovery in stroke: A pilot study. *British Journal of Occupational Therapy, 81*(11), 641–648. https://doi.org/10.1177/0308022618770141

Lee, D.-H., Kim, W.-J., Oh, J.-S., & Chang, M. (2015). Taping of the elbow extensor muscle in chronic stroke patients: Comparison between before and after three-dimensional motion analysis. *Journal of Physical Therapy Science, 27*(7), 2101–2103. https://doi.org/10.1589/jpts.27.2101

Lee, M.-J., Lee, J.-H., & Lee, S.-M. (2018). Effects of robot-assisted therapy on upper extremity function and activities of daily living in hemiplegicpatients: A single-blinded, randomized, controlled trial. *Technology and Health Care, 26*(4), 659–666. https://doi.org/10.3233/THC-181336

Lee, M.-J., Lee, J.-H., Koo, H.-M., & Lee, S.-M. (2017). Effectiveness of bilateral arm training for improving extremity function and activities of daily living performance in hemiplegic patients. *Journal of Stroke and Cerebrovascular Diseases, 26*(5), 1020–1025. https://doi.org/10.1016/j.jstrokecerebrovasdis.2016.12.008

Liao, W.-W., Wu, C.-Y., Hsieh, Y. W., Lin, K. C., & Chang, W. Y. (2012). Effects of robot-assisted upper limb rehabilitation on daily function and real-world arm activity in patients with chronic stroke: A randomized controlled trial. *Clinical Rehabilitation, 26*(2), 111–120. https://doi.org/10.1177/0269215511416383

Lin, K.-C., Chen, Y.-A., Chen, C.-L., Wu, C.-Y., & Chang, Y.-F. (2010). The effects of bilateral arm training on motor control and functional performance in chronic stroke: A randomized controlled study. *Neurorehabilitation and Neural Repair, 24*(1), 42–51. https://doi.org/10.1177/1545968309345268

Lin, K.-C., Chen, Y.-T., Huang, P.-C., Wu, C.-Y., Huang, W.-L., Yang, H.-W., Lai, H.-T., & Lu, H.-J. (2014). Effect of mirror therapy combined with somatosensory stimulation on motor recovery and daily function in stroke patients: A pilot study. *Journal of the Formosan Medical Association, 113*(7), 422–428. https://doi.org/10.1016/j.jfma.2012.08.008

Lu, E. C., Wang, R. H., Hebert, D., Boger, J., Galea, M. P., & Mihailidis, A. (2011). The development of an upper limb stroke rehabilitation robot: Identification of clinical practices and design requirements through a survey of therapists. *Disability and Rehabilitation Assistive Technology, 6*(5), 420–431. https://doi.org/10.3109/17483107.2010.544370

Marquez-Chin, C., Bagher, S., Zivanovic, V., & Popovic, M. R. (2017). Functional electrical stimulation therapy for severe hemiplegia: Randomized control trial revisited. *Canadian Journal of Occupational Therapy, 84*(2), 87–97. https://doi.org/10.1177/0008417416668370

McCall, M., McEwen, S., Colantonio, A., Streiner, D., & Dawson, D. R. (2011). Modified constraint-induced movement therapy for elderly clients with subacute stroke. *American Journal of Occupational Therapy, 65*(4), 409–418. https://doi.org/10.5014/ajot.2011.002063

Mishra, N. (2015). Comparison of effects of motor imagery, cognitive and motor dual task training methods on gait and balance of stroke survivors. *Indian Journal of Occupational Therapy, 47*(2), 46–57.

Murdolo, Y., Brown, T., Fielding, L., Elliott, S., & Castles, E. (2017). Stroke survivors' experiences of using the Graded Repetitive Arm Supplementary Program (GRASP) in an Australian acute hospital setting: A mixed-methods pilot study. *Australian Occupational Therapy Journal, 64*(4), 305–313. https://doi.org/10.1111/1440-1630.12363

Nilsen, D. M., Gillen, G., & Gordon, A. M. (2010). Use of mental practice to improve upper-limb recovery after stroke: A systematic review. *American Journal of Occupational Therapy, 64*(5), 695–708. https://doi.org/10.5014/ajot.2010.09034

O'Toole, M. T. (Ed.). (2017). *Mosby's dictionary of medicine, nursing & health professions* (10th ed.). Elsevier.

Page, S. J., Dunning, K., Hermann, V., Leonard, A., & Levine, P. (2011). Longer versus shorter mental practice sessions for affected upper extremity movement after stroke: A randomized controlled trial. *Clinical Rehabilitation, 25*(7), 627–637. https://doi.org/10.1177/0269215510395793

Page, S. J., Fulk, G. D., & Boyne, P. (2012). Clinically important differences for the upper-extremity Fugl-Meyer Scale in people with minimal to moderate impairment due to chronic stroke. *Physical Therapy, 92*(6), 791–798. https://doi.org/10.2522/ptj.20110009

Paik, Y. R., Kim, S. K., Lee, J. S., & Jeon, B. J. (2014). Simple and task-oriented mirror therapy for upper extremity function in stroke patients: A pilot study. *Hong Kong Journal of Occupational Therapy, 24*(1), 6–12. https://doi.org/10.1016/j.hkjot.2014.01.002

Pandian, S., & Arya, K. N. (2012). Relation between the upper extremity synergistic movement components and its implication for motor recovery in poststroke hemiparesis. *Topics in Stroke Rehabilitation, 19*(6), 545–555. https://doi.org/10.1310/tsr1906-545

Pandian, S., Arya, K. N., & Davidson, E. W. R. (2012). Comparison of Brunnstrom movement therapy and Motor Relearning Program in rehabilitation of post-stroke hemiparetic hand: A randomized trial. *Journal of Bodywork and Movement Therapies, 16*(3), 330–337. https://doi.org/10.1016/j.jbmt.2011.11.002

Pandian, S., Arya, K. N., & Kumar, D. (2014). Does motor training of the nonparetic side influences balance and function in chronic stroke? A pilot RCT. *Scientific World Journal, 2014*, Article 769726. https://doi.org/10.1155/2014/769726

Park, J. H. (2019). Dual task training effects on upper extremity functions and performance of daily activities of chronic stroke patients. *Osong Public Health and Research Perspectives, 10*(1), 2–5. https://doi.org/10.24171/j.phrp.2019.10.1.02

Park, J.-Y., Chang, M., Kim, K.-M., & Kim, H.-J. (2015). The effect of mirror therapy on upper-extremity function and activities of daily living in stroke patients. *Journal of Physical Therapy Science, 27*(6), 1681–1683. https://doi.org/10.1589/jpts.27.1681

Park, Y., Chang, M., Kim, K.-M., & An, D.-H. (2015). The effects of mirror therapy with tasks on upper extremity function and self-care in stroke patients. *Journal of Physical Therapy Science, 27*(5), 1499–1501. https://doi.org/10.1589/jpts.27.1499

Pérez-Cruzado, D., Merchán-Baeza, J. A., González-Sánchez, M., & Cuesta-Vargas, A. I. (2017). Systematic review of mirror therapy compared with conventional rehabilitation in upper extremity function in stroke survivors. *Australian Occupational Therapy Journal, 64*(2), 91–112. https://doi.org/10.1111/1440-1630.12342

Pila, O., Duret, C., Gracies, J.-M., Francisco, G. E., Bayle, N., & Hutin, É. (2018). Evolution of upper limb kinematics four years after subacute robot-assisted rehabilitation in stroke patients. *International Journal of Neuroscience, 128*(11), 1030–1039. https://doi.org/10.1080/0020745 4.2018.1461626

Poole, J. L., Carbajal, T., Cole, A., Ginther, A., Streng, S., Quinlan, J., Rouw, M., Singleton, S. L., & Skipper, B. (2019). In-home, client-based intensive therapy intervention for upper extremity hemiparesis after stroke. *Annals of International Occupational Therapy, 2*(1), 7–15. https://doi .org/10.3928/24761222-20180723-01

Poole, J. L., Sadek, J., & Haaland, K. Y. (2011). Meal preparation abilities after left or right hemisphere stroke. *Archives of Physical Medicine and Rehabilitation, 92*(4), 590–596. https://doi.org/ 10.1016/j.apmr.2010.11.021

Porter, R. S. (Ed.). (2018). *The Merck manual of diagnosis and therapy* (20th ed.). Merck Sharp & Dohme.

Prager, E. M., Birkenmeier, R. L., & Lang, C. E. (2011). Exploring expectations for upper-extremity motor treatment in people after stroke: A secondary analysis. *American Journal of Occupational Therapy, 65*(4), 437–444. https://doi.org/10.5014/ajot.2010.000430

Rayegani, S. M., Raeissadat, S. A., Sedighipour, L., Rezazadeh, I. M., Bahrami, M. H., Eliaspour, D., & Khosrawi, S. (2014). Effect of neurofeedback and electromyographic-biofeedback therapy on improving hand function in stroke patients. *Topics in Stroke Rehabilitation, 21*(2), 137–151. https://doi.org/10.1310/tsr2102-137

Royal College of Occupational Therapists. (2015). *Splinting for the prevention and correction of contractures in adults with neurological dysfunction: Practice guidelines for occupational therapists and physiotherapist.*

Sabari, J. S., Capasso, N., & Feld-Glazman, R. (2014). Optimizing motor planning and performance in clients with neurological disorders. In M. V. Radomski & C. A. Trombly Latham (Eds.), *Occupational therapy for physical dysfunction* (7th ed., pp. 614–674). Wolters Kluwer.

Samuelkamaleshkumar, S., Reethajanetsureka, S., Pauljebaraj, P., Benshamir, B., Padankatti, S. M., & David, J. A. (2014). Mirror therapy enhances motor performance in the paretic upper limb after stroke: A pilot randomized controlled trial. *Archives of Physical Medicine and Rehabilitation, 95*(11), 2000–2005. https://doi.org/10.1016/j.apmr.2014.06.020

Saposnik, G., Teasell, R., Mamdani, M., Hall, J., McIlroy, W., Cheung, D., Thorpe, K. E., Cohen, L. G., & Bayley, M. (2010). Effectiveness of virtual reality using Wii gaming technology in stroke rehabilitation: A pilot randomized clinical trial and proof of principle. *Stroke, 41*(7), 1477–1484. https://doi.org/10.1161/STROKEAHA.110.584979

Schmid, A. A., Van Puymbroeck, M., Altenburger, P. A., Schalk, N. L., Dierks, T. A., Miller, K. K., Damush, T., Bravata, D. M., & Williams, L. S. (2012). Poststroke balance improves with yoga: A pilot study. *Stroke, 43*(9), 2402–2407. https://doi.org/10.1161/STROKEAHA.112.658211

Schneider, E. J., Ada, L., & Lannin, N. (2019). Extra upper limb practice after stroke: A feasibility study. *Pilot and Feasibility Studies, 5,* Article 156. https://doi.org/10.1186/s40814-019-0531-5

Schultz-Krohn, W., & Mclaughlin-Gray, J. (2018). Traditional sensorimotor approaches to intervention. In H. M. Pendleton & W. Schultz-Krohn (Eds.), *Pedretti's occupational therapy* (8th ed., pp. 766–797). Elsevier.

Sethy, D., Bajpai, P., Kujur, E. S., Mohakud, K., & Sahoo, S. (2016). Effectiveness of modified constraint induced movement therapy and bilateral arm training on upper extremity function after chronic stroke: A comparative study. *Open Journal of Therapy and Rehabilitation, 4*(1), 1–9. https://doi.org/10.4236/ojtr.2016.41001

Sethy, D., Sahoo, S., Kujur, E. S., & Bajpai, P. (2018). Stroke upper extremity rehabilitation: Effect of bilateral arm training. *International Journal of Health & Allied Sciences, 7*(4), 217–221.

Shirahama, K., Gocyou, M., Morita, T., Kitahashi, T., & Yasuda, T. (2016). Development of a task-specific occupational therapy training menu for the improvement of upper limb function in stroke patients. *Asian Journal Occupational Therapy, 12*(1), 43–51. https://doi.org/10.11596/asiajot.12.43

Simpson, L. A., Eng, J. J., Backman, C. L., & Miller, W. C. (2013). Rating of Everyday Arm-use in the Community and Home (REACH) scale for capturing affected arm-use after stroke: Development, reliability, and validity. *PLOS ONE, 8*(12), Article e83405. https://doi.org/10.1371/journal.pone.0083405

Simpson, L. A., Eng, J. J., & Chan, M. (2017). H-GRASP: The feasibility of an upper limb home exercise program monitored by phone for individuals post stroke. *Disability and Rehabilitation, 39*(9), 874–882. https://doi.org/10.3109/09638288.2016.1162853

Sin, H. H., & Lee, G. C. (2013). Additional virtual reality training using Xbox Kinect in stroke survivors with hemiplegia. *American Journal of Physical Medicine & Rehabilitation, 92*(10), 871–880. https://doi.org/10.1097/PHM.0b013e3182a38e40

Stoykov, M. E., & Stinear, J. W. (2010). Active-passive bilateral therapy as a priming mechanism for individuals in the subacute phase of post-stroke recovery: A feasibility study. *American Journal of Physical Medicine & Rehabilitation, 89*(11), 873–878. https://doi.org/10.1097/PHM.0b013e3181f1c31c

Takahashi, K., Domen, K., Sakamoto, T., Toshima, M., Otaka, Y., Seto, M., Irie, K., Haga, B., Takebayashi, T., & Hachisuka, K. (2016). Efficacy of upper extremity robotic therapy in subacute poststroke hemiplegia: An exploratory randomized trial. *Stroke, 47*(5), 1385–1388. https://doi.org/10.1161/STROKEAHA.115.012520

Tanabe, H., Nagao, T., & Tanemura, R. (2011). Application of constraint-induced movement therapy for people with severe chronic plegic hand. *Asian Journal of Occupational Therapy, 9*(1), 7–14.

Thielbar, K. O., Triandafilou, K. M., Fischer, H. C., O'Toole, J. M., Corrigan, M. L., Ochoa, J. M., Stoykov, M. E., & Kamper, D. G. (2017). Benefits of using a voice and EMG-driven actuated glove to support occupational therapy for stroke survivors. *IEEE Transactions on Neural Systems and Rehabilitation Engineering, 25*(3), 297–305. https://doi.org/10.1109/TNSRE.2016.2569070

Toh, S. F. M., & Fong, K. N. K. (2012). Systematic review on the effectiveness of mirror therapy in training upper limb hemiparesis after stroke. *Hong Kong Journal of Occupational Therapy, 22*(2), 84–95. https://doi.org/10.1016/j.hkjot.2012.12.009

Turville, M., Carey, L. M., Matyas, T. A., & Blennerhassett, J. (2017). Change in functional arm use is associated with somatosensory skills after sensory retraining poststroke. *American Journal of Occupational Therapy, 71*(3), Article 7103190070. https://doi.org/10.5014/ajot.2017.024950

Turville, M., Matyas, T. A., Blennerhassett, J. M., & Carey, L. M. (2018). Initial severity of somatosensory impairment influences response to upper limb sensory retraining post-stroke. *NeuroRehabilitation, 43*(4), 413–423. https://doi.org/10.3233/NRE-182439

Umeki, N., Murata, J., & Higashijima, M. (2019). Effects of training for finger perception on functional recovery of hemiplegic upper limbs in acute stroke patients. *Occupational Therapy International, 2019*, Article 6508261. https://doi.org/10.1155/2019/6508261

Villafañe, J. H., Taveggia, G., Galeri, S., Bissolotti, L., Mullè, C., Imperio, G., Valdes, K., Borboni, A., & Negrini, S. (2018). Efficacy of short-term robot-assisted rehabilitation in patients with hand paralysis after stroke: A randomized clinical trial. *Hand, 13*(1), 95–102. https://doi.org/10.1177/1558944717692096

Wu, A. J., Radel, J., & Hanna-Pladdy, B. (2011). Improved function after combined physical and mental practice after stroke: A case of hemiparesis and apraxia. *American Journal of Occupational Therapy, 65*(2), 161–168. https://doi.org/10.5014/ajot.2011.000786

Wu, C.-Y., Chuang, L.-L., Lin, K.-C., Chen, H.-C., & Tsay, P.-K. (2011). Randomized trial of distributed constraint-induced therapy versus bilateral arm training for the rehabilitation of upper-limb motor control and function after stroke. *Neurorehabilitation and Neural Repair, 25*(2), 130–139. https://doi.org/10.1177/1545968310380686

Wu, C.-Y., Hsieh, Y.-W., Lin, K.-C., Chuang, L.-L., Chang, Y.-F., Liu, H.-L., Chen, C.-L., Lin, K.-H., & Wai, Y.-Y. (2010). Brain reorganization after bilateral arm training and distributed constraint-induced therapy in stroke patients: A preliminary functional magnetic resonance imaging study. *Chang Gung Medical Journal, 33*(6), 628–638.

Wu, C.-Y., Huang, P.-C., Chen, Y.-T., Lin, K.-C., & Yang, H.-W. (2013). Effects of mirror therapy on motor and sensory recovery in chronic stroke: A randomized controlled trial. *Archives of Physical Medicine and Rehabilitation, 94*(6), 1023–1030. https://doi.org/10.1016/j.apmr.2013.02.007

Wu, C.-Y., Yang, C.-L., Chen, M.-D., Lin, K.-C., & Wu, L.-L. (2013). Unilateral versus bilateral robot-assisted rehabilitation on arm-trunk control and functions post stroke: A randomized controlled trial. *Journal of NeuroEngineering and Rehabilitation, 10*, Article 35. https://doi.org/10.1186/1743-0003-10-35

Wu, C.-Y., Yang, C.-L., Chuang, L.-L., Lin, K.-C., Chen, H.-C., Chen, M.-D., & Huang, W.-C. (2012). Effect of therapist-based versus robot-assisted bilateral arm training on motor control, functional performance, and quality of life after chronic stroke: A clinical trial. *Physical Therapy and Rehabilitation Journal, 92*(8), 1006–1016. https://doi.org/10.2522/ptj.20110282

Yamada, N., Kakuda, W., Kondo, T., Mitani, S., Shimizu, M., & Abo, M. (2014). Local muscle injection of botulinum toxin type A synergistically improves the beneficial effects of repetitive transcranial magnetic stimulation and intensive occupational therapy in post-stroke patients with spastic upper limb hemiparesis. *European Neurology, 72*(5-6), 290–298. https://doi.org/10.1159/000365005

Yamada, N., Kakuda, W., Kondo, T., Shimizu, M., Mitani, S., & Abo, M. (2013). Bihemispheric repetitive transcranial magnetic stimulation combined with intensive occupational therapy for upper limb hemiparesis after stroke: A preliminary study. *International Journal of Rehabilitation Research, 36*(4), 323–329. https://doi.org/10.1097/MRR.0b013e3283624907

Yamada, N., Kakuda, W., Senoo, A., Kondo, T., Mitani, S., Shimizu, M., & Abo, M. (2013). Functional cortical reorganization after low-frequency repetitive transcranial magnetic stimulation plus intensive occupational therapy for upper limb hemiparesis: Evaluation by functional magnetic resonance imaging in poststroke patients. *International Journal of Stroke, 8*(6), 422–429. https://doi.org/10.1111/ijs.12056

Yang, C.-L., Lin, K.-C., Chen, H.-C., Wu, C.-Y., & Chen, C.-L. (2012). Pilot comparative study of unilateral and bilateral robot-assisted training on upper-extremity performance in patients with stroke. *American Journal of Occupational Therapy, 66*(2), 198–206. https://doi.org/10.5014/ajot.2012.003103

Yin, C. W., Sien, N. Y., Ying, L. A., Chung, S. F.-C. M., & Leng, D. T. M. (2014). Virtual reality for upper extremity rehabilitation in early stroke: A pilot randomized controlled trial. *Clinical Rehabilitation, 28*(11), 1107–1114. https://doi.org/10.1177/0269215514532851

Yu, G.-H., Lee, J.-S., Kim, S.-K., & Cha, T.-H. (2017). Effects of interactive metronome training on upper extremity function, ADL and QOL in stroke patients. *NeuroRehabilitation, 41*(1), 161–168. https://doi.org/10.3233/NRE-171468

BIBLIOGRAPHY

Ahn, S.-N. (2018). Differences in body awareness and its effects on balance function and independence in activities of daily living for stroke. *Journal of Physical Therapy Science, 30*(11), 1386–1389. https://doi.org/10.1589/jpts.30.1386

Carey, L. M. (Ed.). (2012). *Stroke rehabilitation: Insights from neuroscience and imaging.* Oxford University Press.

Carey, L. M., Abbott, D. F., Harvey, M. R., Puce, A., Seitz, R., & Donnan, G. A. (2011). Relationship between touch impairment and brain activation after lesions of subcortical and cortical somatosensory regions. *Neurorehabilitation and Neural Repair, 25*(5), 443–457. https://doi.org/10.1177/1545968310395777

Carey, L. M., & Matyas, T. A. (2011). Frequency of discriminative sensory loss in the hand after stroke in a rehabilitation setting. *Journal of Rehabilitation Medicine, 43*(3), 257–263. https://doi.org/10.2340/16501977-0662

de Oliverira, M. C., Demartino, A. M., Rodrigues, L. C., Gomes, R. P., & Michaelsen, S. M. (2018). The activity assessment instruments of the upper limbs do contemplate* the most accomplished task at home by people with hemiparesis? *Cadernos Brasileiros de Terapia Ocupacional, 26*(4), 809–827. https://doi.org/10.4322/2526-8910.ctoAO1219

Doyle, S., Bennett, S., & Gustafsson, L. (2013). Occupational therapy for upper limb post-stroke sensory impairment: A survey. *British Journal of Occupational Therapy, 76*(10), 434–442. https://doi.org/10.4276/030802213X13807217284143

Gillen, G. (Ed.). (2016). *Stroke rehabilitation: A function-based approach* (4th ed.). Mosby.

Kisara, Y., Fujita, T., Ohashi, T., Yamane, K., & Sato, A. (2018). Relationship of unaffected grip strength and trunk function with toileting performance in stroke patients. *Asian Journal of Occupational Therapy, 14*(1), 17–21. https://doi.org/10.11596/asiajot.14.17

Miczak, K., & Padova, J. (2018). Muscle overactivity in the upper motor neuron syndrome: Assessment and problem solving for complex cases: the role of physical and occupational therapy. *Physical Medicine and Rehabilitation Clinics of North America, 29*(3), 529–536. https://doi.org/10.1016/j.pmr.2018.03.006

Pollock, A., Farmer, S. E., Brady, M. C., Langhorne, P., Mead, G. E., Mehrholz, J., & van Wijck, F. (2014). Interventions for improving upper limb function after stroke. *Cochrane Database of Systematic Reviews, 11,* Article CD010820. https://doi.org/10.1002/14651858.CD0108 20.pub2

Pumpa, L. U., Cahill, L. S., & Carey, L. M. (2015). Somatosensory assessment and treatment after stroke: An evidence-practice gap. *Australian Occupational Therapy Journal, 62*(2), 93–104. https://doi.org/10.1111/1440-1630.12170

Rand, D. (2018). Proprioception deficits in chronic stroke-Upper extremity function and daily living. *PLOS ONE, 13*(3), Article e0195043. https://doi.org/10.1371/journal.pone.0195043

Salbach, T. R., & Rehabilitation and Recovery Following Stroke Writing Group. (2019). *Management of the arm and hand following stroke.* Heart and Stroke Foundation.

Semenko, B., Thalman, L., Ewert, E., Delorme, R., Hui, S., Flett, H., & Lavoie, N. (2015). *An evidence based occupational therapy toolkit for assessment and treatment of the upper extremity post stroke.* Winnipeg Regional Health Authority. https://professionals.wrha.mb.ca/old/professionals/occupational-therapy/files/Stroke-UEToolkit.pdf

---

*The published article includes this typo.

Swallowing Disorders: Adult

Also called dysphagia or deglutition disorders.

Description

Swallowing disorder, or dysphagia, is difficulty swallowing. The condition results from difficulty transferring or transporting liquids, solids, or both from the mouth (oral cavity or pharynx) to the stomach (Porter, 2018). The disorder may affect mastication, sucking, saliva management, bolus passage, and control through the oral cavity, pharynx, or esophageal entrance and impair airway protection (Swan et al., 2015). (Note: Feeding and eating problems in infants and children are covered under Feeding Disorders in Children in Section 1: Development Disorders. This chapter focuses primarily on adults.)

Cause

Two types and causes: Oropharyngeal dysphagia (OD) is difficulty chewing and emptying material (food or liquids) from the oropharynx into the esophagus, which results from abnormal function proximal to the esophagus, most often occurring in patients with neurologic conditions or muscular disorders that affect skeletal muscles. Esophageal dysphagia (ED) is difficulty passing food down the esophagus, which results from either a motility disorder or a mechanical obstruction (Porter, 2018). Therapists work primarily with oropharyngeal dysphagia.

Phases of Swallowing (Adapted from Avery, 2018)

- *Preoral phase:* Physical and cognitive orientation to eating occurs. Self-feeding occurs during the preoral phase while the client moves food or liquid to the mouth. The preoral phase is mostly voluntary.
- *Oral preparatory phase:* A food or liquid bolus is made by the structures of the oral cavity, which involves tasting, chewing, manipulating, and containing the bolus in the mouth. The oral preparatory phase is also primarily voluntary.
- *Oral phase:* The bolus is propelled toward the pharynx by motion of the tongue against the hard and soft palates. Voluntary and involuntary actions occur during the oral phase.
- *Pharyngeal phase:* The soft palate elevates to close off the nasopharynx. The larynx lifts and protracts. The epiglottis moves posteriorly to cover the opening to the larynx, preventing the food or liquid bolus from entry. The swallow response is initiated as the bolus is propelled through the pharynx during closure of the larynx and the opening of the upper esophageal sphincter. The pharyngeal phase is primarily involuntary, although voluntary controls may alter its motions.
- *Esophageal phase:* The upper esophageal sphincter returns to its closed position to keep food or liquid from entering the pharynx. The bolus travels through the esophagus. The lower esophageal sphincter opens, allowing the bolus to pass into stomach. The esophageal phase is involuntary although body position changes may alter the movement of the bolus through the esophagus.

Evaluation/Assessment

Areas

- Activities of Daily Living/Instrumental ADL: eating foods of different textures, drinking liquids of different consistencies, meal preparation and diet planning, grocery shopping
- Education/Work: may not be directly affected unless the person works as a taste tester
- Play/Leisure: effect, if any, depends on whether leisure occupation includes food or drink, such as going to cooking classes or sampling wines and cheeses
- Rest/Sleep: sleep disturbances

- Social Participation: may limit participation in eating and dining with family and friends at home, on picnics, or at restaurants
- Sensorimotor: swallowing reflexes, tongue and epiglottis mobility, jaw muscle strength, cranial nerve function, palate elevation, hand functions, body positioning and alignment, upper extremity muscle strength, upper extremity joint range of motion, taste, smell, vision, touch, pain
- Cognitive/Perceptual: attention, memory, executive functions
- Psychosocial: depression, anxiety, apathy, quality of life
- Context/Environment: adapted devices, information resources, social support
- Comorbidities: neurological disorders, musculoskeletal disorders, mental health disorders, and systemic disorders

Instruments

Instruments Developed by Occupational Therapy Personnel

- Acute Stroke Dysphagia Screen (ASDS; Edmiaston et al., 2010, in References; also called the Barnes-Jewish Hospital-Stroke Dysphagia Screen [BJH-SDS], Edmiaston et al., 2014, in References)
- Dysphagia Evaluation Protocol (DEP; Avery-Smith et al., 1997)
- McGill Ingestive Skills Assessment (MISA; Lambert et al., 2003; see also Francis-Bacz et al., 2013; and Hansen et al., 2011, in References)
- Occupational Therapy Clinical Dysphagia Assessment (OTCDA; Meriano, 2010, in References; see Latella & Meriano, 2010, in References)
- Three-Step Dysphagia Screen (TSDS; Latella, 2010, in References; see Latella & Meriano, 2010, in References)

Instruments and Procedures Developed by Other Professionals and Used by Occupational Therapy Personnel

- 3-oz Water Swallow Test (3WST; DePippo et al., 1992)
- Bedside Evaluation of Dysphagia (BED; Hardy, 1995)
- Bolus scintigraphy (instrument measurement)
- Burke Dysphagia Screening Tool (BDST; DePippo et al., 1994)
- Caregiver Mealtime and Dysphagia Questionnaire (CDMQ; Colodny, 2008)
- Eating Assessment Tool (EAT-10; Belafsky et al., 2008; see also Cordier et al., 2017, in References)
- Electromyography (instrument measurement)
- Endoscopy (instrument measurement)
- Esophageal manometry (instrument measurement)
- Functional Oral Intake Scale (FOIS; Crary et al., 2005)
- Gugging Swallowing Screen (GSS; Trapl et al., 2007)
- Mann Assessment of Swallowing Ability (MASA; Mann, 2002)
- Mini-Mental State Examination (MMSE; Folstein et al., 1975)
- Modified barium swallow (MBS) procedure
- Northwestern Dysphagia Patient Check Sheet (NDPCS; Logemann et al., 1999; reproduced in Latella & Meriano, 2010; in References)
- Self-Report Symptom Inventory (SRSI: Wallace et al., 2000; reproduced in Latella & Meriano, 2010, in References)
- Standardized Bedside Swallowing Assessment (SBSA; Ellul et al., 1997, in References)
- Successful EATing (Boylston & O'Day, 1999)
- Surface electromyography (instrument measurement)
- Swallowing . . . on a Plate (SOAP; Shanley & O'Loughlin, 1996)
- Swallowing Quality of Life questionnaire (SWAL-QOL; McHorney et al., 2002)
- Ultrasound (instrument measurement)
- Time Test of Swallowing (TTS; Hinds & Wiles, 1998)
- Videofluoroscopic Dysphagia Scale (VDS; Han et al., 2008)
- Videofluoroscopic swallowing study (VFSS; instrument measurement)

Problems/Issues

Activities of Daily Living/Instrumental ADL

- Person may have difficulty chewing foods of certain textures due to weak jaw muscles, lack of teeth, or both.
- Person may have difficulty moving food around mouth to position for chewing or preparing bolus for swallowing.
- Person may have difficulty managing liquids of different consistencies to control liquid in preparation for swallowing.
- Person may have difficulty with swallowing mechanism.
- Person may have difficulty maintaining liquid in center of mouth to align for swallowing.
- Person may lose weight and endanger overall health due to difficulty with swallowing.

Education/Work

- Person may choose not to participate in break times due to difficulties managing swallowing difficulties.

Play/Leisure

- Person may limit engagement in leisure occupations if food or meals are involved.

Rest/Sleep

- Person may have difficulty staying awake long enough to finish eating or drinking.

Social Participation

- Person may be unable to participate or restrict participation in social events that involve eating and drinking, such as going out with family or friends to a restaurant to celebrate a birthday.

Sensorimotor

- Person may have weakened jaw and lip (oropharyngeal) muscles, called presbyphagia.
- Person may have difficulty controlling saliva.
- Person may have difficulty with tongue or epiglottis mobility.
- Person may have tongue tremor.
- Person may have slow or prolonged food bolus flow.
- Person may have delayed swallowing reflex.
- Person may have poor or inadequate palate elevation.
- Person may experience regurgitation.
- Person may experience tracheal penetration or aspiration.
- Person may be missing teeth or have poorly fitting dentures that hinder effective chewing.
- Person may assume poor positioning and alignment while eating or drinking or be unable to assume a good body position and alignment without support.
- Person may lack coordination of upper extremity to retrieve food or drink and bring same to mouth.
- Person may have difficulty holding onto eating or drinking utensils in desired position to insert food or liquid into mouth.
- Person may experience aspiration of foods or liquids.
- Person may experience episodes of coughing.
- Person may experience pain in jaw or throat.
- Person may be unable to taste different types of foods or liquids.
- Person may be unable to smell different types of foods or liquids.

Cognitive/Perceptual

- Person may have difficulty attending to eating and drinking tasks (become easily distracted).
- Person may have difficulty remembering what foods or liquids should be eaten or drunk versus those that are not recommended.
- Person may take extra time to finish eating or drinking, which is calculated into time management allotted for eating and drinking.

Psychosocial
- Person may refuse to eat or drink due to depression.
- Person may have certain attitudes (preferences, religious practices) about food or drink.
- Person may experience decreased quality of life due to difficulties with chewing and swallowing (Carneiro et al., 2013; Hong & Yoo, 2017).

Context/Environment
- Person, family, and caregivers may lack knowledge about dysphagia and its consequences to health and well-being.
- Person, family, and caregivers may lack access to resources to manage dysphagia.
- Person, family, and caregivers may require instruction and training to manage dysphagia.

Intervention/Treatment

Models and programs developed by occupational therapy personnel include bedside self-exercise program (Cho et al., 2017), head extension swallowing exercise (J.-C. Oh, 2016), occupational therapy role (Avery, 2011), and tongue strengthening (J.-S. Park et al., 2015). Models and programs developed by other professionals but used by occupational therapy personnel include case study (Dismukes et al., 2018), chin tuck against resistance exercise (CTAR; J.-S. Park, An, et al., 2018), effortful swallow and electrical stimulation (J.-S. Park, Oh, et al., 2018; J.-S. Park, Oh, Hwang, et al., 2016; J.-W. Park et al., 2012), expiratory muscle strengthening (Eom et al., 2017; Moon et al., 2017; J.-S. Park, Oh, Chang, et al., 2016), head lift exercise (J.-S. Park et al., 2017), high-frequency rTMS (J.-W. Park et al., 2013), jaw opening exercise (D. H. Oh, Won, et al., 2017), Kinesio Taping (Heo & Kim, 2015), manual facilitation (Won, 2012), Mendelsohn maneuver and effortful swallowing (J.-H. Kim et al., 2017), neck exercises (K. D. Kim et al., 2015), neuromuscular electrical stimulation (Choi, 2016; D.-H. Oh, Park, & Kim, 2017; J.-S. Park et al., 2019; J.-S. Park, Oh, Hwang, et al., 2016), Shaker exercise (Choi et al., 2017), and tongue-to-palate resistance raining (H. D. Kim et al., 2017). Team members include physicians, nursing personnel, speech–language pathologists, physical therapy personnel, dieticians and nutritionists, family members, caregivers, and occupational therapy personnel. Goal is to improve preparation and intake of food and drink to support healthy living.

Activities of Daily Living/Instrumental ADL
- Modify diet texture
  - Level 1: pureed, pudding, applesauce (little or no chewing required).
  - Level 2: soft macaroni and cheese, soft cooked vegetables, semisolid foods requiring some chewing.
  - Level 3: soft foods.
- Modify liquid viscosity: thin, nectar thick, honey thick, or spoon thick.
- Schedule more frequent eating times with less food, more snacks.

Education/Work
- Schedule breaks and meals when fewer people are in the break room or cafeteria.
- Bring snacks that client knows can be eaten instead of depending on what is available.

Play/Leisure
- Arrange schedule to reduce eating time during leisure occupation.

Rest/Sleep
- Adjust eating times around sleep schedule. Some clients may prefer to snack before a nap or bedtime while others sleep better after food has been digested.

Social Participation
- Schedule visits to public eating places during quieter, less crowded times.
- Provide meaningful activities during wait times at restaurants.

Sensorimotor

- Provide preparatory exercises prior to eating to facilitate oral and pharyngeal motions.
- Provide stimulation through vibration, tapping, and stretching.
- Provide a sensory diet to heighten tactile and proprioceptive input to stimulate sensation and movement prior to eating.
- Use desensitizing and calming approaches to address hypersensitivities.
- Facilitate optimal digestion of food and drink through optimal positioning.
- Position upper arm for maximum participation in eating process.
- Position body for safety while eating and drinking.
- Reinforce strategies that enhance and improve swallowing safety.

Cognitive/Perceptual

- No information identified.

Psychosocial

- Prepare client for eating by talking about meal 5 to 10 minutes before food is served.

Context/Environment

- Modify mealtime environment including visual presentation of meal to encourage eating, increase opportunity to smell food before eating, provide type of music person enjoys, decrease background noise, and provide a quiet environment.
- Provide adapted eating utensils that create a sense of independence.
- Train family members and caregivers to individualize feeding and swallowing strategies.

Precautions/Safety Considerations

- Aspiration pneumonia (food or liquid going down trachea).
- Choking hazards (food not chewed adequately, bolus too large or in wrong position in mouth, swallowing reflex not working in sequence).
- Obstruction to breathing cycle (swallowing process takes too long and interferes with breathing).
- Thickeners used to change the consistency of food are not liked by clients (make food taste different) and may not provide adequate hydration. Try finding a food of the correct consistency.

Prognosis and Outcome

Variable. Outcome is usually dependent on prognosis of underlying condition.

REFERENCES

Avery, W. (2011). Fact sheet: *Occupational therapy: A vital role in dysphagia care*. American Occupational Therapy Association.

Carneiro, D., Belo, L. R., Coriolano, M. G. W. S., Asano, A. G. C., & Lins, O. G. (2013). Quality of life in dysphagia in Parkinson's disease: A systematic review. *Revista CEFAC, 15*(5), 1347–1356.

Cho, Y. S., Oh, D. H., Paik, Y. R., Lee, J. H., & Park, J. S. (2017). Effects of bedside self-exercise on oropharyngeal swallowing function in stroke patients with dysphagia: A pilot study. *Journal of Physical Therapy Science, 29*(10), 1815–1816. https://doi.org/10.1589/jpts.29.1815

Choi, J.-B. (2016). Effect of neuromuscular electrical stimulation on facial muscle strength and oral function in stroke patients with facial palsy. *Journal of Physical Therapy Science, 28*(9), 2541–2543. https://doi.org/10.1589/jpts.28.2541

Choi, J.-B., Shim, S.-H., Yang, J.-E., Kim, H.-D., Lee, D.-H., & Park, J.-S. (2017). Effects of Shaker exercise in stroke survivors with oropharyngeal dysphagia. *NeuroRehabilitation, 41*(4), 753–757. https://doi.org/10.3233/NRE-172145

Cordier, R., Joosten, A., Clavé, P., Schindler, A., Bülow, M., Demir, N. Arslan, S. S., & Speyer, R. (2017). Evaluating the psychometric properties of the Eating Assessment Tool (EAT-10) using Rasch analysis. *Dysphagia, 32*, 250–260. https://doi.org/10.1007/s00455-016-9754-2

Dismukes, D., Thrush, A., & Copeland, J. M. (2018). Using interprofessional collaboration to help patients with dysphagia. *SIS Quarterly Practice Connections, 3*(1), 21–23.

Edmiaston, J., Connor, L. T., Loehr, L., & Nassief, A. (2010). Validation of a dysphagia screening tool in acute stroke patients. *American Journal of Critical Care, 19*(4), 357–364. https://doi.org/10.4037/ajcc2009961

Edmiaston, J., Connor, L. T., Steger-May, K., & Ford, A. L. O. (2014). A simple bedside stroke dysphagia screen, validated against videofluoroscopy, detects dysphagia and aspiration with high sensitivity. *Journal of Stroke and Cerebrovascular Diseases, 23*(4), 712–716. https://doi.org/10.1016/j.jstrokecerebrovasdis.2013.06.030

Ellul, J., Barer, D., & Fall, S. (1997). Improving detection and management of swallowing problems in acute stroke: A multicenter study. *Cerebrovascular Disease, 7*(Suppl. 4), 18.

Eom, M.-J., Chang, M.-Y., Oh, D.-H., Kim, H.-D., Han, N.-M., & Park, J.-S. (2017). Effects of resistance expiratory muscle strength training in elderly patients with dysphagic stroke. *NeuroRehabilitation, 41*(4), 747–752. https://doi.org/10.3233/NRE-172192

Francis-Bacz, C., Wood-Dauphinee, S., & Gisel, E. (2013). The discriminative validity of the McGill Ingestive Skills Assessment. *Physical & Occupational Therapy in Geriatrics, 31*(2), 148–158. https://doi.org/10.3109/02703181.2013.775689

Hansen, T., Lambert, H. C., & Faber, J. (2011). Content validation of a Danish version of "The McGill Ingestive Skills Assessment" for dysphagia management. *Scandinavian Journal of Occupational Therapy, 18*(4), 282–293. https://doi.org/10.3109/11038128.2010.521949

Heo, S. Y., & Kim, K. M. (2015). Immediate effects of Kinesio Taping on the movement of the hyoid bone and epiglottis during swallowing by stroke patients with dysphagia. *Journal of Physical Therapy Science, 27*(11), 3355–3357.

Hong, D. G., & Yoo, D. H. (2017). A comparison of the swallowing function and quality of life by oral intake level in stroke patients with dysphagia. *Journal of Physical Therapy Science, 29*(9), 1552–1554. https://doi.org/10.1589/jpts.29.1552

Kim, H. D., Choi, J. B., Yoo, S. J., Chang, M. Y., Lee, S. W., & Park, J. S. (2017). Tongue-to-palate resistance training improves tongue strength and oropharyngeal swallowing function in subacute stroke survivors with dysphagia. *Journal of Oral Rehabilitation, 44*(1), 59–64. https://doi.org/10.1111/joor.12461

Kim, J.-H., Kim, Y.-A., Lee, H.-J., Kim, K.-S., Kim, S.-T., Kim, T.-S., & Cho, Y.-S. (2017). Effect of the combination of Mendelsohn maneuver and effortful swallowing on aspiration in patients with dysphagia after stroke. *Journal of Physical Therapy Science, 29*(11), 1967–1969. https://doi.org/10.1589/jpts.29.1967

Kim, K. D., Lee, H. J., Lee, M. H., & Ryu, H. J. (2015). Effects of neck exercises on swallowing function of patients with stroke. *Journal of Physical Therapy Science 27*(4), 1005–1008. https://doi.org/10.1589/jpts.27.1005

Latella, D. (2010). Three-Step Dysphagia Screen. In W. Avery (Ed.), *Dysphagia care and related feeding concerns for adults* (2nd ed., p. 87). AOTA Press.

Latella, D., & Meriano, C. (2010). Clinical evaluation of dysphagia. In W. Avery (Ed.), *Dysphagia care and related feeding concerns for adults* (2nd ed., pp. 83–120). AOTA Press.

Meriano, C. (2010). Occupational Therapy Clinical Dysphagia Assessment. In W. Avery (Ed.), *Dysphagia care and related feeding concerns for adults* (2nd ed., p. 99). AOTA Press.

Moon, J. H., Jung, J.-H., Won, Y. S., Cho, H.-Y., & Cho, K.-H. (2017). Effects of expiratory muscle strength training on swallowing function in acute stroke patients with dysphagia. *Journal of Physical Therapy Science, 29*(4), 609–612. https://doi.org/10.1589/jpts.29.609

Oh, D.-H., Park, J.-S., & Kim, W.-J. (2017). Effect of neuromuscular electrical stimulation on lip strength and closure function in patients with dysphagia after stroke. *Journal of Physical Therapy Science, 29*(11), 1974–1975. https://doi.org/10.1589/jpts.29.1974

Oh, D.-H., Won, J.-H., Kim, Y.-A., & Kim, W.-J. (2017). Effects of jaw opening exercise on aspiration in stroke patients with dysphagia: A pilot study. *Journal of Physical Therapy Science, 29*(10), 1817–1818. https://doi.org/10.1589/jpts.29.1817

Oh, J.-C. (2016). A pilot study of the head extension swallowing exercise: New method for strengthening swallowing-related muscle activity. *Dysphagia, 31*, 680–686. https://doi.org/10.1007/s00455-016-9732-8

Park, J.-S., An, D.-H., Oh, D.-H., & Chang, M.-Y. (2018). Effect of chin tuck against resistance exercise on patients with dysphagia following stroke: A randomized pilot study. *NeuroRehabilitation, 42*(2), 191–197. https://doi.org/10.3233/NRE-172250

Park, J.-S., Hwang, N.-K., Kim, H.-H., Lee, G., & Jung, Y.-J. (2019). Effect of neuromuscular electrical stimulation combined with effortful swallowing using electromyographic biofeedback on oropharyngeal swallowing function in stroke patients with dysphagia: A pilot study. *Medicine, 98*(44), Article e17702. https://doi.org/10.1097/MD.0000000000017702

Park, J.-S., Hwang, N.-K., Oh, D.-H., & Chang, M.-Y. (2017). Effect of head lift exercise on kinematic motion of the hyolaryngeal complex and aspiration in patients with dysphagic stroke. *Journal of Oral Rehabilitation, 44*(5), 385–391. https://doi.org/10.1111/joor.12492

Park, J.-S., Kim, H.-J., & Oh, D.-H. (2015). Effect of tongue strength training using the Iowa Oral Performance Instrument in stroke patients with dysphagia. *Journal of Physical Therapy Science, 27*(12), 3631–3634. https://doi.org/10.1589/jpts.27.3631

Park, J.-S., Oh, D.-H., Chang, M.-Y., & Kim, K.-M. (2016). Effects of expiratory muscle strength training on oropharyngeal dysphagia in subacute stroke patients: A randomised controlled trial. *Journal of Oral Rehabilitation, 43*(5), 364–372. https://doi.org/10.1111/joor.12382

Park, J.-S., Oh, D.-H., Hwang, N.-K., & Lee, J.-H. (2016). Effects of neuromuscular electrical stimulation combined with effortful swallowing on post-stroke oropharyngeal dysphagia: A randomised controlled trial. *Journal of Oral Rehabilitation, 43*(6), 426–434. https://doi.org/10.1111/joor.12390

Park, J.-S., Oh, D.-H., Hwang, N.-K., & Lee, J.-H. (2018). Effects of neuromuscular electrical stimulation in patients with Parkinson's disease and dysphagia: A randomized, single-blind, placebo-controlled trial. *NeuroRehabilitation, 42*(4), 457–463. https://doi.org/10.3233/NRE-172306

Park, J.-W., Oh, J.-C., Lee, J.-W., Yeo, J.-S., & Ryu, K.-H. (2013). The effect of 5Hz high-frequency rTMS over contralesional pharyngeal motor cortex in post-stroke oropharyngeal dysphagia: A randomized controlled study. *Neurogastroenterology & Motility, 25*(4), e224–e250. https://doi.org/10.1111/nmo.12063

Park, J.-W., Kim, Y., Oh, J.-C., & Lee, H.-J. (2012). Effortful swallowing training combined with electrical stimulation in post-stroke dysphagia: A randomized controlled study. *Dysphagia, 27*(4), 521–527. https://doi.org/10.1007/s00455-012-9403-3

Porter, R. S. (Ed.). (2018). *The Merck manual of diagnosis and therapy* (20th ed.). Merck Sharp & Dohme.

Swan, K., Speyer, R., Heijnen, B. J., Wagg, B., & Cordier, R. (2015). Living with oropharyngeal dysphagia: Effects of bolus modification on health-related quality of life—A systematic review. *Quality of Life Research, 24*, 2447–2456. https://doi.org/10.1007/s11136-015-0990-y

Won, Y. S. (2012). Influence of manual facilitation technique on swallowing disorder and aspiration pneumonia caused by severe dysphagia with stroke. *Journal of Physical Therapy Science, 24*(9), 909–913. https://doi.org/10.1589/jpts.24.909

BIBLIOGRAPHY

American Occupational Therapy Association. (2017). The practice of occupational therapy in feeding, eating, and swallowing. *American Journal of Occupational Therapy, 71*(Suppl. 2), Article 7112410015. https://doi.org/10.5014/ajot.2017.716S04

Avery, W. (Ed.). (2010). *Dysphagia care and related feeding concerns for adults* (2nd ed.). AOTA Press.

Avery, W. (2011). Dysphagia management. In G. Gillen (Ed.), *Stroke rehabilitation* (3rd ed., pp. 629–647). Elsevier Mosby.

Avery, W. (2014). Dysphagia. In M. V. Radomski & C. A. Trombly Latham (Eds.), *Occupational therapy for physical dysfunction* (7th ed., pp. 1327–1351). Wolters Kluwer.

Avery, W. (2016). Dysphagia management. In G. Gillen (Ed.), *Stroke rehabilitation* (4th ed., pp. 690–709). Elsevier.

Avery, W. (2018). Dysphagia. In H. Smith-Gabai & S. E. Holm (Eds.), *Occupational therapy in acute care* (2nd ed., pp. 583–598). AOTA Press.

Lee, M. L., Kim, J. U., Oh, D. H., Park, J. Y., & Lee, K. J. (2018). Oropharyngeal swallowing function in patients with presbyphagia. *Journal of Physical Therapy Science, 30*(11), 1357–1358. https://doi.org/10.1589/jpts.30.1357

Martino, R., Beaton, D., & Diamant, N. E. (2010). Perceptions of psychological issues related to dysphagia differ in acute and chronic patients. *Dysphagia, 25*(1), 26–34.

Oh, J.-C., Park, J.-H., Jung, M.-Y., Yoo, E.-Y., Chang, K.-Y., & Lee, T.-Y. (2016). Relationship between quantified instrumental swallowing examination and comprehensive clinical swallowing examination. *Occupational Therapy International, 23*(1), 3–10. https://doi.org/10.1002/oti.1391

Paul, S., & D'Amico, M. (2013). The role of occupational therapy in the management of feeding and swallowing disorders. *New Zealand Journal of Occupational Therapy, 60*(2), 27–31.

Smith, J. (2018). Eating and swallowing. In H. M. Pendleton & W. Schultz-Krohn (Eds.), *Pedretti's occupational therapy* (8th ed., pp. 669–700). Elsevier Mosby.

Cardiopulmonary Disorders

Cardiac Conditions

Description

Several cardiac conditions are combined in this chapter because the issues for occupational therapy are similar.

- *Cardiac arrest* (CA) is the cessation of cardiac mechanical activity resulting in the absence of circulating blood flow. Cardiac arrest stops blood from flowing to vital organs, depriving them of oxygen to meet the metabolic requirements of body tissue (O'Toole, 2017; Porter, 2018).
- *Congestive heart failure* (CHF) describes impaired ability of the heart to pump blood and the inability of the heart to maintain the metabolic needs of the body. Causes include myocardial infarction, ischemic heart disease, and cardiomyopathy (O'Toole, 2017). See also Congenital Heart Disease.
- *Coronary artery disease* (CAD) is an abnormal condition that may affect the heart's arteries and produce various pathological effects, especially the reduced flow of oxygen and nutrients to the myocardium. Also called coronary heart disease (O'Toole, 2017).
- *Coronary artery bypass graft* (CABG) surgery is open heart surgery in which a prosthesis or a section of a vein or internal mammary artery is grafted from the aorta onto one of the coronary arteries, bypassing a narrowing or blockage in the coronary artery (O'Toole, 2017).
- *Heart failure* (HF) is a syndrome of ventricular dysfunction. Left ventricular dysfunction or failure causes shortness of breath (dyspnea) and fatigue. Right ventricular dysfunction or failure causes peripheral and abdominal fluid accumulation (edema). The ventricles can be involved separately or together. Also called cardiac failure (O'Toole, 2017; Porter, 2018).
- *Myocardial infarction* (MI) is necrosis of a portion of the cardiac muscle caused by an obstruction in a coronary artery resulting from atherosclerosis, a thrombus, or a spasm. Also called heart attack (O'Toole, 2017).

Cause

Multiple causes are involved, including hereditary, lifestyle, and environment influences such as cigarette smoking, high blood pressure, diabetes, obesity, high cholesterol level, and lack of routine exercise.

Classification: New York Heart Association (Adapted from Porter, 2018)

- I (None): Ordinary physical activity does not cause undue fatigue, dyspnea, or palpitation.
- II (Mild): Ordinary physical activity causes fatigue, dyspnea, palpitation, or angina.
- III (Moderate): Comfortable at rest, less than ordinary physical activity cause fatigue, dyspnea, palpitation, or angina.
- IV (Severe): Symptoms occur at rest; any physical activity increases discomfort.

Evaluation/Assessment

Areas

- Activities of Daily Living/Instrumental ADL: basic ADLs, mobility, meal planning and preparation, dietary restriction, shopping, medication management
- Education/Work: return to work, retirement
- Play/Leisure: interests, types, frequency, location, structured, unstructured
- Rest/Sleep: sleep disturbance, sleep habits
- Social Participation: type, frequency, location, with whom

- Sensorimotor: endurance (fatigue, lack of energy, activity tolerance), edema management, muscle strength, joint range of motion, fine motor skills (dexterity, coordination), positioning, pain management, visuospatial relations
- Cognitive/Perceptual: attention, memory, executive function (planning, problem-solving, compliance with limitations, judgment of safety, self-management), cognitive impairment, dementia
- Psychosocial: depression, anxiety, emotional distress, role performance, quality of life, sense of well-being, sense of self-efficacy
- Context/Environment: health literacy, patient education, lifestyle modification, environmental modification, resources
- Comorbidities: obesity, diabetes, smoking, mood disorders, hypertension, high cholesterol

Instruments

Instruments Developed by Occupational Therapy Personnel

- Activity Card Sort (2nd ed.; ACS-2; Baum & Edwards, 2008)
- Performance Assessment of Self-Care Skills (Version 4.1; PASS 4.1; Chisholm et al., 2016)

Instruments Developed by Other Professionals and Used by Occupational Therapy Personnel

- Borg Rating of Perceived Exertion Scale (BRPES; Borg, 1982)
- Center for Epidemiologic Studies Depression Scale (CES-D; Radloff, 1977)
- Cerebral Performance Category (CPC; Jennett & Bond, 1975)
- Computer Assessment of Mild Cognitive Impairment (CAMCI; Saxton et al., 2009)
- Extended Glasgow Outcome Scale (GOSE; Wilson et al., 1998)
- Fatigue Impact Scale (FIS; Fisk et al., 1994)
- Fatigue Severity Scale (FSS; Krupp et al., 1989)
- Functional Activities Questionnaire (FAQ; Pfeffer et al., 1982)
- Health Utilities Index (HUI; Furlong et al., 2001)
- Keitel Functional Test (KFT; Holm et al., 2008)
- Media and Technology Usage and Attitudes Scale (MATUAS; Rosen et al., 2013)
- Modified Fatigue Impact Scale (MFIS; Ritvo et al., 1997)
- Modified Rankin Scale (mRS; Lindsay Wilson et al., 2005)
- Participation Objective, Participation Subjective (POPS; Brown et al., 2004)
- Patient Activation Measure (PAM; Hibbard et al., 2004; Insignia Health)
- Patient Activation Measure–Short Form–13 (PAM-SF-13; Hubbard et al., 2005; see also Ngooi et al., 2017, in References)
- Patient-Reported Outcomes Measurement Information Systems Short Form 8a–Fatigue (PROMIS Fatigue 8a; Lai et al., 2011)
- Self-Care of Heart Failure Index (SCHFI; Riegel et al., 2009)
- Short-Form 36 Health Survey (SF-36; Ware et al., 1993)
- Specific Activity Scale (SAS; Goldman et al., 1981)

Problems/Issues

Activities of Daily Living/Instrumental ADL

- Person may not have enough energy to complete morning routine of bathing, grooming, dressing, preparing and eating breakfast, and brushing teeth.
- Person may have difficulty integrating dietary restrictions into meal planning and preparation.
- Person may experience insufficient energy to prepare meals that have been traditionally prepared.
- Person may report that shopping trips are extremely fatiguing.
- Person may find driving or taking public transportation exhausting.

Education/Work

- Person may be unable to work (paid or unpaid) due to fatigue and/or environmental barriers (Nordgren & Söderlund, 2016).

Play/Leisure
- Person may have stopped engaging in favorite leisure occupations.
- Person may have attempted to replace lost leisure occupations with new ones.

Rest/Sleep
- Person may experience sleep disturbance.
- Person may have poor or irregular sleep habits.

Social Participation
- Person may have stopped participating or limited participation in social activities.

Sensorimotor
- Person usually reports a lack of endurance (energy, activity tolerance).
- Person may experience swelling (edema), especially if right ventricular dysfunction has occurred.
- Person may lose muscle strength and joint range of motion due to reduced activity level.
- Person may experience dyspnea (shortness of breath), especially in left ventricular dysfunction has occurred.
- Person and caregivers may need instruction on positioning to support breathing process.

Cognitive/Perceptual
- Person may experience cognitive impairment (Norris, 2020).
  - Persons with heart failure may have problems with attention, memory, and executive dysfunction.
  - Person with coronary artery disease may have problems with memory and executive dysfunction.
  - Person who has had coronary artery bypass graft surgery may experience problems with executive dysfunction.
- Person may experience visuospatial relations problems, especially if coronary artery disease is present.

Psychosocial
- Person may experience depression.
- Person may experience anxiety and emotional distress.
- Person may experience loss of performance of life roles.
- Person may experience decreased quality of life and life satisfaction after cardiac surgery (Oberai, 2014).
- Person may experience decreased sense of self-efficacy.

Context/Environment
- Person may lack knowledge about cardiac conditions including the specific condition(s) the person has.
- Person may lack health literacy.
- Person may need to make lifestyle changes, such as quitting smoking.
- Person may lack knowledge of community and internet resources.

Intervention/Treatment

Models and programs developed by occupational therapy personnel include Energy Conservation Plus Problem Solving (EC + PS; Kim et al., 2019; Kim et al., 2016, 2017), Hear-Happy Occupations (White & Buyting, 2011), left ventricular assistive device intervention model (Padmanabhan & Thankachan, 2011), occupational therapy in a cardiac rehab service (Quinlan, 2015), outpatient cardiac rehabilitation program (White & Buyting, 2011), and self-management through telehealth (Carroll & Nxumalo, 2017). Models and programs developed by other professionals but used by occupational therapy personnel include Actor-Network Theory (ANT; McDougall et al., 2018), energy conservation program (Norberg et al., 2017), presurgery education

(O'Brien et al., 2013), and Total Artificial Heart Implant (Oldenburg et al., 2018). Team members include physicians, cardiologists, nursing personnel, physical therapy personnel, vocational rehabilitation specialists, and occupational therapy personnel. Goals vary depending on the type of cardiac condition. Typical goals are to increase level of independence and improve cognitive function (Tamuleviciute-Prasciene et al., 2018).

Activities of Daily Living/Instrumental ADL

- Suggest client organize daily tasks into units of activity that stay within activity tolerance, such as changing some morning activities to evening. For example, bathing or showering in the evening may reduce energy expenditure in the morning and add to sleep habits and routines. Another example may be change breakfast to foods that are easy to prepare, such as ready-to-eat cereal or microwavable foods as opposed to foods that must be prepared (bacon, eggs, and toast).
- Assist client to modify routines for home management (cleaning, dusting, vacuuming, doing laundry).
- Provide demonstration and training in shower protocol if client has a ventricular assistive device (VAD).

Education/Work

- Review with client work opportunities (paid and unpaid) that fit within the client's work tolerance, especially those than can be done at home or require minimum travel.
- Suggest trying out different work opportunities.
- Recommend to employer modifications that can accommodate client's needs and limitations.

Play/Leisure

- Assist client to select and engage in leisure occupations that are meaningful to the client.
- Assist client to explore adapting existing leisure occupations to adjust to energy level.
- Assist client to explore new leisure occupations that are within the client's functional ability.

Rest/Sleep

- Assist client to identify sleep disturbances and recommend ways to reduce the disturbances, such as reducing environment issues.
- Assist client to establish and maintain sleep habits and routines that allow client to get adequate rest.

Social Participation

- Encourage client to continue participation in social activities adjusting to level of energy.

Sensorimotor

- Instruct client in energy conservation and motion economy.
- Instruct client in fatigue management.
- Instruct client and caregivers on positioning to maintain breathing process.
- Assist client to develop an exercise program to maintain or increase muscle strength and joint range of motion.
- Assist client to select occupations to maintain or increase fine motor skills including hand functions, dexterity, and coordination.

Cognitive/Perceptual

- Assist client to establish goals and priorities.
- Assist client to create an activity schedule that accounts for activity tolerance.
- Provide practice in increasing attention and concentration.
- Consider providing client with memory aids.
- Provide practice in executive functions such as planning, problem solving, and development of self-management program.

Psychosocial

- Discuss with client issues that lead to anxiety and emotional distress.

- Provide client with approaches to reduce stress, such as deep-breathing exercises, relaxation training, imagery, yoga.
- Assist client to develop and implement a plan to improve quality of life and life satisfaction.
- Assist client to increase sense of self-efficacy including self-management programs.

Context/Environment

- Provide client with training and instruction on the use of equipment such as ventricular assistive device (VAD) or CPAP devices.
- Provide instructions that are free of jargon and use language understood at ages 10 and 11 (elementary Grades 5 and 6) with pictures and illustrations.
- Repeat and review instructions frequently, especially if cognitive impairment is present.
- Assist client to participate in patient education programs such as smoking cessation, weight-loss program, or dietary restrictions to decrease edema, cholesterol, and hypertension.
- Assist client to identify and use resources in the community and on the internet.
- Assist client to identify and modify environmental barriers, such as stairs, or use of adapted equipment, such as a scooter for longer trips.

Precautions/Safety Considerations

- Monitor for difficulty breathing, increased heart rate, or increased blood pressure during intervention sessions.
- Intervention sessions may initially range from 15 to 60 minutes to 2 hours as client can tolerate providing 2 to 5 visits per week, depending on goals and training.

Prognosis and Outcome

Prognosis and outcome are variable depending on the type and extent of disease and degree of heart dysfunction as well as age and other comorbidities. Recovery from cardiac arrest is multifaceted and may continue for months (Raina et al., 2015).

Cost Effectiveness

Rogers et al. (2017), reported that increased spending for occupational therapy services reduced readmission rates for heart failure, pneumonia, and acute myocardial infarction. Jianu and Macovei (2012) reported improved quality of life after occupational therapy intervention.

REFERENCES

Carroll, O., & Nxumalo, K. (2017). Improving heart failure self-management through telehealth services. *OT Practice, 22*(19), 18–20.

Jianu, A., & Macovei, S. (2012). The occupational therapy impact on the recovery of convalescent elderly people after an acute myocardial infarction. *Palestrica of the Third Millennium–Civilization and Sport, 13*(1), 23–26.

Kim, Y. J., Radloff, J. C., Crane, P. A., & Bolin, L. P. (2019). Rehabilitation intervention for individuals with heart failure and fatigue to reduce fatigue impact: A feasibility study. *Annals of Rehabilitation Medicine, 43*(6), 686–699. https://doi.org/10.5535/arm.2019.43.6.686

Kim, Y. J., Rogers, J. C., Raina, K. D., Callaway, C. W., Rittenberger, J. C., Leibold, M. L., & Holm, M. B. (2016). An intervention for cardiac arrest survivors with chronic fatigue: A feasibility study with preliminary outcomes. *Resuscitation, 105,* 109–115. https://doi.org/10.1016/j.resuscitation.2016.05.020

Kim, Y. J., Rogers, J. C., Raina, K. D., Callaway, C. W., Rittenberger, J. C., Leibold, M. L., & Holm, M. B. (2017). Solving fatigue-related problems with cardiac arrest survivors living in the community. *Resuscitation, 118,* 70–74. https://doi.org/10.1016/j.resuscitation.2017.07.005

McDougall, A., Kinsella, E. A., Goldszmidt, M., Harkness, K., Strachan, P., & Lingard, L. (2018). Beyond the realist turn: A socio-material analysis of heart failure self-care. *Sociology of Health & Illness, 40*(1), 218–233. https://doi.org/10.1111/1467-9566.12675

Ngooi, B. X., Packer, T. L., Kephart, G., Warner, G., Koh, K. W. L., Wong, R. C. C., & Lim, S. P. (2017). Validation of the Patient Activation Measure (PAM-13) among adults with cardiac conditions in Singapore. *Quality of Life Research, 26*, 1071–1080. https://doi.org/10.1007/s11136-016-1412-5

Norberg, E.-B., Löfgren, B., Boman, K., Wennberg, P., & Brännström, M. (2017). A client-centred progamme focusing energy conservation for people with heart failure. *Scandinavian Journal of Occupational Therapy, 24*(6), 455–467. https://doi.org/10.1080/11038128.2016.1272631

Nordgren, L., & Söderlund, A. (2016). Heart failure clients' encounters with professionals and self-rated ability to return to work. *Scandinavian Journal of Occupational Therapy, 23*(2), 115–126. https://doi.org/10.3109/11038128.2015.1078840

Norris, J. (2020). Cognitive function in cardiac patients: Exploring the occupational therapy role in lifestyle medicine. *American Journal of Lifestyle Medicine, 14*(1), 61–70. https://doi.org/10.1177/1559827618757189

Oberai, S. (2014). Review study of health related quality of life (HROL) among coronary artery disease patients after cardiac surgery. *Indian Journal of Occupational Therapy, 46*(1), 22–26.

O'Brien, L., McKeough, C., & Abbasi, R. (2013). Pre-surgery education for elective cardiac surgery patients: A survey from the patient's perspective. *Australian Occupational Therapy Journal, 60*(6), 404–409. https://doi.org/10.1111/1440-1630.12068

Oldenburg, H., Brannon, C., Luckhardt, A., & Joyce, D. (2018). Occupational and physical therapy outcome measures with a patient implanted with a Total Artificial Heart: A case report. *Journal of Acute Care Occupational Therapy, 1*(1), 1–20. https://jacotorg.files.wordpress.com/2018/10/jacot_case-report_volume1-number1_fall-2018.pdf

O'Toole, M. T. (Ed.). (2017). *Mosby's dictionary of medicine, nursing & health professions* (10th ed.). Elsevier.

Padmanabhan, K., & Thankachan, S. (2011). Occupational therapy in cardiac care left ventricular assistive devices. *OT Practice, 16*(22), 15–20.

Porter, R. S. (Ed.). (2018). *The Merck manual of diagnosis and therapy* (20th ed.). Merck Sharp & Dohme.

Quinlan, S. (2015). Integrating OT into a cardiac rehab service. *OT News, 23*(5), 41.

Raina, K. D., Rittenberger, J. C., Holm, M. B., & Callaway, C. W. (2015). Functional outcomes one year after a cardiac arrest. *BioMed Research International, 2015*, Article 283608. https://doi.org/10.1155/2015/283608

Rogers, A. T., Bai, G., Lavin, R. A., & Anderson, G. F. (2017). Higher hospital spending on occupational therapy is associated with lower readmission rates. *Medical Care Research and Review, 74*(6), 668–686. https://doi.org/10.1177/1077558716666981

Tamuleviciute-Prasciene, E., Drulyte, K., Jurenaite, G., Kubilius, R., & Bjarnason-Wehrens, B. (2018). Frailty and exercise training: How to provide best care after cardiac surgery or intervention for elder patients with valvular heart disease. *BioMed Research International, 2018*, Article 9849475. https://doi.org/10.1155/2018/9849475

White, C. M., & Buyting, P. L. (2011). Heart-happy occupations in a cardiac rehabilitation circuit. *Occupational Therapy Now, 13*(5), 11–13.

BIBLIOGRAPHY

Huntley, N. (2014). Cardiac and pulmonary diseases. In M. V. Radomski & C. A. Trombly Latham (Eds.), *Occupational therapy for physical dysfunction* (7th ed., pp. 1300–1326). Wolters Kluwer.

Martin, R. (2017). Cardiopulmonary disorders. In B. J. Atchison & D. P. Dirette (Eds.), *Conditions in occupational therapy* (5th ed., pp. 329–342). Wolters Kluwer.

Matthews, M. M. (2018). Cardiac and pulmonary disease. In H. M. Pendleton & W. Schultz-Krohn (Eds.), *Pedretti's occupational therapy* (8th ed., pp. 1117–1133). Elsevier.

Smith-Gabai, H., & Holm, S. E. (2017). The cardiac system. In H. Smith-Gabai & S. E. Holm (Eds.), *Occupational therapy in acute care* (2nd ed., pp. 223–247). AOTA Press.

Chronic Obstructive Pulmonary Disease

Also called COPD, chronic obstructive lung disease. Kinds include asthma,
chronic bronchitis, and emphysema.

Description

Chronic obstructive pulmonary disease (COPD) is airflow limitation to the lungs caused by an inflammatory response to inhaled toxins such as cigarette smoke (Porter, 2018). COPD is a progressive and irreversible condition characterized by diminished inspiratory and expiratory capacity of the lungs (O'Toole, 2017). Dyspnea is a symptom used to characterize a subjective experience of breathing discomfort (Fung et al., 2012).

Cause

Etiology includes inhalational exposure (smoking, air pollution, occupational exposures to mineral or cotton dust, or inhaled chemicals such as cadmium) and genetic factors (alpha-1 antitrypsin deficiency; Porter, 2018).

Evaluation/Assessment

Areas

- Activities of Daily Living/Instrumental ADL: basic ADLs (dressing, showering, walking, stair climbing, medication management, child care), advanced ADLs including independent living skills (housekeeping)
- Education/Work: work history, work conditions, work tasks
- Play/Leisure: interests (gardening, sports), types, frequency, location
- Rest/Sleep: sleep disturbances, sleep disorders
- Social Participation: type, frequency, location, with whom
- Sensorimotor: muscle strength, endurance, fatigue, activity tolerance
- Cognitive/Perceptual: executive functions
- Psychosocial: depression, anxiety, self-esteem, self-efficacy
- Context/Environment: environmental modifications, lifestyle modification, health care literacy
- Comorbidity: cardiovascular disease

Instruments

Instruments Developed by Occupational Therapy Personnel

- ADL Interview (ADL-I) based on the ADL Taxonomy (Törnquist & Sonn, 1994; Sonn et al., 1999; see also Bendixen et al., 2014, in References)
- Canadian Occupational Performance Measure (5th ed.; COPM-5; Law et al., 2014)
- Chronic Respiratory Questionnaire Self-Report (CRQ-SR; Williams et al., 2001)
- Extended Activities of Daily Living Scale (EADLS; see Nottingham Extended Activities of Daily Living)
- Milliken Activities of Daily Living Scale (MAS; Seaton et al., 2005)
- Nottingham Extended Activities of Daily Living (NEADL; Nouri & Lincoln, 1987)
- Pulmonary Rehabilitation Adapted Index of Self-Efficacy (PRAISE; Vincent et al., 2011, in References)

Instruments Developed by Other Professionals and Used by Occupational Therapy Personnel

- 6-minute walking distance (6MWD) test (Troosters et al., 1999)
- Activities of Daily Living Simulation Test (ADL-ST; Ries et al., 1988; see also description of use in Çalik Kütükcü et al., 2015, in References)
- Beard Leisure Satisfaction Scale (BLSS; Beard & Ragheb, 1980)
- BODE Index (body-mass index; Celli et al., 2004)
- Borg Rating of Perceived Exertion Scale (BRPES; Borg, 1982)

- Brief Illness Perception Questionnaire (BIPQ; Broadbent et al., 2006)
- Bristol COPD Knowledge Questionnaire (BCKQ; White et al., 2006)
- Capacity of Daily Living during the Morning (CDLM; Partridge et al., 2010)
- COPD Assessment Test (CAT; Jones et al., 2009; see also Chaplin et al., 2015, in References)
- Dynamometer (grip strength; JAMAR Hydraulic, Lafayette Instrument)
- Endurance Shuttle Walking Test (ESWT; Revill et al., 1999)
- Frenchay Activity Index (FAI; Holbrook & Skilbeck, 1983)
- Functional Performance Inventory (FPI; Leidy, 1999)
- Functional Performance Inventory–Short Form (FPI-SF; Leidy et al., 2012)
- General Anxiety Disorder-7 (GAD-7; Spitzer et al., 2006)
- General Self-Efficacy Scale (GSE; Jerusalem & Schwarzer, 1992)
- Glittre Activities of Daily Living Test (GADLT; Skumlien et al., 2006; see also description of use in Çalik Kütükcü et al., 2015, in References)
- Hospital Anxiety and Depression Scale (HADS; Zigmond & Snaith, 1983)
- Incremental Shuttle Walk Test (ISWT; Singh et al., 1992; see also Houchen-Wollofff et al., 2017, in References)
- London Chest Activities of Daily Living (LCADL) scale (Garrod et al., 2000)
- Manchester Respiratory ADL Questionnaire (MRADL; Yohannes et al., 2000)
- Modified Medical Research Council Dyspnea Scale (MMRC-DS; Kim et al., 2013)
- Pittsburgh Sleep Quality Index (PSQI; Buysse et al., 1989)
- Pulmonary function tests such as forced vital capacity (FVC), forced expiratory volume (FEV), residual volume (RV), and total lung capacity (TTLC)
- Pulmonary Functional Status and Dyspnea Questionnaire–Modified (PFSDq-M; Lareau et al., 1998)
- Pulmonary Functional Status Scale–Short Form (PFSS-11; Chen et al., 2010)
- Rosenberg Self-Esteem Scale (RSES; Rosenberg, 1965)
- Spirometer (various sources)
- St. George's Respiratory Questionnaire (SGRQ; Jones et al., 1992)
- University of California at San Diego Shortness of Breath Questionnaire (UCSD SOBQ; Eakin et al., 1998)

Problems/Issues

Activities of Daily Living/Instrumental ADL

- Person may lack energy or endurance to complete dressing tasks, such as putting on socks and shoes or putting on garments that must go over the head.
- Person may be at risk for losing weight due to low activity, tolerance for eating, or becoming overweight due to lack of exercise or poor food choices.
- Person may lack energy or endurance to walk more than a short distance or climb stairs.
- Person may lack energy or endurance to get in and out of a vehicle or get onto or off of a bus or train.
- Person may have difficulty expending energy for reaching overhead to put dishes away or retrieve items from cupboards.
- Person may have difficulty expending energy for doing laundry, including sorting, folding, and putting items away.
- Person may lack activity tolerance to go to the grocery store, select items, return home, and put items into the refrigerator or pantry.
- Person may lack activity tolerance to complete household tasks such as dusting, sweeping, or vacuuming.
- Person may lack activity tolerance to prepare a meal, serve, and clean up afterwards.
- Person may find driving causes fatigue.
- Person may lack activity tolerance to care for children or pets.
- Person may have difficulty remembering to take medication as prescribed.

Education/Work
- Person may lack energy or endurance to complete tasks that require certain physical actions such as frequent reaching overhead, frequent bending and stooping down, sitting for several hours, walking some distance, walking quickly, climbing stairs, or any combination of such movements.
- Person may experience fatigue by getting to and from work by walking, standing, climbing, or sitting for long periods of time.
- Person may be employed in a work setting that emits occupational exposure which aggravate COPD condition.
- Person may have lost a job or retired due to work conditions that aggravated COPD condition.

Play/Leisure
- Person may be unable to engage in favorite activities due lack of energy, endurance, or physical requirements.

Rest/Sleep
- Person may have a sleep disorder, such as apnea.
- Person may have sleep disturbances.

Social Participation
- Person may have limited or stopped participation in social activities due to lack of energy, endurance, or physical requirements.

Sensorimotor
- Person has reduced airflow, with episodes of breathlessness or dyspnea.
- Person has reduced energy level, endurance, and activity tolerance.
- Person usually experiences fatigue with exertion.
- Person may have reduced muscle strength.

Cognitive/Perceptual
- Person may experience loss of or difficulty with memory.
- Person may experience difficulty with executive functions (planning, organizing, problem-solving, making decisions and choices).

Psychosocial
- Person may become depressed.
- Person may experience loss of self-esteem and self-efficacy.
- Person may experience loss of or changes in role performance.
- Person may experience difficulty being motivated to quit smoking.

Context/Environment
- Person may lack information about COPD and its management.
- Person may lack knowledge of available resources in the community or on the internet.
- Person may lack social support.
- Person may need environment modification at home, at work, and in the community.

Intervention/Treatment

Models and programs developed by occupational therapy personnel include the Canadian Model of Occupational Performance and Engagement (Martinsen et al., 2017), energy conservation and work simplification (Alam, 2016), occupational therapy for end of life (Morgan & White, 2012), and personalized pulmonary rehabilitation occupational therapy (PPR-OT; Maekura et al., 2015). Models and programs developed by other professionals but used by occupational therapy personnel include arm strength training (Çalik Kütükcü et al., 2017), care bundle (Sewell et al., 2017), conceptual model for pulmonary rehabilitation (Sully et al., 2012), home-based rehabilitation program (Horton et al., 2018), patient-needs assessment model (Sully et al., 2011), post-exacerbation pulmonary rehabilitation (PEPR; Revitt et al., 2013; Revitt et al., 2018), qigong (Liu et al., 2012; Ng et al., 2011), respiration rehabilitation program (Oh et al., 2016), and Self-Management Programme of Activity, Coping and Education for Chronic Obstructive Pulmonary Disease (SPACE for COPD; Apps et al., 2013; Mitchell et al., 2014). Team members include physicians, pulmonologists and respiratory therapists, nursing personnel, dieticians, social workers, pharmacists, physical therapy personnel, and occupational therapy personnel. The goal is to reduce feeling of breathlessness or dyspnea, maintain cardiopulmonary capacity, improve quality of life, and improve functional ability to perform valued and meaningful everyday life tasks through education, problem-solving, and use of techniques such as energy conservation (Maekura et al., 2015; Singh & Sewell, 2012).

Activities of Daily Living/Instrumental ADL
- Assist client to explore work simplification strategies for dressing, such as sitting rather than standing, wearing shoes without laces (loafers, shoes with Velcro fasteners), cardigans instead of pullover sweaters, loose-fitting rather than form-fitting garments.
- Assist client to organize kitchen cookware and food storage so that frequently used items are within easy reach, including being left on a stove or countertop.
- Assist client to identify tasks (dressing, meal preparation, leisure) that can be done sitting on a stool rather than standing.
- Assist client to modify bathing tasks, such as using a tub chair, handheld shower head, organizing bathing items into a waterproof basket.
- Assist client in identifying easy to prepare meals or sharing meal preparation and cleanup activities with others.
- Assist client to organize shopping list in order of aisles to reduce amount of walking.
- Assist client to identify and plan nutritious meals that maintain appropriate weight for individual's health status.
- Assist client to organize and follow medication program.

Education/Work
- Review work site (paid or unpaid) to organize activities into a routine than requires less energy expenditure.
- Organize work space to reduce need for reaching overhead or stooping down to open drawers and retrieve items from low shelves.
- Consider whether person may need a permit to park vehicle near the entrance to reduce amount of walking or stair climbing.

Play/Leisure
- Explore with client whether modifications can be made to permit continued engagement in favorite leisure occupations, such as indoor gardening or gardening area at waist height to reduce bending and stooping.
- Explore with client whether new or different leisure occupations may be of interest that require less energy expenditure.

Rest/Sleep
- Consider whether person may need to be referred to a sleep specialist for sleep disorder management.
- Assist client to review sleep habits and routines to facilitate more regular sleep patterns including environment adjustments such as light, noise, and temperature.
- Assist client to review bedding and mattress to permit easier bed mobility and better bed positioning.

Social Participation

- Assist person to participate in social activities by suggesting alternatives, such as shorter outings, more at-home events, fewer people, easy access, less action required of client, more passive participation.

Sensorimotor

- Assist team to develop an appropriate exercise and activity management program to maintain optimal health for individual client, including type, duration, and frequency of exercise.
- Assist client to use energy conservation and work simplification principles, such as pacing and avoid rushing, alternating work and rest breaks, prioritizing tasks, seeking assistance from others.
- Assist client to use good posture to promote breathing and lung function, such as sitting when possible and avoiding lifting arms above shoulder height as much as possible.
- Assist client to use correct body mechanics, including keeping posture upright, keeping arms close to body when carrying objects, keeping load between both arms equal.

Cognitive/Perceptual

- Assist client to plan and organize daily routine and tasks.
- Assist client to make choices about occupations in which to engage (Kerr & Ballinger, 2010).

Psychosocial

- Assist client to differentiate between symptoms of anxiety and inadequate air supply or exchange.
- Develop coping strategies to increase self-management, such as guided imagery, relaxation training, mindfulness, pursed lip breathing.
- Provide group interventions for support and education.
- Support and promote sense of self-esteem and self-efficacy (Bonsaksen et al., 2015).

Context/Environment

- Provide information and education about COPD and its management.
- Assist client to access resources in the community and on the internet.
- Assist team to create a behavioral and pharmacological program for smoking cessation.
- Assist client to select and use household or electric appliances that can conserve energy.
- Consider if telemonitoring may be feasible and practical.

Precautions/Safety Considerations

Person may be at risk for falls.

Prognosis and Outcome

Prognosis is poor. About 50% of clients with severe COPD die within 10 years of diagnosis (Porter, 2018). Intervention needs to individualized because research demonstrates a lack of association between problematic ADLs and clinical determinants (Annegarn et al., 2012). An increase in walking distance improves chance of survival (Houchen-Wolloff et al., 2017). Increased exercise capacity may improve performance in ADLs (Tekerlek et al., 2020; Vaes et al., 2019).

REFERENCES

Alam, M. J. (2016). Occupational therapy in respiratory medicine: Global challenge in the 21st century. *International Journal of Respiratory Medicine, 1*(1), 2–5.

Annegarn, J., Meijer, K., Passos, V. L., Stute, K., Wiechert, J., Savelberg, H. H. C. M., Schols, A. M. W. J., Wouters, E. F. M., & Spruit, M. A. (2012). Problematic activities of daily life are weakly associated with clinical characteristics in COPD. *JAMDA: Journal of the American Medical Directors Association, 13*(3), 284–290. https://doi.org/10.1016/j.jamda.2011.01.002

Apps, L. D., Mitchell, K. E., Harrison, S. L., Sewell, L., Williams, J. E., Young, H. M. L., Steiner, M., Morgan, M., & Singh, S. J. (2013). The development and pilot testing of the self-management programme of activity, coping and education for chronic obstructive pulmonary disease (SPACE for COPD). *International Journal of Chronic Obstructive Pulmonary Disease, 8*, 317–327. https://doi.org/10.2147/COPD.S40414

Bendixen, H. J., Wæhrens, E. E., Wilcke, J. T., & Sørensen, L. V. (2014). Self-reported quality of ADL task performance among patients with COPD exacerbations. *Scandinavian Journal of Occupational Therapy, 21*(4), 313–320. https://doi.org/10.3109/11038128.2014.899621

Bonsaksen, T., Fagermoen, M. S., & Lerdal, A. (2015). Factors associated with self-esteem in persons with morbid obesity and in persons with chronic obstructive pulmonary disease: A cross-sectional study. *Psychology, Health & Medicine, 20*(4), 431–442. https://doi.org/10.10 80/13548506.2014.959529

Çalik Kütükcü, E., Arikan, H., Sağlam, M., Vardar Yağli, N., Öksüz, C., İnal İnce, D., Savci, S., Düger, T., & Çöplü, L. (2015). A comparison of activities of daily living in geriatric and non-geriatric patients with chronic obstructive pulmonary disease. *Turkish Journal of Geriatrics, 18*(1), 68–74.

Çalik Kütükcü, E., Arikan, H., Sağlam, M., Vardar Yağli, N., Öksüz, C., İnal İnce, D., Savci, S., Düger, T., & Çöplü, L. (2017). Arm strength training improves activities of daily living and occupational performance in patients with COPD. *Clinical Respiratory Journal, 11*(6), 820–832. https://doi.org/10.1111/crj.12422

Chaplin, E., Gibb, M., Sewell, L., & Singh, S. (2015). Response of the COPD Assessment Tool in stable and postexacerbation pulmonary rehabilitation populations. *Journal of Cardiopulmonary Rehabilitation and Prevention, 35*(3), 214–218. https://doi.org/10.1097/HCR.0000000000000090

Fung, A., Chan, L. C., So, C. T., Chau, S. S. L., Chan, T. M., Chan, C., Chu, A. W. Y., Ng, B. H. P., Cheung, B. Y. H., Chan, A., K. K., Wong, W. K. W., Chu, C. W. H., & Fong, K. N. K. (2012). Reliability and validity of the self-administered Chinese version of the Shortness of Breath Questionnaire (C-SOBQ) in patients with chronic obstructive pulmonary disease. *Hong Kong Journal of Occupational Therapy, 22*(2), 75–83. https://doi.org/10.1016/j.hkjot.2012.12.010

Horton, E. J., Mitchell, K. E., Johnson-Warrington, V., Apps, L. D., Sewell, L., Morgan, M., Taylor, R. S., & Singh, S. J. (2018). Comparison of a structured home-based rehabilitation programme with conventional supervised pulmonary rehabilitation: A randomized non-inferiority trial. *Thorax, 73*(1), 29–36. https://doi.org/10.1136/thoraxjnl-2016-208506

Houchen-Wolloff, L., Williams, J. E. A., Green, R. H., Woltmann, G., Steiner, M. C., Sewell, L., Morgan, M. D. L., & Singh, S. J. (2017). Survival following pulmonary rehabilitation in patients with COPD: The effect of program completion and change in incremental shuttle walking test distance. *International Journal of Chronic Obstructive Pulmonary Disease, 13*, 37–44. https://doi.org/10.2147/COPD.S143101

Kerr, A., & Ballinger, C. (2010). Living with chronic lung disease: An occupational perspective. *Journal of Occupational Science, 17*(1), 34–39. https://doi.org/10.1080/14427591.2010.9686670

Liu, X.-D., Jin, H.-Z., Ng, B. H.-P., Gu, Y.-H., Wu, Y.-C., & Lu, G. (2012). Therapeutic effects of Qigong in patients with COPD: A randomized controlled trial. *Hong Kong Journal of Occupational Therapy, 22*, 38–46. https://doi.org/10.1016/j.hkjot.2012.06.002

Maekura, R., Hiraga, T., Miki, K., Kitada, S., Miki, M., Yoshimura, K., Yamamoto, H., Kawabe, T., & Mori, M. (2015). Personalized pulmonary rehabilitation and occupational therapy based on cardiopulmonary exercise testing for patients with advanced chronic obstructive pulmonary disease. *International Journal of Chronic Obstructive Pulmonary Disease, 10*(1), 1787–1800. https://doi.org/10.2147/COPD.S86455

Martinsen, U., Bentzen, H., Holter, M. K., Nilsen, T., Skullerud, H., Mowinckel, P., & Kjeken, I. (2017). The effect of occupational therapy in patients with chronic obstructive pulmonary disease: A randomized controlled trial. *Scandinavian Journal of Occupational Therapy, 24*(2), 89–97. https://doi.org/10.3109/11038128.2016.1158316

Mitchell, K. E., Johnson-Warrington, V., Apps, L. D., Bankart, J., Sewell, L., Williams, J. E., Rees, K., Jolly, K., Steiner, M., Morgan, M., & Singh, S. J. (2014). A self-management programme for

COPD: A randomized controlled trial. *European Respiratory Journal, 44*, 1538–1547. https://doi.org/10.1183/09031936.00047814

Morgan, D. D., & White, K. M. (2012). Occupational therapy interventions for breathlessness at the end of life. *Current Opinion in Supportive and Palliative Care, 6*(2), 138–143. https://doi.org/10.1097/SPC.0b013e3283537d0e

Ng, B. H. P., Tsang, H. W. H., Jones, A. Y. M., So, C. T., & Mok, T. Y. W. (2011). Functional and psychosocial effects of health *Qigong* in patients with COPD: A randomized controlled trial. *Journal of Alternative and Complementary Medicine, 17*(3), 243–251. https://doi.org/10.1089/acm.2010.0215

Oh, H.-W., Kim, S.-H., & Kim, K.-U. (2016). The effects a respiration rehabilitation program on IADL, satisfaction with leisure, and quality of sleep of patients with chronic obstructive pulmonary disease. *Journal of Physical Therapy Science, 28*(12), 3357–3360. https://doi.org/10.1589/jpts.28.3357

O'Toole, M. T. (Ed.). (2017). *Mosby's dictionary of medicine, nursing & health professions* (10th ed.). Elsevier.

Porter, R. S. (Ed.). (2018). *The Merck manual of diagnosis and therapy* (20th ed.). Merck Sharp & Dohme.

Revitt, O., Sewell, L., Morgan, M. D., Steiner, M., & Singh, S. (2013). Short outpatient pulmonary rehabilitation programme reduces readmission following a hospitalization for an exacerbation of chronic obstructive pulmonary disease. *Respirology, 18*(7), 1063–1068. https://doi.org/10.1111/resp.12141

Revitt, O., Sewell, L., & Singh, S. (2018). Early versus delayed pulmonary rehabilitation: A randomized controlled trial—Can we do it? *Chronic Respiratory Disease, 15*(3), 323–326. https://doi.org/10.1177/1479972318757469

Sewell, L., Schreder, S., Steiner, M., & Singh, S. J. (2017). A strategy to implement a chronic obstructive pulmonary disease discharge care bundle on a large scale. *Future Healthcare Journal, 6*(3), 198–201. https://doi.org/10.7861/futurehosp.4-3-198

Singh, S., & Sewell, L. (2012). Occupational therapy, environmental modifications, and pulmonary rehabilitation. In S. H. Ahmedzai, D. R. Baldwin, & D. C. Currow (Eds.), *Supportive care in respiratory disease*. Oxford Press. https://doi.org/10.1093/acprof:oso/9780199591763.003.0009

Sully, J.-L., Baltzan, M. A., Wolkove, N., & Demers, L. (2012). Development of a patient needs assessment model for pulmonary rehabilitation. *Qualitative Health Research, 22*(1), 76–88. https://doi.org/10.1177/1049732311418246

Tekerlek, H., Cakmak, A., Çalik Kütükcü, E., Arikan, H., Inal-Ince, D., Saglam, M., Vardar-Yagli, N., Oksuz, C., Duger, T., Savci, S., Bozdemir-Ozel, C., Sonbahar, H., Karaduz, B. N., & Coplu, L. (2020). Exercise capacity and activities of daily living are related in patients with chronic obstructive pulmonary disease. *Archivos de Bronconeumología, 56*(4), 208–213. https://doi.org/10.1016/j.arbres.2019.06.015

Vaes, A. W., Delbressine, J. M. L., Mesquita, R., Goertz, Y. M. J., Janssen, D. J. A., Nakken, N., Franssen, F. M. E., Vanfleteren, L. E. G. W., Wouters, E. F. M., & Spruit, M. A. (2019). Impact of pulmonary rehabilitation on activities of daily living in patients with chronic obstructive pulmonary disease. *Journal of Applied Physiology, 126*(3), 607–615. https://doi.org/10.1152/japplphysiol.00790.2018

Vincent, E., Sewell, L., Wagg, K., Deacon, S., Williams, J., & Singh, S. (2011). Measuring a change in self-efficacy following pulmonary rehabilitation: An evaluation of the PRAISE tool. *Chest, 140*, 1534–1539. https://doi.org/10.1378/chest.10-2649

BIBLIOGRAPHY

Dahl-Popolizio, S., Rogers, O., Muir, S. L., Carroll, J., & Manson, L. (2017). Interprofessional primary care: The value of occupational therapy. *Open Journal of Occupational Therapy, 5*(3), Article 11. https://doi.org/10.15453/2168-6408.1363

Goto, Y. (2017). Measurement of activities of daily living in patients with chronic obstructive pulmonary disease. *Pulmonary Research and Respiratory Medicine, 2,* S23–S25. https://doi.org/10.17140/PRRMOJ-SE-2-104

Mitchell, K. E., Johnson V., Houchen-Wolloff, L., Sewell, L., Morgan, M. D., Steiner, M. C., & Singh, S. J. (2018). Agreement between adherences to four physical activity recommendations in patients with COPD: Does the incremental shuttle walk test predict adherence? *Clinical Respiratory Journal, 12*(2), 510–516. https://doi.org/10.1111/crj.12555

Sewell, L. (2018). Occupational therapy and pulmonary rehabilitation. In C. Clini, A. Holland, F. Pitta, & T. Troosters (Eds.), *Textbook of pulmonary rehabilitation* (pp. 159–169). Springer. https://doi.org/10.1007/978-3-319-65888-9_12

Sewell, L., Singh, S. J., Williams, J. E., & Morgan, M. D. (2010). Seasonal variations affect physical activity and pulmonary rehabilitation outcomes. *Journal of Cardiopulmonary Rehabilitation and Prevention, 30*(5), 329–333. https://doi.org/10.1097/HCR.0b013e3181e175f2

Walker, B. A., Breckner, H., Carrier, M., Pullen, W., Reagan, E., Telfer, L., & Zimmerman, T. (2016). An open-access review to determine best evidence-based practice for COPD. *Open Journal of Occupational Therapy, 4*(2), Article 8. https://doi.org/10.15453/2168-6408.1199

Ward, S., Sewell, L., & Singh, S. (2018). Evaluation of multidisciplinary pulmonary rehabilitation education delivered by either DVD or spoken talk. *Clinical Respiratory Journal, 12*(11), 2546–2550. https://doi.org/10.1111/crj.12954

Congenital Heart Disease

Also called CHD, congenital cardiac anomaly, congenital heart defect.
See also Feeding Disorders in Children, Premature Infant.

Description

The term *congenital heart disease* is used to describe any structural or functional abnormality or defect of the heart or great vessels that is present at birth (O'Toole, 2017).

Cause

Congenital heart disease may be inherited or the result of environmental factors such as material infections (rubella, systemic lupus erythematosus), diabetes, exposure to radiation or exposure to noxious substances (teratogenic agents) during pregnancy (O'Toole, 2017; Porter, 2018). A high prevalence of neurodevelopmental impairments is also reported in adolescents and young adults with congenital heart disease, especially in males (Fontes et al., 2019; Majnemer et al., 2012).

Classification

- Cyanotic heart anomalies: Varying amounts of deoxygenated (lack of oxygen) venous blood are shunted to the left heart (right-to-left shunt), reducing systemic arterial oxygen saturation. Conditions include, in order of frequency: Tetralogy of Fallot, transportation of the great arteries, tricuspid atresia, pulmonary atresia, persistent truncus arteriosus, and total anomalous pulmonary venous return.
- Acyanotic
  - Left-to-right shunt: Oxygenated blood from the left atrium or ventricle or aorta shunts to the right atrium or ventricle or pulmonary artery though an opening between the two sides. Conditions include, in order of frequency: ventricular septal defect, atrial septal defect, patent ductus arteriosus, and atrioventricular septal defect.
  - Obstructive lesions: Oxygenated blood flow is obstructed, causing a pressure gradient across the obstruction, which may result in hypertrophy and heart failure. Conditions

include, in order of frequency: pulmonic stenosis, aortic stenosis, aortic coarctation, and hypoplastic left heart syndrome (Porter, 2018).
- Single-ventricle/univentricle physiology (one side of heart involved): Hypoplastic left heart syndrome, tricuspid atresia.
- Biventricular physiology (both sides of heart involved): Tetralogy of Fallot, transposition of the great arteries (Easson et al., 2019).

Evaluation/Assessment
Areas
- Activities of Daily Living/Instrumental ADL:
  - ▶ Infant/Toddler: feeding (oral motor skills: sucking, swallowing, chewing), communication (receptive, expressive)
  - ▶ Child/Adolescent/Adult: All basic ADLs, independent living skills based on appropriate age
- Education/Work:
  - ▶ Child/Adolescent: academic skills, academic achievement, school activities
  - ▶ Adolescent/Adult: work skills, work performance
- Play/Leisure: interests, types, frequency, location
- Rest/Sleep: sleep habits, sleep disturbances
- Social Participation: type, frequency, location, with whom
- Sensorimotor: primitive reflexes, gross motor skills, fine motor skills, manual dexterity, endurance, sensory sensitivities
- Cognitive/Perceptual: attention, memory (working memory), executive function (problem-solving, self-management), visual-spatial skills
- Psychosocial: parent–child bonding, self-advocacy, peer relations, quality of life
- Context/Environment: knowledge of cardiac condition, knowledge of resources
- Development (Infant, Child, Adolescent only): developmental delay, developmental milestones, gross motor delay
- Comorbidities: medical instability, chromosomal abnormalities such as Down syndrome (trisomy 21), attention-deficit/hyperactive disorder, growth failure, diabetes, obesity, seizure disorders, asthma, cardiac surgery (Mackie et al., 2012); allergies, psychiatric conditions (depression, anxiety), specific learning disability, autism spectrum disorder (Majnemer et al., 2017); failure to thrive and feeding intolerance (Coker-Bolt et al., 2013)

Instruments
Instruments Developed by Occupational Therapy Personnel
- Children's Assessment of Participation and Enjoyment and Preferences for Activities of Children (CAPE/PAC; King et al., 2004)
- Infant Feeding & Nutrition Checklist (IFNC; St. Pierre et al., 2010, in References)
- Infant Malnutrition and Feeding Checklist (see Infant Feeding & Nutrition Checklist)
- Interviewer's Guide: Interviews of Adolescents and Young Adults (for ages 13 or older; Mackie et al., 2012, in References)
- Interviewer's Guide: Interviews of Parents (for children aged 6–12; Mackie et al., 2012, in References)
- Leiter International Performance Scale (3rd ed.; Leiter-3; Roid et al., 2013)
- MyHeart Scale (MyHeart; Mackie et al., 2014, in References)

Instruments Developed by Other Professionals and Used by Occupational Therapy Personnel
- Ages and Stages Questionnaire (3rd ed.; ASQ; Squires & Bricker, 2009)
- Aristotle Patient-Adjusted Complexity score (Aristotle Score; Lacour-Gayet et al., 2004; see also Campbell et al., 2017, in References)
- ASEBA Preschool Forms & Profiles (Achenbach & Rescorla, 2000)
- Assessment of General Movements (GMs; Einspieler & Prechtl, 2005)

- Bayley Scales of Infant and Toddler Development (4th ed.; Bayley-4; Bayley & Aylward, 2019)
- Beckman Oral Hypersensitivity Scale (BOHS; Beckman, 2004)
- Beckman Oral Motor Evaluation Protocol (BOME; Beckman, 2006)
- Behavior Rating Inventory of Executive Function–Adult Version (BRIEF-A; Roth et al., 2005)
- Child Behavior Checklist (CBCL; Achenbach, 2001)
- Child Health Questionnaire–Parent Form (CHQ-PF50; Landgraf et al., 1996)
- Dimensions of Mastery Questionnaire 18 (DMQ 18; Morgan et al., 2017)
- Feeding Readiness Assessment (FRA; Ehrmann et al., 2018, in References)
- Functional Independence Measure for Children (Version 5.01; WeeFIM; Uniform Data System for Medical Rehabilitation, 1998)
- Movement Assessment Battery for Children (2nd ed.; M-ABC-2; Henderson et al., 2007)
- Parent Report of Children's Abilities–Revised (PRCA-R; Johnson et al., 2004)
- Parenting Stress Index (4th ed.; PSI-4; Abidin, 2012)
- Peabody Developmental Motor Scales (3rd ed.; PDMS-3; Folio & Fewell, 2023)
- Peabody Picture Vocabulary Test (5th ed.; PPVT-4; Dunn, 2018)
- Strengths and Difficulties Questionnaire (SDQ; Goodman, 1997)
- Test of Infant Motor Performance (3rd ed.; TIMP-3; Campbell et al., 2012)
- Transition Readiness Assessment Questionnaire (TRAQ; Sawicki et al., 2011)
- Vineland Adaptive Behavior Scales (3rd ed.; Vineland-3; Sparrow et al., 2016)
- Wechsler Preschool and Primary Scale of Intelligence (4th ed.; WPPSI-IV; Wechsler, 2012)

Problems/Issues

Activities of Daily Living/Instrumental ADL
- Infants diagnosed with hypoplastic left heart syndrome, long intubation periods, long duration withholding of enteral feeding, and presence of gastroesophageal reflux disease are predictors of poor oral feeding (Indramohan et al., 2017).
- Parents and person may have difficulty with medication management.

Education/Work
- Child/adolescent may have delay or difficulty in performing academic tasks.
- Child/adolescent may exhibit behavioral problems in classroom or school environment.

Play/Leisure
- Adolescents report reduced engagement in leisure occupations due to impaired motor, behavioral and cognitive development (Majnemer et al., 2019).

Rest/Sleep
- Not discussed.

Social Participation
- Adolescents report reduced participation in social activities.

Sensorimotor
- Infant may have low endurance, fatigues quickly.
- Child/adolescent may have delayed or difficulty with gross motor skills such as throwing, aiming, and catching.
- Child/adolescent may have delayed or difficulty with fine motor skills, such as dexterity.

Cognitive/Perceptual
- Child/adolescent may lack a self-management program.

Psychosocial
- Child/adolescent may exhibit behavioral problems.
- Child/adolescent may lack persistence in task performance.
- Child/adolescent may exhibit poor motivation.
- Child/adolescent may lack self-advocacy skills.

Context/Environment
- Parents and caregivers may lack knowledge of feeding techniques for infants with congenital heart disorders or diseases.
- Parents may lack information on developmental progress of children with congenital heart disorders or diseases.
- Parents and clients may lack information about available resources: community, state, national, internet.

Intervention/Treatment

Models and programs developed by occupational therapy personnel: None. Models and programs developed by other professionals but used by occupational therapy personnel include the Beckman method (Indramohan et al., 2017), oral motor stimulation protocol (Coker-Bolt et al., 2013), team approach (Chorna et al., 2016), and transition intervention protocol (Mackie et al., 2014). Team members include pediatricians, neonatologists, pediatric and adult cardiologists, dieticians, dentists, physical therapists, speech–language pathologists, and occupational therapy personnel. Goal is to establish oral feeding.

Activities of Daily Living/Instrumental ADL
- Feeding: Oral motor exercises to stimulate gums, cheeks, and lips by stretching and stroking.
- Develop oral motor skills (sucking, swallowing, chewing).
- Promote nonnutritive sucking.
- Oral motor exercises, which are described as follows:
  - ► Upper and lower lips: Side-to-side stretching is used by pressing lip tissue with finger and moving slowly back and forth across the lips.
  - ► Gum massage: Massaging gum is applied to each tooth using finger in a circular motion starting in the middle of the gum and working outward.
  - ► Biting: Tapping pressure on molars may be used to encourage biting action.
  - ► Cheek stretch (lower and upper): Stretching is performed by using finger inside mouth in front of jawbone and gently pulling cheek skin outward on the upper and lower cheeks.
  - ► Tongue sweep: Gentle pressure is applied to areas of the mouth (roof, both sides, and bottom).
  - ► Sucking: Finger is placed on tongue or a pacifier is used to promote sucking activity.
  - ► For detailed description of actions and recommended number of repetitions see Coker-Bolt et al. (2013).

Education/Work
- Not discussed.

Play/Leisure
- Infant/child: Encourage development of play skills.
- Child/adolescent: Encourage development of leisure occupations.

Rest/Sleep
- See Sleep–Wake Disorders in Section 13: Lifestyle Disorders.

Social Participation
- Child/adolescent: Encourage and support development of and participation in social activities.

Sensorimotor
- Provide opportunity to practice gross and fine motor skills.

Cognitive/Perceptual
- Focus is on improving client's knowledge of cardiac condition, medication schedule, and medical management (surgical procedures).

Psychosocial
- Provide opportunity to develop self-mastery skills.
- Support motivation and persistence in occupational performance.

Context/Environment
- Provide client with access to local cardiac services and resources.

Precautions/Safety Considerations
- Not discussed.

Prognosis and Outcome

Literature suggests that children born with cardiac conditions requiring heart surgery should be followed for subsequent delays in motor, cognition, and psychosocial functions (Campbell et al., 2019). Intervention programs have not been published in the occupational therapy literature.

REFERENCES

Infants and Toddlers

Campbell, M., Rabbidge, B., Ziviani, J., & Sakzewski, L. (2017). Clinical feasibility of pre-operative neurodevelopmental assessment of infants undergoing open heart surgery. *Journal of Paediatrics and Child Health, 53*(8), 794–799. https://doi.org/10.1111/jpc.13565

Campbell, M. J., Ziviani, J. M., Stocker, C. F., Khan, A., & Sakzewski, L. (2019). Neuromotor performance in infants before and after early open-heart surgery and risk factors for delayed development at 6 months of age. *Cardiology in the Young, 29*(2), 100–109. https://doi.org/10.1017/S1047951118001622

Chorna, O., Baldwin, H. S., Neumaier, J., Gogliotti, S., Powers, D., Mouvery, A., Bichell, D., & Maitre, N. L. (2016). Feasibility of a team approach to complex congenital heart defect neurodevelopmental follow-up. *Circulation: Cardiovascular Quality and Outcomes, 9*(4), 432–440. https://doi.org/10.1161/CIRCOUTCOMES.116.002614

Coker-Bolt, P., Jarrard, C., Woodard, F., & Merrill, P. (2013). The effects of oral motor stimulation on feeding behaviors of infants born with univentricle anatomy. *Journal of Pediatric Nursing, 28*(1), 64–71. https://doi.org/10.1016/j.pedn.2012.03.024

Easson, K., Dahan-Oliel, N., Rohlicek, C., Sahakian, S., Brossard-Racine, M., Mazer, B., Riley, P., Maltais, D. B., Nadeau, L., Hatzigeorgiou, S., Schmitz, N., & Majnemer, A. (2019). A comparison of developmental outcomes of adolescent neonatal intensive care unit survivors born with a congenital heart defect or born preterm. *Journal of Pediatrics, 207*, 34–41. https://doi.org/10.1016/j.jpeds.2018.11.002

Ehrmann, D. E., Mulvahill, M., Harendt, S., Church, J., Stimmler, A., Vichayavilas, P., Batz, S., Rodgers, J., DiMaria, M., Jaggers, J., Barrett, C., & Kaufman, J. (2018). Toward standardization of care: The feeding readiness assessment after congenital cardiac surgery. *Congenital Heart Disease, 13*(1), 31–37. https://doi.org/10.1111/chd.12550

Indramohan, G., Pedigo, T. P., Rostoker, N., Cambare, M., Grogan, T., & Federman, M. D. (2017). Identification of risk factors for poor feeding in infants with congenital heart disease and a novel approach to improve oral feeding. *Journal of Pediatric Nursing, 35*, 149–154. https://doi.org/10.1016/j.pedn.2017.01.009

St. Pierre, A., Khattra, P., Johnson, M., Cender, L., Manzano, S., & Holsti, L. (2010). Content validation of the infant malnutrition and feeding checklist for congenital heart disease: A tool to identify risk of malnutrition and feeding difficulties in infants with congenital heart disease. *Journal of Pediatric Nursing, 25*(5), 367–374. https://doi.org/10.1016/j.pedn.2009.04.009

Children, Adolescents, and Young Adults

Easson, K., Dahan-Oliel, N., Rohlicek, C., Sahakian, S., Brossard-Racine, M., Mazer, B., Riley, P., Maltais, D. B., Nadeau, L., Hatzigeorgiou, S., Schmitz, N., & Majnemer, A. (2019). A comparison of developmental outcomes of adolescent neonatal intensive care unit survivors born with a congenital heart defect or born preterm. *Journal of Pediatrics, 207*, 34–41. https://doi.org/10.1016/j.jpeds.2018.11.002

Fontes, K., Rohlicek, C. V., Saint-Martin, C., Gilbert, G., Easson, K., Majnemer, A., Marelli, A., Chakravarty, M. M., & Brossard-Racine, M. (2019). Hippocampal alterations and functional correlates in adolescents and young adults with congenital heart disease. *Human Brain Mapping, 40*(12), 3548–3560. https://doi.org/10.1002/hbm.24615

Mackie, A. S., Islam, S., Magill-Evans, J., Rankin, K. N., Robert, C., Schuh, M., Nicholas, D., Vonder Muhll, I., McCrindle, B. W., Yasui, Y., & Rempel, G. R. (2014). Healthcare transition for youth with heart disease: A clinical trial. *Heart, 100*(14), 1113–1118. https://doi.org/10.1136/heartjnl-2014-305748

Mackie, A. S., Rempel, G. R., Rankin, K. N., Nicholas, D., & Magill-Evans, J. (2012). Risk factors for loss to follow-up among children and young adults with congenital heart disease. *Cardiology in the Young, 22*(3), 307–315. https://doi.org/10.1017/S104795111100148X

Majnemer, A., Dahan-Oliel, N., Rohlicek, C., Hatzigeorgiou, S., Mazer, B., Maltais, D. B., & Schmitz, N. (2017). Educational and rehabilitation service utilization in adolescents born preterm or with a congenital heart defect and at high risk for disability. *Developmental Medicine & Child Neurology, 59*(10), 1056–1062. https://doi.org/10.1111/dmcn.13520

Majnemer, A., Limperopoulos, C., Shevell, M., Rohlicek, C., Rosenblatt, B., & Tchervenkov, C. (2012). Gender differences in the developmental outcomes of children with congenital cardiac defects. *Cardiology in the Young, 22*(5), 514–519. https://doi.org/10.1017/S1047951111002071

Majnemer, A., Rohlicek, C., Dahan-Oliel, N., Sahakian, S., Mazer, B., Maltais, D. B., & Schmitz, N. (2019). Participation in leisure activities in adolescents with congenital heart defects. *Developmental Medicine & Child Neurology, 62*(8). Advance online publication. https://doi.org/10.1111/dmcn.14422

O'Toole, M. T. (Ed.). (2017). *Mosby's dictionary of medicine, nursing & health professions* (10th ed.). Elsevier.

Porter, R. S. (Ed.). (2018). *The Merck manual of diagnosis and therapy* (20th ed.). Merck Sharp & Dohme.

Hand and Wrist Conditions

Arthroplasty: Metacarpophalangeal Joint

Also called joint replacement.

Description

The surgical reconstruction or replacement of the metacarpophalangeal (MCP) joint with a prosthesis (O'Toole, 2017).

Cause

Painful, degenerative, or deformity, including subluxation and ulnar drift in finger joint due to primarily to rheumatoid arthritis or to correct a congenital deformity (O'Toole, 2017).

Evaluation/Assessment

Areas

- Activities of Daily Living/Instrumental ADL: self-maintenance, basic ADLs
- Education/Work: work tasks involving hand and finger motions (keyboarding, making change, assembling small electronics)
- Play/Leisure: leisure interests and occupations, especially those involving hand and finger motions (needlework, building small car or boat kits, examining coins, playing card or board games)
- Rest/Sleep: sleep disturbance
- Social Participation: no information identified
- Sensorimotor: grip and pinch strength, range of motion, ulnar drift of fingers, extensor lag, pain, edema, manipulation of objects (picking up, turning over, stacking, and moving)
- Cognitive/Perceptual: body image
- Psychosocial: depression, anxiety, quality of life, self-efficacy, social roles
- Context/Environment: client education, resources
- Comorbidities: rheumatoid arthritis, joint space narrowing, ulnar drift, volar subluxation or intrinsic tightness (Lubahn et al., 2011)

Instruments

Instruments Developed by Occupational Therapy Personnel

- Arthritis Hand Function Test (AHFT; Backman et al., 1991; Backman & Mackie, 1997)

Instruments Developed by Other Professionals and Used by Occupational Therapy Personnel

- Arthritis Impact Measurement Scales-2 (AIMS2; Meenan et al., 1992)
- Grip strength (dynamometry; JAMAR, Lafayette Instrument; Wang et al., 2018)
- Jebsen-Taylor Hand Function Test (JTHFT; Jebsen et al., 1969)
- Joint range of motion (goniometry; Shurtleff & Kaskutas, 2018)
- Michigan Hand Outcomes Questionnaire (MHQ; Chung et al., 1998)
- Pinch meter (pinch strength, two and three finger, lateral; B&E Engineering; Mathiowetz et al., 1986)
- Sollerman Hand Function Test (SHFT; Sollerman & Ejeskär, 1995)

Problems/Issues

Activities of Daily Living/Instrumental ADL

- Person may experience difficulty performing self-maintenance activities such as buttoning, zipping, fastening.

Education/Work

- Person may experience difficulty performing work tasks involving finger motions such as keyboarding, making change.

Play/Leisure
- Person may have decreased engagement in favorite leisure activities that involve finger motions, such as needlework, playing a musical instrument.

Rest/Sleep
- Not discussed.

Social Participation
- Person may have reduced participation in social activities that involve finger motions, such as playing board or card games.

Sensorimotor
- Person may lack joint flexion and extension.
- Person may have postoperative pain and edema.
- Person may experience rotation of index finger.
- Person may continue to have tendency for ulnar deviation.
- Person may have fragile skin.
- Person may have difficulty applying splint or orthosis due to weakness in nonsurgical hand.

Cognitive/Perceptual
- Cognitive dysfunction is not directly involved. Cognitive impairment may exist from other causes and may require adjustment in intervention plan.

Psychosocial
- Person may experience changes in quality of life.
- Person may express feelings of discomfort about appearance of hands and about wearing a hand splint.

Context/Environment
- Person usually needs education about living with rheumatoid arthritis and joint replacement.
- Person may need information about community and internet resources.

Intervention/Treatment

Models and programs developed by occupational therapy personnel: No information identified. Models and programs developed by other professionals but used by occupational therapy personnel: Postoperative protocols including splinting, activity, and exercises are not well described (Massy-Westropp, 2012). Team members include physicians, surgeons, physical therapists, and occupational therapy personnel. Goals postsurgery are to optimize wound healing; prevent scar adherence; control edema; maintain neutral alignment and desired degree of range of motion at the reconstructed joints; optimize occupational performance of activities of daily living, work, and leisure; and maintain active motion of all nonoperated joints of the upper extremity (Lubahn et al., 2011).

Activities of Daily Living/Instrumental ADL
- Light ADLs usually can be started at about 5 weeks.

Education/Work
- Return to work for light duty or supervisory work can be initiated at about 6 weeks.

Play/Leisure
- Approximate time for light leisure activities, about 5 weeks.

Rest/Sleep
- Time for wearing night splint is variable but may be continued for 2 months or more, depending on daytime response to therapy and functional activity.

Social Participation
- No information identified.

Sensorimotor
- Dressing
  - ▶ Bulky dressing is removed within 2 weeks.
  - ▶ A light compressive dressing is applied.
  - ▶ Dressing is changed at each visit until sutures are remove at 10 to 14 days.
- Edema
  - ▶ Elevate hand to control edema.
  - ▶ Coban bandage may be used to control edema in fingers.
  - ▶ Avoid traction of skin in ulnar direction.
- Exercises
  - ▶ Gentle passive and active range of motion for MCP joint is started as soon as orthosis is applied.
  - ▶ Continue active range of motion exercises for wrist, elbow, shoulder, neck, hips, and knees to prevent deformities related to rheumatoid arthritis.
- Joint alignment
  - ▶ Control alignment whenever movement occurs, whether passive or active.
- Joint protection
  - ▶ Principles of joint protection should be followed at all times.
- Orthotic (splint) positioning
  - ▶ Purpose: Control position and alignment of reconnected joints and allow guided range of motion.
  - ▶ Type: Dynamic dorsal extension outrigger orthosis is applied within 1 week of surgery for day wear. MCP should be at 0 degrees, fingers in neutral. Several variations of outriggers exist.
  - ▶ Alternate type: A static orthosis, without outrigger, but with MCP joint support in neutral or radial alignment may be used at night. An ulnar border or trough or Velcro straps should be used to prevent ulnar drift.
  - ▶ Note: Hayashi and Uchiya (2011) reported static splinting provided positive long-term results as opposed to dynamic in a case study.
- Skin care
  - ▶ Regular, daily inspection of skin should occur, whether by therapist or client.
- Timing
  - ▶ 3 days to 2 weeks: Outrigger orthosis is applied and gentle exercises are started.
  - ▶ 3 weeks
    - o Out of orthosis exercises may be started.
    - o Contrast baths may be started for edema control.
  - ▶ 4 weeks
    - o Coordination and balancing exercises are used to maintain flexion and extension.
    - o Light strengthening exercises may be started.
    - o Review joint protection principles to modify and correct client's behavior and habits.
  - ▶ 5 weeks
    - o Light ADLs and functional activities can be added.
    - o Continue therapy with exercises and light functional strengthening.
    - o Remind client to avoid deformity positions and to respect pain.
    - o Recommend using forearm instead of hand to carry objects.
    - o Orthosis may be continued to control alignment and provide extension assist if extensor lag is present.
  - ▶ 6 weeks
    - o Daytime dynamic orthosis may be discontinued.

○ A small hand-based orthosis may be useful to protect reconstructed joints from undesirable forces.
○ Return to light or supervisory work is allowed.
▶ 8 weeks
○ Scar maturation should be under way.
○ Functional strengthening and night positioning orthosis may be continued.
○ Range of motion should be 40 to 80 degrees of flexion. Functional range for client is most important.
○ Pain and deformity should be decreased.

Cognitive/Perceptual
• Not discussed.

Psychosocial
• Not discussed, except for satisfaction with improved appearance of hand.

Context/Environment
• Client and family education, especially joint protection.

Precautions/Safety Considerations

Continue to stress importance of joint protection. Continue to stress importance of following precautions regarding use of prostheses in MCP joints in everyday activities.

Prognosis and Outcome

Outcome after MCP joint arthroplasty is generally good, although different types of implants tend to result in different results. The NeuFlex implant demonstrated superior range of motion, whereas the Swanson implant received better self-reported function and aesthetics (Escott et al., 2010). Ulnar drift, extensor lag, and arm motion improved, but grip strength and prehension may not improve (Chung et al., 2012). Complications include infection, malpositioning, broken prostheses, and return of ulnar drift (Lubahn et al., 2011). Functional improvement, pain reduction, and hand appearance are ranked highest in level of satisfaction among clients (Bogoch et al., 2011). The necessary joint range of motion of the MCP joints to maintain hand function are flexion range of motion >70 degrees with extension range of motion <30 degrees of extension lag (Hayashi et al., 2014).

REFERENCES

Bogoch, E. R., Escott, B. G., & Ronald, K. (2011). Hand appearance as a patient motivation for surgery and a determinant of satisfaction with metacarpophalangeal joint arthroplasty for rheumatoid arthritis. *Journal of Hand Surgery, 36*(6), 1007–1014. https://doi.org/10.1016/j.jhsa.2011.02.002

Chung, K. C., Burns, P. B., Kim, H. M., Burke, F. D., Shaw Wilgis, E. F., & Fox, D. A. (2012). Long-term followup for rheumatoid arthritis patients in a multicenter outcomes study of silicone metacarpophalangeal joint arthroplasty. *Arthritis Care & Research, 64*(9), 1292–1300. https://doi.org/10.1002/acr.21705

Escott, B. G., Ronald, K., Judd, M. G. P., & Bogoch, E. R. (2010). NeuFlex and Swanson metacarpophalangeal implants for rheumatoid arthritis: Prospective randomized, controlled clinical trial. *Journal of Hand Surgery–American, 35*(1), 44–51. https://doi.org/10.1016/j.jhsa.2009.09.020

Hayashi, H., Shimizu, H., Okumura, S., & Miwa, K. (2014). Necessary metacarpophalangeal joints range of motion to maintain hand function. *Hong Kong Journal of Occupational Therapy, 24*(2), 51–55. https://doi.org/10.1016/j.hkjot.2014.10.001

Hayashi, H., & Uchiya, J. (2011). A 3-year follow-up study on the alternating use of static splints after metacarpophalangeal joint arthroplasty in a patient with rheumatoid arthritis. *Asian Journal of Occupational Therapy, 9*(1), 1–5. https://doi.org/10.11596/asiajot.9.1

Lubahn, J., Wolfe, T., & Feldscher, S. B. (2011). Joint replacement in the hand and wrist: Surgery and therapy. In T. M. Skirven, A. L. Osterman, J. M. Fedorczyk, & P. C. Amadio (Eds.), *Rehabilitation of the hand and upper extremity* (6th ed., pp. 1376–1398). Elsevier/Mosby.

Massy-Westropp, N. (2012). Postoperative therapy for metacarpophalangeal arthroplasty. In S. Fokter (Ed.), *Recent advances in arthroplasty* (pp. 565–576). InTech.

O'Toole, M. T. (Ed.). (2017). *Mosby's dictionary of medicine, nursing & health professions* (10th ed.). Elsevier.

Arthroplasty: Proximal Interphalangeal Joint

Also called joint replacement.

Description

The surgical reconstruction or replacement of the proximal interphalangeal (PIP) joint with a prosthesis (O'Toole, 2017). PIP joint arthroplasty may be indicated if osteoarthritis is present, nonsurgical management of a PIP injury is unsuccessful, if significant radiographic changes in the joint are observed, or if painful degenerative or posttraumatic joint deformities are present (Feldscher, 2010). Joint replacement may be considered if there is "adequate bone stock, soft tissue coverage, absence of infection, intact neurovascular/musculotendinous systems, intact flexor/extensor mechanisms, and proper balance and stability of collateral ligaments" (Feldscher, 2010, p. 315). Three types of implants have been used: Swanson silicone implant, Ascension pyrocarbon implant, and Avanta titanium cobalt chromium implant (Lubahn et al., 2011). Five different surgical procedures are reported (Feldscher, 2010; Tranchida et al., 2019), and a summary of exercise regimes reported from 2006 to 2014 show various therapeutic interventions with no consistency in timing of exercises, use or type of splints, range of motion to be limited or achieved, or grip and pinch strength to be achieved (Downey, 2019). However, problems other than body structure and function are not described in any detail.

Cause

Trauma, degenerative osteoarthritis, or rheumatic disease to the finger(s) and PIP joint(s) (Downey, 2019).

Evaluation/Assessment

Areas

- Activities of Daily Living/Instrumental ADL: basic ADLs and independent living skills, especially functional limitations
- Education/Work: work skills, work location
- Play/Leisure: interests, type, frequency, location
- Rest/Sleep: sleep habits, sleep schedule
- Social Participation: type, frequency, location, with whom
- Sensorimotor: range of motion, grip strength, pain, edema, contractures
- Cognitive/Perceptual: not directly involved. Other comorbidities such as dementia may exist
- Psychosocial: motivation, self-efficacy, social roles, quality of life
- Context/Environment: support system
- Comorbidities: osteoarthritis, rheumatoid arthritis, nonunion fractures

Instruments

Instruments Developed by Occupational Therapy Personnel

- Canadian Occupational Performance Measure (5th ed.; COPM-5; Law et al., 2014)

Instruments Developed by Other Professionals and Used by Occupational Therapy Personnel

- Disabilities of the Arm, Shoulder, and Hand (3th ed.; DASH-3; Kennedy et al., 2011)

- Grip strength (dynamometer; JAMAR, Lafayette Instrument; Wang et al., 2018)
- Jebsen-Taylor Hand Function Test (JTHFT; Jebsen et al., 1969)
- Joint range of motion (goniometry; Shurtleff & Kaskutas, 2018)
- Michigan Hand Outcomes Questionnaire (MHQ; Chung et al., 1998)
- Visual analogue scale (pain scale; scored: 0 = *no pain*, 10 = *worst pain ever*)

Problems/Issues

Activities of Daily Living/Instrumental ADL
- Person may experience functional limitations in performing ADLs.

Education/Work
- Not discussed.

Play/Leisure
- Not discussed.

Rest/Sleep
- Person may have changes in sleep habits due to pain.

Social Participation
- Not discussed.

Sensorimotor
- Person usually has decreased range of motion.
- Person usually has decreased grip and pinch strength.
- Person usually has pain in the joints and hand(s) involved.
- Person may have decreased endurance and activity tolerance due to pain.
- Person may have decreased tactile sensation.

Cognitive/Perceptual
- Not discussed.

Psychosocial
- Person may experience decreased quality of life and life satisfaction due to limitations and pain.
- Person may express decreased sense of self-efficacy due to inability to perform certain tasks or occupations.
- Person may become depressed or anxious about loss of function.
- Person may be unable or have difficulty performing certain social roles such as cooking.

Context/Environment
- Person may lack social support.
- Person may have limited knowledge about joint deformity and dysfunction.
- Person may lack knowledge about the underlying cause.

Intervention/Treatment

Models and programs developed by occupational therapy personnel include postoperative management (Feldscher, 2010). Models and programs developed by other professionals but used by occupational therapy personnel include static versus dynamic splinting (Riggs et al., 2011). Postoperative protocols including splinting, activity, and exercises are not well described (Massy-Westropp, 2012). Team members include physicians, surgeons, rheumatologists, physical therapists, and occupational therapy personnel. Goals are edema, scar, and pain management; prevention of tendon adhesion; promote increased range of motion; and improve functional performance of daily occupations.

Activities of Daily Living/Instrumental ADL
- Light functional activities may be started about 1-month postsurgery.

Education/Work
- Not discussed.

Play/Leisure
- Not discussed.

Rest/Sleep
- Not discussed.

Social Participation
- Not discussed.

Sensorimotor
- Exercises: Use functional activities such as grasping objects large in size and diameter, such as an empty bottle, and progressing to grasping objects that are small in diameter, such as marker (Downey, 2019).
- Timing (Note: Protocols vary widely as reviewed by Downey, 2019, and Feldscher, 2010): Below is a sample protocol summarizing key elements from protocols reviewed by Downey and Feldscher. Specific protocols will depend on physician preference, characteristics of the type of implant, and individual client factors such as age, degree of dysfunction, and type of hand function needed by the client.
  - ▶ 1 day: Forearm-based resting splint provided.
  - ▶ 3–4 days: Forearm-based static splint for nighttime use is applied with wrist at 15 degrees extension, metacarpophalangeal (MCP) joints slightly flexed, and PIP joints near full extension.
  - ▶ 5–7 days: Dynamic splint is applied for daytime wear, with wrist in 15 degrees extension, MCP joints in 20 degrees flexion, and PIP joints near full extension.
  - ▶ 3–7 days: 10–12 repetitions per hour of dynamically assisted PIP extension to neutral and flexion to 30 degrees.
  - ▶ 2 weeks: PIP joint flexion in increased to 45 degrees if there is no extension lag.
  - ▶ 4 weeks: Dynamic splint is discontinued. Buddy taping is initiated. PIP flexion is increased to 60 degrees assuming full PIP extension and light functional activities are initiated.
  - ▶ 6 weeks: Goal is to achieve 0–75 degrees of active range of motion in PIP joint. Gentle stretching may begin to increase range of motion.
  - ▶ 3 months: Splinting may be continued if needed. Activities are performed as tolerated.

Cognitive/Perceptual
- Not discussed.

Psychosocial
- Encourage client to identify and prioritize goals and approaches (choices of activities) to intervention within recommended protocol established for type of implant.
- Encourage client to stay motivated to complete and comply with exercise program.

Context/Environment
- Home exercise program may be provided, including instructions for wound care and edema control.

Precautions/Safety Considerations
Complications reported include squeaking of the prosthesis during movement, dislocation of the prosthesis, and delayed wound healing (Riggs et al., 2011). Motions to be avoided are hyperextension, rotation, deviation, and extension lag (Feldscher, 2010).

Prognosis and Outcome

Wijk et al. (2010) found that a review of outcomes listed decreased pain, but no improvement in range of motion and grip strength. However, one-third of clients reported significant improvement in occupational performance and satisfaction. Thirteen percent of clients required a second surgical procedure. Hendricks et al. (2020) reported that pain was significantly reduced while active range of motion significantly increased following pyrocarbon proximal interphalangeal joint arthroplasty. Adams et al. (2012) concluded in their meta-analysis studies that the effectiveness of PIP joint replacement has not been established.

REFERENCES

Adams, J., Ryall, C., Pandyan, A., Metcalf, C., Stokes, M., Bradley, S., & Warwick, D. J. (2012). Proximal interphalangeal joint replacement in patients with arthritis of the hand: A meta-analysis. *Journal of Bone & Joint Surgery–British, 94B*(10), 1305–1312. https://doi.org/10.1302/0301-620X.94B10.29035

Downey, M. (2019). The effectiveness of exercise following proximal interphalangeal joint replacements: A critical review of the evidence. *Acta Scientific Orthopaedics, 2*(8) 50–58. https://doi.org/10.31080/ASOR.2019.02.0081

Feldscher, S. B. (2010). Postoperative management for PIP joint pyrocarbon arthroplasty. *Journal of Hand Therapy, 23*(3), 315–322. https://doi.org/10.1016/j.jht.2009.10.011

Hendricks, N., Nadasan, T., Olagbegi, O. M., & Chemane, N. (2020). Patient characteristics, therapy service delivery and patient outcomes following pyrocarbon proximal interphalangeal joint arthroplasty. *South African Journal of Occupational Therapy, 50*(1), 3–11. https://doi.org/10.17159/2310-3833/2020/Vol50n1a2

Lubahn, J., Wolfe, T., & Feldscher, S. B. (2011). Joint replacement in the hand and wrist: Surgery and therapy. In T. M. Shriven, A. L. Osterman, J. M. Fedorzyk, & P. C. Amadio (Eds.), *Rehabilitation of the hand and upper extremity* (6th ed., pp. 1376–1398). Elsevier/Mosby.

Massy-Westropp, N. (2012). Postoperative therapy for metacarpophalangeal arthroplasty. In S. Fokter (Ed.), *Recent advances in arthroplasty* (pp. 565–576). Intech.

O'Toole, M. T. (Ed.). (2017). *Mosby's dictionary of medicine, nursing & health professions* (10th ed.). Elsevier.

Riggs, J. M., Lyden, A. K., Chung, K. C., & Murphy, S. L. (2011). Static versus dynamic splinting for proximal interphalangeal joint pyrocarbon implant arthroplasty: A comparison of current and historical cohorts. *Journal of Hand Therapy, 24*(3), 231–239. https://doi.org/10.1016/j.jht.2011.03.003

Tranchida, G. V., Allen, S. T., Moen, S. M., Erickson, L. O., & Ward, C. M. (2019). Comparison of volar and dorsal approach for PIP arthroplasty. *Hand.* Advance online publication. https://doi.org/10.1177/1558944719861718

Wijk, U., Wollmark, M., Kopylov, P., & Tägil, M. (2010). Outcomes of proximal interphalangeal joint pyrocarbon implants. *Journal of Hand Surgery, 35*(1), 38–43. https://doi.org/10.1016/j.jhsa.2009.08.010

Carpal Tunnel Syndrome

Description

Carpal tunnel syndrome (CTS) occurs from compression of the median nerve in the volar aspect of the wrist between the transverse superficial inelastic carpal ligament and the flexor tendons of the forearm muscles. The compression results in paresthesias in the radial-palmar aspect of the hand and pain in the wrist and palm (Porter, 2018). CTS may be unilateral or bilateral. Surgery involves release of the transverse carpal ligament. Nonsurgical intervention includes wrist orthosis, exercises, ultrasound, and steroid injections (Lim et al., 2017).

Cause

Etiology is idiopathic, although risk factors have been identified. CTS is most common in women ages 30–40. Risk factors include rheumatoid arthritis, diabetes mellitus, hypothyroidism, acromegaly, amyloidosis, and pregnancy (Porter, 2018). Symptoms may be caused by trauma, synovitis, or tumor (O'Toole, 2017).

Classification (Lim et al., 2017)

- Mild: paresthesia of palmar aspects of thumb, index finger, middle finger, and radial half of ring finger (median nerve distribution)
- Moderate: similar to mild
- Severe: thenar atrophy, loss of sensibility resulting in weakness and loss of hand function

Evaluation/Assessment

Areas

- Activities of Daily Living/Instrumental ADL: self-maintenance skills
- Education/Work: work tasks (keyboarding or other repetitive motions)
- Play/Leisure: interests, type, frequency, location
- Rest/Sleep: sleep disturbance due to pain
- Social Participation: type, frequency, location, with whom
- Sensorimotor: fine motor skills (holding, manipulating, dexterity), grip strength, thenar atrophy, posture, positioning, pain (especially in opposition of thumb), sensation
- Cognitive/Perceptual: not directly involved; note whether cognitive impairment is present
- Psychosocial: quality of life, anxiety
- Context/Environment: splints, ergonomic design, home and work task modification, social support
- Comorbidities: rheumatoid arthritis, osteoarthritis, diabetes, acromegaly, cancer, manual wheelchair users

Instruments

Instruments Developed by Occupational Therapy Personnel

- Flinn Performance Screening Tool (FPST; Flinn et al., 2012, in References)
- Manual Ability Measure-20 (MAM-20; Hill & Chen, 2012)
- Shape/Texture Identification (STI-test; Rosén & Lundborg, 1998)

Instruments Developed by Other Professionals and Used by Occupational Therapy Personnel

- Boston Carpal Tunnel Questionnaire (BCTQ) Functional Status Scale (FSS) 8 items (Levine et al., 1993)
- Boston Carpal Tunnel Questionnaire (BCTQ) Symptom Severity Scale (SSS), 11 items; Functional Status Scale (FSS), 8 items (Levine et al., 1993)
- Brigham and Woman's Hospital Carpal Tunnel Syndrome Questionnaire (see Boston Carpal Tunnel Questionnaire)
- Canterbury CTS Severity Scale (CSS; Bland, 2000; see Carpal Tunnel Syndrome Assessment Questionnaire)
- Carpal Tunnel Questionnaire (see Boston Carpal Tunnel Questionnaire)
- Carpal Tunnel Syndrome Assessment Questionnaire (Canterbury CTS Severity Scale; CSS; Bland, 2000)
- Disabilities of the Arm, Shoulder, and Hand (3rd ed.; DASH-3; Kennedy et al., 2011)
- European Quality of Life 5-Dimension Scale (EQ-5D; EuroQol Group, 1990)
- Functional Box Scale (FBS; Waterfield & Sim, 1996)
- Functional Status Scale (see Boston Carpal Tunnel Questionnaire)
- Grip strength (dynamometer; JAMAR; Martin vigorimeter)
- Manual Muscle Test (MMT; Kaskutas, 2018)
- Phalen's test (Walsh & Chee, 2018)

- Pittsburgh Sleep Quality Index (PSQI; Buysse et al., 1989)
- Pinch strength—lateral and palmar (pinch meter; B&E Engineering; Mathiowetz et al., 1986)
- Range of motion (goniometer; including Total Active Motion; TAM)
- Semmes-Weinstein Monofilament Test (SWMT; Semmes-Weinstein Aesthesiometer Kit, North Coast Medical)
- State Trait Anxiety Inventory (2nd ed.; STAI-2; Spielberger, 1989)
- Static Two-Point Discrimination Test (STPD; Mackinnon-Dellon Disk-Criminator, Abrams & Ivy, 2018, p. 586)
- Symptom Severity Scale (see Boston Carpal Tunnel Questionnaire)
- Ultrasound scanner (usually requires additional training; available from rehabilitation equipment and supply vendors)
- Visual or verbal analogue scale (VAS) pain scale (scored: 0 = *no pain*, 10 = *severe pain or worst pain ever*)

Problems/Issues

Activities of Daily Living/Instrumental ADL

- Person may have difficulty performing dressing tasks that require finger–thumb opposition, such as buttoning or zipping.
- Person may experience severe pain while performing simple tasks, such as grasping utensils and opening containers.

Education/Work

- Person may experience pain when performing repetitive tasks, such as keyboarding (Toosi et al., 2011).

Play/Leisure

- Person may experience pain when engaged in leisure activities that require finger–thumb opposition such as needlework or holding gardening tools.

Rest/Sleep

- Person may experience wrist pain while sleeping.
- Person may experience decreased manual ability due to decreased sleep quality (Goorman et al., 2019).

Social Participation

- Person may experience pain while participating in social activities especially if finger–thumb opposition is involved, such as playing cards or texting on a smartphone.

Sensorimotor

- Person usually has pain in the hand and wrist associated with tingling (pins and needles sensation) and numbness along the distribution of the median nerve (palmar side of the thumb and index and middle fingers and radial half of the ring finger).
- Person may have pain at night, described as burning or aching.
- Person may experience difficulty with fine motor tasks.
- Person may have thenar atrophy and muscle weakness of thumb opposition and abduction.
- Person may experience changes in sensation, such as burning, tingling, or aching.

Cognitive/Perceptual

- Not directly involved. Check for cognitive impairment.

Psychosocial

- Person may experience decreased quality of life.
- Person may experience anxiety about ability to perform life roles.

Context/Environment

- Person may lack knowledge about carpal tunnel syndrome and intervention.

- Person may lack knowledge about resources to reduce effects of repetitive strain.
- Person may lack social support.
- Person may be using hands to move a manual wheelchair, which requires large forces transmitted through the wrist and an extreme range of wrist motion (Zukowski et al., 2014).

Intervention/Treatment

Models and programs developed by occupational therapy personnel include adapted devices at gas pump (Wong & Rocker, 2018), full-time wrist splinting (Hall et al., 2013), and splinting/stretching program (Baker et al., 2013). Models and programs developed by other professionals but used by occupational therapy personnel include low-level laser therapy (Fusakul et al., 2014), one hand therapy visit (Mack et al., 2017), tendon and nerve guiding exercises (Hirata et al., 2016), wheelchair ergonomics (Zukowski, 2014), and recommended order of intervention: ergonomics, splinting and analgesics, corticosteroid injections, surgical decompression (Porter, 2018). Team members include general physicians, hand surgeons, physical therapists, and occupational therapy personnel. Goal of intervention is to decrease pressure on the median nerve, improve neural circulation, reduce pain and restore wrist and hand function, and occupational performance (Evans, 2011). However, there is insufficient evidence to recommend a specific type of intervention after release of the medium nerve (Cantero-Téllez et al., 2016).

Activities of Daily Living/Instrumental ADL (Hirata et al., 2016)
- Clients may start with light load activities in pain-free range of motion and gradually increase load.
- Clients should hold wrist in neutral position and minimize wrist flexion and extension to reduce numbness.
- Clients should avoid applying pressure or gripping heavy loads involving holding a stretch for 1 month after surgery to prevent palmar dislocation.
- Adapted devices: Dycem pad to assist in opening containers, extended handles to reduce grip force needed to start spray nozzle, using rotary forces to engage levers such as gas-pump handles.
- Education/Work: See instructions above.

Play/Leisure
- No information identified.

Rest/Sleep
- See Sleep–Wake Disorders in Section 13: Lifestyle Conditions.

Social Participation
- No information identified.

Sensorimotor
- Note: Exercises are performed with head in midline, shoulder girdle in neutral position, and forearm placed on table with elbow flexed at 90 degrees. There is no agreement as to which of the mobilization techniques is best (Lim et al., 2017).
- Lumbrical stretches (Baker et al., 2012):
  ▶ Client rests hand, palm down on thigh, with proximal interphalangeal (PIP) and distal interphalangeal (DIP) joints fully flexed.
  ▶ Client presses downward over the metacarpophalangeal (MCP) joints with opposite hand.
  ▶ Client pulls wrist, MCP, PIP, and DIP joints into maximum extension with opposed hand.
- General stretches (Baker et al., 2012):
  ▶ Client holds a position of composite wrist, MCP, PIP and DIP extension.
  ▶ Client rests for 5 seconds with wrist in neutral position.
  ▶ Client makes a composite wrist, MCP, PIP, and DIP full flexion.

- ▶ Client rests for 5 seconds with wrist in neutral position.
- ▶ Exercise schedule: Each stretch held for 7 seconds, 10 times per session, 6 sessions per day.
- Median nerve mobilization technique #1: Nerve gliding exercises (Hirata et al., 2016). Also called distal nerve tensioning (Lim et al., 2017):
  - ▶ Finger and thumb flexion with wrist in neutral position.
  - ▶ Finger and thumb stretches with wrist in neutral position.
  - ▶ Wrist and finger stretches with thumb in neutral position.
  - ▶ Wrist, finger, and thumb stretches.
  - ▶ Forearm supination while performing wrist, finger, and thumb stretches.
  - ▶ Thumb stretches with forearm supination.
  - ▶ Exercise schedule:
    - ○ Each exercise position is maintained for 5 seconds.
    - ○ Three sets of exercises are performed 10 times per day for 1 week.
    - ○ Exercises are stopped immediately if pain is experienced in wound or palm.
- Median nerve mobilization technique #2: Upper quarter nerve tensioning in which affected upper extremity undergoes (Lim et al., 2017):
  - ▶ Slight glenohumeral abduction.
  - ▶ Shoulder girdle depression.
  - ▶ Elbow extension.
  - ▶ Lateral rotation of the whole arm.
  - ▶ Wrist, thumb, and finger extension.
  - ▶ Exercise schedule:
    - ○ 10 repetitions for 3–5 sessions per day.
    - ○ Each stretch is maintained for 5 seconds.
- Median nerve mobilization technique #3: Nerve sliding (Lim et al., 2017):
  - ▶ Affected distal extremity undergoes wrist extension and finger flexion, then alternate wrist flexion and finger extension.
  - ▶ Affected upper extremity undergoes elbow flexion followed by wrist extension, then alternate elbow extension and wrist flexion.
  - ▶ Exercise schedule: 10 repetitions for 10 sessions a day.
- Tendon-gliding exercises (Hirata et al., 2016):
  - ▶ Finger stretches.
  - ▶ Hook fist: MCP extended, PIP and DIP joints flexed.
  - ▶ Full fist: MCP, PIP, and DIP joints fully flexed.
  - ▶ Table top: MCP flexed, PIP and DIP joints extended.
  - ▶ Straight fist: MCP and PIP flexed, DIP joints extended.
- Splints:
  - ▶ Note: no agreement on preferred splint.
  - ▶ Cock-up splint: Wrist at 0 degrees of extension. Finger joints not controlled by splint—allowed to naturally position (Baker et al., 2012).
  - ▶ Lumbrical Positioning splint: Wrist at 0 degrees of extension and MCP joints at 0 to 10 degrees of flexion (Baker et al., 2012).
  - ▶ Wrist control orthosis: Wrist at 2 degrees of flexion and 3 degrees of ulnar deviation. Thumb is not included (Evans, 2011).
  - ▶ Full resting pan splint: Wrist at 0 degrees, MCP at slight flexion and PIP joints at neutral. Thumb is included in its own gutter (Evans, 2011).
- Edema: Tubular compression sleeves may be used.
- Scar management: Needed when open carpal tunnel release surgery is performed.
  - ▶ Scar mobilization massage 3 times per day for 3–5 minutes.
  - ▶ Use of scar pad (Elasto-Gel cast and splint padding worn 8 hours a day once incision is healed).

Cognitive/Perceptual
- No information identified.

Psychosocial
- No information identified.

Context/Environment
- Provide instructions and demonstration of a home exercise program.
- Provide information about managing and reducing wrist pain such as wrist support splint or taping.
- Assist client to review and modify as needed home, work, and leisure occupations to minimize repetitive strain actions.
- Assist client to explore and select ergonomically designed devices and adapted equipment that can minimize repetitive strain actions.

Precautions/Safety Considerations

Stretching exercises should stay within pain limits. Pain may be more severe at night (Porter, 2018). Sensory deficit in palmar aspect of first three fingers may follow (Porter, 2018). Muscles controlling thumb abduction and opposition may become weak and atrophied (Porter, 2018). Trigger finger may occur (see Trigger Finger in this Section).

Prognosis and Outcome

If conservative approaches are not successful, surgery may be required; however, guidelines are lacking as to when conservative approaches should cease and surgery be performed (Baker & Livengood, 2014). Sensory relearning is reported to not be effective for tactile sensory and functional deficits after carpal tunnel decompression (Jerosch-Herold et al., 2016). Only three treatments for CTS are supported by evidence: splining, steroid injections, and surgery (Kaile, 2014).

Costs

Client-reported symptom severity is positively associated with costs (Jerosch-Herold et al., 2017).

REFERENCES

Baker, N. A., & Livengood, H. M. (2014). Symptom severity and conservative treatment for carpal tunnel syndrome in association with eventual carpal tunnel release. *Journal of Hand Surgery, 39*(9), 1792–1798. https://doi.org/10.1016/j.jhsa.2014.04.034

Baker, N. A., Moehling, K. K., Desai, A. R., & Gustafson, N. P. (2013). Effect of carpal tunnel syndrome on grip and pinch strength compared with sex- and age-matched normative data. *Arthritis Care & Research, 65*(12), 2041–2045. https://doi.org/10.1002/acr.22089

Baker, N. A., Moehling, K. K., Rubinstein, E. N., Wollstein, R., Gustafson, N. P. Y., & Baratz, M. (2012). The comparative effectiveness of combined lumbrical muscle splints and stretches on symptoms and function in carpal tunnel syndrome. *Archives of Physical Medicine and Rehabilitation, 93*(1), 1–10. https://doi.org/10.1016/j.apmr.2011.08.013

Cantero-Téllez, R., García-Orza, S., & Cuadros-Romero, M. (2016). Physiotherapy and occupational therapy evidence-based intervention after carpal tunnel release: Literature review. *Journal of Novel Physiotherapies, 6*(3), Article 1000296. https://doi.org/10.4172/2165-7025.1000296

Evans, R. B. (2011). Therapist's management of carpal tunnel syndrome: A practical approach. In T. M. Shirven, A. L. Osterman, J. M. Fedorczyk, & P. C. Amadio (Eds.), *Rehabilitation of the hand and upper extremity* (6th ed., pp. 666–677). Elsevier Mosby.

Flinn, S. R., Pease, W. S., & Freimer, M. L. (2012). Score reliability and construct validity of the Flinn Performance Screening Tool for adults with symptoms of carpal tunnel syndrome. *American Journal of Occupational Therapy, 66*(3), 330–337. https://doi.org/10.5014/ajot.2012.000935

Fusakul, Y., Aranyavalai, T., Saensri, P., & Thiengwittayaporn, S. (2014). Low-level laser therapy with a wrist splint to treat carpal tunnel syndrome: A double-blinded randomized controlled trial. *Lasers in Medical Science, 29*(3), 1279–1287. https://doi.org/10.1007/s10103-014-1527-2

Goorman, A. M., Dawson, S., Schneck, C., & Pierce, D. (2019). Association of sleep and hand function in people with carpal tunnel syndrome. *American Journal of Occupational Therapy, 73*(6), Article 7306205050. https://doi.org/10.5014/ajot.2019.034157

Hall, B., Lee, H. C., Fitzgerald, H., Byrne, B., Barton, A., & Lee, A. H. (2013). Investigating the effectiveness of full-time wrist splinting and education in the treatment of carpal tunnel syndrome: A randomized controlled trial. *American Journal of Occupational Therapy, 67*(4), 448–459. https://doi.org/10.5014/ajot.2013.006031

Hirata, J., Suzuki, T., Yamamoto, T., Miyazaki, Y., Ogasahara, Y., Hashizume, H., & Inoue, K. (2016). Effects of tendon and nerve gliding exercises and instructions in activities of daily living following endoscopic carpal tunnel release. *Asian Journal of Occupational Therapy, 11*(1), 35–41. https://doi.org/10.11596/asiajot.11.35

Jerosch-Herold, C., Houghton, J., Blake, J., Shaikh, A., Wilson, E. C., & Shepstone. L. (2017). Association of psychological distress, quality of life and costs with carpal tunnel syndrome severity: A cross-sectional analysis of the PALMS cohort. *BMJ Open, 7*(11), Article e017732. https://doi.org/10.1136/bmjopen-2017-017732

Jerosch-Herold, C., Houghton, J., Miller, L., & Shepstone, L. (2016). Does sensory relearning improve tactile function after carpal tunnel decompression? A pragmatic, assessor-blinded, randomized clinical trial. *Journal of Hand Surgery European Volume 41*(9), 948–956. https://doi.org/10.1177/1753193416657760

Kaile, E. (2014). An OT by another name? *OT News, 22*(11), 30–31.

Lim, Y. H., Chee, D. Y., Girdler, S., & Lee, H. C. (2017). Median nerve mobilization techniques in the treatment of carpal tunnel syndrome: A systematic review. *Journal of Hand Therapy, 30*(4), 397–406. https://doi.org/10.1016/j.jht.2017.06.019

Mack, E. M., Callinan, N. J., Reams, M., Bohn, D. C., & Chmielewski, T. L. (2017). Patient-reported outcomes after open carpal tunnel release using a standard protocol with 1 hand therapy visit. *Journal of Hand Therapy, 30*(1), 58–64. https://doi.org/10.1016/j.jht.2016.03.007

O'Toole, M. T. (Ed.). (2017). *Mosby's dictionary of medicine, nursing & health professions* (10th ed.). Elsevier.

Porter, R. S. (Ed.). (2018). *The Merck manual of diagnosis and therapy* (20th ed.). Merck Sharp & Dohme.

Toosi, K. K., Impink, B. G., Baker, N. A., & Boninger, M. L. (2011). Effects of computer keyboarding on ultrasonographic measures of the median nerve. *American Journal of Industrial Medicine, 54*(11), 826–833. https://doi.org/10.1002/ajim.20983

Wong, S., & Rocker, J. D. (2018). Helping a client with carpal tunnel syndrome and trigger fingers pump gas. *OT Practice, 23*(18), 29–31.

Zukowski, L. A., Roper, J. A., Shechtman, O., Otzel, D. M., Hovis, P. W., & Tillman, M. D. (2014). Wheelchair ergonomic hand drive mechanism use improves wrist mechanics associated with carpal tunnel syndrome. *Journal of Rehabilitation Research and Development, 51*, 1515–1524. https://doi.org/10.1682/JRRD.2013.09.0211

BIBLIOGRAPHY

Cantero-Téllez, R., Naughton, N., Algar, L., & Valdes, K. (2019). Linking hand therapy outcome measures used after carpal tunnel release to the International Classification of Functioning, Disability and Health: A systematic review. *Journal of Hand Therapy, 32*(2), 233–242. https://doi.org/10.1016/j.jht.2018.02.006

Fernandes, J. G. (2018). Occupational therapists' role in perinatal care: A health promotion approach. *American Journal of Occupational Therapy, 72*(5), Article 7205347010. https://doi.org/10.5014/ajot.2018.028126

Jerosch-Herold, C., Shepstone, L., Houghton, J., Wilson, E. C. F., & Blake, J. (2019). Prognostic factors for response to treatment by corticosteroid injection or surgery in carpal tunnel syndrome (palms study): A prospective multicenter cohort study. *Muscle & Nerve, 60*(1), 32–40. https://doi.org/10.1002/mus.26459

Jerosch-Herold, C., Shepstone, L., & Miller, L. (2012). Sensory relearning after surgical treatment for carpal tunnel syndrome: A pilot clinical trial. *Muscle & Nerve, 46*(6), 879–884. https://doi.org/10.1002/mus.23421

Jerosch-Herold, C., Shepstone, L., Miller, L., & Chapman, P. (2011). The responsiveness of sensibility and strength tests in patients undergoing carpal tunnel decompression. *BMC Musculoskeletal Disorders, 12*, Article 244. https://doi.org/10.1186/1471-2474-12-244

Dupuytren's Disease

Also called Dupuytren's contracture.

Description

Dupuytren's disease, or contracture, is a progressive contracture of the palmar fascial bands, causing flexion deformities of the fingers (Porter, 2018, p. 289). The disease results in thickening and tightening of subcutaneous tissue of the palm, causing the fourth and fifth digits to flex and to resist extension (O'Toole, 2017).

Cause

Dupuytren's is an autosomal dominant condition with variable penetrance. It occurs more commonly among men older than 45, of Celtic descent, and in persons with diabetes, alcoholism, or epilepsy. However, the specific factors that cause the palmar fascia to thicken and contract are unknown (Porter, 2018).

Evaluation/Assessment

Areas

- Activities of Daily Living/Instrumental ADL: eating, bathing, dressing, writing
- Education/Work: keyboarding
- Play/Leisure: types of actions requiring repetitive hand functions such as playing an instrument, frequency, location
- Rest/Sleep: changes in sleep habits related to discomfort or pain
- Social Participation: types of social actions that require repetitive hand function, frequency, location, with whom
- Sensorimotor: finger extension/joint range of motion, hand functions, grip strength, pain, sensibility
- Cognitive/Perceptual: body image
- Psychosocial: anxiety, sense of competence, self-confidence, self-awareness about appearance, role competency, quality of life
- Context/Environment: knowledge of disorder, resources, splints
- Comorbidities: carpal tunnel syndrome, diabetes, triggering digits, abductor digit minimi band

Instruments

Instruments Developed by Occupational Therapy Personnel

- Canadian Occupational Performance Measure (5th ed.; COPD-5; Law et al., 2014; see also van de Ven-Stevens et al., 2015, in References)

Instruments Developed by Other Professionals and Used by Occupational Therapy Personnel
- Circumference (edema) tape measure
- Disabilities of the Arm, Shoulder, and Hand (3rd ed.; DASH-3; Kennedy et al., 2011; see also Forget et al., 2014; Jerosch-Herold, Shepstone, Chojnowski, & Larson, 2011; and Packham, 2011, in References). (Note: The DASH did not measure the severity of flexion contracture and functional disability.)
- Dynamometry (grip strength; JAMAR Hydraulic, Lafayette Instrument; Wang et al., 2018)
- European Quality of Life 5-Dimension Scale (EuroQol 5 Dimension, EQ-5D; EuroQol Group, 1990)
- Joint range of motion (goniometer; Shurtleff & Kaskutas, 2018; see also Engstrand et al., 2012, and Pratt & Ball, 2016, in References)
- Michigan Hand Outcomes Questionnaire (MHQ; Chung et al., 1998)
- Patient Activation Measure (PAM; Hibbard et al., 2004)
- Patient Outcomes of Surgery–Hand/Arm (POS-Hand/Arm; Cano et al., 2004)
- Patient-Rated Wrist/Hand Evaluation (PRWHE; MacDermid & Tottenham, 2004)
- QuickDASH (3rd ed.; DASH-3; Kennedy et al., 2011; see also Budd et al., 2011, in References)
- Volumeter or water displacement (edema; Abrams & Ivy, 2018; Stern, 1991)

Problems/Issues

Activities of Daily Living/Instrumental ADL
(Note: Not all persons with Dupuytren's report difficulty performing everyday tasks.)
- Person may experience difficulty with washing and bathing.
- Person may experience difficulty with dressing tasks, such as buttoning a shirt and dealing with fasteners.
- Person may experience difficulty using eating utensils, especially cutting with a knife.
- Person may experience difficulty manipulating small objects in the hand, such as using a key, turning a doorknob, or pulling off sheets of bathroom tissue.
- Person may experience difficulty writing with a pen or pencil because of the position of the contracture of the fourth and fifth fingers.
- Person may experience difficulty pushing up from a chair using the affected hand.
- Person may experience difficulty carrying objects weighing 10 pounds or more with affected hand.

Education/Work
- Person may experience difficulty with keyboarding on the computer because of the contracture(s).
- Person may experience difficulty with meal preparation, such as carrying a pan of food from the stove to the sink.
- Person may experience difficulty performing household cleaning and maintenance tasks.

Play/Leisure
- Person may experience difficulty playing an instrument with a keyboard, such as the piano.
- Person may experience difficulty gripping handles, such as those of a golf club.

Rest/Sleep
- Person may experience pain in the hand, which interferes with sleep.

Social Participation
- Person may restrict or stop social participation activities because of the appearance of the contractures in the hand.

Sensorimotor (Sweet & Blackmore, 2014)
- Person usually has reduced active range of motion of the fingers (usually the fourth and/or fifth) on the affected hand.

- Person usually cannot fully extend the involved proximal interphalangeal joint (PIPJ) of the finger(s) because of the flexion contracture.
- Person may show lateral band migration volar to the axis of the PIPJ contracture.
- Person may have shortening of the collateral ligament.
- Person may have digital nerve shortening and digital nerve entrapment within the Dupuytren's cord.
- Person may have vascular shortening.
- Person may have lumbrical and interosseus muscle shortening.

Cognitive/Perceptual
- Person may experience changes in body image.

Psychosocial
- Person may be self-conscious about appearance of the hand.
- Person may resist participating in certain social rituals, such as shaking hands, because one or more fingers cannot be fully extended.
- Person may feel the quality of life has been reduced.

Context/Environment
- Person may lack knowledge of the disorder and its management.
- Person may lack information about available resources.
- Person may need splints to maintain extension.

Intervention/Treatment

Intervention is based on remedial approaches, but wound management and tissue viability are considered before increasing range of motion. Models and programs developed by occupational therapy personnel include hand therapist-based protocol (Malafa et al., 2016) and nighttime splinting (Jerosch-Herold, Shepstone, Chojnowski, Larson, et al., 2011). Models and programs developed by other professionals but used by occupational therapy personnel include the wide-awake approach (Nelson et al., 2010). Team members include physicians, hand surgeons, physical therapy personnel, and occupational therapy personnel. Goal is to enable person to return to previous level of occupational performance and be able to perform the valued and meaningful occupations of the person's choice.

Activities of Daily Living/Instrumental ADL
- No information identified.

Education/Work
- No information identified.

Play/Leisure
- No information identified.

Rest/Sleep
- Issues related to comfort while sleeping with a night splint should be addressed.

Social Participation
- No information identified.

Sensorimotor
- Nonoperative or conservative approaches: Includes enzymatic fasciotomy (collagenase injection), skeletal traction, use of progressive mechanical tension orthoses, radiation, dimethyl sulfoxide, vitamin E, allopurinol, ultrasound therapy, steroid injections, interferon, and various orthotic devices.
- General goals (Evans, 2011)
  - ▶ Minimize inflammation associated with edema, hematoma, infection, or neural tension.

▶ Maximize tissue nutrition and oxygenation. (Note: Avoid early stretching, stressful splinting, and exercise techniques that may contribute to edema and increased capillary pressure.)
▶ Promote wound healing and scar reorganization by limiting tension to incision sites and avoiding opening wound sites.
▶ Improve joint motion with attention to proximal interphalangeal (PIP) extension, distal interphalangeal (DIP) flexion (Note: without increasing inflammation).

- Postsurgery (Malafa et al., 2016)
  ▶ Client's forearm is placed in neutral position with wrist in full flexion.
  ▶ Metacarpophalangeal joint (MCP) joint of affected digit is fully flexed.
  ▶ Passive wrist and MCP flexion are maintained while PIP and DIP joints are brought slowly into maximum extension.
  ▶ Next, MCP extension is added until digit is in maximum extension.
  ▶ Cord should release.
  ▶ If cord does not release, client-controlled wrist extension is added with palm flat on table while asking client to raise the elbow until the wrist is extended.
  ▶ Position maintained for 15–20 seconds.
- Postoperative early phase, no tension protocol (Evans, 2011)
  ▶ Wound healing (excluding skin grafts)
    ○ Wash with soap and water (Ivory or Dove pump soap recommended).
    ○ Use dressing to maintain humidity to speed cellular growth.
    ○ Use agents to control potential infection.
  ▶ Edema control
    ○ Use 2-inch Coban (self-adhesive bandage), single layer on diagonal for fingers.
    ○ If edema or hematoma is observed, reapply hand dressing.
    ○ Maintain elevation.
    ○ Cool compresses may be used if there are no vascular issues.
  ▶ Splinting
    ○ Tension should be avoided to reduce mechanical stress to the healing tissues.
    ○ A dorsal block splint is used to include affected digits and neighboring digits. Wrist in neutral, MCP joints at 40–50 degrees flexion, IP joints in neutral. Splint should allow digital flexion but prevent MCP extension.
  ▶ Exercise
    ○ No exercises during early inflammatory state (1–3 days).
    ○ Gentile flexion within limits of splint (3–7 days).
    ○ Monitor skin flaps and skin nutrition.
    ○ Continuous passive motion (CPM) is not considered useful.
- Postoperative weeks 2–3
  ▶ Wound management
    ○ Continue dressing until incision line has closed.
    ○ Use soap and water only (avoid prepared washes or alcohol).
  ▶ Scar management
    ○ Tension reduced splinting and gentle exercise to minimize scarring.
    ○ Micropore paper tape applied above and below incision placed longitudinally in lines of tension may be applied to dry skin.
  ▶ Splinting
    ○ Continue dorsal block splint with MCP joints at 45 degrees.
    ○ At Week 2, start volar PIP digital extension splint.
    ○ Volar static PIP splint with DIP joint free can be used as a night splint for PIP extension.
    ○ Avoid aggressive extension splinting that may contribute to tissue anoxia.
    ○ A dynamic flexion splint is usually not needed unless a flare develops.
  ▶ Modalities
    ○ Cool compresses to start, progressing to warm compresses to control inflammation.

- o High volt galvanic stimulation may be used for edema.
- o Function electric simulation (FES) may be used to facilitate flexion.
- o Iontophoresis with dexamethasone may be used for digital nerve pain or burning session.
  - ► Exercise
    - o Gentle joint blocking to facilitation flexor digitorum profundus (FDP) and flexor digitorum sublimis (FDS) tension guide.
    - o Avoid composite extension of all joints.
    - o PIP can be extended gently with MCP flexed.
    - o MCP can be extend gently with wrist in neutral and PIP flexed.
    - o Avoid using therapy equipment such as exercise putty, sponges, squeeze balls, hand grippers.
- • Postoperative weeks 3–6
  - ► Scar management
    - o For flat, nonpainful scar, use paper tape longitudinally for 2 months.
    - o For hypertrophic scar, use ultrasound and silicone gel sheeting for 10 to 12 hours per day.
    - o For burning or painful scar, use iontophoresis with dexamethasone, 6 treatments.
    - o General: gentle massage.
  - ► Splinting
    - o Provide prolonged gentle stress using nighttime composite extension splint.
    - o Use PIP digital extension splints intermittently 5 times per day for 15 20 minutes.
    - o Serial casting may be used for inflamed PIP joints with flexion contracture.
    - o Dynamic flexion splint with 200–250 grams of pressure may be used to improve composite flexion.
    - o Composite dynamic extension may be used for extrinsic flexor tightness and limited composite flexion.
  - ► Modalities
    - o Heat or FES may be used for joint stiffness.
    - o Cold or high voltage galvanic stimulation may be used for inflammation.
    - o Ultrasound may be used for hypertrophic scarring.
    - o Iontophoresis may be used for painful or burning scarring.
    - o Manual massage may be used to soften scarring and reduce edema.
  - ► Exercise
    - o Continue gentle blocking, emphasizing PIP extension and DIP flexion.
    - o During DIP exercises position finger to stretch the oblique retinacular ligament.
    - o Light strengthening with isometric exercise for gross grasp using cylindrical objects 2 to 3 inches in diameter to avoid repetitive full-fisting.
- • Complications: watch for infection, flap necrosis, white finger, nerve damage, sympathetic flare, hypertrophic scarring, joint stiffness, recurrence, or disease extension.
- • High risk for complications: client with more than two involved digits, radial nerve disease, PIP joint flexion contracture greater than 45 to 60 degrees, and ruddy type complexion (Evans, 2011).

Cognitive/Perceptual
- • Not discussed; consider body image changes.

Psychosocial
- • Not discussed; consider self-efficacy, role performance.

Context/Environment
- • Written home program with illustrations/drawing should be provided.
- • Provide copy to spouse, family member, or caregiver as well as to client.
- • Provide information on disorder and its management.
- • Provide access to resources in the community and on the internet.

Precautions/Safety Considerations

- Observe female clients carefully (higher risk of complications if have ruddy complexion).
- Observe clients with more than three fingers involved (higher risk of complications).
- Observe clients with PIP joint release in addition to MCP release for complications.
- Observe clients with additional diagnoses, such as carpal tunnel syndrome or diabetes, for complications.
- Caution clients to follow instructions as written (men may tend to overdo exercises and have complications).
- Watch for signs of complex regional pain syndrome (CRPS; see Section 2: Sensory Disorders, for details).

Prognosis and Outcome

In general, prognosis and outcome are favorable. Many clients achieve full occupational performance of their previous occupations. However, nonsurgical intervention should include both static splints (extension orthosis) and hand therapy exercises (home program; Pashmdarfard et al., 2019; Sweet & Blackmore, 2014). Clients report fear of hurting the hand, anxiety about ability to cope with daily life, ability to handle occupational demands, and overall quality of life (Engstrand et al., 2015; Engstrand et al., 2014; Engstrand et al., 2016).

REFERENCES

Budd, H. R., Larson, D., Chojnowski, A., & Shepstone, L. (2011). The QuickDASH score: A patient-reported outcome measure for Dupuytren's surgery. *Journal of Hand Therapy*, 24(1), 15–20. https://doi.org/10.1016/j.jht.2010.08.006

Engstrand, C., Krevers, B., & Kvist, J. (2012). Brief report: Interrater reliability in finger joint goniometer measurement in Dupuytren's disease. *American Journal of Occupational Therapy*, 66(1), 98–103. https://doi.org/10.5014/ajot.2012.001925

Engstrand, C., Krevers, B., & Kvist, J. (2015). Factors affecting functional recovery after surgery and hand therapy in patients with Dupuytren's disease. *Journal of Hand Therapy*, 28(3), 255–259. https://doi.org/10.1016/j.jht.2014.11.006

Engstrand, C., Krevers, B., Nylander, G., & Kvist, J. (2014). Hand function and quality of life before and after fasciectomy for Dupuytren contracture. *Journal of Hand Surgery*, 39(7), 1333–1343. https://doi.org/10.1016/j.jhsa.2014.04.029

Engstrand, C., Kvist, J., & Krevers, B. (2016). Patients' perspective on surgical intervention for Dupuytren's disease—Experiences, expectations and appraisal of results. *Disability and Rehabilitation*, 38(26), 2538–2549. https://doi.org/10.3109/09638288.2015.1137981

Evans, R. B. (2011). Therapeutic management of Dupuytren's contracture. In T. M. Shirven, A. L. Osterman, J. M. Fedorczyk, & P. C. Amadio (Eds.), *Rehabilitation of the hand and upper extremity* (6th ed., pp. 281–288). Elsevier/Mosby.

Forget, N. J., Jerosch-Herold, C., Shepstone, L., & Higgins, J. (2014). Psychometric evaluation of the Disabilities of the Arm, Shoulder and Hand (DASH) with Dupuytren's contracture: Validity evidence using Rasch modeling. *BMC Musculoskeletal Disorders*, 15, Article 361. https://doi.org/10.1186/1471-2474-15-361

Jerosch-Herold, C., Shepstone, L., Chojnowski, A., & Larson, D. (2011). Severity of contracture and self-reported disability in patients with Dupuytren's contracture referred for surgery. *Journal of Hand Therapy*, 24(1), 6–10. https://doi.org/10.1016/j.jht.2010.07.006

Jerosch-Herold, C., Shepstone, L., Chojnowski, A., Larson, D., Barrett, E., & Vaughan, S. P. (2011). Night-time splinting after fasciectomy or dermo-fasciectomy for Dupuytren's contracture: A pragmatic, multi-centre, randomised controlled trial. *BMC Musculoskeletal Disorders*, 12, Article 136. https://doi.org/10.1186/1471-2474-12-136

Malafa, M. M., Lehrman, C., Criley, J. W., & Amirlak, B. (2016). Collagenase Dupuytren contracture: Achieving single treatment success with a hand therapist-based protocol. *Plastic and Reconstructive Surgery–Global Open, 4*(2), Article e629. https://doi.org/10.1098/GOX .0000000000000565

Nelson, R., Higgins, A., Conrad, J, Bell, M., & Lalonde, D. (2010). The wide-awake approach to Dupuytren's disease: Fasciectomy under local anesthetic with epinephrine. *Hand, 5*(2), 117–124. https://doi.org/10.1007/s11552-009-9239-y

O'Toole, M. T. (Ed.). (2017). *Mosby's dictionary of medicine, nursing & health professions* (10th ed.). Elsevier.

Packham, T. (2011). Clinical commentary in response to: Severity of contracture and self-reported disability in patients with Dupuytren's contracture referred for surgery. *Journal of Hand Therapy, 24*(1), 12–14. https://doi.org/10.1016/j.jht.2010.10.001

Pashmdarfard, M., Azad, A., Amini, M., & Golabi, G. (2019). The effect of splinting after Dupuytren's contracture operation: A systematic review. *Iranian Rehabilitation Journal, 17*(4), 297–304. https://doi.org/10.32598/irj.17.4.297

Porter, R. S. (Ed.). (2018). *The Merck manual of diagnosis and therapy* (20th ed.). Merck Sharp & Dohme.

Pratt, A. L., & Ball, C. (2016). What are we measuring? A critique of range of motion methods currently in use for Dupuytren's disease and recommendations for practice. *BMC Musculo-skeletal Disorders, 17*, Article 20. https://doi.org/10.1186/s12891-016-0884-3

Sweet, S., & Blackmore, S. (2014). Surgical and therapy update on the management of Dupuytren's disease. *Journal of Hand Therapy, 27*(2), 77–84. https://doi.org/10.1016/j.jht.2013.10.006

van de Ven-Stevens, L. A. W., Graff, M. J. L., Peters, M. A. M., van der Linde, H., & Geurts, A. C. H. (2015). Construct validity of the Canadian Occupational Performance Measure in participants with tendon injury and Dupuytren disease. *Physical Therapy, 95*(5), 750–757. https://doi .org/10.2522/ptj.20130590

BIBLIOGRAPHY

Cooper, C. (2014). Dupuytren's disease. In C. Cooper (Ed.), *Fundamentals of hand therapy* (2nd ed., pp. 542–550). Mosby/Elsevier.

Larson, D. (2012). The relative responsiveness of patient-rated outcome measures in evaluating clinical change after Dupuytren's surgery: A literature review and prospective observational pilot study. *Hand Therapy, 17*(3), 52–59. https://doi.org/10.1258/ht.2012.012008

Turesson, C. (2018). The role of hand therapy in Dupuytren disease. *Hand Clinics, 34*(3), 395–401. https://doi.org/10.1016/j.hcl.2018.03.008

Turesson, C., Kvist, J., & Krevers, B. (2020). Experiences of men living with Dupuytren's disease—Consequences of the disease for hand function and daily activities. *Journal of Hand Therapy, 33*(3), 386–393. https://doi.org/10.1016/j.jht.2019.04.004

Extensor Tendon Injuries

Also called extensor tendon lacerations.
See also Mallet Finger Injury.

Description

Extensor tendon injuries affect the tendons and related structures of the extensor muscles on the dorsum (posterior surface) of the hand and the wrist. The extensor muscles include the extensor digitorum communis (EDC), extensor indicis proprius (EIP), extensor digiti minimi (EDM), extensor pollicis longus (EPL), extensor pollicis brevis (EPB), and abductor pollicis longus (APL). The lumbrical and interosseous muscles may also be involved. Related structures include the juncturae tendinum fibers, central slip, sagittal band, lateral band, triangular ligament and Landsmeer ligament, nerves, synovial fluid, and blood supply (Klein, 2014). Injuries are described based on assigned zones of the hand.

Cause

Laceration (knife, sharp object), rupture (torsion, tearing force, rheumatoid arthritis), fraying, crush injury, blunt force trauma. Causes can be grouped as open or closed. Open injuries occur most often from sharp objects. Closed injuries occur most often as a rupture due to friction on a bony prominence or weakening of a tendon due to disease process (Klein, 2014).

Extensor Tendon Zones (Cooper, 2014)
- Zone 1: Distal interphalangeal joint (DIP) joints of digits two to five and distal phalanx
- Zone 2: Middle phalanx of digits two to five
- Zone 3: Proximal interphalangeal (PIP) joints of digits two to five
- Zone 4: Proximal phalanx of digits two to five
- Zone 5: Metacarpophalangeal (MCP) joints of digits two to five
- Zone 6: Metacarpal bones of digits two to five
- Zone 7: Carpal bones of the wrist joint
- Zone T1: Interphalanx joint of the thumb
- Zone T2: Proximal phalanx bone of the thumb
- Zone T3: MCP joint of the thumb
- Zone T4: Metacarpal bone of the thumb
- Zone T5: Carpometacarpal (CMC) joint of the thumb

Extensor Zone Injuries
- Zones I and II (see Mallet Finger Injury, this Section)
- Zones III and IV: Common injury is a rupture of the EDC tendon from its attachment on the middle phalanx
- Zones V, VI, and VII: Common injury is due to laceration with a sharp object or disease process such as arthritis resulting in rupture or fraying

Evaluation/Assessment

Areas
- Activities of Daily Living/Instrumental ADL: normally performed ADLs and IADLs
- Education/Work: work tasks, work conditions/environment
- Play/Leisure: type, location, frequency
- Rest/Sleep: sleep disturbance
- Social Participation: type, location, frequency, with whom
- Sensorimotor: fine and gross motor skills, hand grasp and release functions, grip strength, pinch strength, range of motion, dexterity, manipulation, pain, edema
- Cognitive/Perceptual: dementia, executive dysfunction that may interfere with cooperating in intervention or following instructions for exercises and wearing splint
- Psychosocial: coping and stress, body image, quality of life
- Context/Environment: information resources

Instruments

Instruments Developed by Occupational Therapy Personnel
- Canadian Occupational Performance Measure (5th ed.; COPM-5; Law et al., 2014; see also van de Ven-Stevens et al., 2015, in References)

Instruments Developed by Other Professionals and Used by Occupational Therapy Personnel
- Disabilities of Arm, Shoulder, and Hand (3rd ed.; DASH-3; Kennedy et al., 2011)
- Grip/hand strength (JAMAR dynamometer; Wang et al., 2018)
- Joint range of motion (goniometer; Shurtleff & Kaskutas, 2018)

- Michigan Hand Outcomes Questionnaire (MHQ; Chung et al., 1998)
- Miller's criteria (Miller, 1942)
- Patient Evaluation Measure (PEM; Macey et al., 1995)
- Pinch meter (pinch strength; Mathiowetz et al., 1985)

Problems/Issues

Problems are not discussed in detail under extensor tendon injuries (see Flexor Tendon Injuries in Section 5 for a list of additional possible problems).

Activities of Daily Living/Instrumental ADL
- Person may report difficulty performing specific ADL or IADL tasks that involve the injured digit and hand.

Education/Work
- Person may report difficulty performing specific work-related tasks that involve the injured digit or hand.

Play/Leisure
- Person may be unable to perform or experience difficulty performing specific tasks related to preferred leisure activities that involve the injured digit or hand.

Rest/Sleep
- Person may find wearing a night splint uncomfortable or report pain.

Social Participation
- Person may be sensitive to wearing a splint in public.

Sensorimotor
- Person may experience loss of pinch strength if radial digits (thumb, index, and middle fingers) are involved, especially on dominant hand.
- Person may experience loss of ability to grasp objects depending on digits involved, and type of activity performed with involved hand.
- Person may experience decreased grip strength depending on digit(s) involved and type of activity performed with involved hand.
- Person may experience decreased dexterity and speed of movement depending on digit(s) involved and type of activity performed with involved hand.
- Person may experience swelling of injured digit or hand.
- Person may experience pain in involved digit(s) or hand.

Cognitive/Perceptual
- Person may forget or fail to perform prescribed exercises.

Psychosocial
- Person may report difficulty coping with wearing splint as specified.
- Person may feel splint draws unwanted attention to injury by others.

Context/Environment
- Person may not understand nature of injury or need for rehabilitation services.

Complications
- Person may experience attenuation, extension lag on MCP movement, extrinsic tightness, adhesions, or rupture.

Intervention/Treatment

Models and programs developed by occupational therapy personnel include active motion program (Svens et al., 2015). Models and programs developed by other professionals but used by occupational therapy personnel include early controlled passive motion regime for zone II (Gangatharam & Le Blanc, 2011), postoperative treatment protocols for zones V and VI (Hall et al., 2010), relative motion orthoses for zones III and IV (Hirth et al., 2017), and relative motion orthoses for zones V and VI (Hirth et al., 2011; Lutz et al., 2015). Team members include physicians, hand surgeons, plastic surgeons, physical therapy personnel, and occupational therapy personnel. Goals are restoration of function, minimizing disability, and decreasing the risk of complications (Lutz et al., 2015).

Activities of Daily Living/Instrumental ADL
- Light activities of daily living restarted at about 6 weeks postsurgery after splint is removed.
- At 10–12 weeks, all activities can be restarted.

Education/Work
- At 10–12 weeks, person can return to work except for heavy manual labor jobs, which are delayed until 12 weeks plus.

Play/Leisure
- Same as for Education/Work.

Rest/Sleep
- See Sleep–Wake Disorders in Section 13: Lifestyle Conditions.

Social Participation
- No information identified.

Sensorimotor
- Immobilization protocol (Hall et al, 2010)
  - ▸ Weeks 1–2: Immobilize hand in splint with wrist at 40–45 degrees extension, MCP at 0–20 degrees flexion, and interphalangeal (IP) at 0 degrees.
  - ▸ Weeks 3–6: Begin graded mobilization program.
  - ▸ Weeks 6–10: Splint discontinued and graded mobilization program continued.
  - ▸ Weeks 10–12: Gradually increase resistive activities and return to work/regular activities.
  - ▸ Week 12+: Return to heavy manual labor.
- Early passive motion protocol (adapted from Hall et al., 2010)
  - ▸ Weeks 1–2
    - ○ Passive motion is started on days 1–5 after surgery in a dynamic splint with wrist immobilized at 40–45 degrees extension, MCP at 0 degrees and palmar block allowing 30–40 degrees of MCP active flexion and passive extension.
    - ○ Exercise 20 times per hour in the splint: active MCP flexion, passive MP extension with IP extended.
    - ○ Supervised exercise with therapist: passive wrist tenodesis and IP joint motion.
  - ▸ Weeks 3–6: Palmar block removed and full active flexion started. By 6th week splint discontinued and graded mobilization program started.
  - ▸ Weeks 6–10: Graded exercise program completed and light activities of daily living started.
  - ▸ Weeks 10–12: Gradually increase resistive activities and return to work or regular activities.
- Early active motion protocol (adapted from Hall et al, 2010)
  - ▸ Weeks 1–2
    - ○ Active motion started on days 1–5 after surgery. Palmar blocking splint extended to the IP joint, with wrist immobilized at 30 degrees extension, MCP blocked at 45 degrees flexion, and IP joints free to move.
    - ○ Exercise 10 times per hour in the splint.
    - ○ Active MCP flexion and extension with IP extended.
    - ○ Composite active flexion and extension in the splint within limits of splint block.
  - ▸ Weeks 3–6
    - ○ Splint adjusted to allow 70 degrees of MCP flexion.

   ○ Active hook fists started (extensor digitorum tendon glides).
   ▸ Weeks 6–12: Same as above.

Cognitive/Perceptual
- No information identified.

Psychosocial
- No information identified.

Context/Environment
- Client should be instructed regarding purpose of exercises and may need visual and auditory instructions to comply.
- Client should be instructed in purpose of splints and proper care and maintenance.
- Client should be instructed to inspect digits and hand regularly for skin irritation.

Precautions/Safety Considerations

Splints should be monitored for proper fit and skin irritation or breakdown.

Prognosis and Outcome

Generally good outcome after 3 months.

REFERENCES

Cooper, C. (2014). *Fundamentals of hand therapy* (2nd ed.). Elsevier.

Gangatharam, S., & Le Blanc, M. (2011). Early controlled passive motion regime for zone II extensor tendon injury: A case report. *Techniques in Hand & Upper Extremity Surgery*, *15*(2), 72–74. https://doi.org/10.1097/BTH.0b013e3181ebe693

Hall, B., Lee, H., Page, R., Rosenwax, L., & Lee, A. H. (2010). Comparing three postoperative treatment protocols for extensor tendon repair in zones V and VI of the hand. *American Journal of Occupational Therapy*, *64*(5), 682–688. https://doi.org/10.5014/ajot.2010.09091

Hirth, M. J., Bennett, K., Mah, E., Farrow, H. C., Cavallo, A. V., Ritz, M., & Findlay, M. W. (2011). Early return to work and improved range of motion with modified relative motion splinting: A retrospective comparison with immobilization splinting for zones V and VI extensor tendon repairs. *Hand Therapy*, *16*(4), 86–94. https://doi.org/10.1258/ht.2011.011012

Hirth, M. J., Howell, J. W., & O'Brien, L. (2017). Two case reports—Use of relative motion orthoses to manage extensor tendon zones III and IV and sagittal band injuries in adjacent fingers. *Journal of Hand Therapy*, *30*(4), 546–557. https://doi.org/10.1016/j.jht.2017.04.006

Klein, L. J. (2014). Extensor tendon injury. In C. Cooper (Ed.), *Fundamentals of hand therapy* (2nd ed., pp. 426–437). Elsevier Mosby. https://doi.org/10.1016/B978-0-323-09104-6.00031-6

Lutz, K., Pipicelli, J., & Grewal, R. (2015). Management of complications of extensor tendon injuries. *Hand Clinics*, *31*(2), 301–310. https://doi.org/10.1016/j.hcl.2014.12.006

Svens, B., Ames, E., Burford, K., & Caplash, Y. (2015). Relative active motion programs following extensor tendon repair: A pilot study using a prospective cohort and evaluating outcomes following orthotic interventions. *Journal of Hand Therapy*, *28*(1), 11–19. https://doi.org/10.1016/j.jht.2014.07.006

van de Ven-Stevens, L. A. W., Graff, M. J. L., Peters, M. A. M., van der Linde, H., & Geurts, A. C. H. (2015). Construct validity of the Canadian Occupational Performance Measure in participants with tendon injury and Dupuytren disease. *Physical Therapy*, *95*(5), 750–757. https://doi.org/10.2522/ptj.20130590

BIBLIOGRAPHY

Chinchalkar, S. J., & Pipicelli, J. G. (2010). Complications of extensor tendon repairs at the extensor retinaculum. *Journal of Hand and Microsurgery*, *2*(1), 3–12. https://doi.org/10.1007/s12593-010-0008-5

Evans, R. B. (2011). Clinical management of extensor tendon injuries: The therapist's perspective. In T. M. Skirven, A. L. Osterman, J. M. Fedorczyk, & P. C. Amadio (Eds.), *Rehabilitation of the hand and upper extremity* (6th ed., pp. 521–554). Elsevier/Mosby.

Evans, R. B. (2017). *Rehabilitation following extensor tendon injuries.* http://handfoundation.org/wp-content/uploads/2015/02/820am_evans.pdf

Hirth, M. J., Howell, J. W., & O'Brien, L. (2016). Relative motion orthoses in the management of various hand conditions: A scoping review. *Journal of Hand Therapy, 29*(4), 405–432. https://doi.org/10.1016/j.jht.2016.07.001

Ng, C. Y., Chalmer, J., Macdonald, D. J. M., Mehta, S. S., Nuttall, D., & Watts, A. C. (2012). Rehabilitation regimens following surgical repair of extensor tendon injuries of the hand: A systematic review of controlled trials. *Journal of Hand and Microsurgery, 4*(2), 65–73. https://doi.org/10.1007/s12593-012-0075-x

Flexor Tendon Injuries

Description

Flexor tendon injuries involve the flexor digitorum superficialis (FDS) for each finger, the flexor digitorum profundus (FDP) for each finger, and the flexor pollicis longus for the thumb, and their related structures including ligaments, pulleys, bands, nerves, synovial fluid, and blood supply (Klein, 2014). The flexor carpi radialis (FCR) and flexor carpi ulnaris (FCU) muscles may also be involved. This chapter focuses on adults with flexor tendon injuries. For children, see article by von der Heyde (2015).

Cause

The most common causes are traumatic injury either by open lacerations (cuts) or closed rupture (Klein, 2014).

Flexor Tendon Zones

- Zone I: Boundaries are from the tip of the finger to the middle of the middle phalanx. Zone 1 contains only the FDP. Common injury called Jersey finger.
- Zone II: Boundaries are from the middle of the middle phalanx to the distal palmar crease in the palm. Zone 2 includes the A1 through A3 pulleys as well as both tendons for the FDS and the FDP. At the level of the proximal third of the proximal phalanx, the FDS tendons split into two slips called Camper's chiasm, which then divide around the FDP tendon and reunite at the dorsal aspect of the FDP, inserting into the distal end of the middle phalanx (Frost & Schepis, 2011). Because of the complex anatomy, historically, Zone 2 has been called "No Man's Land" because successful repair has been difficult and functional recovery poor.
- Zone III: Boundaries are the distal border of the transverse carpal ligament and the proximal educe of the fibrosseus sheath in the palm (Chinchalkar et al., 2015).
- Zone IV: Boundaries are from the carpal ligament to the carpal tunnel.
- Zone V: Boundaries are from the carpal tunnel to forearm.

Evaluation/Assessment

Areas

- Activities of Daily Living/Instrumental ADL: self-care, care of others, driving
- Education/Work: household management, computer keyboarding
- Play/Leisure: sports, games, musical instruments
- Rest/Sleep: discomfort, pain
- Social Participation: type, location
- Sensorimotor: grip and pinch strength, joint range of motion, pain, edema, sensation

- Cognitive/Perceptual: not directly involved; level of knowledge and understanding may affect choice of intervention program
- Psychosocial: quality of life, life roles
- Context/Environment: social support, adapted devices, community resources
- Comorbidity: dementia

Instruments

Instruments Developed by Occupational Therapy Personnel
- Canadian Occupational Performance Measure (5th ed.; COPM-5; Law et al., 2014)
- Interview questions (Kaskutas & Powell, 2013)

Instruments Developed by Other Professionals and Used by Occupational Therapy Personnel
- Disabilities of the Arm, Shoulder, and Hand (3rd ed.; DASH-3; Kennedy et al., 2011)
- Grip strength (dynamometer; JAMAR, Lafayette Instrument; Wang et al., 2018; Note: Do not test until tendon repair is fully healed.)
- Joint range of motion (goniometry; Shurtleff & Kaskutas, 2018; Note: Do not test until tendon repair is fully healed.)
- Pinch meter (pinch strength; B&E Engineering; Mathiowetz et al., 1985; Note: Do not test until tendon repair is fully healed.)

Problems/Issues

Activities of Daily Living/Instrumental ADL
- Person usually has difficulty washing hands when orthosis is worn.
- Person may have difficulty cutting meat with knife and fork.
- Person may have difficulty applying makeup.
- Person may have difficulty fastening pants or buttoning a shirt.
- Person may have difficulty bathing or showering.
- Person may have difficulty with toileting.
- Person may have difficulty brushing hair.
- Person may have difficulty with dressing tasks such as fastening a bra or putting on pantyhose.
- Person may have difficulty pulling up pants.
- Person may have difficulty putting on a coat.
- Person may have difficulty driving.
- Person may have difficulty carrying groceries.
- Person may have difficulty doing laundry.
- Person may have difficulty manipulating money.
- Person may have difficulty mowing the lawn or doing other yard work.
- Person may have difficulty with cooking tasks.
- Person may have difficulty opening jars.
- Person may have difficulty caring for pets.
- Person may have difficulty with child caring tasks, including dressing, bathing, diapering, and lifting the child.
- Person may have difficulty with house cleaning chores.
- Person may have difficulty making a bed.
- Person may have difficulty opening doors or manipulating keys.

Education/Work
- Person may have difficulty keyboarding or handwriting.
- Person may have difficulty performing work tasks requiring hand functions.

Play/Leisure
- Person may have difficulty playing games, including video games.
- Person may have difficulty playing a musical instrument, such as a guitar.
- Person may have difficulty engaging in sports activities, such as basketball.

Rest/Sleep
- Person may experience sleep disturbance due to pain or positioning to accommodate orthosis.

Social Participation
- Person may limit social participation activities because of limitations related to hand function.

Sensorimotor
- Person has restricted hand function due to the splint.
- Person has decreased range of motion.
- Person has decreased hand strength.
- Person may have pain.
- Person may have edema.
- Person may experience sensory loss if nerves are severed.

Cognitive/Perceptual
- Person may not comply with wearing instructions for orthosis because splint interferes with completing daily tasks.
- Person may refuse to wear orthosis in public because of the splint's appearance and unwanted attention from others regarding the appearance.

Psychosocial
- Person may express concern about loss of independence and need to rely on others to complete tasks.
- Person may experience difficulty fulfilling expected life roles.

Context/Environment
- Family members or caregivers may have to perform or help perform tasks usually done independently by the person.
- Person, family members, and caregivers may lack knowledge about one-handed techniques or adapted devices.

Intervention/Treatment

Models and programs developed by occupational therapy personnel include Zone III modification (Chinchalkar et al., 2015). Models and programs developed by other professionals but used by occupational therapy personnel include flexor tendon repair protocols (Frost & Schepis, 2011), Zone II flexor tendon repairs (Kannas et al., 2015), and wide-awake flexor tendon repair (Safdar, 2015). Team members include general physicians, hand surgeons, physical therapists, and occupational therapy personnel. Goals are to promote functional range of motion while safely mobilizing repaired tendon(s) and to prevent gapping, rupture, or adhesions (Kannas et al., 2015).

Activities of Daily Living/Instrumental ADL
- Client may benefit from being taught to use one-handed techniques during recovery time.
- Client may benefit from instruction and use of selected adapted devices during recovery time that facilitate one-handed approaches, such as electric can opener, universal cuff with an opening into which eating utensils will fit when facing toward thumb, or turned around so opening faces little finger and a peg or dowel with rubber tip can be inserted for keyboarding.

Education/Work
- Assist client with work station modification during recovery time.
- Consider if adapted devices would be useful, such as electric staplers or carts to move items that are usually carried.
- Client may need to change work assignments during recovery time.

Play/Leisure

- Assist client to modify approaches to engage in leisure occupations during recovery time.
- Client may be interested in exploring and learning new leisure occupations that can be performed within compliance instruction.

Rest/Sleep

- Assist client to address sleep issues: pain, discomfort, positioning orthosis during sleep.

Social Participation

- Assist client to modify participation in social activities that are acceptable to the client during recovery time.

Sensorimotor

- There are three rehabilitation programs for flexor tendon repair: delayed immobilization, early passive mobilization, and early active mobilization. Factors influencing choice include repair technique, associated tendon healing, passive versus active range of motion, edema, tendon adhesions, and physician preference (Frost & Schepis, 2011; Kannas et al., 2015).
- Delayed immobilization (usually reserved for clients who are too young or might not have the cognitive ability to understand the precautions according to Frost & Schepis, 2011).
  - ▶ Weeks 1–3
    - ○ Wrist and hand are immobilized in a dorsal cast or orthosis with wrist in 30 degrees of flexion and metacarpophalangeal (MCP) joints in 40 degrees of flexion; interphalangeal (IP) joints are in complete extension.
    - ○ At 3 weeks, cast or orthosis is removed to begin exercises.
    - ○ Client begins active and passive motion of the wrist and digits, including tendon-gliding exercises in hook, straight distal interphalangeal (DIP), or fist positions.
    - ○ Orthosis is modified to place wrist in neutral position. Orthosis is worn between exercises.
  - ▶ Weeks 4–6
    - ○ Cast or orthosis is discontinued.
    - ○ Active and passive differential tendon gliding exercises and synergistic wrist motion are initiated.
    - ○ Synergistic wrist motion (SWM) or tenodesis permits wrist extension while the digits flex and vice versus (Pettengill & Van Strien, 2011).
  - ▶ Weeks 6–8
    - ○ At 6 weeks, light resistive exercise is started.
    - ○ At 8 weeks, client should progress to moderate to heavy resistive activities.
  - ▶ Weeks 8–12
    - ○ Client continues moderate to heavy resistive activities.
    - ○ At Week 12, client is allowed unrestricted use and function of the hand.
- Early passive motion (modifications of Kleinert protocol and Duran and Houser protocol; Frost & Schepis, 2011; Pettengill & Van Strien, 2011).
  - ▶ Weeks 0–3
    - ○ Forearm dorsal block wrist and hand orthosis used to immobilize the wrist between neutral and 20 degrees of flexion, with MCP joints placed in 40 degrees of flexion, and IP joints completely extended to the dorsal block.
    - ○ In the Kleinert protocol, client extends against resistance provided by rubber bands or elastic thread that is attached proximal to the wrist.
    - ○ Client actively extends against the resistance and then relaxes to allow the rubber band to fix the digit into the palm.
    - ○ Exercise occurs every hour.
    - ○ In the Duran protocol, client actively extends again the dorsal block splint without resistance.

○ Client then passively flexes the digit into the palm.
○ Exercise is performed 3 to 4 times per day.
► Weeks 3–6
○ Physician assesses the quality of tendon glide to determine if active flexion exercises should be initiated while continuing use of dorsal block splint.
► Weeks 6–8
○ Splint is discontinued at 6 weeks depending the quality of the tendon glide.
○ Light functional activities of daily living such as brushing teeth, feeding self, holding an 8-ounce cup or phone can be initiated.
► Weeks 8–12
○ Heavy lifting may be initiated.
○ At 12 weeks, activities unrestricted.
○ Note: Results are better if client lacks full range of motion than if a tendon ruptures from overexercising.
• Early active motion: Strickland and Cannon protocol; Evans and Thompson protocol (Frost & Schepis, 2011; Pettengill & Van Strien, 2011; Safdar, 2015).
► Time periods and tasks vary.
► Splint: A dorsal block protective splint is worn from 1 to 7 weeks. Wrist position may vary from 20 degrees of wrist flexion to 20 degrees of wrist extension. Position of MCP joints may vary from 40 degrees of flexion to 70 or 90 degrees of flexion. The IP joints usually are strapped to the dorsal block in full extension when not being exercised.
► Exercises: Active tendon gliding exercise is not permitted during Weeks 1–3. At Week 4, active mobilization exercises and passive flexion and extension exercises are done every hour for 4 weeks. At 5 to 6 weeks, differential tendon gliding and active fisting exercises are initiated
► Functional activities: At Week 7, dorsal block splint is discontinued. Participation in functional activities and performance of progressive resistive exercises are started.
► Variation in protocols: Strickland and Cannon protect wrist movement using a dorsal block wrist hinge splint that limits wrist extension beyond 30 degrees and allows the client to perform exercises at home. Evans and Thompson do not use a hinge splint and limit client to performing place-hold exercises in therapy session.

Cognitive/Perceptual
• Provide verbal information at level of client's learning ability and written instruction at reading level.

Psychosocial
• Allow client to express concerns and problems in regard to complying with instructions and restrictions.

Context/Environment
• Provide instruction in use of adaptive strategies such as one-hand techniques and use of adapted devices that meet the needs of the client to perform everyday occupations.
• Provide resources to acquire adapted devices.
• Provide instruction on wearing and caring for orthotic device.

Precautions/Safety Considerations (Kaskutas & Powell, 2013)

Noncompliance with wearing instructions is a frequent problem. Therapists can assist by helping clients to use adapted techniques and devices during recovery time to facilitate safety in occupational performance of daily activities and life role tasks while complying with rehabilitation program. Do not allow client to stretch or move the hand when postoperative dressing or orthoses are removed. Client should be instructed to maintain position in which the hand is positioned to avoid tendon rupture. When fabricating an orthosis do not stretch repaired tendon to avoid possible tendon rupture. Do not measure grip or pinch strength following tendon repair until after full 12- to-14-week healing period has occurred.

Prognosis and Outcome

Formula for determining results of flexor tendon repair: (PIP + DIP flexion) – (Loss of PIP extension + loss of DIP extension) – 175 × 100 = % of normal. Excellent: 85%–100%. Good: 70%–84%. Fair: 50%–69%. Poor: Less than 50%.

REFERENCES

Chinchalkar, S. J., Pipicelli, J. G., Agur, A., & Athwal, G. S. (2015). Zone III flexor tendon injuries—A proposed modification to rehabilitation. *Journal of Hand Therapy, 28*(3), 319–324. https://doi.org/10.1016/j.jht.2014.11.008

Frost, L., & Schepis, K. M. (2011). A review of three flexor tendon repair protocols. *Physical Disabilities Special Interest Section Quarterly, 34*(4), 1–4.

Kannas, S., Jeardeau, T. A., & Bishop, A. T. (2015). Rehabilitation following zone II flexor tendon repairs. *Techniques in Hand & Upper Extremity Surgery, 19*(1), 2–10. https://doi.org/10.1097/BTH.0000000000000076

Kaskutas, V., & Powell, R. (2013). The impact of flexor tendon rehabilitation restrictions on individuals' independence with daily activities: Implications for hand therapists. *Journal of Hand Therapy, 26*(1), 22–29. https://doi.org/10.1016/j.jht.2012.08.004

Klein, L. J. (2014). Flexor tendon injury. In C. Cooper (Ed.), *Fundamentals of hand therapy* (2nd ed., pp. 412–425). Elsevier Mosby.

Pettengill, K., & Van Strien, G. (2011). Postoperative management of flexor tendon injuries. In T. M. Shirven, A. L. Osterman, J. M. Fedorczyk, & P. C. Amadio (Eds.), *Rehabilitation of the hand and upper extremity* (6th ed., pp. 457–478). Elsevier/Mosby.

Safdar, S. (2015). Wide-awake flexor tendon repair. *OT Practice, 20*(8), 7–16.

von der Heyde, R. (2015). Flexor tendon injuries in children: Rehabilitative options and confounding factors. *Journal of Hand Therapy, 28*(2), 195–200. https://doi.org/10.1016/j.jht.2014.12.002

BIBLIOGRAPHY

Powell, R. K., & von der Heyde, R. L. (2014). The inclusion of activities of daily living in flexor tendon rehabilitation: A survey. *Journal of Hand Therapy, 27*(1), 23–29. https://doi.org/10.1016/j.jht.2013.09.007

von der Heyde, R. L. (2013). Clinical commentary in response to "The impact of flexor tendon rehabilitation restrictions on individuals' independence with daily activities: Implications for hand therapists." *Journal of Hand Therapy, 26*(1), 30–31. https://doi.org/10.1016/j.jht.2012.10.003

Hand Fractures

Description

Hand fractures include fractures to the metacarpal and phalange bones. Metacarpal fracture sites can be located in the head, neck, shaft, and base. The most common metacarpal fracture is to the fifth or little finger (Boxer's fracture; Porter, 2018). The second most common is a fracture at the first metacarpal base (thumb), known as a Bennett's fracture. Another fracture is called the Rolando's fracture, which occurs at the first metacarpal base (thumb) but presents with a "T" or a "Y" fracture pattern that splits the articular surface of the base of the metacarpal (Varney,

2014). Reduction is not recommended if dorsal or volar angulation is less than 35 degrees for fourth metacarpal or 45 degrees for fifth metacarpal. Reduction is recommended if the angulation is greater than stated previously, if a rotation deformity is present, or if the second and third metacarpals are also fractured with angulation (Porter, 2018).

Fracture sites in the phalanges most often occur in the shaft of the proximal phalanx (P1), proximal distal one third of the middle phalanx (P2), and shaft or tuft (end) of the distal phalanx (P3; Varney, 2014).

Cause

Metacarpal and phalange fractures usually result from an axial load, such as punching with a clenched fist (Porter, 2018). Other causes are crush injury, torsion, or compression (Varney, 2014). The reason the first and fifth digits are most often involved is that they are "border digits" on the medial and lateral sides of the hands and thus are most exposed, and in addition, those digits are the most mobile (Varney, 2014).

Evaluation/Assessment

Areas

- Activities of Daily Living/Instrumental ADL: self-maintenance (Note: Fractures of fourth and fifth digits do not limit performance of most daily activities.)
- Education/Work: work tasks and equipment
- Play/Leisure: interests and values, frequency, location
- Rest/Sleep: sleep habits
- Social Participation: type, frequency, location, with whom
- Sensorimotor: grip strength, range of motion, dexterity, pain, edema, joint lag, peripheral nerve damage, ligament injury, tendon injury, skin
- Cognitive/Perceptual: not directly involved (note comorbidities)
- Psychosocial: quality of life
- Context/Environment: information, resources, social support
- Comorbidities: osteoarthritis, dementia, history of previous hand injuries

Instruments

Instruments Developed by Occupational Therapy Personnel
- Arthritis Hand Function Test (AHFT; Backman et al., 1991)
- Hand Function Survey (HFS; Blennerhassett et al., 2008)

Instruments Developed by Other Professionals and Used by Occupational Therapy Personnel
- Disabilities of the Arm, Shoulder, and Hand (3rd ed.; DASH-3; Kennedy et al., 2011; see also Weinstock-Zlotnick et al., 2015, in References)
- Edema (circumferential gauge or tape measure)
- Functional Independence Measure (FIM; Uniform Data System for Medical Rehabilitation, 1997)
- Grip strength (dynamometer; JAMAR, Lafayette Instrument; Wang et al., 2018)
- Jebsen-Taylor Hand Function Test (JTHFT; Jebsen et al., 1969)
- Joint range of motion (goniometry; Shurtleff & Kaskutas, 2018)
- Michigan Hand Outcomes Questionnaire (MHQ; Chung et al., 1998; see also Weinstock-Zlotnick et al., 2015, in References)
- Minnesota Rate of Manipulation Test (MRMT; Lafayette Instrument)
- Motor Assessment Scale (MAS; Carr et al., 1985)
- Patient-Rated Wrist/Hand Evaluation (PRWHE; MacDermid & Tottenham, 2004; see also Weinstock-Zlotnick et al., 2015, in References)
- QuickDASH (Kennedy et al., 2011)
- Upper Limb Functional Index (ULFI; Gabel, Michener, Burkett, & Neller, 2006)

Problems/Issues

Activities of Daily Living/Instrumental ADL

- Person may have difficulty performing self-maintenance occupations depending on the location of the fracture, stabilization approach (splint, hardware), and hand dominance.

Education/Work

- Person may have difficulty performing work tasks depending on type of work performed, location of the fracture, stabilization approach, and hand dominance.

Play/Leisure

- Person may be unable to engage in favorite leisure occupations or require modification.

Rest/Sleep

- Person may experience sleep disturbance due to pain or required positioning for external fixator hardware.

Social Participation

- Person may restrict or stop participation in social activities because of appearance of hand or restricted hand use due to stabilization that interferes with social performance.

Sensorimotor

- Person usually experiences loss of grip strength.
- Person usually experiences pain and tenderness.
- Person may experience loss of range of motion. Note: Always compare range of motion (ROM) to opposite side when reporting results.
- Person may experience swelling.
- Person may experience deformity, including limitation of motion and visual appearance.
- Person may experience loss of sensation due to nerve injury or impairment.
- Person may have soft tissue injury in addition to fracture.

Cognitive/Perceptual

- Person may need to be aware of hand placement if an external fixator or splint is applied.

Psychosocial

- Person may have concerns about appearance of hand with an external fixator attached and/or about wearing a splint in public.

Context/Environment

- Person may need instructions and training in cleaning pins if percutaneous pins are applied to stabilize fracture site.
- Person may need instructions on splint application, wearing time, and care.

Intervention/Treatment

Models or programs developed by occupational therapy personnel include the hand arc splint (Baier & Szekeres, 2010) and swing traction splinting (Hirth et al., 2013). Models or programs developed by other professionals but used by occupational therapy personnel include bivalve finger orthosis (Monasterio et al., 2015), distraction splinting (O'Brien & Presnell, 2010), immediate proximal phalangeal mobilization program (Byrne et al., 2020), metacarpal fracture patient pathway (Toemen & Midgley, 2010), patient pathway programs (Midgley & Toemen, 2011), and swing traction protocol (O'Brien et al., 2014). Team members include physicians, hand surgeons, physical therapists, and occupational therapy personnel. Goals are to ensure fracture and wound healing; reduce or control pain, edema, and stiffness; improve range of motion and muscle strength; maintain arches of the hand, joint stability, alignment, and tendon length; and promote occupational performance of daily activities. Healing occurs in three stages: inflammatory, repair, and remodeling.

Activities of Daily Living/Instrumental ADL
- Generally, client can resume light ADLs between 5 and 6 weeks.

Education/Work
- Return to work depends on type of work demanded of the hands (e.g., office work is less demanding on fracture site than construction work).

Play/Leisure
- No information identified.

Rest/Sleep
- No information identified.

Social Participation
- No information identified.

Sensorimotor
- Note: Detailed intervention tables for metacarpal and phalangeal fractures plus intervention for soft tissue injury are provided in Gallagher and Blackmore (2011).
- Early mobilization: Subject continues to be controversial. Timing of exercises depends on physician preference, fracture location, fracture displacement, type of reduction and hardware used, soft tissue injury, client's daily functional demands, and stage of healing (Varney, 2014).
- Splints according to location of metacarpal fractures (Midgley & Toemen, 2011).
  - ▶ Base of first metacarpal: Forearm based thermoplastic wrist splint.
  - ▶ Shaft of metacarpal with stable fracture: Three-point fixation splint that is hand-based, circumferential, and provides a three-point pressure—one point on the apex of the fracture dorsally and two volar pressure points on either side of the fracture.
  - ▶ Shaft of metacarpal fixated with open reduction internal fixation (ORIF): "Sandwich splint" hand-based circumferential splint that does not apply any pressure on the fracture site.
  - ▶ Shaft of metacarpal that is unstable fracture or stabilized with Kirschner wire (K-wire) fixation: Forearm-based wrist splint with wrist extension at 20 degrees and dorsal hood metacarpophalangeal joint in 70 degrees flexion.
  - ▶ Neck or head of metacarpal that is stable or unstable with K-wire of ORIF fixation: Hand-based dorsal gutter splint with metacarpophalangeal joints in 70 degrees of flexion.
  - ▶ Ulnar gutter splint: For children, hand-based splints result in earlier improved in range of motion and grip strength (Davison et al., 2016).
- Strengthening: Avoid until fracture is healed as demonstrated radiographically.
- Timetable (general)
  - ▶ 3–7 weeks: Metacarpal bone should heal.
  - ▶ 5–6 weeks: Controlled active range of motion (AROM) of joints just proximal and distal to fracture site.
  - ▶ 5–6 weeks: Light ADLs may begin.
  - ▶ 7–8 weeks: Passive range of motion (PROM) may begin including static progressive or dynamic splinting.
  - ▶ 8–10 weeks: Resistive exercises may be started.

Cognitive/Perceptual
- Not directly affected. Consider whether dementia or visual impairment may affect intervention plan, especially home exercise program.

Psychosocial
- No information identified.

Context/Environment
- Provide instructions and training of pin sites if a fixator device is applied, which has external parts such as pins.

- Provide instructions, training, and care of splint or splints.
- Provide information and recommendation if adapted devices might be useful during time fracture site is healing.
- Provide instruction and training in home exercise program.

Precautions/Safety Considerations

If fracture was the result of punching someone else in the mouth, client should be monitored for infection, especially if soft tissue injury occurred in addition to fracture. If fracture site was reduced with percutaneous pins, watch for signs of infection. Clean each pin with a separate cotton swab. Observe and treat nerve and soft tissue injury as well as bone fracture or fractures. The force needed to break a bone or bones may have damaged nerve, skin, tendon, and ligament as well. During healing watch for signs of tendon adhesions and flexor tenosynovitis. Do not begin strengthening exercises until fracture site shows solid internal healing as demonstrated by radiography. Unrecognized fracture may result in deformity such as angulation or reduced motion and strength.

Prognosis and Outcome

Good for younger clients and for clients who comply with rehabilitation program (Fok et al., 2013). Current review of traction orthoses provides limited data due to small- and low-quality studies (Packham et al., 2016).

REFERENCES

Baier, S., & Szekeres, M. (2010). The hand arc—A hand-based splint design for intraarticular fractures. *Journal of Hand Therapy, 23*(1), 73–76. https://doi.org/10.1016/j.jht.2009.07.006

Byrne, B., Jacques, A., & Gurfinkel, R. (2020). Non-surgical management of isolated proximal phalangeal fractures with immediate mobilization. *Journal of Hand Surgery (European Volume), 45*(2), 126–130. https://doi.org/10.1177/1753193419881086

Davison, P. G., Boudreau, N., Burrows, R., Wilson, K. L., & Bezuhly, M. (2016). Forearm-based ulnar gutter versus hand-based thermoplastic splint for pediatric metacarpal neck fractures: A blinded, randomized trial. *Plastic and Reconstructive Surgery, 137*(3), 908–916. https://doi.org/10.1097/01.prs.0000479974.45051.78

Fok, M. W. M., Ip, W. Y., Fung, B. K. K., Chan, R. K., & Chow, S. P. (2013). Ten-year results using a dynamic treatment for proximal phalangeal fractures of the hands. *Orthopedics, 36*(3), e348–e352. https://doi.org/10.3928/01477447-20130222-25

Gallagher, K. G., & Blackmore, S. M. (2011). Intra-articular hand fractures and joint injuries: Part II—Therapist's management. In T. M. Skirven, A. L. Osterman, J. M. Fedorczyk, & P. C. Amadio (Eds.), *Rehabilitation of the hand and upper extremity* (6th ed., pp. 417–435). Elsevier Mosby.

Hirth, M. J., Jacobs, D. J., & Sleep, K. (2013). Hand-based swing traction splinting for intra-articular proximal interphalangeal joint fractures. *Hand Therapy, 18*(2), 42–56. https://doi.org/10.1177/1758998313490856

Midgley, R., & Toemen, A. (2011). Evaluation of an evidence-based patient pathway for non-surgical and surgically managed metacarpal fractures. *Hand Therapy, 16*(1), 19–25. https://doi.org/10.1258/ht.2010.010026

Monasterio, M., Longsworth, K. A., & Viegas, S. (2015). Use of a bivalve finger fracture orthosis for a new treatment protocol of a PIP comminuted fracture and dorsal dislocation. *Journal of Hand Therapy, 28*(1), 77–81. https://doi.org/10.1016/j.jht.2014.08.002

O'Brien, L., & Presnell, S. (2010). Patient experience of distraction splinting for complex finger fracture dislocations. *Journal of Hand Therapy, 23*(3), 249–259. https://doi.org/10.1016/j.jht.2010.01.002

O'Brien, L. J., Simm, A. T., Loh, I. W. H., & Griffiths, K. M. (2014). Swing traction versus no-traction for complex intra-articular proximal inter-phalangeal fractures. *Journal of Hand Therapy, 27*(4), 309–316. https://doi.org/10.1016/j.jht.2014.07.003

Packham, T. L., Ball, P. D., MacDermid, J. C., Bain, J. R., & DalCin, A. (2016). A scoping review of applications and outcomes of traction orthoses and constructs for the management of intra-articular fractures and fracture dislocations in the hand. *Journal of Hand Therapy, 29*(3), 246–268. https://doi.org/10.1016/j.jht.2016.04.001

Porter, R. S. (Ed.). (2018). *The Merck manual of diagnosis and therapy* (20th ed.). Merck Sharp & Dohme.

Toemen, A., & Midgley, R. (2010). Hand therapy management of metacarpal fractures: An evidence-based patient pathway. *Hand Therapy, 15*(4), 87–93. https://doi.org/10.1258/ht.2010.010018

Varney, A. C. (2014). Hand fractures, In C. Cooper (Ed.), *Fundamentals of hand therapy* (2nd ed., pp. 361–382). Elsevier.

Weinstock-Zlotnick, G., Page, C., Ghomrawi, H. M., & Wolff, A. L. (2015). Responsiveness of three Patient Report Outcome (PRO) measures in patients with hand fractures: A preliminary cohort study. *Journal of Hand Therapy, 28*(4), 403–411. https://doi.org/10.1016/j.jht.2015.05.004

Hand Injuries and Impairments

See also Carpal Tunnel Syndrome, Complex Regional Pain Syndrome, Dupuytren's Disease, Extensor Tendon Lacerations, Flexor Tendon Injuries, Hand Fractures, Mallet Finger Injury, Osteoarthritis of the Hand, Osteoarthritis of the Thumb, Peripheral Nerve Injuries, Stiff Hand, Trigger Finger.

Description

Hand injuries and impairments interfere with or reduce functions of the hand, including flexion, extension, opposition, abduction, adduction, and grasp or grip, which decreases effectiveness or prevents the performance of daily activities. In addition, sensory input in the hand provides feeling without looking, provides protection from injury, and facilitates object manipulation. Finally, the hand can touch others, be a source of beauty or handsomeness, gives comfort, and expresses emotions and gestures (Walsh & Chee, 2018). This chapter focuses on hand injuries in adults as a general topic, but does not discuss specific types of hand injuries.

Cause

Congenital anomalies (missing or deformed parts), congenital disorders (cerebral palsy), disease related (infection, deformities, degenerative), accidents (motor vehicle, sports, home, community, or work related), and bites (insect, dog, or other animal).

Evaluation/Assessment

Areas

- Activities of Daily Living/Instrumental ADL: basic ADLs (eating, dressing, grooming, bathing, toileting, brushing teeth, brushing and combing hair, putting on makeup, shaving, dialing or pressing keypads); independent living (meal preparation, housekeeping choices, doing laundry, home maintenance, shopping, driving, using public transportation, sexual function, child care, pet care)
- Education/Work: handwriting; cutting; turning pages; keyboarding; grasping, holding, positioning, and releasing objects/tools; lifting; carrying; turning knobs; opening and closing doors/drawers/cabinets/boxes

- Play/Leisure: interests, location, frequency, hand-use demands
- Rest/Sleep: sleep disturbance due to pain in hands
- Social Participation: type, frequency, location, with whom, hand-use demands, social activity withdrawal
- Sensorimotor: active and passive joint range of motion, joint mobility, joint stiffness, muscle strength (grip and pinch), hand functions (grasp, grip, pinch), dexterity (accuracy, speed), two-hand coordination, eye–hand coordination, in-hand object manipulation, sensation and sensibility (tactile, pressure, mechanical, temperature, haptic, stereognosis), pain
- Cognitive/Perceptual: executive function (problem solving)
- Psychosocial: depression, anxiety, anger, guilt, role performance, self-esteem, self-efficacy, social isolation
- Context/Environment: adapted devices, splints and orthotic devices, patient/client education, resources

Instruments
Instruments Developed by Occupational Therapy Personnel
- Canadian Occupational Performance Measure (5th ed.; COPM-5; Law et al., 2014)
- Nine Hole Peg Test (NHPT, 9HPT; Keller et al., 1971; Grice et al., 2003, adult norms)

Instruments Developed by Other Professionals and Used by Occupational Therapy Personnel
- Cold Sensitivity Severity (CSS; McCabe et al., 1991)
- Disabilities of the Arm, Shoulder, and Hand (3rd ed.; DASH-3; Kennedy et al., 2011)
- Edema (circumferential, tape measure, volumeter, Figure 8 measure; see Klein, 2014; and Nadar et al., 2013, in References)
- Global Wrist Impairment Score (GWIS; MacDermid et al., 2007)
- Grip strength (dynamometer; JAMAR dynamometer, Lafayette Instrument; Wang et al., 2018)
- Hand Assessment Tool (HAT; Naidu et al., 2009)
- Impact of Event Scale (IES; Schwarzwald et al., 1987)
- Jebsen-Taylor Hand Function Test (JTHFT; Jebsen et al., 1969)
- Joint range of motion (goniometry; Shurtleff & Kaskutas, 2018; see also Klein, 2014; and de Klerk et al., 2015, in References)
- Manual Muscle Test (MMT; Kaskutas, 2018; see also de Klerk et al., 2015, in References)
- Modified Hand Injury Severity Scale (MHISS; Urso-Baiarda et al., 2008)
- Occupational Hand Use Questionnaire (OHUQ; Nathan et al., 1993)
- Occupational Stress Questionnaire (OSQ; Karasek & Theorell, 1990)
- Pinch meter (pinch strength; B&E Engineering; Mathiowetz et al., 1985)
- QuickDASH (Kennedy et al., 2011)
- Semmes-Weinstein Monofilaments (SWMs; Bell-Krotoski, 2011; see Klein, 2014, in References)
- Sense of Coherence Scale (SOC; Antonovsky, 1993)
- Short-Form Health Survey (SF-12; Ware et al., 1996)
- Short-Form 36 Health Survey (SF-36; Ware et al., 1993)
- Total active range of motion (TAM; Klein, 2014, in References)
- Touch pressure (sensibility; see Semmes-Weinstein Monofilaments)
- Two-point discrimination (sensibility; Klein, 2014, in References)
- Visual analogue scale (pain scale; scored 0 = *no pain*, 10 = *worst pain ever*)
- Visual analogue scale (sleep disturbance; 1 = *no sleep disturbance*, 10 = *unable to sleep*)
- World Health Organization Disability Assessment Schedule 2.0 (WHODAS 2.0; WHO, 1985)

Problems/Issues
Activities of Daily Living/Instrumental ADL
- Person may have difficulty holding eating utensils or using both hands to cut food.
- Person may have difficulty with dressing skills (buttoning, snapping, zipping, tying, two-hand coordination to hold items).

- Person may have difficulty with meal preparation (such as opening cans or jars, cutting, slicing, mixing, stirring).
- Person may have difficulty pressing keypads or on/off switches on phone or electric applications.
- Person may experience financial restrictions and loss of paid work.
- Person may be unable to drive independently and require assistance from others.
- Person may experience difficulty shopping for groceries and other supplies due to limitations in hand functions.
- Person may experience difficulty with child and pet care due to limitations in hand function.
- Person may experience sexual dysfunctions due to changes in hand function.

Education/Work

- Person may have difficulty holding a pen or pencil to write, holding crayons or paint bushes to color or paint, cutting with scissors, molding clay, pasting items together.
- Person may have difficulty keyboarding or pressing keypad.
- Person may have difficulty picking up, lifting, carrying, placing objects.
- Person may have difficulty opening or closing doors, including those with keypad entrance.
- Person may be unable to work (paid or unpaid) or need to change work setting while hand injury heals.
- Loss of grip strength, reduced total active range of motion, pain, and psychosocial factors may reduce ability to return to work (Chang et al., 2011; Marom et al., 2019; Ramel et al., 2013).

Play/Leisure

- Person may not be able to engage in leisure occupations that require specific hand functions, such as grasp, pinch, press, cut, manipulate, place, hold tools in specific position to sew, knit, crochet, embroider, saw, nail, carve, glue together, place game pieces in position, dig in garden, trim plants.
- Person may be unable to engage in sports activities due to specific finger injuries (Netscher et al., 2017).

Rest/Sleep

- Person may experience sleep disturbance due to pain or discomfort.
- Person may experience nightmares.

Social Participation

- Person may limit or stop participation in social activities due to difficulty with or loss of hand functions.

Sensorimotor

- Person may experience loss of active and/or passive joint range of motion.
- Person may experience decreased joint flexibility and/or increased joint stiffness.
- Person may experience loss of hand functions (reach, grasp, and release).
- Person may experience loss of hand skills (dexterity, accuracy, speed, object manipulation, two-hand coordination, eye–hand coordination).
- Person may experience decreased grip and/or pinch strength.
- Person may experience pain or pain catastrophizing (MacDermid et al., 2018).
- Person may experience sensory loss (desensitization) or sensory hyperesthesia.

Cognitive/Perceptual

- Person may have difficulty concentrating, paying attention.
- Person may experience catastrophic thinking.
- Person may experience changes in perception of body image.

Psychosocial

- Person may experience depression and anxiety.

- Person may experience feelings of anger or guilt related to hand injury.
- Person may experience stress and difficulty coping.
- Person may experience flashbacks reliving injury in total or in part including replaying (experiences accident again in the mind), appraisal (visualizes extent of injury), or projection (see scenes that never actually occurred).
- Person may experience loss of or changes in sense of self-esteem, self-confidence, or self-worth.
- Person may experience decreased quality of life and life satisfaction.
- Person may experience decreased ability to perform role performance tasks.
- Person may become dependent on others to perform certain tasks resulting in changes in role performance.

Context/Environment
- Person (family, caregivers) may lack knowledge about hand rehabilitation and recovery.
- Person may lack knowledge and information about adaptive devices or assistive technology.
- Person may lack knowledge and information about available rehabilitation programs and other community or internet resources.

Intervention/Treatment

Models and programs developed by occupational therapy personnel include the Canadian Model of Occupational Performance; occupation-based approaches; occupational adaptation and occupation as means/ends models of practice with examples that include biomedical, biomechanical, and biopsychosocial models with examples that include desensitization program (Göransson & Cederlund, 2011); handy tips for hurting hands (Baptista et al., 2018); home-based exercises (Ganjiwale & Ganjiwale, 2014); instruction on DVD (Kingston et al., 2014); occupational coaching (Garren, 2019); occupation-based intervention (Che Daud et al., 2016); and splinting (Ganjiwale & Ganjiwale, 2014). Models and programs developed by other professionals but used by occupational therapy personnel include computer gaming (Ganjiwale et al., 2019; Proffitt et al., 2015), sense of coherence (Cederlund, Ramel, et al., 2010), and telehealth (Worboys et al., 2018). Team members include physicians, nursing personnel, orthotists, prosthetists, physical therapy personnel, and occupational therapy personnel. Goals are to ensure that the rehabilitation process promotes healing while also enabling the client to perform meaningful or purposeful activities in their daily lives. Positive outcomes include enhancing satisfaction with the therapy experiences and results, maintaining or improving ability to engage in desired roles with the family and community, and to experience a quality of life as the client defines it (American Occupational Therapy Association, 2016).

Activities of Daily Living/Instrumental ADL
- Techniques for opening jars and bottles.
- Use built-up or enlarged handles on eating utensils, toothbrush and hairbrush, comb.

Education/Work
- Provide opportunity to increase grip strength to degree required for job performance.
- Provide opportunity to practice actions and motions required for job performance such as carrying, lifting, placing, pulling, pushing, turning hand/wrist over, keyboarding, pressing individual buttons or keypads.
- Explore whether job modification or workplace redesign may enable return to work.
- Explore whether work tasks or work environment could be made safer to reduce injury potential to client in future.
- Explore with client if other jobs or work conditions may be suitable alternatives.

Play/Leisure
- Suggest modifications to leisure occupations such as doing indoor gardening or in a terrarium while hand heals (e.g., being scorekeeper or referee rather than active player).

- Explore with client whether new leisure occupations may be better suited to current level of hand function and interest level.
- Use of sports activities provides an occupation focused approach (Jepsen & Hunt, 2019).

Rest/Sleep

- See Sleep–Wake Disorders in Section 13: Lifestyle Conditions.

Social Participation

- Encourage client to continue participation in social activities.
- Suggest modifications of social activities that may support participation, such as shorter outings, more passive participation, use of adapted devices, or explaining limitations to friends in advance.

Sensorimotor

- Energy conservation and work simplification (e.g., make cupcakes for birthday party instead of baking a cake; tools and technique are easier to manage).
- Exercises: tendon gliding exercises, forearm stretches, opposition exercise, postural exercises using hand exerciser, Chinese balls, pegboards, paper wadding (page or card).
- Turning, manipulating buttons, pinching beads in putty.
- Joint protection.
- One-handed techniques: compensatory strategies while injured hand is in splint or bandages.
- Pain management: contrast baths, taping.
- Splints for thumb, fingers, and wrist (e.g., thumb spica, finger extension, wrist cock-up; Ganjiwale & Ganjiwale, 2014; Hirth et al., 2016; Li & Li-Tsang, 2010; Russell, 2015).

Cognitive/Perceptual

- Education about ergonomically designed workplace and tools.
- Education about proper pinch pattern, basic hand and forearm anatomy.
- Assist client to problem solve situations in client's daily life that prevent client from performing important tasks.
- Encourage self-management program.

Psychosocial

- Discuss with client fears and anxieties about hand function and appearance.
- Promote resilience to enable client to demonstrate positive adaptive behaviors.
- Increase stress management and coping skills that support active engagement strategies to managing stress and coping while discouraging disengagement strategies (helplessness, lack of control, catastrophizing, distancing, avoidance). Examples include the following (Bates & Mason, 2014; Cederlund, Thorén-Jönsson, & Dahlin, 2010; Hannah, 2011):
  ▸ Accept situation and try to make the most of it as a learning experience.
  ▸ Actively process traumatic experience to explain how and why it happened.
  ▸ Compare to something worse to change the meaning of the situation.
  ▸ Distract attention from negative aspects of situation by staying busy.
  ▸ Maintain as much control as possible within one's own capacities.
  ▸ Seek social support from others with a social network.
  ▸ Solve practical problems by self to build confidence in one's own capacity.
  ▸ Take pain relieving actions to distract from focus on pain and discomfort.
  ▸ Use positive thinking to focus on positive aspects of situation.
- Support role identity and performance of role tasks.
- Facilitate client to identify occupations that contribute to increased quality of life.

Context/Environment

- Assistive devices to open jars and bottles, using built-up handles.
- Provide information on available community and internet resources.

Precautions/Safety Considerations

Depending on type of injury and surgical procedures, certain restrictions in movement and motions may be necessary to project tissue healing process, which client and therapist must observe. Monitor for signs of infections or additional injury.

Prognosis and Outcome

Hand injuries often are slow to heal and may result in disability for several weeks or months. Sensitivity of cold may persist (Vaksvik et al., 2016). Occupational therapy personnel continue to be slow to integrate the occupational perspective into hand therapy practice, which focuses on human as occupational beings who perform and engage in occupation that impacts health and well-being within the context of the person's environment (Burley, Cox, et al., 2018; Burley, Di Tommaso, et al., 2018; Colaianni & Provident, 2010; Colaianni et al., 2015; Dapito & Bondoc, 2018; Grice, 2015; Jack & Estes, 2010).

REFERENCES

American Occupational Therapy Association. (2016). *Fact sheet: Occupational therapy's role with rehabilitation of the hand.*

Baptista, M., Kugel, J., Javaherian, H., & Krpalek, D. (2018). Functional outcomes of a community occupation-based hand therapy class for older adults. *Physical & Occupational Therapy in Geriatrics, 36*(4), 380–398. https://doi.org/10.1080/02703181.2018.1556230

Bates, E., & Mason, R. (2014). Coping strategies used by people with a major hand injury: A review of the literature. *British Journal of Occupational Therapy, 77*(6), 289–295. https://doi.org/10.4276/030802214X14018723137995

Burley, S., Cox, R., Di Tommaso, A., & Molineux, M. (2018). Primary contact occupational therapy hand clinics: The pull of an occupational perspective. *Australian Occupational Therapy Journal, 65*(6), 533–543. https://doi.org/10.1111/1440-1630.12507

Burley, S., Di Tommaso, A., Cox, R., & Molineux, M. (2018). An occupational perspective in hand therapy: A scoping review. *British Journal of Occupational Therapy, 81*(6), 299–318. https://doi.org/10.1177/0308022617752110

Cederlund, R. I., Ramel, E., Rosberg, H.-E., & Dahlin, L. B. (2010). Outcome and clinical changes in patients 3, 6, 12 months after a severe or major hand injury—Can sense of coherence be an indicator for rehabilitation focus? *BMC Musculoskeletal Disorders, 11*, Article 286. https://doi.org/10.1186/1471-2474-11-286

Cederlund, R., Thorén-Jönsson, A.-L., & Dahlin, L. B. (2010). Coping strategies in daily occupations 3 months after a severe or major hand injury. *Occupational Therapy International, 17*(1), 1–9. https://doi.org/10.1002/oti.287

Chang, J.-H., Wu, M., Lee, C.-L., Guo, Y.-L., & Chiu, H.-Y. (2011). Correlation of return to work outcomes and hand impairment measures among workers with traumatic hand injury. *Journal of Occupational Rehabilitation, 21*(1), 9–16. https://doi.org/10.1007/s10926-010-9246-4

Che Daud, A. Z., Yau, M. K., Barnett, F., Judd, J., Jones, R. E., & Nawawi, R. F. M. (2016). Integration of occupation based intervention in hand injury rehabilitation: A randomized controlled trial. *Journal of Hand Therapy, 29*, 30–40. https://doi.org/10.1016/j.jht.2015.09.004

Colaianni, D., & Provident, I. (2010). The benefits of and challenges to the use of occupation in hand therapy. *Occupational Therapy in Health Care, 24*(2), 130–146. https://doi.org/10.3109/07380570903349378

Colaianni, D., Provident, I., DiBartola, L., & Wheeler, S. (2015). A phenomenology of occupation-based hand therapy. *Australian Occupational Therapy Journal, 62*(3), 177–186. https://doi.org/10.1111/1440-1630.12192

Dapito, D. H., & Bondoc, S. (2018). A qualitative approach to the use of occupational based practice in hand therapy. *Journal of Hand Therapy, 31*(1), 149–150. https://doi.org/10.1016/j.jht.2017.11.015

de Klerk, S., Buchanan, H., & Pretorius, B. (2015). Occupational therapy hand assessment practices: Cause for concern? *South African Journal of Occupational Therapy, 45*(2), 43–50. https://doi.org/10.17159/2310-3833/2015/v45n2a7

Ganjiwale, D., & Ganjiwale, J. (2014). Occupational therapy rehabilitation of post operative hand injury cases using modified low cost splints and home based exercises: A rural Indian experience. *Indian Journal of Physiotherapy & Occupational Therapy, 8*(3), 208–213. https://doi.org/10.5958/0973-5674.2014.00383.9

Ganjiwale, D., Pathak, R., Dwivedi, A., Ganjiwale, J., & Parekh, S. (2019). Occupational therapy rehabilitation of industrial setup hand injury cases for functional independence using modified joystick in interactive computer gaming in Anand, Gujarat. *National Journal of Physiology, Pharmacy and Pharmacology, 9*(2), 111–116. https://doi.org/10.5455/njppp.2019.9.06202112018001

Garren, K. R. (2019). A woodworker's hand injury. In B. A. Boyt Schell & G. Gillen (Eds.), *Willard and Spackman's occupational therapy* (13th ed., pp. 1047–1054). Wolters Kluwer.

Göransson, I., & Cederlund, R. (2011). A study of the effect of desensitization on hyperaesthesia in the hand and upper extremity after injury or surgery. *Hand Therapy, 16*(1), 12–18. https://doi.org/10.1258/ht.2010.010023

Grice, K. O. (2015). The use of occupation-based assessments and intervention in the hand therapy setting—A survey. *Journal of Hand Therapy, 28*(3), 300–306. https://doi.org/10.1016/j.jht.2015.01.005

Hannah, S. D. (2011). Psychosocial issues after a traumatic hand injury: Facilitating adjustment. *Journal of Hand Therapy, 24*(2), 95–103. https://doi.org/10.1016/j.jht.2010.11.001

Hirth, M. J., Howell, J. W., & O'Brien, L. (2016). Relative motion orthoses in the management of various hand conditions: A scoping review. *Journal of Hand Therapy, 29*(4), 405–432. https://doi.org/10.1016/j.jht.2016.07.001

Jack, J., & Estes, R. I. (2010). Documenting progress: Hand therapy treatment shift from biomechanical to occupational adaptation. *American Journal of Occupational Therapy, 64*(1), 82–87. https://doi.org/10.5014/ajot.64.1.82

Jepsen, J., & Hunt, L. A. (2019). Hand rehabilitation and the athlete: Getting the ball rolling with occupational centered interventions. *OT Practice, 24*(5), 13–15.

Kingston, G. A., Williams, G., Gray, M. A., & Judd, J. (2014). Does a DVD improve compliance with home exercise programs for people who have sustained a traumatic hand injury? Results of a feasibility study. *Disability and Rehabilitation Assistive Technology, 9*(3), 188–194. https://doi.org/10.3109/17483107.2013.806600

Klein, L. J. (2014). Evaluation of the hand and upper extremity. In C. Cooper (Ed.), *Fundamentals of hand therapy* (2nd ed., pp. 67–86). Elsevier.

Li, H. C. K., & Li-Tsang, C. W. P. (2010). Sports related hand injuries in Hong Kong. *Hong Kong Journal of Occupational Therapy, 20*(1), 13–18. https://doi.org/10.1016/S1569-1861(10)70053-X

MacDermid, J. C., Valdes, K., Szekeres, M., Naughton, N., & Algar, L. (2018). The assessment of psychological factors on upper extremity disability: A scoping review. *Journal of Hand Therapy, 31*(4), 511–523. https://doi.org/10.1016/j.jht.2017.05.017

Marom, B. S., Ratzon, N. Z., Carel, R. S., & Sharabi, M. (2019). Return-to-work barriers among manual workers after hand injuries: 1-year follow-up cohort study. *Archives of Physical Medicine and Rehabilitation, 100*(3), 422–432. https://doi.org/10.1016/j.apmr.2018.07.429

Nadar, M. S., Al-Kandari, D., & Taaqi, M. (2013). Reliability of occupational therapy students using the figure-of-eight technique of measuring hand volume. *Hong Kong Journal of Occupational Therapy, 23*(1), 20–25. https://doi.org/10.1016/j.hkjot.2013.04.001

Netscher, D. T., Pham, D. T., & Staines, K. G. (2017). Finger injuries in ball sports. *Hand Clinics, 33*(1), 119–139. https://doi.org/10.1016/j.hcl.2016.08.018

Proffitt, R., Sevick, M., Chang, C.-Y., & Lange, B. (2015). User-centered design of a controller-free game for hand rehabilitation. *Games for Health Journal, 4*(4), 259–264. https://doi.org/10.1089/g4h.2014.0122

Ramel, E., Rosberg, H.-E., Dahlin, L. B., & Cederlund, R. I. (2013). Return to work after a serious hand injury. *Work, 44*(4), 459–469. https://doi.org/10.3233/WOR-2012-1373

Russell, C. R. (2015). Therapy challenges for athletes: Splinting options. *Clinics in Sports Medicine, 34*(1), 181–191. https://doi.org/10.1016/j.csm.2014.09.012

Vaksvik, T., Røkkum, M., Haugstvedt, J. R., & Holm, I. (2016). Small-to-moderate decreases in cold hypersensitivity up to 3 years after severe hand injuries: A prospective cohort study. *Journal of Plastic Surgery and Hand Surgery, 50*(2), 74–79. https://doi.org/10.3109/20006 56X.2015.1089877

Walsh, J. M., & Chee, N. (2018). Hand and upper extremity injuries. In H. M. Pendleton & W. Schultz-Krohn (Eds.), *Pedretti's occupational therapy* (8th ed., pp. 972–1003). Mosby.

Worboys, T., Brassington, M., Ward, E. C., & Cornwell, P. L. (2018). Delivering occupational therapy hand assessment and treatment sessions via telehealth. *Journal of Telemedicine and Telecare, 24*(3), 185–192. https://doi.org/10.1177/1357633X17691861

BIBLIOGRAPHY

Amini, D. (2011). Occupational therapy interventions for work-related injuries and conditions of the forearm, wrist, and hand: A systematic review. *American Journal of Occupational Therapy, 65*(1), 29–36. https://doi.org/10.5014/ajot.2011.09186

Ammann, B., Satink, T., & Andresen, M. (2012). Experiencing occupations with chronic hand disability: Narratives of hand-injured adults. *Hand Therapy, 17*(4), 87–94. https://doi.org/ 10.1177/1758998312471253

Bell, J., Gray, M., & Kingston, G. (2011). The longer term functional impact of a traumatic hand injury on people living in a regional metropolitan Australian location. *International Journal of Therapy and Rehabilitation, 18*(7), 370–381. https://doi.org/10.12968/ijtr.2011.18.7.370

Brown, C. (2019). Occupation-based interventions in hand rehabilitation: Stamp collecting. *OT Practice, 24*(5), 14.

Cabral, L. H. A., Sampaio, R. F., Figueiredo, I. M., & Mancini, M. C. (2010). Factors associated with return to work following a hand injury: A qualitative/quantitative approach. *Brazilian Journal of Physical Therapy, 14*(2), 149–157. http://dx.doi.org/10.1590/S1413-35552010005000004

Che Daud, A. Z., Yau, M. K., Barnett, F., & Judd, J. (2016). Occupation-based intervention in hand injury rehabilitation: Experiences of occupational therapists in Malaysia. *Scandinavian Journal of Occupational Therapy, 23*(1), 57–66. https://doi.org/10.3109/11038128.2015.10 62047

Cooper, C. (2014). Fundamentals: Hand therapy concepts and treatment techniques. In C. Cooper (Ed.), *Fundamentals of hand therapy* (2nd ed., pp. 1–14). Elsevier.

Cooper, C. (2014). Hand impairments. In M. V. Radomski & C. A. Trombly Latham (Eds.), *Occupational therapy for physical dysfunction* (7th ed., pp. 1129–1167). Wolters-Kluwer.

Dorich, J., & Harpster, K. (2015). Pediatric hand therapy. In J. Case-Smith & J. C. O'Brien (Eds.), *Occupational therapy for children and adolescents* (7th ed., pp. 812–838). Mosby.

Fitinghoff, H., Lindqvist, B., Nygård, L., Ekholm, J., & Schult, M.-L. (2011). The ICF and post-surgery occupational therapy after traumatic hand injury. *International Journal of Rehabilitation Research, 34*(1), 79–88. https://doi.org/10.1097/MRR.0b013e328341946c

Kingston, G. A., Judd, J., & Gray, M. A. (2014). The experience of living with a traumatic hand injury in a rural and remote location: An interpretative phenomenological study. *Rural and Remote Health, 14*(3), Article 2764.

Kingston, G. A., Judd, J., & Gray, M. A. (2015). The experience of medical and rehabilitation intervention for traumatic hand injuries in rural and remote North Queensland: A qualitative study. *Disability and Rehabilitation, 37*(5), 423–429. https://doi.org/10.3109/09638288.20 14.923526

Kingston, G. A., Tanner, B., & Gray, M. A. (2010). The functional impact of a traumatic hand injury on people who live in rural and remote locations. *Disability and Rehabilitation, 32*(4), 326–335. https://doi.org/10.3109/09638280903114410

Kingston, G., Williams, G., Judd, J., & Gray, M. (2016). The functional impact of a traumatic hand injury: A comparison of rural/remote and metropolitan/regional populations. *International Journal of Therapy and Rehabilitation, 23*(9), 406–413. https://doi.org/10.12968/ijtr.2016.23.9.406

Lashgari, D., Arkins, M., & Baumgarten, J. (2018). Orthotics. In H. M. Pendleton & W. Schultz-Krohn (Eds.), *Pedretti's occupational therapy* (8th ed., pp. 728–765). Mosby.

Seu, M., & Pasqualetto, M. (2012). Hand therapy for dysfunction of the intrinsic muscles. *Hand Clinics, 28*(1), 87–100. https://doi.org/10.1016/j.hcl.2011.09.001

Takata, S. C., Wade, E. T., & Roll, S. C. (2019). Hand therapy interventions, outcomes, and diagnoses evaluated over the last 10 years: A mapping review linking research to practice. *Journal of Hand Therapy, 32*(1), 1–9. https://doi.org/10.1016/J.JHT.2017.05.018

Mallet Finger Injury

Also called mallet deformity, hammer finger.

Description

Mallet finger is a flexion deforming of the fingertip with or without fracture, at the proximal end of the distal phalanx (Porter, 2018). The injury occurs when there is a disruption of the extensor tendon mechanism of the hand (Minchin & Spirtos, 2012). The result is a loss of the ability to extend the distal joint of the finger (O'Toole, 2017). Mallet finger injury is classified as a Zone 1 hand injury (Lutz et al., 2015).

Cause

The cause is avulsion of the extensor tendon usually the result of forced flexion of the distal phalanx, typically when hit with a ball or similar object (Porter, 2018). However, the injury can occur as a result of a laceration (Minchin & Spirtos, 2012). Mallet finger injuries commonly occur during sports activities or minor incidents, including baseball, basketball, football, skiing, rugby, bed making, and donning socks (Devan, 2014; Minchin & Spirtos, 2012; Netscher et al., 2017).

Evaluation/Assessment

Areas

- Activities of Daily Living/Instrumental ADL: basic ADLs
- Education/Work: keyboarding, bed making
- Play/Leisure: sports activities, type, frequency, location
- Rest/Sleep: sleep disturbance
- Social Participation: type, frequency, location, with whom
- Sensorimotor: finger range of motion, extensor lag, joint stiffness, pinch grips (thumb-index, tripod), pain, edema
- Cognitive/Perceptual: not directly involved
- Psychosocial: quality of life
- Context/Environment: information resources, splinting
- Comorbidities: existing upper extremity conditions, arthritis, swan neck deformity

Instruments

Instruments Developed by Occupational Therapy Personnel
- No information identified

Instruments Developed by Other Professionals and Used by Occupational Therapy Personnel
- Disabilities of Arm, Shoulder, and Hand (3rd ed.; DASH-3; Kennedy et al., 2011)

- Grip strength (dynamometry; Wang et al., 2018)
- Joint range of motion (goniometry; Shurtleff & Kaskutas, 2018)
- Michigan Hand Outcomes Questionnaire (MHQ; Chung et al., 1998)
- Pinch meter/pinch strength (tip to tip; Mathiowetz et al., 1985)
- Visual analogue scale (pain scale; scored: 0 = *no pain*, 10 = *worst pain ever*)

Problems/Issues

Activities of Daily Living/Instrumental ADL
- Person may experience difficulty performing tasks, such as buttoning, depending on which finger is involved.
- Person may experience difficulty putting on gloves.
- Person may experience difficulty putting on socks.
- Person may experience difficulty reaching into a pants pocket.

Education/Work
- Person may be unable to keyboard using the involved finger.
- Person may be unable to perform selected household tasks using the involved finger, such as opening a jar.

Play/Leisure
- Person may be unable to engage in sports activities due to injured finger.

Rest/Sleep
- No information identified.

Social Participation
- Person may restrict participation in social activities due to injury.

Sensorimotor
- Person cannot actively extend the distal joint of the involved finger, but can passively extend the joint.
- Person lacks full range of motion of the involved finger.
- Person may experience pain in the involved finger and hand.
- Person may experience edema/swelling in the involved finger.
- Person may experience extensor lag of greater than 10 degrees.
- Person may experience joint stiffness.

Cognitive/Perceptual
- Not directly affected.

Psychosocial
- Person may experience decreased quality of life.

Context/Environment
- Person may lack knowledge about mallet finger injury and its management.

Intervention/Treatment

Intervention is based on wound healing and tissue repair followed by biomechanical-based exercises related to body structure and function (Valdes et al., 2016). Models or programs developed by occupational therapy personnel include mallet finger orthosis (Harte, 2016). Models or programs developed by other professionals but used by occupational therapy personnel include elastic tape (Mak et al., 2016) and two-step orthosis protocol (Saito & Kihara, 2016a, 2016b). Team members include physicians, physical therapy personnel, and occupational therapy personnel. The goal of intervention is to closely approximate the extensor tendon ends so that primary healing of the tendon can occur (Tocco et al., 2013).

Activities of Daily Living/Instrumental ADL
- No information identified.

Education/Work
- No information identified.

Play/Leisure
- No information identified.

Rest/Sleep
- No information identified.

Social Participation
- No information identified.

Sensorimotor
- Conservative (Saito & Kihara, 2016a, 2016b; Valdes et al., 2015)
  - ► Weeks 1–6
    - ○ Maintain distal interphalangeal (DIP) in extension or slight hyperextension. Splinting may involve one splint only or time may be divided between two different types of splint; Kinesio Taping may be used after a period of thermoplastic splint use, and casting has been used as opposed to thermoplastic splints.
    - ○ Maintain skin integrity.
    - ○ If proximal interphalangeal (PIP) develops hyperextension, it should be splinted at 30–45 degree of flexion.
    - ○ Splint type: There is no evidence that one type of splinting material (aluminum, thermoplastic, or tape) is better than another or that combining thermoplastic splint and Kinesio Taping improves outcome (Devan, 2014; Harte, 2016; Mak et al., 2016; Minchin & Spirtos, 2012; Saito & Kihara, 2016a, 2016b; Valdes et al., 2015, 2016).
    - ○ Casting may provide better results, but studies are limited (Tocco et al., 2013).
  - ► Weeks 6–8
    - ○ If extensor lag is present, continue splinting for 2 additional weeks.
    - ○ Night splint may be worn for up to 4 weeks following original device removal.
    - ○ Taping may replace day splint.
    - ○ Active range of motion exercises should be started using blocking technique so that full range of extension of finger joints is not permitted.
  - ► Weeks 8–12
    - ○ Passive range of motion exercise started.
    - ○ Stretching exercise started.
    - ○ Muscle strengthening exercises started.
    - ○ At 12 weeks, no restrictions.
- Postsurgery: No discussion

Cognitive/Perceptual
- No information identified.

Psychosocial
- No information identified.

Context/Environment
- Home instruction: Provide written instructions with drawings.
- Client compliance: Major issue related to poor outcome.

Precautions/Safety Considerations
No information identified.

Prognosis and Outcome

Generally good outcome. Problems included extensor lag. Increased edema, age, and decreased client adherence negatively influence outcome (Valdes et al., 2015).

REFERENCES

Devan, D. (2014). A novel way of treating mallet finger injuries. *Journal of Hand Therapy, 27*(4), 325–329. https://doi.org/10.1016/j.jht.2014.02.005

Harte, D. (2016). The challenge of the mallet orthosis: A simple solution. *Journal of Hand Therapy, 29*(3), 348–351. https://doi.org/10.1016/j.jht.2016.01.001

Lutz, K., Pipicelli, J., & Grewal, R. (2015). Management of complications of extensor tendon injuries. *Hand Clinics, 31*(2), 301–310. https://doi.org/10.1016/j.hcl.2014.12.006

Mak, L., Aitkens, L. D., & Novak, C. B. (2016). Mallet finger injuries—A new method to maintain distal interphalangeal joint extension. *Journal of Hand Therapy, 29*(3), 352–355. https://doi.org/10.1016/j.jht.2016.01.002

Minchin, P., & Spirtos, M. (2012). Investigation of the conservative management of mallet injury in Irish acute hospitals. *Hand Therapy, 17*(2), 28–36. https://doi.org/10.1258/ht.2012.012004

Netscher, D. T., Pham, D. T., & Staines, K. G. (2017). Finger injuries in ball sports. *Hand Clinics, 33*(1), 119–139. https://doi.org/10.1016/j.hcl.2016.08.018

O'Toole, M. T. (Ed.). (2017). *Mosby's dictionary of medicine, nursing & health professions* (10th ed.). Elsevier.

Porter, R. S. (Ed.). (2018). *The Merck manual of diagnosis and therapy* (20th ed.). Merck Sharp & Dohme.

Saito, K., & Kihara, H. (2016a). A randomized controlled trial of the effect of 2-step orthosis treatment for a mallet finger of tendinous origin. *Journal of Hand Therapy, 29*(4), 433–439. https://doi.org/10.1016/j.jht.2016.07.005

Saito, K., & Kihara, H. (2016b). Therapeutic value of using two-step splinting for mallet finger. *Asian Journal of Occupational Therapy, 12*(1), 23–28. https://doi.org/10.11596/asiajot.12.23

Tocco, S., Boccolari, P., Landi, A., Leonelli, C., Mercanti, C., Pogliacomi, F., Sartini, S., Zingarello, L., & Nedelec, B. (2013). Effectiveness of cast immobilization in comparison to the gold-standard self-removal orthotic intervention for closed mallet fingers: A randomized clinical trial. *Journal of Hand Therapy, 26*(3), 191–201. https://doi.org/10.1016/j.jht.2013.01.004

Valdes, K., Naughton, N., & Algar, L. (2015). Conservative treatment of mallet finger: A systematic review. *Journal of Hand Therapy, 28*(3), 237–246. https://doi.org/10.1016/j.jht.2015.03.001

Valdes, K., Naughton, N., & Algar, L. (2016). ICF components of outcome measures for mallet finger: A systematic review. *Journal of Hand Therapy, 29*(4), 388–395. https://doi.org/10.1016/j.jht.2016.06.005

Osteoarthritis of the Hand

See also Osteoarthritis of the Thumb.

Description

Osteoarthritis of the hand is a joint disease that causes pain, stiffness, deformity, and loss of mobility in the hands. The disorder has a functional and negative impact on the person's quality of life by making everyday occupations difficult to perform (da Silva Santos et al., 2018). Osteoarthritis of the hand is characterized by progressive loss of articular cartilage, deformities in the distal (DIP) and proximal (PIP) interphalangeal joints called, respectively, Heberden's nodes and Bouchard's nodes (Poole et al., 2010).

Cause

Early onset osteoarthritis is usually caused by trauma, but the cause of most osteoarthritis is unknown. Factors include chemical, emotional stress, endocrine, genetic, or mechanical (O'Toole, 2017). There are no significant differences between women and men in terms of daily functioning and health status (Stamm et al., 2011).

Evaluation/Assessment

Areas

- Activities of Daily Living/Instrumental ADL: self-maintenance
- Education/Work: work or volunteer tasks
- Play/Leisure: interests, values, type, frequency, level of satisfaction
- Rest/Sleep: sleep disturbance
- Social Participation: type, frequency, location, with whom
- Sensorimotor: grip and pinch strength, range of motion of digits, functional grasp patterns, stiffness (especially in the morning), deformities of distal and proximal interphalangeal joints, fine motor skills, dexterity, hand pain
- Cognitive/Perceptual: ask person what he or she regards as being most important problem; also consider whether cognitive impairment may be a factor in planning and implementing intervention program
- Psychosocial: motivation, depression, anxiety, quality of life, self-efficacy, role performance
- Context/Environment: social support, home- and work-site modification, adapted devices
- Comorbidities: osteoarthritis of the thumb and carpal tunnel syndrome (see chapters in this Section), dementia

Instruments

Instruments Developed by Occupational Therapy Personnel

- Arthritis Hand Function Test (AHFT; Backman & Mackie, 1997)
- Canadian Occupational Performance Measure (5th ed.; COPM-5; Law et al., 2014)
- Evaluation of Daily Activity Questionnaire (EDAQ; Hammond et al., 2017)
- Measure of Activity Performance of the Hand (MAP-Hand; Paulsen et al., 2010; see also Fernandes et al., 2012, in References)

Instruments Developed by Other Professionals and Used by Occupational Therapy Personnel

- Australian/Canadian Osteoarthritis Hand Index (AUSCAN; Bellamy et al., 2002; see also Moe et al., 2010, and Poole, 2011, in References)
- Cochin Scale or Cochin Hand Function Scale (see Hand Function Disability Scale)
- Disabilities of the Arm, Shoulder, and Hand (3rd ed.; DASH-3; Kennedy et al., 2011)
- Dreiser's Functional Index (DFI; see Functional Index for Hand Osteoarthritis)
- Duruöz Hand Index (see Hand Function Disability Scale)
- Functional Index for Hand Osteoarthritis (FIHOA; Dreiser et al., 1995; see also Moe et al., 2010; Poole, 2011, and Poole et al., 2010, in References)
- Grip Ability Test (GAT; Dellhag & Bjelle, 1995; see also Poole, 2011, in References)
- Hand Function Disability Scale (HFDS; Duruöz et al., 1996; see Poole, 2011, and Poole et al., 2010, in References)
- Hand Functional Index (HFI; see Keitel Functional Test)
- Jebsen-Taylor Hand Function Test (JTHFT; Jebsen et al., 1969; see also Poole, 2011, in References)
- Keitel Functional Test (KFT; Holm et al., 2008)
- Michigan Hand Outcomes Questionnaire (MHQ; Chung et al., 1998; see also Poole, 2011, and Poole et al., 2010, in References)
- Moberg Picking-Up Test (MPUT; Moberg, 1958; see also Silva et al., 2017, in References)
- Numeric rating scale (NRS; scored 0–10 for pain or stiffness)

- Patient-Specific Functional Scale (PSFS; Stratford et al., 1995; see also Wright et al., 2017, in References)
- Visual analogue scale (VAS; scored 0–10 for pain or stiffness)

Problems/Issues

Activities of Daily Living/Instrumental ADL
- Person may have difficulty performing self-maintenance occupations.

Education/Work
- Person may have difficulty performing work-related tasks.

Play/Leisure
- Person may be unable to engage in favorite leisure occupations due to pain, decreased grip, or pinch strength and joint mobility.
- Person may choose to limit engagement in leisure occupations to avoid pain and limited strength and joint mobility in hand.

Rest/Sleep
- Person may experience sleep disturbance due to pain.

Social Participation
- Person may restrict or stop participation in social activities due to pain, physical appearance of hand(s), or difficulty with mobility and strength.

Sensorimotor
- Person may experience decreased grip and pinch strength.
- Person may experience stiffness and difficulty flexing and extending the fingers, especially in the morning (joint mobility).
- Person may have loss of range of motion in the fingers.
- Person may experience decreased fine motor skills, including dexterity (speed and accuracy).
- Person may experience decreased in-hand manipulation and two-handed coordination.
- Person may have nodes on the finger joints (Heberden's nodes and Bouchard's nodes).
- Person may experience joint pain in hand and fingers.

Cognitive/Perceptual
- Not directly affected. Check for cognitive impairment.

Psychosocial
- Person may experience decreased quality of life.
- Person may become depressed.
- Person may be anxious about changes in body image.
- Person may be unable to perform certain role performance tasks.

Context/Environment
- Person may lack information about osteoarthritis and its management.
- Person may lack information and resources about adapted equipment.
- Person may lack social support.

Intervention/Treatment

Models and programs developed by occupational therapy personnel include assistive technology (da Silva Santos et al., 2018; Kjeken et al., 2011) and joint protection (McGee & Mathiowetz, 2017; Oppong et al., 2015). Models and programs developed by other professionals but used by occupational therapy personnel include compression gloves (Hammond et al., 2016), exercise program (Kjeken et al., 2015), grip strength exercises (Stoffer-Marx et al., 2018), hand exercises (Kjeken, 2011), multidimensional intervention (Stukstette et al., 2012), self-management

(Dziedzic et al., 2011; Dziedzic et al., 2015; Kjeken et al., 2013), and therapeutic exercise guidelines (Brosseau et al., 2018). Team members include general physicians, rheumatologists, psychologists, physical therapists, and occupational therapy personnel. Goals are to decrease pain and increase occupational performance.

Activities of Daily Living/Instrumental ADL
- Practice in performing daily activities as part of range of motion program.
- Discussion and practice of daily activities as part of joint protection, pain and fatigue management programs, and use of adapted devices (ergonomically designed, electronic).

Education/Work
- Explore with client whether adapted devices and work site modification (work simplification, better ergonomic design) might permit person to continue working or volunteering.

Play/Leisure
- Explore with client important leisure occupations and whether adapted devices or techniques would permit person to continue to enjoy doing the occupation.

Rest/Sleep
- See Sleep–Wake Disorders in Section 13: Lifestyle Conditions.

Social Participation
- Explore with client whether adapted devices or modified techniques would permit person to continue to participate in valued social occupations.

Sensorimotor
- Compression gloves: May be useful at night to reduce swelling and edema (see Hammond et al., 2016).
- Energy conservation and work simplification: Provide information and practice on ways to conserve energy and simplify tasks based on what the client does every day.
- Fatigue management: Provide fatigue management program (discuss and try out ways to make more effective use of energy, such as breaking up tasks into work and rest cycles).
- Heat and cold modalities: Paraffin has been used.
- Joint protection: Provide instruction and demonstration of joint protection strategies.
  - ▶ Distribute weight of what is lifted over several joints, such as lifting with both hands instead of one, or dividing the weight equally and lift half the load using each hand.
  - ▶ Avoid prolonged grips in any one position (holding smartphone in one hand for 15 minutes while reading and answering email or playing online game for 30 minutes).
  - ▶ Use the largest grip and largest joint possible (e.g., carry purse on forearm or shoulder, not hand).
  - ▶ Reduce the effort needed to do a task (use labor-saving gadgets, slide instead of lifting, reduce the weight of what is lifted; e.g., divide the sack of groceries into two before carrying into house).
- Range of motion and joint mobility: Provide exercises (isometric, isotonic, and functional) to increase flexion and extension, abduction and adduction, and opposition with thumb; Stukstette et al., 2012).
  - ▶ Mobility of wrist and fingers
    - ○ Put arms outstretched on a table with palms together. Move wrists as far as possible toward the body by bending elbows. Keep hands together and fingers extended.
    - ○ Hold a stick loosely in the hands. Create a wringing movement with wrist. Make movements with wrists as large as possible. Do not pinch the stick.
  - ▶ Mobility of finger joints: Close fingertips as far as possible into palm of hand (make a small fist). Stretch fingers and a normal fist, stretch fingers completely and repeat.
- Pain management: Provide pain management program (discuss and demonstrate ways to reduce pain while performing everyday activities).

- Splints: Resting splint worn at night.
- Stiffness: Provide exercises to reduce morning stiffness.
- Strengthening: Provide exercises to increase grip and pinch strength: elastic bands, play-dough, bean or rice bags, rubber balls (see Kjeken et al., 2015; Stoffer-Marx et al., 2018).
  - ▶ Hand exercises
    - ○ Small fist: Flex DIP and PIP joints of second to fifth finger while metacarpophalangeal (MCP) joints remain straight (extended).
    - ○ Build a housetop: Flex MCP of second to fifth fingers. DIP and PIP joint remain straight (extended).
    - ○ Make O sign: Form a round ring by touching thumb to each of fingertips.
    - ○ Spread fingers: Lay hand on table and spread fingers as far apart as possible while fingers stay in touch with the surface and stay extended.
    - ○ Lateral pinch: Hand is positioned in medial position. Touch the tip of the thumb to the side of the index finger near the PIP—alternately press thumb against side of index finger and relax.
  - ▶ Exercises with therapy putty
    - ○ Create a ball with therapy putty with one hand.
    - ○ Roll therapy putty with one hand into a long rope.
    - ○ Squeeze the rope with the thumb and index finger.
    - ○ With thumb and index fingertips touching, wrap the rope around all fingers to form a ring.
    - ○ Put hand through ring and open hand against resistance of the therapy putty.
- Spring-loaded weights.
- Tendon gliding exercises (see range of motion exercises for full fist, hook fist, and tabletop plus straight fist; MCP and PIP flexed with DIP extended).

Cognitive/Perceptual

- Client may benefit from exploring better time-management strategies.
- Consider whether cognitive impairment is present when providing home instructions and access to other resources.

Psychosocial

- Facilitate discussion with client regarding living with and managing chronic osteoarthritis to reduce anxiety and depression.
- Improve self-efficacy by providing information about coping with pain, fatigue, activity limitations and participation, ergonomics and exercises to strengthen and improve mobility, plus adapted equipment and splint/orthotics if needed.
- Encourage client to explore approaches and new ideas for maintaining and improving quality of life.

Context/Environment

- Provide information and resources in the community or on the internet about living with hand osteoarthritis and its management.
- Provide instructions for wear and care of splints or orthotic devices.
- Provide home exercise program with instructions and demonstration (see Hennig et al., 2015; Stoffer-Marx et al., 2018).
- Discuss, demonstrate, and provide resources for adapted devices.
  - ▶ Electric versus manual (electric can opener, blender, chopper).
  - ▶ Elongated handles (increase leverage).
  - ▶ Enlarged handles (increase grip potential).
  - ▶ Vertical handles (permits downward pressure, takes advantage of gravity).
  - ▶ Nonskid/nonslip matting (decrease need to hold items).
  - ▶ Specially designed openers: buttonhook (decrease need for fine motor skills).

- Discuss with client the advantages of using ergonomically designed devices to reduce pain and effective use of limited grip and pinch strength.
- Explore whether home modification might be useful, such as better organization of kitchen items to reduce fatigue.

Precautions/Safety Considerations

A review of joint protection programs found no evidence that such programs were superior to usual care and control of pain, although studies were of low quality (Bobos et al., 2019).

Prognosis and Outcome

Currently, there is no cure for osteoarthritis of the hand. The disorder remains a chronic condition. Intervention mostly addresses symptoms using a combination of pharmacologic and nonpharmacologic approaches, including occupational therapy.

Cost Effectiveness

Self-managed hand exercise programs are cost-effective (Oppong et al., 2015). However, overall evidence about effectiveness of exercise remains unclear (Østerås et al., 2017).

REFERENCES

Bobos, P., Nazari, G., Szekeres, M., Lalone, E. A., Ferreira, L., & MacDermid, J. C. (2019). The effectiveness of joint-protection programs on pain, hand function, and grip strength levels in patients with hand arthritis: A systematic review and meta-analysis. *Journal of Hand Therapy, 32*(2), 194–211. https://doi.org/10.1016/j.jht.2018.09.012

Brosseau, L., Thevenot, O., MacKiddie, O., Taki, J., Wells, G. A. Guitard, P., Léonard, G., Paquet, N. Aydin, S. Z., Toupin-April, K., Cavallo, S., Moe, R. H., Shaikh, K., Gifford, W., Loew, L., De Angelis, G., Shallwani, S. M., Aburub, A. S., Mizusaki Imoto, A., . . . Longchamp. G. (2018). The Ottawa Panel guidelines on programmes involving therapeutic exercise for the management of hand osteoarthritis. *Clinical Rehabilitation, 32*(11), 1449–1471. https://doi.org/10.1177/0269215518780973

da Silva Santos, P., Macêdo Martins, N., Moura Moreira Leite, V., Carneiro de Menezes Sanguinetti, D., Porto Amorim Paixão, L. K., Lopes Marques, C. D., & Salgado Amaral, D. (2018). Use of assistive devices by individuals with hands osteoarthritis. *Brazilian Journal of Occupational Therapy, 26*(1), 145–152. https://doi.org/10.4322/2526-8910.ctoAO0999

Dziedzic, K. S., Hill, S., Nicholls, E., Hammond, A., Myers, H., Whitehurst, T., Bailey, J., Clements, C., Whitehurst, D. G. T., Jowett, S., Handy, J., Hughes, R. W., Thomas, E., & Hay, E. M. (2011). Self-management, joint protection and exercises in hand osteoarthritis: A randomised controlled trial with cost effectiveness analyses. *BMC Musculoskeletal Disorders, 12*, Article 156. https://doi.org/10.1186/1471-2474-12-156

Dziedzic, K., Nicholls, E., Hill, S., Hammond, A., Handy, J., Thomas, E., & Hay, E. (2015). Self-management approaches for osteoarthritis in the hand: A 2 × 2 factorial randomised trial. *Annals of the Rheumatic Diseases, 74*(1), 108–118. https://doi.org/10.1136/annrheumdis-2013-203938

Fernandes, L., Grotle, M., Darre, S., Nossum, R., & Kjeken, I. (2012). Validity and responsiveness of the Measure of Activity Performance of the Hand (MAP-Hand) in patients with hand osteoarthritis. *Journal of Rehabilitation Medicine, 44*(10), 869–876. https://doi.org/10.2340/16501977-1035

Hammond, A., Jones, V., & Prior, Y. (2016). The effects of compression gloves on hand symptoms and hand function in rheumatoid arthritis and hand osteoarthritis: A systematic review. *Clinical Rehabilitation, 30*(3), 213–224. https://doi.org/10.1177/0269215515578296

Hennig, T., Hæhre, L., Hornburg, V. T., Mowinckel, P., Norli, E. S., & Kjeken, I. (2015). Effect of home-based hand exercises in women with hand osteoarthritis: A randomised controlled trial. *Annals of the Rheumatic Diseases, 74*(8), 1501–1508. http://dx.doi.org/10.1136/annrheumdis -2013-204808

Kjeken, I. (2011). Occupational therapy-based and evidence-supported recommendations for assessment and exercises in hand osteoarthritis. *Scandinavian Journal of Occupational Therapy, 18*(4), 265–281. https://doi.org/10.3109/11038128.2010.514942

Kjeken, I., Darre, S., Slatkowsky-Cristensen, B., Hermann, M., Nilsen, T., Eriksen, C. S., & Nossum, R. (2013). Self-management strategies to support performance of daily activities in hand osteoarthritis. *Scandinavian Journal of Occupational Therapy, 20*(1), 29–36. https://doi .org/10.3109/11038128.2012.661457

Kjeken, I., Darre, S., Smedslund, G., Hagen, K. B., & Nossum, R. (2011). Effect of assistive technology in hand osteoarthritis: A randomised controlled trial. *Annals of the Rheumatic Diseases, 70*(8), 1447–1452. https://doi.org/10.1136/ard.2010.148668

Kjeken, I., Grotle, M., Hagen, K. B., & Østerås, N. (2015). Development of an evidence-based exercise programme for people with hand osteoarthritis. *Scandinavian Journal of Occupational Therapy, 22*(2), 103–116. https://doi.org/10.3109/11038128.2014.941394

McGee, C., & Mathiowetz, V. (2017). Evaluation of hand forces during a joint-protection strategy for women with hand osteoarthritis. *American Journal of Occupational Therapy, 71*(1), Article 7101190020. https://doi.org/10.5014/ajot.2017.022921

Moe, R. H., Garratt, A., Slatkowsky-Christensen, B., Maheu, E., Mowinckel, P., Kvien, T. K., Kjeken, I., Hagen, K. B., & Uhlig, T. (2010). Concurrent evaluation of data quality, reliability and validity of the Australian/Canadian Osteoarthritis Hand Index and the Functional Index for Hand Osteoarthritis. *Rheumatology, 49*(12), 2327–2336. https://doi.org/10.1093/ rheumatology/keq219

Oppong, R., Jowett, S., Nicholls, E., Whitehurst, D. G. T., Hill, S., Hammond, A., Hay, E. M., & Dziedzic, K. (2015). Joint protection and hand exercises for hand osteoarthritis: An economic evaluation comparing methods for the analysis of factorial trials. *Rheumatology, 54*(5), 876–883. https://doi.org/10.1093/rheumatology/keu389

Østerås, N., Kjeken, I., Smedslund, G., Moe, R. H., Slatkowsky-Christensen, B., Uhlig, T., & Hagen, K. B. (2017). Exercise for hand osteoarthritis: A Cochrane systematic review. *Journal of Rheumatology, 44*(12), 1850–1858. https://doi.org/10.3899/jrheum.170424

O'Toole, M. T. (Ed.). (2017). *Mosby's dictionary of medicine, nursing & health professions* (10th ed.). Elsevier.

Poole, J. L. (2011). Measures of hand function. *Arthritis Care & Research, 63*(S11), S189–S199. https://doi.org/10.1002/acr.20631

Poole, J. L., Lucero, S. L., & Mynatt, R. (2010). Self-reports and performance-based tests of hand function in persons with osteoarthritis. *Physical & Occupational Therapy in Geriatrics, 28*(3), 249–258. https://doi.org/10.3109/02703181.2010.504960

Silva, P. G., Jones, A., da Rocha Correa Fernandes, A., & Natour, J. (2017). Moberg Picking-Up Test in patients with hand osteoarthritis. *Journal of Hand Therapy, 30*(4), 522–528. https:// doi.org/10.1016/j.jht.2016.10.005

Stamm, T. A., Machold, K., Sahinbegovic, E., Haider, S., Ernst, M., Binder, A., Dallos, T., Zwerina, J., & Smolen, J. (2011). Daily functioning and health status in patients with hand osteoarthritis: Fewer differences between women and men than expected. *Wiener Klinische Wochenschrift, 123*(19-20), 603–606. https://doi.org/10.1007/s00508-011-1597-0

Stoffer-Marx, M. A., Klinger, M., Luschin, S., Meriaux-Kratochvila, S., Zettel-Tomenendal, M., Nell-Duxneuner, V., Zwerina, J., Kjeken, I., Hackl, M. Öhlinger, S., Woolf, A., Redlich, K., Smolen, J. S., & Stamm, T. A. (2018). Functional consultation and exercises improve grip strength in osteoarthritis of the hand—a randomised controlled trial. *Arthritis Research and Therapy, 20*(1), Article 253. https://doi.org/10.1186/s13075-018-1747-0

Stukstette, M. J. P. M., Hoogeboom, T. J., de Ruiter, R., Koelmans, P., Veerman, E., den Broeder, A. A., Cats, H., Bijlsma, J. W., Dekker, J., & van den Ende, C. H. M. (2012). A multidisciplinary and multidimensional intervention for patients with hand osteoarthritis. *Clinical Rehabilitation, 26*(2), 99–110. https://doi.org/10.1177/0269215511417739

Wright, H. H., O'Brien, V., Valdes, K., Koczan, B., MacDermid, J., Moore, E., & Finley, M. A. (2017). Relationship of the Patient-Specific Functional Scale to commonly used clinical measures in hand osteoarthritis. *Journal of Hand Therapy, 30*(4), 538–545. https://doi.org/10.1016/j.jht.2017.04.003

BIBLIOGRAPHY

Bukhave, E. B., la Cour, K., & Huniche, L. (2014). The meaning of activity and participation in everyday life when living with hand osteoarthritis. *Scandinavian Journal of Occupational Therapy, 21*(1), 24–30. https://doi.org/10.3109/11038128.2013.857428

Kjeken, I., Smedslund, G., Moe, R. H., Slatkowsky-Christensen, B., Uhlig, T., & Birger Hagen, K. (2011). Systematic review of design and effects of splints and exercise programs in hand osteoarthritis. *Arthritis Care & Research, 63*(6), 834–848. https://doi.org/10.1002/acr.20427

Kloppenburg, M., Kroon, F. P., Blanco, F. J., Doherty, M., Dziedzic, K. S., Greibrokk, E., Haugen, I. K., Herrero-Beaumont, G., Jonsson, H., Kjeken, I., Maheu, E., Ramonda, R., Ritt, M. J., Smeets, W., Smolen, J. S, Stamm, T. A., Szekanecz, Z., Wittoek, R., & Carmona. L. (2019). 2018 update of the EULAR recommendations for the management of hand osteoarthritis. *Annals of the Rheumatic Diseases, 78*(1), 16–24. https://doi.org/10.1136/annrheumdis-2018-213826

Poole, J. L., Santhanam, D. D., & Latham, A. L. (2013). Hand impairment and activity limitations in four chronic diseases. *Journal of Hand Therapy, 26*(3), 232–237. https://doi.org/10.1016/j.jht.2013.03.002

Valdes, K., & Marik, T. (2010). A systematic review of conservative interventions for osteoarthritis of the hand. *Journal of Hand Therapy, 23*(4), 334–351. https://doi.org/10.1016/j.jht.2010.05.001

Osteoarthritis of the Thumb

Also called carpometacarpal (CMC) osteoarthritis, carpometacarpal joint osteoarthritis, trapeziometacarpal osteoarthritis, CMC joint osteoarthritis, CMC1 osteoarthritis, basal joint osteoarthritis, thumb arthritis, thumb osteoarthritis.

See also Osteoarthritis of the Hand.

Description

Progressive instability and loss of mobility of the carpometacarpal joint of the thumb (CMC1) causing pain, deformity, and decreased ability to oppose thumb and finger for pinch and grasp. The CMC1 joint is composed of two bones (trapezium, a carpal bone in wrist, and the first metacarpal of the thumb), which form a biconcave/biconvex articulating surface; five ligaments, which provide most of the stability (anterior oblique, posterior oblique, radial collateral, ulnar collateral, and intermetacarpal); and eight muscles, which primarily serve to position the thumb for motion (flexor pollicis longus and brevis, adductor pollicis, abductor pollicis longus and brevis, extensor pollicis longus and brevis, and opponens pollicis). The flexor pollicis longus and brevis and adductor pollicis provide the most force during grasp and pinch activities (Gustafson et al., 2014). In later stages a third bone, the scaphoid carpal bone, may be a factor if the index finger becomes involved.

Cause

Two causes are discussed: an insufficiency or laxity of the anterior oblique ligament, or deterioration of the cartilage layers between the articulating surfaces of the trapezium and first metacarpal bone (Grenier et al., 2016). The loss of a stable base of control of the thumb at the CMC joint is considered the core concept that results in the progressing imbalance of forces around the joint, subluxation, and functional deformity (DeMott, 2017). Intervention depends on which cause is accepted or advanced as the rationale for treatment. Therefore, a variety of interventions are presented in the literature, focused on ligaments versus bones, nonsurgery (conservative approach) versus surgical approach, single versus multimodal intervention, and best evidence for type of intervention to be used. For example, there is disagreement as to whether joint instability is best modified by increasing muscle strength (remedial approach) or whether intervention should focus on compensating for instability (Jansen et al., 2017).

Stages

- Stage 1: Radiographic evidence of joint widening but articular surfaces are normal in appearance and less than one-third subluxation of metacarpal base is observed.
- Stage 2: Radiographic evidence of significant joint capsule laxity. At least one-third subluxation of metacarpal base is present. Small bone or calcific fragments may be present.
- Stage 3: Radiographic evidence shows greater than one-third subluxation of metacarpal base is present. Bone or calcific fragments, and slight joint space narrowing is observed.
- Stage 4: Radiographic evidence of major subluxation is present, and joint space is very narrow. Subchondral bone changes are observed. Osteophyte formation and significant erosion of dorsal facet of the trapezium is present (adapted from Grenier et al., 2016). The so-called zig-zag deformity (between thumb metacarpal, proximal and distal phalanxes) may be seen in advanced stage.

Classification (adapted from Grenier et al., 2016)

- Stage 1: Pain, positive grind test, ligamentous laxity and dorsoradial subluxation of CMC1.
- Stage 2: Instability, chronic subluxation, radiographic degenerative changes.
- Stage 3: Involvement of scaphotrapezial joint or trapeziometacarpal joint of index finger.
- Stage 4: Stages 2 and 3 plus degenerative changes at the metacarpophalangeal (MCP) joint.

Evaluation/Assessment

Areas

- Activities of Daily Living/Instrumental ADL: ability to perform everyday tasks person typically performed
- Education/Work: ability to perform work tasks
- Play/Leisure: ability to perform favorite leisure activities, interests, frequency, location
- Rest/Sleep: sleep disturbances
- Social Participation: ability to perform tasks associated with person's social activities, type, frequency, location
- Sensorimotor: grasp and pinch strength, joint mobility (thumb and index finger), joint range of motion (thumb and fingers), hand stiffness, hand dexterity, pressure pain threshold, fatigue, proprioception (joint position sense)
- Cognitive/Perceptual: problem solving
- Psychosocial: quality of life, self-efficacy, coping skills
- Context/Environment: client and family education, adapted devices
- Comorbidities: osteoarthritis of the hand, knee, or hip

Instruments

Instruments Developed by Occupational Therapy Personnel

- Activities of Daily Living Questionnaire (ADLQ; Weiss et al., 2000)
- Canadian Occupational Performance Measure (5th ed.; COPM-5; Law et al., 2014)
- Green "Hand Assessment" Test (Green, 1974)

Instruments Developed by Other Professionals and Used by Occupational Therapy Personnel

- Australian/Canadian Osteoarthritis Hand Index (AUSCAN; Bellamy et al., 2002)

- Cochin Hand Function Scale (CHFS; see Hand Function Disability Scale [HFDS])
- Disabilities of the Arm, Shoulder, and Hand (3rd ed.; DASH-3; Kennedy et al., 2011)
- Finger to palm distance test (FPD; finger is flexed into palm; finger should flex into palmar crease; distance is measured with a short ruler from fingertip to crease if finger does not flex into crease)
- Functional Index for Hand Osteoarthritis (FIHOA; Dreiser et al., 2000)
- Grind test (compressing the CMC joint while gently rotating the head of the metacarpal on the trapezium; crating or crepitus is evidence of damaged cartilage; Beasley, 2014, p. 458, in References)
- Grip Ability Test (GAT; Dellhag & Bjelle, 1995)
- Grip strength (dynamometry; JAMAR dynamometer; Grippit; Wang et al., 2018; see also Villafañe, Valdes, Angulo-Diaz-Parreño, et al., 2015; Villafañe et al., 2017; Villafañe, Valdes, Vanti, et al., 2015, in References)
- Hand Function Disability Scale (HFDS; Duruöz et al., 1996)
- Joint Position Sense Test (JPST; Kalisch et al., 2012)
- Joint range of motion (goniometry; Shurtleff & Kaskutas, 2018; see also Villafañe & Valdes, 2013, in References)
- Kellgren-Lawrence Grade/Grading System (KLG; Kellgren & Lawrence, 1957)
- Modified Kapandji Index (MFI; Lefevre-Colau et al., 2003)
- Numeric pain scale (NPS; 0–10: 0 = *no pain*, 10 = *severe pain*)
- Numeric rating scale (NRS; 0–10, stiffness)
- O'Connor Finger Dexterity Test (OFDT; O'Connor, 1926)
- Patient-Reported Wrist/Hand Evaluation (PRWHE; MacDermid & Tottenham, 2004)
- Pinch strength test (B&E Pinch Meter, Grippit electronic instrument; Mathiowetz et al., 1985; see also Villafañe & Valdes, 2014; Villafañe et al., 2017, in References)
- Pollexograph (de Kraker et al., 2009)
- Purdue Pegboard Test (PPT; Tiffin, 1948)
- QuickDASH (Kennedy et al., 2011)
- Stanford Health Assessment Questionnaire (SHAQ; Bruce & Fries, 2003)
- Visual analogue scale (VAS; 0–10 cm, pain or stiffness)

Problems/Issues

Activities of Daily Living/Instrumental ADL
- Person may have difficulty grasping or gripping objects used in daily life.
- Person may experience pain in CMC joint when grasping or gripping objects.

Education/Work
- Person may have difficulty performing work tasks that require thumb and fingers to grasp or grip objects.
- Person may experience pain, especially if force or grip strength is required.

Play/Leisure
- Person may limit or cease engagement in leisure activities that require grasp or grip due to lack of strength or pain or both.

Rest/Sleep
- No information identified.

Social Participation
- Person may limit or stop participation in social activities due to decreased grip strength or pain or both.

Sensorimotor
- Person may have reduced joint range of motion of thumb.

- Person may have contracture of soft tissue in the web space between thumb and index finger (first web space), which limits thumb mobility in extension, abduction and opposition.
- Person may be using a poor pinch pattern (typically CMC flexion with metacarpophalangeal hyperextension and interphalangeal hyperflexion).
- Person may have difficulty with opposition or use an adapted pattern (index finger touches lateral border of thumb instead of pad due to reduced rotation of the thumb).
- Person may experience reduced hand grip and pinch strength.
- Person may experience difficulty rotating the thumb at the CMC thumb joint to oppose the fingers.
- Person may exhibit deformity in the thumb due to subluxation of the CMC joint (zig-zag deformity).
- Person often experiences pain, especially if force is applied in gripping or pinching an object or pressure is applied into the CMC joint.
- Person may have decreased sense of proprioception in the CMC (Ouegnin & Valdes, 2020).

Cognitive/Perceptual
- Cognition is not affected directly by osteoarthritis of the thumb, but consideration should be given to intervention planning if cognitive impairment or uncorrected visual limitations are present.

Psychosocial
- Person may experience decreased quality of life related to limitations.
- Person may experience decreased sense of self-efficacy due to limitations of grasp, pinch, or pain.

Context/Environment
- Person may lack knowledge about osteoarthritis of the thumb or its management.
- Person may lack knowledge of community or internet resources.

Intervention/Treatment

Models and programs developed by occupational therapy personnel include the lisent-centered approach (Shankland & Nedelec, 2018), dynamic stability program (DeMott, 2017; O'Brien & Giveans, 2013), exercise program (Valdes & von der Heyde, 2012), home exercise program (Scott, 2018), making a difference (Roundtree, 2011), multimodal treatment (Shankland et al., 2017), nonsurgical treatment (Gustafson et al., 2014), occupational therapy intervention (Teuchert et al., 2017), and splints (Cantero-Téllez, Valdes, et al., 2018; Sillem et al., 2011). Models and programs developed by other professionals but used by occupational therapy personnel include elastic tape (Villafañe & Valdes, 2015), immobilization (Cantero-Téllez, Villafañe et al., 2018), surgery (Richard et al., 2014; van der Veen et al., 2013; Yao & Lashgari, 2014), and therapeutic exercise guidelines (Brosseau et al., 2018). Team members include general physicians, rheumatologists, physical therapists, and occupational therapy personnel. Goals are to provide pain relief and improve hand function through a multifaceted intervention approach (Roundtree, 2011).

Activities of Daily Living/Instrumental ADL
- Encourage client to continue performing ADLs with modifications to decrease stress and pain on CMC joint.

Education/Work
- Encourage client to continue work if client desires; identify work tasks that may need modification or elimination.

Play/Leisure
- Encourage client to continue engagement in favorite leisure activities; identify actions or motions that may need modification.

Rest/Sleep

- Client may need instruction on wearing a night splint.

Social Participation

- Encourage client to continue participation in social activities with suggestions for modifications if needed.

Sensorimotor

- Ergonomics
  - ▶ Purpose: Reduce stress on CMC joint.
  - ▶ Technique: Use objects designed to make use of full hand grasp rather than pincher grasp: right angle knives, use electric can opener.
- Exercise (Note: Exercises should be limited to pain-free range. Limit or discontinue if inflammation is present.)
  - ▶ Purpose: Rebalance and restabilize muscle forces, improve range of motion, soft tissue release in first web space.
  - ▶ Technique:
    - ○ General stretching, isotonic and isometric exercises.
    - ○ Use of functional hand exercises: tasks involving pinching or grasping using opposition such as picking up coins, putting dishes and utensils in a drawer, squeezing a sponge, twisting a washcloth.
- Joint protection
  - ▶ Purpose: Reduce stress on CMC joint.
  - ▶ Technique:
    - ○ Use palm to turn knobs or lids of jars rather than thumb and fingers.
    - ○ Use larger joints rather than smaller joint.
- Massage (self-applied)
  - ▶ Purpose: Relieve soft tissue contractures and trigger points.
  - ▶ Technique:
    - ○ Set hand on a tennis ball and then use flexed proximal interphalangeal (PIP) joint of middle finger to apply pressure to web space between thumb and index finger.
    - ○ Use empty roll-on deodorant boot as a massage tool applied to first web space and base of CMC joint.
    - ○ Use of opposite hand is not recommended because condition may be bilateral and cause further damage to other thumb.
- Needling or acupuncture
  - ▶ Purpose: Reduce pain.
  - ▶ Technique: Not described. Would require addition training beyond entry-level education.
- Pain management
  - ▶ Purpose: Manage pain.
  - ▶ Technique: Identify situations and activities that cause most pain and suggest methods to reduce the actions and movements that cause the pain.
- Physical modalities
  - ▶ Purpose: Pain relief.
  - ▶ Technique: Paraffin, laser, iontophoresis with dexamethasone.
  - ▶ Time: 3 to 6 sessions.
- Positioning
  - ▶ Purpose: Maintain resting or neutral position: CMC joint is in abduction and slight extension, metacarpophalangeal joint is flexed.
  - ▶ Technique: See orthoses or splints.
- Orthoses and splints
  - ▶ Purpose: Reduce pain, maintain functional position, promote normal movement pattern.

▶ Type: Ballena or Whale (which includes the metacarpophalangeal joint); Colditz (metacarpophalangeal joint is excluded); Comfort Coll orthosis (North Coast Medical), Thumb Spica orthosis.

▶ Wearing time: Full time 3–4 weeks; nighttime thereafter or when used for stressful activities.

▶ Caution: One splint type does not fit all. Splint fabrication may require multiple attempts to identify client's thumb and hand function requirements. A different splint may be needed for day use versus nighttime.

- Stiffness: Use static progressive splinting (Wang et al., 2014).
- Surgery: Use of Artelon CMC Spacer not recommended (Richard et al., 2014).

Cognitive/Perceptual

- Not discussed (see Precautions/Safety Considerations).

Psychosocial

- Discuss with client issues important to client's quality of life and recommend compensatory approaches as needed.

Context/Environment

- Provide client education on abnormal pinch biomechanics, training in joint protection techniques, and information on wearing and caring for a splint.
- Provide a home program of exercises.
- Provide knowledge about community and internet resources. (Note: The YouTube videos on thumb exercises for carpometacarpal osteoarthritis have a low level of evidence to support their use; Villafañe et al., 2018.)
- Suggest and provide training in use of adaptive devices and equipment (Roundtree, 2011).
  ▶ Paint can opener to release air seal on new jars.
  ▶ Nonslip material for opening or turning caps, bottles, knobs, lids.
  ▶ Spring-loaded scissors.
  ▶ "Dumbbell" keyholder (small rod with balls that twist on and off at either end to hold keys and provide turning leverage).
  ▶ Electric can opener and toothbrush.
  ▶ Cylindrical tubing to build up handles on eating utensils, toothbrush.

Precautions/Safety Considerations

Recommendation in literature is for supervised exercise under therapist direction rather than depending on a home exercise program. Cognitive impairment may limit client's ability to identify problems and problem solve. Therapist may need to complete more observation of functional performance.

Prognosis and Outcome

Osteoarthritis of the thumb is a chronic condition, but clients can learn to manage their pain, reduce stress on the CMC joint, and continue daily occupational performance (Roundtree, 2011). Occupational therapy may delay or reduce the need for CMC joint surgery (Gravås, Østerås, et al., 2019; Gravås, Tveter, et al., 2019).

REFERENCES

Beasley, J. (2014). Arthritis. In C. Cooper (Ed.), *Fundamentals of hand therapy* (2nd ed., pp. 457–478). Elsevier.

Brosseau, L., Thevenot, O., MacKiddie, O., Taki, J., Wells, G. A. Guitard, P., Léonard, G., Paquet, N., Aydin, S. Z., Toupin-April, K., Cavallo, S., Moe, R. H., Shaikh, K., Gifford, W., Loew, L., De Angelis, G., Shallwani, S. M., Aburub, A. S., Mizusaki Imoto, A., . . . Longchamp. G.

(2018). The Ottawa Panel guidelines on programmes involving therapeutic exercise for the management of hand osteoarthritis. *Clinical Rehabilitation, 32*(11), 1449–1471. https://doi.org/10.1177/0269215518780973

Cantero-Téllez, R., Valdes, K., Schwartz, D. A., Medina-Porqueres, I., Arias, J. C., & Villafañe, J. H. (2018). Necessity of immobilizing the metacarpophalangeal joint in carpometacarpal osteoarthritis: Short-term effect. *Hand, 13*(4), 412–417. https://doi.org/10.1177/1558944717708031

Cantero-Téllez, R., Villafañe, J. H., Valdes, K., & Berjano, P. (2018). Effect of immobilization of metacarpophalangeal joint in thumb carpometacarpal osteoarthritis on pain and function: A quasi-experimental trial. *Journal of Hand Therapy, 31*(1), 68–73. https://doi.org/10.1016/j.jht.2016.11.005

DeMott, L. (2017). Novel isometric exercises for the dynamic stability programs for thumb carpal metacarpal joint instability. *Journal of Hand Therapy, 30*(3), 372–375. https://doi.org/10.1016/j.jht.2016.09.005

Gravås, E. M. H., Østerås, N., Nossum, R., Eide, R. E. M., Klokkeide, Å., Matre, K. H., Olsen, M., Andreassen, O., Haugen, I. K., Tveter, A. T., & Kjeken, I. (2019). Does occupational therapy delay or reduce the proportion of patients that receives thumb carpometacarpal joint surgery? A multicentre randomised controlled trial. *RMD Open, 5*, Article e001046. https://doi.org/10.1136/rmdopen-2019-001046

Gravås, E. M. H., Tveter, A. T., Nossum, R., Eide, R. E. M., Klokkeide, Å., Matre, K. H., Olsen, M., Andreassen, Ø., Østerås, N., Haugen, I. K., & Kjeken, I. (2019). Non-pharmacological treatment gap preceding surgical consultation in thumb carpometacarpal osteoarthritis—A cross-sectional study. *BMC Musculoskeletal Disorders, 20*(1), Article 180. https://doi.org/10.1186/s12891-019-2567-3

Grenier, M.-L., Mendonca, R., & Dalley, P. (2016). The effectiveness of orthoses in the conservative management of thumb CMC joint osteoarthritis: An analysis of functional pinch strength. *Journal of Hand Therapy, 29*(3), 307–313. https://doi.org/10.1016/j.jht.2016.02.004

Gustafson, N. P., Jacobs, B. M., & Baker, N. A. (2014). Nonsurgical treatments can relieve pain, improve hand function in thumb carpometacarpal joint osteoarthritis. *The Rheumatologist, 8*(3), 31–33.

Jansen, V., Hendrick, P., & Ellis, J. (2017). Therapy management of thumb carpometacarpal osteoarthritis: Exploring UK therapists' perceptions of joint instability. *Hand Therapy, 22*(3), 118–128. https://doi.org/10.1177/1758998317698099

O'Brien, V. H., & Giveans, M. R. (2013). Effects of a dynamic stability approach in conservative intervention of the carpometacarpal joint of the thumb: A retrospective study. *Journal of Hand Therapy, 26*(1), 44–52. https://doi.org/10.1016/j.jht.2012.10.005

Ouegnin, A., & Valdes, K. (2020). Joint position sense impairments in older adults with carpometacarpal osteoarthritis: A descriptive comparative study. *Journal of Hand Therapy, 33*(4), 547–552. https://doi.org/10.1016/j.jht.2019.01.006

Richard, M. J., Lunich, J. A., & Correll, G. R. (2014). The use of the Artelon CMC Spacer for osteoarthritis of the basal joint of the thumb. *Journal of Hand Therapy, 27*(2), 122–126. https://doi.org/10.1016/j.jht.2013.12.001

Roundtree, L. C. (2011). Making a difference: Hand therapy. *Rehab Management, 24*(3), 10–13.

Scott, A. (2018). Is a joint-specific home exercise program effective for patients with first carpometacarpal joint osteoarthritis? A critical review. *Hand Therapy, 23*(3), 83–94. https://doi.org/10.1177/1758998318774815

Shankland, B., Beaton, D., Ahmed, S., & Nedelec, B. (2017). Effects of client-centered multimodal treatment on impairment, function, and satisfaction of people with thumb carpometacarpal osteoarthritis. *Journal of Hand Therapy, 30*(3), 307–313. https://doi.org/10.1016/j.jht.2017.03.004

Shankland, B., & Nedelec, B. (2018). A client-centered approach for thumb carpometacarpal joint osteoarthritis pain: Two case studies. *Journal of Hand Therapy, 31*(2), 265–270. https://doi.org/10.1016/j.jht.2018.01.005

Sillem, H., Backman, C. L., Miller, W. C., & Li, L. C. (2011). Comparison of two carpometacarpal stabilizing splints for individuals with thumb osteoarthritis. *Journal of Hand Therapy*, *24*(3), 216–226. https://doi.org/10.1016/j.jht.2010.12.004

Teuchert, R., de Klerk, S., Nieuwoudt, H. C., Otero, M., van Zyl, N., & Coetzé, M. (2017). Occupational therapy intervention into osteo-arthritis of the carpometacarpal joint of the thumb in the South African context. *South African Journal of Occupational Therapy*, *47*(1), 41–45. http://dx.doi.org/10.17159/2310-3833/2017/v47n1a8

Valdes, K., & von der Heyde, R. (2012). An exercise program for carpometacarpal osteoarthritis based on biomechanical principles. *Journal of Hand Therapy*, *25*(3), 251–263. https://doi.org/10.1016/j.jht.2012.03.008

van der Veen, F. J., White, D. N., Dapper, M. M., Griot, J. P., & Ritt, M. P. (2013). Clinical evaluation of the Articulinx Intercarpometacarpal Cushion for the first CMC joint: A feasibility study. *Journal of Wrist Surgery*, *2*(3), 276–281. https://doi.org/10.1055/s-0033-1353243

Villafañe, J. H., Cantero-Téllez, R., Valdes, K., Usuelli, F. G., & Berjano, P. (2018). Educational quality of YouTube videos in thumb exercises for carpometacarpal osteoarthritis: A search on current practice. *Hand*, *13*(6), 715–719. https://doi.org/10.1177/1558944717726139

Villafañe, J. H., & Valdes, K. (2013). Combined thumb abduction and index finger extension strength: A comparison of older adults with and without thumb carpometacarpal osteoarthritis. *Journal of Manipulative & Physiological Therapy*, *36*(4), 238–244. https://doi.org/10.1016/j.jmpt.2013.05.004

Villafañe, J. H., & Valdes, K. (2014). Reliability of pinch strength testing in elderly subjects with unilateral thumb carpometacarpal osteoarthritis. *Journal of Physical Therapy Science*, *26*(7), 993–995. https://doi.org/10.1589/jpts.26.993

Villafañe, J. H., & Valdes, K. (2015). Mobilization with movement and elastic tape application for the conservative management of carpometacarpal joint osteoarthritis. *Journal of Hand Therapy*, *28*(1), 82–85. https://doi.org/10.1016/j.jht.2014.08.001

Villafañe, J. H., Valdes, K., Angulo-Diaz-Parreño, S., Pillastrini P., & Negrini, S. (2015). Ulnar digits contribution to grip strength in patients with thumb carpometacarpal osteoarthritis is less than in normal controls. *Hand*, *10*(2), 191–196. https://doi.org/10.1007/s11552-014-9682-2

Villafañe, J. H., Valdes, K., Bertozzi, L., & Negrini, S. (2017). Minimal clinically important difference of grip and pinch strength in women with thumb carpometacarpal osteoarthritis when compared to healthy subjects. *Rehabilitation Nursing*, *42*(3), 139–145. https://doi.org/10.1002/rnj.196

Villafañe, J. H., Valdes, K., Vanti, C., Pillastrini, P., & Borboni, A. (2015). Reliability of handgrip strength test in elderly subjects with unilateral thumb carpometacarpal osteoarthritis. *Hand*, *10*(2), 205–209. https://doi.org/10.1007/s11552-014-9678-y

Wang, J., Erlandsson, G., Rui, Y.-J., & Li-Tsang, C. (2014). Efficacy of static progressive splinting in the management of metacarpophalangeal joint stiffness: A pilot clinical trial. *Hong Kong Journal of Occupational Therapy*, *24*(2), 45–50. https://doi.org/10.1016/j.hkjot.2014.07.001

Yao, J., & Lashgari, D. (2014). Thumb basal joint: Utilizing new technology for the treatment of a common problem. *Journal of Hand Therapy*, *27*(2), 127–133. https://doi.org/10.1016/j.jht.2013.12.012

BIBLIOGRAPHY

Aebischer, B., Elsig, S., & Taeymans, J. (2016). Effectiveness of physical and occupational therapy on pain, function and quality of life in patients with trapeziometacarpal osteoarthritis—A systematic review and meta-analysis. *Hand Therapy*, *21*(1), 5–15. https://doi.org/10.1177/1758998315614037

Bertozzi, L., Valdes, K., Vanti, C., Negrini, S., Pillastrini, P., & Villafañe, J. H. (2015). Investigation of the effect of conservative interventions in thumb carpometacarpal osteoarthritis:

Systematic review and meta-analysis. *Disability and Rehabilitation, 37*(22), 2025–2043. https://doi.org/10.3109/09638288.2014.996299

O'Brien, V. H., & McGaha, J. L. (2014). Current practice patterns in conservative thumb CMC joint care: Survey results. *Journal of Hand Therapy 27*(1), 14–22. https://doi.org/10.1016/j.jht.2013.09.001

Valdes, K., Naughton, N., & Algar, L. (2016). Linking ICF components to outcome measures for orthotic intervention for CMC OA: A systematic review. *Journal of Hand Therapy, 29*(4), 396–404. https://doi.org/10.1016/j.jht.2016.06.001

Villafañe, J. H., Valdes, K., O'Brien, V., Seves, M., Cantero-Téllez, R., & Berjano, P. (2018). Conservative management of thumb carpometacarpal osteoarthritis: An Italian survey of current clinical practice. *Journal of Bodywork and Movement Therapies, 22*(1), 37–39. https://doi.org/10.1016/j.jbmt.2017.03.015

Wolfe, T., Chu, J. Y., Woods, T., & Lubahn, J. D. (2014). A systematic review of postoperative hand therapy management of basal joint arthritis. *Clinical Orthopaedics and Related Research, 472*(4), 1190–1197. https://doi.org/10.1007/s11999-013-3285-z

Stiff Hand

Description

Stiff means difficult to bend or rigid and is used to describe hand joints that lack motion and provide resistance to movement (Colditz, 2011; Colditz, 2014). Stiffness refers to difficulty in moving a joint. Stiffness may result from direct injury to the hand or secondarily due to disuse after trauma (Seu & Pasqualetto, 2012). Separation should be made between the inability to move a joint as opposed to reluctance to move a joint because of pain. Characteristics of stiffness may be caused by the following:

- Discomfort that occurs with motion when attempting to move a joint (such as in the hand) after a period of rest, which occurs in rheumatic arthritis.
- Stiffness is more severe and prolonged with increasing severity of joint inflammation in rheumatoid disease.
- Morning stiffness in peripheral joints that lasts more than 1 hour can be an important early symptom of joint inflammation, such as rheumatoid arthritis, psoriatic arthritis, or chronic viral arthritis (Porter, 2018).

Cause

Cause may be the result of tight connective tissue, by arthritis or by other rheumatic disorders (O'Toole, 2017). Joints may become stiff during the healing process following trauma, as new collagen develops, which is relatively disorganized and thus resistant to movement. A second cause may occur when uninjured, immobilized joints undergo stress deprivation, triggering excessive collagen cross-linking (Colditz, 2014). Risk factors include multiple tissue trauma, prolonged immobilization, infection, and a decrease in tissue elasticity seen in older persons (Gangatharam, 2018). Colditz (2014) suggested stiffness itself may cause a change in motor representation in the brain. The example is a client who initiated finger flexion with the metacarpophalangeal joint rather than the interphalangeal joints following immobilization for a distal radius fracture.

Terminology

- *AROM:* Active range of motion of a joint.
- *Creep-based loading:* Force is applied as a constant force and the displacement of the limb varies (principle of dynamic orthoses; Schwartz, 2012).
- *Daily TERT:* Refers to total number of hours per day that a splint is used to hold a joint at the end of available ROM (Glasgow, Fleming Tooth, & Peters, 2012).

- *Elastic deformation:* Tissue reverts back to its original length when the force on it is removed (Schwartz, 2012).
- *Plastic deformation:* Tissue maintains its new length, even when the force is removed (Schwartz, 2012).
- *PROM:* Passive range of motion of a joint.
- *Stress relaxation loading:* Displacement is constant and applied force varies. Principle of static progressive orthoses (Schwartz, 2012).
- *TAC:* Torque angle curve.
- *TERT:* Total end range of time. Term used to describe the number of hours a joint is held at the end of available ROM under light tension (Glasgow, Fleming, Tooth, & Hockey, 2012; Glasgow, Fleming, Tooth, & Peters, 2012).
- *TROM:* Torque range of motion.

Evaluation/Assessment

Areas
- Activities of Daily Living/Instrumental ADL: dressing, eating
- Education/Work: work-related activities
- Play/Leisure: interests, frequency, location
- Rest/Sleep: sleep habits, sleep disturbances
- Social Participation: type, frequency, location, with whom
- Sensorimotor: joint range of motion (passive and active), edema (pitting and nonpitting), hand functions, physical activity/fitness, contractures, pain, overprotection of injured joint leading to nonmovement
- Cognitive/Perceptual: understanding and compliance with instructions for intervention instructions
- Psychosocial: self-efficacy, anxiety, depression, sense of helplessness
- Context/Environment: knowledge of injury and healing process, social and family support, available transportation and resources
- Comorbidities: distal radius fracture, any previous hand injury

Instruments
Instruments Developed by Occupational Therapy Personnel
- None

Instruments Developed by Other Professionals and Used by Occupational Therapy Personnel
- Disabilities of the Arm, Shoulder, and Hand (3rd ed.; DASH-3; Kennedy et al., 2011)
- Haldex tension gauge (available from rehabilitation equipment and supply vendors)
- Joint range of motion (goniometry; Shurtleff & Kaskutas, 2018)
- Modified Weeks Test (MWT; Flowers, 2002; see Gangatharam, 2018, in References)

Problems/Issues

Activities of Daily Living/Instrumental ADL
- Person may have difficulty performing certain ADL tasks due to decreased or limited range of motion in one or more fingers.

Education/Work
- Person may have difficulty performing work tasks due to decreased or limited range of motion in the hand and fingers.

Play/Leisure
- No information identified.

Rest/Sleep
- No information identified.

Social Participation
- No information identified.

Sensorimotor
- Person usually has reduced joint range of motion and joint mobility due to stiffness or contracture.
- Person usually has reduced hand functions (grasp, grip, manipulation, dexterity, coordination).
- Person may reduce physical activity to guard or protect injured joint.
- Person may have reduced sensation (tactile, proprioception, pressure).

Cognitive/Perceptual
- Person may have difficulty understanding or following intervention instructions for wearing splint or performing exercises.

Psychosocial
- Person may experience anxiety and depression.
- Person may be fearful of moving injured joint because of pain.
- Person may have low self-efficacy and sense of helplessness to change outcome.
- Person may not be motivated to overcome hand or upper extremity dysfunction.

Context/Environment
- Person may lack social and family support.
- Person may lack information about progression of stiffness and lack of joint mobility.
- Person may lack transportation to seek intervention.
- Person may follow instructions for wearing splint or use of adapted devices.

Intervention/Treatment

Models and programs developed by occupational therapy personnel include active redirection (Colditz, 2014); Capener splinting (Glasgow, Fleming, Tooth, & Peters, 2012), casting motion to mobilize stiffness (CMMS; Midgley, 2016), dual orthosis (Harte & Porter-Armstrong, 2012), extension orthoses (Glasgow & Peters, 2016), and target-focused exercise regime (Gangatharam, 2018). Models and programs developed by other professionals but used by occupational therapy personnel include dynamic splinting (Glasgow et al., 2011; Nakayama et al., 2016) and static progressive splinting (Wang et al., 2014). Team members include physicians, hand surgeons, physical therapy personnel, and occupational therapy personnel. Goals are to facilitate restoration of function and regain range of motion and movement of the affected joints to facilitate independent performance of everyday activities (Glasgow et al., 2011; Wang et al., 2014).

Activities of Daily Living/Instrumental ADL
- No information identified.

Education/Work
- No information identified.

Play/Leisure
- No information identified.

Rest/Sleep
- No information identified.

Social Participation
- No information identified.

Sensorimotor
- Cast
  - Limits all active flexion and extension to finger interphalangeal joint(s) until motion is regained (Colditz, 2014).

- Edema
  - ▶ Reduce edema, to increase potential for movement.
  - ▶ Edema control techniques include elevation, active motion, compression, and gentle external massage (Colditz, 2011).
- Exercises/mobilization
  - ▶ Increase movement to decrease stiffness and tissue adherence.
  - ▶ Early mobility (Colditz, 2011).
  - ▶ Tendon gliding (Colditz, 2011).
- Orthoses
  - ▶ Dynamic proximal interphalangeal (PIP) joint extension orthosis to passively extend the PIP joint (Colditz, 2014). Materials may include elastic bands, springs, coils, or Lycra (Glasgow et al., 2011).
  - ▶ Static metacarpophalangeal joint extension blocking orthosis for stiffer PIP joint (Colditz, 2014).
    - ○ Static progressive: Consists of a stable base and an element of mobility using an inelastic material, which holds the joint at the end range of available extension (Young et al., 2018).
    - ○ Serial static: Holds the joint at the available end range of passive extension (Young et al., 2018).

Cognitive/Perceptual
- Provide explicit verbal instructions, check for recall, and support with written instructions.
- With client input, set treatment goals and action plans.

Psychosocial
- Use motivation techniques including counseling session, positive feedback, rewards, contracts, exercise diaries.
- Instruction in stress management: coping strategies, relaxation techniques, yoga, mindfulness.

Context/Environment
- Provide client with regular schedule of follow-up visits to monitor progress and modify splint as needed.

Precautions/Safety Considerations

Maximal tolerable stress level should not be exceeded because result could lead to tissue failure (Schwartz, 2012). Dynamic orthoses using creep loading may be painful to wear, and joint may be damaged by prolonged compression (Schwartz, 2012).

Prognosis and Outcome

Variable. Stiffness or contracture to the proximal interphalangeal (PIP) joint is particularly challenging to treat effectively to regain functional range of motion. Theory and research findings support use of mobilizing splinting and active and passive exercises as the best choices to decrease contracture and mobilize the stiff hand (Glasgow et al., 2010).

REFERENCES

Colditz, J. C. (2011). Therapist's management of the stiff hand. In T. M. Skirven, A. L. Osterman, J. Fedorczyk, & P. Amadio (Eds.), *Rehabilitation of the hand and upper extremity* (6th ed., pp. 894–921). Mosby.

Colditz, J. C. (2014). Active redirection instead of passive motion for joint stiffness. *ASHT Times*, *21*(3), 6–9. https://bracelab.com/media/magefan_blog/PDFs/Active-Redirection-ASHT-Times_1.pdf

Gangatharam, S. (2018). Target-focused exercise regime to improve patient compliance and range of motion in the stiff hand. *Journal of Hand Therapy*, *31*(4), 568–571. https://doi.org/10.1016/j.jht.2018.07.003

Glasgow, C., Fleming, J., Tooth, L. R., & Hockey, R. L. (2012). The long-term relationship be-tween duration of treatment and contracture resolution using dynamic orthotic devices for the stiff proximal interphalangeal joint: A prospective cohort study. *Journal of Hand Therapy, 25*(1), 38–46. https://doi.org/10.1016/j.jht.2011.09.006

Glasgow, C., Fleming, J., Tooth, L. R., & Peters, S. (2012). Randomized controlled trial of daily total end range time (TERT) for Capener splinting of the stiff proximal interphalangeal joint. *American Journal of Occupational Therapy, 66*(2), 243–248. https://doi.org/ 10.5014/ ajot.2012.002816

Glasgow, C., & Peters, S. (2016). Extension orthoses and the stiff proximal interphalangeal joint following hand trauma: A review of current clinical practice in the Australian context. *Hand Therapy, 21*(3), 77–84. https://doi.org/ 10.11771758998316644275

Glasgow, C., Tooth, L. R., & Fleming, J. (2010). Mobilizing the stiff hand: Combining the-ory and evidence to improve clinical outcomes. *Journal of Hand Therapy, 23*(4), 392–400. https://doi.org/10.1016/j.jht.2010.05.005

Glasgow, C., Tooth, L. R., Fleming, J., & Peters, S. (2011). Dynamic splinting for the stiff hand after trauma: Predictors of contracture resolution. *Journal of Hand Therapy, 24*(3), 195–205. https://doi.org/10.1016/j.jht.2011.03.001

Harte, D., & Porter-Armstrong, A. (2012). Managing the stiff hand: Dual orthosis innovation. *Journal of Hand Therapy, 25*(3), 342–344. https://doi.org/10.1016/j.jht.2012.03.002

Midgley, R. (2016). Case report: The casting motion to mobilize stiffness technique for reha-bilitation after a crush and degloving injury of the hand. *Journal of Hand Therapy, 29*(3), 323–333. https://doi.org/10.1016/j.jht.2016.03.013

Nakayama, J., Horiki, M., Denno, K., Ogawa, K., Oka, H., & Domen, K. (2016). Clinical response of dynamic splint using functional scales for the extension contracture of the metacarpopha-langeal joint. *Asian Journal of Occupational Therapy, 12*(1), 85–91. https://doi.org/10.11596/ asiajot.12.85

O'Toole, M. T. (Ed.). (2017). *Mosby's dictionary of medicine, nursing & health professions* (10th ed.). Elsevier.

Porter, R. S. (Ed.). (2018). *The Merck manual of diagnosis and therapy* (20th ed.). Merck Sharp & Dohme.

Schwartz, D. A. (2012). Static progressive orthoses for the upper extremity: A comprehensive literature review. *Hand, 7*(1), 10–17. https://doi.org/10.1007/s11552-011-9380-2

Seu, M., & Pasqualetto, M. (2012). Hand therapy for dysfunction of the intrinsic muscles. *Hand Clinics, 28*(1), 87–100. https://doi.org/10.1016/j.hcl.2011.09.001

Wang, J., Erlandsson, G., Rui, Y.-J., & Li-Tsang, C. (2014). Efficacy of static progressive splinting in the management of metacarpophalangeal joint stiffness: A pilot clinical trial. *Hong Kong Journal of Occupational Therapy, 24*(2), 45–50. https://doi.org/10.1016/j.hkjot.2014.07.001

Young, N., Terrington, N., Francis, D., & Robinson, L. S. (2018). Orthotic management of fixed flexion deformity of the proximal interphalangeal joint following traumatic injury: A systematic review. *Hong Kong Journal of Occupational Therapy, 31*(1), 3–13. https://doi.org/ 10.1177/1569186118764067

Trigger Finger

Also called stenosing tenosynovitis (ST), stenosing flexor tenosynovitis (SFT), volar flexor tenosynovitis, digital flexor tendinitis, or jerk finger.

Description

Trigger finger is a phenomenon in which the movement of a finger is halted momentarily in flexion or extension and then continues with a jerk (O'Toole, 2017). When trigger finger oc-curs, the finger flexors contract but are unable to reextend due to a nodule within the tendon sheath or sheath constriction (*Stedman's*, 2011). Triggering of the digital flexor tendons most commonly occurs at the fibro-osseous tunnel formed by the metacarpal neck dorsally and the A1 pulley volar to the metacarpophalangeal (MCP) joint at the distal palmar crease (Langer et al., 2014; Lee et al., 2011). Tenosynovitis is an inflammatory condition, sometimes with subsequent fibrosis of tendons and tendon sheaths of the digit or digits (Porter, 2018).

Cause

Cause is idiopathic. People whose work or hobbies require repetitive gripping actions are at high risk of developing trigger finger. Trigger finger is more common and a higher risk factor in women and in anyone with diabetes or rheumatoid arthritis (Langer et al., 2016; Porter, 2018).

Classification Systems

Amsterdam Severity Scale in Stenosing Tenosynovitis (ASSiST; Peter et al., 2009)
- Grade 0   No impairment
- Grade 1   Palpable nodule or crepitation, with a normal active range of motion (AROM)
- Grade 2   A perceptible click or a reduced tempo of active finger flexion with a full AROM (determined by the maximum passive range of motion)
- Grade 3   Restriction in AROM by a tendon obstruction under the pulley or within the tendon sheath

Froimson Classification (Tung et al., 2010)
- Grade I   Pretriggering, pain: tenderness over A1 pulley; history of catching but not demonstrable on physical examination
- Grade II   Triggering: demonstrable catching, patient can actively extend
- Grade III   Triggering: demonstrable catching requiring passive extension or inability to actively flex
- Grade IV   Contracture: demonstrable catching, with a fixed flexion proximal interphalangeal (PIP) joint contracture

Quinnell System (Langer et al., 2015)
- 1 Uneven movement
- 2 Actively correctable locking of the digit
- 3 Passively correctable locking
- 4 Fixed deformity

Evaluation/Assessment

Areas
- Activities of Daily Living/Instrumental ADL: eating and drinking, dressing (fasteners)
- Education/Work: work tasks (repetitive hand gripping movements)
- Play/Leisure: leisure activities (repetitive hand gripping movements), frequency, location
- Rest/Sleep: sleep habits, sleep disturbance
- Social Participation: type, location, frequency, with whom
- Sensorimotor: finger movement (active, passive), grip and pinch strength, adjustment of grip force, joint range of motion, contracture, palpation for nodule (volar aspect of MCP

and PIP joints), inflammation, swelling or tenderness (flexor tendon), pain (wrist, hand), sensation
- Cognitive/Perceptual: not directly related
- Psychosocial: depression, quality of life, role performance
- Context/Environment: knowledge of condition and intervention options
- Comorbidities: rheumatoid arthritis, diabetes, carpal tunnel syndrome
- Differential diagnosis: Dupuytren's contracture, flexor tendon or sheath tumors, MCP joint acute inflammation, de Quervain's tenosynovitis, sesamoid bone abnormalities

Instruments

Instruments Developed by Occupational Therapy Personnel
- Box and Block Test (BBT; Mathiowetz et al., 1985)
- Canadian Occupational Performance Measure (5th ed.; COPM-5; Law et al., 2014)
- Functional Dexterity Test (FDT; Aaron & Jansen, 2003)
- Nine Hole Peg Test (NHPT; Mathiowetz et al., 1985)

Instruments Developed by Other Professionals and Used by Occupational Therapy Personnel
- Disabilities of the Arm, Shoulder, and Hand (3rd ed.; DASH-3; Kennedy et al., 2011; see also Langer et al., 2015, in References)
- Grip strength (dynamometry; JAMAR Hydraulic Hand Dynamometer; Wang et al., 2018; see also Langer et al., 2017, in References)
- Jebsen-Taylor Hand Function Test (JTHFT; Jebsen et al., 1969)
- Joint range of motion (goniometry; Shurtleff & Kaskutas, 2018)
- Modified Kapandji Index (MKI; Lefevre-Colau et al., 2003)
- Open and Close Hand Test (OCHT; Mary Pack Arthritis Program, 2015)
- Pinch meter (pinch strength; B&L Engineering; Mathiowetz et al., 1985)
- Purdue Pegboard Test (PPT; Tiffin, 1947; see also Langer et al., 2017, in References)
- Semmes-Weinstein Monofilaments (measurement instruments)
- Two-Point Discrimination (TPD; Disk-Criminator or Boley Gauge; measurement instrument)
- Ultrasound imaging (see Chuang et al., 2017, in References)
- Visual analogue scale (pain scale; scored: 0 = *no pain*, 10 = *worst pain ever*)
- World Health Organization Quality of Life (WHOQOL-BREF; The WHOQOL Group, 1998; see also Langer et al., 2015, in References)

Problems/Issues

Activities of Daily Living/Instrumental ADL
- Person has difficulty applying proper force to grasp a water bottle (i.e., squeezing it or letting it slip).

Education/Work
- Person may experience symptoms due to work-related activities that require frequent gripping actions (e.g., cutting using scissors, using wire cutters).

Play/Leisure
- Person may experience symptoms due to engagement in hobby or sports activities that require frequent and repeated gripping actions (e.g., holding a racket, cutting equipment).

Rest/Sleep
- Sleep disturbance.

Social Participation
- No information identified.

Sensorimotor
- Person may experience finger/thumb stiffness, especially in the morning.
- Person may notice a popping, clicking, or snapping sensation when the finger is moved.

- Person may notice that a finger/thumb catches or locks in flexed position, which suddenly pops when extended.
- Person may notice that a finger/thumb catches or locks in flexed position, which cannot be straightened without assistance.
- Person may have difficulty adjusting amount of grip strength (force) to hold or release objects in hand (lack of smooth coordination in picking up, holding, and releasing objects).
- Person may have difficulty with force coordination, even if only one digit is affected by trigger finger (Chen et al., 2013).
- Person may experience tenderness or a bump (nodule) at the base of the affected finger in the palm of the hand.
- Person may experience swelling, tenderness, or thickening along flexor tendon sheath.
- Person may have a distinct nodule on volar aspect of the MCP and PIP joints that can be felt by palpation.
- Person may experience pain in hand or wrist during activity or resting near palmar crease (A1 pulley) or near PIP joint (A3 pulley).

Cognitive/Perceptual
- No information identified.

Psychosocial
- No information identified.

Context/Environment
- Person may not be aware of conditions or actions that aggravate symptoms.
- Person may not know the disorder can be treated and managed.

Intervention/Treatment

Models and programs developed by occupational therapy personnel include splint adaptation (Wong & Rocker, 2018). Models and programs developed by other professionals but used by occupational therapy personnel include combined therapy (Choudhury & Tay, 2014), Isoforce outrigger orthosis (Marrel et al., 2016), laser therapy and massage (Aranyavalai et al., 2014), night splinting (Drijkoningen et al., 2018), postoperative rehabilitation (Lu et al., 2015), and splint designs (Tarbhai et al., 2012). Team members include physicians, hand surgeons, nursing personnel, psychologists, physical therapy personnel, and occupational therapy personal. Goals are to relieve symptoms and assist client to regain function to perform daily activities. (Note: There are no suggestions for intervention in any area except Sensorimotor.)

Activities of Daily Living/Instrumental ADL
- No information identified.

Education/Work
- No information identified.

Play/Leisure
- No information identified.

Rest/Sleep
- No information identified.

Social Participation
- No information identified.

Sensorimotor
- Heat therapy
  - ▶ Equipment: Hot packs, paraffin wax, or hot water bath.
  - ▶ Time: 10–14 minutes each application, 2–3 times a day.

- Low-level laser (Note: requires training beyond typical occupational therapy education).
  - ▶ Equipment: Laser class 3B (789–860 mm GaAIAs Laser) 8 Joules (2–3 points).
- Ultrasound
  - ▶ Equipment: Ultrasound machine.
  - ▶ Method: Under water or direct contact with ultrasound gel. Use pulsed ultrasound in acute stage. Use continuous ultrasound for thermal effect to decrease pain.
  - ▶ Time: 2 times a week for 3 weeks.
- Cryotherapy
  - ▶ Equipment: Cold packs, ice cube massage.
  - ▶ Method: Apply cryotherapy to affected area where pain occurs.
  - ▶ Time: 20 minutes each application 2–3 times a day.
  - ▶ Precaution: Cold may "mask" pain and should be monitored closely if Raynaud's phenomenon is present.
- Contrast bath
  - ▶ Equipment: Hot and cold towels, pans, or tanks.
  - ▶ Method: Alternate hot (5 seconds) and cold (10 seconds).
  - ▶ Repetitions and time: Repeat alternating hot and cold for 20 minutes, 2–3 times a day.
  - ▶ Temperature: According to client's tolerance.
- Massage
  - ▶ Method: Massage entire tendon sheath and adjacent area using Cyrriax popularized transverse friction massage (move over client's skin perpendicular to tendon fiber orientation with increasing pressure).
  - ▶ Time: Up to 15 minutes.
  - ▶ Note: If tendon and pulley are involved, the tendon should be held taut and mobilized perpendicular to the sheath.
- Exercise (range of motion)
  - ▶ Method: Tendon gliding exercise using hook fist in an MCP blocking splint or passive full fist without splint.
  - ▶ Repetition: 5 repetitions each exercise, 3 times a day.
  - ▶ Precaution: Avoid full and repetitive fisting while symptoms persist.
- Taping (Kinesio Taping)
  - ▶ Method 1: Tape is attached proximal to the dorsal surface of the PIP joint down to dorsal aspect of metacarpal.
  - ▶ Method 2: Middle part of tape is applied to palmar aspect of base of affected proximal phalange. The two ends of the tape are crossed over to the dorsal aspect of MCP joint attaching proximally to dorsal aspect of metacarpal forming a V. A second tape is applied, as per Method 1.
- Compression
  - ▶ Method: Use Digi-Sleeve for single finger swelling, and compression glove for multiple fingers or palmar swelling.
  - ▶ Wearing: Can be worn under a splint, provided it does not compromise splint fit for day or night use.
  - ▶ Precaution: Resize or discontinue use if numbness or tingling occurs in the fingers or skin irritation occurs.
- Joint protection
  - ▶ Client should avoid:
    - ○ Activities that require tight, prolonged, repetitive grip.
    - ○ Full or repetitive fist position when symptoms are present.
    - ○ Prolonged, forceful tip-to-tip pinch (opposition) with affected finger.
    - ○ Power tools that cause vibration.
    - ○ Pressure in palm of hand, such as holding grocery bags by handles or suitcase handles.

- ▶ Client should:
  - ○ Use padded steering wheel cover for driving and padded gloves for prolonged, repetitive grip tools.
  - ○ Use compensatory approaches, including use of other fingers or other hand or vice to hand object normally held with fingers.
  - ○ Use padded straps on handles, use shoulder straps, use suitcases with wheels, carry grocery bags in arms.
- • Splinting
  - ▶ MCP blocking splints
    - ○ Purpose: Reduce pain and swelling due to diffuse tenosynovitis or triggering.
    - ○ Description: Splint holds MCP joint in 0–15 degrees flexion, but allows full PIP movement.
      - ▷ Palmar ring splint
        - • Advantage: Splint allows tip-to-tip prehension and full thenar motion.
        - • Material: Customized from low temperature thermoplastic material, with plastic disc extending beyond palmar crease or metal triangular bar.
        - • Options: Dorsal part of ring can have a separation to permit ease of putting splint on and off. A strap can be added to maintain contact of splint with palm to ensure correct MCP position with A1 pulley.
        - • Wearing time: Metal type should be worn during day only. Total time 8–10 weeks most common. Variable 3–12 weeks.
      - ▷ Dorsal ring splint
        - • Advantage: Splint leaves palm free for gripping.
        - • Material: Customized from low temperature thermoplastic material by creating a strip of plastic in which the midpoint is applied to ventral surface of proximal end of interphalangeal (IP) joint and wrapped around proximal finger down the dorsal side. A strap around the palm and dorsal surface is required to maintain contact of splint with dorsal aspect of hand.
        - • Option: Splint may be padded over MCP joint dorsally to reduce pressure.
        - • Wearing: Use for daytime only. Total time 8–10 weeks most commonly recommended. Range 3–12 weeks.
      - ▷ Hand-based palmar splint
        - • Advantage: Useful when more than one finger is involved.
        - • Method: Customized from low temperature thermoplastic to encompass involved fingers at proximal ends into palm of hand with a strap that wraps around the dorsum of the hand. Splint should allow full thumb opposition avoiding thenar crease.
  - ▶ PIP joint/thumb IP blocking splint
    - ○ Advantage: Used to control pain, swelling, or triggering due to a nodule at A3 in a single finger or at A1 pulley in thumb. Also used with A1 pulley triggering if a less restrictive splint is required. Splint allows optimal hand function for gripping because only one joint of affected finger is splinted.
    - ○ Method: Customized thermoplastic cylinder splint holds PIP joint in full extension, limiting flexor tendon excursion through affected pulley.
    - ○ Types include cylinder, metal ring, or PIP volar gutter for fingers and a reverse oval-8 for thumb.
  - ▶ MCP/PIP limiting splint
    - ○ Advantage: Less restriction with ring type splints allowing more hand function.
    - ○ Type: Anti-swan neck splint positioned upside down on finger with central bar proximal to PIP joint. Objective is to significantly limit pip joint flexion and partially limit MCP flexion.
  - ▶ Hand resting splint
    - ○ Advantage: General use for flexor tenosynovitis, pain at night and problematic finger locking in the morning.

○ Type: Splint typically supports MCP joints in 15–20 degrees flexion but should be reduced to 0 to 5 degrees flexion to decrease force at A1 pulley. PIP joints should be positioned at 20 degrees flexion and DIP points at 10 degrees.
○ Wearing time: Generally, nighttime. Daily range of motion exercise is recommended to prevent joint stiffness.
- Corticosteroid injections
  ▶ Advantage: Quick, no therapy may be needed, success rate 50% to 90%.
  ▶ Disadvantage: High rate of recurrence, less successful in clients with triggering for more than 6 months or people with diabetes mellitus.
  ▶ Method: Lack of improvement after 2 or 3 injections usually indicates failure.
  ▶ Options: Combined injections with other interventions such as splinting can improve success rate.

Cognitive/Perceptual
- No information identified.

Psychosocial
- No information identified.

Context/Environment
- No information identified.

Precautions/Safety Considerations
- Precautions if splints are used (Mary Pack Arthritis Program, 2015).
  ▶ Thickness of ring splints should not facilitate ulnar drift in adjacent fingers.
  ▶ Split should be monitored to ensure it does not aggravate PIP joint inflammation.
  ▶ Split may impair hand function if PIP joint flexion is limited resulting in noncompliance with wearing instructions.
  ▶ Daily range of motion exercises are recommended to prevent joint stiffness.
  ▶ Always check for pressure areas on skin; avoid splints that are too tight fitting.
  ▶ Always check for pressure areas on skin regularly, especially if splint is worn overnight.

Prognosis and Outcome
Generally, outcome is good but may come back. In follow-up study, clients continued to report disability in activities requiring strength and more severe pain than control subjects (Langer et al., 2018). Orthotic devices (splinting) have been found to be effective in reducing pain when worn for 6–10 weeks (Lunsford et al., 2019; Valdes, 2012).

REFERENCES
Aranyavalai, T., Kusakul, Y., & Saensri, P. (2014). Treatment of trigger fingers associated with carpal tunnel syndrome by low-level laser therapy and specific hand massage: A case report. *Vajira Medical Journal, 58*(1), 59–65.
Chen, P.-T., Lin, C.-J., Jou, I.-M., Chieh, H.-F., Su, F.-C., & Kuo, L.-C. (2013). One digit interruption: The altered force patterns during functionally cylindrical grasping tasks in patients with trigger digits. *PLOS ONE, 8*(12), Article e83632. https://doi.org/10.1371/journal.pone.0083632
Choudhury, M. M., & Tay, S. C. (2014). Prospective study on the management of trigger finger. *Hand Surgery, 19*(3), 393–397. https://doi.org/10.1142/S0218810414500336
Chuang, B.-I., Kuo, L.-C., Yang, T.-H., Su, F.-C., Jou, I.-M., Lin, W.-J., & Sun, Y.-N. (2017). A medical imaging analysis system for trigger finger using an adaptive texture-based active shape model (ATASM) in ultrasound images. *PLOS ONE, 12*(10), Article e0187042. https://doi.org/10.1371/journal.pone.0187042
Drijkoningen, T., van Berckel, M., Becker, S. J. E., Ring, D. C., & Mudgal, C. S. (2018). Night splinting for idiopathic trigger digits. *Hand, 13*(5), 558–562. https://doi.org/10.1177/1558944717725374

Langer, D., Luria, S., Bar-Haim Erez, A., Michailevich, M., Rogev, N., & Maeir, A. (2015). Stenosing flexor tenosynovitis: Validity of standard assessment tools of daily functioning and quality of life. *Journal of Hand Therapy, 28*(4), 384–387. https://doi.org/10.1016/j.jht.2015.04.005

Langer, D., Luria, S., Maeir, A., & Erez, A. (2014). Occupation-based assessments and treatments of trigger finger: A survey of occupational therapists from Israel and the United States. *Occupational Therapy International, 21*(4), 143–155. https://doi.org/101002/oti.1372

Langer, D., Luria, S., Michailevich, M., & Maeir, A. (2018). Long-term functional outcome of trigger finger. *Disability and Rehabilitation, 40*(1), 90–95. https://doi.org/10.1080/0963828 8.2016.1243161

Langer, D., Maeir, A., Michailevich, M., Applebaum Y., & Luria, S. (2016). Using the international classification of functioning to examine the impact of trigger finger. *Disability and Rehabilitation, 38*(26), 2530–2537. https://doi.org/10.3109/09638288.2015.1137980

Langer, D., Maeir, A., Michailevich, M., & Luria, S. (2017). Evaluating hand function in clients with trigger finger. *Occupational Therapy International, 2017*, Article 9539206. https://doi.org/10.1155/2017/9539206

Lee, M. P., Biafora, S. J., & Zelouf, D. S. (2011). Management of hand and wrist tendinopathies. In T. M. Shireven, A. L. Osterman, J. M. Fedorczyk, & P. C. Amadio (Eds.), *Rehabilitation of the hand and upper extremity* (6th ed., pp. 569–588). Mosby.

Lu, S.-C., Kuo, L.-C., Hsu, H.-Y., Jou, I.-M., Sun, Y.-N., & Su, F.-C. (2015). Finger movement function after ultrasound-guided percutaneous pulley release for trigger finger: Effects of postoperative rehabilitation. *Archives of Physical Medicine & Rehabilitation, 96*(1), 91–97. https://doi.org/10.1016/j.apmr.2014.09.001

Lunsford, D., Valdes, K., & Hengy, S. (2019). Conservative management of trigger finger: A systematic review. *Journal of Hand Therapy, 32*(2), 212–221. https://doi.org/10.1016/j.jht.2017.10.016

Marrel, M., Jörn, G. U., Marks, M., Herren, D. B., & Goldhahn, J. (2016). Isoforce: A new outrigger system for static progressive orthotic interventions of the proximal interphalangeal joint with constant force transmission—Results of a biomechanical study. *Journal of Hand Therapy, 29*(4), 451–458. https://doi.org/10.1016/j.jht.2016.05.002

Mary Pack Arthritis Program. (2015). *Best practice recommendations for management of flexor tenosynovitis of the RA hand*. Vancouver Coastal Health.

O'Toole, M. T. (Ed.). (2017). *Mosby's dictionary of medicine, nursing & health professions* (10th ed.). Elsevier.

Peter, W. F. H., Steultjens, M. P., Mesman, T., Dekker, J., & Hoeksma, A. F. (2009). Interobserver reliability of the Amsterdam Severity Scale in Stenosing Tenosynovitis (ASSiST). *Journal of Hand Therapy, 22*(4), 355–359. https://doi.org/10.1016/j.jht.2009.06.004

Porter, R. S. (Ed.). (2018). *The Merck manual of diagnosis and therapy* (20th ed.). Merck Sharp & Dohme.

Stedman's medical dictionary for the health professions and nursing (7th ed.). (2011). Wolters Kluwer.

Tarbhai, K., Hannah, S., & von Schroeder, H. P. (2012). Trigger finger treatment: A comparison of 2 splint designs. *Journal of Hand Surgery American, 37*(2), 243–249. https://doi.org/10.1016/j.jhsa.2011.10.038

Tung, W.-L., Kuo, L.-C., Lai, K.-Y., Jou, I.-M., Sun, Y.-N., & Su, F.-C. (2010). Quantitative evidence of kinematics and functional differences in different graded trigger fingers. *Clinical Biomechanics, 25*(6), 535–540. https://doi.org/10.1016/j.clinbiomech.2010.02.009

Valdes, K. (2012). A retrospective review to determine the long-term efficacy of orthotic devices for trigger finger. *Journal of Hand Therapy, 25*(1), 89–96. https://doi.org/10.1016/j.jht.2011.09.005

Wong, S., & Rocker, J. D. (2018). Helping a client with carpal tunnel syndrome and trigger fingers pump gas. *OT Practice, 23*(18), 29–31.

Injuries

Amputation: Lower Extremity

Also called lower limb amputation (LLA), above knee amputation (AKA),
below knee amputation (BKA).

Description

The surgical removal of a part of the body, such as a limb or part of limb, to treat a disease, disorder, or condition (O'Toole, 2017). Eight levels are recognized: hemipelvectomy, hip disarticulation, transfemoral (above knee; AKA), knee disarticulation, transtibial (below knee; BKA), Syme's amputation (all of foot below tibia), transmetatarsal (through the metatarsal bones), ray (all bones of one toe), and toe (proximal and/or distal phalanx). Generally, the more proximal an amputation occurs, the greater the functional challenge for the person to overcome (Orr et al., 2018). The occupational therapy evaluation of a lower extremity amputee should include assessment of upper extremity range of motion and grip and pinch strength. Upper extremity weakness or injury can impact ability to ambulate with crutches or propel a wheelchair prior to receiving a prosthesis (Klarich & Brueckner, 2014).

Cause

Four major causes are peripheral vascular disease (PVD), such as caused by atherosclerosis or diabetes mellitus; trauma, due to environmental hazards; malignancy (cancer); or birth defect (Orr et al., 2018; Porter, 2018).

Evaluation/Assessment

Areas
- Activities of Daily Living/Instrumental ADL: basic ADL, independent living skills
- Education/Work: work skills, work tasks, work environment
- Play/Leisure: interests, location, frequency
- Rest/Sleep: sleep disturbance
- Social Participation: type, location, frequency, with whom
- Sensorimotor: muscle strength, range of motion, endurance, balance, posture and postural control, coordination, stump care and management, skin and wound care, edema, scar management, pain (including phantom pain), sensation
- Cognitive/Perceptual: functional cognition, body image (Note: Cognition is not affected directly unless brain injury also occurred, but functional cognition affects type and extent of intervention planning.)
- Psychosocial: depression, anxiety, self-image, self-efficacy, self-confidence, self-worth, role performance, quality of life
- Context/Environment: social support, adapted devices and equipment (orthoses, prostheses), home or work station modification, available resources, prosthesis issues (choice, use, comfort, tolerance, care, and cosmesis)
- Development (Infant, Child, Adolescent only): no information identified
- Comorbidities: diabetes, cancer, infection, fractures of other bones, brain injury

Instruments
Instruments Developed by Occupational Therapy Personnel
- No information identified

Instruments Developed by Other Professionals and Used by Occupational Therapy Personnel
- Activities-Specific Balance Confidence (ABC) Scale (Powell & Myers, 1995; see also Sakakibara et al., 2011, in References)
- Barthel Index (BI; Mahoney & Barthel, 1965)
- Beck Depression Inventory (2nd ed.; BDI-II; Beck et al., 1996)

- Body Image Questionnaire (BIQ; Bruchon-Schweitzer, 1987)
- Functional Autonomy Measurement System–Revised (SMAF; Desrosiers et al., 1995)
- Ways of Coping Questionnaire–Revised (WCQ-R; Folkman et al., 1986)

Problems/Issues

Activities of Daily Living/Instrumental ADL

- Person may experience difficulty with mobility, including bed mobility, transfers, sit to stand, moving about the house and yard, stepping up and down curbs, getting in and out of a vehicle and wheelchair.
- Person may experience loss of income due to inability to work.
- Person may experience difficulty performing independent living skills, such as driving, shopping, and child or pet care.

Education/Work

- Person may experience difficulty performing specific work tasks, such as lifting or carrying.
- Person may experience difficulty negotiating around work environment.
- Person may have difficulty getting to work setting if transportation is required.

Play/Leisure

- Person may have difficulty engaging in or be unable to engage in favorite leisure occupations.

Rest/Sleep

- Person may experience sleep disturbance due to pain.

Social Participation

- Person may be unable to participate in some social activities.
- Person may restrict participation in social activities.

Sensorimotor

- Person may experience reduced joint range of motion.
- Person may have reduced muscle strength.
- Person may experience difficulty with standing balance and postural control.
- Person may experience difficulty with positioning body.
- Person may experience increased fatigue.
- Person may need residual-limb shaping.
- Person may experience pain including phantom limb pain.

Cognitive/Perceptual

- Person may experience changes in cognitive function due to medications (to manage pain, or treat cancer).
- Person usually experiences a change in body image.

Psychosocial

- Person may experience depression due to loss of limb.
- Person may express fear and anxiety about ability to deal with the future.
- Person may express decreased sense of self-esteem, self-confidence, self-efficacy, self-worth.
- Person may experience changes in role performance.
- Person may face discrimination and stereotyping as disabled.

Context/Environment

- Person and significant others may lack information about care and management of stump.
- Person may lack information about selection, availability, and use of adapted devices.
- Person may lack information about selection, use, and care of prosthetic devices.
- Person may lack knowledge of support groups and other community and internet resources.
- Person may need training in use of walking aids.

Intervention/Treatment

Models and programs developed by occupational therapy personnel: No information identified. Models and programs developed by other professionals but used by occupational therapy personnel include commercial games (Imam et al., 2018), preprosthetic ADL program (De-Rosende Celeiro et al., 2017), preprosthetic care (Klarich & Brueckner, 2014), and Wii Fit (Imam et al., 2017). Team members include physicians, orthopedic surgeons, prosthetists and orthotists, psychologists, physical therapy personnel, vocational rehabilitation specialists, social workers, and occupational therapy personnel. Goals are to facilitate independence in self-care activities and use of adaptations and technology (De-Rosende Celeiro et al., 2017).

Activities of Daily Living/Instrumental ADL

- Provide training and practice in transfers: bed, chair, toilet, tub and shower, wheelchair, and vehicle (car, truck, bus, train).
- Provide practice in dressing, toileting, bathing/showering, grooming.
- Provide practice in moving safely about environments, including home, yard, stairs, uneven ground, using walking aids and prosthesis.
- Consider whether medication management may be needed to manage concurrent medical problems (diabetes, cancer, pain).
- Consider whether driving retraining will be needed.
- Consider whether caregiving counseling will be needed.
- Provide information and practice in stump care and scar management.
- Assist in shaping and shrinking stump with team members.
- Provide information on prevention or delay of skin breakdown (Porter, 2018).
  - ▶ Be aware of pressure-sensitive areas (see chart in Porter, 2018, pp. 3202–3203).
  - ▶ Have interface that fits well.
  - ▶ Maintain stable body weight.
  - ▶ Eat healthy diet and drink water.
  - ▶ Monitor and control blood sugar if diabetic.
  - ▶ Avoid changes in body alignment, such wearing different shoes.
- Provide practice in putting on and taking off prosthesis.

Education/Work

- Provide access to information about employment rights of disabled persons (laws, policies, and regulations).

Play/Leisure

- Assist person to engage in favorite leisure occupations with modifications if needed.
- Assist person to explore new or novel leisure occupations, especially if some previously enjoyed leisure occupations must be discontinued or curtailed.

Rest/Sleep

- Discuss with client better positioning for sleep.

Social Participation

- Encourage client to participate in social activities with modifications, such as shorter outings to reduce fatigue, making sure friends understand limitations.

Sensorimotor

- Provide muscle strengthening for remaining musculature in lower extremity and increased strengthening of upper extremities to assist in mobility.
- Provide exercises to maintain or increase joint range of motion.
- Increase endurance and general conditioning (e.g., walking with a prosthesis requires more energy than walking on two legs).
- Provide practice in balance and postural control.

- Provide education in energy conservation in daily activities.
- Provide stump desensitization.

Cognitive/Perceptual

- Discuss with client issues related to body image, and make recommendations as needed.

Psychosocial

- Assist client to develop coping skills, such as self-control, seeking social support, problem solving, learning new things, and positive reappraisal (Couture et al., 2012).

Context/Environment

- Provide safety education in fall prevention.
- Provide training in care and maintenance of adapted equipment and prosthesis.
- Provide information on home modification to increase accessibility.
- Assist client in deciding which foot prostheses to select (solid ankle, single axis, multiple axis, stored-energy [dynamic response], and/or sport-specific).
- Assist team members to ensure prosthesis fits properly and provides maximum benefit to client in performing daily activities.
- Assist client to become an advocate on behalf of self and others (Frederiks & Visagie, 2013).

Precautions/Safety Considerations

Person is at increased risk for falls. Person is at increased risk for injury from architectural barriers. Person needs to maintain core strength and general conditioning (Klarich & Brueckner, 2014).

Prognosis and Outcome

Variable depending on factors such as management of diabetes, cancer treatment, or reduction of risk factors that contributed to trauma incidence. Spiliotopoulou and Atwal (2012) state the gaps and limited published evidence of occupational therapy with lower limb amputations.

REFERENCES

Couture, M., Desrosiers, J., & Caron, C. D. (2012). Coping with a lower limb amputation due to vascular disease in the hospital, rehabilitation, and home setting. *International Scholarly Research Network, 2012*, Article 179878. https://doi.org/10.5402/2012/179878

De-Rosende Celeiro, I., Simón Sanjuán, L., & Santos-del-Riego, S. (2017). Activities of daily living in people with lower limb amputation: Outcomes of an intervention to reduce dependence in pre-prosthetic phase. *Disability and Rehabilitation, 39*(18), 1799–1806. https://doi.org/10.1080/09638288.2016.1211757

Frederiks, J. P., & Visagie, S. (2013). The rehabilitation programme and functional outcomes of persons with lower limb amputations at a primary level rehabilitation centre. *South African Journal of Occupational Therapy, 43*(3), 18–27.

Imam, B., Miller, W. C., Finlayson, H., Eng, J. J., & Jarus, T. (2017). A randomized controlled trial to evaluate the feasibility of the Wii Fit for improving walking in older adults with lower limb amputation. *Clinical Rehabilitation, 31*(1), 82–92. https://doi.org/10.1177/0269215515623601

Imam, B., Miller, W. C., Finlayson, H., Eng, J. J., & Jarus, T. (2018). A clinical survey about commercial games in lower limb prosthetic rehabilitation. *Prosthetics and Orthotics International, 42*(3), 311–317. https://doi.org/10.1177/0309364617740238

Klarich, J., & Brueckner, I. (2014). Amputee rehabilitation and preprosthetic care. *Physical Medicine and Rehabilitation Clinics of North America, 25*(1), 75–91. https://doi.org/10.1016/j.pmr.2013.09.005

Orr, A. E., Glover, J. S., & Cook, C. L. (2018). Amputations and prosthetics: Section 3: Lower limb amputations. In H. M. Pendleton & W. Schultz-Krohn (Eds.), *Pedretti's occupational therapy* (8th ed., pp. 1107–1116). Elsevier.

O'Toole, M. T. (Ed.). (2017). *Mosby's dictionary of medicine, nursing & health professions* (10th ed.). Elsevier.

Porter, R. S. (Ed.). (2018). Limb prosthetics. *The Merck manual of diagnosis and therapy* (20th ed., pp. 3197–3205). Merck Sharp & Dohme.

Sakakibara, B. M., Miller, W. C., & Backman, C. L. (2011). Rasch analyses of the Activities-specific Balance Confidence Scale with individuals 50 years and older with lower-limb amputations. *Archives of Physical Medicine and Rehabilitation, 92*(8), 1257–1263. https://doi.org/10.1016/j.apmr.2011.03.013

Spiliotopoulou, G., & Atwal, A. (2012). Is occupational therapy practice for older adults with lower limb amputations evidence-based? A systematic review. *Prosthetics and Orthotics International, 36*(1), 7–14. https://doi.org/10.1177/0309364611428662

Amputation: Upper Extremity

See also Amputation: Lower Extremity.

Description

The surgical removal of a part of the body, such as a limb or part of limb, to treat a disease, disorder, or condition (O'Toole, 2017). Nine levels of amputation are recognized: interscapular thoracic, shoulder disarticulation, transhumeral (short), transhumeral (long), elbow disarticulation, transradial (short), transradial (long), wrist disarticulation, and transmetacarpal (Orr et al., 2018). Disarticulations are amputations occurring through or at the level of a specific joint (shoulder, elbow, or wrist). The other amputations cut through (trans) sections of bone. This chapter focuses on adults with upper extremity amputation. One article on children with congenital amputation was identified (Zuniga et al., 2018).

Cause

Diseases involving compromised blood circulation, infections, peripheral vascular disease, tumors, traumatic injuries, or birth defects (O'Toole, 2017; Porter, 2018).

Evaluation/Assessment

Areas

- Activities of Daily Living/Instrumental ADL: basic ADLs (eating, dressing, grooming, toileting, brushing teeth, medications); independent living (meal preparation, shopping, housekeeping, laundry, child care, pet care, financial management, driving, transportation)
- Education/Work: work skills and work tasks
- Play/Leisure: type, location, frequency
- Rest/Sleep: sleep disturbances
- Social Participation: type, location, frequency, with whom
- Sensorimotor: muscle strength, range of motion, endurance, balance, posture and postural control, dexterity, accuracy, stump care and management, skin and wound care, edema, scar management, pain (including phantom pain), sensation
- Cognitive/Perceptual: functional cognition, body image (Note: Cognition is not affected directly unless brain injury also occurred, but functional cognition affects type and extent of intervention planning.)
- Psychosocial: depression, anxiety, self-image, self-efficacy, self-confidence, self-worth, role performance, quality of life
- Context/Environment: social support, adapted devices and equipment (orthoses, prostheses), home or work station modification, available resources, prosthesis issues (choice, use, comfort, tolerance, care, and cosmesis)

- Development (Infant, Child, Adolescent only): no information identified
- Comorbidities: diabetes, cancer, infection, fractures of other bones, brain injury

Instruments
Instruments Developed by Occupational Therapy Personnel
- Assessment of Capacity of Myoelectric Control (ACMC; Hermansson et al., 2005)
- Assessment of Motor and Process Skills (8th ed.; AMPS-8; Fisher & Bray Jones, 2016)
- Box and Block Test (BBT; Mathiowetz et al., 1985)
- ICF-Based Questionnaire on Activities, Participation and Environmental Factors (Frederiks & Visagie, 2013, in References)
- Klein-Bell ADL Scale (Klein-Bell, KB, KB-ADL; Klein & Bell, 1982)
- Kohlman Evaluation of Living Skills (4th ed.; KELS-4; Kohlman-Thomson & Robnett, 2016)
- Nine Hole Peg Test (NHPT; Mathiowetz et al., 1985)
- Performance and Satisfaction in Activities of Daily Living (PS-ADL; Archenholtz & Dellhag, 2008)

Instruments Developed by Other Professionals and Used by Occupational Therapy Personnel
- Activities-Specific Balance Confidence (ABC) Scale (Powell & Myers, 1995)
- Barthel Index (BI; Mahoney & Barthel, 1965)
- Functional Independence Measure (FIM; Uniform Data System for Medical Rehabilitation, 1997)
- Grip strength (dynamometry; JAMAR Hydraulic, Lafayette Instrument; Wang et al., 2018)
- Instrumental Activities of Daily Living Scale (IADL; Lawton & Brody, 1969)
- Jebsen-Taylor Hand Function Test (JTHFT; Jebsen et al., 1969)
- Manual Muscle Test (MMT; Kaskutas, 2018)
- Orthotics and Prosthetics User Survey (OPUS; Heinemann et al., 2003)
- Purdue Pegboard Test (PPT; Tiffin, 1948)
- QuickDASH (Kennedy et al., 2011)
- Short-Form 36 Health Survey (SF-36; Ware et al., 1993)
- Visual analogue scale (pain scale: scored 0 = *no pain*, 10 = *worst pain ever*)
- Ways of Coping Questionnaire–Revised (WCQ-R; Folkman et al., 1986)

Problems/Issues
Activities of Daily Living/Instrumental ADL
- Person usually experiences difficulty performing basic ADLs, especially tasks involving the dominant hand or typically performed with two hands (e.g., cutting meat, peeling vegetables, trimming nails, fastening buttons, serving food, tying trash bag ties, cutting toenails, opening packages, washing glasses, and carrying bulky items; Whelan et al., 2014).
- Person may experience difficulty performing independent living skills.

Education/Work
- Person may experience difficulty performing specific work tasks.
- Person may have difficulty getting to work setting if transportation is required.

Play/Leisure
- Person may be unable to engage in favorite leisure occupations.

Rest/Sleep
- Person may experience sleep disturbance.

Social Participation
- Person may resist or restrict participation in social activities.

Sensorimotor
- Person usually experiences loss of muscle strength depending on level of amputation.

- Person usually experiences decreased or loss of range of motion depending on level of amputation.
- Person may experience decreased endurance and activity tolerance.
- Person may experience changes in postural control, especially if amputation occurred at shoulder level.
- Person always experiences loss of tactile (light and deep pressure) and proprioception sensation below the level of the amputation (sensation of forearm and upper arm is less acute than in hand and finger pads).
- Person may experience real pain and phantom pain (pain experience in the area of the amputation).
- Person may experience phantom sensation (as though the amputated limb is still there).

Cognitive/Perceptual
- Person may experience changes in cognitive function due to medications (to manage pain, or treat cancer).
- Person usually experiences a change in body image.

Psychosocial
- Person may experience depression due to loss of limb.
- Person may express fear and anxiety about ability to deal with the future.
- Person may express decreased sense of self esteem, self-confidence, self-efficacy, self-worth.
- Person may experience changes in role performance.

Context/Environment
- Person and significant others may lack information about care and management of stump.
- Person may lack information about selection, availability, and use of adapted devices.
- Person may lack information about selection, use, and care of prosthetic devices.
- Person may lack knowledge of support groups and other community and internet resources.

Intervention/Treatment

Models and programs developed by occupational therapy personnel include gardening (Cook & Scoble, 2019), hand rehabilitation (Whelan et al., 2014), managing daily activities (Fletchall & Atkins, 2011), prosthesis training (Gulick, 2016; Johnson & Mansfield, 2014), and sample goals and interventions (Weimer & Chung, 2016). Models and programs developed by other professionals but used by occupational therapy personnel include finger rehabilitation (Stapanian et al., 2010), mirror therapy (Finn et al., 2017), powered shoulder prosthesis (Resnik et al., 2014), preprosthetic care and treatment (Klarich & Brueckner, 2014; Weimer & Chung, 2016), prosthetic training (Johnson & Mansfield, 2014; Weimer & Chung, 2016), and SmartHand tactile display (Antfolk, Balkenius, Lundborg, et al., 2010; Antfolk, Balkenius, Rosén, et al., 2010; Antfolk et al., 2012; Antfolk et al., 2013; Björkman et al., 2016; Wijk et al., 2019). Team members include physicians, orthopedic surgeons, prosthetists and orthotists, psychologists, physical therapy personnel, vocational rehabilitation specialists, social workers, and occupational therapy personnel. Goal is to provide the client with adaptive techniques and strategies that enable the person to regain functional independence, the ability to participate in all desired life tasks, to use a prosthetic device if prescribed, and to optimize quality of life (Gulick, 2016; Weimer & Chung, 2016).

Activities of Daily Living/Instrumental ADL
- Provide instruction and training on compensatory techniques, including use of other body parts (feet, chin, knees, and teeth), use of a prosthesis, adapted devices or environment modifications to perform basic ADL tasks.
- Provide information on prevention or delay of skin breakdown (Porter, 2018).
  - ▶ Be aware of pressure-sensitive areas (see chart in Porter, 2018, pp. 3202–3203).
  - ▶ Have interface that fits well.

- ► Maintain stable body weight.
- ► Eat healthy diet and drink water.
- ► Monitor and control blood sugar if diabetic.
- Discuss different ways to manage independent living tasks, including use of adapted device, use of a prosthesis, environment modifications, changes in role performance tasks, and hiring others to perform certain tasks.
- Provide instruction in using one-handed techniques as well as bilateral techniques with residual part of limb or when a prosthesis is worn.

Education/Work
- Explore with client what adaptations or modifications are needed to facilitate work performance (paid and unpaid).
- Assist client to explore issues that may facilitate or hinder return to work or to plan for retirement.

Play/Leisure
- Explore with client compensatory strategies to allow client to engage in favorite leisure occupations.
- Explore with client new leisure occupations that client can perform.

Rest/Sleep
- See Sleep–Wake Disorders in Section 13: Lifestyle Conditions.

Social Participation
- Encourage client to participate in social activities.

Sensorimotor
- Provide therapeutic exercises to maintain or regain muscle strength in remaining muscle groups and encourage client to use residual limb in daily activities for bilateral tasks as tolerated.
- Provide therapeutic activities to maintain joint range of motion in remaining joints to avoid contractures, using active range of motion first, then passive range of motion (moist heat pack can be used to increase tissue elasticity prior to stretching exercises).
- Assist client to increase endurance and activity tolerance; instruction in energy conservation and motion economy may be useful.
- Assist in team management instruction for wound management, such as daily washing and drying limb and stump with a mild soap, cleaning and debridement as needed, visual inspection to monitor for skin breakdown, and massage creams for scar management.
- Provide information and practice in managing stump, including wound healing, stump shrinkage, and stump wrapping.
- Assist in instructing client in learning to wrap by demonstrating use of figure-eight wrapping or use of compression aid (always wrap proximal to distal; apply bandage in a smooth, even fashion; remove bandage 2–3 times per day to inspect for skin breakdown; apply clean bandage every other day; hand wash bandages with soap and lie flat to dry).
- Instruct client in edema and scar management, such as self-massage, proper position, and avoiding prolonged dependent positioning, using elastic bandaging or rigid dressing, and wrapping using figure eights.
- Assist in instructing client to use prosthesis to perform ADL, work, and leisure tasks.
- Assist in desensitizing residual limb using textures such as rice, clay, and felt, with the client pushing the limb into texture in 5-second intervals; other texture may include terrycloth, silk, or cotton; use massage, vibration, tapping, and rubbing.

Cognitive/Perceptual
- Assist client to compensate for lack of tactile sense, especially in protecting from injury (visual inspection is usually needed as a compensatory strategy).
- Discuss with client effect amputation has on body and self-image.

Psychosocial
- Discuss with client feelings of depression, anxiety, and fear about being an amputee and functioning at home, at work, and in the community.
- Prioritize goals based on client's interests and goals.
- Assist client to regain sense of self-efficacy, self-confidence, self-worth.
- Provide positive feedback when tasks or goals are accomplished.

Context/Environment (Widehammar et al., 2018)
- Provide information, training, and care for adapted devices and prosthetic device if used.
- Examples of useful adapted devices include universal cuff, loops added to socks and towels, swivel spoons, oversized grips, long-handled sponges, reachers or grabbers, elastic shoelaces, suction brush sponge, rocker knife, electric can opener.
- Assist client in determining what type of prosthesis to get: body-powered, externally powered, myoelectric, cosmetic, or hybrid and what hand prostheses to include (pincher/precision grip, tripod/palmar grip, lateral/key pinch, hook, spherical, sport-specific, or myoelectric).
- If a prosthesis is used, client should be trained to put the prosthesis on and take it off and be able to wear the prosthesis comfortably for 4–6 hours. Client should know the parts of the prosthesis by name: socket, harness, cable, terminal device, wrist unit, and sock. Useful objects for training use of prosthesis include plastic cups, blocks, sponges, weights, bolts, glass jars, and ping pong balls (Weimer & Chung, 2016).
- Provide information on support groups, community and internet resources.

Precautions/Safety Considerations
Stump shrinkage occurs over time, affecting effective use of prosthesis. Additional stockings may be needed to fill space between stump and prosthesis or prosthesis may need to be remodeled or replaced. Avoid wrapping limb in a circular pattern. Prosthesis should not be immersed in water.

Prognosis and Outcome
Person can return to productive and satisfying life at home, at work, and within community. Knowledge and use of adapted devices and environment modifications often improve occupational performance and quality of life.

REFERENCES
Antfolk, C., Balkenius, C., Lundborg, G., Rosén, B., & Sebelius, F. (2010). Design and technical construction of a tactile display for sensory feedback in a hand prosthesis system. *Biomedical Engineering Online*, 9, Article 50. https://doi.org/10.1186/1475-925X-9-50

Antfolk, C., Balkenius, C., Rosén, B., Lundborg, G., & Sebelius, F. (2010). SmartHand tactile display: A new concept for providing sensory feedback in hand prostheses. *Journal of Plastic Surgery and Hand Surgery*, 44(1), 50–53. https://doi.org/10.3109/02844310903259090

Antfolk, C., Björkman, A., Frank, S. O., Sebelius, F., Lundborg, G., & Rosén, B. (2012). Sensory feedback from a prosthetic hand based on air-mediated pressure from the hand to the forearm skin. *Journal of Rehabilitation Medicine*, 44(8), 702–707. https://doi.org/10.2340/16501977-1001

Antfolk, C., Cipriani, C., Carrozza, M. C., Balkenius, C., Björkman, A., Lundborg, G., Rosén, B., & Sebelius, F. (2013). Transfer of tactile input from an artificial hand to the forearm: Experiments in amputees and able-bodied volunteers. *Disability and Rehabilitation: Assistive Technology*, 8(3), 249–254. https://doi.org/10.3109/17483107.2012.713435

Björkman, A., Wijk, U., Antfolk, C., Björkman-Burtscher, I., & Rosén, B. (2016). Sensory qualities of the phantom hand map in the residual forearm of amputees. *Journal of Rehabilitation Medicine*, 48(4), 365–370. https://doi.org/10.2340/16501977-2074

Cook, S., & Scoble, J. (2019). Occupation as rehabilitation. *OT News*, 27(1), 42–43.

Finn, S. B., Perry, B. N., Clasing, J. E., Walters, L. S., Jarzombek, S. L., Curran, S., Rouhanian, M., Keszler, M. S., Hussey-Andersen, L. K., Weeks, S. R., Pasquina, P. F., & Tsao, J. W. (2017). A randomized, controlled trial of mirror therapy for upper extremity phantom limb pain in male amputees. *Frontiers in Neurology, 8.* Article 267. https://doi.org/10.3389/fneur.2017.00267

Fletchall, S., & Atkins, D. J. (2011). Managing daily activities in adults with upper-extremity amputations. In C. H. Christiansen & K. M. Matuska (Eds.), *Ways of living* (4th ed., pp. 315–347). AOTA Press.

Frederiks, J. P., & Visagie, S. (2013). The rehabilitation programme and functional outcomes of persons with lower limb amputations at a primary level rehabilitation centre. *South African Journal of Occupational Therapy, 43*(3), 18–27.

Gulick, K. L. (2016). *Fact Sheet: The occupational therapy role in rehabilitation for the person with an upper-limb amputation.* American Occupational Therapy Association.

Johnson, S. S., & Mansfield, E. (2014). Prosthetic training: Upper limb. *Physical Medicine and Rehabilitation Clinics of North America, 25*(1), 133–151. https://doi.org/10.1016/j.pmr.2013.09.012

Klarich, J., & Brueckner, I. (2014). Amputee rehabilitation and preprosthetic care. *Physical Medicine and Rehabilitation Clinics of North America, 25*(1), 75–91. https://doi.org/10.1016/j.pmr.2013.09.005

Orr, A. E., Glover, J. S., & Cook, C. L. (2018). Amputations and prosthetics: Sections 1 & 2. In H. M. Pendleton & W. Schultz-Krohn (Eds.), *Pedretti's occupational therapy* (8th ed., pp. 1083–1107). Elsevier.

O'Toole, M. T. (Ed.). (2017). *Mosby's dictionary of medicine, nursing & health professions* (10th ed.). Elsevier.

Porter, R. S. (Ed.). (2018). Limb prosthetics. In *The Merck manual of diagnosis and therapy* (20th ed., pp. 3197–3205). Merck Sharp & Dohme.

Resnik, L., Klinger, S. L., Korp, K., & Walters, L. S. (2014). Training protocol for powered shoulder prosthesis. *Journal of Rehabilitation Research and Development, 51*(8), vii–xvi. https://doi.org/10.1682/JRRD.2014.07.0162

Stapanian, M. A., Stapanian, A. M. P., & Staley, K. E. (2010). Case report: Rehabilitation for bilateral amputation of fingers. *American Journal of Occupational Therapy, 64*(6), 923–928. https://doi.org/10.5014/ajot.2010.09153

Weimer, H., & Chung, A. (2016). *Clinical review: Amputation, upper extremity, in adults: Occupational therapy.* EBSCO Information Services, CINAHL Information Systems.

Whelan, L., Flinn, S., & Wagner, N. (2014). Individualizing goals for users of externally powered partial hand prostheses. *Journal of Rehabilitation Research and Development, 51*(6), 885–894. https://doi.org/10.1682/JRRD.2013.08.0181

Widehammar, C., Pettersson, I., Janeslätt, G., & Hermansson, L. (2018). The influence of environment: Experiences of users of myoelectric arm prosthesis—A qualitative study. *Prosthetics and Orthotics International, 42*(1), 28–36. https://doi.org/10.1177/0309364617704801

Wijk, U., Svensson, P., Antfolk, C., Carlsson, I. K., Björkman, A., & Rosén, B. (2019). Touch on predefined areas on the forearm can be associated with specific fingers: Towards a new principle for sensory feedback in hand prostheses. *Journal of Rehabilitation Medicine, 51*(3), 209–216. https://doi.org/10.2340/16501977-2518

Zuniga, J. M., Dimitrios, K., Peck, J. L., Srivastava, R., Pierce, J. E., Dudley, D. R., Salazar, D. A., Young, K. J., & Knarr, B. (2018). Coactivation index of children with congenital upper limb reduction deficiencies before and after using a wrist-driven 3D printed partial hand prosthesis. *Journal of NeuroEngineering and Rehabilitation, 15,* Article 48. https://doi.org/10.1186/s12984-018-0392-9

BIBLIOGRAPHY

Antfolk, C., D'Alonzo, M., Controzzi, M., Lundborg, G., Rosén, B., Sebelius, F., & Cipriani, C. (2013). Artificial redirection of sensation from prosthetic fingers to the phantom hand map on transradial amputees: Vibrotactile versus mechanotactile sensory feedback. *IEEEE Transactions on Neural Systems and Rehabilitation Engineering, 21*(1), 112–120. https://doi.org/10.1109/TNSRE.2012.2217989

Antfolk, C., D'Alonzo, M., Rosén, B., Lundborg, G., Sebelius, F., & Cipriani, C. (2013). Sensory feedback in upper limb prosthetics. *Expert Review of Medical Devices, 10*(1), 45–54. https://doi.org/10.1586/erd.12.68

Björkman, A., Weibull, A., Olsrud, J., Ehrsson, H. H., Rosén, B., & Björkman-Burtscher, I. M. (2012). Phantom digit somatotopy: A functional magnetic resonance imaging study in forearm amputees. *European Journal of Neuroscience, 36*(1), 2098–2106. https://doi.org/10.1111/j.1460-9568.2012.08099.x

Butkus, J., Dennison, C., Orr, A., & St. Laurent, M. (2014). Occupational therapy with the military upper extremity amputee: Advances and research implications. *Current Physical Medicine and Rehabilitation Reports, 2*, 255–262. https://doi.org/10.1007/s40141-014-0065-y

Cipriani, C., Antfolk, C., Controzzi, M., Lundborg, G., Rosén, B., Carrozza, M. C., & Sebelius, F. (2011). Online myoelectric control of a dexterous hand prosthesis by transradial amputees. *IEEE Transactions on Neural Systems and Rehabilitation Engineering, 19*(3), 260–270. https://doi.org/10.1109/TNSRE.2011.2108667

Mitsch, S., Walters, L. S., & Yancosek, K. (2014). Amputations and prosthetics. In M. V. Radomski & C. A. Trombly Latham (Eds.), *Occupational therapy for physical dysfunction* (7th ed., pp. 1266–1299). Wolters Kluwer.

Svensson, P., Wijk, U., Björkman, A., & Antfolk, C. (2017). A review of invasive and non-invasive sensory feedback in upper limb prostheses. *Expert Review of Medical Devices, 14*(6), 439–447. https://doi.org/10.1080/17434440.2017.1332989

Wijk, U., & Carlsson, I. (2015). Forearm amputees' views of prosthesis use and sensory feedback. *Journal of Hand Therapy, 28*(3), 269–278. https://doi.org/10.1016/j.jht.2015.01.013

Brain Injuries: Adult

Also called traumatic brain injury (TBI), acquired brain injury (ABI).

See also Brain Injuries: Child and Adolescent, Cognitive Impairment, Concussion and Post-Concussion, Executive Dysfunction, Memory Impairment.

Description

Traumatic or acquired brain injury is described as physical injury to brain tissue that temporarily or permanently impairs brain function. Injuries may be described as open or closed. Open injuries usually involve penetration of the scalp and skull and may include the meninges and underlying brain tissue. Closed injuries usually occur when the head is struck, strikes an object, or is shaken violently, causing rapid acceleration and deceleration of brain tissue. Common types include basilar skull fracture, brain contusion, concussion, diffuse axonal injury, epidural hematoma, subarachnoid hemorrhage, or subdural hematoma. Clinical manifestations vary depending on the severity and type of injury. A score on the Glasgow Coma Scale of 14–15 is classified as mild, 9–13 moderate, and 3–8 severe (Porter, 2018).

Cause

Motor vehicle accidents (MVA) and other transportation-related accidents (bicycle, all-terrain vehicles [ATVs], snowmobiles, golf carts, wheelchairs), falls (especially in the elderly), violence (including assaults and gunshot wounds to the head), or sports injuries to the head (Porter, 2018).

Evaluation/Assessment

Areas

- Activities of Daily Living/Instrumental ADL: dysphagia, dress (outdoors clothes), functional mobility, transfers, home management, shopping, meal preparation and cleanup, financial planning, driving

- Education/Work: return to work or school
- Play/Leisure: type, frequency, interests, level of satisfaction
- Rest/Sleep: sleep disturbances, sleep routine
- Social Participation: type, frequency, location, with whom
- Sensorimotor: fatigue, joint range of motion, muscle strength, bilateral integration of two sides of body, sensory impairment, headaches, dizziness, pain, joint stiffness
- Cognitive/Perceptual: level of arousal, attention and concentration, amnesia, memory and prospective memory, executive function (planning, problem solving, mental flexibility, judgment of safety)
- Psychosocial: self-awareness, self-regulation, self-efficacy, anxiety, depression, emotional lability, aggression, impulsivity, disinhibition, irritability, personality change, apathy, motivation, quality of life
- Context/Environment: social support, adapted equipment, orthotic devices, home modification
- Comorbidities: diabetes, hypertension, fractures, hydrocephalus, substance abuse

Instruments

Instruments Developed by Occupational Therapy Personnel

- ADL Profile (Activities of Daily Living Profile; Dutil et al., 2005; see also Dutil et al., 2017, in References)
- Adult Subjective Assessment of Participation (ASAP; Jarus et al., 2006)
- Allen Cognitive Level Screen (5th ed.; ACLS-5; Allen et al., 2007; see also Toneman et al., 2010, in References)
- Assessment of Military Multitasking Performance (AMMP; Radomski et al., 2013, in References)
- Assessment of Motor and Process Skills (8th ed.; AMPS-8; Fisher & Bray Jones, 2016)
- Behavioural Dysregulation Rating Scale (BDRS; McKeon et al., 2017, and McKeon et al., 2018, in References)
- Canadian Occupational Performance Measure (COPM-5; Law et al., 2014)
- Cognitive Assessment of Minnesota (CAM; Rustad et al., 1993)
- Dynamic Loewenstein Occupational Therapy Cognitive Assessment (DLOTCA; Katz et al., 2012)
- Flow State Scale for Occupational Tasks (FSSOT; Yoshida et al., 2013)
- Instrumental Activities of Daily Living Profile (IADL Profile; Bottari et al., 2009; see Bottari et al., 2010a, 2010b; and Le Dorze et al., 2014, in References)
- Reintegration to Normal Living Index (RNLI; Wood-Dauphine et al., 1988)
- Weekly Calendar Planning Activity (WCPA; Toglia, 2015; see also Ko, 2019, in References)

Instruments Developed by Other Professionals and Used by Occupational Therapy Personnel

- Abdel-Khalek Happiness Scale (AHKS; Abdel-Khalek, 2006)
- Colour Trails Test (CTT; D'Elia et al., 1996)
- Community Integration Questionnaire (CIQ; Willer et al., 1993)
- Continuous Performance Test (CPT; Rosvold et al., 1956)
- Depression Anxiety Stress Scales-21 (DASS-21; Lovibond & Lovibond, 1995)
- Disability Rating Scale (DRS; Rappaport et al., 1982; see also Conti, 2017, in References)
- Frontal Assessment Battery (FAB; Dubois et al., 2000)
- Glasgow Coma Scale (GCS; Teasdale & Jennett, 1974)
- Goal Attainment Scaling (GAS; Kiresuk & Sherman, 1968)
- Instrumental Activities of Daily Living Scale (IADL; Lawton & Brody, 1969)
- Levels of Cognitive Functioning Scale (see Rancho Levels of Cognitive Functioning; see also Conti, 2017, in References)
- Life Habits Questionnaire (LIFE-H 3.1; Noreau et al., 2002)
- Mini-Mental State Examination (MMSE; Folstein et al., 1975)
- Modified Barthel Index (MBI; Collin et al., 1988)
- Montreal Cognitive Assessment (MoCA; Nasreddine et al., 2005)

- Moss Attention Rating Scale (MARS; Whyte et al., 2003)
- National Institutes of Health Toolbox Cognition Battery (NIHTB-CB; Gershon et al., 2013; see Tulsky et al., 2017, in References)
- Neurobehavioral Cognitive Status Examination (NCSE, Cognistat; Kiernan et al., 1987)
- Patient Competency Rating Scale (PCRS; Prigatano & Fordyce, 1986; see also Sveen et al., 2015, in References)
- Primary Care Evaluation of Mental Disorders (PRIME-MD; Spitzer et al., 1994)
- Quality of Life and Health Questionnaire (QLHQ; Hadorn & Uebersax, 1995)
- Rancho Levels of Cognitive Functioning (3rd ed.; RLCF-3; Hagen, 1998)
- Rancho Los Amigos Cognitive Scale (RLAS; see Rancho Levels of Cognitive Functioning)
- Rivermead Behavioural Memory Test (3rd ed.; RBMT-3; Wilson et al., 2008)
- Rowland Universal Dementia Assessment Scale (RUDAS; Storey et al., 2004)
- Satisfaction with Life Scale (SWLS; Diener et al., 1985)
- Self-Regulation Skills Interview (SRSI; Ownsworth et al., 2000)
- Social Provisions Scale (SPS; Cutrona & Russell, 1987)
- Stroop Color and Word Test (SCWT; Golden, 1978)
- Symbols Digit Modalities Test (SDMT; Smith, 1973)
- Symptom Checlist-90-Revised (SCL-90-R; Derogatis, 1994)
- UCLA Loneliness Scale (Russell et al., 1978)
- Ways of Coping Questionnaire–Revised (WoC-R; Folkman et al., 1986)

Problems/Issues

Activities of Daily Living/Instrumental ADL

- Person may have difficulty performing basic ADLs such as eating, dressing, grooming, bathing/showering, toileting, transfers, mobility, communication.
- Person may have difficulty with independent living skills such as meal planning, preparation, and cleanup, shopping for groceries and household supplies.
- Person may have difficulty with home management and home maintenance activities (doing laundry, vacuuming, dusting, sewing on a missing button).
- Person may need assistance in transitioning from home life to independent living.
- Person may experience difficulty with financial management including budgeting, making correct change, writing a check, balancing a checkbook, accessing and using electronic banking including online banking, automatic teller/banking machine (ATM).
- Person may have difficulty driving safely or using public transportation.

Education/Work

- Person may experience discrimination or stigma in the workplace environment, including social exclusion, hiring discrimination, denial of promotion and demotion, harassment, and failure to provide reasonable accommodation.
- Person may need workplace accommodation for physical, cognitive, sensory, or psychological issues.
- Person may need individualized placement and supported employment to resume or change employment.
- Person and health-care team must determine carefully what information to disclose to employer/supervisor to reduce impact of discrimination (Stergiou-Kita et al., 2017).
- Person's degree of fatigue, difficulty thinking and concentrating, and inability to maintain previous workload or standards are barriers to return to work (Colantonio et al., 2016; Cooksley et al., 2018).

Play/Leisure

- Person may restrict or eliminate previously enjoyed leisure activities.
- Person may be unable to enjoy engagement in leisure activities due to physical, cognitive, sensory, or psychological issues.

Rest/Sleep

- Person may experience sleep disturbances (falling asleep, staying asleep).
- Person may experience difficulty maintaining sleep habits and routines due to pain or side effects of medication.

Social Participation

- Person may restrict or stop participation in social activities.
- Person may have difficulty participating in social conversation and communication.

Sensorimotor

- Person may experience fatigue, loss of energy, and low level of endurance.
- Person may have loss of joint range of motion.
- Person may have muscle weakness.
- Person may experience reduced or lost sensory discrimination such as inability to smell or taste different odors or types of foods.
- Person may experience pain, stiffness, and aching in or around joints as part of a long-term, chronic response to traumatic brain injury (TBI).
- Person may experience visual problems such as diplopia, increased sensitivity to light and glare, decreased contrast sensitivity.
- Person may experience difficulty screening out background noise from foreground speech or sounds.

Cognitive/Perceptual

- Person may have difficulty maintaining a level of arousal and alertness necessary to participate in daily activities or interact with family and caregivers on a minimum level of cooperation.
- Person may have difficulty maintaining attention and concentration long enough to accomplish daily routines, following simple instructions, or participate in social activities.
- Person may have difficulty with short-term memory.
- Person may have difficulty deciding and selecting appropriate outdoors clothing for temperature and weather conditions (cold, hot, snow, rain, wind).
- Person may be unable to remember information from one day to the next.
- Person may have difficulty with prospective memory.
- Person may have difficulty with executive functions, including planning ahead, problem solving, making decisions, judgment of safety, mental flexibility.

Psychosocial

- Person may have difficulty with emotional regulation.
- Person may experience emotional lability.
- Person may be impulsive and engage in behavior that constitutes danger to self or others.
- Person may be easily irritated.
- Person may express anger that is not appropriate for the situation.
- Person may become aggressive.
- Person may express and display symptoms of anxiety. Family members and caregivers may also express and display symptoms of anxiety.
- Person may become depressed.

Context/Environment

- Person may have limited social support.
- Person may need assistive or orthotic devices.
- Person may need home accommodation.
- Person, family, caregivers, and employers may need information about brain injury and its effects on daily activities during both the acute and chronic phase.
- Person may need referral to community resources.
- Public beliefs about brain injury may shape policy that is not consistent with known facts about TBI in the acute or chronic phase.

Intervention/Treatment

Models and programs developed by occupational therapy personnel include actual reality (Goverover & DeLuca, 2015), attention training (Yoshida et al., 2014), clinical reasoning (Bottari et al., 2014), community-based interventional programs for family caregivers (Suzuki & Tanemura, 2011), community-based program (White et al., 2018), financial management activity process (Engel et al., 2019), goal setting (Hunt, Le Dorze, Polatajko, et al., 2015; Hunt, Le Dorze, Trentham, et al., 2015), multicontextual approach (Toglia et al., 2011; Toglia et al., 2010), occupation-based intervention (Miyahara et al., 2018), occupation-based strategy training (Dawson et al., 2013), and occupational performance coaching (Lum et al., 2018). Models and programs by other professionals but used by occupational therapy personnel include the citizen accompaniment project for community integration (Therriault et al., 2016), cognitive behavior therapy (Arundine et al., 2012), leisure education program (Carbonneau et al., 2011), Life Skills Group (Foxhall & Gurr, 2014), neurofunctional approach (Giles, 2018), practice guidelines–OT (Wheeler & Acord-Vira, 2016), practice guidelines–vocational (Stergiou-Kita et al., 2012), Rehabilitation Toolkit (Weightman et al., 2014), and self-generation learning and memory (Goverover et al., 2010). Team members include physicians, nurses and nursing practitioners, psychologists, physical therapists, and occupational therapy practitioners. Intervention is usually multidisciplinary and interdisciplinary, focused on client's goals, is activity based, in relevant environmental context, and designed to improve occupational performance. When setting goals, acknowledge and affirm the client's goals. Use open-ended questioning about specific tasks and reflective listening to identify problems that can become goals (Hunt, Le Dorze, Polatajko, et al., 2015). Use of compensatory approaches is important, especially in the area of cognitive functioning.

Activities of Daily Living/Instrumental ADL
- Provide opportunity to practice deciding what garments and footwear would be necessary for different types of weather conditions and practice in putting clothing items on and removing them.
- Provide opportunity to practice meal planning, meal preparation, and cleanup.
- Provide opportunity to practice home management skills (doing laundry, vacuuming, dusting, washing and putting dishes and eating utensils away).
- Provide practice in making lists of grocery items and shopping online or in a grocery store.
- Provide practice in financial management including budgeting, writing checks, and counting change.
- Provide practice in driving using virtual reality programs to simulate driving performance.
- Consider if practice is needed to use public transportation safely and effectively.

Education/Work
- Consider modification of number of work hours (part-time, fewer days), work shift (day, evening, night), location of work (on-site versus home), working conditions (office, warehouse, outside), physical demands (sitting, standing, climbing), interaction with others (minimum, some, a lot).
- Consider if changing or modifying work tasks or assignments would permit person to work more successfully.
- Consider whether changing to a different vocation would better suit the person's abilities.
- Consider whether job coaching or shadowing would assist person to better perform job duties.

Play/Leisure
- Encourage client to renew interest in previous leisure activities, suggesting modifications to permit engagement using current level of ability.
- Explore with client new leisure activities.

Rest/Sleep
- Review sleep protocol including sleep habits including sleep preparation, amount of sleep usually obtained or needed, during which hours of day.

- Review and modify sleeping environment (sheets, mattress, blankets, pillows, external room noises, darkness of room, schedule).
- Review effect of medications on sleep and make recommendations to modify to extent possible in relation to positive value of medication to health conditions.

Social Participation

- Encourage person to participate in social activities by grading participation in terms of amount of time activity requires, number of people involved, family versus strangers, location nearby versus distance away from home base, and amount of passive versus active participation required.
- Provide opportunity to practice socializing (social training) in various environments consistent with the client's lifestyle.

Sensorimotor

- Provide exercise program to improve motor function including joint range of motion, muscle strengthening, and endurance. Integrate exercise into daily activities as much as possible.
- Qigong may be useful to increase physical activity, strengthening, and balance.
- Provide instruction in energy conservation: pacing, taking breaks, division of labor with others, organizing activities according to energy level during the day.
- Provide pain management program.
- Provide practice in visually scanning to improve search skills using digits, letters, symbols, pictures of objects, real objects, computer tests, virtual reality.

Cognitive/Perceptual

- Multimodal stimulation (vision, auditory, tactile, smell, movement) may increase arousal and alertness.
- Consider use of pictures or auditory reminders to facilitate following instructions for daily activities such as brushing teeth or grooming tasks.
- Auditory reminders using a familiar voice may be useful to support attention and encourage performance.
- Use paper calendars or smartphone calendars and auditory reminders to help person keep track of appointments or upcoming events.
- Increase complexity of task, but not intensity of sensory stimulation (not brighter light and not louder sound) as ability level increases.
- Suggest compensatory strategies for memory such as pacing, chunking, and self-talk.
- Provide opportunity to practice problem solving and decision making.
- Provide practice in using judgment of safety and awareness of danger.
- Provide practice in visual perception tasks such as figure–ground, contrast sensitivity, moving from far to near and vice versa, reading instructions or directions, looking for a distant target (building, road sign), visual field awareness.

Psychosocial

- Provide instruction in stress management techniques: relaxation training, deep breathing, yoga.
- Provide social training to recognize and identify ability to name basic emotions, interpret comments, and determine whether a person is lying or being sarcastic.
- Provide opportunity to engage in activities to increase self-esteem and self-confidence.
- Provide social skills training to manage emotional regulation including different social behaviors and practice in decoding emotions.
- Peer mentoring programs with other TBI clients can be useful to improve emotional awareness, decrease avoidance behavior, decrease chaos in the home environment, deal with somatic symptoms, and decrease substance abuse.

Context/Environment

- Consider using environmental cues to encourage behavior: opening shades and turning on lights in morning to signal time to get out of bed, smell of coffee to encourage eating breakfast, running water in shower to encourage bathing/showering, lay out clothes for dressing.
- Provide opportunity to practice cognitive and psychosocial skills in community and other relevant environments.
- Assist family and caregivers to understand rationale for performing certain caregiving tasks and provide practice in actually performing the tasks important or essential to managing individual client, especially in the home environment.
- Provide family, friends, colleagues, coworkers, and caregivers with information about managing a person with a traumatic brain injury as a chronic condition.
- Provide family with information about community resources.
- Consider use of adaptive devices.
- Consider recommending home modifications such as grab bars or porch railing.
- Consider whether visual aids may be needed, such as magnifying glasses, prisms, enlarged font size on computer screen.
- Provide practice for client to physically be in and participate in the community.
- Use of landmark-based directions (concrete) rather than right–left or north–south (abstract) directions may maximize performance when walking in the community.

Precautions/Safety Considerations

Monitor for seizures, especially in sitting and standing positions. Do not use intervention activities that are nonpurposeful such as cones, pegs, shoulder arc equipment, or arm bikes unless the items such as cones or pegs can be constructed into a purposeful activity, such as a game of tic-tac-toe.

Prognosis and Outcome

Outcome varies with severity of injury. Most progress is seen within 6 months, and improvement can occur over several years (Porter, 2018). Return to work is possible but is dependent on services such as job development, job coaching, case management, and job retention (Grigorovich et al., 2017).

REFERENCES

Arundine, A., Bradbury, C. L., Dupuis, K., Dawson, D. R., Ruttan, L. A., & Green, R. E. A. (2012). Cognitive behavior therapy after acquired brain injury: Maintenance of therapeutic benefits at 6 months posttreatment. *Journal of Head Trauma Rehabilitation, 27*(2), 104–112. https://doi.org/10.1097/HTR.0b013e3182125591

Bottari, C., Dassa, C., Rainville, C., & Dutil, É. (2010a). A generalizability study of the Instrumental Activities of Daily Living Profile. *Archives of Physical Medicine and Rehabilitation, 91*(5), 734–742. https://doi.org/10.1016/j.apmr.2009.12.023

Bottari, C., Dassa, C., Rainville, C., & Dutil, É. (2010b). The IADL Profile: Development, content, validity, intra- and interrater agreement. *Canadian Journal of Occupational Therapy, 77*(2), 90–100. https://doi.org/10.2182/cjot.2010.77.2.5

Bottari, C., Iliopoulos, G., Shun, W., Lam, P., & Dawson, D. R. (2014). The clinical reasoning that guides therapists in interpreting errors in real-world performance. *Journal of Head Trauma Rehabilitation, 29*(6), E18–E30. https://doi.org/10.1097/HTR.0000000000000029

Carbonneau, H., Martineau, É., Andre, M., & Dawson, D. (2011). Enhancing leisure experiences post traumatic brain injury: A pilot study. *Brain Impairment, 12*(2), 140–151. https://doi.org/10.1375/brim.12.2.140

Colantonio, A., Salehi, S., Kristman, V., Cassidy, J. D., Carter, A., Vartanian, O., Bayley, M., Kirsh, B., Hébert, D., Lewko, J., Kubrak, O., Mantis, S., & Vernich, L. (2016). Return to work

after work-related traumatic brain injury. *NeuroRehabilitation, 39*(3), 389–399. https://doi
.org/10.3233/NRE-161370

Conti, G. E. (2017). Acquired brain injury. In B. J. Atchison & D. P. Dirette (Eds.), *Conditions in
occupational therapy* (5th ed., pp. 363–386). Wolters Kluwer.

Cooksley, R., Maguire, E., Lannin, N. A., Unsworth, C. A., Farquhar, M., Galea C., Mitra, B., &
Schmidt, J. (2018). Persistent symptoms and activity changes three months after mild traumatic brain injury. *Australian Occupational Therapy Journal, 65*(3), 168–175. https://doi.org/
10.1111/1440-1630.12457

Dawson, D. R., Binns, M. A., Hunt, A., Lemsky, C., & Polatajko, H. J. (2013). Occupation-based
strategy training for adults with traumatic brain injury: A pilot study. *Archives of Physical Medicine and Rehabilitation, 94*(10), 1959–1963. https://doi.org/10.1016/j.apmr.2013.05.021

Dutil, É., Bottari, C., & Auger, C. (2017). Test–retest reliability of a measure of independence in
everyday activities: The ADL Profile. *Occupational Therapy International, 2017*, Article 3014579.
https://doi.org/10.1155/2017/3014579

Engel, L. L., Beaton, D. E., Green, R. E., & Dawson, D. R. (2019). Financial Management Activity
Process: Qualitative inquiry of adults with acquired brain injury. *Canadian Journal of Occupational Therapy, 86*(3), 196–208. https://doi.org/10.1177/0008417419833839

Foxhall, M., & Gurr, B. (2014). Skills for life—Evaluation of a group intervention for brain
injury survivors. *Social Care & Neurodisability, 5*(4), 214–222. https://doi.org/10.1108/SCN
-07-2014-0013

Giles, G. M. (2018). Neurofunctional approach to rehabilitation after brain injury. In N. Katz &
J. Toglia (Eds.), *Cognition, occupation, and participation across the lifespan* (4th ed., pp. 419–442).
AOTA Press.

Goverover, Y., Chiaravalloti, N., & DeLuca, J. (2010). Pilot study to examine the use of self-
generation to improve learning and memory in people with traumatic brain injury. *American
Journal of Occupational Therapy, 64*(4), 540–546. https://doi.org/10.5014/ajot.2010.09020

Goverover, Y., & DeLuca, J. (2015). Actual reality: Using the Internet to assess everyday functioning after traumatic brain injury. *Brain Injury, 29*(6), 715–721. https://doi.org/10.3109/
02699052.2015.1004744

Grigorovich, A., Stergiou-Kita, M., Damianakis, T., Le Dorze, G., Lemsky, C., & Hebert, D.
(2017). Persons with brain injury and employment supports: Long-term employment outcomes and use of community based services. *Brain Injury, 31*(5), 607–619. https://doi.org/
10.1080/02699052.2017.1280855

Hunt, A. W., Le Dorze, G., Polatajko, H., Bottari, C., & Dawson, D. R. (2015). Communication
during goal-setting in brain injury rehabilitation: What helps and what hinders? *British Journal of Occupational Therapy, 78*(8), 488–498. https://doi.org/10.1177/0308022614562784

Hunt, A. W., Le Dorze, G., Trentham, B., Polatajko H. J., & Dawson, D. R. (2015). Elucidating
a goal-setting continuum in brain injury rehabilitation. *Qualitative Health Research, 25*(8),
1044–1055. https://doi.org/10.1177/1049732315588759

Ko, C. (2019). Using the Weekly Calendar Planning Activity with clients with acquired brain
injuries. *SIS Quarterly Practice Connections, 4*(4), 27–29.

Le Dorze, G., Villeneuve, J., Zumbansen, A., Masson-Trottier, M., & Bottari, C. (2014). Verbal
assistance within the context of an IADL evaluation. *Open Journal of Therapy and Rehabilitation, 2*(4), 182–198. https://doi.org/10.4236/ojtr.2014.24024

Lum, A. R., Anderson, M., & Dean, E. (2018). Using occupational performance coaching in mild
traumatic brain injury rehabilitation. *SIS Quarterly Practice Connections, 3*(2), 29–30.

McKeon, A., Terhorst, L., Ding, D., Cooper, R., & McCue, M. (2018). Naturalistic physiological
monitoring as an objective approach for detecting behavioral dysregulation after traumatic
brain injury: A pilot study. *Journal of Vocational Rehabilitation, 49*(3), 379–388. https://doi
.org/10.3233/JVR-180981

McKeon, A., Terhorst, L., Skidmore, E., Ding, D. Cooper, R., & McCue, M. (2017). A novel tool for naturalistic assessment of behavioural dysregulation after traumatic brain injury: A pilot study. *Brain Injury, 31*(13-14), 1781–1790. https://doi.org/10.1080/02699052.2017.1388444

Miyahara, T., Shimizu, H., Yamane, S., & Hanaoka, H. (2018). Occupation-based intervention to improve self-awareness in persons with acquired brain injury: A single-case experimental design. *Asian Journal of Occupational Therapy, 14*(1), 33–41. https://doi.org/10.11596/asiajot.14.33

Porter, R. S. (Ed.). (2018). *The Merck manual of diagnosis and therapy* (20th ed.). Merck Sharp & Dorme.

Radomski, M. V., Weightman, M. M., Davidson, L. F., Finkelstein, M., Goldman, S., McCulloch, K., Roy, T. C., Scherer, M., & Stern, E. B. (2013). Development of a measure to inform return-to-duty decision making after mild traumatic brain injury. *Military Medicine, 178*(3), 246–253. https://doi.org/10.7205/MILMED-D-12-00144

Stergiou-Kita, M., Dawson, D., & Rappolt, S. (2012). Inter-professional clinical practice guideline for vocational evaluation following traumatic brain injury: A systematic and evidence-based approach. *Journal of Occupational Rehabilitation, 22*(2), 166–181. https://doi.org/10.1007/s10926-011-9332-2

Stergiou-Kita, M., Grigorovich, A., Damianakis, T., Le Dorze, G., David, C., Lemsky, C., & Hebert, D. (2017). The big sell: Managing stigma and workplace discrimination following moderate to severe brain injury. *Work, 57*(2), 245–258. https://doi.org/10.3233/WOR-172556

Suzuki, Y., & Tanemura, R. (2011). Community-based interventional programmes for family caregivers of persons with traumatic brain injury. *Asian Journal of Occupational Therapy, 9*(1), 15–22.

Sveen, U., Andelic, N., Bautz-Holter, E., & Røe, C. (2015). Self-reported competency—Validation of the Norwegian version of the patient competency rating scale for traumatic brain injury. *Disability and Rehabilitation, 37*(3), 239–246. https://doi.org/10.3109/09638288.2014.913706

Therriault, P. Y., Lefebvre H., Guindon, A., Levert, M. J., Briand, C., & Lord, M. M. (2016). Accompanying citizen of persons with traumatic brain injury in a community integration project: An exploration of the role. *Work, 54*(3), 591–600. https://doi.org/10.3233/WOR-162342

Toglia, J., Goverover, Y., Johnston, M. V., & Dain, B. (2011). Application of the multicontextual approach in promoting learning and transfer of strategy use in an individual with TBI and executive dysfunction. *OTJR: Occupation, Participation, and Health, 31*(Suppl. 1), S53–S60. https://doi.org/10.3928/15394492-20101108-09

Toglia, J., Johnston, M. V., Goverover, Y., & Dain, B. (2010). A multicontext approach to promoting transfer of strategy use and self regulation after brain injury: An exploratory study. *Brain Injury, 24*(4), 664–677. https://doi.org/10.3109/02699051003610474

Toneman, M., Brayshaw, J., Lange, B., & Trimboli, C. (2010). Examination of the change in Assessment of Motor and Process Skills performance in patients with acquired brain injury between the hospital and home environment. *Australian Occupational Therapy Journal, 57*(4), 246–252. https://doi.org/10.1111/j.1440-1630.2009.00832.x

Tulsky, D. S., Holdnack, J. A., Cohen, M. L., Heaton, R. K., Carlozzi, N. E., Wong, A. W. K., Boulton, A. J., & Heinemann, A. W. (2017). Factor structure of the NIH Toolbox Cognition Battery in individuals with acquired brain injury. *Rehabilitation Psychology, 62*(4), 435–442. https://doi.org/10.1037/rep0000183

Weightman, M., Radomski, M., Mashima, P., & Roth, C. (Eds.). (2014). *Mild traumatic brain injury rehabilitation toolkit.* Government Publishing Office.

Wheeler, S., & Acord-Vira, A. (2016). *Occupational therapy practice guidelines for adults with traumatic brain injury.* American Occupational Therapy Association.

White, B. P., Brinkman, A. K., Kresge, B. P., & Couture, L. (2018). Quality of life, stress perception: An quality of social networks in persons living and brain injury: an exploration of the effectiveness of a community-based program. *Open Journal of Occupational Therapy, 6*(4), Article 4. https://doi.org/10.15453/2168-6408.1428

Yoshida, K., Sawamura, D., Ogawa, K., Ikoma, K., Asakawa, K., Yamauchi, T., & Sakai, S. (2014). Flow experience during attentional training improves cognitive functions in patients with traumatic brain injury: An exploratory case study. *Hong Kong Journal of Occupational Therapy*, 24(2), 81–87. https://doi.org/10.1016/j.hkjot.2015.01.001

BIBLIOGRAPHY

Andelic, N., Bautz-Holter, E., Ronning, P., Olafsen, K., Sigurdardottir, S., Schanke, A. K., Sveen, U., Tornas, S., Sandhaug, M., & Røe, C. (2012). Does an early onset and continuous chain of rehabilitation improve the long-term functional outcome of patients with severe traumatic brain injury? *Journal of Neurotrauma*, 29(1), 66–74. https://doi.org/10.1089/neu.2011.1811

Andelic, N., Perrin, P. B., Forslund, M. V., Soberg, H. L. Sigurdardottir, S., Sveen, U., Jerstad, T., & Roe, C. (2015). Trajectories of physical health in the first 5 years after traumatic brain injury. *Journal of Neurology*, 262(3), 523–531. https://doi.org/10.1007/s00415-014-7595-1

Andelic, N., Sigurdardottir, S., Schanke, A. K., Sandvik, L., Sveen, U., & Røe, C. (2010). Disability, physical health and mental health 1 year after traumatic brain injury. *Disability and Rehabilitation*, 32(13), 1122–1131. https://doi.org/10.3109/09638280903410722

Barrie, D., Franzsen, D., & Gradidige, K. (2014). Anxiety and the perceived adequacy of information received by family members during the in-patient rehabilitation of patients with brain injury. *South African Journal of Occupational Therapy*, 44(1), 31–35.

Bottari, C., & Dawson, D. R. (2011). Executive functions and real-world performance: How good are we at distinguishing people with acquired brain injury from healthy controls? *OTJR: Occupation, Participation, and Health*, 31(Suppl. 1), S61–S68. https://doi.org/10.3928/153944 92-20101108-10

Bottari, C., Gosselin, N., Chen, J. K., & Ptito, A. (2017). The impact of symptomatic mild traumatic brain injury on complex everyday activities and the link with alterations in cerebral functioning: Exploratory case studies. *Neuropsychological Rehabilitation*, 27(5), 871–890. https://doi.org/10.1080/09602011.2015.1110528

Bottari, C., Gosselin, N., Guillemette, M., Lamoureux, J., & Ptito, A. (2011). Independence in managing one's finances after traumatic brain injury. *Brain Injury*, 25(13/14), 1306–1317. https://doi.org/10.3109/02699052.2011.624570

Brown, S., Hawker, G., Beaton, D., & Colantonio, A. (2011). Long-term musculoskeletal complaints after traumatic brain injury. *Brain Injury*, 25(5), 453–461. https://doi.org/10.3109/02699052.2011.556581

Chan, V., Stock, D., Jacob, B., Cullen, N., & Colantonio, A. (2018). Readmission following hypoxic ischemic brain injury: A population-based cohort study. *CMAJ Open*, 6(4), E568–E574. https://doi.org/10.9778/cmajo.20180080

Cogan, A. M. (2014). Occupational needs and intervention strategies for military personnel with mild traumatic brain injury and persistent post-concussion symptoms: A review. *OTJR: Occupation, Participation and Health*, 34(3), 150–159. https://doi.org/10.3928/15394492 -20140617-01

Dillahunt-Aspillaga, C., Smith, T. J., Hanson, A., Ehlke, S., Stergiou-Kita, M., Dixon, C. G., & Quichocho, D. (2015). Exploring vocational evaluation practice following traumatic brain injury. *Behavioral Neurology*, 2013, Article 924027. https://doi.org/10.1155/2015/924027

Fogelberg, D. J., Hoffman, J. M., Dikmen, S., Temkin, N. R., & Bell, K. R. (2012). Association of sleep and co-occurring psychological conditions at 1 year after traumatic brain injury. *Archives of Physical Medicine and Rehabilitation*, 93(8), 1313–1318. https://doi.org/10.1016/j.apmr.2012.04.031

Gagnon, A., Lin, J., & Stergiou-Kita, M. (2016). Family members facilitating community reintegration and return to productivity following traumatic brain injury—motivations, roles and challenges. *Disability and Rehabilitation*, 38(5), 433–441. https://doi.org/10.3109/0963 8288.2015.1044035

Gosselin, N., Chen, J.-K., Bottari, C., Petrides, M., Jubault, T., Tinawi, S., de Guise, E., & Ptito, A. (2012). The influence of pain on cerebral functioning after mild traumatic brain injury. *Journal of Neurotrauma, 29*(17), 2625–2634. https://doi.org/10.1089/neu.2012.2312

Gosselin, N., Bottari, C., Chen, J.-K., Petrides, M., Tinawi, S., de Guise, É., & Ptito, A. (2011). Electrophysiology and functional MRI in post-acute mild traumatic brain injury. *Journal of Neurotrauma, 28*(3), 329–341. https://doi.org/10.1089/neu.2010.1493

Gourdeau, J., Fingold, A., Colantonio, A., Mansfield, E., & Stergiou-Kita, M. (2020). Workplace accommodations following work-related mild traumatic brain injury: What works? *Disability and Rehabilitation, 42*(4), 552–561. https://doi.org/10.1080/09638288.2018.1503733

Goverover, Y., Genova, H., Smith, A., Chiaravalloti, N., & Lengenfelder, J. (2017). Changes in activity participation following traumatic brain injury. *Neuropsychological Rehabilitation, 27*(4), 472–485. https://doi.org/10.1080/09602011.2016.1168746

Guerriero, E. N., Smith, P. M., Stergiou-Kita, M., & Colantonio, A. (2016). Rehabilitation utilization following a work-related traumatic brain injury: A sex-based examination of workers' compensation claims in Victoria, Australia. *PLOS ONE, 11*(3), Article e0151462. https://doi.org/10.1371/journal.pone.0151462

Haffejee, S., Ntsiea, V., & Mudzi, W. (2013). Factors that influenced functional mobility outcomes of patients after traumatic brain injury. *Hong Kong Journal of Occupational Therapy, 23*(1), 39–44. https://doi.org/10.1016/j.hkjot.2013.08.001

Haveraaen, L., Brouwers, E. P. M., Sveen, U., Skarpaas, L. S., Sagvaag, H., & Aas, R. W. (2017). The first six years of building and implementing a return-to-work service for patients with acquired brain injury: The rapid-return-to-work cohort study. *Journal of Occupational Rehabilitation, 27*(4), 623–632. https://doi.org/10.1007/s10926-016-9693-7

Hellweg, S. (2012). Effectiveness of physiotherapy and occupational therapy after traumatic brain injury in the intensive care unit. *Critical Care Research and Practice, 2012*, Article 768456. https://doi.org/10.1155/2012/768456

Juengst, S. B., Arenth, P. M., Whyte, E. M., & Skidmore, E. R. (2014). Brief report of affective state and depression status after traumatic brain injury. *Rehabilitation Psychology, 59*(2), 242–246. https://doi.org/10.1037/a0036294

Kendrick, D., Silverberg, N. D., Barlow, S., Miller, W. C., & Moffat, J. (2012). Acquired brain injury self-management programme: A pilot study. *Brain Injury, 26*(10), 1243–1249. https://doi.org/10.3109/02699052.2012.672787

Kim, H., & Colantonio, A. (2010). Effectiveness of rehabilitation in enhancing community integration after acute traumatic brain injury: A systematic review. *American Journal of Occupational Therapy, 64*(5), 709–719. https://doi.org/10.5014/ajot.2010.09188

Kim, H., Colantonio, A., Dawson, D. R., & Bayley, M. T. (2013). Community integration outcomes after traumatic brain injury due to physical assault. *Canadian Journal of Occupational Therapy, 80*(1), 49–58. https://doi.org/10.1177/0008417412473262

Koller, K., Woods, L., Engel, L., Bottari, C., Dawson, D. R., & Nalder, E. (2016). Loss of financial management independence after brain injury: Survivors' experiences. *American Journal of Occupational Therapy, 70*(3), Article 7003180070. https://doi.org/10.5014/ajot.2016.020198

Lamontagne, M. E., Poncet, F., Careau, E., Sirois, M. J., & Boucher, N. (2013). Life habits performance of individuals with brain injury in different living environments. *Brain Injury, 27*(2), 135–144. https://doi.org/10.3109/02699052.2012.722253

Lefaivre, A. (2014). *Traumatic brain injury rehabilitation: The Lefaivre rainbow effect.* CRC Press.

Mansfield, E., Stergiou-Kita, M., Cassidy, J. D., Bayley, M., Mantis, S., Kristman, V., Kirsh, B., Gomez, M., Jeschke, M. G., Vartanian, O., Moody, J., & Colantonio, A. (2015). Return-to-work challenges following a work-related mild TBI: The injured worker perspective. *Brain Injury, 29*(11), 1362–1369. https://doi.org/10.3109/02699052.2015.1053524

Marshall, C. A., Nalder, E., Colquhoun, H., Lenton, E., Hansen, M., Dawson, D. R., Zabjek, K., & Bottari, C. (2019). Interventions to address burden among family caregivers of persons

aging with TBI: A scoping review. *Brain Injury, 33*(3), 255–265. https://doi.org/10.1080/02
699052.2018.1553308

McLean, A. M., Jarus, T., Hubley, A. M., & Jongbloed, L. (2012). Differences in social participation between individuals who do and do not attend brain injury drop-in centres: A preliminary study. *Brain Injury, 26*(1), 83–94. https://doi.org/10.3109/02699052.2011.635353

McLean, A. M., Jarus, T., Hubley, A. M., & Jongbloed, L. (2014). Associations between social participation and subjective quality of life for adults with moderate to severe traumatic brain injury. *Disability and Rehabilitation, 36*(17), 1409–1418. https://doi.org/10.3109/09638288
.2013.834986

Mollayeva, T., Mollayeva, S., & Colantonio, A. (2018). Traumatic brain injury: Sex, gender and intersecting vulnerabilities. *Nature Reviews Neurology, 14*(12), 711–722. https://doi.org/10.1038/
s41582-018-0091-y

Moller, C. L., Lingah, T., & Phehlukwayo, S. M. (2017). "We all need employment"—An exploration of the factors which influence the return-to-work after a severe traumatic brain injury. *South African Journal of Occupational Therapy, 47*(3), 17–24. https://doi.org/10.17159/
2310-3833/2017/v47n3a4

Nadeau, B. (2016). *Fact sheet: Occupational therapy and community reintegration of persons with brain injury.* American Occupational Therapy Association.

Nalder, E., & Fleming, J. (2018). Transition to community integration for people with acquired brain injury. In N. Katz & J. Toglia (Eds.), *Cognition, occupation, and participation across the lifespan* (4th ed., pp. 173–188). AOTA Press.

Ocampo-Chan, S., Badley, E., Dawson, D. R., Ratcliff, G., & Colantonio, A. (2014). Factors associated with self-reported arthritis 7 to 24 years after a traumatic brain injury. *Perceptual and Motor Skills, 118*(1), 274–292. https://doi.org/10.2466/15.PMS.118k12w2

Powell, J. (2014). Traumatic brain injury. In M. V. Radomski & C. A. Trombly Latham (Eds.), *Occupational therapy for physical dysfunction* (7th ed., pp. 1042–1075). Wolters Kluwer.

Powell, J. M., Rich, T. J., & Wise, E. K. (2016). Effectiveness of occupation- and activity-based interventions to improve everyday activities and social participation for people with traumatic brain injury: A systematic review. *American Journal of Occupational Therapy, 70*(3), Article 7003180040. https://doi.org/10.5014/ajot.2016.020909

Soberg, H. L., Røe, C., Anke, A., Arango-Lasprilla, J. C., Skandsen, T., Sveen, U., von Steinbüchel, N., & Andelic, N. (2013). Health-related quality of life 12 months after severe traumatic brain injury: A prospective nationwide cohort study. *Journal of Rehabilitation Medicine, 45*(8), 785–791. https://doi.org/10.2340/16501977-1158

Stergiou-Kita, M., Dawson, D. R., & Rappolt, S. G. (2011). An integrated review of the processes and factors relevant to vocational evaluation following traumatic brain injury. *Journal of Occupational Rehabilitation, 21*(3), 374–394. https://doi.org/10.1007/s10926-010-9282-0

Stergiou-Kita, M., Mansfield, E., Sokoloff, S., & Colantonio, A. (2016). Gender influences on return to work after mild traumatic brain injury. *Archives of Physical Medicine and Rehabilitation, 97*(2 Suppl.), S40–S45. https://doi.org/10.1016/j.apmr.2015.04.008

Stergiou-Kita, M., Rappolt, S., & Dawson, D. (2012). Towards developing a guideline for vocational evaluation following traumatic brain injury: The qualitative synthesis of clients' perspectives. *Disability and Rehabilitation, 34*(3), 179–188. https://doi.org/10.3109/09638
288.2011.591881

Stergiou-Kita, M., Yantzi, A., & Wan, J. (2010). The personal and workplace factors relevant to work readiness evaluation following acquired brain injury: Occupational therapists' perceptions. *Brain Injury, 24*(7-8), 948–958. https://doi.org/10.3109/02699052.2010.491495

Sveen, U., Bautz-Holter, E., Sandvik, L., Alvsåker, K., & Røe, C. (2010). Relationship between competency in activities, injury severity, and post-concussion symptoms after traumatic brain injury. *Scandinavian Journal of Occupational Therapy, 17*(3), 225–232. https://doi.org/10.31
09/11038120903171295

Sveen, U. Østensjø, S., Laxe, S., & Soberg, H. L. (2013). Problems in functioning after a mild traumatic brain injury within the ICF framework: The patient perspective using focus groups. *Disability and Rehabilitation, 35*(9), 749–757. https://doi.org/10.3109/09638288.2012.707741

Sveen, U., Røe, C., Sigurdardottir, S., Skandsen, T., Andelic, N., Manskow, U., Berntsen, S. A., Soberg, H. L., & Anke, A. (2016). Rehabilitation pathways and functional independence one year after severe traumatic brain injury. *European Journal of Physical and Rehabilitation Medicine, 52*(5), 650–661.

Sveen, U., Søberg, H. L., & Østensjø, S. (2016). Biographical disruption, adjustment and reconstruction of everyday occupations and work participation after mild traumatic brain injury: A focus group study. *Disability and Rehabilitation, 38*(23), 2296–2304. https://doi.org/10.3109/09638288.2015.1129445

Tan-Rapues, C. (2018). Mild traumatic brain injury: A review of current occupational therapy practice in Aotearoa New Zealand's acute settings. *New Zealand Journal of Occupational Therapy, 65*(1), 28–35.

Terry, D. P., Iverson, G. L., Panenka, W., Colantonio, A., & Silverberg, N. D. (2018). Workplace and non-workplace mild traumatic brain injuries in an outpatient clinic sample: A case-control study. *PLOS ONE, 13*(6), Article e0198128. https://doi.org/10.1371/journal.pone.0198128

Tipton-Burton, M. (2013). Traumatic brain injury. In H. M. Pendleton & W. Schultz-Krohn (Eds.), *Pedretti's occupational therapy* (7th ed., pp. 841–879). Elsevier.

Wang, J., Mahajan, H. P., Toto, P. E., McCue, M. P., & Ding, D. (2019). The feasibility of an automatic prompting system in assisting people with traumatic brain injury in cooking tasks. *Disability and Rehabilitation: Assistive Technology, 14*(8), 817–825. https://doi.org/10.1080/17483107.2018.1499144

Wheeler, S., Acord-Vira, A., & Davis, D. (2016). Effectiveness of interventions to improve occupational performance for people with psychosocial, behavioral, and emotional impairments after brain injury: A systematic review. *American Journal of Occupational Therapy, 70*(3), Article 7003180060. https://doi.org/10.5014/ajot.115.020677

Wheeler, S., Acord-Vira, A., Arbesman, M., & Lieberman, D. (2017). Occupational therapy interventions for adults with traumatic brain injury. *American Journal of Occupational Therapy, 71*(3), Article 7103395010. https://doi.org/10.5014/ajot.2017.713005

Zarshenas, S., Colantonio, A., Alavinia, S. M., Jaglal, S., Tam, L., & Cullen, N. (2019). Predictors of discharge destination from acute care in patients with traumatic brain injury: A systematic review. *Journal of Head Trauma Rehabilitation, 34*(1), 52–64. https://doi.org/10.1097/HTR.0000000000000403

Brain Injuries: Child and Adolescent

Also called head injuries, acquired brain injury, traumatic brain injury.

See also Brain Injuries: Adult, Cognitive Impairment, Concussion and Post-Concussion, Executive Dysfunction, Memory Impairment.

Description

Brain injury is brain damage to the brain that occurs after birth from a traumatic or nontraumatic cause. Brain injury is a complex condition that can impair motor, cognitive, social, and behavioral functions (Lindsay et al., 2015).

Cause

Brain injury may be traumatic as a result of trauma to the head such as a blow to the head, fall, motor vehicle accident, or sports injury, or nontraumatic caused by cerebral anoxia, brain tumor, stroke, toxic or metabolic damage, or brain infection (Austin et al., 2018).

Evaluation/Assessment
Areas
- Activities of Daily Living/Instrumental ADL: basic ADLs (eating, swallowing, dressing, grooming, toileting), transfers (bed, toilet, tub or shower, car), communication skills (speech intelligibility, perceive, interpret and respond), locomotion (walking, wheelchair, stairs), community mobility (bus, taxis, train), independent living (meal preparation, housework, shopping, finances)
- Education/Work: academic performance (reading, writing, mathematics), work habits and skills
- Play/Leisure: play skills (cooperative play, taking turns), leisure interests, values, frequency, location, level of satisfaction
- Rest/Sleep: sleep disturbance, sleep habits and routine, sleep disorders
- Social Participation: type, frequency, location, with whom
- Sensorimotor: gross and fine motor skills, muscle tone, reflexes, balance and coordination, positioning, joint range of motion, muscle strength, visual functions (acuity, perception, binocularity, eye–hand coordination, scanning), sensory registration (auditory, gustatory, olfactory, proprioception, tactile, visual)
- Cognitive/Perceptual: level of consciousness, attention and orientation, memory, executive functions (problem solving, safety awareness)
- Psychosocial: quality of life, social skills (awareness of social rules and boundaries, processing and interpreting emotions conveyed by facial expressions, listening and working with others to solve conversational tasks), self-esteem, self-awareness, emotional regulation, adjustment to limitations, motivation, quality of life
- Context/Environment: adapted devices (walker, helmets, scooter, cane, wheelchair), home modification, family and social support, education about brain injury (client, family, caregiver), knowledge about resources (community, internet)
- Development (Infant, Child, Adolescent only): developmental milestones, regression following injury

Instruments
Instruments Developed by Occupational Therapy Personnel
- Assessment of Motor and Process Skills (8th ed.; AMPS-8; Fisher & Bray Jones, 2016)
- Canadian Occupational Performance Measure (5th ed.; COPM-5; Law et al., 2014)
- Child and Adolescent Scale of Participation–Youth Version Revised (CASP-YR; McDougall et al., 2013; see also Golos & Bedell, 2016, 2018, in References)
- Child Occupational Self-Assessment (Version 2.2; COSA; Kramer et al., 2014)
- Children's Assessment of Participation and Enjoyment and Preferences for Activities of Children (CAPE/PAC; King et al., 2004)
- Dynamic Loewenstein Occupational Therapy Cognitive Assessment (DLOTCA; Katz et al., 2012)
- Evaluation of Social Interaction (3rd ed.; ESI-3; Fisher & Griswold, 2015)
- Pediatric Evaluation of Disability Inventory (PEDI; Haley et al., 1992)
- Pediatric Evaluation of Disability Inventory—Computer Adaptive Test (PEDI-CAT; Kramer et al., 2016)
- Perceived Efficacy and Goal Setting (PEGS; Missiuna & Pollock, 2000)
- Revised Knox Preschool Play Scale (RKPPS; Knox, 2008)
- School Assessment of Motor and Process Skills (2nd ed.; ScAMPS-2; Fisher et al., 2007; see also Sakzewski et al., 2017, in References)
- School Function Assessment (SFA; Coster et al., 1998)
- Sensory Profile (2nd ed.; SP-2; Dunn, 2014)
- Sensory Processing Measure (SPM; Parham et al., 2007)
- Test of Playfulness (Version 4.2; ToP 4.2; Bundy, 2010)
- Weekly Calendar Planning Activity (WCPA; Toglia, 2015)

Instruments Developed by Other Professionals and Used by Occupational Therapy Personnel

- Accelerometry (instrument; see Baque, Sakzewski, et al., 2017, in References)
- Beery-Buktenica Developmental Test of Visual-Motor Integration (6th ed.; Beery VMI-6; Beery et al., 2010)
- Behavioural Assessment of the Dysexecutive Syndrome in Children (BADS-C; Emslie et al., 2003)
- Children's Orientation and Amnesia Test (COAT; Ewing-Cobbs et al., 1990)
- Detailed Assessment of Speed of Handwriting (DASH; Barnett et al., 2007)
- Developmental Test of Visual Perception (3rd ed.; DTVP-3; Hammill et al., 2014)
- Disability Rating Scale (DRS; Rapaport et al., 1982)
- Functional Independence Measure (FIM; Uniform Data System for Medical Rehabilitation, 1997)
- Functional Independence Measure for Children (Version 5.01; WeeFIM; Uniform Data System for Medical Rehabilitation, 1998)
- Functional Independence Measure–Functional Assessment Measure (FIM+FAM; Turner-Stokes et al., 1999; see also Austin et al., 2018, in References)
- Glasgow Coma Scale (GCS; Teasdale & Jennett, 1974)
- Goal Attainment Scaling (GAS; Kiresuk & Sherman, 1968; Kiresuk et al., 1994)
- Hypertonia Assessment Tool (HAT; Jethwa et al., 2010)
- Modified Ashworth Scale (MAS; Bohannon & Smith, 1987)
- Modified Tardieu Scale (MTS; Haugh et al., 2006)
- Motor-Free Visual Perception Test (4th ed.; MVPT-4; Colarusso & Hammill, 2015)
- Neurological Impairment Scale (NIS; Turner-Stokes et al., 2013)
- Profile of Pragmatic Impairments in Communication (PPIC; Linscott et al., 1996)
- Q-sort method (to sort statements regarding barriers and facilitators to community participation; see Thompson et al., 2016, in References)
- Rancho Levels of Cognitive Functioning (3rd ed.; RLCF-3; Hagen, 1998)
- Rancho Los Amigos–Revised (see Rancho Levels of Cognitive Functioning)
- Rivermead Behavioural Memory Test for Children (RBMT-C; Wilson et al., 1991)
- Rosenberg Self-Esteem Scale (RSES; Rosenberg, 1965)
- Social Networks Inventory (SNI; Treadwell et al., 1993)
- Test of Everyday Attention for Children (2nd ed.; TEA-Ch2; Manley et al, 2016)
- Test of Visual Perceptual Skills (4th ed.; TVPS-4; Martin, 2017)
- Videofluoroscopic or flexible endoscopic evaluation for swallowing (procedure)
- Wessex Head Injury Matrix (WHIM; Shiel et al., 2000)
- Wide Range Assessment of Visual Motor Abilities (WRAVMA; Adams & Sheslow, 1995)

Problems/Issues

Activities of Daily Living/Instrumental ADL

- Child or adolescent may be unable to eat or drink independently and require tube feeding or assistance to get food from plate to mouth.
- Child or adolescent may be incontinent in bladder and bowel functions.
- Child or adolescent may have a tracheostomy tube to facilitate breathing.
- Child or adolescent may have reduced communication skills relative to age.
- Child or adolescent may have difficulty performing basic ADLs, including eating, dressing, toileting, bathing or showering, brushing teeth, grooming, transfers, functional communication.
- Child or adolescent may have difficulty with mobility such as moving about the home, yard, school, or community.
- Child or adolescent may have difficulty using public transportation such as a taxi, school bus, or train system, including getting in/on or out/off the transport.
- Child or adolescent may have difficulty performing household chores such as washing dishes, loading and unloading the dishwasher, setting the table, cleaning up after a meal, watering

plants, feeding/grooming/walking pets, dusting or straightening up rooms, doing laundry, making simple meals, taking out trash.
- Child or adolescent may have difficulty walking about the community, riding a scooter or tricycle, riding a bike or modified wheelchair.

Education/Work
- Child or adolescent may have difficulty completing assignments and projects.
- Child or adolescent may have difficulty participating in physical education or sports activities.
- Child or adolescent may have difficulty keeping a desk or backpack organized and accessible.
- Child or adolescent may experience difficulty creating a routine to get ready for school.
- Child or adolescent may have difficulty arriving at school and leaving as per routine schedule and time.
- Adolescent may not have explored work activities.

Play/Leisure
- Child may not have developed play skills (cooperative play, taking turns, sharing objects).
- Child or adolescent may not have developed leisure interests or skills such as reading a book, listening to music.
- Child or adolescent may have difficulty engaging in sport activities such as playing a sport, going swimming, going to the gym.

Social Participation
- Child or adolescent may not participate or lack skills in social activities.
- Child or adolescent may have difficulty going to a movie or shopping with friends.
- Child or adolescent may experience difficulty participating in special school events or trips.

Rest/Sleep
- Child or adolescent may experience sleep disturbance.
- Child or adolescent may not have an established sleep (go to bed) routine.

Sensorimotor
- Child or adolescent may have difficulty gaining and maintaining head and trunk control.
- Child or adolescent may have difficulty with balance and coordination.
- Child or adolescent may have loss of gross and fine motor skills.
- Child or adolescent may have reduced endurance and activity tolerance.
- Child or adolescent may experience pain.
- Child or adolescent may have reduced or lost sensory registration.
- Child or adolescent may have loss of skin sensation and be at risk for pressure sores.

Cognitive/Perceptual
- Child or adolescent may experience difficulty with paying attention.
- Child or adolescent may have difficulty following directions to complete an assignment or activity.
- Child or adolescent may have difficulty with simple problem solving (two choice).
- Child or adolescent may make unsafe decisions and lack judgment of safety.
- Child or adolescent may experience loss of visual spatial relations.

Psychosocial
- Child or adolescent may have limited self-awareness.
- Child or adolescent may have low self-esteem.
- Child or adolescent may have limited coping skills.
- Child or adolescent may have poor quality of life.
- Child or adolescent may have limited social skills, including social integration.
- Child or adolescent may have poor emotional regulation.
- Child or adolescent may have low motivation.

Context/Environment

- Family or caregivers may have limited information or understanding of effects of brain injury in a child or adolescent.
- Child or adolescent may lack family or social support.
- Child or adolescent may lack access to adaptive devices and equipment.

Developmental skills

- Child may not have achieved or have loss of functional gross motor skills (rolling over, supine to sit, sitting, sit to stand, stand, gait pattern, stair climbing, jumping, hopping, running, standing on one foot, standing with eyes closed).

Intervention/Treatment

Models and programs developed by occupational therapy personnel include case review (Titchener et al., 2018) and Cognitive Orientation to daily Occupational Performance (CO-OP; Jackman et al., 2018; Missiuna et al., 2010). Models and programs developed by other professionals but used by occupational therapy personnel include arts-based programs (Agnihotri et al., 2012, 2014), Social Participation and Navigation (SPAN) app-based coaching intervention (Bedell et al., 2017; Narad et al., 2018; Wade et al., 2018), initiation of therapy (Bennett et al., 2013), web-based multimodal therapy (Baque, Barber, et al., 2017; Sakzewski et al., 2016), music therapy (Twyford & Watters, 2016), Nintendo Wii (Tatla et al., 2014), virtual reality (Bart et al., 2011), virtual reality–balance (Cheung et al., 2013), virtual supermarket (Erez et al., 2013), and Xbox Kinect (Cheung et al., 2013). Team members include physicians (physiatrist, neurologist), nursing personnel, psychologists, neuropsychologists, social workers, physical therapists, speech–language pathologists, therapeutic recreational specialists or recreational therapists, social workers, educators, parents, caregivers, and occupational therapy personnel. The goal of intervention is to return the child or adolescent to school and community living.

Activities of Daily Living/Instrumental ADL

- An augmentative communication system may be needed to facilitate communication, such as gestures, alphabet board, picture board, phrase board, app on cell phone.
- Adjustments may be needed for eating such as bolus modification (changing texture, viscosity, volume, or temperature), postural modification (seated or reclined, chin down, head rotated), behavioral adjustments (rate of administrating bites of food), modification of administration (special nipples, bottles), oral sensitivity (texture, placement of bolus, type of feeding device).
- Retraining of basic ADLs may be needed for eating, bathing/showering, dressing and undressing, toileting, grooming, transfers.
- Adolescents who are driving age may need driver evaluation and training.
- Adolescents may need practice in planning and preparing meals, managing finances, finding an apartment, living in a school dormitory, living with roommates, shopping.

Education/Work

- Provide assistance in modifying academic tasks as needed, such as enlarging print, using computer-assisted programs, reducing need for written responses, increasing computer-assisted responses or verbal responses, recommending use of a teacher's aide.
- Provide assistance in school-related activities such as navigating about the school building and classroom, navigating the cafeteria or canteen with a food tray, using the library, organizing a locker or cubby space, engaging in school sports or special activities.
- Adolescent may need opportunity to work on basic job skills (exploring vocational interests, practicing for an interview, preparing a resume, volunteering to gain real-life experience, arranging for transportation).

Play/Leisure

- Provide opportunity to interact with other peers or age-appropriate children in games and activities.

- Provide opportunity to explore leisure activities that can be done with others and those that can be done alone.

Rest/Sleep
- Consider whether environmental modifications may be useful, such as blackout curtain, turning off the TV, using earplugs, night-lights.

Social Participation
- Encourage participation in social activities such as going to movies, going out to eat, attending a concert or sporting event, going to a party.

Sensorimotor
- Art-based media such as theater, music, or dance may assist in development of balance, exercise, or coordination.
- Provide instruction on energy conservation such as pacing (work and rest breaks).
- Provide bimanual training that requires repetitive practice using two-handed tasks that are within ability level and as close to age-appropriate level as possible.
- Provide strength training activities that involve repetitive, effortful muscle contraction (may include electric stimulation, biofeedback, or mental imagery).
- Motor imagery may be useful such as visualization, kinesthetic, auditory, or visual imagery of movement.
- Mirror therapy may be useful where hemiplegia is involved.
- Casting or splinting may be useful to reduce spasticity, improve joint range, and improve function.

Cognitive/Perceptual
- Token economy (behavior modification) may work well for some clients.
- Provide training in self-management, including goal setting and self-monitoring behaviors.
- Provide information on memory-assisting devices (calendars, notebooks, journals, daily planners) and electronic memory devices (alarms, cell phone apps, personal digital assistant).
- Provide opportunity to use executive functioning skills such as problem solving, using judgment of safety, planning a schedule, making a grocery list, following directions to complete a project.

Psychosocial
- Art-based media such as theater, music, painting, sculpture, and dance/movement may be useful to develop psychological and social skills such as group dynamics and self-awareness.
- The Wii program may be useful with some clients (Tatla et al., 2014).

Context/Environment
- Assistive devices may be useful with basic ADLs (built up or elongated handles, reachers/grabbers, buttonhooks, plate guards, sporks, sock aids).
- Virtual reality may useful in developing ability to move about community.
- Family or other caregivers may need information about home modification such as ramps, wider aisles to accommodate a wheelchair, grab bars, device management.
- Family or other caregivers may need information about community resources.

Precautions/Safety Considerations
Monitor for physical safety. Check for risk of seizures. Check for skin integrity to prevent pressure sores. Check for risk of deep venous thromboembolism risk.

Prognosis and Outcome
Variable depending on extent of injury and availability of rehabilitation services.

REFERENCES

Agnihotri, S., Gray, J., Colantonio, A., Polatajko, H., Cameron, D., Wiseman-Hakes, C., Rumney, P., & Keightley, M. (2012). Two case study evaluations of an arts-based social skills intervention for adolescents with childhood brain disorder. *Developmental Neurorehabilitation, 15*(4), 284–297. https://doi.org/10.3109/17518423.2012.673178

Agnihotri, S., Gray, J., Colantonio, A., Polatajko, H., Cameron, D., Wiseman-Hakes, C., Rumney, P., & Keightley, M. (2014). Arts-based social skills interventions for adolescents with acquired brain injuries: Five case reports. *Developmental Neurorehabilitation, 17*(1), 44–63. https://doi.org/10.1177/0308022617735036

Austin, D., Frater, T., Wales, L., & Dunford, C. (2018). Measuring changes in functional ability in older children and young people with acquired brain injury using the UK FIM+FAM. *British Journal of Occupational Therapy, 81*(2), 74–81. https://doi.org/10.1177/1308022617735036

Bart, O., Agam, T., Weiss, P., & Kizony, R. (2011). Using video-capture virtual reality for children with acquired brain injury. *Disability and Rehabilitation, 33*(17-18), 1579–1586. https://doi.org/10.3109/09638288.2010.540291

Baque, E., Barber, L., Sakzewski, L., & Boyd, R. N. (2017). Randomized controlled trial of web-based multimodal therapy for children with acquired brain injury to improve gross motor capacity and performance. *Clinical Rehabilitation, 31*(6), 722–732. https://doi.org/10.1177/0269215516651980

Baque, E., Sakzewski, L., Trost, S. G., Boyd, R. N., & Barber, L. (2017). Validity of accelerometry to measure physical activity intensity in children with an acquired brain injury. *Pediatric Physical Therapy, 29*(4), 322–329. https://doi.org/10.1097/PEP.0000000000000439

Bedell, G. M., Wade, S. L., Turkstra, L. S., Haarbauer-Krupa, J., & King, J. A. (2017). Informing design of an app-based coaching intervention to promote social participation of teenagers with traumatic brain injury. *Developmental Neurorehabilitation, 20*(7), 408–417. https://doi.org/10.1080/17518423.2016.1237584

Bennett, T. D., Niedzwecki, C. M., Korgenski, E. K., & Bratton, S. L. (2013). Initiation of physical, occupational, and speech therapy in children with traumatic brain injury. *Archives of Physical Medicine and Rehabilitation, 94*(7), 1268–1276. https://doi.org/10.1016/j.apmr.2013.02.021

Cheung, J., Maron, M., Tatla, S., & Jarus, T. (2013). Virtual reality as balance rehabilitation for children with brain injury: A case study. *Technology and Disability, 25*(3), 207–219. https://doi.org/10.3233/TAD-130383

Erez, N., Weiss, P. L., Kizony, R., & Rand, D. (2013). Comparing performance within a virtual supermarket of children with traumatic brain injury to typically developing children: A pilot study. *OTJR: Occupation, Participation and Health, 33*(4), 218–227. https://doi.org/10.3928/15394492-20130912-04

Golos, A., & Bedell, G. (2016). Psychometric properties of the Child and Adolescent Scale of Participation (CASP) across a 3-year period for children and youth with traumatic brain injury. *NeuroRehabilitation, 38*(4), 311–319. https://doi.org/10.3233/NRE-161322

Golos, A., & Bedell, G. (2018). Responsiveness and discriminant validity of the Child and Adolescent Scale of Participation across three years for children and youth with traumatic brain injury. *Developmental Neurorehabilitation, 21*(7), 431–438. https://doi.org/10.1080/17518423.2017.1342711

Jackman, M., Novak, I., Lannin, N. Froude, E., Miller, L., & Galea, C. (2018). Effectiveness of Cognitive Orientation to daily Occupational Performance over and above functional hand splints for children with cerebral palsy or brain injury: A randomized controlled trial. *BMC Pediatrics, 18*(1), Article 248. https://doi.org/10.1186/s12887-018-1213-9

Lindsay, S., Hartman, L. R., Reed, N., Gan, C., Thomson, N., & Solomon, B. (2015). A systematic review of hospital-to-school reintegration interventions for children and youth with acquired brain injury. *PLOS ONE, 10*(4), Article e0124679. https://doi.org/10.1371/journal.pone.0124679

Missiuna, C., DeMatteo, C., Hanna, S., Mandich, A., Law, M., Mahoney, W., & Scott, L. (2010). Exploring the use of cognitive intervention for children with acquired brain injury. *Physical & Occupational Therapy in Pediatrics, 30*(3), 205–219. https://doi.org/10.3109/01942631003761554

Narad, M. E., Bedell, G., King, J. A., Johnson, J., Turkstra, L. S., Haarbauer-Krupa, J., & Wade S. L. (2018). Social Participation and Navigation (SPAN): Description and usability of app-based coaching intervention for adolescents with TBI. *Developmental Neurorehabilitation, 21*(7), 439–448. https://doi.org/10.1080/17518423.2017.1354092

Sakzewski, L., Lewis, M. J., McKinlay, L., Ziviani, J., & Boyd, R. N. (2016). Impact of multi-modal web-based rehabilitation on occupational performance and upper limb outcomes: Pilot randomized trial in children with acquired brain injuries. *Developmental Medicine & Child Neurology, 58*(12), 1257–1264. https://doi.org/10.1111/dmcn.13157

Sakzewski, L., Lewis, M., & Ziviani, J. (2017). Test–retest reproducibility of the Assessment of Motor and Process Skills for school-aged children with acquired brain injuries. *Scandinavian Journal of Occupational Therapy, 24*(3), 161–166. https://doi.org/10.3109/11038128.2016.1152296

Tatla, S. K., Radomski, A., Cheung, J., Maron, M., & Jarus, T. (2014). Wii-habilitation as balance therapy for children with acquired brain injury. *Developmental Neurorehabilitation, 17*(1), 1–15. https://doi.org/10.3109/17518423.2012.740508

Thompson, M., Elliott, C., Willis, C., Ward, R., Falkmer, M., Falkmer, T., Gubbay, A., & Girdler, S. (2016). Can, want and try: Parents' viewpoints regarding the participation of their child with an acquired brain injury. *PLOS ONE, 11*(7), Article e0157951. https://doi.org/10.1371/journal.pone.0157951

Titchener, A., Dunford, C., & Wales, L. (2018). A reflective case review: Relearning handwriting after a traumatic brain injury. *British Journal of Occupational Therapy, 81*(5), 290–293. https://doi.org/10.1177/0308022617752066

Twyford, K., & Watters, S. (2016, February 9). In the groove: An evaluation to explore a joint music therapy and occupational therapy intervention for children with acquired brain injury. *Voices, 16*(1). https://doi.org/10.15845/voices.v16i1.851

Wade, S. L., Bedell, G., King, J. A., Jacquin, M., Turkstra, L. S., Haarbauer-Krupa, J., Johnson, J., Salloum, R., & Narad, M. E. (2018). Social Participation and Navigation (SPAN) program for adolescents with acquired brain injury: Pilot findings. *Rehabilitation Psychology, 63*(3), 327–337. https://doi.org/10.1037/rep0000187

BIBLIOGRAPHY

Agnihotri, S., Keightley, M. L., Colantonio, A., Cameron, D., & Polatajko, H. (2010). Community integration interventions for youth with acquired brain injuries: A review. *Developmental Neurorehabilitation, 13*(5), 369–382. https://doi.org/10.3109/17518423.2010.499409

Anaby, D., Law, M., Hanna, S., & Dematteo, C. (2012). Predictors of change in participation rates following acquired brain injury: Results of a longitudinal study. *Developmental Medicine & Child Neurology, 54*(4), 339–346. https://doi.org/10.1111/j.1469-8749.2011.04204.x

Baque, E., Barber, L., Sakzewski, L., & Boyd, R. N. (2016). Reproducibility in measuring physical activity in children and adolescents with an acquired brain injury. *Brain Injury, 30*(13-14), 1692–1698. https://doi.org/10.1080/02699052.2016.1201594

Baque, E., Barber, L., Sakzewski, L., & Boyd, R. N. (2016). Test–re-test reproducibility of activity capacity measures for children with an acquired brain injury. *Brain Injury, 30*(9), 1143–1149. https://doi.org/10.3109/02699052.2016.1165869

Baque, E., Barber, L., Sakzewski, L., Ware, R., & Boyd, R. N. (2017). Characteristics associated with physical activity capacity and performance in children and adolescents with an acquired brain injury. *Brain Injury, 31*(5), 667–673. https://doi.org/10.1080/02699052.2017.1291990

Chan, V., Mann, R. E., Pole, J. D., & Colantonio, A. (2015). Children and youth with "unspecified injury to the head": Implications for traumatic brain injury research and surveillance. *Emerging Themes in Epidemiology, 12*, Article 9. https://doi.org/10.1186/s12982-015-0031-x

Chan, V., Pole, J. D., Mann, R. E., & Colantonio, A. (2015). A population based perspective on children and youth with brain tumours. *BMC Cancer, 15*, Article 1007. https://doi.org/10.1186/s12885-015-2016-0

Chan, V., Thurairajah, P., & Colantonio, A. (2013). Defining traumatic brain injury in children and youth using International Classification of Diseases Version 10 codes: A systematic review protocol. *Systematic Reviews, 2*, Article 102. https://doi.org/10.1186/2046-4053-2-102

College of Occupational Therapists. (2015). *Children and young people with acquired brain injury: Current practice in occupational therapy.*

Dunford, C., Bannigan, K., & Wales, L. (2013). Measuring activity and participation outcomes for children and young people with acquired brain injury: An occupational therapy perspective. *British Journal of Occupational Therapy, 76*(2), 67–76. https://doi.org/10.4276/030802213X13603244419158

Galvin, J., Froude, E., & McAleer, J. (2010). Children's participation in home, school and community life after acquired brain injury. *Australian Occupational Therapy Journal, 57*(2), 118–126. https://doi.org/10.1111/j.1440-1630.2009.00822.x

Gordon, A. L., & di Maggio, A. (2012). Rehabilitation for children after acquired brain injury: Current and emerging approaches. *Pediatric Neurology, 46*(6), 339–344. https://doi.org/10.1016/j.pediatrneurol.2012.02.029

Jones, M., Hocking, C., & McPherson, K. (2017). Communities with participation-enabling skills: A study of children with traumatic brain injury and their shared occupations. *Journal of Occupational Science, 24*(1), 88–104. https://doi.org/10.1080/14427591.2016.1224444

Lindsay, S., Proulx, M., Maxwell, J., Hamdani, Y., Bayley M., Macarthur, C., & Colantonio, A. (2016). Gender and transition from pediatric to adult health care among youth with acquired brain injury: Experiences in a transition model. *Archives of Physical Medicine and Rehabilitation, 97*(2, Suppl.), S33–S39. https://doi.org/10.1016/j.apmr.2014.04.032

Peranich, L., Reynolds, K. B., O'Brien, S., Bosch, J., & Cranfill, T. (2010). The roles of occupational therapy, physical therapy, and speech/language pathology in primary care. *Journal for Nurse Practitioners, 6*(1), 36–43. https://doi.org/10.1016/j.nurpra.2009.08.021

Rivara, F. P., Ennis, S. K., Mangione-Smith, R., MacKenzie, E. J., Jaffe, K. M., & National Expert Panel for the Development of Pediatric Rehabilitation Quality Care Indicators. (2012). Quality of care indicators for the rehabilitation of children with traumatic brain injury. *Archives of Physical Medicine and Rehabilitation, 93*(3), 381–385. https://doi.org/10.1016/j.apmr.2011.08.015

Sakzewski, L., Lewis, M. J., McKinlay, L., Ziviani, J., & Boyd, R. N. (2017). Sakzewski et al. reply. *Developmental Medicine & Child Neurology, 59*(3), 336–337. https://doi.org/10.1111/dmcn.13235

Tatla, S. K., Sauve, K., Jarus, T., Virji-Babul, N., & Holsti, L. (2014). The effects of motivating interventions on rehabilitation outcomes in children and youth with acquired brain injuries: A systematic review. *Brain Injury, 28*(8), 1022–1035. https://doi.org/10.3109/02699052.2014.890747

Tousignant, B., Jackson, P. L., Massicotte, E., Beauchamp, M. H., Achim, A. M., Vera-Estay, E., Bedell, G., & Sirois, K. (2018). Impact of traumatic brain injury on social cognition and adolescents in contribution of other higher order cognitive functions. *Neuropsychological Rehabilitation, 28*(3), 429–447. https://doi.org/10.1080/09602011.2016.1158114

Wales, L., Hawley, C., & Sidebotham, P. (2013). How an occupational therapist should conceptualise self-awareness following traumatic brain injury in childhood—A literature review. *British Journal of Occupational Therapy, 76*(7), 325–332. https://doi.org/10.4276/030802213X13729279115013

Wiseman-Hakes, C., Saleem, M., Poulin, V., Nalder, E., Balachandran, P., Gan, C., & Colantonio, A. (2020). The development of intimate relationships in adolescent girls and women with traumatic brain injury: A framework to guide gender specific rehabilitation and enhance positive social outcomes. *Disability and Rehabilitation, 42*(24), 3559–3565. https://doi.org/10.1080/09638288.2019.1597180

Ziviani, J., Desha, L., Feeney, R., & Boyd, R. (2010). Measures of participation outcomes and environmental considerations for children with acquired brain injury: A systematic review. *Brain Impairment, 11*(2), 93–112. https://doi.org/10.1375/brim.11.2.93

Concussion and Post-Concussion

Also called mild brain injury, mild head injuries.
See also Brain Injuries: Adult, Brain Injuries: Child and Adolescent.

Description

A concussion is a transient and reversible posttraumatic alteration in mental status, such as loss of consciousness or memory, or confusion, lasting from seconds to minutes but less than 6 hours. Gross structural brain lesions and serious neurologic residua are not part of concussion, although temporary disability can occur due to symptoms such as nausea, headache, dizziness, memory disturbance, and difficulty concentrating (post-concussion syndrome) that usually resolve within weeks (Porter, 2018). Persistent symptoms exist when neurologic or psychiatric conditions were present before the concussion (Finn, 2019).

Cause

Etiology includes violent shaking or jarring as might occur as a result of a motorized vehicle crash (cars, trucks, vans, buses, motorcycles, sports carts), nonmotorized transportation crash (bicycles, scooters, collision with pedestrians), fall (especially in older adults and young children), assault, and sports activities (Porter, 2018).

Evaluation/Assessment

Areas
- Activities of Daily Living/Instrumental ADL: basic and independent living
- Education/Work: academic performance, work requirements, reading comprehension
- Play/Leisure: child—stages of play development; adult—interests, frequency, location
- Rest/Sleep: sleep disturbance
- Social Participation: type, frequency, location, with whom (family, friends, peers, colleagues)
- Sensorimotor: dizziness, fatigue, headache, visual, vestibular, auditory, sensory processing
- Cognitive/Perceptual: attention and concentration, memory especially working memory, executive functions (time management, problem solving, decision making, judgment of safety)
- Psychosocial: nervousness, worry, depression, anxiety, role performance, quality of life
- Context/Environment: environmental modifications, knowledge/education of resources, social support
- Comorbidities: existing health conditions, depression, anxiety

Instruments
Instruments Developed by Occupational Therapy Personnel
- Assessment of Motor and Process Skills (8th ed.; AMPS-8; Fisher & Bray Jones, 2016)
- Canadian Occupational Performance Measure (5th ed.; COPM-5; Law et al., 2014)
- Charge of Quarters (CQ) Duty Task (Smith et al., 2014, in References)
- National Institutes of Health (NIH) Activity Record (ACTRE) (NIH-ACTRE; Gerber & Furst, 1992)
- Occupational Domains (OD; Harris et al., 2019, in References)
- Occupational Gaps Questionnaire (OGQ; Eriksson et al., 2013, in References)
- Weekly Calendar Planning Activity (WCPA; Toglia, 2015)

Instruments Developed by Other Professionals and Used by Occupational Therapy Personnel
- Acute Concussion Evaluation (ACE; Gioia, 2019)
- Concussion Symptom Inventory (CSI; Randolph et al., 2009)
- Convergence Insufficiency Symptom Survey–Revised (CISS; Rouse et al., 2004)
- Developmental Eye Movement Test (DEMT; Garzia et al., 1990)
- Developmental Test of Visual Perception–Adolescent and Adult (2nd ed.; DTVP-A:2; Reynolds et al., 2021)
- Dynavision (D2; Dynavision International, 2016)
- Fatigue Severity Scale (FSS; Krupp et al., 1989)
- Functional Outcomes of Sleep Questionnaire (FOSQ; Weaver et al., 1997)
- Glasgow Coma Scale (GCS; Teasdale & Jennett, 1974; see https://www.glasgowcomascale.org)
- Injury Severity Score (ISS; Baker et al., 1974)
- King-Devick Test (KDT; King-Devick Technologies)
- Military Acute Concussion Evaluation (MACE; French et al., 2008)
- Patient Competency Rating Scale (PCRS; Prigatano & Fordyce, 1986)
- Pittsburgh Sleep Quality Index (PSQI; Buysse et al., 1989)
- Postconcussion Symptom Inventory (PCSI; Sady et al., 2014)
- Rivermead Post Concussion Symptoms Questionnaire (RPCSQ; King et al., 1995)
- Short-Form 36 Health Survey (SF-36; Ware et al., 1993)
- Sport Concussion Assessment Tool (5th ed., SCAT-5; Echemendia et al., 2017)

Problems/Issues

Activities of Daily Living/Instrumental ADL
- Child may experience nausea and vomiting.

Education/Work
- Child may be unable to complete assignments that involve reading (visual attention, visual tracking).
- Child may be unable to concentrate to complete tests.
- Child may have reduced reading speed and accuracy.

Play/Leisure
- Child may be limited by physician on amount of screen time (TV, computer, tablet, phone) during initial time period after concussion (1 to 2 weeks).
- Child usually is restricted on engagement in active sports until symptoms clear.

Rest/Sleep
- Child may experience excessive daytime sleepiness even with normal sleep schedule.
- Child may sleep more or less than normal.
- Child may be drowsy.
- Child may have difficulty falling asleep or staying asleep.

Social Participation
- Child may experience difficulty participating in social occupations due to physical, cognitive, and/or psychological symptoms such as blurred vision, balance problems, difficulty concentrating, fatigue, confusion, irritability, anxiety, and others.
- Child may prefer to avoid crowds or events that are noisy.

Sensorimotor
- Child often has headache.
- Child may report more fatigue than usual.
- Child may have balance problems.
- Child may experience sense of dizziness (spinning or movement sensation).
- Child may experience numbness or tingling.

- Child may have visual problems, such as decreased contrast sensitivity or increased sensitivity to light and glare.
- Child may have ocular motor dysfunction such as impaired fixation, saccadic eye movement, or smooth pursuits.
- Child may have binocular vision disorders such as convergence insufficiency or excess.
- Child may have accommodative insufficiency that impacts focusing ability, especially when transitioning gaze from near to far or vice versa.
- Child may experience eye strain, visual fatigue, blurry vision, diplopia (double vision).
- Child may have auditory problems such as increased sensitivity to noise or sounds.
- Child or adult may experience "ringing in the ears" (tinnitus).

Cognitive/Perceptual

- Child may have difficulty paying attention and maintaining concentration.
- Child may have difficulty remembering, or forgets recent information.
- Child may be confused about recent events.
- Child may answer questions slowly.
- Child may ask to have questions repeated.
- Child may have visual perceptual dysfunction resulting in poor visual motor integration, impaired visual spatial skills such as poor peripheral awareness, impaired figure–ground ability, or decreased reaction time and processing speed.

Psychosocial

- Child/adult may experience a loss of identity as a team member (military or sport) because he or she cannot participate as planned.
- Child/adult may feel he or she has "let the team down" because he or she cannot participate as planned.
- Child may report feeling nervous or be worried or anxious more than usual.
- Child may be more irritable than normal.
- Child may experience feelings of sadness or show signs of depression (Stazyk et al., 2017).
- Child may be more emotional than usual.
- Child may report feeling as though in a fog.
- Child may be reluctant (lack motivation) to reengage in activities and occupations.

Context/Environment

- Child, family, friends, and peers may lack information, knowledge, and understanding about the effects of a concussion and post-concussion symptoms.

Intervention/Treatment

Models and programs developed by occupational therapy practitioners include case study (Colbourn, 2017), client-centered, occupation-based model (Finn, 2019), Return to School (RTS) protocol (DeMatteo et al., 2015), return to work (Acord-Vira et al., 2018), and stages of change model of behavior modification (Brayton-Chung et al., 2016). Models and programs developed by other professionals but used by occupational therapy personnel include hand self-shiatsu (Qin et al., 2019), mindfulness-based yoga (Paniccia et al., 2019), multimodal approach (Reed et al., 2014), and patrol-exertion multitask (Scherer et al., 2018). Current general guidelines for treating concussion deemphasize the complete rest approach recommended in the past, and "highlight the importance of a graded return to activity that does not significantly provoke or exacerbate symptoms" referred to as a "symptom-limited approach" where activity is terminated if symptoms worsen (Finn, 2019, p. 2). Team members include physicians, nursing personnel, psychologists, athletic trainers, recreation specialists, speech–language pathologists or speech therapists, physical therapy personnel, and occupational therapy personnel. The focus of occupational therapy is to address occupational performance skills and patterns that will promote the return to engagement and participation in meaningful and purposeful activities as quickly as symptom abatement occurs (Brayton-Chung et al., 2016).

Activities of Daily Living/Instrumental ADL
- No information identified.

Education/Work
- Return-to-school protocol adapted (DeMatteo et al., 2015)
  - ► Stage 1: Brain Rest–No School (timetable about 1 week).
    - o No school for at least 1 week.
    - o Cognitive rest: No TV, video games, testing, reading.
    - o When symptom free, move to Stage 2.
  - ► Stage 2: Getting Ready to Go Back (timetable about 2 weeks post-concussion).
    - o Start this stage 2 days prior to going back to school.
    - o Begin grade activity guided by symptoms (walking, 15 minutes of screen time twice daily, begin reading).
    - o If symptoms worsen, reduce activity.
    - o When symptom free, move to Stage 3.
  - ► Stage 3: Back to School/Modified Academics (timetable may last days or months).
    - o Have a quiet retreat space at school and get lots of sleep at home.
    - o Modify academics.
      - ▷ Attendance: Start attendance with 1 hour, then half days, then every other day.
      - ▷ Curriculum: Attend less stressful classes, no tests, homework in 15-minute blocks up to a maximum of 45 minutes daily.
      - ▷ Environment: Preferential seating, avoid music class, gym class, cafeteria, taking the bus, carrying heavy books.
      - ▷ Activities: Limit screen/TV time into 15-minute blocks up to 1 hour daily.
    - o When symptom free, move to Stage 4.
    - o If symptoms persist past 4 weeks recovery, an Individualized Education Program (IEP) may be needed.
  - ► Stage 4: Nearly Normal Routines
    - o Attend full day of school but may attend less than 5 days per week.
    - o Complete as much homework as possible and a maximum of one test per week.
    - o When symptom free, move to Stage 5.
  - ► Stage 5: Full Activation
    - o Gradual return to normal routines, including attendance, homework, tests, and extra-curricular activities.
- Return-to-work protocol (Acord-Vira et al., 2018)
  - ► Rest: Avoid activities in all environments (home, work, leisure) that are known to exacerbate signs and symptoms such as long hours, stressful projects or situations, overstimulating environments, strenuous physical or cognitive activities.
  - ► Light duty physical or cognitive job-related tasks: Focus on implementing strategies and accommodations to facilitate a gradual, progressive plan to engage in work-related activities while managing symptoms.
  - ► Job-specific activities: Focus on adapting the work environment and essential job functions such as taking rest breaks, shorting time frames, working in quieter environment, wearing a cap to reduce glare from overhead lights and consideration for potential concerns such as preventing further injury on the job, or inability to perform at preinjury status.
  - ► Return to full work duty: Focus on implementing individualized plan including educating coworkers and supervisor regarding employee's status.

Play/Leisure
- Return-to-play protocol (as summarized in Finn, 2019)
  - ► Stage 1: Symptom-free activity: Engage in activity of daily living not causing symptoms with goal of returning to work and school activities as tolerated.
  - ► Stage 2: Light aerobic exercise: Stationary bicycle or walking with goal to raise heart rate.

- ▶ Stage 3: Sport-specific activities: Running, swimming, with goal to incorporate movement.
- ▶ Stage 4: Noncontact practice: Resistance training, sports simulation without potential of head injury with goal of providing exercises requiring coordination and thinking.
- ▶ Stage 5: Full contact practice: Simulation of sport activities, normal training activities with goal of building confidence and allowing assessment by athletic staff.
- ▶ Stage 6: Return to sport: Game play.

Rest/Sleep

- When symptoms are present, daytime naps and rest periods are needed. As symptoms are reduced and physical activity increases, decrease daytime napping and encourage return to nighttime sleeping.
- Suggest limiting screen usage in bed.
- Recommend light-blocking curtains.
- Provide instruction in sleep hygiene (see Sleep–Wake Disorders in Section 13: Lifestyle Conditions).

Social Participation

- No information identified.

Sensorimotor

- Provide energy (conservation) management strategies.
- Provide aerobic physical exercise.
- Provide sport coordination drills.
- Adaptive devices for visual deficit may include use of various colored overlaps and filters such as amber or blue transparencies to decrease brightness and increase contrast.
- Blue-light filters may be used with cell phones and computer screens.
- Dimming the room lights and dimming the computer screen display may reduce glare.
- Consider if a sensory diet would facilitate management of sensory sensitivities.

Cognitive/Perceptual

- Create a balanced activity schedule that may include environmental modifications, assistive technology, activity modifications, and strategies for pacing and energy conservation.
- Client-centered, occupation-based model (Finn, 2019)
  - ▶ Recognition and evaluation (focus on how activity demands or environmental factors may have contributed to symptoms).
    - ○ Recognize and identify symptoms and impact on occupational performance.
    - ○ Recognize internal and external factors that contribute to symptoms.
  - ▶ Rest (relative rest: stop any activity that increases symptoms).
    - ○ Rest-cognitive.
    - ○ Recommendations for strategic rest.
  - ▶ Resume activity with recommendations (focus on establishing parameters to ensure activity challenges are below or at the subsymptom threshold).
    - ○ Return to activity with graduated approach.
    - ○ Recommendation for subsymptom threshold activity.
  - ▶ Reflect and reevaluation (focus on developing awareness of how strategies or other factors may influence participation, engagement, and overall satisfaction with occupational performance).
    - ○ Reflect on activity level and associated symptoms.
    - ○ Reevaluate occupational performance.
    - ○ Recalibrate as needed.
  - ▶ Resume all activities: Restriction free.

Psychosocial

- Reengagement in activity to promote self-confidence.
- Mindfulness-based techniques for stress reduction and relaxation training.

Context/Environment
- Include family and caregivers in intervention program plan and goals.
- Provide information to family and caregivers as to what to expect during recovery.

Precautions/Safety Considerations

Red flag warnings: headaches worsen, seizure occurs, repeated vomiting, slurred speech, cannot be awakened, cannot recognize people or places, increasing confusion or irritability, neck pain, weakness in arms or legs, unusual behavioral change, change in state of consciousness, focal neurologic signs (Porter, 2018).

Prognosis and Outcome

Symptoms usually resolve within 3 months but some individuals may experience continuing impairment (Cogan et al., 2019).

REFERENCES

Acord-Vira, A., Davis, D., Wheeler, S., & Cannoy, A. (2018). Occupational therapy's role in return to work after a concussion. *SIS Quarterly Practice Connections, 3*(2), 31–33.

Brayton-Chung, A., Finch, N., & Keilty, K. D. (2016). Back in action: The role of occupational therapy in concussion rehabilitation. *OT Practice, 21*(21), 8–12.

Cogan, A. M., Haines, C. E., Devore, M. D., Lepore, K. M., & Ryan, M. (2019). Occupational challenges in military service members with chronic mild traumatic brain injury. *American Journal of Occupational Therapy, 73*(3), Article 7303205040. https://doi.org/10.5014/ajot.2019.027599

Colbourn, J. (2017). Lived experience of an occupational therapist living with post-concussion symptoms. *Occupational Therapy Now, 19*(3), 20–21.

DeMatteo, C., Stazyk, K., Giglia, L., Mahoney, W., Singh, S. K., Hollenberg, R., Harper, J. A., Missiuna, C., Law, M., McCauley, D., & Randall, S. (2015). A balanced protocol for return to school for children and youth following concussive injury. *Clinical Pediatrics, 54*(8), 783–792. https://doi.org/10.1177/0009922814567305

Eriksson, G., Tham, K., & Kottorp, A. (2013). A cross-diagnostic validation of an instrument measuring participation in everyday occupations: The Occupational Gaps Questionnaire (OGQ). *Scandinavian Journal of Occupational Therapy, 20*(2), 152–160. https://doi.org/10.3109/11038 128.2012.749944

Finn, C. (2019). An occupation-based approach to management of concussion: Guidelines for practice. *Open Journal of Occupational Therapy, 7*(2), Article 11. https://doi.org/10.15453/2168 -6408.1550

Harris, M. B., Rafeedie, S., McArthur, D., Babikian, T., Snyder, A., Polster, D., & Giza, C. C. (2019). Addition of occupational therapy to an interdisciplinary concussion clinic improves identification of functional impairments. *Journal of Head Trauma Rehabilitation, 34*(6), 425–432. https://doi.org/10.1097/htr.0000000000000544

Paniccia, M., Knafo, R., Thomas, S., Taha, T., Ladha, A., Thompson, L., & Reed, N. (2019). Mindfulness-based yoga for youth with persistent concussion: A pilot study. *American Journal of Occupational Therapy, 73*(1), Article 7301205040. https://doi.org/10.5014/ajot.2019.027672

Porter, R. S. (Ed.). (2018). *The Merck manual of diagnosis and therapy* (20th ed.). Merck Sharp & Dohme.

Qin, P., Dick, B. D., Leung, A., & Brown, C. A. (2019). Effectiveness of hand self-shiatsu to improve sleep following sport-related concussion in young athletes: A proof-of-concept study. *Journal of Integrative Medicine, 17*(1), 24–29. https://doi.org/10.1016/j.joim.2018.11.002

Reed, N., Murphy, J., Dick, T., Mah, K., Paniccia M., Verweel, L., Dobney, D., & Keightley, M. (2014). A multi-modal approach to assessing recovery in youth athletes following concussion. *Journal of Visualized Experiments, 91*, Article e51892. https://doi.org/10.3791/51892

Scherer, M. R., Weightman, M. M., Radomski, M. V., Smith, L., Finkelstein, M., Cecchini, A. Heaton, K. J., & McCulloch, K. (2018). Measuring soldier performance during the Patrol-Exertion Multitask: Preliminary validation of a postconcussive functional return-to-duty metric. *Archives of Physical Medicine and Rehabilitation, 99*(2, Suppl.), S79–S85. https://doi.org/10.1016/j.apmr.2017.04.012

Smith, L. B., Radomski, M. V., Davidson, L. F., Finkelstein, M., Weightman, M. M., McCulloch, K. L., & Scherer, M. R. (2014). Development and preliminary reliability of a multitasking assessment for executive functioning after concussion. *American Journal of Occupational Therapy, 68*(4), 439–443. https://doi.org/10.5014/ajot.2014.012393

Stazyk, K., DeMatteo, C., Moll, S., & Missiuna, C. (2017). Depression in youth recovering from concussion: Correlates and predictors. *Brain Injury, 31*(5), 631–638. https://doi.org/10.1080/02699052.2017.1283533

BIBLIOGRAPHY

Cogan, A. M. (2014). Occupational needs and intervention strategies for military personnel with mild traumatic brain injury and persistent post-concussion symptoms: A review. *OTJR: Occupation, Participation & Health, 34*(3), 150–159. https://doi.org/10.3928/15394492-20140617-01

Cogan, A. M., Huang, J., & Philip, J. (2019). Military service member perspectives about occupational therapy treatment in a military concussion clinic. *OTJR: Occupation, Participation and Health, 39*(4), 232–238. https://doi.org/10.1177/1539449218813849

DeMatteo, C., McCauley, D., Stazyk, K., Harper, J., Adamich, J., Randall, S., & Missiuna, C. (2015). Post-concussion return to play and return to school guidelines for children and youth: A scoping methodology. *Disability and Rehabilitation, 37*(12), 1107–1112. https://doi.org/10.3109/09638288.2014.952452

DeMatteo, C., Stazyk, K., Singh, S. K., Giglia, L., Hollenberg, R., Malcolmson, C. H., Mahoney, W., Harper, J. A., Missiuna, C., Law, M., & McCauley, D. (2015). Development of a conservative protocol to return children and youth to activity following concussive injury. *Clinical Pediatrics, 54*(2), 152–163. https://doi.org/10.1177/0009922814558256

Finn, C., & Waskiewicz, M. (2015). The role of occupational therapy in managing post-concussive syndrome. *Physical Disabilities Special Interest Section Quarterly, 38*(1), 1–4.

Gauvin-Lepage, J., Friedman, D., Grilli, L., Sufrategui, M., De Matteo, C., Iverson, G. L., & Gagnon, I. (2020). Effectiveness of an exercise-based active rehabilitation intervention for youth who are slow to recover after concussion. *Clinical Journal of Sport Medicine, 30*(5), 423–432. https://doi.org/10.1097/JSM.0000000000000634

Gosselin, N., Saluja, R. S., Chen, J. K., Bottari, C., Johnston, K., & Ptito, A. (2010). Brain functions after sports-related concussion: Insights from event-related potentials and functional MRI. *Physician and Sportsmedicine, 38*(3), 27–37. https://doi.org/10.3810/psm.2010.10.1805

Hunt, A. W., De Feo, L., Macintyre, J., Greenspoon, D., Dick, T., Mah, K., Paniccia, M., Providenza, C., & Reed, N. (2016). Development and feasibility of an evidence-informed self-management education program in pediatric concussion rehabilitation. *BMC Health Services Research, 16*, Article 400. https://doi.org/10.1186/s12913-016-1664-3

Hunt, A. W., Laupacis, D., Kawaguchi, E., Greenspoon, D., & Reed, N. (2018). Key ingredients to an active rehabilitation programme post-concussion: Perspectives of youth and parents. *Brain Injury, 32*(12), 1534–1540. https://doi.org/10.1080/02699052.2018.1502894

Hunt, A. W., Paniccia, M., Mah, K., Dawson, D., & Reed, N. (2019). Feasibility and effects of the CO-OP Approach in postconcussion rehabilitation. *American Journal of Occupational Therapy, 73*(1), Article 7301205060. https://doi.org/10.5014/ajot.2019.027995

Hunt, A. W., Paniccia, M., Reed, N., & Keightley, M. (2016). Concussion-like symptoms in child and youth athletes at baseline: What is "typical"? *Journal of Athletic Training, 51*(10), 749–757. https://doi.org/10.4085/1062-6050-51.11.12

Jaber, A. F., Hartwell, J., & Radel, J. D. (2019). Interventions to address the needs of adults with postconcussion syndrome: A systematic review. *American Journal of Occupational Therapy, 73*(1), Article 7301205030. https://doi.org/10.5014/ajot.2019.028993

Keightley, M. L., Côté, P., Rumney, P., Hung, R., Carroll, L. J., Cancelliere, C., & Cassidy, J. D. (2014). Psychosocial consequences of mild traumatic brain injury in children: Results of a systematic review by the International Collaboration on Mild Traumatic Brain Injury Prognosis. *Archives of Physical Medicine and Rehabilitation, 95*(3, Suppl.), S192–S200. https://doi.org/10.1016/j.apmr.2013.12.018

Lax, I. D., Paniccia, M., Agnihotri, S., Reed, N., Garmaise, E., Azadbakhsh, M., Ng, J., Monette, G., Wiseman-Hakes, C., Taha, T., & Keightley, M. (2015). Developmental and gender influences on executive function following concussion in youth hockey players. *Brain Injury, 29*(12), 1409–1419. https://doi.org/10.3109/02699052.2015.1043344

McDonald, T., Burghart, M. A., & Nazir, N. (2016). Underreporting of concussions and concussion-like symptoms in female high school athletes. *Journal of Trauma Nursing, 23*(5), 241–246. https://doi.org/10.1097/JTN.0000000000000227

McInnes, K., Friesen, C. L., MacKenzie, D. E., Westwood, D. A., & Boe, S. G. (2017). Mild traumatic brain injury (mTBI) and chronic cognitive impairment: A scoping review. *PLOS ONE, 12*(4), Article e0174847. https://doi.org/10.1371/journal.pone.0174847

Mollayeva, T., Cassidy, J. D., Shapiro, C. M., Mollayeva, S., & Colantonio, A. (2017). Concussion/mild traumatic brain injury-related chronic pain in males and females: A diagnostic modelling study. *Medicine, 96*(7), Article e5917. https://doi.org/10.1097/MD.0000000000005917

Mollayeva, T., Stock, D., & Colantonio, A. (2019). Physiological and pathological covariates of persistent concussion-related fatigue: Results from two regression methodologies. *Brain Injury, 33*(4), 463–479. https://doi.org/10.1080/02699052.2019.1566833

Mortenson, P., Singhal, A., Hengel, A. R., & Purtzki, J. (2016). Impact of early follow-up intervention on parent-reported postconcussion pediatric symptoms: A feasibility study. *Journal of Head Trauma and Rehabilitation, 31*(6), E23–E32. https://doi.org/10.1097/HTR.0000000000000223

Paniccia, M., & Reed, N. P. (2017). Dove and hawk profiles in youth concussion: Rethinking occupational performance. *Canadian Journal of Occupational Therapy, 84*(2), 111–118. https://doi.org/10.1177/0008417416688302

Paniccia, M., Taha, T., Keightley, M., Thomas, S., Verweel, L., Murphy, J., Wilson, K., & Reed, N. (2018). Autonomic function following concussion in youth athletes: An exploration of heart rate variability using 24-hour recording methodology. *Journal of Visualized Experiments, 139*, e58203. https://doi.org/10.3791/58203

Paniccia, M., Verweel, L., Thomas, S. G., Taha, T., Keightley, M., Wilson, K. E., & Reed, N. (2018). Heart rate variability following youth concussion: How do autonomic regulation and concussion symptoms differ over time postinjury? *BMJ Open Sport & Exercise Medicine, 4*(1), Article e000355. https://doi.org/10.1136/bmjsem-2018-000355

Reed, N. (2011). Sport-related concussion and occupational therapy: Expanding the scope of practice. *Physical & Occupational Therapy in Pediatrics, 31*(3), 222–224. https://doi.org/10.3109/01942638.2011.589719

Reed, N., Greenspoon, D., Iverson, G. L., DeMatteo, C., Fait, P., Gauvin-Lepage, J., Hunt, A., & Gagnon, I. J. (2015). Management of persistent postconcussion symptoms in youth: A randomised control trial protocol. *BMJ Open, 5*(7), Article e008468. https://doi.org/10.1136/bmjopen-2015-008468

Reed, N., Leeder, K., & Zemek, R. (2018). Patient engagement in pediatric concussion research. *CMAJ, 190*(Suppl.), S28–S30. https://doi.org/10.1503/cmaj.180450

Reed, N. P. (2012). Concussion in hockey: Taking an occupational perspective on risk in sports. *Canadian Journal of Occupational Therapy, 79*(1), 5–6. https://doi.org/10.1177/000841741207900101

Sang, R. C., Vawda, Y., Greenspoon, D., Reed, N., & Hunt, A. W. (2020). An innovative approach to measuring youth concussion recovery. Occupational performance. *British Journal of Occupational Therapy, 83*(4), 220–227. https://doi.org/10.1177/0308022619851415

Schmidt, J., Hayward, K. S., Brown, K. E., Zwicker, J. G., Ponsford, J., van Donkelaar, P., Babul, S., & Boyd, L. A. (2018). Imaging in pediatric concussion: A systematic review. *Pediatrics, 141*(5), Article e20173406. https://doi.org/10.1542/peds.2017-3406

Simpson-Jones, M. E., & Hunt, A. W. (2019). Vision rehabilitation interventions following mild traumatic brain injury: A scoping review. *Disability and Rehabilitation, 41*(18), 2206–2222. https://doi.org/10.1080/09638288.2018.1460407

Stephens, J. A., Davies, P. L., Gavin, W. J., Mostofsky, S. H., Slomine, B. S., & Suskauer, S. J. (2020). Evaluating motor control improves discrimination of adolescents with and without sports related concussion. *Journal of Motor Behavior, 52*(1), 13–21. https://doi.org/10.1080/002228 95.2019.1570908

Sutton, M., Chan, V., Escobar, M., Mollayeva, T., Hu, Z., & Colantonio, A. (2019). Neck injury comorbidity in concussion-related emergency department visits: A population-based study of sex differences across the life span. *Journal of Women's Health, 28*(4), 473–482. https://doi .org/10.1089/jwh.2018.7282

Sveen, U., Bautz-Holter, E., Sandvik, L., Alvsåker, K., & Røe, C. (2010). Relationship between competency in activities, injury severity, and post-concussion symptoms after traumatic brain injury. *Scandinavian Journal of Occupational Therapy, 17*(3), 225–232. https://doi.org/10 .3109/11038120903171295

Wiseman-Hakes, C., Gosselin, N., Sharma, B., Langer, L., & Gagnon, I. (2019). A longitudinal investigation of sleep and daytime wakefulness in children and youth with concussion. *ASN Neuro, 11*. https://doi.org/10.1177/1759091418822405

Distal Radial Fracture

Also called Colles' fracture, Smith's fracture, Barton's fracture, DRF.
See also Complex Regional Pain Syndrome, Peripheral Nerve Injuries, Stiff Hand.

Description

Distal fracture of the radius usually results in dorsal displacement or angulation of the fractured section of the radius wrist bone (Colles' fracture). Volar or palmar displacement of the fractured section is called a Smith's fracture. The ulnar styloid process may also be fractured (R. S. Porter, 2018). Barton's fracture is an intra-articular fracture of the distal radius with dislocation of the radiocarpal joint. Chauffeur's fracture is a fracture of the radial styloid process. Monteggia fracture is an unstable fracture of the ulnar shaft and radial head dislocation (Moscony & Shank, 2014). Distal radial fractures are more common in young children due to high impact sports and in older women due to loss of bone density. Associated soft tissue injuries may include triangular fibrocartilage complex (TFCC), peripheral nerve injury, ligament sprain or tear, and aggravation of preexisting osteoarthritis.

Cause

The most common cause is a fall in which the person attempts to stop the fall (or forward motion) by extending the upper extremity and hyperextending the wrist and hand (Colles' fracture). Cause is also described as a "fall on outstretched hand" (FOOSH). In the case of Smith's fracture, the wrist was flexed during the injury (R. S. Porter, 2018). Barton's fracture is caused by shearing forces from the proximal carpus translating across the radius (Moscony & Shank, 2014).

Evaluation/Assessment

Areas
- Activities of Daily Living/Instrumental ADL: self-maintenance skills
- Education/Work: work tasks, equipment used
- Play/Leisure: interests and values
- Rest/Sleep: sleep habits
- Social Participation: type and location
- Sensorimotor: muscle and grip strength, range of motion, stiffness, fine motor skills, dexterity, pain, sensation (tactile, proprioceptive or joint positioning)
- Cognitive/Perceptual: not directly affected (check for dementia or visual impairment)
- Psychosocial: quality of life, life roles
- Context/Environment: adapted devices, splinting, home and community safety
- Comorbidities: osteoporosis, osteoarthritis, postural instability/postural sway, visual impairment, dementia, complex regional pain syndrome (CRPS-Type 1), median nerve injury, stiff hand, depression, diabetes, hypertension

Instruments

Instruments Developed by Occupational Therapy Personnel
- Canadian Occupational Performance Measure (5th ed.; COPM-5; Law et al., 2014)
- Criterion-Based Numeric Pain Scale (CR12; Wilson et al., 2014, in References)
- Global Rate of Change (GROC) Scale (Wilson et al., 2014, in References)
- Wrist Performance Test (WPT; Bemgård & Archenholtz, 2018, in References)

Instruments Developed by Other Professionals and Used by Occupational Therapy Personnel
- Disabilities of the Arm, Shoulder, and Hand (3rd ed.; DASH-3; Kennedy et al., 2011)
- Grip strength (dynamometer; JAMAR, Lafayette Instrument; Wang et al., 2018)
- Joint range of motion (goniometer; Shurtleff & Kaskutas, 2018)
- Michigan Hand Outcomes Questionnaire (MHQ; Chung et al., 1998)
- Moberg Picking-Up Test (MPUT; Moberg, 1958)
- Patient-Rated Wrist/Hand Evaluation (PRWHE; MacDermid & Tottenham, 2004)
- Pinch strength (pinch meter; B&E Engineering; Mathiowetz et al., 1985)
- Push-off test (bear weight through palm: e.g., a door or push up from a chair; dynamometer placed on a surface)
- Quick Disabilities of the Arm, Shoulder, and Hand (QuickDASH; Kennedy et al., 2011; see also Smith-Forbes et al., 2018, in References)
- Semmes-Weinstein Monofilaments (Bell-Krotoski, 2011)
- Sollerman Hand Function Test (SHFT; Sollerman & Ejeskär, 1995)
- Visual analogue scale (VAS; numerical pain scale: 0 = *no pain* to 10 = *severe/worst ever pain*)

Problems/Issues

Activities of Daily Living/Instrumental ADL
- Person may have difficulty performing self-maintenance tasks, especially if the wrist of dominant hand is involved.
- Person may lose independence and may become dependent on others.
- Person may be unable to drive a vehicle.

Education/Work
- Person may have difficulty performing work or volunteer tasks.

Play/Leisure
- Person may not be able to engage in favorite leisure occupations, such as needlework.

Rest/Sleep
- Person may experience sleep disturbance due to pain.

Social Participation
- Person may be limited in participation of social activities where hand function is expected, such as eating at a restaurant.

Sensorimotor
- Person usually has pain in the wrist and hand; pain in forearm and shoulder is also reported.
- Person usually experiences reduced grip strength due to changes in the biomechanical integrity of the wrist (Mifsud & Drew, 2015).
- Person may experience loss of range of motion in wrist and fingers.
- Person may experience edema (swelling).
- Person may experience stiffness in hand and fingers.
- Person may experience pain.
- Person may experience loss of tactile or proprioceptive (joint positioning) sensation.

Cognitive/Perceptual
- Not directly affected. (Consider whether dementia or visual impairment exists.)

Psychosocial
- Person may become depressed or anxious about appearance of hand after healing has occurred.
- Person may be unable to perform expected social roles.
- Person may become dependent on others for care.
- Person may experience decreased quality of life.
- Person may experience changes in role expectations and performance.

Context/Environment
- Person may need instruction in wearing and caring for a cast and/or splint.
- Person may need instruction in home exercise program.
- Person may need adaptive devices.
- Person may have limited social support.

Intervention/Treatment

Models and programs developed by occupational therapy personnel include distal radioulnar joint orthosis (V. H. O'Brien & Thurn, 2013), Functional Capacity Evaluation Protocol (Cheng & Cheng, 2011); home-based exercise program (Sen & Mohapatra, 2014), and occupational performance intervention (Dahlqvist & Rosén, 2016). Models and programs developed by other professionals but used by occupational therapy personnel include combined physical and occupational therapy (Filipova et al., 2015), compression gloves (Miller-Shahabar et al., 2018), mirror therapy (Bayon-Calatayud et al., 2016), modified manual edema mobilization (Knygsand-Roenhoej & Maribo, 2011), progressive early digit mobilization (Kuo et al., 2013), repetitive wrist extension exercise (Mitsukane et al., 2015), and sensorimotor proprioception protocol (Wollstein et al., 2019). Team members include physicians, nursing personnel, physical therapists, and occupational therapy personnel. Goals include reducing pain and edema, regaining motion and strength, and improving occupational performance in daily activities. Type of intervention significantly changes timing of rehabilitation. Range of motion exercises after stabilization surgery can occur after 7 to 10 days, whereas the same exercises may not be possible in a cast for up to 6 weeks.

Activities of Daily Living/Instrumental ADL
- If cast is applied, limited to assist until cast is removed.
- External fixation: activities as tolerated.
- Dorsal or volar plating: usually after 6 weeks.
- Provide basic training in one-handed techniques.

Education/Work
- Variable, depending on type of work tasks involved.

Play/Leisure
- Variable, depending on type of leisure activities in which client engages.

Rest/Sleep
- Pain management may be needed.
- Adjustment in sleep positions may be helpful.

Social Participation
- Variable, depending on type and location of social activities.

Sensorimotor
- Cast: Used for nonoperated (nonreduced) fractures for 4–6 weeks. Activities will be limited by cast, but noninvolved joints should be used to avoid stiffness and loss of range of motion from disuse.
- Desensitization: May be needed for irritated radial nerve when external fixation is used.
- Edema control: Use positioning (elevation of extremity), retrograde massage, compression wraps or gloves, and active range of motion of uninvolved joint.
- Pain management: Ice packs, functional activities.
- Range of motion
  - Cast: Immediate active range of motion (AROM) of uninvolved joints (expect limitation in forearm rotation). Begin AROM of wrist after cast is removed.
  - External fixation: Immediate AROM of uninvolved joints. After hardware is removed, active and passive range of motion to wrist and forearm (focus on flexion of digits, wrist extension ulnar deviation and supination).
  - Dorsal and volar plating: Immediate AROM of all uninvolved joints. Use place and hold for wrist extension for 4–6 weeks if extensor digitorum communis (EDC) is compromised.
  - Hot packs and therapeutic whirlpool provide positive results for active wrist range of motion (Szekeres et al., 2018).
- Scar management: Important when dorsal or volar plating are used.
- Splint
  - Resting splint for comfort when cast is removed or between exercise sessions for fixation or plating.
  - Static progressive splinting, such as a circumferential wrist orthosis, is used to regain range of motion once healing has occurred.
  - For volar plating, a wrist extension immobilized splint may be used for 4–6 weeks.
- Stiffness and tightness
  - Encourage client to maintain motion and movement in all uninvolved joints.
  - If external fixator is used, exercises should focus on metacarpophalangeal (MPC), proximal interphalangeal (PIP), and distal interphalangeal (DIP) flexion and PIP and DIP flexion with MPC extended. Pay close attention to index finger in particular.
- Strengthening: Should not be started until fracture is healed, at approximately 8 weeks.
- Timing
  - Protective phase: 1–6 weeks
    - Protect fracture site, control swelling and pain, avoid pin-site infection.
    - Cast, orthoses, stabilizers, edema control, wound care, exercises.
  - Motion/mobilization phase
    - Noninvolved joints: motion begins immediately.
    - Involved wrist joint: depends on type of immobilization device.
  - Strengthening phase
    - Full engagement in daily activities.
    - Increase range of motion.
    - Isometric progressing to isotonic exercises: free weights, TheraBand, Theraputty, grip exerciser.

- Wound care: Important if external fixation or subcutaneous pinning is used to avoid infection (bacteria have direct access to subcutaneous tissue and healing bone). If using cotton swabs, use only one per pin.

Cognitive/Perceptual
- Assist client in self-management skills.
- Note whether dementia and visual impairment may require adjustments in home instructions and management of wound care.

Psychosocial
- Provide opportunity for client to discuss concerns about ability to perform life roles.
- Provide motivation to engage in rehabilitation and return to performing daily occupations.

Context/Environment
- Provide client with home instructions and demonstration regarding exercises to maintain range of motion in uninvolved joints.
- Provide client with instructions and demonstration regarding exercises to regain range of motion after fracture has healed.
- Provide client with instructions and training to manage wound care if external fixation or subcutaneous pinning is used.
- Provide client with instructions on use and care of cast and splints.
- If a fall was the cause of fracture, fall prevention program may be initiated.

Precautions/Safety Considerations
- Avoid strengthening occupations until fracture site has completely healed.
- Minimize stiffness by maintaining active motion in all uninvolved joints.
- Watch for signs of dislocation, tendinitis, or ligament sprains.
- Person may continue to be at risk for falls due to postural instability (postural sway).
- Person may incur rupture of the flexor pollicis longus (FPL) due to improper plate placement, screw back-out, or chronic use of steroids (Valdes, 2011).

Prognosis and Outcome

Generally, outcome is good. Most clients should be able to resume normal occupations after 6 weeks if healing is complete. Some clients continue to have pain, which may be diagnosed as complex regional pain syndrome (Nielsen & Dekkers, 2013; R. S. Porter, 2018; Yang et al., 2018). Core outcome measurement should include evaluation of pain, function, and complications (Goldhahn et al., 2014). Major complication is contracture, limiting total active motion (TAM) of the digits or total active motion of the forearm (Kirby & Sparrow, 2018); carpal instability is another complication (L. O'Brien et al., 2018). Clients may continue to experience difficulty with certain tasks, such as picking up nuts and putting on bolts, turning screws with a screwdriver, buttoning buttons, and picking up wooden blocks, lifting them over a table edge, and placing them on the table (S. Porter, 2013) using Sollerman Hand Function Test.

Cost Effectiveness

Cost for OT in nonoperative cases was $1,070, or 17% of total, because OT is one of the major cost items. Cost of OT in operative cases was $750, or 4.9% of total, because cost of surgery, anesthesiology, radiology, and bed and room costs are added to total (Swart et al., 2017).

REFERENCES
Bayon-Calatayud, M., Benavente-Valdepeñas, A. M., & del Prado Vazquez-Muñoz, M. (2016). Mirror therapy for distal radial fractures: A pilot randomized controlled study. *Journal of Rehabilitation Medicine, 48*(9), 829–832. https://doi.org/10.2340/16501977-2130

Bemgård, M., & Archenholtz, B. (2018). Developing an instrument for the measurement of grip ability after distal radius fracture. *Scandinavian Journal of Occupational Therapy, 25*(6), 466–474. https://doi.org/10.1080/11038128.2017.1323950

Cheng, A. S. K., & Cheng, S. W. C. (2011). Use of job-specific functional capacity evaluation to predict the return to work of patients with a distal radius fracture. *American Journal of Occupational Therapy, 65*(4), 445–452. https://doi.org/10.5014/ajot.2011.001057

Dahlqvist, Å., & Rosén, B. (2016). Early occupational performance intervention enhances outcome after distal radius fracture: A nonrandomized controlled trial. *Hand Therapy, 21*(3), 100–109. https://doi.org/10.1177/1758998316656019

Filipova, V., Lonzarić, D., & Papež, B. (2015). Efficacy of combined physical and occupational therapy in patients with conservatively treated distal radius fracture: Randomized controlled trial. *Wiener Klinische Wochenschrift, 127*(Suppl. 5), 282–287. https://doi.org/10.1007/s00508-015-0812-9

Goldhahn, J., Beaton, D., Ladd, A., Macdermid, J., & Hoang-Kim, A. (2014). Recommendation for measuring clinical outcome in distal radius fractures: A core set of domains for standardized reporting in clinical practice and research. *Archives of Orthopaedic and Trauma Surgery, 134*(2), 197–205. https://doi.org/10.1007/s00402-013-1767-9

Kirby, E., & Sparrow, S. (2018). A retrospective analysis of the number of therapy visits after distal radius fractures using a new provider-scored clinical severity scale. *Journal of Hand Therapy, 31*(4), 480–485. https://doi.org/10.1016/j.jht.2017.06.008

Knygsand-Roenhoej, K., & Maribo, T. (2011). A randomized clinical controlled study comparing the effect of modified manual edema mobilization treatment with traditional edema technique in patients with a fracture of the distal radius. *Journal of Hand Therapy, 24*(3), 184–194. https://doi.org/10.1016/j.jht.2010.10.009

Kuo, L.-C., Yang, T.-H., Hsu, Y.-Y., Wu, P.-T., Lin, C.-L., Hsu, H.-Y., & Jou, I.-M. (2013). Is progressive early digit mobilization intervention beneficial for patients with external fixation of distal radius fracture? A pilot randomized controlled trial. *Clinical Rehabilitation, 27*(11), 983–993. https://doi.org/10.1177/0269215513487391

Mifsud, C., & Drew, T. (2015). Pathomechanics of the wrist following fractures of the distal radius. *Hand Therapy, 20*(1), 11–23. https://doi.org/10.1177/1758998315574352

Mitsukane, M., Sekiya, N., Himei, S., & Oyama, K. (2015). Immediate effects of repetitive wrist extension on grip strength in patients with distal radial fracture. *Archives of Physical Medicine and Rehabilitation, 96*(5), 862–868. https://doi.org/10.1016/j.apmr.2014.09.024

Miller-Shahabar, I., Schreuer, N., Katsevman, H., Bernfeld, B., Cons, A., Raisman, Y., & Milman, U. (2018). Efficacy of compression gloves in rehabilitation of distal radius fractures: Randomized controlled study. *American Journal of Physical Medicine & Rehabilitation, 97*(12), 904–910. https://doi.org/10.1097/PHM.0000000000000998

Moscony, A. M. B., & Shank, T. (2014). Wrist fractures. In C. Cooper (Ed.), *Fundamentals of hand therapy* (2nd ed., pp. 312–335). Elsevier. https://doi.org/10.1016/B978-0-323-09104-6.00025-0

Nielsen, T. L., & Dekkers, M. K. (2013). Progress and prediction of occupational performance in women with distal radius fractures: A one-year follow-up. *Scandinavian Journal of Occupational Therapy, 20*(2), 143–151. https://doi.org/10.3109/11038128.2012.748823

O'Brien, L., Robinson, L., Lim, E., O'Sullivan, H., & Kavnoudias, H. (2018). Cumulative incidence of carpal instability 12–24 months after fall onto outstretched hand. *Journal of Hand Therapy, 31*(3), 282–286. https://doi.org/10.1016/j.jht.2017.08.006

O'Brien, V. H., & Thurn, J. (2013). A simple distal radioulnar joint orthosis. *Journal of Hand Therapy, 26*(3), 287–290. https://doi.org/10.1016/j.jht.2013.04.004

Porter, R. S. (Ed.). (2018). *The Merck manual of diagnosis and therapy* (20th ed.). Merck Sharp & Dohme.

Porter, S. (2013). Occupational performance and grip function following distal radius fracture: A longitudinal study over a six-month period. *Hand Therapy, 18*(4), 118–128. https://doi.org/10.1177/1758998313512280

Sen, R., & Mohapatra, J. (2014). Home-based exercise program (HEP) vs. institution-based occupational therapy (IOT) in improving hand skills in post Collies'* fractures: A comparative study. *Indian Journal of Occupational Therapy, 46*(3), 90–97.

Smith-Forbes, V., Howell, D. M., Willoughby, J., Pitts, D. G., & Uhl, T. L. (2018). A retrospective cohort study of QuickDASH scores for three hand therapy acute upper limb conditions. *Military Medicine, 183*(Suppl. 1), 522–529. https://doi.org/10.1093/milmed/usx199

Swart, E., Tulipan, J., & Rosenwasser, M. P. (2017). How should the treatment costs of distal radius fractures be measured? *American Journal of Orthopedics, 46*(1), e54–e59.

Szekeres, M., MacDermid, J. C., Grewal, R., & Birmingham, T. (2018). The short-term effects of hot packs vs therapeutic whirlpool on active wrist range of motion for patients with distal radius fracture: A randomized controlled trial. *Journal of Hand Therapy, 31*(3), 276–281. https://doi.org/10.1016/j.jht.2017.08.003

Valdes, K. (2011). Rehabilitation of flexor tendon ruptures after volar plate fixation of the distal radius: A case series. *Hand, 6*(4), 429–437. https://doi.org/10.1007/s11552-011-9360-6

Wilson, K., von der Heyde, R., Sparks, M., Hammerschmidt, K., Pleimann, D., Ranz, E., Rector, J., & Sniezak, D. (2014). The impact of demographic factors and comorbidities on distal radius fracture outcomes. *Hand, 9*(1), 80–86. https://doi.org/10.1007/s11552-013-9559-9

Wollstein, R., Harel, H., Lavi, I., Allon, R., & Michael, D. (2019). Postoperative treatment of distal radius fractures using sensorimotor rehabilitation. *Journal of Wrist Surgery, 8*(1), 2–9. https://doi.org/10.1055/s-0038-1672151

Yang, Z., Lim, P. P. H., Teo, S. H., Chen, H., Qiu, H., & Pua, Y. H. (2018). Association of wrist and forearm range of motion measures with self-reported functional scores amongst patients with distal radius fractures: A longitudinal study. *BMC Musculoskeletal Disorders, 19*, Article 142. https://doi.org/10.1186/s12891-018-2065-z

BIBLIOGRAPHY

Bamford, R., & Walker, D. M. (2010). A qualitative investigation into the rehabilitation experience of patients following wrist fracture. *Hand Therapy, 15*(3), 54–61.

Farzad, M., Layeghi, F., Hosseini, A., Dianat, A., Ahrari, N., Rassafiani, M., & Mirzaei, H. (2018). Investigate the effect of psychological factors in development of complex regional pain syndrome Type I in patients with fracture of the distal radius: A prospective study. *Journal of Hand Surgery (Asian-Pacific Volume), 23*(4), 554–561. https://doi.org/10.1142/S2424835518500571

Marik, T. (2017). Clinical relevance commentary in response to: Repositioning the scapula with taping following distal radius fracture: Kinematic analysis using 3-dimensional motion system. *Journal of Hand Therapy, 30*(4), 483–484. https://doi.org/10.1016/j.jht.2017.09.001

Michlovitz, S., & Festa, L. (2011). Therapist's management of distal radius fractures. In T. M. Skirven, A. L. Osterman, J. M. Fedorczyk, & P. C. Amadio (Eds.), *Rehabilitation of the hand and upper extremity* (6th ed., pp. 949–962). Mosby.

Souer, J. S., Buijze, G., & Ring, D. (2011). A prospective randomized controlled trial comparing occupational therapy with independent exercises after volar plate fixation of a fracture of the distal part of the radius. *Journal of Bone and Joint Surgery, 93*(19), 1761–1766. https://doi.org/10.2106/JBJS.J.01452

Taghavi Azar Sharabiani, P., Jafari, D., Mehdizadeh, H., Brumagne, S., Davoudi, M., Mazhar, F. N., Rostami, S., Jamali, S., Parnianpour, M., Taghizadeh, G., & Khalaf, K. (2019). Can postural instability in individuals with distal radius fractures be alleviated by concurrent cognitive tasks? *Clinical Orthopaedics and Related Research, 477*(7), 1659–1671. https://doi.org/10.1097/CORR.0000000000000788

Valdes, K., Naughton, N., & Burke, C. J. (2015). Therapist-supervised hand therapy versus home therapy with therapist instruction following distal radius fracture. *Journal of Hand Surgery, 40*(6), 1110e1–1116e1. https://doi.org/10.1016/j.jhsa.2015.01.036

---

* The published article includes this typo.

Valdes, K., Naughton, N., & Michlovitz, S. (2014). Therapist supervised clinic-based therapy versus instruction in a home program following distal radius fracture: A systematic review. *Journal of Hand Therapy, 27*(3), 165–174. https://doi.org/10.1016/j.jht.2013.12.010

Waljee, J. F., Zhong, L., Shauver, M., & Chung, K. C. (2014). Variation in the use of therapy following distal radius fractures in the United States. *Plastic and Reconstructive Surgery–Global Open, 2*(4), e130. https://doi.org/10.1097/GOX.0000000000000019

Ydreborg, K., Engstrand, C., Steinvall, I., & Larsson, E. L. (2015). Hand function, experienced pain, and disability after distal radius fracture. *American Journal of Occupational Therapy, 69*(1), Article 6901290030. https://doi.org/10.5014/ajot.2015.013102

Hip Arthroplasty

Also called hip replacement, total hip replacement (THR), joint replacement of the hip, total hip arthroplasty (THA).

Description

Hip arthroplasty or hip replacement is surgery in which all or part of the hip joint is removed and replaced with an artificial ball and socket joint implant (O'Toole, 2017). The primary rationale for hip precautions and modified techniques for daily living activities is to prevent dislocation of the implant during specific hip movements in relation to the surgical site. Newer surgery technique and modification of the implant have reduced the need for some hip precautions (Kerrigan & Saltzman, 2017). Thus, surgeons vary in their recommendations or requirements for specific hip precautions and may not prescribe any for some clients. The recommendations listed below provide examples for clients who do need to follow hip precautions and modify their lifestyle as a result of the hip replacement surgery.

Cause

Primary reasons for hip arthroplasty are advanced osteoarthritis, rheumatoid arthritis, other degenerative joint disease or a hip fracture that does not heal (O'Toole, 2017).

Hip Movement Precautions Based on Location of Surgical Incision Site (Kerrigan & Saltzman, 2017)

- Posterior incision: No hip flexion beyond 90 degrees, no hip adduction past neutral, and no hip internal rotation.
- Anterior incision: No hip extension and no hip external rotation.
- Both posterior and anterior incisions (global): No hip flexion beyond 90 degrees, no hip adduction past neutral, no hip internal or external rotation, no hip prone lying, and no bridging.
- Trochanteric incision (for trochanteric osteotomy and hip replacement): No active hip abduction.

Evaluation/Assessment

Areas

- Activities of Daily Living/Instrumental ADL: self-maintenance skills with adapted devices and modified techniques
- Education/Work: work requirements
- Play/Leisure: interests and values
- Rest/Sleep: sleep disturbances, sleep modifications
- Social Participation: type, frequency, location
- Sensorimotor: joint range of motion, muscle strength, endurance and activity tolerance, pain and pain tolerance

- Cognitive/Perceptual: not directly affected; monitor for cognitive impairment due to other causes
- Psychosocial: depression, anxiety, quality of life, fear of resuming normal activities, social roles
- Context/Environment: adapted devices, client and family education, community resources, hip precautions, joint protection, fall prevention, social support
- Comorbidities: osteoarthritis, rheumatoid arthritis, obesity, fractures, urinary incontinence

Instruments

Instruments Developed by Occupational Therapy Personnel

- Nottingham Extended Activities of Daily Living (NEADL; Nouri, & Lincoln, 1987)
- Westmead Home Safety Assessment (WeHSA; Clemson et al., 1997)

Instruments Developed by Other Professionals and Used by Occupational Therapy Personnel

- Aberdeen Impairment Activity Limitation and Participation Restriction (AIALPR; Pollard et al., 2009)
- Barthel ADL Index (Collin et al., 1988)
- Client Service Receipt Inventory (CSRI; Beecham & Knapp, 2001)
- European Quality of Life 5-Dimension Scale (EuroQol 5 or EQ-5D; EuroQol Group, 1990)
- Grip strength (dynamometer; JAMAR, Lafayette Instrument; Wang et al., 2018)
- Hospital Anxiety and Depression Scale (HADS; Zigmond & Snaith, 1983)
- Inpatient Rehabilitation Facility Patient Assessment Instrument (IRF-PAI; Department of Health and Human Services, Centers for Medicare and Medicaid Services, 2006)
- Knowledge Inventory (KI; Keaney & Lawdis, 2017, in References)
- Muscle strength (manual muscle testing; Nicholas Manual Muscle Tester, Lafayette Instrument)
- Oxford Hip Score (OHS; Dawson et al., 1996)
- State Trait Anxiety Inventory (STAI; Spielberger et al., 1983)
- Western Ontario and McMaster Universities Osteoarthritis Index (WOMAC; Bellamy et al., 1988)
- Visual analogue scale (VAS; 10-point numeric scale for pain: 0 = *no pain*, 10 = *worst pain ever*)

Problems/Issues

Activities of Daily Living/Instrumental ADL

- Person will have limitations regarding performance of daily living activities (see Precautions/ Safety Considerations).
- Person will have restrictions on some activities, such as driving.
- Person may experience loss of independence during the recovery time and restrictions on independence following recovery.

Education/Work

- Person may be unable to perform certain job tasks because of restrictions or limitations due to existing osteoarthritis and hip prosthesis, such as those involving extensive physical or repetitive movement (climbing, stooping, crouching, walking on uneven surfaces, getting in and out of vehicles, standing for long periods of time).

Play/Leisure

- Person may experience restrictions on engagement in favorite leisure occupations during recovery time, especially those involving lower extremity, such as sports.
- Person may be advised to discontinue engagement in some leisure occupations.
- Person may need to explore new leisure occupations or modify engagement in previous activities.

Rest/Sleep

- Person may experience restrictions in sleep position during recovery period.
- Person may need to modify sleep positions or habits to accommodate hip prosthesis.

Social Participation
- Person may experience restrictions on participation in social occupations if those activities include extensive or prolonged use of lower extremities.
- Person may need to modify participation in some social occupations to accommodate hip prosthesis restrictions.
- Person may need to explore new social activities if participation in previous social occupations and events are restricted due to hip prosthesis.

Sensorimotor
- Person usually will have restrictions on hip range of motion during recovery time.
- Person may have reduced muscle strength.
- Person may experience reduced endurance and activity tolerance.
- Person usually has some pain during recovery time.

Cognitive/Perceptual
- Not directly involved, but cognitive impairment may be present due to comorbidities and may determine intervention plan, especially ability to understand and follow precautions.

Psychosocial
- Person may experience depression and anxiety regarding loss of independence or loss of ability to engage and participate in favorite leisure and social occupations.
- Person may experience decreased quality of life and sense of self-efficacy due to restrictions that limit role functions the person previously fulfilled.

Context/Environment
- Person usually needs education and training in selection and use of adapted devices.
- Person may need education and training on hip precautions following surgery.
- Person may need information and access to resources about living with a hip prosthesis such as joint protection and fall prevention.
- Person may lack social support or social support may be inadequate. Postsurgery some assistance is required for most people.

Intervention/Treatment

Models and programs developed by occupational therapy personnel include Pre-Operative Occupational Therapy (PreOpOTed; Keaney & Lawdis, 2017), Quick Reference Guide (Royal College of Occupational Therapists, 2017), and telehealth (Cason & Richmond, 2016). Models and programs developed by other professionals but used by occupational therapy personnel include adaptive device training (Bozorgi et al., 2016), Pre-operative Occupational Therapy to Optimise Recovery (PROOF-THR; Jepson et al., 2016), patient education (Drummond et al., 2013), preoperative home-based program (Orpen & Harris, 2010), and RESTORE Programme (Blom, 2016). Team members include general physicians, surgeons, rheumatologists, nursing personnel, psychologists, physical therapists, and occupational therapy personnel. Goal is to restore physical function and independence and prevent future injury.

Activities of Daily Living/Instrumental ADL
- Dressing with aids (reacher, grabber, dressing stick)
  - Designate a sturdy chair, bench, or stool that does not require bending hips at more than 90 degrees, and sit to begin dressing.
  - Always dress operated leg first and undress it last.
  - Organize clothes within easy reach before sitting in a chair.
  - When using dressing aids, always use them on outside (lateral side) of operated leg to avoid twisting hip.
  - Gather leg hole of pants/jeans/trousers and grip the hole with helping hand.
  - Use helping hand to lower pants to floor and hook them over the foot of operated leg.

- ▶ Keeping hold of pants with helping hand, pull the pants up the leg, over the knee, so they can be held without overstretching.
- ▶ Then, grip the unoperated leg hole of the pants with helping hand and pull it over the unoperated foot. Once pants are positioned at knees, stand to pull them up over buttocks, and fasten.
- ▶ Skirts can be pulled over head.
- Shoehorn
  - ▶ Place shoe on ground in front of foot (footwear must slip on without requiring tying shoe laces; elastic shoe laces may be used; loafers are usually best).
  - ▶ Place end of shoehorn into the shoe and press to shoe bottom.
  - ▶ Guide foot into shoe until shoe is on the foot (do not bend over).
  - ▶ Pull shoehorn out of shoe.
  - ▶ Repeat for other shoe and foot.
- Sock aid
  - ▶ Place sock aid between thighs, with rope end in lap.
  - ▶ Put sock on aid, keeping heel of sock at bottom of aid.
  - ▶ Pull sock all the way down until it touches the rope knots, but not over the rope knots.
  - ▶ Hold one rope in each hand and drop sock aid to floor in front of operated leg.
  - ▶ Pull ropes to pull sock over foot; keep pulling until aid comes out of sock.
  - ▶ Repeat for other foot.
- Washing hair
  - ▶ Wash hair while standing in shower or leaning backwards, not forwards.
- Bed transfer
  - ▶ When getting into bed, lead with unoperated leg, and when getting out of bed, lead with operated leg.
- Driving and car transfers
  - ▶ Plan on not driving for about 6 weeks or until physician gives permission.
  - ▶ Insurance company may need to be notified about hip surgery.
  - ▶ Car transfer technique
    - ○ Before entering car, position it away from curb to reduce amount of drop into car seat.
    - ○ Move passenger seat back as far as possible and angle seat back so it is partially reclined.
    - ○ Open passenger door completely and back body to door opening, using walking aid for support.
    - ○ Keep walking back until the seat can be felt on back of knees.
    - ○ Before sitting down, put hand on the passenger seat for support.
    - ○ Roll window down and grip open door window frame with other hand.
    - ○ Gently lower buttocks down, remembering to keep operated leg extended.
    - ○ Carefully lift operated leg and slide into car and face forward.
    - ○ A plastic bag may make transfer easier by providing a slippery surface.
    - ○ When transferring out of car ensure operated leg is out before standing up.
- Sit on high furniture, pushing up from the arms and keeping operated leg out in front of body.
- Sit and walk for short periods of time. Create and use rest breaks.
- Use walking aids and adapted equipment as supplied.
- During sexual activity, be the passive partner for about 3 months after operation.

Education/Work

- Earlier return-to-work time is associated with less pain and fewer functional limitations in everyday activities (Sankar et al., 2013).
- Early return to work is more feasible for clients whose job task requires low physical demand.

Play/Leisure

- Occupations requiring primarily upper extremity can continue as per the client's interest. New activities can be explored and added. Caution about prolonged sitting should be observed.

- Occupations such as swimming and walking on flat surfaces are encouraged. Caution about amount of time should be observed.
- Engagement in occupations such as jogging, hiking, mountain biking, and snow or water skiing may need to be limited or stopped because they endanger the integrity of the prosthetic components.
- Other limitations are sports requiring speed and high joint impact, load, or stress, such as football, soccer, basketball, and handball (Schmidt Hanson, 2014).

Rest/Sleep

- Assist client in complying with sleep-on-back requirement. Adjustments in mattress and bedding materials may be helpful. Adding restful sounds and decreasing lighting may be useful.

Social Participation

- Assist client to modify participation in social events during postsurgery recovery to comply with hip precautions.

Sensorimotor

- Increase upper extremity muscle strength to assist with transfers.

Cognitive/Perceptual

- Asking questions of client can be helpful to determine what information has been learned about hip replacement surgery and what issues remain (see Knowledge Index in Keaney & Lawdis, 2017, in References).
- Time management may be important because hip precautions typically are in force for 6 weeks to 3 months, depending on progress of recovery.

Psychosocial

- Not discussed.

Context/Environment

- Consider preoperative education and training program (Keaney & Lawdis, 2017).
- Adapted equipment: Provide instruction in use and care.
  - ► Abduction pillow
  - ► Bedside and/or toilet commode chair (frames and rails)
  - ► Chair riser
  - ► Cushion seat
  - ► Elevated toilet seat
  - ► Long-handled shoehorn
  - ► Reacher or grabber
  - ► Rolling cart (trolley)
  - ► Sock aid
  - ► Sturdy chair, stool, or bench
  - ► Tub bench/shower chair
- Community and internet resources: Provide information about and instruction if needed.

Precautions/Safety Considerations

- Hip precautions (Note: There are various views regarding the need, type, and usefulness of hip precautions; Coole et al., 2013; Drummond et al., 2012; Fox et al., 2011; Lightfoot et al., 2018; Smith & Sackley, 2016). Contrary views state that no precautions are needed (Barnsley et al., 2015; McQuaid et al., 2014).
  - ► Do not cross legs, even at the ankles. Keep legs apart.
  - ► Do not turn operated leg in or out. Keep feet pointed forward.
  - ► Do not sleep on side of body. Use a pillow between knees to prevent turning on side of body.
  - ► Do not bend down to the feet from waist, whether sitting or standing.
  - ► Do not get in or out of the bathtub without using equipment, including tub seat.

► Avoid bending hip or lifting leg more than 90 degrees.
► Avoid bending to floor.
► Avoid twisting at hip when lying down, sitting, or standing.
► Avoid putting hands beyond knees.
► Avoid bringing knee of operated leg up toward chest while sitting.
► Avoid sitting on low furniture where hip is lower than knee.
► Avoid straining hips during sexual intercourse.
• Adapted devices: Major reasons for not using adapted devices was lack of choice in selection and lack of training in proper use (Thomas et al., 2010).

Prognosis and Outcome

Variable. Some clients are able to return to work and daily life within 1 month while others may take 12 months. Previous health status, age, amount of pain, amount or number of physical limitations, and type of work are all factors in recovery (Sankar et al., 2013).

REFERENCES

Barnsley, L., Barnsley, L., & Page, R. (2015). Are hip precautions necessary post total hip arthroplasty? A systematic review. *Geriatric Orthopaedic Surgery & Rehabilitation, 6*(3), 230–235. https://doi.org/10.1177/2151458515584640

Blom, A. W. (2016). Occupational therapy in total hip replacement: Systematic review and feasibility randomized controlled trial. In A. W. Blom, N. Artz, A. D. Beswick, A. Burston, P. Dieppe, K. T. Elvers, R. Gooberman-Hill, J. Horwood, P. Jepson, E. Johnson, E. Lenguerrand, E. Marques, S. Noble, M. Pyke, C. Sackley, G. Sands, A. Sayers, V. Wells, & V. Wylde (Eds.), *Improving patients' experience and outcome of total joint replacement: The RESTORE programme* (pp. 281–300). NIHR Journals Library.

Bozorgi, A. A. J., Ghamkhar, L., Kahlaee, A. H., & Sabouri, H. (2016). The effectiveness of occupational therapy supervised usage of adaptive devices on functional outcomes and independence after total hip replacement in Iranian elderly: A randomized controlled trial. *Occupational Therapy International, 23*, 143–153. https://doi.org/10.1002/oti.1419

Cason, J., & Richmond, T. (2016). Innovative occupational therapy practice for patients with lower extremity joint replacement. *SIS Quarterly Practice Connections, 1*(1), 10–11.

Coole, C., Edwards, C., Brewin, C., & Drummond, A. (2013). What do clinicians think about hip precautions following total hip replacement? *British Journal of Occupational Therapy, 76*(7), 300–307. https://doi.org/10.4276/030802213X13729279114898

Drummond, A., Coole, C., Brewin, C., & Sinclair, E. (2012). Hip precautions following primary total hip replacement: A national survey of current occupational therapy practice. *British Journal of Occupational Therapy, 75*(4), 164–170. https://doi.org/10.4276/030802212X1333 6366278059

Drummond, A., Edwards, C., Coole, C., & Brewin, C. (2013). What do we tell patients about elective total hip replacement in the UK? An analysis of patient literature. *BMC Musculoskeletal Disorders, 14*, Article 152. https://doi.org/10.1186/1471-2474-14-152

Fox, R., Halliday, R., Barnfield, S., Roxburgh, J., Dunford, J., & Chesser, T. J. S. (2011). Hip precautions after hemiarthroplasty: What is happening in the UK and at what cost? *Annals of the Royal College of Surgeons of England, 93*(5), 396–397. https://doi.org/10.1308/003588411 X581376

Jepson, P., Sands, G., Beswick, A. D., Davis, E. T., Blom, A. W., & Sackley, C. M. (2016). A feasibility randomised controlled trial of pre-operative occupational therapy to optimise recovery for patients undergoing primary total hip replacement for osteoarthritis (PROOF-THR). *Clinical Rehabilitation, 30*(2), 156–166. https://doi.org/10.1177/0269215515576811

Keaney, K., & Lawdis, K. (2017). Pre-operative occupational therapy for patients having total hip replacements. *Journal of Community Medicine & Health Education, 7*(5), Article 100563. https://doi.org/10.4172/2161-0711.1000563

Kerrigan, D. A., & Saltzman, K. N. (2017). Orthopedics and musculoskeletal disorders: Surgical interventions. In H. Smith-Gabai & S. E. Holm (Eds.), *Occupational therapy in acute care* (2nd ed., pp. 441–469). AOTA Press.

Lightfoot, C., Sehat, K., Drury, G., Brewin, C., Coole, C., & Drummond, A. (2018). Hip precautions after hip operation (HippityHop): Protocol for a before and after study evaluating hip precautions following total hip replacement. *British Journal of Occupational Therapy, 81*(6), 319–325. https://doi.org/10.1177/0308022618757183

McQuaid, L., Cope, J., & Fenech, A. (2014). Occupational therapy in orthopaedics: An alternative to hip precautions? *International Journal of Therapy and Rehabilitation, 21*(11), 508–510. https://doi.org/10.12968/ijtr.2014.21.11.508

Orpen, N., & Harris, J. (2010). Patients' perceptions of preoperative home-based occupational therapy and/or physiotherapy interventions prior to total hip replacement. *British Journal of Occupational Therapy, 73*(10), 461–469. https://doi.org/10.4276/030802210X12865330218267

O'Toole, M. T. (Ed.). (2017). *Mosby's dictionary of medicine, nursing & health professions* (10th ed.). Elsevier.

Royal College of Occupational Therapists. (2017). *Occupational therapy for adults undergoing total hip replacement: Quick reference guide.*

Sankar, A., Davis, A. M., Palaganas, M. P., Beaton, D. E., Badley, E. M., & Gignac, M. A. (2013). Return to work and workplace activity limitations following total hip or knee replacement. *Osteoarthritis and Cartilage, 21*(10), 1485–1493. https://doi.org/10.1016/j.joca.2013.06.005

Schmidt Hanson, C. (2014). Restoring competence in leisure pursuits. In M. V. Radomski & C. A. Trombly Latham (Eds.), *Occupational therapy for physical dysfunction* (7th ed., pp. 909–924). Wolters Kluwer.

Smith, T. O., & Sackley, C. M. (2016). UK survey of occupational therapists' and physiotherapists' experiences and attitudes towards hip replacement precautions and equipment. *BMC Musculoskeletal Disorders, 17*, Article 228. https://doi.org/10.1186/s12891-016-1092-x

Thomas, W. N., Pinkelman, L. A., & Gardine, C. J. (2010). The reasons for noncompliance with adaptive equipment in patients returning home after a total hip replacement. *Physical & Occupational Therapy in Geriatrics, 28*(2), 170–180. https://doi.org/10.3109/02703181003698593

BIBLIOGRAPHY

Dorsey, J., & Bradshaw, M. (2017). Effectiveness of occupational therapy interventions for lower-extremity musculoskeletal disorders: A systematic review. *American Journal of Occupational Therapy, 71*(1), Article 7101180031. https://doi.org/10.5014/ajot.2017.023028

Mallinson, T. R., Bateman, J., Tseng, H. Y., Manheim, L., Almagor, O., Deutsch, A., & Heinemann, A. W. (2011). A comparison of discharge functional status after rehabilitation in skilled nursing, home health, and medical rehabilitation settings for patients after lower-extremity joint replacement surgery. *Archives of Physical Medicine and Rehabilitation, 92*(5), 712–720. https://doi.org/10.1016/j.apmr.2010.12.007

Murphy, L. F., & Lawson, S. (2018). Orthopedic conditions: Hip fractures and hip, knee, and shoulder replacements. Section 2: Hip joint replacements. In H. M. Pendleton & W. Schultz-Krohn (Eds.), *Pedretti's occupational therapy* (8th ed., pp. 1007–1016). Mosby.

Westby, M. D., & Backman, C. L. (2010). Patient and health professional views on rehabilitation practices and outcomes following total hip and knee arthroplasty for osteoarthritis: A focus group study. *BMC Health Services Research, 10*, Article 119. https://doi.org/10.1186/1472-6963-10-119

Westby, M. D., Brittain, A., & Backman, C. L. (2014). Expert consensus on best practices for post-acute rehabilitation after total hip and knee arthroplasty: A Canada and United States Delphi study. *Arthritis Care & Research, 66*(3), 411–423. https://doi.org/10.1002/acr.22164

Hip Fracture

See also Hip Arthroplasty.

Description

Fractures of the hip bone (femur) occur in the femoral head, femoral neck, between the trochanters or prominences (intertrochanter), or subtrochanter (below the trochanters) of the femur (Porter, 2018).

Cause

The most common cause is a fall, but in the elderly minimal forces such as rolling over in bed, getting up from a chair, or walking may result in a fracture because of underlying conditions such as osteoporosis (Porter, 2018).

Weight Bearing Percentages (Maher, 2014; Murphy & Lawson, 2018)
- Non–weight bearing (NWB): 0% weight on operated limb: Use walker or crutches.
- Touchdown weight bearing (TDWB): 10%–15% weight on operated limb: Use walker or crutches.
- Partial weight bearing (PWB): 30% weight on operated limb; Use walker or crutches.
- 50% weight bearing (50WB): 50% weight on operated limb: Use cane.
- Weight bearing as tolerated (WBAT): Use cane if needed.
- Full weight bearing (FWB): 70%–100% weight on operated limb: Use cane or no device.

Evaluation/Assessment

Areas
- Activities of Daily Living/Instrumental ADL: self-maintenance skills (dressing lower extremities, toileting, transfers, mobility), community transportation (car, bus, taxi, train)
- Education/Work: paid work and volunteer occupations
- Play/Leisure: interests and values, frequency, location
- Rest/Sleep: sleep habits, sleep disturbances
- Social Participation: type, frequency, location, with whom
- Sensorimotor: muscle strength, range of motion, pain, posture, balance
- Cognitive/Perceptual: cognitive status especially evidence of dementia, health literacy
- Psychosocial: depression, self-efficacy, quality of life
- Context/Environment: home safety, home modification, adapted devices, fall risk and prevention, social support
- Comorbidities: osteoporosis, osteoarthritis, sarcopenia or presarcopenia, decreased grip strength, dementia, visual impairment, frailty, weight loss, urinary tract infection

Instruments
Instruments Developed by Occupational Therapy Personnel
- Activity Card Sort (2nd ed.; ACS-2; Baum & Edwards, 2008)

Instruments Development by Other Professionals and Use by Occupational Therapy Personnel
- Barthel Index (BI; Mahoney & Barthel, 1965)
- Berg Balance Scale (BBS; Berg et al., 1989)
- Falls Efficacy Scale (FES; Hellström & Lindmark, 1999)
- Functional Independence Measure (FIM; Uniform Data System for Medical Rehabilitation, 1997)

- General Health Questionnaire (GHQ; Goldberg & Williams, 1988)
- Goldberg Anxiety and Depression Scale (GADS; Goldberg et al., 1988)
- Grip strength (dynamometer; JAMAR, Lafayette Instrument; Wang et al., 2018)
- Harris Hip Score (HHS; Harris, 1969)
- Home Safety Checklist (Centers for Disease Control, n.d.)
- Index of Activities of Daily Living (Index of ADL; Katz Index; Katz et al., 1963; Katz et al., 1970)
- Modified Barthel Index (MBI; Shaw et al., 1989)
- Short-Form Health Survey (SF-12; Ware et al., 1996)
- Short Physical Performance Battery (SPPB; Guralnik et al., 1994)
- Short Portable Mental Status Questionnaire (SPMSQ; Pfeiffer, 1975)
- Timed Up and Go test (TUG; Podsiadlo & Richardson, 1991)
- Traffic Light System–Basic Activities of Daily Living (TLS-BasicADL; Asplin et al., 2014)

Problems/Issues
Activities of Daily Living/Instrumental ADL
- Person may have difficulty performing activities that involve lower extremity such as dressing lower extremity, toileting, bathing/showering, sit to stand, climbing stairs, walking on uneven surfaces.
- Note that upper extremity grip strength is critical to performing self-maintenance activities including safe transfers and use of mobility devices (Di Monaco, Castiglioni, De Toma, Gardin, Giordano, & Tappero, 2015).

Education/Work
- Person may have stopped or restricted work or volunteering.

Play/Leisure
- Person may have stopped or limited engagement in favorite leisure occupations.

Rest/Sleep
- Person may have difficulty sleeping due to pain or discomfort.

Social Participation
- Person may have restricted participation in social occupations.

Sensorimotor
- Person frequently has pain.
- Person may experience discomfort when lying down, sitting, standing, or climbing stairs.
- Person may have reduced range of motion, especially in the lower extremities.
- Person may have muscle weakness which includes upper and lower extremities.
- Person may have reduced endurance and activity tolerance.
- Person may have reduced muscle mass in lower extremities.
- Person may have reduced grip strength compared to persons of equal age.

Cognitive/Perceptual
- Not directly affected but comorbidities such as dementia or visual impairment may need to be considered in intervention plan.

Psychosocial
- Person may experience reduced quality of life.
- Person may experience depression or anxiety.

Context/Environment
- Person will need instruction on hip precautions.
- Person may need information and instruction on use of adapted devices.
- Person may need information on community and internet resources.

Intervention/Treatment

Models and programs developed by occupational therapy personnel include home visits (Lockwood et al., 2017), occupation-based intervention (Wong et al., 2018), occupational therapy intervention (Segev-Jacubovski et al., 2019), and reducing emotional distress (Martín-Martín, Valenza-Demet, Ariza-Vega, et al., 2014; Martín-Martín, Valenza-Demet, Jiménez-Moleón, et al., 2014). Models and programs developed by other professionals but used by occupational therapy personnel include community rehabilitation (Roberts et al., 2017), coordinated rehabilitation (Asplin et al., 2017), and prioritized care processes (Kim & Leland, 2016). Team members may include physicians, nursing personnel, physical therapists, and occupational therapy personnel. Goals are to return the client to home and community able to perform occupations of daily living safely and effectively with as much independence as possible, including use of adapted devices as needed.

Activities of Daily Living/Instrumental ADL
- Provide instructions on managing self-maintenance activities within hip precaution limitations, including use of adapted devices.
- Provide instructions on safe transfers: bed to chair, getting up from a chair, getting in and out of tub or shower, getting in and out of the car.
- Provide assistance in learning to manage medications and side effects.
- Discuss with client appropriate means of community mobility and problem solve barriers.

Education/Work
- If client is volunteering, assist client to review volunteer tasks and discuss what modifications may be needed. Example: Could some be done via smartphone apps?

Play/Leisure
- Discuss with client engagement in favorite leisure occupations and any modifications that may be needed.
- Discuss with client exploring and engaging in new leisure interests and occupations.

Rest/Sleep
- Discuss sleep habits with client and suggest modifications if needed.

Social Participation
- Encourage client to participate in social activities within functional limitations and safety precautions.

Sensorimotor
- Mobilization usually should begin within 24 hours of surgery.
- Body mechanics and joint protection: Assist client to use body mechanics to avoid injury.
- Pain management: Collaborate with client and rehabilitation staff to identify optimal times for rehabilitation based on pain medication schedule, monitor pain during therapy sessions and determine when pain interferes with client's ability to participate in therapy.
- Precautions: Assist client (family, caregivers) to learn and observe hip precautions.
- Positioning: Including standing, in bed, in a chair, on a sofa and on the toilet.
- Mobility: Including bed mobility, sitting up, lying down, moving from side to side, sitting on bed's edge.
- Muscle strengthening: Provide resistive exercises and activities to increase strength.
- Transferring: See ADL/IADL.
- Techniques for sitting, standing, dressing and undressing, bathing, walking, and going up and down stairs.

Cognitive/Perceptual
- Develop meaningful goals and achievable outcomes with client and caregiver input.
- Assist client and caregivers to understand "new self" with functional limitations.

- Assist client to problem solve about goals or tasks important to client.
- Assist client to learn and follow fall prevention program.
- Provide instruction at level client (family or caregiver) can comprehend including demonstration, hand-over-hand assistance, verbal cues, illustrated handouts.

Psychosocial
- Address client's concerns about surgery and recovery, including fear of falling.
- Provide stress management and coping strategies (also used for pain management) techniques such as deep breathing, playing relaxing music, doing meditation.
- Provide opportunity to express feelings of depression, especially regarding loss of functions client used to take for granted.
- Assist client to explore issues related to improving health status and quality of life.

Context/Environment
- Provide information on home safety modifications including grab bars, railings, decluttering, lighting, etc. If possible, arrange a home visit.
- Provide information, selection, acquisition, and training in use of assistive devices for dressing, walking, bathing, and toileting.
- Provide information, outpatient classes, and internet resources about fall prevention.
- Assist in discharge planning so client has needed information, made home modifications, and obtained equipment/devices before being discharged.

Precautions/Safety Considerations

Client may remain at risk for falls even after a comprehensive rehabilitation program (Asplin et al., 2017). Adherence to recommendations for fall prevention significantly reduces risk of falling (Di Monaco et al., 2012), but telephone call reminders do not reduce risk (Di Monaco, De Toma, et al., 2015).

Prognosis and Outcome

Better outcomes are associated with facilities that do more hip fracture repair surgeries (Gozalo et al., 2015; Teppala et al., 2017). Overall outcome is dependent on degree of disability and sensitivity of measurement instrument to evaluate the disability (Hershkovitz et al., 2015; Hoang-Kim et al., 2013). Handgrip strength at admission and at discharge is an independent predictor of functional outcome (Di Monaco et al., 2014; Di Monaco, Castiglioni, De Toma, Gardin, Giordano, De Monaco, et al., 2015). Presence of sarcopenia reduces functional ability in activities of daily living (Di Monaco, Castiglioni, De Toma, Gardin, Giordano, De Monaco, & Tappero, 2015). Occupational therapy improved health perceptions and patient emotions (Lee et al., 2019). Clients whose facture occurred in a skilled nursing facility (SNF) usually returned to the same facility following surgery (Leland et al., 2015). Pain is associated with poor outcomes (Leland et al., 2018). A discharge motor rating of 58 on the Functional Independence Measure yielded the best balance of sensitivity and specificity for setting discharge level (Wang et al., 2014). Treatment for hip fracture improves survival for clients on hospice care (Leland et al., 2012).

REFERENCES

Asplin, G., Carlsson, G., Zidén L., & Kjellby-Wendt, G. (2017). Early coordinated rehabilitation in acute phase after hip fracture—A model for increased patient participation. *BMC Geriatrics*, *17*(1), 240. https://doi.org/10.1186/s12877-017-0640-z

Di Monaco, M., Castiglioni, C., De Toma, E., Gardin L., Giordano, S., Di Monaco, R., & Tappero, R. (2014). Handgrip strength but not appendicular lean mass is an independent predictor of functional outcome in hip-fracture women: A short-term prospective study. *Archives of Physical Medicine and Rehabilitation*, *95*(9), 1719–1724. https://doi.org/10.1016/j.apmr.2014.04.003

Di Monaco, M., Castiglioni, C., De Toma, E., Gardin L., Giordano, S., Di Monaco, R., & Tappero, R. (2015). Presarcopenia and sarcopenia in hip-fracture women: Prevalence and association with ability to function in activities of daily living. *Aging in Clinical and Experimental Research*, 27(4), 465–472. https://doi.org/10.1007/s40520-014-0306-z

Di Monaco, M., Castiglioni, C., De Toma, E., Gardin L., Giordano, S., & Tappero, R. (2015). Handgrip strength is an independent predictor of functional outcome in hip-fracture women: A prospective study with 6-month follow-up. *Medicine*, 94(6), e542. https://doi.org/10.1097/MD.0000000000000542

Di Monaco, M., De Toma, E., Gardin L., Giordano, S., Castiglioni, C., & Vallero, F. (2015). A single postdischarge telephone call by an occupational therapist does not reduce the risk of falling in women after hip fracture: A randomized controlled trial. *European Journal of Physical and Rehabilitation Medicine*, 51(1), 15–22.

Di Monaco, M., Vallero, F., De Toma, E., Castiglioni, C., Gardin, L., Giordano, S., & Tappero, R. (2012). Adherence to recommendations for fall prevention significantly affects the risk of falling after hip fracture: Post-hoc analyses of a quasi-randomized controlled trial. *European Journal of Physical and Rehabilitation Medicine*, 48(1), 9–15.

Gozalo, P., Leland, N. E., Christian, T. J., Mor, V., & Teno, J. M. (2015). Volume matters: Returning home after hip fracture. *Journal of the American Geriatrics Society*, 63(10), 2043–2051. https://doi.org/10.1111/jgs.13677

Hershkovitz, A., Brown, R., Burstin, A., & Brill, S. (2015). Measuring rehabilitation outcome in post-acute hip fractured patients. *Disability and Rehabilitation*, 37(2), 158–164. https://doi.org/10.3109/09638288.2014.911968

Hoang-Kim, A., Beaton, D., Bhandari, M., Kulkarni, A., & Schemitsch, E. (2013). The need to standardize functional outcome in randomized trials of hip fracture: A review using the ICF framework. *Journal of Orthopaedic Trauma*, 27(1), e1–e8. https://doi.org/10.1097/BOT.0b013e318252d3c4

Kim, L. H., & Leland, N. E. (2016). Rehabilitation practitioners' prioritized care processes in hip fracture post-acute care. *Physical & Occupational Therapy in Geriatrics*, 34(2-3), 155–168. https://doi.org/10.1080/02703181.2016.1267295

Lee, S. Y., Jung, S. H., Lee, S.-U., Ha, Y.-C., & Lim, J.-Y. (2019). Is occupational therapy after hip fracture surgery effective in improving function? A systematic review and meta-analysis of randomized controlled studies. *American Journal of Physical Medicine & Rehabilitation*, 98(4), 292–298. https://doi.org/10.1097/PHM.0000000000001069

Leland, N. E., Gozalo, P., Bynum, J., Mor, V., Christian, T. J., & Teno, J. M. (2015). What happens to patients when they fracture their hip during a skilled nursing facility stay? *Journal of the American Medical Directors Association*, 16(9), 767–774. https://doi.org/10.1016/j.jamda.2015.03.026

Leland, N. E., Lepore, M., Wong, C., Chang, S. H., Freeman, L., Crum, K., Gillies, H., & Nash, P. (2018). Delivering high quality hip fracture rehabilitation: The perspective of occupational and physical therapy practitioners. *Disability and Rehabilitation*, 40(6), 646–654. https://doi.org/10.1080/09638288.2016.1273973

Leland, N. E., Teno, J., Gozalo, P., Bynum, J., & Mor, V. (2012). Decision making and outcomes of a hospice patient hospitalized with a hip fracture. *Journal of Pain and Symptom Management*, 44(3), 458–465. https://doi.org/10.1016/j.jpainsymman.2011.09.011

Lockwood, K. J., Taylor, N. F., Boyd, J. N., & Harding, K. E. (2017). Pre-discharge home visits by occupational therapists completed for patients following hip fracture. *Australian Occupational Therapy Journal*, 64(1), 41–48. https://doi.org/10.1111/1440-1630.12311

Maher, C. (2014). Orthopaedic conditions: Hip fractures. In M. V. Radomski & C. A. Trombly Latham (Eds.), *Occupational therapy for physical dysfunction* (7th ed., pp. 1114–1119). Wolters Kluwer.

Martín-Martín, L. M., Valenza-Demet, G., Ariza-Vega, P., Valenza, C., Castellote-Caballero, Y., & Jiménez-Moleón, J. J. (2014). Effectiveness of an occupational therapy intervention in reducing emotional distress in informal caregivers of hip fracture patients: A randomized controlled trial. *Clinical Rehabilitation, 28*(8), 772–783. https://doi.org/10.1177/0269215513519343

Martín-Martín, L. M., Valenza-Demet, G., Jiménez-Moleón, J. J., Cabrera-Martos, I., Revelles-Moyano, F. J., & Valenza, M. C. (2014). Effect of occupational therapy on functional and emotional outcomes after hip fracture treatment: A randomized controlled trial. *Clinical Rehabilitation, 28*(6), 541–551. https://doi.org/10.1177/0269215513511472

Murphy, L. F., & Lawson, S. (2018). Orthopedic conditions: Hip fractures and hip, knee, and shoulder replacements. Section 1: Hip fractures and replacements. In H. M. Pendleton & W. Schultz-Krohn (Eds.), *Pedretti's occupational therapy* (8th ed., pp. 1007–1017). Mosby.

Porter, R. S. (Ed.). (2018). *The Merck manual of diagnosis and therapy* (20th ed.). Merck Sharp & Dohme.

Roberts, J. L., Din, N. U., Williams, M., Hawkes, C. A., Charles, J. M., Hoare, Z., Morrison, V., Alexander, S., Lemmey, A., Sackley, C., Logan, P., Wilkinson, C., Rycroft-Malone, J., & Williams, N. H. (2017). Development of an evidence-based complex intervention for community rehabilitation of patients with hip fracture using realist review, survey and focus groups. *BMJ Open, 7*(10), e014362.

Segev-Jacubovski, O., Magen, H., & Maeir, A. (2019). Functional ability, participation, and health-related quality of life after hip fracture. *OTJR: Occupation Participation and Health, 39*(1), 41–47. https://doi.org/10.1177/1539449218796845

Teppala, S., Ottenbacher, K. J., Eschbach, K., Kumar, A., Al Snih, S., Chan, W. J., & Reistetter, T. A. (2017). Variation in functional status after hip fracture: Facility and regional influence on mobility and self-care. *Journals of Gerontology: Series A, 72*(10), 1376–1382. https://doi.org/10.1093/gerona/glw249

Wang, C. Y., Graham, J. E., Karmarkar, A. M., Reistetter, T. A., Protas, E., & Ottenbacher, K. J. (2014). FIM motor scores for classifying community discharge after inpatient rehabilitation for hip fracture. *PM&R, 6*(6), 493–497. https://doi.org/10.1016/j.pmrj.2013.12.008

Wong, C., Fagan, B., & Leland, N. E. (2018). Occupational therapy practitioners' perspectives on occupation-based interventions for clients with hip fracture. *American Journal of Occupational Therapy, 72*(4), Article 720405050. https://doi.org/10.5014/ajot.2018.026492

BIBLIOGRAPHY

Dorsey, J., & Bradshaw, M. (2017). Effectiveness of occupational therapy interventions for lower-extremity musculoskeletal disorders: A systematic review. *American Journal of Occupational Therapy, 71*(1), Article 7101180031. https://doi.org/ 10.5014/ajot.2017.023028

Leland, N., Gozalo, P., Christian, T. J., Bynum, J., Mor, V., Wetle, T. F., & Teno, J. (2015). An examination of the first 30 days after patients are discharged to the community from hip fracture post-acute care. *Medical Care, 53*(10), 879-887. https://doi.org/10.1097/MLR.0000000000000419

Wang, A. Q.-L., Ng, B. H.-P., Cheug, L. P.-C., & Chin, R. P.-H. (2017). Factors affecting mortality and hospital admission after hip surgery among elderly patients with hip fracture in Hong Kong—Review of a three-year follow-up. *Hong Kong Journal of Occupational Therapy, 30*(1), 6–13. https://doi.org/10.1016/j.hkjot.2017.10.004

Knee Arthroplasty

Also called knee replacement, total knee replacement (TKR), joint replacement of the knee, unicompartmental knee arthroplasty (UKA), total knee arthroplasty (TKA).

Description

Surgical insertion of a hinged prosthesis performed to relieve pain and restore motion and mobility to a knee (O'Toole, 2017). The need for a knee replacement occurs when the menisci deteriorate as a result of changes due to disease, trauma, or aging. As the cartilage deteriorates, the articulation between the tibia and femur is not smooth. When the bones rub together, pain increases as does inflammation in the tendons, ligaments, and synovial lining of the joint (Kerrigan & Saltzman, 2017). A partial or unicompartmental knee arthroplasty (UKA) may be used if there is medial or lateral compartmental damage between the femur and tibia. Surgery for UKA is minimally invasive and allows for greater knee flexion more quickly after surgery with increased stability. Total knee replacement (TKR) is indicated when two or more compartments of the knee are damaged. Various prosthetic devices are available.

Cause

Osteoarthritis, rheumatoid arthritis, or trauma.

Evaluation/Assessment

Areas

- Activities of Daily Living/Instrumental ADL: functional mobility prior to surgery, including daily activity routine and performance of ADL/IADL tasks
- Education/Work: work requirements if client is still working (paid or unpaid)
- Play/Leisure: interests, type, location, frequency
- Rest/Sleep: sleep disturbance
- Social Participation: type, location, frequency, with whom
- Sensorimotor: joint range of motion, muscle strength (both upper extremity and lower extremity), endurance and activity tolerance, coordination and balance, sensation, pain
- Cognitive/Perceptual: cognitive functioning (memory, problem solving, sequencing, following instructions)
- Psychosocial: stress management, quality of life, fear of falling, hesitation about resuming activities following surgery
- Context/Environment: adapted equipment, home safety, social support, community resources
- Comorbidities: obesity, osteoarthritis

Instruments

Instruments Developed by Occupational Therapy Personnel

- None identified

Instruments Developed by Other Professionals and Used by Occupational Therapy Personnel

- Functional Independence Measure (FIM; Uniform Data System for Medical Rehabilitation, 1997)
- Inpatient Rehabilitation Facility Patient Assessment Instrument (IRF-PAI; Department of Health and Human Services, Centers for Medicare and Medicaid Services, 2006)
- Joint range of motion (goniometer; Shurtleff & Kaskutas, 2018)
- Manual Muscle Test (MMT; Kaskutas, 2018)
- Short-Form 36 Health Survey (SF-36; Ware et al., 1993)
- Western Ontario & McMaster Universities Osteoarthritis Index (WOMAC; Bellamy et al., 2010)

Problems/Issues

Activities of Daily Living/Instrumental ADL

- Person has difficulty with functional mobility (bed mobility, sit to stand, standing, stand to sit, walking, climbing stairs).

Education/Work

- No information identified.

Play/Leisure

- Person may have limited or stopped engaging in favorite leisure activities.

Rest/Sleep
- Person may report difficulty getting a good night's sleep due to limited mobility or pain.

Social Participation
- Person may have restricted participation in social activities due to pain.

Sensorimotor
- Person may have decreased range of motion in the knee.
- Person may have decreased muscle strength in knee and lower extremity.
- Person may have decreased endurance and activity tolerance.
- Person usually has pain.

Cognitive/Perceptual
- Not involved directly; consider possible comorbidities.

Psychosocial
- Person may experience decreased quality of life.

Context/Environment
- Person may lack knowledge and information about knee replacement surgery and post-discharge management.
- Person may need adapted equipment.
- Person may lack social support.

Intervention/Treatment

Models and programs developed by occupational therapy personnel include telehealth (Cason & Richmond, 2016). Models and programs developed by other professionals but used by occupational therapy: None identified. Team members include physicians, surgeons, rheumatologists, physical therapists, and occupational therapy personnel. Goal is to restore functional mobility, increase joint motion, alleviate pain, maintain joint alignment and stability, and increase occupational performance (Murphy & Lawson, 2018).

Activities of Daily Living/Instrumental ADL
- Out-of-bed activities typically start on 1st day after surgery. General health of client and physiological response to surgery may limit initial activities.
- Dressing
  - ▶ Purpose: Compensate for limited range of motion or decreased balance.
  - ▶ Technique: Use footstool to reach feet, sit to dress lower extremities, long-handled shoehorn, avoid twisting and rotation motions of the knees.
- Car seats and driving
  - ▶ Caution: Driving should not be attempted until person is off narcotic medications.
  - ▶ After right-side knee replacement, physician should give OK for driving to resume after motor control is considered adequate to control pedals.
  - ▶ Bucket type seats should be avoided if possible. A twist-turn pad may be used to fill in bucket seat space. Bench style seats are preferred.
  - ▶ Technique: Move the seat as far back as it will go, back up to seat, hold onto a stable part of the car; extend operated leg and slowly slide into car seat; lean forward for clearance from top of car and then move body and head into car.
  - ▶ Caution: Prolonged sitting is not recommended. Take frequent breaks (every 2 hours) if long trips are necessary.
- Ambulatory assistance
  - ▶ Purpose: Provide greater stability as prescribed by physician.
  - ▶ Technique: Walker, crutches, canes. Scooter may be useful for longer distances. A temporary sticker for disabled parking may be useful.

- Transfer techniques
  - ▶ Purpose: Safe transfer from bed to chair, sit to stand, toileting, tub or shower to dry surface.
  - ▶ Technique
    - ○ Commode chair
      - ▷ Sit down: Use chair with armrests, back up to chair, extend operated leg forward, reach for armrests, place hands on armrests, slowly lower body to sitting position.
      - ▷ Stand up: Place hands on armrests, place both feet on floor, lean forward maintaining contact with armrests, slowing rise to standing position and release grip on armrests.
    - ○ Tub/shower
      - ▷ Note: Tub bathing or showering may not be permitted until surgery site is healed. Sponge baths may be needed initially.
      - ▷ Seated: Use tub transfer seat as per commode and flexible shower hose.
      - ▷ Standing: Place walker beside tub, place hands on grab bars, lift one leg into tub, transfer weight, lift other leg into tub or shower. Walker may be transferred into shower for added stability.
- Homemaking: Avoid prolonged static positions, use stools at sink, sit when possible.
- Sexual activity: Generally avoid during healing process, side-lying on nonoperated side may reduce knee pain, kneeling position should be avoided.

Education/Work

- Earlier return-to-work time is associated less pain and fewer functional limitations in everyday activities (Sankar et al., 2013).

Play/Leisure

- Activities requiring primarily upper extremity should continue as per the client's interest. New activities can be explored and added. Caution about prolonged sitting should be observed.
- Activities such as swimming, cycling, and walking are encouraged.
- Engagement in activities such as jogging, hiking, mountain biking, and snow or water skiing may need to limited or stopped because they endanger the integrity of the prosthetic components.
- Other limitations are sports requiring speed and high joint impact, load, or stress such as football, soccer, basketball, and handball (Schmidt Hanson, 2014).

Rest/Sleep

- Person should sleep with legs extended while healing occurs. A small pillow may be placed between extended legs for comfort if physician approves.

Social Participation

- Person can resume participation in social activities as soon as healing occurs; caution against standing or sitting for long periods of time is advised.

Sensorimotor

- Exercise: Focus on encouraging activities that require normal knee joint flexion and extension.
- Muscle strengthening: Slowly increase amount of activity starting with ADLs.
- Pain management: Use of superficial cold modalities, proper positioning during transitional movements, engage client in deep breathing, and balance of rest and activity.
- Positioning
  - ▶ In bed: Keep knees fully extended. If on side a small cushion or pillow may be placed between ankles, not knees until completely healed.
  - ▶ Sitting: Elevate feet so knees are extended.
  - ▶ Standing: Stand straight looking ahead, not at feet.
- Swelling: Slowly increasing activity should not increase swelling.
- Weight bearing: Start by sitting on side of bed and placing both feet on floor; therapist may need to provide support on side of surgery.

Cognitive/Perceptual
- Preoperative program should include preparing for surgery, what to expect while in the hospital, the recovery process, realistic information regarding pain after surgery, expected functional levels postsurgery, when to resume normal activities at home, available adaptive equipment and techniques, functional mobility, home safety, precaution, caregiver training, exercise before and after surgery, and anatomy of the knee joint (Causey-Upton et al., 2019).

Psychosocial
- Coping and stress management: deep breathing, relaxation training, yoga.

Context/Environment
- Medical equipment
  - ▶ Antiembolism hose
    - ○ Purpose: Assist in circulation, prevent edema, and reduce risk of deep-vein thrombosis (DVT).
    - ○ Technique: Elastic hosiery extended up to knee or over knee to thigh worn 24 hours a day, except for bathing.
  - ▶ Continuous passive motion (CPM) machine
    - ○ Purpose: CPM device may be prescribed by physician to improve functional range of motion and reduce postsurgical edema. There is limited evidence of long-term effectiveness (Murphy & Lawson, 2018)
    - ○ Technique: Mechanical device supports joint and is set to move slowly through a designated range of motion.
  - ▶ Commode chair
    - ○ Purpose: Aids in safe transfer and allows client to limit knee flexion during toileting.
    - ○ Technique: Chair is placed over the toilet.
  - ▶ Hemovac
    - ○ Purpose: Assist with postoperative drainage of blood.
    - ○ Technique: Plastic drainage tube is inserted in surgical site during surgery. Tube may be connected to a potable suction machine, which remains for 1 to 2 days. Tube should be disconnected during activity to avoid blockage.
  - ▶ Incentive spirometer
    - ○ Purpose: To encourage deep breathing and prevent development of postoperative pneumonia.
    - ○ Technique: Client blows into the portable breathing apparatus, which records volume of air blown from lungs.
  - ▶ Orthoses (knee immobilizer or brace)
    - ○ Purpose: May be prescribed by physician if knee joint is unstable following surgery.
    - ○ Technique: Consult with physician regarding wearing instructions and when immobilizer or brace can be removed for therapist supervised activities. Note whether wearing instructions are being followed.
  - ▶ Sequential compressive device (SCD)
    - ○ Purpose: Reduce risk of DVT.
    - ○ Technique: Inflatable, external leggings that provide intermittent pneumatic compression of the legs.
- Adapted equipment: Provide instruction, training, and care/maintenance.
  - ▶ Commode chair or raised toilet seat: Provides armrests for stability and reduces amount of muscle strength needed to rise from seat.
  - ▶ Reacher: Reduces need to bend over and stoop to pick up or put down objects.
  - ▶ Walker or cane: Increases stability.
- Fall prevention
  - ▶ Hospital should have a fall prevention program that is followed.
  - ▶ Home evaluation to assess for risk of falls is useful.

- Home modification
  - ▶ Grab bars and nonskid stickers or strips in shower and tub.
  - ▶ Remove throw rugs from pathway.
- Home and community safety
  - ▶ Remove throw rugs.
  - ▶ Organize kitchen and cooking items so frequently used items are easy to reach and minimize need for bending, stooping or crouching.

Precautions/Safety Considerations

- Client should avoid rotation of the knee for about 12 weeks following surgery, but no restriction on flexion and extension.
- Clients who have both knee replacements done in one surgery will have slower recovery because there is no nonoperated leg to assist with walking, transition from sit to stand, or perform daily occupations; positive side is only one hospitalization.
- Observe for signs of dislocation of the prosthesis, degeneration of prosthetic parts, fractures of bone next to implantation, loosening of prosthesis or prosthetic parts, infection, increased swelling, or increased pain at joint site (Murphy & Lawson, 2018).

Prognosis and Outcome

Generally, knee replacement is successful and mobility is improved, although limitations on strenuous and high-impact activities may be limited (Causey-Upton et al., 2019). Prosthesis should last 10 to 15 years, depending on client's level and type of activity. Persons who had higher preoperative functional limitations; were single, separated, divorced, or widowed; were unemployed or retired; had a long wait time for surgery; or had a number of complications had worse functional limitations at 6 months postsurgery (Desmeules et al., 2013; Desmeules et al, 2012). Readiness for discharge was increased if the client had prior knowledge of others who had a positive experience, had attended a preoperative education program, had interacted with knowledgeable staff, and had support at home (Causey-Upton & Howell, 2017). Primary reasons for readmission to a hospital are infection, joint stiffness, and respiratory or cardiovascular events (Welsh et al., 2017).

REFERENCES

Cason, J., & Richmond, T. (2016). Innovative occupational therapy practice for patients with lower extremity joint replacement. *SIS Quarterly Practice Connections, 1*(1), 10–11.

Causey-Upton, R., & Howell, D. M. (2017). Patient experiences when preparing for discharge home after total knee replacement. *Internet Journal of Allied Health Sciences and Practice, 15*(1), Article 5.

Causey-Upton, R., Howell, D. M., Kitzman, P. H., Custer, M. G., & Dressler, E. (2019). Factors influencing discharge readiness after total knee replacement. *Orthopedic Nursing, 38*(1), 6–14. https://doi.org/10.1097/NOR.0000000000000513

Desmeules, F., Dionne, C. E., Belzile, E. L., Bourbonnais, R., Champagne, F., & Frémont, P. (2013). Determinants of pain, functional limitations and health-related quality of life six months after total knee arthroplasty: Results from a prospective cohort study. *BMC Sports Science, Medicine and Rehabilitation, 5*, Article 2. https://doi.org/10.1186/2052-1847-5-2

Desmeules, F., Dionne, C. E., Belzile, E. L., Bourbonnais, R., & Frémont, P. (2012). The impacts of pre-surgery wait for total knee replacement on pain, function and health-related quality of life six months after surgery. *Journal of Evaluation in Clinical Practice, 18*(1), 111–120. https://doi.org/10.1111/j.1365-27532010.01541.x

Kerrigan, D. A., & Saltzman, K. H. (2017). Orthopedics and musculoskeletal disorders. In H. Smith-Gabai & S. E. Holm (Eds.), *Occupational therapy in acute care* (2nd ed., pp. 441–469). AOTA Press.

Murphy, L. F., & Lawson, S. (2018). Orthopedic conditions: Hip fractures and hip, knee, and shoulder replacements. Section 2: Knee joint replacements. In H. M. Pendleton & W. Schultz-Krohn (Eds.), *Pedretti's occupational therapy* (8th ed., pp. 1017–1021). Mosby.

O'Toole, M. T. (Ed.). (2017). *Mosby's dictionary of medicine, nursing & health professions* (10th ed.). Elsevier.

Sankar, A., Davis, A. M., Palaganas, M. P., Beaton, D. E., Badley, E. M., & Gignac, M. A. (2013). Return to work and workplace activity limitations following total hip or knee replacement. *Osteoarthritis and Cartilage, 21*(10), 1485–1493. https://doi.org/10.1016/j.joca.2013.06.005

Schmidt Hanson, C. (2014). Restoring competence in leisure pursuits. In M. V. Radomski & C. A. Trombly Latham (Eds.), *Occupational therapy for physical dysfunction* (7th ed., pp. 909–924). Wolters Kluwer.

Welsh, R. L., Graham, J. E., Karmarkar, A. M., Leland, N. E., Baillargeon, J. G., Wild, D. L., & Ottenbacher, K. J. (2017). Effects of postacute settings on readmission rates and reasons for readmission following total knee arthroplasty. *Journal of the American Medical Directors Association, 18*(4), 367.e1–367.e10. https://doi.org/10.1016/j.jamda.2016.12.068

BIBLIOGRAPHY

Mallinson, T. R., Bateman, J. Tseng, H. Y. Manheim, L., Almagor, O., Deutsch, A., & Heinemann A. W. (2011). A comparison of discharge functional status after rehabilitation in skilled nursing, home health, and medical rehabilitation settings for patients after lower-extremity joint replacement surgery. *Archives of Physical Medicine and Rehabilitation, 92*(5), 712–720. https://doi.org/10.1016/j.apmr.2010.12.007

Westby, M. D., & Backman, C. L. (2010). Patient and health professional views on rehabilitation practices and outcomes following total hip and knee arthroplasty for osteoarthritis: A focus group study. *BMC Health Services Research, 10*, Article 119. https://doi.org/10.1186/1472-6963-10-119

Westby, M. D., Brittain, A., & Backman, C. L. (2014). Expert consensus on best practices for postacute rehabilitation after total hip and knee arthroplasty: A Canada and United States Delphi study. *Arthritis Care & Research, 66*(3), 411–423. https://doi.org/10.1002/acr.22164

Lateral Epicondylitis

Also called tennis elbow, lateral humeral epicondylitis, lateral epicondylalgia, lateral epicondylosis, tendinitis.

Description

Lateral epicondylitis is the result of inflammation and microtearing of fibers in the extensor tendons of the forearm. A common symptom is pain at the lateral epicondyle of the elbow, which radiates into the forearm (Porter, 2018). The extensor carpi radialis brevis (ECRB) muscle is most often involved, followed by the extensor digitorum communis (EDC; Cooper, 2014). Both attach to the lateral epicondyle of the humerus.

Cause

Theories about the cause include occupational and nonathletic activities that require repetitive and forceful forearm supination and pronation, or overuse or weakness of the ECRB and longus muscles of the forearm (Porter, 2018). The use of awkward wrist postures such as wrist deviation, combined with extension and movement velocity, may induce lateral epicondylitis (Lee et al., 2016).

Evaluation/Assessment

Areas

- Activities of Daily Living/Instrumental ADL: basic ADLs, independent living skills
- Education/Work
  - ▸ Work activities that require repetitive grasping and twisting of the elbow, such as turning a screwdriver
  - ▸ Use of work benefits such as sick leave
- Play/Leisure: sports activities such as tennis or racquetball, frequency, location
- Rest/Sleep: sleep disturbance
- Social Participation: type, frequency, location, with whom
- Sensorimotor: grip strength, joint range of motion, edema, pain
- Cognitive/Perceptual: not directly affected
- Psychosocial: role performance, quality of life
- Context/Environment: knowledge of source of injury, social support, community or internet resources
- Development (Infant, Child, Adolescent only): no information identified
- Comorbidities: no information identified

Instruments

Instruments Developed by Occupational Therapy Personnel

- Occupational Self-Assessment (Version 2.2; OSA 2.2; Baron et al., 2006)

Instruments Development by Other Professionals and Used by Occupational Therapy Personnel

- Disabilities of the Arm, Shoulder, and Hand (3rd ed.; DASH-3; Kennedy et al., 2011)
- Grip strength/dynamometer (Jamar Dynamometer, Lafayette Instrument; Wang et al., 2018)
- Jebsen-Taylor Hand Function Test (JTHFT; Jebsen et al., 1969)
- Joint range of motion (goniometry; Shurtleff & Kaskutas, 2018)
- Patient-Rated Tennis Elbow Evaluation (PRTEE; MacDermid, 2005)
- Pinch strength/pinch meter (B&E Engineering; Mathiowetz et al., 1985)
- Provocative testing (Cooper, 2014, in References)
  - ▸ Cozen's test: Examiner's thumb stabilizes client's elbow at the lateral epicondyle with the forearm pronate. Client makes a fist and then actively extends and radially deviates wrist while examiner resists the motion.
  - ▸ Mill's test: Client's shoulder is placed in neutral position. The examiner palpates tender area at or near the lateral epicondyle and then pronates forearm and fully flexes the wrist while moving elbow from flexion to extension.
- QuickDASH (QDASH; Kennedy et al., 2011; see also Smith-Forbes et al., 2016, 2018, in References)
- Short-Form 36 Health Survey (SH-36; Ware et al., 1993)
- Total Active Motion: (metacarpophalangeal [MCP] + proximal interphalangeal [PIP] + distal interphalangeal [DIP] flexion) – (MCP + PIP + DIP extension loss) = total active motion (TAM)
- Visual analogue scale (pain scale; scored: 0 = *no pain*, 10 = *worst pain ever*)

Problems/Issues

Education/Work

- Person may be unable to keyboard or experience limitations in keyboarding.
- Person may be unable to perform or experience limitations in performing work activities related to upper extremity movement of the elbow, including limitations of range of motion, strength and endurance, and increased pain.

Play/Leisure
- Person may be unable to engage or experience limitations in engaging in leisure activities that require upper extremity movements such as tennis or racquetball.
- Person may experience pain while engaging in repetitive activities, such as knitting.

Rest/Sleep
- Person may experience aching pain, which interferes with sleep.

Social Participation
- Person may limit or stop participation in social activities because of pain or limited strength.

Sensorimotor
- Person has reduced grip strength, especially when elbow is extended.
- Person experiences pain when gripping objects with affected extremity.
- Person has inflammation of tissue in the forearm.
- Person experiences tenderness in the extensor muscle mass near the lateral epicondyle or anterior or distal to it (Cooper, 2014).
- Person may limit upper extremity range of motion to avoid pain; range of motion may become limited due to disuse.
- Person may experience morning stiffness when moving elbow.
- Person may experience tightness of the extrinsic upper extremity extensors and stretching of the extensor muscles causes pain.

Cognitive/Perceptual
- No information identified.

Psychosocial
- Person may limit or stop engaging in social roles because of feelings of not being able to "keep up" or "share the load of expectations."

Context/Environment
- No information identified.

Complications
- Subperiosteal hemorrhage calcification, spur formation, tendon degeneration.

Intervention/Treatment

Models and programs developed by occupational therapy personnel include biomechanical and occupational adaptation (Bachman, 2016) and elastic therapeutic tape (Wegener et al., 2015, 2016). Models and programs developed by other professionals but used by occupational therapy personnel include counterforce forearm brace (Saurabh & Snehal, 2017; Shamsoddini et al., 2010), interdisciplinary cooperation (Nilsson, Lindgren, & Månsson, 2012), and structured program (Nilsson, Baigi, et al., 2012). Team members include physicians, orthopedic surgeons, nursing personnel, physical therapy personnel, and occupational therapy personnel. Goals are to reduce pain, increase strength, and improve function (Bachman, 2016).

Activities of Daily Living/Instrumental ADL
- Not discussed.

Education/Work
- Therapist and client can discuss pacing, activity modification, ergonomics approaches to facilitate work activity (Bachman, 2016).

Play/Leisure
- Not discussed.

Rest/Sleep
- Not discussed.

Social Participation
- Therapist and client can discuss different approaches to participating in social activity (Bachman, 2016).

Sensorimotor
- Nonintervention treatment is rest, ice, and NSAIDs.
- Conservative
  - ▶ Activity modification: Reducing number of steps in process, dividing activity tasks into smaller or more steps.
  - ▶ Compensatory techniques: Use more one-handed approaches.
  - ▶ Ergonomics: Optimizing work and leisure occupations to person's ability and limitations to promote safety and return potential reinjury.
  - ▶ Exercises: Extensor muscle strengthening.
  - ▶ Pain management: Pacing focusing on alternate cycles of rest and activity.
  - ▶ Posture: Maintaining good posture, providing a pillow or other support for affected arm.
  - ▶ Splinting/bracing: Night resting splint, Kinesio Taping or bandaging (Wegener et al., 2015, 2016), counterforce brace (Shamsoddini et al., 2010).

Cognitive/Perceptual
- Not discussed.

Psychosocial
- Life roles: Person may need to explore with the therapist's assistance novel or revised methods of accomplishing life roles, such as dividing role with other family members or changing role expectations with others in social situations.

Context/Environment
- Ergonomics: Person may benefit from learning ways to reduce the stress and movement of the affected extremity, such as using a wrist support when keyboarding, putting objects in pockets as opposed to carrying them, sliding as opposed to lifting, using a cart to move objects rather than carrying (Nilsson, Baigi, et al., 2012; Nilsson, Lindgren, & Månsson, 2012).
- Adaptive devices: Person may benefit from using adaptive devices that reduce the need for grip strength.

Precautions/Safety Considerations

Avoid overuse syndrome, which may contribute to tissue damage. Do not use heat modalities if inflammation or swelling is present in or around the elbow.

Prognosis and Outcome

Condition is chronic but can be managed using a variety of intervention approaches.

REFERENCES

Bachman, S. (2016). Evidence-based approach to treating lateral epicondylitis using the occupational adaptation model. *American Journal of Occupational Therapy, 70*(2), Article 7002360010. https://doi.org/10.5014/ajot.2016.016972

Cooper, C. (2014). Elbow, wrist, and hand tendinopathies. In C. Cooper (Ed.), *Fundamentals of hand therapy* (2nd ed., pp. 383–393). Elsevier.

Lee, S.-Y., Chieh, H.-F., Lin, C.-J., Jou, I.-M., Kuo, L.-C., & Su, F.-C. (2016). The potential risk factors relevant to lateral epicondylitis by wrist coupling posture. *PLOS ONE, 11*(5), Article e0155379. https://doi.org/10.1371/journal.pone.0155379

Nilsson, P., Baigi, A., Swärd, L., Möller, M., & Månsson, J. (2012). Lateral epicondylalgia: A structured programme better than corticosteroids and NSAID. *Scandinavian Journal of Occupational Therapy, 19*(5), 404–410. https://doi.org/10.3109/11038128.2011.620983

Nilsson, P., Lindgren, E.-C., & Månsson, J. (2012). Lateral epicondylalgia: A quantitative and qualitative analysis of interdisciplinary cooperation and treatment choice in the Swedish health care system. *Scandinavian Journal of Caring Science, 26*(1), 28–37. https://doi.org/10.1111/j.1471-6712.2011.00899.x

Porter, R. S. (Ed.). (2018). *The Merck manual of diagnosis and therapy* (20th ed.). Merck Sharp & Dohme.

Saurabh, P., & Snehal, D. (2017). Effectiveness of Kinesiotape versus Counterforce brace as an adjunct to occupational therapy in lateral epicondylitis. *Indian Journal of Physiotherapy and Occupational Therapy, 11*(2), 42–46.

Shamsoddini, A., Hollisaz, M. T., Hafezi, R., & Amanellahi, A. (2010). Immediate effects of counterforce forearm brace on grip strength and wrist extension force in patients with lateral epicondylosis. *Hong Kong Journal of Occupational Therapy, 20*(1), 8–12. https://doi.org/10.1016/S1569-1861(10)70052-8

Smith-Forbes, E. V., Howell, D. M., Willoughby, J., Pitts, D. G, & Uhl, T. L. (2016). Specificity of the minimal clinically important difference of the quick Disabilities of the Arm Shoulder and Hand (QDASH) for distal upper extremity conditions. *Journal of Hand Therapy, 29*(1), 81–88. https://doi.org/10.1016/j.jht.2015.09.003

Smith-Forbes, E. V., Howell, D. M., Willoughby, J., Pitts, D. G, & Uhl, T. L. (2018). A retrospective cohort study of QuickDASH scores for three hand therapy acute upper limb conditions. *Military Medicine, 183*(Suppl. 1), 522–529. https://doi.org/10.1093/milmed/usx199

Wegener, R. L., Brown, T., & O'Brien, L. (2015). The use of elastic therapeutic tape and eccentric exercises for lateral elbow tendinosis: A case series. *Hand Therapy, 20*(2), 56–63. https://doi.org/10.1177/1758998315580823

Wegener, R. L., Brown, T., & O'Brien, L. (2016). A randomized controlled trial of comparative effectiveness of elastic therapeutic tape, sham tape or eccentric exercises along for lateral elbow tendinosis. *Hand Therapy, 21*(4), 131–139. https://doi.org/10.1177/1758998316656660

Peripheral Nerve Injuries

Also called peripheral nerve disorders, peripheral nerve lesions, mononeuropathies.

Description

Peripheral nerve injuries to the median, radial, or ulnar nerve are characterized by sensory disturbances and muscle weakness in the distribution of the affected nerve (Porter, 2018). The median nerve exits the brachial plexus from C6–T1, the radial nerve exits from C5–C8, and the ulnar nerve exits from C8–T1. The median nerve innervates the pronator teres, flexor digitorum sublimis (FDS), flexor carpi radialis (FCR), palmaris longus, flexor digitorum profundus (FDP), flexor pollicis longus (FPL), pronator quadratus, abductor pollicis brevis (APB), opponens pollicis, superficial head of flexor pollicis brevis, and first and second lumbricals. The radial nerve innervates the triceps (lateral, long, and medial heads), anconeus, brachioradialis (BR), extensor carpi radialis longus (ECRL), extensor carpi radialis brevis (ECRB), supinator, extensor digitorum (ED), extensor digiti quinti (EDQ), extensor carpi ulnaris (ECU), abductor pollicis longus (APL), extensor pollicis longus (EPL), extensor pollicis brevis (EPB), and extensor indicis proprius (EIP). The ulnar nerve innervates the flexor carpi ulnaris (FCU), palmaris brevis, abductor digiti minimi, adductor pollicis, palmar and dorsal interosseus, flexor digiti minimi brevis, flexor pollicis brevis, and third and fourth lumbricals (Moscony, 2014). This chapter focuses on peripheral nerve injuries in adults. For pediatric injuries, see Ho (2015).

Cause

Trauma is the most common cause leading to bone fracture, joint dislocation, nerve compression, or skin lacerations. Other causes are violent muscular activity, forcible overextension of a joint, prolonged uninterrupted pressure at bony prominence, or nerve compression by a tumor, hyperostosis, a cast, crutches, prolonged cramped posture, or hemorrhage (Porter, 2018).

Characteristics of Dysfunction (Duff & Estilow, 2011)

- *Median:* Classic deformity is the sign of "benediction," with thumb in adduction and index and long fingers in extension and adduction while ring and little fingers are flexed. Sensation includes anterior (palmar) surface of thumb, index, long, and lateral one half of ring fingers, and the dorsal joints on the posterior side.
- *Radial:* Characteristic position: forearm pronation, wrist flexion (dropped wrist), thumb flexion and abduction, slight metacarpophalangeal (MCP) and interphalangeal (IP) extension. The person is unable to extend wrist and fingers simultaneously or abduct the extended thumb. Sensation includes posterior (dorsal) surface of thumb, index, long and lateral one half of ring fingers except for distal joint.
- *Ulnar:* Classic deformity is "claw hand deformity" or "partial intrinsic minus" deformity (hyperextension of ulnar metacarpophalangeal joints) due to loss of interossei and lumbricals III and IV with less posturing in the index and long fingers (lumbricals intact). Sensation includes posterior and anterior surfaces of medial one half of ring finger and all of little finger.

Evaluation/Assessment

Areas

- Activities of Daily Living/Instrumental ADL: basic ADLs involving grasp and release
- Education/Work: work history, work status, work tasks (job duties), handwriting, keyboarding
- Play/Leisure: interests, type, frequency, location
- Rest/Sleep: sleep disturbance
- Social Participation: type, frequency, location, with whom
- Sensorimotor: joint range of motion, muscle strength (grip and pinch), muscle atrophy, positioning of hand, hand functions (grasp, hook, pinch), edema management, scar management, sensation (touch, pain, proprioception, temperature)
- Cognitive/Perceptual: executive functions, stereognosis, graphesthesia
- Psychosocial: depression, anxiety, role performance, interpersonal relations, quality of life
- Context/Environment: adapted devices, splints, knowledge of peripheral nerve injury (PNI) and hand dysfunction, resources
- Comorbidities: fractures, dislocations, compression syndrome, nerve entrapment, soft tissue injury, vascular injury

Instruments

Instruments Developed by Occupational Therapy Personnel

- Adolescent/Adult Sensory Profile (AASP; Brown & Dunn, 2002)
- Canadian Occupational Performance Measure (COPM-5; Law et al., 2014)
- Impact of a Hand Nerve Disorder (I-HaND; Ashwood et al., 2018, in References)
- Manual Tactile Test (MTT; Hsu et al., 2013; see also Hsu et al., 2017, and Hsu et al., 2016, in References)
- Nine Hole Peg Test (NHPT; Mathiowetz et al., 1985 [adult]; Poole et al., 2015 [child])
- Pain Questionnaire (PQ; Wojtkiewicz et al., 2015, in References)
- Rosén Score (RS; Rosén & Lundborg, 2000)
- Shape/Texture Identification (STI-test; Rosén & Lundborg, 1998; see also Linnertz et al., 2019, in References)

Instruments Developed by Other Professionals and Used by Occupational Therapy Personnel
- Disabilities of the Arm, Shoulder, and Hand (3rd ed.; DASH-3; Kennedy et al., 2011; see also Yazdani & Dehkordi, 2013, in References)
- Dellon-McKinnon Disk-Criminator (Commercial instrument)
- Dynamic Two-Point Discrimination (see Two-Point Discrimination Test)
- Froment's Sign/Froment's Paper Sign (see Ho, 2015, in References)
- Grip strength (dynamometry; JAMAR Dynamometer, Lafayette Instrument; Wang et al., 2018)
- Illness Intrusiveness Scale (IIS; also called the Impact of Illness Scale; Klimidis et al., 2001)
- Jebsen-Taylor Hand Function Test (JTHFT; Jebsen et al., 1969)
- Joint range of motion (goniometry; Shurtleff & Kaskutas, 2018)
- Manual Muscle Test (MMT; Kaskutas, 2018)
- McGill Pain Questionnaire (MPQ; Melzack, 1975)
- Michigan Hand Outcomes Questionnaire (MHQ; Chung et al., 1998)
- Minnesota Manual Dexterity Test (MMDT; Lafayette Instrument)
- Moberg Picking-Up Test (MPUT; Moberg, 1958)
- Pain Disability Index (PDI; Tait et al., 1987)
- Patient Evaluation Measure (PEM; Macey et al., 1995)
- Pinch-holding-up activity (PHUA) test (Chiu et al., 2014)
- Pinch meter (B&E Engineering; Mathiowetz et al., 1985)
- Purdue Pegboard Test (PPT; Tiffin, 1948)
- QuickDASH (Kennedy et al., 2011)
- Scale for Muscle Strength (Medical Research Council [MRC], 1976)
- Semmes-Weinstein Monofilaments (SWMs) Test (Bell-Krotoski, 2011)
- Short-Form McGill Pain Questionnaire (2nd ed.; SF-MPQ-2; Dworkin et al., 2009)
- Sollerman Hand Function Test (SHFT; Sollerman & Ejeskär, 1995)
- Static Two-Point Discrimination (STPD; Abrams & Ivy, 2018; see Two-Point Discrimination Test)
- Ten Test (TT; Strauch & Lang, 2003)
- Tinel's Sign (see Ho, 2015, in References)
- Touch/Pressure Threshold (Weinstein enhanced sensory test [WEST]; commercially available)
- Two-Point Discrimination Test (Disk-Criminator or Boley Gauge)
- Vibration (tuning forks)
- Visual analogue scale (pain scale; 0–10 scale: 0 = *no pain*, 10 = *worst pain ever*)
- Wrinkle Test (O'Riain Test; O'Riain, 1973; see also Ho, 2015, in References)
- Note: Useful differences in test results between normal and injured hands (listed in Valdes, 2017)

Problems/Issues
Activities of Daily Living/Instrumental ADL
- Person may have difficulty performing basic ADLs, especially if radial and medial nerves are involved and the task requires two hands, such as difficulty with fasteners, cutting with knife and fork, opening jars, putting toothpaste on a toothbrush, cutting nails, wringing out a washcloth.
- Person may have difficulty performing tasks usually done with dominant hand if that is the injured hand, such as opening and closing doors, turning on or off electronic devices, hand-writing, turning pages in a book or magazine, handling small coins, using various controls in the vehicle.
- Person may have difficulty holding onto objects and complains they slip out of the injured hand.
- Person may have difficulty performing child care activities such as dressing and washing.

Education/Work

- Person may have difficulty performing work tasks such as keyboarding, lifting, carrying, placing items requiring two hands.

Play/Leisure

- Person may be unable to engage in favorite leisure occupations requiring two hands or use of injured hand.

Rest/Sleep

- Person may have sleep disturbances due to pain.

Social Participation

- Person may restrict or limit participation in social activities, such as eating out due to loss of hand functions (playing golf, tennis, racquetball, volleyball, basketball, sewing, knitting, crocheting, needlework).

Sensorimotor

- Person usually experiences muscle paralysis and muscle weakness of muscles innervated by the specific nerve.
- Person may develop abnormalities of the hand caused by muscle imbalance between the intrinsic and extrinsic muscles such as a claw hand (Seu & Pasqualetto, 2012).
- Person usually experiences loss of range of motion of actions controlled by muscles innervated by the specific nerve.
- Person usually experiences loss of touch (tactile) sensation below the level of injury during period of nerve regeneration.
- Person with an ulnar nerve injury may develop
  - a postural abnormality in which the small/little finger is in an abducted position;
  - difficulty opening and closing the hand because the extrinsic flexors act first on the IPs and lastly on the MCPs, resulting in the flexed fingers pushing an object away before it can be secured in the palm of the hand;
  - difficulty grasping large objects because of loss of abduct and adduct of the digits;
  - decreased grip strength to inability to activate lumbricals;
  - decreased coordination due to inability to activate lumbricals; and
  - decreased ability or weakness with lateral pinch due to reduced palmar adduction (Seu & Pasqualetto, 2012).
- Person may experience pain.
- Person may experience hypersensitivity (including hyperesthesia and allodynia).
- Person may become sensitive to cold temperatures.
- Person may experience loss of proprioception.
- Person may experience astereognosis (inability to identify objects by touch alone without visual assistance).
- Person may experience tactile gnosis (limited ability to distinguish shapes and textures).
- Person may not be able to localize correctly site of sensory stimulus (localization).
- Person may experience limited protective touch.
- Person may experience impaired light touch perception.

Cognitive/Perceptual

- Person may have difficulty with tactile perception and stereognosis.

Psychosocial

- Person may experience symptoms of depression and/or anxiety.
- Person may experience changes in role performance due to lack of hand functions.
- Person may experience unwanted changes in interpersonal relations, including intimate relations.
- Person may experience decreased quality of life, especially females (Wojtkiewicz et al., 2015).

Context/Environment
- Person may lack knowledge about PNI and its management.
- Person may need adapted devices.
- Person may need splints.
- Person may lack information about available resources.

Intervention/Treatment

Models and programs developed by occupational therapy personnel include radial nerve palsy orthosis (Peck & Ollason, 2015). Models and programs developed by other professionals but used by occupational therapy personnel include adaptive process (Ashwood et al., 2019), constraint-induced movement therapy (Rostami et al., 2017; Rostami et al., 2015), guided plasticity training (Rosén et al., 2015), sensory reeducation (Rosén & Lundborg, 2011), touch-observation and mirror therapy (Hsu et al., 2019), and mirror therapy (Paula et al., 2016). Team members include physicians, neurologists, surgeons, physical therapy personnel, and occupational therapy personnel. Goals include restoring motor and sensory function to perform everyday tasks of living and to maintain quality of life, including meaningful work and household roles, intimate relationships, sleep habits, and control of pain (Stonner et al., 2017).

Activities of Daily Living/Instrumental ADL
- Assist in suggesting compensatory techniques to accomplish everyday tasks while nerve regeneration is occurring.

Education/Work
- Assist person to continue working with environmental modifications as needed, such as an arm support on a chair.
- Assist person to explore with employer whether a less demanding job (use of injured hand and arm) is temporarily available if usual work assignment requires use of hand and arm that would endanger healing, such as requiring lifting heavy loads or finger dexterity.

Play/Leisure
- Encourage person to continue to engage in leisure occupations within safe limits of nerve repair.
- Suggest modifications that may be helpful (such as a slotted tray to hold cards needed to play a card game).

Rest/Sleep
- Assist person to use or adapt sleeping positions (such as resting injured hand/arm on a pillow) and equipment (such as night splint) that provide maximum sleep and rest.

Social Participation
- Encourage person to participate in social activities and cultural events within safe limits of nerve repair.
- Suggest modifications that may be helpful, such as use of adapted devices (universal cuff for lack of grip or enlarged handles for decreased grip).

Sensorimotor
- Provide range of motion (tendon) exercises specific to injury.
- Provide nerve gliding or nerve sliding program to prevent adhesions and enhance blood flow.
  - Forearm supination produces the most distally oriented median nerve gliding.
  - Full finger flexion produces the proximally oriented median nerve gliding.
  - Motion should be slow and steady.
  - Exercise should be stopped if numbness, discomfort, or pain increases.
- Provide tendon glide exercise following surgery.
  - Straight hand (full extension of wrist and finger joints).
  - Tabletop (wrist extended, MCP joints flexed, proximal and distal joints extended).

▶ Hook (wrist and MCP joints extended, proximal and distal joints flexed).

▶ Straight (wrist extended; MCP and proximal joints flexed, distal joints extended).

▶ Fist (wrist extended; MCP, proximal, and distal joints in full flexion).

- Provide exercises and occupations specific to loss hand functions.
- Assist client to use injured hand within safe limits to avoid disuse syndrome leading to atrophy.
- Provide sensory reeducation program, especially for median and ulnar nerve injuries, that provide sensory input to the volar (palmar) surface of the hand, such as agnosia, astereognosis, inability to localize sensory stimulus, limited protective touch, impaired light touch perception, numbness (Jerosch-Herold, 2011).
- Provide a pain desensitization program for hypersensitivity, including hyperesthesia and allodynia.
- Provide edema management, such as retrograde massage using Coban.

Cognitive/Perceptual

- Provide practice in tactile perception and stereognosis of fingers and palm of hand.

Psychosocial

- Assist client to address changes in role performance that may be temporary versus those that may be more permanent.
- Assist client to counteract feelings of depression and withdrawal by supporting continuing engagement and participation in daily occupations.
- Assist client in maintaining (or improving) quality of life.

Context/Environment

- Provide information on disorder and its management.
- Provide access to resources in the community and on the internet.
- Provide access to adapted devices as useful to client.
- Provide splinting as needed.
  ▶ Radial: Low profile radial nerve palsy orthosis that dynamically holds the MCP joints in extension but allows full digit flexion and leaves palmar surface free.
  ▶ Radial: Colditz radial nerve palsy splint does not immobilize wrist, but moves with natural tenodesis effect.
  ▶ Radial: Wrist cock-up splint positions wrist in extension and is useful as a night splint but blocks access to palmar sensation useful during the day.
  ▶ Interosseous palsy: Ring splint in figure eight; cross-over bar positioned at joint to prevent hyperextension.
  ▶ Median nerve palsy: Static thenar web spacer to prevent adduction contracture.
  ▶ Ulnar nerve palsy: Anti-claw splint to maintain MCP flexion, proximal and distal joint extension.

Precautions/Safety Considerations

Client is at risk for injuries (such as cuts, abrasions, and burns) due to decreased sensation.

Prognosis and Outcome

Pain and disability may continue for many months or years postinjury (Novak et al., 2010, 2011). Recovery of touch (tactile sensation) is affected by the number and function of regenerated fibers and mechanoreceptors. Tactile perception (gnosis) depends on the input and plasticity of the central nervous system. Recovery of one or both is variable (Krarup et al., 2017).

REFERENCES

Ashwood, M., Jerosch-Herold, C., & Shepstone, L. (2018). Development and validation of a new patient-reported outcome measure for peripheral nerve disorders of the hand, the I-HaND

Scale. *Journal of Hand Surgery European Volume, 43*(8), 864–874. https://doi.org/10.1177/17 53193418780554

Ashwood, M., Jerosch-Herold, C. & Shepstone, L. (2019). Learning to live with a hand nerve disorder: A constructed grounded theory. *Journal of Hand Therapy, 32*(3), 334–344. https://doi.org/10.1016/j.jht.2017.10.015

Duff, S. V., & Estilow, T. (2011). Therapist's management of peripheral nerve injury. In T. M. Skirven, A. L. Osterman, J. M. Fedorczyk, & P. C. Amadio (Eds.), *Rehabilitation of the hand and upper extremity* (6th ed., pp. 619–633). Mosby.

Ho, E. S. (2015). Evaluation of pediatric upper extremity peripheral nerve injuries. *Journal of Hand Therapy, 28*(2), 135–143. https://doi.org/10.1016/j.jht.2014.09.003

Hsu, H.-Y., Chen, P.-T., Kuan, T.-S., Yang, H.-C., Shieh, S.-J., & Kuo, L.-C. (2019). A touch-observation and task-based mirror therapy protocol to improve sensorimotor control and functional capability of hands for patients with peripheral nerve injury. *American Journal of Occupational Therapy, 73*(2), Article 7302205020. https://doi.org/10.5014/ajot.2018.027763

Hsu, H.-Y., Kuo, L.-C., Kuan, T.-S., Yang, H.-C., Su, F.-C., Chiu, H.-Y., & Shieh, S.-J. (2017). Determining the functional sensibility of the hand in patients with peripheral nerve repair: Feasibility of using a novel manual tactile test for monitoring the progression of nerve regeneration. *Journal of Hand Therapy, 30*(1), 65–73. https://doi.org/10.1016/j.jht.2016.03.004

Hsu, H.-Y., Shieh, S.-J., Kuan, T.-S, Yang, H.-C., Su, F.-C., Chiu, H.-Y., & Kuo, L.-C. (2016). Manual tactile test predicts sensorimotor control capability of hands for patients with peripheral nerve injury. *Archives of Physical Medicine and Rehabilitation, 97*(6), 983–990. https://doi.org/10.1016/j.apmr.2016.01.008

Jerosch-Herold, C. (2011). Sensory relearning in peripheral nerve disorders of the hand: A web-based survey and Delphi consensus method. *Journal of Hand Therapy, 24*(4), 292–298. https://doi.org/10.1016/j.jht.2011.05.002

Krarup, C., Rosén, B., Boeckstyns, M., Ibsen Sørensen, A., Lundborg, G., Moldovan, M., & Archibald, S. J. (2017). Sensation, mechanoreceptor, and nerve fiber function after nerve regeneration. *Annals of Neurology, 82*(6), 940–950. https://doi.org/10.1002/ana.25102

Linnertz, P., Ek, J. P., & Rosén, B. (2019). Shape-texture-identification—STI—A test for tactile gnosis: Concurrent validity of STI2. *Journal of Hand Therapy, 32*(4), 470–475. https://doi.org/10.1016/j.jht.2018.05.004

Moscony, A. M. B. (2014). Peripheral nerve problems. In C. Cooper (Ed.), *Fundamentals of hand therapy* (2nd ed., pp. 272–311). Elsevier.

Novak, C. B., Anastakis, D. J., Beaton, D. E., Mackinnon, S. E., & Katz, J. (2010). Relationships among pain disability, pain intensity, illness intrusiveness, and upper extremity disability in patients with traumatic peripheral nerve injury. *Journal of Hand Surgery, 35*(10), 1633–1639. https://doi.org/10.1016/j.jhsa.2010.07.018

Novak, C. B., Anastakis, D. J., Beaton, D. E., Mackinnon, S. E., & Katz, J. (2011). Biomedical and psychosocial factors associated with disability after peripheral nerve injury. *Journal of Bone and Joint Surgery, 93*(10), 929–936. https://doi.org/10.2106/JBJS.J.00110

Paula, M. H., Barbosa, R. I., Marcolino, A. M., Elui, V. M., Rosén, B., & Fonseca, M. C. R. (2016). Early sensory re-education of the hand after peripheral nerve repair based on mirror therapy: A randomized controlled trial. *Brazilian Journal of Physical Therapy, 20*(1), 58–65. https://doi.org/10.1590/bjpt-rbf.2014.0130

Peck, J., & Ollason, J. (2015). Low profile radial nerve palsy orthosis with radial and ulnar deviation. *Journal of Hand Therapy, 28*(4), 421–424. https://doi.org/10.1016/j.jht.2014.11.007

Porter, R. S. (Ed.). (2018). *The Merck manual of diagnosis and therapy* (20th ed.). Merck Sharp & Dohme.

Rosén, B., & Lundborg, G. (2011). Sensory reeducation. In T. M. Skirven, A. L. Osterman, J. M. Fedorczyk, & P. C. Amadio (Eds.), *Rehabilitation of the hand and upper extremity* (6th ed., pp. 634–645). Mosby.

Rosén, B., Vikström, P., Turner, S., McGrouther, D. A., Selles, R. W., Schreuders, T. A. R., & Björk-man, A. (2015). Enhanced early sensory outcome after nerve repair as a result of immediate post-operative re-learning: A randomized controlled trial. *Journal of Hand Surgery, European, 40*(6), 598–606. https://doi.org/10.1177/1753193414553163

Rostami, H. R., Akbarfahimi, M., Hassani Mehraban, A., Akbarinia, A. R., & Samani, S. (2017). Occupation-based intervention versus rote exercise in modified constraint-induced move-ment therapy for patients with median and ulnar nerve injuries: A randomized controlled trial. *Clinical Rehabilitation, 31*(8), 1087–1097. https://doi.org/10.1177/0269215516672276

Rostami, H. R., Khayatzadeh Mahany, M., & Yarmohammadi, N. (2015). Feasibility of the modified constraint-induced movement therapy in patients with median and ulnar nerve injuries: A single-subject A-B-A design. *Clinical Rehabilitation, 29*(3), 277–284. https://doi.org/10.1177/0269215514542357

Seu, M., & Pasqualetto, M. (2012). Hand therapy for dysfunction of the intrinsic muscles. *Hand Clinics, 28*(1), 87–100. https://doi.org/10.1016/j.hcl.2011.09.001

Stonner, M. M., Mackinnon, S. E., & Kaskutas, V. (2017). Predictors of disability and quality of life with an upper-extremity peripheral nerve disorder. *American Journal of Occupational Therapy, 71*(1), Article 7101190050. https://doi.org/10.5014/ajot.2017.022988

Valdes, K. (2017). Clinical relevance commentary in response to: The sensory function of the un-injured nerve in patients after median and ulnar nerve injury. *Journal of Hand Therapy, 30*(1), 104–105. https://doi.org/10.1016/j.jht.2016.12.002

Wojtkiewicz, D. M., Saunders, J., Domeshek, L., Novak, C. B., Kaskutas, V., & Mackinnon, S. E. (2015). Social impact of peripheral nerve injuries. *Hand, 10*(2), 161–167. https://doi.org/10.1007/s11552-014-9692-0

Yazdani, F., & Dehkordi, F. (2013). Occupational therapy intervention in combination flexor tendon and peripheral nerve injury: 10 patients with disabilities of arm shoulder and hand. *Iranian Rehabilitation Journal, 11*, 21–26.

BIBLIOGRAPHY

Miller, L. K., Chester, R., & Jerosch-Herold, C. (2012). Effects of sensory reeducation programs on functional hand sensibility after median and ulnar repair: A systematic review. *Journal of Hand Therapy, 25*(3), 297–307. https://doi.org/10.1016/j.jht.2012.04.001

Rosén, B., & Björkman, A. (2010). Momentary improvement of hand sensibility by excluding vision. *Journal of Plastic Surgery and Hand Surgery, 44*(6), 302–305. https://doi.org/10.3109/2000656X.2010.535284

Rosén, B., Chemnitz, A., Weibull, A., Andersson, G., Dahlin, L. B., & Björkman, A. (2012). Ce-rebral changes after injury to the median nerve: A long-term follow up. *Journal of Plastic Sur-gery and Hand Surgery, 46*(2), 106–112. https://doi.org/10.3109/2000656X.2011.653257

Valdes, K., Naughton, N., & Algar, L. (2014). Sensorimotor interventions and assessments for the hand and wrist: A scoping review. *Journal of Hand Therapy, 27*(4), 272–286. https://doi.org/10.1016/j.jht.2014.07.002

Vikström, P., Björkman, A., Carlsson, I. K., Olsson, A.-K., & Rosén, B. (2018). Atypical sensory processing pattern following median or ulnar nerve injury—A case-control study. *BMC Neu-rology, 18*, Article 146. https://doi.org/10.1186/s12883-018-1152-y

Vikström, P., Carlsson, I., Rosén, B., & Björkman, A. (2018). Patients' views on early sensory relearning following nerve repair—A Q-methodology study. *Journal of Hand Therapy, 31*(4), 443–450. https://doi.org/10.1016/j.jht.2017.07.003

Vikström, P., Rosén, B., Carlsson, I. K., & Björkman, A. (2018). The effect of early relearning on sensory recovery 4 to 9 years after nerve repair: A report of a randomized controlled study. *Journal of Hand Surgery (European Volume), 43*(6), 626–630. https://doi.org/10.1177/1753193418767024

Zink, P. J., & Philip, B. A. (2020). Cortical plasticity in rehabilitation for upper extremity peripheral nerve injury: A scoping review. *American Journal of Occupational Therapy, 74*(1), Article 7401205030. https://doi.org/10.5014/ajot.2020.036665

Polytrauma
Also called major trauma, multiple trauma.

Description

Polytrauma involves injuries to multiple body parts and organs that result in physical, cognitive, psychological, or psychosocial impairments and functional disability (Yamkovenko, 2011). One or more of the injuries may be life threatening. Polytrauma includes such diagnoses as traumatic brain injury (TBI), amputations, spiral cord injury (SCI), fractures, posttraumatic stress disorder (PTSD), and visual and auditory impairments when seen in combinations at the same time (Barnett, 2014). Nerve and blood vessel damage, unhealed wounds, and infections may add to the list of conditions and possible complications. Care usually requires more than 6 months (Yamkovenko, 2011). Interventions may include a stay in the intensive care unit (ICU), inpatient rehabilitation, outpatient rehabilitation, and community reintegration.

Cause

Fall injuries, traffic accidents, violence, and fire may result in polytrauma. The most common cause in war is an explosion or blast-related incident.

Evaluation/Assessment

Areas

- Activities of Daily Living/Instrumental ADL: self-care, sexual health, meal preparation, budgeting, mobility (wheelchair, driving)
- Education/Work: no information identified
- Play/Leisure: interests, values, hobbies, frequency, location
- Rest/Sleep: sleep disturbance
- Social Participation: type, frequency, location, with whom
- Sensorimotor: range of motion, strength, physical endurance, visual impairment
- Cognitive/Perceptual: mental flexibility, fatigue, visual perception, auditory perception
- Psychosocial: depression, anxiety, self-image, interpersonal relations, motivation
- Context/Environment: adapted equipment, social support, environmental barriers
- Comorbidities: amputation, fractures, posttraumatic stress disorder, spinal cord injury, traumatic brain injury, visual and auditory impairments

Instruments

Instruments Developed by Occupational Therapy Personnel
- None identified

Instruments Developed by Other Professionals and Used by Occupational Therapy Personnel
- Abbreviated Injury Scale (AIS; Association for the Advancement of Automotive Medicine, 2015; sample in Sharma & Ranford, 2017, p. 525, in References)
- Behavioral Pain Scale (BPS; Payen et al., 2001; sample in Sharma & Ranford, 2017, p. 535, in References)
- Blood pressure (blood pressure cuff)
- Confusion Assessment Method for the Intensive Care Unit (CAM-ICU; Ely et al., 2001; sample in Sharma & Ranford, 2017, p. 538, in References)

- Critical-Care Pain Observation Tool (CPOT; Gélinas et al., 2006; sample in Sharma & Ranford, 2017, p. 537, in References)
- Galveston Orientation and Amnesia Test (GOAT; Levin et al., 1979; sample in Sharma & Ranford, 2017, p. 533, in References)
- Heart rate (manual or electronic)
- Injury Severity Score (ISS; Baker et al., 1974; sample in Sharma & Ranford, 2017, p. 526, in References)
- Intensive Care Delirium Screening Checklist (ICDSC; Bergeron et al., 2001)
- JFK Coma Recovery Scale–Revised (CRS-R; Giacino et al., 2004; sample in Dekelboum & Parecki, 2018, p. 1189, and Sharma & Ranford, 2017, p. 534, in References)
- Richmond Agitation–Sedation Scale (RASS; Sessler et al. 2002)
- Riker Sedation-Agitation Scale (RikerSAS; Riker et al., 1999)

Problems/Issues

Activities of Daily Living/Instrumental ADL
- Person may have difficulty performing basic self-care skills due to injury to one or both upper extremities.
- Person may be unable to perform instrumental activities due to brain injury or loss of physical mobility.

Education/Work
- Person may be unable to return to original employment due to injury or loss of function or require modifications to the job site.
- Person may need opportunity to explore work settings and decide on vocational choice.

Play/Leisure
- Person may be unable to engage in favorite leisure activities due to injury and need to explore new activities.
- Person may need modification of equipment to engage in previously enjoyed leisure activities.

Rest/Sleep
- Person may experience sleep disturbances.
- Person may have a sleep disorder related to body injury or injuries.

Social Participation
- Person may resist engagement in activities with family and friends in social and community events.
- Person may need modifications in order to participate in social and community events.

Sensorimotor
- Person often has lost range of motion, muscle strength, and physical endurance due to injuries.
- Person may have visual impairment, especially if brain injury is involved.
- Person may have sensory impairment to other senses.

Cognitive/Perceptual
- Person usually experiences pain.
- Person may experience post-concussion syndrome.
- Person may have decreased attending behaviors: focused, divided.
- Person may have decreased memory: immediate, short term, long term.
- Person may have decreased executive function skills, including problem solving, decision making, judgment of safety.

Psychosocial
- Person may demonstrate signs of delirium especially during time in ICU.
- Person may become agitated.

- Person may develop signs of posttraumatic stress disorder (see Posttraumatic Stress Disorder [PTSD] in Section 12: Mental and Behavioral Disorders).
- Person may become depressed as knowledge of disability is gained and understood.
- Person may express anxiety about self, especially in the future.
- Person may express feelings of loss of self-esteem, self-worth, self-image.
- Person may become apathetic and lack motivation.

Context/Environment
- Family and friends may have difficulty understanding what has happened to the person, and thus social support is reduced.
- Environment such as home may not be accessible without modification.

Intervention/Treatment

No specific occupational therapy model of practice is mentioned in the references. Models developed by others include damage control orthopedics (DCO) used by physicians to support survival after severe trauma. There are four phases: (1) lifesaving procedures only are performed, (2) temporary stabilization of major skeletal injuries is done, (3) optimal time is determined for repair of fractures, and (4) focus is on definitive fracture fixation (Sharma & Ranford, 2017). Team members include physicians, nursing personnel, psychologists, vocational counselors, social workers, physical therapy personnel, and occupational therapy personnel. Goals are to maximize (improve, regain) occupational (functional) performance, to participate in valued, purposeful, and necessary activities and roles, and to minimize occupational disruption (Quick et al., 2014).

Activities of Daily Living/Instrumental ADL
- Self-management skills for independent living including shopping, financial management, home management.
- Driver rehabilitation to reestablish driving ability. Focus on road conditions that are perceived as threatening such as being "boxed in" by other cars, loud noises, or unexpected item in or on the side of road (Classen, Monahan, et al., 2014).
- Driver evaluation to determine driving errors such as lane maintenance, vehicle positioning, signaling, speed regulation, gap acceptance between vehicles, visual scanning for traffic signs or potential danger (Classen, Cormack, et al., 2014; Classen, Monahan, et al., 2014).

Education/Work
- Facilitate opportunities to restore income and economic stability.

Play/Leisure
- Encourage engagement in adapted sports activities if needed.

Rest/Sleep
- Establish a normal sleep–wake cycle for client (also see Sleep–Wake Disorders in Section 13: Lifestyle Conditions).

Social Participation
- Encourage participation in family, social, community, and professional activities.

Sensorimotor
- Use wound-care management, manual therapy, and therapeutic exercise to increase motion, strength, and activity tolerance.
- Encourage mobilization as early as possible.
- Provide fine and gross motor coordination and dexterity activities such as fastening buttons, using a computer, or retrieving dishes from cabinets.
- Provide oculomotor and binocular vision training.

Cognitive/Perceptual

- Create a daily schedule of activity when client is in the ICU to reduce delirium.
- Provide cognitive training to enhance executive function, such as strategies to improve attention span and memory and practice in problem solving.
- Provide visual perceptual training.

Psychosocial

- Initiate coping skills such as relaxation training, breathing exercises, mindfulness training.
- Promote sense of belonging and locus of control to restore self-worth, purpose, and intrinsic motivation.
- Reestablish role performance.

Context/Environment

- Adapted equipment or modification of orthotics for ADL performance or leisure activities.
- Client, family, caregiver education to learn and incorporate new strategies into habits, routines, and lifestyles.
- Environmental modification of living environment may be needed.

Precautions/Safety Considerations

Be alert for signs of multiple organ dysfunction syndrome (MODS), such as changes in blood pressure, heart rate, oxygen level, and laboratory tests including red and white blood cell (MODS is a leading cause of death). Be alert to what medications persons is taking and what effect the meds may have on performance, such as sedatives that may increase risk of falling. Be aware that equipment such as splints, braces, casts, and external fixators can act as barriers to early mobilization; examine ways to minimize the barrier(s). Therapy personnel should read the chart regularly to update information on surgeries done or planned. Person may develop polytrauma clinical triad (chronic pain, posttraumatic stress disorder, and post-concussion syndrome [dizziness, nausea, vomiting, headache, diplopia, irritability, cognitive deficits]).

Prognosis and Outcome

Person is at high risk for long-term cognitive impairment, especially in the area of executive functioning.

REFERENCES

Barnett, F. (2014). Running the gamut: Polytrauma occupational therapy services at Walter Reed National Military Medical Center. *OT Practice, 19*(8), 14–19.

Classen, S., Cormack, N. L., Winter, S. M., Monahan, M., Yarney, A., Lutz, A. L., & Platek, K. (2014). Efficacy of an occupational therapy driving intervention for returning combat veterans. *OTJR: Occupation, Participation and Health, 34*(4), 176–182. https://doi.org/10.3928/15394492-20141006-01

Classen, S., Monahan, M., Canonizado, M., & Winter, S. (2014). Utility of an occupational therapy driving intervention for a combat veteran. *American Journal of Occupational Therapy, 68*(4), 405–411. https://doi.org/10.5014/ajot.2014.010041

Dekelboum, S., & Parecki, K. (2018). Polytrauma and occupational therapy. In H. M. Pendleton & W. Schultz-Krohn (Eds.), *Pedretti's occupational therapy* (8th ed., pp. 1184–1194). Elsevier.

Quick, C., Judkins, J., Prudencio, T., Ryan, D., Hawkins, R., Larres, D. Yeager, A., Welsh, A., & Hackett, L. (2014). *Fact sheet: Occupational therapy in polytrauma.* American Occupational Therapy Association.

Sharma, L., & Ranford, J. (2017). Trauma. In H. Smith-Gabai & S. E. Holm (Eds.), *Occupational therapy in acute care* (2nd ed., pp. 511–538). American Occupational Therapy Association.

Yamkovenko, S. (2011). The new wounds of ward: Polytrauma care and occupational therapy. *OT Practice, 6*(21), 12–18.

Rotator Cuff Disorders

Also called rotator cuff impingement syndrome, rotator cuff tendinopathy.

Description

Rotator cuff disorders include tendinitis and partial or complete tears of the muscles that form the rotator cuff: the supraspinatus, infraspinatus, teres minor, and subscapularis muscles and tendons. The supraspinatus provides shoulder elevation (overhead reach), the infraspinatus and teres minor provide external rotation, and subscapularis performs internal rotation. In addition to movement, the rotator cuff muscles also provide a force to control the head of the humerus in the glenoid fossa (Maher, 2014). Disorders include shoulder impingement syndrome, tendinitis, bursitis, and tears. Shoulder impingement syndrome occurs as a result of compression of the structures located in the subacromial space including the subacromial bursa, supraspinatus, joint capsule, and long head of the biceps. Tendinitis usually occurs as a result of overuse and overhead arm activity and causes pain during active shoulder elevation. Bursitis is inflammation of the subacromial bursa causing pain during passive shoulder elevation, but not during active elevation (Maher, 2014). Tears usually occur in the supraspinatus tendon.

Cause

Rotator cuff disorders may be acute or chronic conditions associated with sports injuries that require overhead arm motions, but also occur for reasons unrelated to sports activities or people without a history of shoulder overuse (Porter, 2018). Pathology may be the consequence of tendon degeneration as a result of microtrauma (repetitive motion or overload) or tendon tear from acute trauma, such as a fall on the outstretched hand with the shoulder in external rotation and abduction (Ratte-Larouche et al., 2017).

Evaluation/Assessment

Areas
- Activities of Daily Living/Instrumental ADL: activities requiring overhead arm use or behind the back
- Education/Work: work absenteeism, work tasks requiring overhead arm use
- Play/Leisure: sports activities, other interests, frequency, location
- Rest/Sleep: sleep disturbance (related to pain and discomfort)
- Social Participation: type, frequency, location, with whom
- Sensorimotor: joint range of motion, muscle strength, pain
- Cognitive/Perceptual: memory, executive function
- Psychosocial: quality of life, role performance
- Context/Environment: client education, accessibility, resources
- Comorbidities: falls, fractures

Instruments
Instruments Developed by Occupational Therapy Personnel
- None listed

Instruments Developed by Other Professionals and Used by Occupational Therapy Personnel
- American Shoulder and Elbow Surgeons Assessment (ASESA; American Shoulder and Elbow Surgeons Research Committee, 1994; see also St-Pierre et al., 2015, in References)
- Constant-Murley Shoulder Scoring System (Constant & Murley, 1987)
- Disabilities of the Arm, Shoulder, and Hand (3rd ed.; DASH-3; Kennedy et al., 2011)
- Drop Arm Test (Dropping sign, Dropping Test [supraspinatus and infraspinatus muscles]; Neer & Demarest, 1990; see also Roy et al., 2017, in References)
- Empty Can Test (see Jobe Test)

- European Quality of Life 5-Dimension Scale (EuroQol 5 Dimension, EQ-5D; EuroQol Group, 1990)
- External rotation lag sign (ERLS; supraspinatus or infraspinatus tear; see Roy et al., 2017, in References)
- Full Can Test (Kelly et al., 1996; tests supraspinatus)
- Functional Shoulder Elevation Test (FSET; Hollinshead et al., 2000)
- Gerber's test (see Lift-off Test)
- Global Rating of Change Scale (GRCS; Kamper et al., 2009)
- Hawkins-Kennedy Test (Hawkins Test; Hawkins & Kennedy, 1980 [supraspinatus tendon, impingement syndrome]; see also Roy et al., 2017, and Villafañe et al., 2015, in References)
- Hornblower's sign (Walch et al., 1998 [infraspinatus, teres minor])
- Isokinetic Muscle Performance Test (IMPT; Oh et al., 2010)
- Jobe Test (Empty Can Test; Jobe & Moynes, 1982 [supraspinatus and infraspinatus]; see also Roy et al., 2017, and Villafañe et al., 2015, in References)
- Lift-Off Test (Gerber & Krushell, 1991; test for subscapularis muscle; see also Roy et al., 2017, in References)
- Neer Impingement Test (Neer's sign; Neer, 1972; subacromial impingement; see also Villafañe et al., 2015, in References)
- Numerical Pain Rating Scales (NPRS; visual analogue scale)
- Painful Arc of Movement Test (Impingement Test; see Roy et al., 2017, in References)
- Patte Test (Patte; Patte & Gerber, 1987; infraspinatus; see also Villafañe et al., 2015, in References)
- Penn Shoulder Score (PSS; Leggin et al., 2006)
- Rotator Cuff Quality of Life Scale (RC-QOL; Hollinshead et al., 2000)
- Shoulder Disability Questionnaire (SDQ; van der Heijden et al., 2000)
- Shoulder Pain and Disability Index (SPADI; Roach et al., 1991)
- Simple Shoulder Test (SST; Lippitt et al., 1993)
- University of California Los Angeles Shoulder Scale (UCLA Shoulder Scale; Roddey et al., 2000)
- Upper Extremity Functional Index (UEFI; Stratford et al., 2001; see also St-Pierre et al., 2016, in References)
- Upper Limb Functional Index (ULFI; Gabel et al., 2006)
- Western Ontario Rotator Cuff (WORC) index (Kirkley et al., 2003; see also St-Pierre et al., 2015, in References)
- Yocum Test (YT; Yocum, 1983; see also Villafañe et al., 2015, in References)

Problems/Issues

Activities of Daily Living/Instrumental ADL
- Person may have difficulty putting on items of clothing that must be slipped over the head such as a T-shirt, sweatshirt, or sweater.
- Person may have difficulty brushing, combing, or washing hair.
- Person may have difficulty hooking a bra, zipping a back-facing zipper, retrieving a wallet from a back pocket, or pulling down a back side of a garment.

Education/Work
- Person may be absent from work for an extended period of time.
- Person may be unable to work because of work demands that require shoulder function.
- Person may be afraid to go to work for fear of additional injury.

Play/Leisure
- Person may be unable to engage in favorite leisure occupations due to shoulder dysfunction.
- Person may need to avoid engagement in leisure occupations that could cause or aggravate shoulder injury, such as sports activities requiring shoulder function (tennis, golf, volleyball, basketball, baseball, bowling).

Rest/Sleep
- Person may experience pain if sleeping with arm above shoulder level.
- Person may experience pain if sleeping with shoulder in adducted and internally rotated position.

Social Participation
- Person may be unable to participate in social activities that require use of shoulder, such as team sports.

Sensorimotor
- Person may experience loss of shoulder joint range of motion.
- Person may experience loss of shoulder and upper extremity muscle strength.
- Person may experience pain in the shoulder, which may radiate down the arm.
- Person may experience stiffness in shoulder and upper extremity.

Cognitive/Perceptual
- Person may experience cognitive impairment, especially if shoulder injury was the result of a fall in which the head also struck a hard surface.

Psychosocial
- Person may become depressed.
- Person may be fearful or anxious about returning to work.
- Person may experience a change in role performance.
- Person may become dependent on others for assistance.
- Person may experience reduced quality of life.

Context/Environment
- Person may lack knowledge of risk of injury to shoulder.
- Person may be unaware of potential community or internet resources.
- Person may be unaware of laws requiring accommodation and accessibility in the workplace.

Intervention/Treatment

Models and programs developed by occupational therapy personnel: None. Models and programs developed by other professionals but used by occupational therapy personnel include manual therapy (Desjardins-Charbonneau et al., 2015) and range of motion exercises (Shimo et al., 2016). Team members include physicians (orthopedists, hand surgeons), nursing personnel, physical therapy personnel, and occupational therapy personnel. Goals are to reduce pain, increase range of motion, and improve functional performance (Desjardins-Charbonneau et al., 2015).

Activities of Daily Living/Instrumental ADL
- Practice in performing ADLs with postsurgical guidelines regarding restricted range of motion.

Education/Work
- Consider with client whether accommodations in workplace would facilitate return to work.
- Consider with client whether redesign of workstation based on ergonomic principles would facilitate return to work.
- Consider with client whether accessibility to workplace (transportation needs including disabled parking) and accessibility within workplace (open doors, stairs, elevators, access to restroom and breakroom/cafeteria) would facilitate return to work.
- Consider with client whether planning for retirement is an option.

Play/Leisure
- Assist client to reengage in favorite leisure occupations, with restrictions on shoulder functions as warranted.
- Assist client to develop new or novel leisure occupations with less demand on shoulder functions.

Rest/Sleep
- Person should be instructed to avoid sleeping with the arm above shoulder level.
- Person should be instructed to avoid sleeping with arm in an adducted and internally rated position to reduce risk of compromising blood supply to the supraspinatus tendon.

Social Participation
- Assist client to continue participation in social occupations with modifications if needed for reduced shoulder function demands.
- Suggest modifications in social participation while shoulder actions are restricted, such as more passive participation (scorekeeper, umpire).

Sensorimotor
- Conservative management: Activity modification to avoid above shoulder level activities, rest, heat or cold applications, nonsteroidal anti-inflammatory drugs (NSAIDs), cortisone injections, electrical stimulation, ultrasound, and exercise.
- Manual therapy: May be used to decrease pain. May not improve function (Desjardins-Charbonneau et al., 2015).
- Pain management: Use of cryotherapy (cold).
- Therapeutic exercise
  - ▶ Focus on pain-free range of motion activities.
  - ▶ Begin with passive range of motion (PROM), moving to active range of motion (AROM), and then to strengthening using isometric and isotonic exercises.
  - ▶ Towel slides: Towel is held with noninvolved hand overhead behind back with involved hand behind back at hip. Noninvolved hand pulls involved hand–arm into internal rotation (Ratte-Larouche et al., 2017).
  - ▶ Overhead pulley: Noninvolved hand pulls involved hand–arm into forward elevation above head (Ratte-Larouche et al., 2017).
  - ▶ Ball rolling against a wall: Using a 12–16 in. diameter ball, client rolls ball with involved hand–arm up wall and from side to side (Ratte-Larouche et al., 2017).
- Therapeutic ultrasound is not recommended (Desmeules et al., 2015).

Cognitive/Perceptual
- Not addressed.

Psychosocial
- Not addressed.

Context/Environment
- Client education to protect the surgical site, promote healing, and prevent recurrence of trauma or slow degenerative process.
- Client education may be needed on donning and doffing a sling if one is used during rehabilitation period.
- Client education may be needed regarding legal rights as a worker or employee.
- Client education may be needed regarding resources available in the community or on the internet.

Precautions/Safety Considerations
Monitor for signs of impingement syndrome.

Prognosis and Outcome
Variable, depending in part on initial cause and in part on adherence to intervention techniques. Surgery may be necessary to remove excess bone and decrease impingement or to repair a complete tear.

REFERENCES

Desjardins-Charbonneau, A., Roy, J. S., Dionne, C. E., Frémont, P., MacDermid, J. C., & Desmeules, F. (2015). The efficacy of manual therapy for rotator cuff tendinopathy: A systematic review and meta-analysis. *Journal of Orthopaedic & Sports Physical Therapy, 45*(5), 330–350. https://doi.org/10.2519/jospt.2015.5455

Desmeules, F., Boudreault, J., Roy, J. S., Dionne, C., Frémont, P., & MacDermid, J. C. (2015). The efficacy of therapeutic ultrasound for rotator cuff tendinopathy: A systematic review and meta-analysis. *Physical Therapy in Sport, 16*(3), 276–284. https://doi.org/10.1016/j.ptsp.2014.09.004

Maher, C. (2014). Orthopaedic conditions. In M. V. Radomski & C. A. Trombly Latham (Eds.), *Occupational therapy for physical dysfunction* (7th ed., pp. 1103–1126). Wolters Kluwer.

Porter, R. S. (Ed.). (2018). *The Merck manual of diagnosis and therapy* (20th ed.). Merck Sharp & Dohme.

Ratte-Larouche, M., Szekeres, M., Sadi, J., & Faber, K. J. (2017). Rotator cuff tendon surgery and postoperative therapy. *Journal of Hand Therapy, 30*(2), 147–157. https://doi.org/10.1016/j.jht.2017.05.008

Roy, J.-S., Desmeules, F., Frémont, P., Dionne, C. E., & MacDermid, J. C. (2017). *Clinical evaluation, treatment and return to work of workers suffering from rotator cuff disorder: A knowledge review.* IRSST.

Shimo, S., Sakamoto, Y., Tokiyoshi, A., & Yamamoto, Y. (2016). Early rehabilitation affects functional outcomes and activities of daily living after arthroscopic rotator cuff repair: A case report. *Journal of Physical Therapy Science, 28*(2), 714–717. https://doi.org/10.1589/jpts.28.714

St-Pierre, C., Desmeules, F., Dionne, C. E., Frémont, P., MacDermid, J. C., & Roy, J. S. (2016). Psychometric properties of self-reported questionnaires for the evaluation of symptoms and functional limitations in individuals with rotator cuff disorders: A systematic review. *Disability and Rehabilitation, 38*(2), 103–122. https://doi.org/10.3109/09638288.2015.1027004

St-Pierre, C., Dionne, C. E., Desmeules, F., & Roy, J. S. (2015). Reliability, validity and responsiveness of a Canadian French adaptation of the Western Ontario Rotator Cuff (WORC) index. *Journal of Hand Therapy, 28*(3), 292–299. https://doi.org/10.1016/j.jht.2015.02.001

Villafañe, J. H., Valdes, K., Anselmi, F., Pirali, C., & Negrini, S. (2015). The diagnostic accuracy of five tests for diagnosing partial-thickness tears of the supraspinatus tendon: A cohort study. *Journal of Hand Therapy, 28*(3), 247–252. https://doi.org/10.1016/j.jht.2015.01.011

BIBLIOGRAPHY

Krischak, G., Gebhard, F., Reichel, H., Friemert, B., Schneider, F., Fisser, C., Kaluscha, R., & Kraus, M. (2013). A prospective randomized controlled trial comparing occupational therapy with home-based exercises in conservative treatment of rotator cuff tears. *Journal of Shoulder and Elbow Surgery, 22*(9), 1173–1179. https://doi.org/10.1016/j.jse.2013.01.008

von der Heyde, R. L. (2011). Occupational therapy interventions for shoulder conditions: A systematic review. *American Journal of Occupational Therapy, 65*(1), 16–23. https://doi.org/10.5014/ajot.2011.09184

Spinal Cord Injuries: Complete (Adult)

Also called paraplegia, quadriplegia, tetraplegia, SCI (Note: paraplegia, quadriplegia, and tetraplegia are used to describe types of neurological involvement in the spinal cord. Terms are not limited to describing spinal cord injuries.).

Description

Spinal cord injuries occur when a blunt physical force damages the vertebrae, ligaments, or disks of the spinal column, causing bruising, crushing, or tearing of the spinal cord tissue, or when the spinal cord is penetrated by a bullet or cut into with a sharp instrument such as a knife blade. The injury may also cause vascular damage resulting in ischemia or hematoma leading to additional damage (Porter, 2018). The injury may result in complete cord injury (no motor or sensory function) or incomplete cord injury (some motor or sensation retained). The cardinal sign of spinal cord injury is a discrete injury level in which neurological function above the injury is intact, and function below the injury is absent or markedly diminished (Porter, 2018).

Cause

The most common causes are motor vehicle crashes in young people and falls in older individuals. Other causes are violence (gunshot injury, stabbings), sports activities, and work-related accidents. About 80% of spinal cord injuries occur in males. In older individuals, osteoporosis and degenerative joint disease may increase the risk of injury (Porter, 2018).

Spinal Injury Impairment Scale
(Adapted from American Spinal Injury Association, 2013)

- A = Complete: There is no motor or sensory function, including in the sacral segments S4–S5.
- B = Sensory incomplete: Sensory but not motor function is preserved below the spinal cord level, including in the sacral segments S4–S5.
- C = Motor incomplete: Motor function is preserved below the neurologic level, and more than half of key muscles below the spinal cord level have a muscle strength grade of less than grade 3.
- D = Motor incomplete: Motor function is preserved below the neurologic level, and at least half of key muscles below the spinal cord level have a muscle grade of equal to or above grade 3.
- E = Normal: Motor and sensory functions are normal.

Key and Non-Key Muscle Function, Upper Extremity
(Summarized from American Spinal Injury Association, 2013)

- Key = C5: Elbow flexors: Non-key = Shoulder flexion, elevation, abduction, adduction, internal and external rotation, and elbow/forearm supination
- Key = C6: Wrist extensors: Non-key = Wrist/forearm pronation and wrist flexion
- Key = C7: Elbow extensors: Non-key = Finger flexion and extension of proximal joints (PIP), thumb flexion extension, abduction in plane of thumb
- Key = C8: Finger flexors: Non-key = Flexion of metacarpophalangeal (MCP) joint and thumb opposition, adduction and abduction perpendicular to palm
- Key = T1: Finger abductors: Non-key = Adduction of index finger

Functional Performance by Level of Injury (Hamby, 2018)

- C1–C3: Dependent with all ADLs, can use electronic activated devices with adapted controls (sip and puff, chin control, head array), no sensation except for face, ventilator dependent and usually has a tracheostomy, incontinent, wears a catheter and has a regimented bowel and bladder program administered by caregiver.
- C4: Dependent with all ADLs, no sensation below level of lesion, may or may not be able to breathe without a ventilator, incontinent, wears a catheter and has a regimented bowel and bladder program administered by caregiver.
- C5: Moderate to maximal assistance needed for functional mobility, minimal to moderate assistance need to perform basic ADLs with adaptive devices, no sensation below level of lesion, regimented bowel and bladder program.
- C6: Moderate assist to independent with basic ADLs with use of adaptive equipment, mobility unsafe on uneven surfaces, may need assistance with transfers, no sensation below level of lesion, regimented bowel and bladder program.

- C7–C8: Able to independently transfer, independent with all basic ADLs with adaptive equipment and durable medical equipment (wheelchair, scooter, hoist), no sensation below level of lesion, may continue to need a bowel and bladder program.
- T1 & below: Independent with all ADLs, may have bowel and bladder dysfunction but can manage program independently.

Evaluation/Assessment

Areas
- Activities of Daily Living/Instrumental ADL: self-maintenance skills (eating, dressing, grooming, bathing/showering, toileting), functional mobility, meal preparation, shopping, driving
- Education/Work: vocational planning and choice, work tolerance, workplace modification
- Play/Leisure: interests, values, location
- Rest/Sleep: sleep habits, sleep disturbances
- Social Participation: type, location, frequency, with whom
- Sensorimotor: muscle strength (stability), muscle tone (spasticity), joint range of motion (flexibility), endurance (tolerance, fatigue), sensation (feeling, discrimination), pain (discomfort)
- Cognitive/Perceptual: attention, memory, executive function, body image
- Psychosocial: depression, anxiety, self-concept, quality of life, interpersonal relations
- Context/Environment: social support, resources, adapted devices
- Comorbidities: osteoporosis, obesity, fractures, pressure ulcers, urinary tract infections, concussion, brain injury

Instruments
(For lists of more assessments, see Jones et al., 2018; Marino et al., 2018.)

Instruments Developed by Occupational Therapy Personnel
- ADL Habits Survey (ADLHS; Bryden & Bezruczko, 2011, in References)
- Functional Task List (FTL; Cornwell et al., 2012, in References)
- Graded Redefined Assessment of Strength Sensibility and Prehension (GRASSP; Kalsi-Ryan et al, 2012; see also Kalsi-Ryan et al., 2016; Kalsi-Ryan et al., 2014; Kalsi-Ryan et al., 2012; Marino et al., 2018; and Velstra et al., 2018, in References)
- Pittsburgh Rehabilitation Participation Scale (PRPS; Lenze et al., 2004)
- Wheelchair Outcome Measure (WhOM; Miller et al., 2011, in References)

Instruments Developed by Other Professionals and Used by Occupational Therapy Personnel
- Capabilities of Upper Extremities-Questionnaire, Revised (CUE-Q; Oleson & Marino, 2014)
- Capabilities of Upper Extremities Test (CUE-T; Marino et al., 1998; see also Marino et al., 2015; Marino et al., 2012; and Marino et al., 2018, in References)
- Community Integration Questionnaire (CIQ; Willer et al., 1993)
- Grasp and Release Test (GRT; Wuolle et al., 1994)
- Jebsen-Taylor Hand Function Test (JTHFT; Jebsen et al., 1969)
- Modified Fatigue Impact Scale (MFIS; Ritvo et al., 1997; see also telephone version by Imam et al., 2012, in References)
- Neuromuscular Recovery Scale (NRS; Behrman et al., 2012; see also Basso et al., 2015; Behrman et al., 2015; and Velozo et al., 2015, in References)
- Participation Measure for Post-Acute Care (PM-PAC; Gandek et al., 2007)
- Physical Activity Wearable Measures (Schneider et al., 2018)
- Spinal Cord Ability Ruler (SCAR; Reed et al., 2017)
- Spinal Cord Independence Measure (Version III; SCIM-III; Itzkovich et al., 2007)
- Spinal Cord Injury Ability Realization Measurement Index (SCIARMI; Catz et al., 2004)
- Spinal Cord Injury-Functional Index (SCI-FI; Tulsky et al., 2012)

Problems/Issues

Activities of Daily Living/Instrumental ADL
- Person with a cervical-level injury will have difficulty performing self-maintenance activities; person with a thoracic or lower-level injury may have difficulty performing self-maintenance activities, especially bathing/showering and toileting.
- Person with a cervical level injury will have difficulty performing meal preparation tasks, home management (cleaning, dusting, doing laundry), child care, pet care, shopping, and driving; person with a thoracic or lower-level injury may have less difficulty performing the same tasks.

Education/Work
- Person will have difficulty commuting to work (paid or unpaid).
- Person may have difficulty working at home depending on the tasks required and technology available.

Play/Leisure
- Person may have difficulty engaging in favorite leisure occupations if motor skills and sensory awareness are involved.

Rest/Sleep
- Person may experience sleep disturbances.

Social Participation
- Person may have difficulty participating in social activities, especially where transport and mobility are involved.

Sensorimotor
- Person may have muscle weakness above level of injury as well as paralysis below level of injury (weakness may include respiration and breathing).
- Person may have reduced range of motion due to loss or weakness of muscle action.
- Person may have changes in muscle tone due to loss or weakness of muscle action.
- Person may have reduced endurance and increased sense of fatigue.
- Person may experience edema or swelling.
- Person may have decreased fine motor skills including coordination and dexterity.
- Person may have decreased sensation (tactile, deep pressure, temperature).
- Person may experience pain.

Cognitive/Perceptual
- Person may have experienced a concussion or a brain injury resulting in cognitive impairment or dysfunction in addition to the spinal cord injury.
- Person may have little knowledge and understanding of the nature of the spinal cord injury that has occurred.
- Person may have a distorted or unrealistic body image.
- Person many have difficulty with visual perception (when concussion also occurred).

Psychosocial
- Person may become depressed as reality of injury is understood.
- Person will experience change in quality of life.
- Person may experience a change in interpersonal relations.
- Person may experience changes in role perform and functions.

Context/Environment
- Person may experience changes in social support.
- Person may need adapted equipment including training (application, putting on and taking off) and care.
- Person may need a splint or splints to improve hand function.

- Person may need home modification.
- Person and caregivers may need training in care of skin to prevent pressure ulcers.
- Person and caregivers may need training in managing mobility including a hoist, wheelchair, or scooter.

Intervention/Treatment

Models and programs developed by occupational therapy personnel include aquatic therapy (Silvestri & Perone, 2015), amount of occupational therapy time (Foy et al., 2011), dynamic splinting (Kimbler & Willis, 2010), ecology of human performance (Silvestri, 2017), enabling performance (Gregorio-Torres et al., 2011), standing tall (Doolin-Carver, 2012), and wheelchair skill training program (Desai et al., 2013). Models and programs developed by other professionals but used by occupational therapy personnel include aerobic exercise (Tawashy et al., 2010), bariatric positioning program (Ardanowski & Pasch, 2011), functional electrical stimulation (Martin, 2011), group therapy (Zanca et al., 2013), multidisciplinary outpatient program (Derakhshanrad et al., 2015), neuroprosthetic approaches (Kilgore et al., 2018; Memberg et al., 2014), robotic therapy (Kim et al., 2019; Sledziewski et al., 2012), wheelchair prescription guidelines (Lukersmith et al., 2013), wheeled mobility training (Taylor et al., 2015), and work and spinal-cord-injury resource program (Dorstyn et al., 2019). Team members including physicians, nursing personnel, psychologists, respiratory or inhalation therapists, physical therapy personnel, and occupational therapy personnel. Goals in therapy are dependent on the level of injury. Long-term goals must take into account the remaining level of functional performance assisted by adapted devices and equipment.

Activities of Daily Living/Instrumental ADL

- Clients with injuries from C2–C4 will need maximum assistance to perform all ADL and IADL tasks.
- Beginning with injuries at C5, clients can practice performing basic ADL skills independently using adapted devices as needed such as eating and washing face and hands, putting on a T-shirt.
- Beginning with injuries at C7–C8, hand function is sufficient for most basic ADLs, and many IADL tasks requiring hand function.
- Promote healthy lifestyle and eating habits to prevent complications.
- Assist client to consider developing intimate and/or sexual relations, such as selecting a sling to allow a person to maintain a sexual position.
- Conduct driving evaluations and training and recommend adaptations to vehicles to ensure driver and passenger safety such as hand controls, lift accessible.
- If young children or pets are part of the household, special training may be needed to manage care from a wheelchair.

Education/Work

- Facilitate education and work opportunities including exploring career opportunities.
- Assist in recommending workstation modification to increase safety and accessibility.

Play/Leisure

- Assist client to identify, explore, and practice leisure occupations that are already known and meaningful to the individual.
- Assist client to identify, explore, and practice leisure occupations that are novel or new to the client but are of interest.

Rest/Sleep

- Assist in identifying bedding that can be used to help turn the client for repositioning but does not increase shear forces; a hoist may be needed.
- Assist in creating a schedule that can be followed at home or other nonhospital environment.

Social Participation
- Encourage and facilitate participation in social activities.
- Assist client to reduce negative attitudes and increase social opportunities.

Sensorimotor
- Provide motor-based interventions by level of injury (Hamby, 2018).
  - ▶ C1–C3-level injury
    - ○ Assist client to increase skills needed to control a wheelchair (blowing paper with a straw for sip and puff); moving chin up, down, and sideways for chin control; moving head right and left for head array.
    - ○ Maintain passive range of motion of upper and lower extremities to maintain flexibility and prevent contractures and deformities.
    - ○ Maintain neck flexibility using isometric exercises if fracture site is stable.
    - ○ Practice moving client in and out of bed using a lift to access wheelchair. Note that client needs to be able to instruct a caregiver on safe lifting.
    - ○ Note positioning time schedule for rolling over or shifting weight while sitting. Client need to be aware of time schedule and instruct a caregiver to change positions.
  - ▶ C4-level injury
    - ○ Increase strength of scapula and trapezius muscles to improve positioning and aid in respiration.
    - ○ Increase strength of accessory and diaphragmatic muscles to improve respiration.
    - ○ Provide practice in "quad coughing."
    - ○ Provide daily passive range of motion to arms and legs to maintain flexibility and prevent deformities.
    - ○ Practice moving client in and out of bed using a lift to access wheelchair (note that client needs to be able to instruct a caregiver on safe lifting).
    - ○ Note positioning time schedule for rolling over or shifting weight while sitting (client needs to be aware of time schedule and instruct a caregiver to change positions).
    - ○ Monitor vital signs.
    - ○ Consider need for splints to facilitate wrist extension.
  - ▶ C5-level injury
    - ○ Increase strength of scapular motions including external rotation.
    - ○ Maintain range of motion especially of elbow extension.
    - ○ Practice ADLs with adapted devices: eating, washing face and hands, upper body dressing.
    - ○ Consider need for splints to facilitate wrist extension.
    - ○ Practice moving client in and out of bed using a lift to access wheelchair.
    - ○ Note positioning time schedule.
    - ○ Monitor vital signs.
  - ▶ C6-level injury
    - ○ Increase strength of scapular motions including depression with lower trapezius.
    - ○ Practice moving from bed to chair and back using a lift.
    - ○ Practice basic ADLs with adapted devices as needed.
    - ○ Focus on use of wrist to maximize tenodesis grasp.
    - ○ Consider use of a short opponens splint.
    - ○ Teach client how to provide effective caregiver instructions.
    - ○ Note positioning time schedule.
    - ○ Monitor vital signs.
  - ▶ C7–C8-level injury
    - ○ Increase strengthening upper extremity muscles including intrinsic hand muscles for opposition.
    - ○ Practice moving from bed to chair using a transfer board.
    - ○ Practice basic ADLs with adapted devices as needed.

- Begin practicing IADLs such as meal preparation, doing laundry, light housekeeping, keyboarding.
- Teach client how to provide effective caregiver instructions.
- Note positioning time schedule.
- Monitor vital signs.
  - ▶ T1-level and below injury
    - Practice moving from bed to chair safely including toilet seat.
    - Practice basic ADLs with or without adapted devices.
    - Focus on IADLs including community skills.
    - Practice independent management of bowel and bladder program.
    - Teach client how to provide effective caregiver instructions.
    - Note positioning time schedule.
    - Monitor vital signs.
- Provide sensory reeducation: Assist client to identify risks for skin injuries.
- Instruct client and caregivers in energy conservation and fatigue management.
- Instruct client in pain management.

Cognitive/Perceptual
- Assist client to problem solve to identify when changes are needed and incorporate new routines as the person ages.

Psychosocial
- Encourage client to express concerns about abilities and limitations.
- Encourage client to identify activities that will improve quality of life.

Context/Environment
- Assist in providing adapted and durable medical equipment and training by level of injury (Hamby, 2018).
  - ▶ C1–C3: Hospital bed, electronic control unit (ECU), power tilt-in-space wheelchair with adapted controls such as sip and puff, chin or head control, and portable ventilator.
  - ▶ C4: Hospital bed, ECU, power tilt-in-space wheelchair, mouth stick.
  - ▶ C5: Hospital bed, mobile arm support, adapted feeding devices such as a universal cuff, hand splints, power tilt-in-space wheelchair, Hoyer lift, roll-in shower chair.
  - ▶ C6: Hospital bed, manual wheelchair with rim projections or electric wheelchair with power lift, adapted equipment for basic ADLs, tub bench or roll-in shower chair.
  - ▶ C7–C8: Hospital or standard bed, sliding/transfer board, manual wheelchair with hand rims, push gloves to protect hands, adapted devices for ADLs, tub bench, adapted seat for bowel program.
- Provide family and caregivers information and training on care of person with a spinal cord injury.
- Provide client and family with information on hiring and training a personal care assistant.
- Provide consultation and recommendation on wheelchair seating and positioning systems to optimize function, mobility, and participation in home and community.
- Provide consultation and training in the use of low- and high-tech assistive technology such as adapting a smartphone, using voice recognition software.
- Provide information and resources on home modification and accessibility.
- Provide information on available community accessibility.
- Educate client to be an advocate for persons with disabilities including laws, transportation, and accessibility.

Precautions/Safety Considerations
- Monitor vital signs regularly (blood pressure, heart and breathing rate, oxygen saturation).
- Monitor skin condition daily to prevent pressure ulcers. Monitor positioning schedule (lying down and sitting) to prevent pressure ulcers.

Prognosis and Outcome

If lesion or injury results in complete loss of motor and sensory function, condition is chronic. Use of adapted and durable medical equipment must be used. Health care needs change with age and should be monitored as the person ages (Kern et al., 2019; Sakakibara et al., 2012).

REFERENCES

American Spinal Injury Association. (2013). *International standards for neurological classification of spinal cord injury.* (See chart in Hamby, 2018, Appendix 18E, pp. 288–289)

Ardanowski, C., & Pasch, P. (2011). Spinal cord injury and the bariatric patient. *Rehab Management, 24*(6), 18–21

Basso, D. M., Velozo, C., Lorenz, D., Suter, S., & Behrman, A. L. (2015). Interrater reliability of the Neuromuscular Recovery Scale for spinal cord injury. *Archives of Physical Medicine and Rehabilitation, 96*(8), 1397–1403. https://doi.org/10.1016/j.apmr.2014.11.026

Behrman, A. L., Velozo, C., Suter, S., Lorenz, D., & Basso, D. M. (2015). Test-retest reliability of the Neuromuscular Recovery Scale. *Archives of Physical Medicine and Rehabilitation, 96*(8), 1375–1384. https://doi.org/10.1016/j.apmr.2015.03.022

Bryden, A., & Bezruczko, N. (2011). An ADL measure for spinal cord injury. *Journal of Applied Measurement, 12*(3), 279–297.

Cornwell, A. S., Liao, J. Y., Bryden, A. M., & Kirsch, R. F. (2012). Standard task set for evaluating rehabilitation intervention for individuals with arm paralysis. *Journal of Rehabilitation Research and Development, 49*(3), 395–403. https://dx.doi.org/10.1682/jrrd.2011.03.0040

Derakhshanrad, N., Vosoughi, F., Yekaninejad, M. S. Moshayedi, P., & Saberi, H. (2015). Functional impact of multidisciplinary outpatient program on patients with chronic complete spinal cord injury. *Spinal Cord, 53*(12), 860–865. https://doi.org/10.1038/sc.2015.136

Desai, R., Jayavant, S., & Varshneya, H. (2013). To investigate the immediate and short term effects of wheelchair skill training program (WSTP) on participation in patients with spinal cord involvement. *Indian Journal of Occupational Therapy, 45*(2), 9–14.

Doolin-Carver, A. J. (2012). Standing tall post-injury. *Rehab Management, 25*(9), 32–35.

Dorstyn, D., Roberts, R., Murphy, G. Craig, A., Kneebone, I., Stewart, P., Chur-Hansen, A., Marshall, R., Clark, J., & Migliorini, C. (2019). Work and SCI: A pilot randomized controlled study of an online resource for job-seekers with spinal cord dysfunction. *Spinal Cord, 57*(3), 221–228. https://doi.org/10.1038/s41393-018-0200-1

Foy, T., Perritt, G., Thimmaiah, D., Heisler, L., Offutt, J. L., Cantoni, K., Hseih, C.-H., Gassaway, J., Ozelie, R., & Backus, D. (2011). Occupational therapy treatment time during inpatient spinal cord injury rehabilitation. *Journal of Spinal Cord Medicine, 34*(2), 162–175. https://doi.org/10.1179/107902611X12971826988093

Gregorio-Torres, T., Laredo, R., & Krenek Andrews, S. (2011). Enabling performance and participation following spinal cord injury. In C. H. Christiansen & K. M. Matuska (Eds.), *Ways of living* (4th ed., pp. 239–280). AOTA Press.

Hamby, J. R. (2018). The nervous system—Spinal cord injuries. In H. Smith-Gabai & S. E. Holm (Eds.), *Occupational therapy in acute care* (2nd ed., pp. 331–339). AOTA Press.

Imam, B., Anton, H. A., & Miller W. C. (2012). Measurement properties of a telephone version of the Modified Fatigue Impact Scale among individuals with a traumatic spinal cord injury. *Spinal Cord, 50*(12), 920–924. https://doi.org/10.1038/sc.2012.79

Jones, L. A. T., Bryden, A., Wheeler, T. L., Tansey, K. E., Anderson, K. D., Beattie, M. S., Blight, A., Curt, A., Field-Fote, E., Guest, J. D., Hseih, J., Jakeman, L. B., Kalsi-Ryan, S., Krisa, L., Lammertse, D. P., Leiby, B., Marino, R., Schwab, J. M., Scivoletto, G., . . . Steeves, J. D. (2018). Considerations and recommendations for selection and utilization of upper extremity clinical outcome assessments in human spinal cord injury trials. *Spinal Cord, 56*, 414–425. https://doi.org/10.1038/s41393-017-0015-5

Kalsi-Ryan, S., Beaton, D., Ahn, H., Askes, H., Drew, B., Curt, A., Popovic, M. R., Wang, J., Verrier, M. C., & Fehlings, M. G. (2016). Responsiveness, sensitivity, and minimally detectable difference of the Graded and Redefined Assessment of Strength, Sensibility, and Prehension, Version 1.0. *Journal of Neurotrauma, 33*(3), 307–314. https://doi.org/10.1089/neu.2015.4217

Kalsi-Ryan, S., Beaton, D., Curt, A., Duff, S., Jiang, D., Popovic, M. R., Rudhe, C., Fehlings, M. G., & Verrier, M. C. (2014). Defining the role of sensation, strength, and prehension for upper limb function in cervical spinal cord injury. *Neurorehabilitation and Neural Repair, 28*(1), 66–74. https://doi.org/10.1177/1545968313490998

Kalsi-Ryan, S., Beaton, D., Curt, A., Duff, S., Popovic, M. R., Rudhe, C., Fehlings, M. G., & Verrier, M. C. (2012). The Graded Redefined Assessment of Strength Sensibility and Prehension: Reliability and validity. *Journal of Neurotrauma, 29*(5), 905–914. https://doi.org/10.1089/neu.2010.1504

Kern, S. B., Hunter, L. N., Sims, A. C., Berzins, D., Riekena, H., Andrews, M. L., Alderfer, J. K., Nelson, K., & Kushner, R. (2019). Understanding the changing health care needs of individuals aging with spinal cord injury. *Topics in Spinal Cord Injury Rehabilitation, 25*(1), 62–73. https://doi.org/10.1310/sci2501-62

Kilgore, K. L., Bryden, A., Keith M. W., Hoyen, H. A., Hart, R., Nemunaitis, G. A., & Peckham, P. H. (2018). Evolution of neuroprosthetic approaches to restoration of upper extremity function in spinal cord injury. *Topics in Spinal Cord Injury Rehabilitation, 24*(3), 252–264. https://doi.org/10.1310/sci2403-252

Kim, J., Lee, B. S., Lee, H.-J., Kim, H.-R., Cho, D.-Y., Lim, J.-E., Kim, J.-J., Kim, H. Y., & Han, Z.-A. (2019). Clinical efficacy of upper limb robotic therapy in people with tetraplegia: A pilot randomized controlled trial. *Spinal Cord, 57*(1), 49–57. https://doi.org/10.1038/s41393-018-0190-z

Kimbler, T. S., & Willis, F. B. (2010). Dynamic splinting for pronation contracture following a spinal cord injury. *Hand Therapy, 15*(1), 20–22. https://doi.org/10.1258/ht.2009.010001

Lukersmith, S., Radbron, L., & Hopman, K. (2013). Development of clinical guidelines for the prescription of a seated wheelchair or mobility scooter for people with traumatic brain injury or spinal cord injury. *Australian Occupational Therapy Journal, 60*(6), 378–386. https://doi.org/10.1111/1440-1630.12077

Marino, R. J., Kern, S. B., Leiby, B., Schmidt-Read, M., & Mulcahey, M. J. (2015). Reliability and validity of the capabilities of upper extremity test (CUE-T) in subjects with chronic spinal cord injury. *Journal of Spinal Cord Medicine, 38*(4), 498–504. https://doi.org/10.1179/2045772314Y.0000000272

Marino, R. J., Patrick, M., Albright, W., Leiby, B. E., Mulcahey, M. J., Schmidt-Read, M., & Kern, S. B. (2012). Development of an objective test of upper-limb function in tetraplegia: The capabilities of upper extremity test. *American Journal of Physical Medicine & Rehabilitation, 91*(6), 478–486 https://doi.org/10.1097/PHM.0b013e31824fa6cc

Marino, R. J., Sinko, R., Bryden, A., Backus, D., Chen, D., Nemunaitis, G. A., & Leiby, B. E. (2018). Comparison of responsiveness and minimal clinically important difference of the Capabilities of Upper Extremity Test (CUE-T) and the Graded Redefined Assessment of Strength, Sensibility and Prehension (GRASSP). *Topics in Spinal Cord Injury Rehabilitation, 24*(3), 227–238. https://doi.org/10.1310/sci2403-227

Martin, R. (2011). Therapy following spinal cord injury. *Rehab Management, 24*(6), 22–23.

Memberg, W. D., Polasek, K. H., Hart, R. L., Bryden, A. M., Kilgore, K. L., Nemunaitis, G. A., Hoyen, H. A., Keith, M. W., & Kirsch, R. F. (2014). Implanted neuroprosthesis for restoring arm and hand function in people with high level tetraplegia. *Archives of Physical Medicine and Rehabilitation, 95*(6), 1201–1211. https://doi.org/10.1016/j.apmr.2014.01.028

Miller, W. C., Garden, J., & Mortenson, W. B. (2011). Measurement properties of the wheelchair outcome measure in individuals with spinal cord injury. *Spinal Cord, 49*(9), 995–1000. https://doi.org/10.1038/sc.2011.45

Porter, R. S. (Ed.). (2018). *The Merck manual of diagnosis and therapy* (20th ed.). Merck Sharp & Dohme.

Sakakibara, B. M., Hitzig, S. L., Miller, W. C., Eng, J. J., & the SCIRE Research Team. (2012). An evidence-based review on the influence of aging with a spinal cord injury on subjective quality of life. *Spinal Cord, 50*(8), 570–578. https://doi.org/10.1038/sc.2012.19

Silvestri, J. (2017). Effects of chronic shoulder pain on quality of life and occupational engagement in the population with chronic spinal cord injury: Preparing for the best outcomes with occupational therapy. *Disability and Rehabilitation, 39*(1), 82–90. https://doi.org/10.3109/09638288.2016.1140829

Silvestri, J. L., & Perone, K. (2015). Aquatic therapy in spinal cord injury. *Rehab Management, 28*(5), 8–13.

Sledziewski, L., Schaaf, R. C., & Mount, J. (2012). Use of robotics in spinal cord injury: A case report. *American Journal of Occupational Therapy, 66*(1), 51–58. https://doi.org/10.5014/ajot.2012.000943

Tawashy, A. E., Eng, J. J., Krassioukov, A. V., Miller, W. C., & Sproule, S. (2010). Aerobic exercise during early rehabilitation for cervical spinal cord injury. *Physical Therapy, 90*(3), 427–437. https://doi.org/10.2522/ptj.20090023

Taylor, S., Gassaway, J., Heisler-Varriale, L. A., Kozlowski, A., Teeter, L., Labarbera, J., Vargas, C., Natale, A., & Swirsky, A. (2015). Patterns in wheeled mobility skills training, equipment evaluation, and utilization: Findings from the SCIRehab project. *Assistive Technology, 27*(2), 59–68. https://doi.org/10.1080/10400435.2014.978511

Velozo, C., Moorhouse, M., Ardolino, E., Lorenz, D., Suter, S., Basso, D. M., & Behrman, A. L. (2015). Validity of the Neuromuscular Recovery Scale: A measurement model approach. *Archives of Physical Medicine and Rehabilitation, 96*(8), 1385–1396. https://doi.org/10.1016/j.apmr.2015.04.004

Velstra, I.-M., Fellinghauer, C., Abel, R., Kalsi-Ryan, S., Rupp, R., & Curt, A. (2018). The Graded and Redefined Assessment of Strength, Sensibility, and Prehension Version 2 provides interval measure properties. *Journal of Neurotrauma, 35*(6), 854–863. https://doi.org/10.1089/neu.2017.5195

Zanca, J. M., Dijkers, M. P., Hsieh, C.-H., Heinemann, A. W., Horn, S. D., Smout, R. J., & Backus, D. (2013). Group therapy utilization in inpatient spinal cord injury rehabilitation. *Archives of Physical Medicine and Rehabilitation, 94*(4, Suppl.), S145–S153. https://doi.org/10.1016/j.apmr.2012.11.049

BIBLIOGRAPHY

Alve, Y. A., & Bontje, P. (2019). Factors influencing participation in daily activities by persons with spinal cord injury: Lessons learned from an international scoping review. *Topics in Spinal Cord Injury Rehabilitation, 25*(1), 41–61. https://doi.org/10.1310/sci2501-41

Anton, H. A., Miller, W. C. Townson, A. F., Imam, B., Silverberg, N., & Forwell, S. (2017). The course of fatigue after acute spinal cord injury. *Spinal Cord, 55*(1), 94–97. https://doi.org/10.1038/sc.2016.102

Atkins, M. S. (2014). Spinal cord injury. In M. V. Radomski & C. A. Thrombly Latham (Eds.), *Occupational therapy for physical dysfunction* (7th ed., pp. 1168–1214). Wolters Kluwer.

Atkins, M. S., & Bashar, J. C. (2015). *Fact sheet: Occupational therapy and the care of individuals with spinal cord injury.* American Occupational Therapy Association.

Atrice, M. B., Morrison, S. A., McDowell, S. L., Ackerman, P. M., Foy, T. A., & Tefertiller, C. (2013). Traumatic spinal cord injury. In D. A. Umphred, G. U. Burton, R. T. Lazaro, & M. L. Roller (Eds.), *Umphred's neurological rehabilitation* (6th ed., pp. 459–520). Elsevier.

Barclay, L., McDonald, R., Lentin, P., & Bourke-Taylor, H. (2016). Facilitators and barriers to social and community participation following spinal cord injury. *Australian Occupational Therapy Journal, 63*(1), 19–28. https://doi.org/10.1111/1440-1630.12241

Barshar, J., & Hughes, C. A. (2018). Spinal cord injury. In H. M. Pendleton & W. Schultz-Krohn (Eds.), *Pedretti's occupational therapy* (8th ed., pp. 904–928). Elsevier.

Brogioli, M., Schneider, S., Popp, W. L., Albisser, U., Brust, A. K. I., Velstra, I. M., Gassert, R., Curt, A., & Starkey, M. L. (2016). Monitoring upper limb recovery after cervical spinal cord injury: Insights beyond assessment scores. *Frontiers in Neurology, 7*, Article 142. https://doi.org/10.3389/fneur.2016.00142

Bryden, A., Kilgore, K. L., & Nemunaitis, G. A. (2018). Advanced assessment of the upper limb in tetraplegia: A three-tiered approach to characterizing paralysis. *Topics in Spinal Cord Injury Rehabilitation, 24*(3), 206–216. https://doi.org/10.1310/sci2403-206

Bryden, A. M., Hoyen, H. A., Keith, M. W., Mejia, M., Kilgore, K. L., & Nemunaitis, G. A. (2016). Upper extremity assessment in tetraplegia: The importance of differentiating between upper and lower motor neuron paralysis. *Archives of Physical Medicine and Rehabilitation, 97*(6, Suppl.), S97–S104. https://doi.org/10.1016/j.apmr.2015.11.021

Callaway, L., Enticott, J., Farnworth, L., McDonald, R., Migliorini, C., & Willer, B. (2017). Community integration outcomes of people with spinal cord injury and multiple matched controls: A pilot study. *Australian Occupational Therapy Journal, 64*(3), 226–234. https://doi.org/10.1111/1440-1630.12350

Chan, C. W. L., Miller, W. C., Quérée, M., Noonan, V. K., Wolfe, D. L., & the SCIRE Research Team. (2017). The development of an outcome measures toolkit for spinal cord injury rehabilitation. *Canadian Journal of Occupational Therapy, 84*(2), 119–129. https://doi.org/10.1177/0008417417690170

Chang, F. H., Ni, P., Coster, W. J., Whiteneck, G. G., & Jette, A. M. (2016). Measurement properties of a modified measure of participation for persons with spinal cord injury. *Journal of Spinal Cord Medicine, 39*(4), 476–483. https://doi.org/10.1080/10790268.2016.1157956

Cohen, M. L., Tulsky, D. S., Holdnack, J. A., Carlozzi, N. E., Wong, A., Magasi, S., Heaton, R. K., & Heinemann, A. W. (2017). Cognition among community-dwelling individuals with spinal cord injury. *Rehabilitation Psychology, 62*(4), 425–434. https://doi.org/10.1037/rep0000140

DeJong, G., Tian, W., Hsieh, C. H., Junn, C., Karam, C., Ballard, P. H., Smout, R. J., Horn, S. D., Zanca, J. M., Heinemann, A. W., Hammond, F. M., & Backus, D. (2013). Rehospitalization in the first year of traumatic spinal cord injury after discharge from medical rehabilitation. *Archives of Physical Medicine and Rehabilitation, 94*(4, Suppl.), S87–S97. https://doi.org/10.1016/j.apmr.2012.10.037

Ford, S., Keay, A., & Skipper, D. (2014). *Occupational therapy interventions for adults with a spinal cord injury: An overview.* Agency for Clinical Innovation. https://aci.health.nsw.gov.au/__data/assets/pdf_file/0004/155191/occupational-therapy-interventions.pdf

Hardwick, D., Bryden, A., Kubec, G., & Kilgore, K. (2018). Factors associated with upper extremity contractures after cervical spinal cord injury: A pilot study. *Journal of Spinal Cord Medicine, 41*(3), 337–346. https://doi.org/10.1080/10790268.2017.1331894

Haywood, C., Pyatak, E., Leland, N., Henwood, B., & Lawlor, M. C. (2019). A qualitative study of caregiving for adolescents and young adults with spinal cord injuries: Lessons from lived experiences. *Topics in Spinal Cord Injury Rehabilitation, 25*(4), 281–289. https://doi.org/10.1310/sci2504-281

Hill, M. R., Noonan, V. K., Sakakibara, B. M., Miller, W. C., & the SCIRE Research Team. (2010). Quality of life instruments and definitions in individuals with spinal cord injury: A systematic review. *Spinal Cord, 48*(6), 438–450. https://doi.org/10.1038/sc.2009.164

Hitzig, S. L., Eng, J. J., Miller, W. C., Sakakibara, B. M., & the SCIRE Research Team. (2011). An evidence-based review of aging of the body systems following spinal cord injury. *Spinal Cord, 49*(6), 684–701. https://doi.org/10.1038/sc.2010.178

Hwang, E. J., Groves, M. D., Sanchez, J. N., Hudson, C. E., Jao, R. G., & Kroll, M. E. (2016). Barriers to leisure-time physical activities in individuals with spinal cord injury. *Occupational Therapy in Health Care, 30*(3), 215–230. https://doi.org/10.1080/07380577.2016.1183180

Kalsi-Ryan, S., Beaton, D., Curt, A., Popovic, M. R., Verrier, M. C., & Fehlings, M. G. (2014). Outcome of the upper limb in cervical spinal cord injury: Profiles of recovery and insights for clinical studies. *Journal of Spinal Cord Medicine, 37*(5), 503–510. https://doi.org/10.1179/20 45772314Y.0000000252

Kumar, S. K., Kumar, V., & Praveenraj, J. D. (2012). Community reintegration and quality of life in rehabilitated south Indian persons with spinal cord injury. *Indian Journal of Occupational Therapy, 44*(3), 11–16.

Lee, A. K., Miller, W. C., Townson, A. F., Anton, H. A., & the F2N2 Research Group. (2010). Medication use is associated with fatigue in a sample of community-living individuals who have a spinal cord injury: A chart review. *Spinal Cord, 48*(5), 429–433. https://doi.org/10.1038/sc.20 09.145

Lundström, U., Lilja, M., Gray, D., & Isaksson, G. (2015). Experiences of participation in everyday occupations among persons aging with a tetraplegia. *Disability and Rehabilitation, 37*(11), 951–957. https://doi.org/10.3109/09638288.2014.948139

Machacova, K., Lysack, C., & Neufeld, S. (2011). Self-rated health among persons with spinal cord injury: What is the role of physical ability? *Journal of Spinal Cord Medicine, 34*(3), 265–272. https://doi.org/10.1179/107902610X12883422813660

Mortenson, W. B., Demers, L., Rushton, P. W., Auger, C., Routhier, F., & Miller, W. C. (2015). Exploratory validation of a multidimensional power wheelchair outcomes toolkit. *Archives of Physical Medicine and Rehabilitation, 96*(12), 2184–2193. https://doi.org/10.1016/j.apmr.20 15.08.430

Mortenson, W. B., Noreau, L., & Miller, W. C. (2010). The relationship between and predictors of quality of life after spinal cord injury at 3 and 15 months after discharge. *Spinal Cord, 48*(1), 73–79. https://doi.org/10.1038/sc.2009.92

Ozelie, R., Gassaway, J., Buchman, E., Thimmaiah, D., Heisler, L., Cantoni, K., Foy, T., Hsieh, C.-H., Smout, R. J., Kreider, S. E. D., & Whiteneck, G. (2012). Relationship of occupational therapy inpatient rehabilitation interventions and patient characteristics to outcomes following spinal cord injury: The SCIRehab project. *Journal of Spinal Cord Medicine, 35*(6), 527–546. https:// doi.org/10.1179/2045772312Y.0000000062

Peljovich, A. E., Bryden, A. M., Malone, K., Hoyen, H., Hernandez-Gonzalez, E., & Keith, M. W. (2011). Rehabilitation of the hand and upper extremity in tetraplegia. In T. M. Skirven, A. L. Osterman, J. M. Fedorczyk, & P. C. Amadio (Eds.), *Rehabilitation of the hand and upper extremity* (6th ed., pp. 1684–1705). Elsevier Mosby.

Price, P., Stephenson, S., Krantz, L., & Ward, K. (2011). Beyond my front door: The occupational and social participation of adults with spinal cord injury. *OTJR: Occupation, Participation and Health, 31*(2), 81–88. https://doi.org/10.3928/15394492-20100521-01

Robinson, J., Forrest, A., Pope-Ellis, C., & Hargreaves, A. T. (2011). A pilot study on sexuality in rehabilitation of the spinal cord injured: Exploring the woman's perspective. *South African Journal of Occupational Therapy, 41*(2), 13–17.

Rushton, P. W., Miller, W. C., Mortenson, W. B., & Garden, J. (2010). Satisfaction with participation using a manual wheelchair among individuals with spinal cord injury. *Spinal Cord, 48*(9), 691–696. https://doi.org/10.1038/sc.2009.197

Schneider, S., Popp, W. L., Brogioli, M., Albisser, U., Demkó, L., Debecker, I., Velstra, I.-M., Gassert, R., & Curt, A. (2018). Reliability of wearable-sensor-derived measures of physical activity in wheelchair-dependent spinal cord injured patients. *Frontiers in Neurology, 9*, Article 1039. https://doi.org/10.3389/fneur.2018.01039

Smith, E. M., Boucher, N., & Miller, W. C. (2016). Caregiving services in spinal cord injury: A systematic review of the literature. *Spinal Cord, 54*(8), 562–569. https://doi.org/10.1038/sc .2016.8

Smith, E. M., Imam, B., Miller, W. C., Silverberg, N. D., Anton, H. A., Forwell, S. J., & Townson, A. F. (2016). The relationship between fatigue and participation in spinal cord injury. *Spinal Cord, 54*(6), 457–462. https://doi.org/10.1038/sc.2015.149

Teo, S. H. J., Sew, S., Backman, C., Forwell, S., Lee, W. K., Chan, P. L., & Dean, E. (2011). Health of people with spinal cord injury in Singapore: Implications for rehabilitation planning and implementation. *Disability and Rehabilitation, 33*(15-16), 1460–1474. https://doi.org/10.31 09/09638288.2010.533812

Thielen, C. C., Marino, R. J., Duff, S., Kaplan, G., & Mulcahey, M. J. (2018). Activity-based rehabilitation interventions of the neurologically impaired upper extremity: Description of a scoping review protocol. *Topics in Spinal Cord Injury Rehabilitation, 24*(3), 239–251. https://doi .org/10.1310/sci2403-288

Trenaman, L., Miller, W. C., Quérée, M., Escorpizo, R., & the SCIRE Research Team. (2015). Modifiable and non-modifiable factors associated with employment outcomes following spinal cord injury: A systematic review. *Journal of Spinal Cord Medicine, 38*(4), 422–431. https://doi .org/10.1179/2045772315Y.0000000031

Trenaman, L. M., Miller, W. C., Escorpizo, R., & the SCIRE Research Team. (2014). Interventions for improving employment outcomes among individuals with spinal cord injury: A systematic review. *Spinal Cord, 52*(11), 788–794. https://doi.org/10.1038/sc.2014.149

Vagal, M. R., & Bijani, J. (2011). Effect of rehabilitation interventions on quality of life (QOL) in patients with thoracic and lumbar level spinal cord dysfunction. *Indian Journal of Occupational Therapy, 43*(2), 16–24.

Van de Velde, D., Bracke, P., Van Hove, G., Josephsson, S., & Vanderstraeten, G. (2013). How do men with paraplegia choose activities in the light of striving for optimal participation? A qualitative study, based on a phenomenological-hermeneutical method. *Disability & Society, 28*(5), 645–659. https://doi.org/10.1080/09687599.2012.728795

Velstra, I.-M., Ballert, C. S., & Cieza, A. (2011). A systematic literature review of outcome measures for upper extremity function using the International Classification of Function, Disability and Health as reference. *PM&R, 3*(9), 846–860. https://doi.org/10.1016/j.pmrj.2011.03.014

Velstra, I.-M., Bolliger, M., Baumberger, M., Rietman, J. S., & Curt, A. (2013). Epicritic sensation in cervical spinal cord injury: Diagnostic gains beyond testing light touch. *Journal of Neurotrauma, 30*(15), 1342–1348. https://doi.org/10.1089/neu.2012.2828

Velstra, I.-M., Bolliger, M., Krebs, J., Rietman, J. S., & Curt, A. (2016). Predictive value of upper limb muscles and grasp patterns on functional outcome in cervical spinal cord injury. *Neurorehabilitation and Neural Repair, 30*(4), 295–306. https://doi.org/10.1177/1545968315593806

Velstra, I. M., Bolliger, M., Tanadini, L. G., Baumberger, M., Abel, R., Rietman, J. S., & Curt, A. (2014). Prediction and stratification of upper limb function and self-care in acute cervical spinal cord injury with the Graded Redefined Assessment of Strength, Sensibility, and Prehension (GRASSP). *Neurorehabilitation and Neural Repair, 28*(7), 632–642. https://doi.org/10.11 77/1545968314521695

Velstra, I.-M., Curt, A., Frotzler, A., Abel, R., Kalsi-Ryan, S., Rietman, J. S., & Bolliger, M. (2015). Changes in strength, sensation and prehension in acute cervical spinal cord injury: European multicenter responsiveness study of the GRASSP. *Neurorehabilitation and Neural Repair, 29*(8), 755–766. https://doi.org/10.1177/1545968314565466

Wong, A. W. K., Chen, C., Baum, M. C., Heaton, R. K., Goodman, B., & Heinemann, A. W. (2019). Cognitive, emotional, and physical functioning as predictors of paid employment in people with stroke, traumatic brain injury, and spinal cord injury. *American Journal of Occupational Therapy, 73*(2), Article 7302205010. https://doi.org/10.5014/ajot.2019.031203

Zbogar, D., Eng, J. J., Noble, J. W., Miller, W. C., Krassioukov, A. V., & Verrier, M. C. (2017). Cardiovascular stress during inpatient spinal cord injury rehabilitation. *Archives of Physical Medicine and Rehabilitation, 98*(12), 2449–2456. https://doi.org/10.1016/j.apmr.2017.05.009

Zbogar, D., Eng, J. J., Miller, W. C., Krassioukov, A. V., & Verrier, M. C. (2017). Movement repetitions in physical and occupational therapy during spinal cord injury rehabilitation. *Spinal Cord, 55*, 172–179. https://doi.org/10.1038/sc.2016.129

Zbogar, D., Eng, J. J., Miller, W. C., Krassioukov, A. V., & Verrier, M. C. (2016). Physical activity outside of structured therapy during inpatient spinal cord injury rehabilitation. *Journal of*

NeuroEngineering and Rehabilitation, 13, Article 99. https://doi.org/10.1186/s12984-016-0208-8

Zbogar, D., Eng, J. J., Miller, W. C., Krassioukov, A. V., & Verrier, M. C. (2016). Reliability and validity of daily physical activity measures during inpatient spinal cord injury rehabilitation. *SAGE Open Medicine, 4*. https://doi.org/10.1177/2050312116666941

Spinal Cord Injuries: Complete (Children and Adolescents)

Also called pediatric spinal cord injury.

See also Spinal Cord Injury: Complete (Adult), Spinal Cord Injury: Incomplete, Pressure Ulcers, Cognitive Impairment, Memory Impairment, Executive Dysfunction.

Description

Spinal cord injury occurring to persons between the ages of 0 to 18. A suggested classification system categorizes clients into four groups: primary ambulators (PrimA), unplanned ambulators (UnPA), planned ambulators (PlanA), and nonambulators (Chafetz et al., 2013).

Cause

The most common cause of pediatric spinal cord injury is motor vehicle accidents. Other traumatic causes are violence, child abuse, falls, and sports injuries from gymnastics, diving, horseback riding, football, and wrestling. Nontraumatic causes include spinal tumor, spinal procedure, or disease such as transverse myelitis (Lowe et al., 2015; Porter, 2018). Cervical level injuries are more common in children under age 8, but thoracic level injuries are more common overall in children and youth. In children under 13 the incidence is equal among boys and girls, but in the teen years the incidence is more frequent in boys (Strenk, 2014).

Evaluation/Assessment

Areas

- Activities of Daily Living/Instrumental ADL: self-maintenance skills, chores (making bed, taking out garbage, cleaning room), transfers, mobility, respiratory status
- Education/Work: education, vocational choice
- Play/Leisure: interests, values, hobbies
- Rest/Sleep: sleep habits
- Social Participation: type, frequency, location, with whom
- Sensorimotor: muscle tone, muscle weakness, paralysis below level of lesion, joint range of motion including reaching, functional skills including hand, autonomic dysreflexia, spasticity, loss of sensation (tactile, deep pressure), temperature regulation, pain
- Cognitive/Perceptual: attention, concentration, memory, executive function
- Psychosocial: anxiety, quality of life, interpersonal relations
- Context/Environment: client, family and caregiver education and training related to management of spinal cord injury (SCI), home modification, adapted devices (selection, use, care), social support, community and internet resources
- Comorbidities: fractures, pressure ulcers, osteoporosis, scoliosis, increased blood pressure, deep vein thrombosis, heterotopic ossification

Instruments

Instruments Developed by Occupational Therapy Personnel

- Graded Redefined Assessment of Strength Sensibility and Prehension (GRASSP; Kalsi-Ryan et al., 2012; see also Mulcahey, Calhoun Thielen, et al., 2018, in References)

- International Spinal Cord Injury Pediatric Activity and Participation Basic Data Set (Hwang et al., 2019, in References)
- Patient-Reported Outcome Measure (PROM; Mulcahey et al., 2010, in References)
- Pediatric Measure of Participation (PMoP; Mulcahey et al., 2012, in References)
- Pediatric Neuromuscular Recovery Scale (PNRS; Ardolino et al., 2016, in References; see also Behrman et al., 2019, in References)
- Pediatric Spinal Cord Injury Activity Measure (PEDI-SCI AM; Slavin et al., 2016, in References)
- Walking Index for Spinal Cord Injury (WISCI-II; see Calhoun & Mulcahey, 2012, and Calhoun Thielen et al., 2017, in References)

Instruments Developed by Other Professionals and Used by Occupational Therapy Personnel
- Capabilities of Upper Extremities Test (CUE-T; Marino et al., 1998; see also Dent et al., 2018, in References)
- International Standards for Neurological Classification of Spinal Cord Injury (ISCOS; American Spinal Injury Association, 2013; see also Mulcahey et al., 2011, in References)
- Kidcope (Spirito et al., 1988)
- Spinal Cord Independence Measure (Version III; SCIM-III) Self-Report (SCIM-III SR; Fekete et al., 2013; see also Mulcahey, Calhoun Thielen, et al., 2018; Mulcahey, Thielen, et al., 2018, in References)

Problems/Issues
Activities of Daily Living/Instrumental ADL
- Child usually has difficulty performing self-maintenance skills.
- Child may have difficulty performing instrumental skills such as chores.
- Child may have difficulty with transfer skills (bed, chair, toilet, vehicle).
- Child may have difficulty with mobility (walking, wheelchair, scooter).
- Child may be ventilator dependent if lesion is at C4 or above.

Education/Work
- Child may need adapted equipment to participate in educational activities such as modification of computer to use voice activation or eye-gaze technology.
- Child may need modification to access school building and classrooms (alternate may be home schooling).

Play/Leisure
- Child may be unable or have difficulty engaging in favorite leisure occupations.
- Child may need to acquire new leisure activities that are within skill level.

Rest/Sleep
- Child may experience decreased quality of sleep due to pain or decreased bed mobility.

Social Participation
- Child may be unable to participate in social activities with friends and family.

Sensorimotor
- Child usually has decreased muscle strength near the site of the lesion and loss of muscle strength below the level of the lesion.
- Child may have decreased joint range of motion.
- Child usually has decreased endurance and increased sense of fatigue.
- Child usually has decreased sense of balance (sitting and standing).
- Child may develop a neuromuscular scoliosis (Mulcahey et al., 2013).
- Child usually has loss of sensation (tactile, deep pressure, temperature, proprioception) below level of lesion.

Cognitive/Perceptual

- Child may have decreased attention span and concentration, especially if head and neck were involved in traumatic injury.
- Child may experience difficulty with memory, especially if traumatic injury occurred.
- Child may have difficulty with executive functions such as problem solving and judgment; skill set may be below age-appropriate level.
- Child may have difficulty with perceptual tasks such as visual perception and spatial relations, especially if traumatic injury occurred.

Psychosocial

- Child may express feelings of anxiety or fear about life situation.
- Child may use cognitive, avoidant, active, or ineffective coping strategies (Russell et al., 2015).
- Child may experience changes in life roles.
- Child may experience changes in social relations.
- Child may experience decreased quality of life.
- Caregiver may lack effective coping skills (Dasch et al., 2011).

Context/Environment

- Child usually needs to learn to use a wheelchair or scooter.
- Child may need home and school modifications.
- Child may need assistance to reintegrate into home, school, and community.
- Parents and caregivers need information and training on managing a person with an SCI.
- Child and caregiver may lack knowledge about the severity of injury (Schottler et al., 2010).
- Child, parents, and caregivers may lack information on available community and internet resources.

Intervention/Treatment

Models and programs developed by occupational therapy personnel: None identified. Models and programs developed by other professionals but used by occupational therapy personnel include computer adaptive testing (Bent et al., 2013) and technology (Bryden et al., 2012). Team members include physicians, nursing personnel, physical therapists, psychologists, educators and special educators, parents and caregivers, and occupational therapy personnel. Goals are to improve functional independence in daily occupations, reduce dependency on caregiver assistance, improve muscle strength in remaining enervated muscles, maintain or improve range of motion, increase endurance, and improve quality of life (Strenk, 2014).

Activities of Daily Living/Instrumental ADL

- Assist child to increase functional ability in basic ADLs to age-appropriate level (self-feeding, grooming, bathing, dressing, toileting (managing clothes and hygiene).
- Assist child to manage bowel and bladder functions.
- Assist child and caregivers on skin care to prevent pressure ulcers.
- Assist child to participate in home management activities through doing chores.
- Assist child in learning transfer and mobility skills (bed, chair, toilet, wheelchair, vehicle).

Education/Work

- Assist child to participate in classroom and school activities using adapted devices and classroom.
- Assist educators to modify school building as needed, such as access to an elevator or keeping child's classes on first floor.
- Assist with lunch activities such as permitting child to leave classroom a few minutes early to go to cafeteria or arranging for child to eat in the classroom.

Play/Leisure

- Assist child to engage in favorite leisure occupations with modifications, if needed.
- Assist child to develop new or expanded leisure occupations that are age appropriate.

Rest/Sleep

- No information identified.

Social Participation

- Encourage participation in social occupations.

Sensorimotor

- Provide therapeutic activities to increase muscle strength in remaining enervated muscles especially shoulder.
- Provide therapeutic activities to increase endurance and manage fatigue.
- Provide therapeutic activities to increase and maintain joint range of motion and stretching.
- Provide therapeutic activities to increase balance (sitting and standing).
- Assist in pain management, if needed.

Cognitive/Perceptual

- No information identified.

Psychosocial

- Assist child to express anxiety and fears so they can be addressed.
- Assist child to develop social interaction skills that may require interaction from a wheelchair.
- Assist child to maintain or improve quality of life.
- Provide stress management and coping skills to caregivers.

Context/Environment

- Provide practice in using wheelchair safely in home, school, and community.
- Provide instruction in selection and maintenance of adapted devices.
- Provide hand splints, if needed, for nighttime (static) and daytime use (static and dynamic).
- Provide information and resources for home and school modification (may need bathroom and bedroom modifications).
- Provide training to family and caregivers on management of a child with spinal cord injury.
- Provide access to community resources and internet sites.
- Provide training in community reintegration.

Precautions/Safety Considerations

Ventilator-dependent child will require additional services including respiratory therapy. Mobility devices (wheelchair, scooter) will need to be changed as the child grows.

Prognosis and Outcome

Complete spinal cord injury is a lifelong disorder. The nature of the issues and concerns change as the child or youth grows and develops. Adapted devices must be modified to accommodate a larger individual. Social behaviors include sexuality. School behaviors change to vocational planning and implementation. Homemaking and independent living need to be addressed. Medical issues such as scoliosis and osteoporosis may need to be considered. Psychosocial health should also be considered (Kelly et al., 2012).

REFERENCES

Ardolino, E. M., Mulcahey, M. J., Trimble, S., Argetsinger, L., Bienkowski, M., Mullen, C., & Behrman, A. L. (2016). Development and initial validation of the Pediatric Neuromuscular Recovery Scale. *Pediatric Physical Therapy, 28*(4), 416–426. https://doi.org/10.1097/PEP.0000000000000285

Bent, L. M., Mulcahey, M. J., Kelly, E. H., Calhoun, C. L. Tian, F., Ni, P. Vogel, L. C., & Haley, S. M. (2013). Validity of computer adaptive tests of daily routines for youth with spinal cord injury. *Topics in Spinal Cord Injury Rehabilitation, 19*(2), 104–113. https://doi.org/10.1310/sci1902-104

Behrman, A. L., Trimble, S. A., Argetsinger, L. C., Roberts, M. T., Mulcahey, M. J., Clayton, L., Gregg, M. E., Lorenz, D., & Ardolino, E. M. (2019). Interrater reliability of the Pediatric Neuromuscular Recovery Scale for spinal cord injury. *Topics in Spinal Cord Injury Rehabilitation, 25*(2), 121–131. https://doi.org/10.1310/sci2502-121

Bryden, A. M., Ancans, J., Mazurkiewicz, J., McKnight, A., & Scholtens, M. (2012). Technology for spinal cord injury rehabilitation and its application to youth. *Journal of Pediatric Rehabilitation Medicine, 5*(4), 287–299. https://doi.org/10.3233/PRM-2012-00227

Calhoun, C. L., & Mulcahey, M. J. (2012). Pilot study of reliability and validity of the Walking Index for Spinal Cord Injury II (WISCI-II) in children and adolescents with spinal cord injury. *Journal of Pediatric Rehabilitation Medicine, 5*(4), 275–279. https://doi.org/10.3233/PRM-2012-00224

Calhoun Thielen, C., Sadowsky, C., Vogel L. C., Taylor, H., Davidson, L., Bultman, J., Gaughan, J., & Mulcahey, M. J. (2017). Evaluation of the Walking Index for Spinal Cord Injury (WISCI-II) in children with spinal cord injury (SCI). *Spinal Cord, 55*(5), 478–482. https://doi.org/10.1038/sc.2016.142

Chafetz, R. S., Gaughan, J. P., Calhoun, C., Schottler, J., Vogel, L. C., Betz, R., & Mulcahey, M. J. (2013). Relationship between neurological injury and patterns of upright mobility in children with spinal cord injury. *Topics in Spinal Cord Injury Rehabilitation, 19*(1), 31–41. https://doi.org/10.1310/sci1901-31

Dasch, K. B., Russell, H. F., Kelly E. H, Gorzkowski, J. A., Mulcahey, M. J., Betz, R. R., & Vogel, L. C. (2011). Coping in caregivers of youth with spinal cord injury. *Journal of Clinical Psychology in Medical Settings, 18*(4), 361–371. https://doi.org/10.1007/s10880-011-9258-z

Dent, K., Grampurohit, N., Thielen, C. C., Sadowsky, C., Davidson, L., Taylor, H. B., Bultman, J., Gaughan, J., Marino R. J., & Mulcahey, M. J. (2018). Evaluation of the Capabilities of Upper Extremity Test (CUE-T) in children with tetraplegia. *Topics in Spinal Cord Injury Rehabilitation, 24*(3), 239–251. https://doi.org/10.1310/sci2403-239

Hwang, M., Augutis, M., Sadowsky, C., Höfers, W., Vogel, L. C., Post, M., Charlifue, S., New, P. W., Fisher, R., Carney, J., Dent, K., & Mulcahey, M. J. (2019). The international spinal cord injury pediatric activity and participation basic data set. *Spinal Cord Series and Cases, 5,* Article 91. https://doi.org/10.1038/s41394-019-0230-8

Kelly, E. H., Mulcahey, M. J., Klaas, S. J., Russell, H. F., Anderson, C. J., & Vogel, L. C. (2012). Psychosocial outcomes among youth with spinal cord injury and their primary caregivers. *Topics in Spinal Cord Injury Rehabilitation, 18*(1), 67–72. https://doi.org/10.1310/sci1801-67

Lowe, A., Sharp, P., Thelen, C., & Warnken, B. (2015). Trauma-induced conditions. In J. Case-Smith & J. Clifford O'Brien (Eds.), *Occupational therapy for children and adolescents* (7th ed., pp. 839–862). Elsevier.

Mulcahey, M. J., Calhoun Thielen, C., Dent, K., Sinko, R., Sadowsky, C., Martin, R., Vogel, L. C., Davidson, L., Taylor, H., Bultman, J., & Gaughan, J. (2018). Evaluation of the Graded Refined Assessment of Strength, Sensibility and Prehension (GRASSP) in children with tetraplegia. *Spinal Cord, 56*(8), 741–749. https://doi.org/10.1038/s41393-018-0084-0

Mulcahey, M., Calhoun, C. L., Tian, F., Ni, P., Vogel, L. C., & Haley, S. M. (2012). Evaluation of newly developed item banks for child-reported outcomes of participation following spinal cord injury. *Spinal Cord, 50*(12), 915–919. https://doi.org/10.1038/sc.2012.80

Mulcahey, M. J., DiGiovanni, N., Calhoun, C., Homko, E., Riley, A., & Haley, S. M. (2010). Children's and parents' perspectives about activity performance and participation after spinal cord injury: Initial development of a patient-reported outcome measure. *American Journal of Occupational Therapy, 64*(4), 605–613. https://doi.org/10.5014/ajot.2010.08148

Mulcahey, M. J., Gaughan, J. P., Betz, R. R., Samdani, A. F., Barakat, N., & Hunter, L. N. (2013). Neuromuscular scoliosis in children with spinal cord injury. *Topics in Spinal Cord Injury Rehabilitation, 19*(2), 96–103. https://doi.org/10.1310/sci1902-96

Mulcahey, M. J., Gaughan, J. P., Chafetz, R., Vogel, L. C., Samdani, A. F., & Betz, R. R. (2011). Interrater reliability of the International Standards for Neurological Classification of Spinal Cord Injury in youths with chronic spinal cord injury. *Archives of Physical Medicine & Rehabilitation, 92*(8), 1264–1269. https://doi.org/10.1016/j.apmr.2011.03.003

Mulcahey, M. J., Thielen, C. C., Sadowsky, C., Silvestri, J. L., Martin, R., White, L., Cagney, J. A., Vogel, L. C., Schottler, J., Davidson, L., Parry, I., Taylor, H. B., Higgins, K., Feltz, M. L., Sinko, R., Bultman, J., Mazurkiewicz, J., & Gaughan, J. (2018). Despite limitations in content range, the SCIM-III is reproducible and a valid indicator of physical function in youths with spinal cord injury and dysfunction. *Spinal Cord, 56*(4), 332–340. https://doi.org/10.1038/s41393-017-0036-0

Porter, R. S. (Ed.). (2018). *The Merck manual of diagnosis and therapy* (20th ed.). Merck Sharp & Dohme.

Russell, H. F., January, A. M., Kelly, E. H., Mulcahey, M. J., Betz, R. R., & Vogel L. C. (2015). Patterns of coping strategy use and relationships with psychosocial health in adolescents with spinal cord injury. *Journal of Pediatric Psychology, 40*(5), 535–543. https://doi.org/10.1093/jpepsy/jsu159

Schottler, J., Vogel, L., Chafetz, R. S., & Mulcahey, M. J. (2010). Patient and caregiver knowledge of severity of injury among youth with spinal cord injury. *Spinal Cord, 48*(1), 34–38. https://doi.org/10.1038/sc.2009.74

Slavin, M. D., Mulcahey, M. J. Calhoun Thielen, C., Ni, P., Vogel, L. C., Haley, S. M., & Jette, A. M. (2016). Measuring activity limitation outcomes in youth with spinal cord injury. *Spinal Cord, 54*(7), 546–552. https://doi.org/10.1038/sc.2015.194

Strenk, M. (2014, September 5). *Early physical therapy/occupational therapy specific interventions for traumatic spinal cord injury (SCI)* [Best evidence statement]. Cincinnati Children's Hospital Medical Center.

BIBLIOGRAPHY

Carroll, A., Vogel, L. C., Zebracki, K., Noonan, V. K., Biering-Sørensen, F., & Mulcahey, M. J. (2017). Relevance of the international spinal cord injury basic data sets to youth: An interprofessional review with recommendations. *Spinal Cord, 55*, 875–881. https://doi.org/10.1038/sc.2017.14

Lindwall, J. J., Russell, H. F., Kelly, E. H., Klaas, S. J., Mulcahey, M. J., Betz, R. R., & Vogel, L. C. (2012). Coping and participation in youth with spinal cord injury. *Topics in Spinal Cord Injury Rehabilitation, 18*(3), 220–231. https://doi.org/10.1310/sci1803-220

Mulcahey, M. J., Calhoun, C. L., Sinko, R., Kelly, E. H., & Vogel, L. C. (2016). The Spinal Cord Independence Measure (SCIM)-III self-report for youth. *Spinal Cord, 54*(3), 204–212. https://doi.org/10.1038/sc.2015.103

Mulcahey, M. J., Slavin, M. D., Ni, P., Vogel, L. C., Thielen, C. C., Coster, W. J., & Jette, A. M. (2016). The Pediatric Measure of Participation (PMoP) short forms. *Spinal Cord 54*(12), 1183–1187. https://doi.org/10.1038/sc.2016.68

Mulcahey, M. J., Vogel, L. C., Sheikh, M., Arango-Lasprilla, J. C., Augutis, M., Garner, E., Hagen, M., Jakeman, L. B., Kelly, E., Martin, R., Odenkirchen, J., Scheel-Sailer, A., Schottler, J., Taylor, H. Thielen, C. C., & Zebracki, K. (2017). Recommendations for the National Institute for Neurologic Disorders and Stroke spinal cord injury common data elements for children and youth with SCI. *Spinal Cord, 55*(4), 331–340. https://doi.org/10.1038/sc.2016.139

Smith, T. F., Russell, H. F., Kelly, E. H., Mulcahey, M. J., Betz, R. R., & Vogel, L. C. (2013). Examination and measurement of coping among adolescents with spinal cord injury. *Spinal Cord, 51*(9), 710–714. https://doi.org/10.1038/sc.2013.65

Tian, F., Ni, P., Mulcahey, M., Hambleton, R., Tulsky, D., Haley, S., & Jette, A. M. (2014). Tracking functional status across the spinal cord injury lifespan: Linking pediatric and adult patient-reported outcome scores. *Archives of Physical Medicine and Rehabilitation, 95*(11), 2078–2085. https://doi.org/10.1016/j.apmr.2014.05.023

Vogel, L. C., Betz, R. R., & Mulcahey, M. J. (2012). Spinal cord injuries in children and adolescents. In J. Verhaagen & J. W. McDonald, III (Eds.), *Handbook of clinical neurology* (Vol. 109, pp. 131–148). Elsevier. https://doi.org/10.1016/B978-0-444-52137-8.00008-5

Vogel, L. C., Zebracki, K., Betz, R. R., & Mulcahey, M. J. (Eds.). (2014). *Spinal cord injury in the child and young adult.* Mac Keith Press.

Spinal Cord Injury: Incomplete

Description

The American Spinal Injury Association (2013) recognizes three types of incomplete spinal cord injuries:

- B = Sensory incomplete: Sensory is preserved below the neurological level of injury, but no motor function is preserved.
- C = Motor incomplete: Motor function is preserved at the most caudal sacral segments for voluntary anal contraction.
- D = Motor incomplete: Status as defined above, with at least half of key muscle functions below single level of injury having a muscle grade at or greater than 3 (active movement, full range of motion against gravity).

Cause

The most common causes of spinal cord injuries are motor vehicle crashes and falls (Porter, 2018). For older individuals, the most common cause of incomplete spinal cord injury is falls (Hsieh et al., 2013). Other causes include sports injuries, stab or gunshot injuries to the spine, congenital disorders, and sequela to disease of the central nervous system.

Types

- *Brown-Séquard syndrome:* Results from unilateral hemisection of the cord resulting in ipsilateral spastic paralysis and loss of position sense below the level of the lesion and contralateral loss of pain and temperature sensation (Porter, 2018).
- *Anterior cord syndrome:* Results from direct injury to the anterior spinal cord or to the anterior spinal arteries resulting in loss of motor and pain sensation bilaterally below the level of the lesion; posterior cord function such as vibration sense and proprioception remain intact (Porter, 2018).
- *Central cord syndrome:* Usually occurs in persons with a narrowed spinal canal due to congenital or degenerative changes after a hyperextension injury. Motor function in the arms is impaired more than in the legs. If the posterior columns are affected, posture, vibration, and light touch are lost. If the spinothalamic tracts are affected, pain, temperature, and touch are lost. Hemorrhage in the spinal cord that results from trauma is usually confined to the cervical central gray matter, resulting in signs of lower motor neuron damage such as muscle weakness and wasting, fasciculations, and diminished tendon reflexes in the arms (Porter, 2018).
- *Cauda equina lesions:* Motor or sensory loss or both, usually partial, occurs in the distal region of the legs. Sensation is usually diminished in the perineal region, called saddle anesthesia. Bowel and bladder dysfunction, either incontinence or retention, may occur (Porter, 2018).

Evaluation/Assessment

Areas

- Activities of Daily Living/Instrumental ADL: basic ADLs (eating, dressing, bathing/showering, grooming, toileting, transfers, skin care), meal preparation, housekeeping, laundry, shopping, driving, yard maintenance, functional mobility, child/pet care

- Education/Work: accessibility, scheduling, workstation organization
- Play/Leisure: type, location, interests
- Rest/Sleep: sleep disturbance
- Social Participation: type, location, with whom
- Sensorimotor: gross motor mobility, hand functions (dexterity, manipulation, coordination), spasticity, fatigue
- Cognitive/Perceptual: may need consideration if spinal cord injury also included a head injury
- Psychosocial: anxiety, stress, role performance, quality of life, self-efficacy
- Context/Environment: accessibility, home modification, durable medical equipment, adapted devices
- Comorbidities: pressure ulcers, urinary tract infections, deep vein thrombosis (DVT)

Instruments

Instruments Developed by Occupational Therapy Personnel
- Box and Block Test (BBT; Holser & Fuchs, 1957; Mathiowetz, Volland, et al., 1985)
- Graded Redefined Assessment of Strength Sensibility and Prehension (GRASSP; Kalsi-Ryan et al., 2012)
- Impact on Participation and Autonomy (IPA) questionnaire (Cardol et al., 1999)
- Manual Function Test (MFT; Moriyama, 1987)
- Reintegration to Normal Living Index (RNLI; Wood-Dauphinee et al., 1988)

Instruments Developed by Other Professionals and Used by Occupational Therapy Personnel
- 6-minute walk test (6MWT; Ditunno et al., 2007)
- 10-Meter-Walk Test (10MWT; Bohannon, 1997; also called Gait Speed Test)
- Activities-Specific Balance Confidence (ABC) Scale (Powell & Myers, 1995)
- Craig Handicap Assessment and Reporting Technique (CHART; Whiteneck, Charlifue, et al., 1992)
- Functional Independence Measure (FIM; Uniform Data System for Medical Rehabilitation, 1997)
- Instrumental Activities of Daily Living (IADL or LIADL; Lawton & Brody, 1969)
- Life Satisfaction Questionnaire (LSQ; Post et al., 1998)
- Satisfaction with Life Scale (SWLS; Diener et al., 1895)
- Spinal Cord Independence Measure (Version III; SCIM-III). Itzkovich et al., 2007)
- Spinal Cord Injury Functional Ambulation Profile (SCI-FAP; Musselman et al., 2011)
- Timed Up and Go test (TUG; Podsiadlo & Richardson, 1991)
- Toronto Rehabilitation Institute Hand Function Test (TRIHFT; Kapadia et al., 2012; see also Kapadia et al., 2011, in References)

Problems/Issues

Activities of Daily Living/Instrumental ADL
- Person may be unable to access bathroom due to narrow doorway.
- Person may experience urinary tract infections.
- Person may experience deep vein thrombosis.
- Person may need assistance in performing homemaking tasks, including meal preparation, housekeeping, shopping, yard maintenance.
- Person may need modification of vehicle to facilitate driving independence.

Education/Work
- Person may be unable to continue education without modifications.
- Person may be unable to continue current line of work.
- Person may need modification to workstation, schedule, job duties, or transportation to continue in present line of work.

Play/Leisure
- Person is unable to engage in gardening at ground level.

Rest/Sleep
- Person may experience sleep disturbance due to pain.

Social Participation
- Person may be unable to participate in social activities.

Sensorimotor
- Person usually experiences fatigue during task management and performance.
- Person may have difficulty maintaining standing balance as a perquisite to walking.
- Person may have loss of upper extremity range of motion, depending on remaining motor function.
- Person may experience difficulty with upper extremity motions (reach, grasp and release), depending on remaining motor function.
- Person may experience difficulty with hand functions (grip strength, dexterity, manipulation, and coordination), depending on remaining motor function.
- Person may experience loss of sensory function, depending on type of injury, including touch or feeling, vibratory sense, temperature, pain, and proprioception.
- Person may experience pressure ulcers (see Pressure Ulcers in Section 10: Skin Disorders).

Cognitive/Perceptual
- Person usually does not experience reduced cognitive function unless brain injury is also present.
- Person may experience changes in or loss of perception in sensory systems affected by the level and type of injury.

Psychosocial
- Person may experience anxiety.
- Person may experience depression and lack of motivation (apathy).
- Person may experience changes in role functions and performance.
- Person may experience changes in sense of self-efficacy.
- Person may experience changes in quality of life and life satisfaction.

Context/Environment
- Person may be unable to move about the home due to architectural barriers (stairs to entrance, doorways too narrow, kitchen and bathroom not wheelchair accessible).
- Person may need adaptive devices and durable medical equipment.
- Person may lack knowledge of available resources.
- Person may lack social support.

Intervention/Treatment

Models and programs developed by occupational therapy personnel include bladder and bowel management (Gallagher & Bell, 2016) and home modification (Backner, 2015). Models and programs developed by other professionals but used by occupational therapy personnel include adult learning theory (Gallagher & Bell, 2016), bimanual training (Kim et al., 2015), functional electrical stimulation therapy (Hitzig et al., 2013; Kapadia et al., 2014; Kapadia et al., 2011; Kapadia et al., 2013; Popovic et al., 2011), gait adaptability retraining approach (Fox et al., 2017), modified constraint-induced movement therapy (Kim et al., 2015), sensory tongue stimulation (Chisholm et al., 2014), task-specific therapy (Chisholm et al., 2014), and whole-body vibration training (In et al., 2018 [Note: No mention of occupational therapist's role]). Team members include physicians, nursing personnel, psychologists, physical therapy personnel, and occupational therapy personnel. Goals are to increase and improve the person's ability to participate in everyday life in the home and community and return to productive living (Gallagher & Bell, 2016).

Activities of Daily Living/Instrumental ADL

- Provide practice in basic ADLs as needed including safe transfer and functional mobility; focus on use of compensatory strategies as needed.
- Provide program in bladder and bowel management.
- Encourage use of a schedule to maintain self-care activities such as self-catherization.
- Consider if instrumental ADLs in the home could be facilitated by home modification (see Context/Environment).

Education/Work

- Support engagement in education or work activities using problem-solving approach to address issues and concerns.

Play/Leisure

- Raised garden beds allow client to continue gardening.

Rest/Sleep

- No information identified.

Social Participation

- Support participation in social activities using problem-solving approach to suggest solutions to situations that may arise in social outings.

Sensorimotor

- Portable neuromodulation stimulator used on the tongue's surface with light pressure to roof of mouth may provide brain activation (Chisholm et al., 2014).
- Body-weight support harness for safety can be used during practice in standing balance training.
- Walking exercise can decrease spasticity and improve balance (In et al., 2018).
- Consider whether a fatigue-management program may be useful.
- Provide muscle strengthening and range of motion exercises for upper extremity.
- Provide opportunity to practice fine motor skills (dexterity, manipulation, coordination).
- Provide task-specific, repetitive hand function training (reach, grasp, release) using full power/circular hand grip, handle grip, two or three finger grip, opposition finger and thumb, and lateral pinch; include heavier objects for power grip (water bottles, coffee mugs) and lighter objects for lateral pinch (keys, holding paper).
- Consider adding functional electrical stimulation for muscle strengthening (Kapadia et al., 2014).

Cognitive/Perceptual

- Adult learning theory may be useful to instruct clients in self-management programs, which focuses on the client as an active learner.
- Use problem-solving approach to everyday life situations including assessment of risk factors.

Psychosocial

- Encourage client to discuss issues of concern that contribute to anxiety and depression.
- Assist client to participate in activities and occupations that improve client's life satisfaction and quality of life.

Context/Environment

- Assist with home modification (ramps or platform lift to entrance, widening doors to 32 inches, appliances reachable via wheelchair, roll in shower or tub bench, toilet commode, ceiling lift, tilting mirrors).
- Assist with instruction for wheelchair maintenance and repair.

- Assist in selection of adaptive devices to facilitate performance of self-care and everyday activities.
- Provide education on risk factors and complications such as pressure ulcers, deep vein thrombosis, and urinary tract infections.
- Assist client to learn advocacy skills related to function and need for assistance.
- Assist in providing caregiver education (family, friends, or personal care attendant).

Precautions/Safety Considerations

- See Precautions/Safety Consideration in Spinal Cord Injury: Complete (Adult).

Prognosis and Outcome

Brain adaptation for persons with incomplete spinal cord injury (SCI) differs sharply from complete SCI, is related to functional behavioral status, and evolves with increasing time postinjury. Rehabilitation programs can take advantage of changes to improve the quality of life for persons with incomplete SCI (Sharp et al., 2017). Prognosis and outcome depend in part on level of injury, amount of sensory and/or motor function remaining intact, and motivation of client to participate in intervention and self-management strategies. Older adults with incomplete spinal cord injury require a different clinical pathway than younger clients, including higher severity of illness score, lower admission and discharge motor scores on the FIM, retirement or unemployment issues, and Medicare insurance (Hsieh et al., 2013).

REFERENCES

American Spinal Injury Association. (2013). *International standards for neurological classification of spinal cord injury.*

Backner, S. (2015). Easy come. Easy go! Easy everything in-between! Part II. *Rehab Management, 28*(6), 26–31.

Chisholm, A. E., Malik, R. N., Blouin, J. S., Borisoff, J., Forwell, S., & Lam, T. (2014). Feasibility of sensory tongue stimulation combined with task-specific therapy in people with spinal cord injury: A case study. *Journal of NeuroEngineering and Rehabilitation, 11,* Article 96. https://doi .org/10.1186/1743-0003-11-96

Fox, E. J., Tester, N. J., Butera, K. A., Howland, D. R., Spiess, M. R., Castro-Chapman, P. L., & Behrman, A. L. (2017). Retraining walking adaptability following incomplete spinal cord injury. *Spinal Cord Series and Cases, 3,* Article 17091. https://doi.org/10.1038/s41394-017-0003-1

Gallagher, G., & Bell, A. (2016). Combining adult learning theory with occupational therapy intervention for bladder and bowel management after spinal cord injury: A case report. *Occupational Therapy in Health Care, 30*(2), 202–209. https://doi.org/10.3109/07380577.2015 .1116130

Hitzig, S. L., Craven, B., Panjwani, A., Kapadia, N., Giangregorio, L. M., Richards, K., Masani, K., & Popovic, M. R. (2013). Randomized trial of functional electrical stimulation therapy for walking in incomplete spinal cord injury: Effects on quality of life and community participation. *Topics in Spinal Cord Injury Rehabilitation, 19*(4), 245–258. https://doi.org/10.1310/ sci1904-245

Hsieh, C., DeJong, G., Groah, S., Ballard, P. H., Horn, S. D., & Tian, W. (2013). Comparing rehabilitation services and outcomes between older and younger people with spinal cord injury. *Archives of Physical Medicine and Rehabilitation, 94*(4, Suppl.) S175–S186. https://doi .org/10.1016/j.apmr.2012.10.038

In, T., Jung, K., Lee, M. G., & Cho, H. Y. (2018). Whole-body vibration improves ankle spasticity, balance, and walking ability in individuals with incomplete cervical spinal cord injury. *NeuroRehabilitation, 42*(4), 491–497. https://doi.org/10.3233/NRE-172333

Kapadia, N. M., Bagher, S., & Popovic, M. R. (2014). Influence of different rehabilitation therapy models on patient outcomes: Hand function therapy in individuals with incomplete SCI.

Journal of Spinal Cord Medicine, 37(6), 734–743. https://doi.org/10.1179/2045772314Y.0000 000203

Kapadia, N. M., Zivanovic, V., Furlan, J. C., Craven, B. C., McGillivray, C., & Popovic, M. R. (2011). Functional electrical stimulation therapy for grasping in traumatic incomplete spinal cord injury: Randomized control trial. *Artificial Organs, 35*(3), 212–216. https://doi.org/ 10.1111/j.1525-1594.2011.01216.x

Kapadia, N., Zivanovic, V., & Popovic, M. R. (2013). Restoring voluntary grasping function in individuals with incomplete chronic spinal cord injury: Pilot study. *Topics in Spinal Cord Injury Rehabilitation, 19*(4), 279–287. https://doi.org/10.1310/sci1904-279

Kim, Y.-J., Kim, J.-K., & Park, S.-Y. (2015). Effects of modified constraint-induced movement therapy and functional bimanual training on upper extremity function and daily activities in a patient with incomplete spinal cord injury: A case study. *Journal of Physical Therapy Science, 27*(12), 3945–3946. https://doi.org/10.1589/jpts.27.3945

Popovic, M. R., Kapadia, N., Zivanovic, V., Furlan, J. C., Craven, B. C., & McGillivray, C. (2011). Functional electrical stimulation therapy of voluntary grasping versus only conventional rehabilitation for patients with subacute incomplete tetraplegia: A randomized clinical trial. *Neurorehabilitation and Neural Repair, 25*(5), 433–442. https://doi.org/10.1177/15459683 10392924

Porter, R. S. (Ed.). (2018). *The Merck manual of diagnosis and therapy* (20th ed.). Merck Sharp & Dohme.

Sharp, K. G., Gramer, R., Page, S. J., & Cramer, S. C. (2017). Increased brain sensorimotor network activation after incomplete spinal cord injury. *Journal of Neurotrauma, 34*(3), 623–631. https://doi.org/10.1089/neu.2016.4503

Musculoskeletal Disorders

Arthritis and Work

Description

Arthritis and rheumatic disease are a complex family of musculoskeletal disorders consisting of more than 100 different diseases or conditions that can affect people of all ages, races, and genders (O'Toole, 2017). The term *arthritis* encompasses conditions that have joint inflammation as a component (Allaire, Keysor, & AlHeresh, 2013). Examples include ankylosing spondylitis, fibromyalgia, gout, juvenile idiopathic arthritis, osteoarthritis, psoriatic arthritis, rheumatoid (inflammatory) arthritis, Sjögren syndrome, systemic lupus erythematosus, and systemic sclerosis/scleroderma (Allaire, Keysor, & AlHeresh, 2013).

Cause

Different forms of arthritis or rheumatic disease have different causations, which may include genetic factors, prior injury especially to joints, disease process, aging process, or lifestyle choices.

Terminology

- *Presenteeism:* Reduced capacity to work while at work due to health (Allaire, AlHeresh, & Keysor, 2013).
- *Work functioning:* An umbrella term that encompasses work activity (execution of work-related tasks) and work participation (involvement in work roles or the lived experience of work; AlHeresh et al., 2017, p. 2).
- *Work status:* Working full-time paid work, part-time paid work, or short-term leave of absence (Allaire, AlHeresh, & Keysor, 2013).

Evaluation/Assessment

Areas

- Activities of Daily Living/Instrumental ADL: mobility, transportation, driving
- Education/Work: job/work characteristics, job satisfaction, job/workplace modification and accommodation, job/work tasks, job loss, job retention, job/work history, work-related equipment/supplies, absenteeism, job/work performance and productivity standards, policies, and procedures,
- Play/Leisure: interests, frequency, location
- Rest/Sleep: sleep habits, sleep disturbance
- Social Participation: interaction with coworkers (colleagues), employee assistance, consultation with others, frequency, location
- Sensorimotor: physical requirements (lifting, carrying, bending, stooping, stepping, climbing), muscle strength, range of motion, endurance, hand functions (grasp, grip strength, dexterity, coordination), fatigue, pain
- Cognitive/Perceptual: attention, memory, executive functions (scheduling, time management, priorities, planning
- Psychosocial: stress, sense of self-efficacy, work performance, depression, anxiety, dissatisfaction with worker role, homemaking role
- Context/Environment: ergonomic design, social support from family and coworkers
- Comorbidities: back pain, diabetes

Instruments

Instruments Developed by Occupational Therapy Personnel

- Ergonomic Assessment Tool for Arthritis (EATA; Backman et al., 2008)

Instruments Developed by Other Professionals and Used by Occupational Therapy Personnel

- Arthritis Impact Measurement Scales 2–Short Form (AIMS2-SF; Guillemin et al., 1997)
- Arthritis Self-Efficacy Scale (ASES; Lorig et al., 1989)

- Career Satisfaction Scale (CSS; Hofmans et al., 2008)
- Endicott Work Productivity Scale (EWPS; Endicott & Nee, 1997; see also AlHeresh et al., 2016; Beaton et al., 2010; and Tang et al., 2013, in References)
- Health and Labor Questionnaire (HLQ; van Roijen et al., 1996; see also World Health Organization Health and Labor Questionnaire)
- Health and Work Performance Questionnaire (HPQ; see World Health Organization Health and Work Performance Questionnaire)
- Health Assessment Questionnaire (HAQ; see Stanford Health Assessment Questionnaire; Bruce & Fries, 2003)
- Hospital Anxiety and Depression Scale (HADS; Zigmond & Snaith, 1983)
- Lubben Social Network Scale–Short Form (LSNS-SF; Lubben et al., 2006)
- Multidimensional Fatigue Inventory (MDFI; Smets et al., 1995)
- Profile of Mood States–Fatigue Subscale (POMS; MacNair et al., 1971)
- RA Work Instability Scale (see Work Instability Scale for Rheumatoid Arthritis; RA-WIS)
- Rheumatoid Arthritis Disease Activity Index (RADAI; Fransen et al., 2000)
- Stanford Presenteeism Scale (SPS-6; Koopman et al., 2002; see also AlHeresh et al., 2016; Beaton et al., 2010; and Tang et al., 2013, in References)
- Valuation of Lost Productivity Questionnaire (VOLP; Zhang et al., 2011; see also AlHeresh et al., 2016, in References)
- Work Experience Survey (WES; Roessler et al., 1995)
- Work Instability Scale for Rheumatoid Arthritis (RA-WIS; Gilworth et al., 2003; see also AlHeresh et al., 2016; Beaton et al., 2010; Tang et al., 2013; and Tang et al., 2010, in References)
- Work Limitations Questionnaire (WLQ; Lerner et al., 2001; see also AlHeresh et al., 2016; Beaton et al., 2010; Tang et al., 2013; and Zhang et al., 2010 in References)
- Work Osteoarthritis or Joint Replacement Questionnaire (WOJRQ; Kievit et al., 2014; see also AlHeresh et al., 2016, in References)
- Work Productivity and Activity Impairment Questionnaire (WPAI; Reilly et al., 1993; see also AlHeresh et al., 2016, and Zhang et al., 2010, in References)
- Work Productivity Survey for Rheumatoid Arthritis (WPS-RA; Zhang et al., 2010; see also AlHeresh et al., 2016, in References)
- Work Role Functioning Questionnaire (Version 2.0; WRFQ; Abma et al., 2018)
- Workplace Activity Limitation Scale (WALS; Gignac et al., 2004; see AlHeresh et al., 2016; Beaton et al., 2010; and Tang et al., 2013, in References)
- World Health Organization Health and Labor Questionnaire (HLQ; van Roijen et al., 1996; see also Zhang et al., 2010, in References)
- World Health Organization Health and Work Performance Questionnaire (WHO-HPQ; Kessler et al., 2003; see also AlHeresh et al., 2017, and Zhang et al., 2010, in References)

Problems/Issues

Activities of Daily Living/Instrumental ADL
- Person may have difficulty with functional mobility.
- Person may lack adequate means of transportation including public and/or individual.

Education/Work
- Person may have difficulty performing job tasks due to limitations in hand functions.
- Person may be unable to maintain productivity standards, such as rate of work or number of units produced in a set time period.
- Person may have difficulty with posture and positioning at work station.
- Person may be dismissed for excessive absences or unauthorized break times.
- Person may experience absenteeism, job disruption, and productivity loss (Jetha et al., 2015).
- Person may have limited work experience due to repeated dismissals.

- Person's choice of work positions may be contributing to increased pain and decreased occupational performance.
- Person may need assistance to transition to another work environment or from work to retirement.

Play/Leisure

- Consider if choice of leisure occupations may be negatively affecting ability to function in work environment. Factors to consider include degree or amount of physical requirements needed to perform leisure occupations or amount of time spent engaged in leisure occupations versus need for rest and sleep.

Rest/Sleep

- Consider if rest and sleep habits may be a factor in limiting job performance and work effectiveness.

Social Participation

- Person may have difficulty coordinating with work peers (keeping up the work activity pace).

Sensorimotor

- Person may have decreased muscle strength in joints affected by the arthritic or rheumatic disease process.
- Person may have limited range of motion in certain joints related to the arthritic or rheumatic disease process.
- Person may have limited or reduced endurance.
- Person may experience joint stiffness, which varies depending on the time of day, static positioning, or degree of increased or decreased level of activity.
- Person may experience increased frequency and degree of fatigue.
- Person may experience pain, especially in joints affected by arthritic or rheumatic disease condition.

Cognitive/Perceptual

- Person may experience cognitive impairment depending on the type of arthritic or rheumatic disease.
- Person may have a history of poor time processing and management, such as difficulty planning ahead to get to work on time.

Psychosocial

- Person may avoid or decrease interaction with coworkers.
- Person may lack social skills to interact effectively with coworkers and supervisors.
- Person may have a history of being dissatisfied with job situation or work conditions.

Context/Environment

- Person may lack information or resources designed to assist workers with physical limitations, including laws such as the Americans With Disabilities Act.
- Person may experience accessibility barriers.
- Person may encounter work stations or environments with poor ergonomic design.
- Person may experience overprotection and unwanted social support while transitioning to employment (Jetha et al., 2014).

Intervention/Treatment

Models and programs developed by occupational therapy personnel include work rehabilitation program (Prior et al., 2017). Models and programs developed by other professionals but used by occupational therapy personnel include ergonomic intervention (Allaire, Backman, et al., 2013), fatigue management program (FAME-W; McCormack et al., 2018), job-retention program (Hammond et al., 2017), and Work-IT Study program (Keysor et al., 2016; Keysor et al., 2018). Team members include physicians, rheumatologists, psychologists, vocational rehabilitation counselors, physical therapy personnel, and occupational therapy personal. Goals are to reduce work limitations and work loss among clients with arthritic, rheumatic, and musculoskeletal conditions (Keysor et al., 2018).

Activities of Daily Living/Instrumental ADL
- Explore with client mobility needs such as a walker, scooter, wheelchair.
- Explore with client transportation needs, such as train, bus, taxi, private car, including parking closer to work station, getting a handicapped parking sticker.

Education/Work
- Provide practice sessions for preparing job resumes, job interviewing, and completing job applications.
- Explore with client interests and activities that might create job opportunities including self-employment as well as working for others.

Play/Leisure
- Assist client to create a balance of occupations (work, play, rest, and sleep) that includes consideration of the demands of the disease condition.

Rest/Sleep
- See Sleep–Wake Disorders in Section 13: Lifestyle Conditions.

Social Participation
- Provide opportunities to participate in work-related situations with coworkers (simulated or real).

Sensorimotor
- Energy conservation: Explore with client which job duties or work station arrangements could be performed with less energy expenditure, including work station redesign and adjustment in job performance duties.
- Work simplification: Explore with client which job duties could be eliminated or redesigned for greater efficiency.
- Exercise: Wrist, hand, upper extremity exercises to maintain range of motion and reduce pain from static positioning.
- Fatigue management: Control the pace or speed of work; alternate or rotate the type of work done; adjust the work and rest periods.
- Pain management: Adjust medication to better accommodate work schedule.

Cognitive/Perceptual
- Assist client to develop a time schedule and provide practice in following the schedule.

Psychosocial
- Provide opportunity to share ideas with client and coworkers about better approaches to accomplish work tasks with defined time periods.

Context/Environment
- Orthotic devices: Consider if an orthotic device such as resting splint or wrist support may improve function and reduce pain.
- Ergonomic adjustments to work station: Use lightweight headset or speaker phone, add footstool, use slanted work table, use ergonomically designed keyboard, use word-prediction software, use bookstands to prop up heavier materials such as manuals or clip board for single or a few pages, temperature control, noise control.
- Client education: Provide client and social support system with information and access to resources that may improve client's ability to find and maintain employment.

- Joint client/employer education: With client's permission visit the work site to observe job duties and work environment to make feasible suggestions for improving work productivity and job satisfaction.
- Employer education: Provide information to employers about job/work accommodation and ergonomically designed work stations.
- Career counseling: Consider referring client to a vocational counselor or vocational rehabilitation counselor for career exploration and evaluation.

Precautions/Safety Considerations

Overuse syndrome or attempting to compensate to the point of causing additional pain and joint damage. Equipment with poor ergonomic design may increase risk of injury or aggravate existing conditions.

Prognosis and Outcome

Variable. Most arthritic and rheumatic diseases are or become chronic conditions even if the degree of chronicity may vary with age or type of disorder. Adjustment to accommodate work conditions with disease/disorder is an ongoing issue that may need to be addressed throughout a client's working years. Working provides different benefits and challenges for men versus women, requiring different long-range plans (Gignac et al., 2014).

REFERENCES

AlHeresh, R., LaValley, M. P., Coster, W., & Keysor, J. J. (2017). Construct validity and scoring methods of the World Health Organization: Health and Work Performance Questionnaire among workers with arthritis and rheumatological conditions. *Journal of Occupational and Environmental Medicine, 59*(6), e112–e118. https://doi.org/10.1097/JOM.0000000000 001044

AlHeresh, R., Vaughan, M., LaValley, M. P., Coster, W., & Keysor, J. J. (2016). Critical appraisal of the quality of literature evaluating psychometric properties of arthritis work outcome assessments: A systematic review. *Arthritis Care & Research, 68*(9), 1354–1370. https://doi .org/10.1002/acr.22814

Allaire, S. J., AlHeresh, R., & Keysor, J. J. (2013). Risk factors for work disability associated with arthritis and other rheumatic conditions. *Work, 45*(4), 499–503. https://doi.org/10.3233/ WOR-131667

Allaire, S. J., Backman, C. L., AlHeresh, R., & Baker, N. A. (2013). Ergonomic intervention for employed persons with rheumatic conditions. *Work, 46*, 355–361. https://doi.org/10.3233/ WOR-131761

Allaire, S. J., Keysor, J. J., & AlHeresh, R. (2013). Effect of arthritis and other rheumatic conditions on employment. *Work, 45*(3), 417–420. https://doi.org/10.3233/WOR-131629

Beaton, D. E., Tang, K., Gignac, M. A. M., Lacaille, D., Badley, E. M., Anis, A. H., & Bombardier, C. (2010). Reliability, validity, and responsiveness of five at-work productivity measures in patients with rheumatoid arthritis or osteoarthritis. *Arthritis Care & Research, 62*(1), 28–37. https://doi.org/10.1002/acr.20011

Gignac, M. A. M., Lacaille, D., Beaton, D. E., Backman, C. L., Cao, X., & Badley, E. M. (2014). Striking a balance: Work-health-personal life conflict in women and men with arthritis and its association with work outcomes. *Journal of Occupational Rehabilitation, 24*, 573–584. https://doi.org/10.1007/s10926-013-9490-5

Hammond, A., O'Brien, R., Woodbridge, S., Bradshaw, L., Prior, Y., Radford, K., Culley, J., Whitham, D., & Pulikottil-Jacob, R. (2017). Job retention vocational rehabilitation for employed people with inflammatory arthritis (WORK-IA): A feasibility randomized controlled trial. *BMC Musculoskeletal Disorders, 18*, Article 315. https://doi.org/10.1186/s12891 -017-1671-5

Jetha, A., Badley, E., Beaton, D., Fortin, P. R., Shiff, N. J., & Gignac, M. A. M. (2015). Unpacking early work experiences of young adults with rheumatic disease: An examination of absenteeism, job disruptions, and productivity loss. *Arthritis Care & Research, 67*(9), 1246–1254. https://doi.org/10.1002/acr.22601

Jetha, A., Badley, E., Beaton, D., Fortin, P. R., Shiff, N. J., Rosenberg, A. M., Tucker, L. B., Mosher D. P., & Gignac, M. A. M. (2014). Transitioning to employment with a rheumatic disease: The role of independence, overprotection and social support. *Journal of Rheumatology, 41*(12), 2386–2394. https://doi.org/10.3899/jrheum.140419

Keysor, J. J., AlHeresh, R., Vaughan, M., LaValley, M. P., & Allaire, S. (2016). The Work-It Study for people with arthritis: Study protocol and baseline sample characteristics. *Work, 54*(2), 473–480. https://doi.org/10.3233/WOR-162331

Keysor, J. J., LaValley, M. P., Brown, C., Felson, D. T., AlHeresh, R. A., Vaughan, M. W., Yood, R., Reed, J. I., & Allaire, S. J. (2018). Efficacy of a work disability prevention program for people with rheumatic and musculoskeletal conditions: A single-blind parallel-arm randomized controlled trial. *Arthritis Care & Research, 70*(7), 1022–1029. https://doi.org/10.1002/acr.23423

McCormack, R. C., O'Shea, F., Doran, M., & Connolly, D. (2018). Impact of a fatigue management in work programme on meeting work demands of individuals with rheumatic diseases: A pilot study. *Musculoskeletal Care, 16*(3), 398–404. https://doi.org/10.1002/msc.1237

O'Toole, M. T. (Ed.). (2017). *Mosby's Dictionary of medicine, nursing & health professions* (10th ed.). Elsevier.

Prior, Y., Amanna, A. E., Bodell, S. J., & Hammond, A. (2017). A qualitative evaluation of occupational therapy-led work rehabilitation for people with inflammatory arthritis: Patients' views. *British Journal of Occupational Therapy, 80*(1), 39–48. https://doi.org/10.1177/0308 022616672666

Tang, K., Beaton, D. E., Lacaille, D., Gignac, M. A. M., Bombardier, C., & Canadian Arthritis Network (CAN) Work Productivity Group. (2013). Sensibility of five at-work productivity measures was endorsed by patients with osteoarthritis or rheumatoid arthritis. *Journal of Clinical Epidemiology, 66*(5), 546–556. https://doi.org/10.1016/j.jclinepi.2012.12.009

Tang, K., Beaton, D. E., Lacaille, D., Gignac, M. A. M., Zhang, W., Anis, A. H., Bombardier, C., & Canadian Arthritis Network Work Productivity Group. (2010). The Work Instability Scale for Rheumatoid Arthritis (RA-WIS): Does it work in osteoarthritis? *Quality of Life Research, 19*, 1057–1068. https://doi.org/10.1007/s11136-010-9656-y

Zhang, W., Gignac, M. A. M., Beaton, D., Tang, K., Anis, A. H., & Canadian Arthritis Network Work Productivity Group. (2010). Productivity loss due to presenteeism among patients with arthritis: Estimates from 4 instruments. *Journal of Rheumatology, 37*(9), 1805–1814. https://doi.org/10.3899/jrheum.100123

BIBLIOGRAPHY

Backman, C. L. (2011). Enabling performance and participation for persons with rheumatic diseases. In C. H. Christiansen & K. M. Matuska (Eds.), *Ways of living* (4th ed., pp. 213–238). AOTA Press.

Gignac, M. A. M., Cao, X., Tang, K., & Beaton, D. E. (2011). Examination of arthritis-related work place activity limitations and intermittent disability over four-and-a-half years and its relationship to job modifications and outcomes. *Arthritis Care & Research, 63*(7), 953–962. https://doi.org/10.1002/acr.20456

Kaptein, S. A., Backman, C. L., Badley, E., Lacaille, D., Beaton, D. E., Hofstetter, C., & Gignac, M. A. M. (2013). Choosing where to put your energy: A qualitative analysis of the role of physical activity in the lives of working adults with arthritis. *Arthritis Care & Research, 65*(7), 1070–1076. https://doi.org/10.1002/acr.21957

Tang, K., Escorpizo, R., Beaton, D. E., Bombardier, C., Lacaille, D., Zhang, W., Anis, A. H., Boonen, A., Verstappen, S. M. M., Buchbinder, R., Osborne, R. H., Fautrel, B., Gignac, M. A. M.,

& Tugwell, P. S. (2011). Measuring the impact of arthritis on worker productivity: Perspectives, methodologic issues, and contextual factors. *Journal of Rheumatology, 38*(8), 1776–1790. https://doi.org/10.3899/jrheum.110405

Cumulative Trauma Disorders

Also called work-related musculoskeletal disorders (WRMSD),
work-related upper limb disorder (WRULD),
repetitive strain injuries (RSI), repetitive stress disorders (RSD).

Description

A cumulative trauma disorder (CTD) is a soft tissue condition that develops in muscles, tendons, and nerve tissues that exceeds the ability to heal. The condition is not a specific disorder, but rather a collection of musculoskeletal disorders characterized by chronic discomfort, pain, and possible functional limitations and impairments. Symptoms tend to fluctuate over time, leading people to disregard the development of a CTD until the injury becomes chronic. Surgery may alleviate some, but not all symptoms, particularly pain. Furthermore, a CTD may result in prolonged disability and delayed return to work (Goodman et al., 2012). Wheelchair users and homemakers (unpaid) are at risk for CTD (Sabari et al., 2016; Yang & Cheung, 2016). CTD can occur in the lower extremities, but most of the literature in occupational therapy is focused on upper extremity conditions.

Cause

The cause is most often due to wear and tear in the muscles, tendons, and nerve tissues as a result of repetitive actions that overload certain soft tissues in static or constrained positions (Cheung et al., 2018; Goodman et al., 2012).

Types (Raheem & Buckshee, 2014)
- Type 1: Refers to localized, clearly defined syndromes, such as carpal tunnel syndrome, de Quervain syndrome, and lateral epicondylitis.
- Type 2: Defined as nontraumatic upper limb pain of unclear cause, such as regional allodynia or hyperalgesia.

Evaluation/Assessment

Areas
- Activities of Daily Living/Instrumental ADL: meal preparation (chopping, cutting, slicing)
- Education/Work: educational or work tasks (computing, carrying, lifting, sorting, shoveling), work positions (bending, stooping, crouching), work locations (crawling under or into a space, climbing over or onto a surface)
- Play/Leisure: types that require repetitive action (gripping, grasping, fingering, throwing, tossing, swinging, hitting), such as playing an instrument or engaging in a sports activity; frequency, location
- Rest/Sleep: sleep disturbance due to pain
- Social Participation: frequency, type, location, with whom (such as a sports activity)
- Sensorimotor: grip strength, joint range of motion, posture, pain
- Cognitive/Perceptual: problem solving, decision making
- Psychosocial: self-efficacy, role performance, quality of life
- Context/Environment: assistive devices
- Comorbidities: carpal tunnel syndrome, cubital tunnel syndrome, de Quervain's tenosynovitis, lateral epicondylitis (tennis elbow), medial epicondylitis, flexor or extensor tendinitis

Instruments
Instruments Developed by Occupational Therapy Personnel
- None

Instruments Developed by Other Professionals and Used by Occupational Therapy Personnel
- Circumference measurement (for edema) tape measure
- Grip strength (dynamometry; JAMAR dynamometer, Lafayette Instrument; Wang et al., 2018)
- Health Assessment Questionnaire (HAQ; Bruce & Fries, 2003)
- Joint range of motion (goniometry; Shurtleff & Kaskutas, 2018)
- Speed of keyboarding/typing test (number of characters typed per minute)
- Visual analogue scale (VAS; pain scale: 0 = *no pain*, 10 = *worst ever*)

Problems/Issues
Education/Work
- Person may experience pain or discomfort while performing work task in the hand, wrist, forearm, shoulder, or back.
- Person may be unable to maintain speed of performance (number of keystrokes per minute).
- Person may be unable to maintain or have difficulty maintaining position needed to accomplish work task.

Play/Leisure
- Person may experience pain or discomfort while engaged in favorite leisure activity.
- Person may have stopped or reduced engagement in leisure activity due to pain or discomfort.

Rest/Sleep
- Person may experience pain that reduces quality and quantity of sleep and rest.

Social Participation
- Person may have stopped or reduced participation in social activities due to pain or discomfort, such playing a round of golf with friends or a game of tennis.

Sensorimotor
- Person may experience decreased grip strength.
- Person may have decreased joint range of motion.
- Person may experience decreased dexterity and speed (characters typed per minute).
- Person may experience numbness or tingling sensation in the fingers, hand, or forearm.
- Person may experience edema or swelling in upper extremity.
- Person may experience pain in the fingers, hand, forearm, shoulder, or back.

Cognitive/Perceptual
- No information identified.

Psychosocial
- Person may report reduced quality of life due to pain and discomfort experienced while engaged or participating in certain activities.
- Person may report changes in role performance.
- Person may report reduced sense of self-efficacy.

Context/Environment
- Person may lack knowledge about the disorder.
- Person may lack knowledge about community or internet resources.

Intervention/Treatment
Models and programs developed by occupational therapy personnel include constructivist-grounded theory (Cheung et al., 2016, 2018), treatment protocol (Raheem & Buckshee, 2014), and therapeutic workshop (Alencar, 2015). Models and programs developed by other professionals

but used by occupational therapy personnel include computer mouse positions (Sako et al., 2017) and ergonomic interventions (Goodman & Flinn, 2015). Team members include physicians, surgeons, psychologists, physical therapy personnel, physical trainers, and occupational therapy personnel. Goals are to improve occupational performance and decrease pain and functional limitation.

Activities of Daily Living/Instrumental ADL
- Suggest home (especially kitchen) modification and workspace adaptations to reduce repetitive actions and use of poor posture positions.
- Explore use of electronic aids to replace manual actions, such as use of ergonomically designed utensils and equipment for meal preparation and housecleaning.

Education/Work
- Suggest workplace modification and workstation adaptations to reduce repetitive actions and poor posture positions.
- Explore use of ergonomically designed tools to be used such as forearm supports, ergonomically designed keyboard and mouse.

Play/Leisure
- Identify leisure activities that may be contributing to cumulative trauma such as throwing, tossing, hitting, swinging a club or racket.
- Assist client to modify position, frequency of engagement, or use of adapted equipment.
- Assist client to explore leisure activities that may require less repetitive actions or poor posture positions.

Rest/Sleep
- See Sleep–Wake Disorders in Section 13: Lifestyle Conditions.

Social Participation
- No information identified.

Sensorimotor
- Fitness training: Provide exercises for stretching, strengthening, and joint mobilization.
- Heat or ice: Provide temporary reduction in pain.
- Posture reeducation: Use audio, visual, and proprioceptive feedback from muscles and joint to maintain good posture and body alignment.
- Pain management: Assist client to explore and implement fitness, activity tolerance activities, and improved ergonomic designed workstation and tools to provide pain relief and reduced discomfort.
- Wrist and forearm supports/splinting: Consider if a wrist or forearm support may assist in maintaining joint alignment and reduce pain.

Cognitive/Perceptual
- Energy conservation education, including planning of activities including breaks (work/rest cycles).
- Ergonomic education: Information on safe handling, good posture, and good tool design based on ergonomic principles.
- Self-management program: Assist client to develop and implement program to reduce or eliminate repetitive motions and poor posture positions.

Psychosocial
- Provide opportunity to discuss changes in quality of life and possible modifications to improve.

Context/Environment
- Provide information on CTD, ergonomic design and workplace modification.
- Provide information on use of ergonomically designed tools and equipment.

Precautions/Safety Considerations

Monitor signs of swelling, inflammation, or pain during use of physical exercises. Avoid stretching nerve if nerve gliding exercises are used. If heat is used, watch for redness, hot-to-touch skin, or swelling in joints. If ice is used, watch for sensory or vascular problems; skin should be checked every few minutes for redness. If vibration is used, lubricate skin to protect.

Prognosis and Outcome

Outcome is variable, depending on client's ability and willingness to self-manage behavior or change work situation, and willingness of employer to make modifications to workplace or work station.

REFERENCES

Alencar, M. D. B. (2015). Occupational therapy interventions to subjects away from work due to RSI/WMSD. *Cadernos de Terapia Ocupacional da UFSCar, 21*(4), 889–898. https://doi.org/10.4322/0104-4931.ctoRE0493

Cheung, T. W. C., Clemson, L., O'Loughlin, K., & Shuttleworth, R. (2016). Understanding decision-making towards housework among women with upper limb repetitive strain injury. *Australian Occupational Therapy Journal, 63*(1), 37–46. https://doi.org/10.1111/1440-1630.12254

Cheung, T. W. C., Clemson, L., O'Loughlin, K., & Shuttleworth, R. (2018). Erognomic* education on housework for women with upper limb repetitive strain injury (RSI): A conceptual representation of therapists' clinical reasoning. *Disability and Rehabilitation, 40*(26), 3136–3146. https://doi.org/10.1080/09638288.2017.1378928

Goodman, G., & Flinn, S. (2015). Ergonomic interventions for computer users with cumulative trauma disorders. In I. Söderback (Ed.), *International handbook of occupational therapy interventions*. Springer. https://doi.org/10.1007/978-3-319-08141-0_15

Goodman, G., Kovach, L., Fisher, A., Elsesser, E., Bobinski, D., & Hansen, J. (2012). Effective interventions for cumulative trauma disorders of the upper extremity in computer users: Practice models based on systematic review. *Work, 42*(1), 153–172. https://doi.org/10.3233/WOR-2012-1341

Raheem, T. A., & Buckshee, R. N. (2014). Occupational therapy management for work related upper limb disorders in computer users. *Indian Journal of Physiotherapy & Occupational Therapy, 8*(2), 130–135. https://doi.org/10.5958/j.0973-5674.8.2.074

Sabari, J., Shea, M., Chen, L., Laurenceau, A., & Leung, E. (2016). Impact of wheelchair seat height on neck and shoulder range of motion during functional task performance. *Assistive Technology, 28*(3), 183–189. https://doi.org/10.1080/10400435.2016.1140692

Sako, S., Sugiura, H., Tanoue, H., Kojima, M., Kono, M., & Inaba, R. (2017). Electromyographic analysis of relevant muscle groups during completion of computer tasks using different computer mouse positions. *International Journal of Occupational Safety and Ergonomics, 23*(2), 267–273. https://doi.org/10.1080/10803548.2016.1275140

Yang, Z., & Cheung, T. W. C. (2016). The inclusion of homemakers as an occupation amongst people with upper limb repetitive stress injuries. *Work, 55*(1), 181–186. https://doi.org/10.3233/WOR-162372

BIBLIOGRAPHY

Roll, S. C., & Hardison, M. E. (2017). Effectiveness of occupational therapy interventions for adults with musculoskeletal conditions of the forearm, wrist, and hand: A systematic review. *American Journal of Occupational Therapy, 71*(1), Article 7101180010. https://doi.org/10.5014/ajot.2017.023234

---

*The published article includes this typo.

Fibromyalgia

Description

Fibromyalgia is a form of nonarticular rheumatism characterized by generalized aching; widespread tenderness of muscles areas around tendon insertions and adjacent soft tissues; muscle stiffness; muscle pain, spasms, fatigue; cognitive deficits, mood swings, sleep disorders; and various other somatic systems, including irritable bowel syndrome and paresthesia. Frequent sites of pain and stiffness are the lower back, neck, should region, arms, hands, knees, hips thighs, legs, and feet. The disorder is more common in women (O'Toole, 2017; Porter, 2018). This chapter focuses on adults with fibromyalgia. One article on juvenile fibromyalgia was identified (Sherry et al., 2015).

Cause

Etiology is unknown.

Evaluation/Assessment

Areas

- Activities of Daily Living/Instrumental ADL: functional performance in self-maintenance skills, nutrition and health, eating, health status, financial resources and management, transportation
- Education/Work: work history, knowledge of worker rights (sick leave, disability insurance)
- Play/Leisure: interests and values
- Rest/Sleep: sleep habits, sleep dysfunction
- Social Participation: frequency, type, location
- Sensorimotor: endurance and activity tolerance, daily exercising, muscle pain
- Cognitive/Perceptual: awareness of impact of diagnosis, attention and concentration, memory, executive functions (problem solving, time management), speed of processing information
- Psychosocial: depression, stress triggers, coping strategies, quality of life, self-efficacy
- Context/Environment: knowledge about chronic disease, social support, adapted devices, resources
- Comorbidities: irritable bowel syndrome, interstitial cystitis, migraine, tension headaches, paresthesias, and depression (Porter, 2018)

Instruments

Instruments Developed by Occupational Therapy Personnel

- Assessment of Motor and Process Skills (8th ed.; AMPS-8; Fisher & Bray Jones, 2016)
- Canadian Occupational Performance Measure (5th ed.; COPM-5; Law et al., 2014)
- Computer Problems Survey (ComPS; Baker et al., 2009)
- Note: Use of observation-based assessment of activities of daily living ability is recommended because self-report instruments do not appear to capture differences in process ability (von Bülow et al., 2015)

Instruments Developed by Other Professionals and Used by Occupational Therapy Personnel

- 6-Minute Walk Test (6MWT; American Thoracic Society, 2002)
- Arthritis Self-Efficacy Scale (ASES; Long et al., 1989)
- Barthel Index (BI; Mahoney & Barthel, 1965)
- Beck Depression Inventory (2nd ed.; BDI-II; Beck et al., 1996)
- Coping Strategies Questionnaire (CSQ; Rosenstiel & Keefe, 1983)
- Effective Musculoskeletal Consumer Scale (EC-17; Kristiansson et al., 2007)
- Fatigue Severity Scale (FSS; Krupp et al., 1989)
- Fibromyalgia Impact Questionnaire Revised (FIQ-R; also called Revised Fibromyalgia Impact Questionnaire; Bennett et al, 2009; original scale by Burckhardt et al., 1991)

- Five Facet Mindfulness Questionnaire–Short Form (FFMQ-SF; Bohlmeijer et al., 2011)
- Functional Independence Measure (FIM; Uniform Data System for Medical Rehabilitation, 1997)
- General Health Questionnaire (GHQ-30; Goldberg & Williams, 1988)
- Generalized Anxiety Disorder Self-Assessment Questionnaire (GAD-10; developed from the Hamilton Anxiety Rating Scale, below; see also Wæhrens et al., 2015, in References)
- Grip strength (dynamometer; JAMAR, Lafayette Instrument; Wang et al., 2018)
- Hamilton Anxiety Rating Scale (HARS; Hamilton, 1959)
- Instrumental Activities of Daily Living Scale (Lawton & Brody, 1969)
- Major Depression Inventory (MDI; Bech et al., 2001)
- Pain Coping Inventory (PCI; Kraaimaat & Evers, 2003)
- painDETECT Questionnaire (PD-Q; Freynhagen et al., 2006)
- Quality of Life Scale (QOLS; Flanagan, 1978, 1982; see also Liedberg et al., 2012, in References)
- Revised Fibromyalgia Impact Questionnaire (FIQ-R; also called Fibromyalgia Impact Questionnaire–Revised; Bennett et al., 2009)
- Short-Form Health Measure/Survey (SF-36; Ware et al., 1993)
- Tampa Scale of Kinesiophobia (TSK; Miller et al., 1991)
- Visual Analogue Scale (VAS) Numeric Rating Scale (NRS) pain scale (scored: 0 = *no pain*, 10 = *worst pain ever*)

Problems/Issues

Activities of Daily Living/Instrumental ADL

- Person may have difficulty performing self-maintenance skills with accuracy and normal speed such as eating, dressing, grooming, bathing, toileting, transfers, going up and down stairs, understanding communication and ability to express oneself.
- Person may have become dependent on others to assist in performing self-maintenance tasks.
- Person may have poor nutritional habits.
- Person may experience difficulty managing finances.
- Person may experience difficulty in driving related to issues with speed and accurate responses.

Education/Work

- Person may be unable to work away from home.
- Person may experience difficulty with work station due to lack of modifications and ergonomically designed workplace.
- Person may lack knowledge about worker rights.
- Person may experience difficulty using computer equipment at work.

Play/Leisure

- Person may be unable to engage or restrict engagement in favorite leisure activities.

Rest/Sleep

- Person may experience sleep disturbance related to pain.
- Person may have developed poor sleep habits and routine.

Social Participation

- Person may have reduced or stopped participation in social activities.

Sensorimotor

- Person may have difficulty moving, bending, and reaching, as demonstrated on the AMPS.
- Person always experiences pain.
- Person usually has reduced amount of endurance and activity tolerance.

Cognitive/Perceptual

- Person may have more difficulty attending to task, make more errors and take longer to complete task than a healthy person would take to perform same task.

- Person may make more execution errors and take longer to complete task when performing from memory than a healthy person would make performing same task.
- Person may have difficulty with executive functions including planning ahead, problem solving, and time management.
- Person may have difficulty with calibrating and pacing according to the AMPS.
- Person may take longer to complete tasks and make more errors involving visual perception than a healthy person would take to perform same task.

Psychosocial
- Person may have difficulty with stress management and coping strategies.
- Person may experience depression and anxiety.

Context/Environment
- Person may lack information about managing disease, including use of adapted devices.
- Person may lack information about available community and internet resources.

Intervention/Treatment

Models and programs developed by occupational therapy personnel include occupational therapy intervention (Siegel et al., 2018). Models and programs developed by other professionals but used by occupational therapy personnel include brief interdisciplinary treatment program (Oh et al., 2010), cognitive performance (Pérez de Heredia-Torres, Huertas Hoyas, Máximo-Bocanegra, et al., 2016), IMPROvE program (von Bülow et al., 2017), multicomponent therapy (Ollevier et al., 2020), multidisciplinary approach (Gonzalez et al., 2015), and multidisciplinary in-patient self-management program (Hamnes et al., 2012). Team members include general physicians, physiatrists, rheumatologists, nursing personnel, psychologists, physical therapy personnel, and occupational therapy personnel. Goals include addressing the physical and psychological aspects of the impact of chronic pain in all occupational performance areas, including self-care, work, leisure, and family life (McVeigh & O'Brien, 2010).

Activities of Daily Living/Instrumental ADL
- Assist client to review and adapt performance of self-maintenance skills to improve performance (accuracy and speed) and minimize pain.
- Assist client to review nutritional choices and food preparation to maintain healthy eating habits.
- Assist client in home management activities focused on joint protection, energy conservation, activity modification, work simplification, and time management.

Education/Work
- Assist client to review work station for better ergonomic design and work efficiency.
- Assist client to organize and modify work tasks to conserve energy, reduce pain, and alleviate stress.

Play/Leisure
- Assist client to engage in leisure occupations of interest and value.

Rest/Sleep
- Assist client to review and revise sleep habits and hygiene.

Social Participation
- Assist client to participate in social activities with family and friends.

Sensorimotor
- Provide instruction in pain management techniques.
- Provide instruction in energy conservation and fatigue management such as pacing, alternating work and rest breaks, scheduling important activities at time person has most energy and less pain.
- Encourage use of good body mechanics and joint protection principles.

- Provide low impact exercise program (pool exercises, walking, cycling) to increase physical fitness.
- Provide activities and exercises to increase grip strength.

Cognitive/Perceptual

- Assist client to use time management techniques to determine where and when energy is being expended.
- Assist client to prioritize occupations to be completed during a day and week.
- Assist client to learn to "grade" occupations according to such parameters as energy requirements, amount of pain, and resulting stress.
- Have client keep a journal to track success of plan to achieve objectives and goals.

Psychosocial

- Provide instruction and practice in stress management and coping techniques such as deep breathing, relaxation training, mindfulness, yoga.
- Provide opportunity to express and talk about feelings of depression.

Context/Environment

- Provide information, selection, and use of adaptive devices.
- Provide information about community and internet resources.

Precautions/Safety Considerations

Cognitive deficits contribute to safety concerns.

Prognosis and Outcome

Condition is chronic. No cure in known. Management of symptoms is important to decrease the severity of disability. Women may continue to have a high level of disability, require a greater level of assistance, and have a reduced quality of life (Pérez, de Heredia-Torres, Huertas-Hoyas, Sánchez-Camarero, et al., 2016).

REFERENCES

Gonzalez, J. G., Rubio, M., Paniagua, C. N. W., Criado-Alvarez, J. J., & Holgado, J. S. (2015). Symptomatic pain and fibromyalgia treatment through multidisciplinary approach for primary care. *Reumatología Clínica, 11*(1), 22–26. https://doi.org/10.1016/j.reuma.2014.03.005

Hamnes, B., Mowinckel, P., Kjeken, I., & Hagen, K. B. (2012). Effects of a one week multidisciplinary inpatient self-management programme for patients with fibromyalgia: A randomised controlled trial. *BMC Musculoskeletal Disorders, 13*, Article 189. https://doi.org/10.1186/14 71-2474-13-189

Liedberg, G. M., Eddy, L. L., & Burckhardt, C. S. (2012). Validity testing of the Quality of Life Scale, Swedish version: Focus group interviews of women with fibromyalgia. *Occupational Therapy International, 19*(4), 167–175. https://doi.org/10.1002/oti.1329

McVeigh, J. G., & O'Brien, R. (2010). Fibromyalgia syndrome and chronic widespread pain. In K. Dziedzic & A. Hammond (Eds.), *Rheumatology evidence-based practice for physiotherapists and occupational therapists* (pp. 255–272). Churchill Livingstone.

Oh, T. H., Stueve, M. H., Hoskin, T. L., Luedtke, C., Vincent, A., Moder, K. G., & Thompson, J. M. (2010). Brief interdisciplinary treatment program for fibromyalgia: Six to twelve months outcome. *American Journal of Physical Medicine & Rehabilitation, 89*(2), 115–124. https://doi .org/10.1097/PHM.0b013e3181c9d817

Ollevier, A., Vanneuville, I., Carron, P., Baetens, T., Goderis, T., Gabriel, L., & Van de Velde, D. (2020). A 12-week multicomponent therapy in fibromyalgia improves health but not in concomitant moderate depression, an exploratory pilot study. *Disability and Rehabilitation, 42*(13), 1886–1893. https://doi.org/10.1080/09638288.2018.1543361

O'Toole, M. T. (Ed.). (2017). *Mosby's dictionary of medicine, nursing & health professions* (10th ed.). Elsevier.

Pérez de Heredia-Torres, M., Huertas-Hoyas, E., Máximo-Bocanegra, N., Palacios-Ceña, D., & Fernández-de-las-Peñas, C. (2016). Cognitive performance in women with fibromyalgia: A case-control study. *Australian Occupational Therapy Journal, 63*(5), 329–337. https://doi.org/10.1111/1440-1630.12292

Pérez de Heredia-Torres, M., Huertas-Hoyas, E., Sánchez-Camarero, C., Pérez-Corrales, J., & Fernández-de-las-Peñas, C. (2016). The occupational profile of women with fibromyalgia syndrome. *Occupational Therapy International, 23*, 132–142. https://doi.org/10.1002/oti.1418

Porter, R. S. (Ed.). (2018). *The Merck manual of diagnosis and therapy* (20th ed.). Merck Sharp & Dohme.

Sherry, D. D., Brake, L., Tress, J. L., Sherker, J., Fash, K., Ferry, K., & Weiss, P. F. (2015). The treatment of juvenile fibromyalgia with an intensive physical and psychosocial program. *Journal of Pediatrics, 167*(3), 731–737. https://doi.org/10.1016/j.jpeds.2015.06.036

Siegel, P., Jones, B. L., & Poole, J. L. (2018). Occupational therapy interventions for adults with fibromyalgia. *American Journal of Occupational Therapy, 72*(5), Article 7205395010. https://doi.org/10.5014/ajot.2018.725002

von Bülow, C., Amris, K., Bandak, E., Danneskiold-Samsøe, B., & Wæhrens, E. E. (2017). Improving activities of daily living ability in women with fibromyalgia: An exploratory, quasi-randomized, phase-two study, IMPROvE trial. *Journal of Rehabilitation Medicine, 49*(3), 241–250. https://doi.org/10.2340/16501977-2198

von Bülow, C., Amris, K., la Cour, K., Danneskiold-Samsøe, B., & Wæhrens, E. E. (2015). Differences in ability to perform activities of daily living among women with fibromyalgia: A cross-sectional study. *Journal of Rehabilitation Medicine, 47*(10), 941–947. https://doi.org/10.2340/16501977-2021

Wæhrens, E. E., Amris, K., Bartels, E. M., Christensen, R., Danneskiold-Samsøe, B., Bliddal, H., & Gudbergsen, H. (2015). Agreement between touch-screen and paper-based patient-reported outcomes for patients with fibromyalgia: A randomized cross-over reproducibility study. *Scandinavian Journal of Rheumatology, 44*(6), 503–510. https://doi.org/10.3109/03009742.2015.1029517

BIBLIOGRAPHY

Amris, K., Luta, G., Christensen, R., Danneskiold-Samsøe, B., Bliddal, H., & Wæhrens, E. E. (2016). Predictors of improvement in observed functional ability in patients with fibromyalgia as an outcome of rehabilitation. *Journal of Rehabilitation Medicine, 48*(1), 65–71. https://doi.org/10.2340/16501977-2036

Baker, N. A., Rubinstein, E. N., & Rogers, J. (2012). Problems and accommodation strategies reported by computer users with rheumatoid arthritis or fibromyalgia. *Journal of Occupational Rehabilitation, 22*(3), 353–362. https://doi.org/10.1007/s10926-012-9353-5

Hammond, A. (2014). Rheumatoid arthritis, osteoarthritis, and fibromyalgia. In M. V. Radomski & C. A. Trombly Latham (Eds.), *Occupational therapy for physical dysfunction* (7th ed., pp. 1215–1243). Wolters Kluwer.

Poole, J. L., & Siegel, P. (2017). Effectiveness of occupational therapy interventions for adults with fibromyalgia: A systematic review. *American Journal of Occupational Therapy, 71*(1), Article 7101180040. https://doi.org/10.5014/ajot.2017.023192

von Bülow, C., Amris, K., La Cour, K., Danneskiold-Samsøe, B., & Wæhrens, E. E. (2016). Ineffective ADL skills in women with fibromyalgia: A cross-sectional study. *Scandinavian Journal of Occupational Therapy, 23*(5), 391–397. https://doi.org/10.3109/11038128.2015.1095237

Wæhrens, E. E., Bliddal, H., Danneskiold-Samsøe, B., Lund, H., & Fisher, A. G. (2012). Differences between questionnaire- and interview-based measures of activities of daily living (ADL) ability and their association with observed ADL ability in women with rheumatoid arthritis, knee osteoarthritis and fibromyalgia. *Scandinavian Journal of Rheumatology, 41*(2), 95–102. https://doi.org/10.3109/03009742.2011.632380

Inflammatory Arthritis

See also Psoriatic Arthritis, Rheumatoid Arthritis.

Description

Inflammatory arthritis is a general or umbrella term for several chronic progressive musculo-skeletal diseases including rheumatoid arthritis (RA), ankylosing spondylitis (AS), connective tissue disease (CTD), psoriatic arthritis (PsA), and systemic lupus erythematosus (SLE; Dures et al., 2014).

Cause

The immune system, the body's defense system, attacks its own tissues, causing pain, stiffness, swelling, tenderness, and joint damage. Surrounding ligaments, tendons, and skin may also be involved (Prior et al., 2017).

Evaluation/Assessment

Areas

- Activities of Daily Living/Instrumental ADL: self-maintenance, functional mobility
- Education/Work: work capacity, work disability, work instability, work productivity absenteeism and presenteeism, work site modification, work site ergonomic design
- Play/Leisure: interests, values, type, frequency
- Rest/Sleep: sleep disturbance
- Social Participation: type, frequency, location, with whom
- Sensorimotor: muscle weakness, joint range of motion, endurance, hand functions, symptom flare-ups, pain, fatigue
- Cognitive/Perceptual: beliefs about illness, body image
- Psychosocial: depression, anxiety, coping strategies, locus of control, avoidance behaviors, sense of helplessness and hopelessness, anhedonia (loss of feeling of pleasure), quality of life, life satisfaction, life and social roles, self-efficacy, self-esteem, self-confidence
- Context/Environment: adapted equipment, home modification, ergonomic design, community resources, social support
- Comorbidity: inflammatory bowel disease (Crohn's disease)

Instruments

Instruments Developed by Occupational Therapy Personnel

- Arthritis Hand Function Test (AHFT; Backman et al., 1991)
- Ergonomic Assessment Tool for Arthritis (EATA; Backman et al., 2008)
- Measure of Activity Performance of the Hand (MAP-HAND; Paulsen et al., 2010)
- Worker Role Interview (Version 10.0; WRI 10.0; Braveman et al., 2005)

Instruments Developed by Other Professionals and Used by Occupational Therapy Personnel

- European Quality of Life 5-Dimension Scale (EQ-5D; EuroQol Group, 1990)
- Grip strength (dynamometer; JAMAR, Lafayette Instrument; Wang et al., 2018)
- Jebsen-Taylor Hand Function Test (JTHFT; Jepsen et al., 1969)
- Michigan Hand Outcomes Questionnaire (MHQ; Chung et al., 1998)
- Multidimensional Health Assessment Questionnaire (MDHAQ; Pincus et al., 1999)
- Purdue Pegboard Test (PPT; Tiffin, 1948)
- RA Work Instability Scale (RA-WIS; Gilworth et al., 2003)
- Short-Form Health Survey 12 (SF-12; Ware et al., 1996)
- Visual Analogue Scale (VAS) Numeric Rating Scale (NRS) pain scale (scored: 0 = *no pain*, 10 = *worst pain ever*)
- Work Activities Limitation Scale (WALS; Gignac et al., 2004)
- Work Experience Survey (WES; Roessler & Gottcent, 1994)
- Work Limitations Questionnaire (WLQ; Lerner et al., 2001)

Problems/Issues

Activities of Daily Living/Instrumental ADL
- No information identified.

Education/Work
- Person may be unable to meet the work demands for productivity required of a job.
- Person may have excessive absences due to flare-ups of the inflammatory process.
- Person may have given up trying to maintain working.

Play/Leisure
- Person may have limited or stopped engagement in favorite leisure occupations.

Rest/Sleep
- Person may experience reduced quality of sleep due to pain or anxiety.

Social Participation
- Person may have restricted participation in social activities.

Sensorimotor
- Person usually experiences acute and chronic pain especially in hand, wrist, and forearm.
- Person usually experiences fatigue, tiredness, and lack of endurance more quickly than would be expected of a person of that age.
- Person may experience muscle weakness.
- Person may experience decreased range of motion.

Cognitive/Perceptual
- No information identified.

Psychosocial
- Person may become depressed.
- Person may express feelings of anxiety, worrying, and psychological distress.
- Person may express feelings of helplessness and hopelessness leading to a lack of motivation.
- Person may express a loss of feeling of pleasure, enjoyment, and reduced quality of life.
- Person may lack a sense of self-efficacy.
- Person may have reduced sense of self-esteem and self-confidence.

Context/Environment
- Person may lack social support.
- Person may lack information about or access to adaptive devices.

Intervention/Treatment

Models and programs developed by occupational therapy personnel include the occupational therapy VR training program for therapists (O'Brien et al., 2013). Models and programs developed by other professions but used by occupational therapy personnel include sample clinical pathway (O'Brien & Backman, 2010), WORK-IA (Hammond et al., 2017), and work rehabilitation program (Prior et al., 2017). Team members include general physicians, rheumatologists, nursing personnel, psychologists, physical therapists, and occupational therapy personnel. Goals are to manage pain and fatigue symptoms; resolve functional limitations; improve connection with family, friends, and community (including roles in housework, leisure, and social activities); reduce depression and anxiety; and assist in engagement in meaningful activities to maintain a sense of identity and positive self-worth (O'Brien & Backman, 2010).

Activities of Daily Living/Instrumental ADL
- Consider with client if use of specific adapted devices such as built-up handles, elongated handles, or electronic devices would make everyday tasks easier.

Education/Work
- Provide review of work station accessibility including ergonomic principles of design.

- Provide review of work demands, including use safe materials handling techniques for lifting, carrying, stooping, climbing, pushing, and pulling.
- Suggest reviewing alternative methods of meeting work demands and productivity standards such as part-time work, working at home, scheduling longer work breaks.

Play/Leisure
- Assist client to explore alternate methods of engaging in favorite leisure occupations.
- Assist client to explore new leisure occupations that may be better suited to degree of disability.

Rest/Sleep
- Assist client to create and follow good sleep hygiene practices.
- Explore with client if changes in sleep arrangements (different bedding, light and noise reduction, location of bed nearer bathroom, addition of a bedside commode) might improve quality of sleep.

Social Participation
- Encourage client to continue or resume participation in social activities with modifications such as outings over shorter periods of time, accessible locations, options for sitting or resting.

Sensorimotor
- Provide instruction in use of energy conservation and work simplification techniques.
- Provide pain-management program.
- Instruct client in joint protection.
- Consider if a hand splint would reduce pain and improve hand function.

Cognitive/Perceptual
- Assist client in learning and practicing self-management strategies.
- Assist client to better understand the body's response to pain, fatigue, and tiredness.
- Instruct client on time management approaches (pacing rest and work cycles, scheduling important activities when person has most energy).

Psychosocial
- Instruct client in stress management and coping techniques (deep breathing exercises, progressive relaxation, mindfulness, yoga).
- Assist client in developing plans and actions that are aimed at staying positive (Macdonald et al., 2018).

Context/Environment
- Assist client to explore and try out adaptive devices (provide instruction in use and care).
- Assist client to identify community resources including services designed for persons with disabilities.
- Telemedicine may be useful for ongoing client education and follow-up.

Precautions/Safety Considerations

Persons with inflammatory arthritis are reported to have problems reading and following written information and instructions. Audiovisual or video communication may be better choices (Hammond et al., 2017; Prior et al., 2017).

Prognosis and Outcome

Inflammatory arthritis is part of a chronic arthritic condition. Supported and compensatory approaches are recommended.

REFERENCES

Dures, E., Almeida, C., Caesley, J., Peterson, A., Ambler, N., Morris, M., Pollock, J., & Hewlett, S. (2014). A survey of psychological support provision for people with inflammatory arthritis in secondary care in England. *Musculoskeletal Care, 12*(3), 173–181. https://doi.org/10.1002/msc.1071

Hammond, A., O'Brien, R., Woodbridge, S., Bradshaw, L., Prior, Y., Radford, K., Culley, J., Whitham, D., & Pulikottil-Jacob, R. (2017). Job retention vocational rehabilitation for employed people with inflammatory arthritis (WORK-IA): A feasibility randomized controlled trial. *BMC Musculoskeletal Disorders, 18,* Article 315. https://doi.org/10.1186/s12891-017-1671-5

Macdonald, G. G., Koehn, C., Attara, G., Stordy, A., Allerdings, M., Leese, J., Li, L. C., & Backman, C. (2018). Patient perspectives on the challenges and responsibilities of living with chronic inflammatory diseases: Qualitative study. *Journal of Participatory Medicine, 10*(4). Article e10815. https://doi.org/10.2196/10815

O'Brien, R., & Backman, C. (2010). Inflammatory arthritis. In K. Dziedzic & A. Hammond (Eds.), *Rheumatology: Evidence-based practice for physiotherapists and occupational therapists* (pp. 211–233). Churchill Livingstone.

O'Brien, R., Woodbridge, S., Hammond, A., Adkin, J., & Culley, J. (2013). The development and evaluation of a vocational rehabilitation training programme for rheumatology occupational therapists. *Musculoskeletal Care, 11*(2), 99–105. https://doi.org/10.1002/msc.1050

Prior, Y., Amanna, A. E., Bodell, S. J., & Hammond, A. (2017). A qualitative evaluation of occupational therapy-led work rehabilitation for people with inflammatory arthritis: Patients' views. *British Journal of Occupational Therapy, 80*(1), 39–48. https://doi.org/10.1177/0308022616672666

BIBLIOGRAPHY

Codd, Y., Stapleton, T., Kane, D., & Mullan, R. (2018). A survey to establish current practice in addressing work participation with inflammatory arthritis in the Irish clinical setting. *Musculoskeletal Care, 16*(1), 158–162. https://doi.org/10.1002/msc.1198

Sarsak, H. I. (2018). Effectiveness of rigid wrist splints on reducing pain and improving hand function in patients with inflammatory arthritis. *Researches in Arthritis & Bone Study, 1*(3), 1–4.

Warmington, K., Flewelling, C., Kennedy, C. A., Shupak, R., Papachristos, A., Jones, C., Linton, D., Beaton, D. E., & Lineker, S. (2017). Telemedicine delivery of patient education in remote Ontario communities: Feasibility of an Advanced Clinician Practitioner in Arthritis Care (ACPAC)-led inflammatory arthritis education program. *Open Access Rheumatology: Research and Reviews, 2017*(9), 11–19. https://doi.org/10.2147/OARRR.S122015

Juvenile Idiopathic Arthritis
Also called juvenile rheumatoid arthritis, JIA, JRA.

Description

Juvenile idiopathic arthritis (JIA) is a group of rheumatic diseases that begins by or before age 16. There are several manifestations, including arthritis, fever, rash, adenopathy, splenomegaly, and iridocyclitis (Porter, 2018). Because bone growth in children is dependent on the epiphyseal plates of the distal epiphyses, skeletal development may be impaired if these structures are damaged (O'Toole, 2017). The most common signs are pain, swelling, and stiffness (Ferdous, 2015).

Cause

The cause is unknown, but there may be a genetic predisposition, and an autoimmune or autoinflammatory pathophysiology. JIA is considered distinct from adult rheumatoid arthritis, although there are some similarities (Porter, 2018).

Classification

Six categories are recognized by the International League of Associations for Rheumatology (Porter, 2018):

- Enthesitis-related arthritis
- Oligoarticular JIA (persistent or extended)
- Polyarticular JIA (rheumatoid factor [RF] negative or positive)
- Psoriatic JIA
- Systemic JIA
- Undifferentiated JIA

Evaluation/Assessment

Areas

- Activities of Daily Living/Instrumental ADL: basic ADLs (eating, dressing, bathing, toileting, functional mobility, medication management); independence (age appropriate)
- Education/Work: academic performance
- Play/Leisure: interests, frequency, location
- Rest/Sleep: habits, routines, sleep disturbances
- Social Participation: type, frequency, location, with whom
- Sensorimotor: range of motion, flexibility, muscle strength, endurance, hand functions (grip strength, grasp, dexterity, coordination, manipulations), fatigue, stiff joints, contractures, general physical fitness, walking speed, edema/swelling, inflammation, pain (soreness, discomfort)
- Cognitive/Perceptual: not affected directly
- Psychosocial: depression, anxiety, irritability, stress and coping skills, motivation, social isolation, quality of life
- Context/Environment: assistive devices and technology, client/family/caregiver/educator education, architectural barriers (home, school, and community accessibility), social support, community and internet resources
- Comorbidities: delayed developmental milestones, growth retardation, osteoporosis, osteonecrosis, skin rash, fever, uveitis (eye inflammation), iridocyclitis, cataracts, glaucoma

Instruments

Instruments Developed by Occupational Therapy Personnel

- Children's Assessment of Participation and Enjoyment and Preferences for Activities of Children (CAPE/PAC; King et al., 2004)

Instruments Developed by Other Professionals and Used by Occupational Therapy Personnel

- Coping Health Inventory for Parents (CHIP; McCubbin et al., 1983)
- Child Health Questionnaire–Parent Form (CHQ-PF50; Landgraf et al., 1996)
- Economic Hardship Questionnaire (EHQ; Lempers et al., 1989)
- Juvenile Arthritis Quality of Life Questionnaire (JAQQ; Duffy et al., 1997)
- Parent Adherence Report Questionnaire (PARQ; De Civita et al., 2005; see also Toupin April et al., 2016, in References)
- Symptom Checklist-90-Revised (SCL-90-R; Derogatis, 1994)

Problems/Issues

Activities of Daily Living/Instrumental ADL

- Child/adolescent may have difficulty performing basic ADLs due to pain, stiffness, physical limitations, or fatigue.
- Child/adolescent may fall behind in developmental milestones.

Education/Work

- Child/adolescent may have difficulty performing some academic skills (holding a pencil, crayon, or paint brush), writing, cutting with scissors, turning pages, carrying books or a food tray.

- Child/adolescent may need seating adaptations, especially if floor activities are part of scheduled academic program.
- Child/adolescent may be unable to participate in physical education or recess activities due to pain and physical limitations.

Play/Leisure
- Child/adolescent may have difficulty handling and manipulating toys due to physical limitations.
- Child/adolescent may limit or stop engaging in play activities that involve physical activity (hopping, jumping, kicking, running).

Rest/Sleep
- Child/adolescent may experience sleeplessness due to pain or discomfort.

Social Participation
- Child/adolescent may be unable to participate in social activities with peers due to physical limitations.

Sensorimotor
- Child/adolescent may experience decreased or limited joint range of motion.
- Child/adolescent may experience stiffness, especially in the morning.
- Child/adolescent may limp when walking and have difficulty climbing stairs.
- Child/adolescent may have reduced walking speed.
- Child/adolescent may experience decreased endurance and increased fatigue.
- Child/adolescent may have activity restrictions due to physical limitations.
- Child/adolescent may have reduced hand functions (grip, grasp, dexterity, coordination, manipulation).
- Child/adolescent may experience recurring pain and soreness, especially in the knees, elbows, and hands, while engaged in physical movements and activities such as walking, getting up or sitting down, hopping, jumping, running, climbing, bending, squatting, lifting, carrying.
- Child/adolescent may have swelling/edema in one or multiple joints.
- Child/adolescent may have inflammation and increased temperature.
- Child/adolescent may have iridocyclitis.

Cognitive/Perceptual
- Not directly affected but pain and fatigue may reduce attention span.

Psychosocial
- Child/adolescent may not be able to interact and socialize with others due to physical limitations (inability to "keep up" with peers).
- Child/adolescent may become socially isolated from peers.
- Child/adolescent may have reduced motivation due to factors such as pain, fatigue, lack of mobility.
- Child/adolescent may have a reduced quality of life.

Context/Environment
- Family, caregivers, and educators may lack information about JIA and its management.
- Family, caregivers, and educators may lack access to community and internet resources.
- Family, caregivers, and educators may lack knowledge of and access to assistive devices and technology.
- Family, caregivers, and educators may lack knowledge about legal supports such as those in the Rehabilitation Act of 1973, Section 504, regulations for accommodations.

Intervention/Treatment
Models and programs developed by occupational therapy personnel include wrist splints (Sarsak, 2018). Models and programs developed by other professionals but used by occupational

therapy personnel include guidelines for foot care (Brosseau et al., 2016), guidelines for structured physical activity (Cavallo et al., 2017), telemedicine delivery (Warmington et al., 2017), and work participation (Codd et al., 2018). Team members include physicians, rheumatologists, ophthalmologists, social workers, educators, physical therapy personnel, and occupational therapy personnel. Goals are to assist client to perform and participate in everyday activities and occupations to the fullest extent possible (Ferdous, 2015).

Activities of Daily Living/Instrumental ADL
- Review daily ADL routine and make recommendations, such as bathing in the morning to reduce stiffness.
- Review and make recommendation for medication management.
- Consider if adapted devices may facilitate performance of ADL tasks.
- Consider if adapted equipment may facilitate mobility (walker, scooter, wheelchair).
- Footwear recommendation by Ottawa Panel (Brosseau et al., 2016).
  ▶ Custom-fitted preformed foot orthotics versus noncustomized leather board control.
  ▶ Custom-made semirigid orthotic versus prefabricated off-the-shelf shoe inserts.
  ▶ Custom-made semirigid orthotics versus new supportive athletic shoes.
  ▶ Prefabricated off-the-shelf shoe inserts versus new supportive athletic shoes.

Education/Work
- Consider if use of a computer with adapted software could improve academic performance.
- Recommend ways to improve access to and reduce barriers at school facilities.

Play/Leisure
- Recommend use of adapted toys.

Rest/Sleep
- See Sleep–Wake Disorders in Section 13: Lifestyle Conditions.

Social Participation
- Encourage participation in social activities within physical limitations.

Sensorimotor
- Aquatic aerobic fitness training: Recommended for long-term management of swollen and tender joints by Ottawa Panel (Cavallo et al., 2017).
- Energy conservation: Determine what actions and activities are essential and whether easier approaches can reduce fatigue, such as sitting for dressing.
- Exercise, structured: Pilates is recommended by Ottawa Panel; fatigue management: activity pacing of alternate rest and activity.
- Home program: Include strengthening, stretching, postural, and functional exercises by Ottawa Panel.
- Muscle strengthening: Therapeutic exercises designed to strengthen core muscle groups and maintain physical fitness.
- Pain management: Techniques to reduce pain and stiffness.
- Range of motion: Stretching exercise of hand and elbows.
- Splints/orthotic devices: Hand splints to maintain extension and prevent flexion contractures.

Cognitive/Perceptual
- Self-management: Assist client to learn to manage daily activity schedule.

Psychosocial
- Stress management: Coping strategies, relaxation training, deep breathing, yoga, mindfulness.

Context/Environment
- Provide information and training to family, caregivers, educators, and other professionals about JIA and management techniques.

- Provide information about access to community and internet resources.
- Provide information about accessibility recommendations including home modification and school and community accessibility available under the (Vocational) Rehabilitation Act, 1973, Section 504 regulations.

Precautions/Safety Considerations

Recommend referral to ophthalmologist if not already evaluated for eye infections (uveitis, iridocyclitis; Porter, 2018).

Prognosis and Outcome

Variable. JIA is a chronic disorder and may evolve into RA or may largely disappear during the adolescent years. Nonsteroidal anti-inflammatory drugs (NSAIDs) reduce symptoms of JIA but do not alter long-term joint disease or prevent complications (Porter, 2018). Children diagnosed at a younger age seem to show better psychosocial adjustment than those diagnosed at an older age (Toupin April et al., 2013). Caregiver financial status and psychological state as well as level of disease activity impacted child's health related quality of life (Toupin April et al., 2013). Adults who adapted to their level of physical function and strength, used assistive devices, adapted their environment, and continued to get support from others were able to maintain good health (Hammar & Håkansson, 2013).

REFERENCES

Brosseau, L., Toupin-April, K., Wells, G., Smith, C. A., Pugh, A. G., Stinson, J. N., Duffy, C. M., Gifford, W., Moher, D., Sherrington, C., Cavallo, S., De Angelis, G., Loew, L., Rahman, P., Marcotte, R., Taki, J., Bisaillon, J., King, J., Coda, A., . . . Bisch, M. (2016). Ottawa panel evidence-based clinical practice guidelines for foot care in the management of juvenile idiopathic arthritis. *Archives of Physical Medicine and Rehabilitation, 97*(7), 1163–1181. https://doi.org/10.1016/j.apmr.2015.11.011

Cavallo, S., Brosseau, L., Toupin-April, K., Wells, G. A., Smith, C. A., Pugh, A. G., Stinson, J., Thomas, R., Ahmed, S., Duffy, C. M., Rahman, P., Àlvarez-Gallardo, I. C., Loew, L., De Angelis, G., Feldman, D. E., Majnemer, A., Gagnon, I. J., Maltais, D., Mathieu, M.-E., Kenny, G. P., . . . Bigford, S. (2017). Ottawa panel evidence-based clinical practice guidelines for structured physical activity in the management of juvenile idiopathic arthritis. *Archives of Physical Medicine and Rehabilitation, 98*(5), 1018–1041. https://doi.org/10.1016/j.apmr.2016.09.135

Codd, Y., Stapleton, T., Kane, D., & Mullan, R. (2018). A survey to establish current practice in addressing work participation with inflammatory arthritis in the Irish clinical setting. *Musculoskeletal Care, 16*(1), 158–162. https://doi.org/10.1002/msc.1198

Ferdous, R. (2015, October). Juvenile rheumatoid arthritis and occupational therapy. *The Independent*. https://m.theindependentbd.com/printversion/details/19885

Hammar, I. O., & Håkansson, C. (2013). The importance for daily occupations of perceiving good health: Perceptions among women with rheumatic diseases. *Scandinavian Journal of Occupational Therapy, 20*(2), 82–92. https://doi.org/10.3109/11038128.2012.699978

O'Toole, M. T. (Ed.). (2017). *Mosby's dictionary of medicine, nursing & health professions* (10th ed.). Elsevier.

Porter, R. S. (Ed.). (2018). *The Merck manual of diagnosis and therapy* (20th ed.). Merck Sharp & Dohme.

Rehabilitation Act of 1973, 29 U.S.C. § 701 *et seq.*

Sarsak, H. I. (2018). Effectiveness of rigid wrist splints on reducing pain and improving hand function in patients with inflammatory arthritis. *Researches in Arthritis & Bone Study, 1*(3), 1–4.

Toupin April, K., Cavallo, S., & Feldman, D. E. (2013). Children with juvenile idiopathic arthritis: Are health outcomes better for those diagnosed younger? *Child: Care, Health and Development, 39*(3), 442–448. https://doi.org/10.1111/j.1365-2214.2012.01386.x

Toupin April, K., Higgins, J., & Feldman, D. E. (2016). Application of Rasch analysis to the parent adherence report questionnaire in juvenile idiopathic arthritis. *Pediatric Rheumatology, 14*(1), Article 45. https://doi.org/10.1186/s12969-016-0105-5

Warmington, K., Flewelling, C., Kennedy, C. A., Shupak, R., Papachristos, A., Jones, C., Linton, D., Beaton, D. E., & Lineker, S. (2017). Telemedicine delivery of patient education in remote Ontario communities: Feasibility of an Advanced Clinician Practitioner in Arthritis Care (ACPAC)-led inflammatory arthritis education program. *Open Access Rheumatology: Research and Reviews, 2017*(9), 11–19. https://doi.org/10.2147/OARRR.S122015

BIBLIOGRAPHY

Cavallo, S., Majnemer, A., Duffy, C. M., & Feldman, D. E. (2015). Participation in leisure activities by children and adolescents with juvenile idiopathic arthritis. *Journal of Rheumatology, 42*(9), 1708–1715. https://doi.org/10.3899/jrheum.140844

Cavallo, S., Toupin April, K., Grandpierre, V., Majnemer, A., & Feldman, D. E. (2014). Leisure in children and adolescents with juvenile idiopathic arthritis: A systematic review. *PLOS ONE, 9*(10), Article 3104642. https://doi.org/10.1371/journal.pone.0104642

Hackett, J., & Johnson, B. (2010). Physiotherapy and occupational therapy for children and young people with juvenile idiopathic arthritis. In K. Dziedzic & A. Hammond (Eds.), *Rheumatology: Evidence-based practice for physiotherapists and occupational therapists* (pp. 323–335). Churchill Livingstone.

Morgan, E. M., Munro, J. E., Horonjeff, J., Horgan, B., Shea, B., Feldman, B. M., Clairman, H., Bingham, C. O., III, Thornhill, S., Strand, V., Alongi, A., Magni-Manzoni, S., van Rossum, M. A. J., Vesely, R., Vojinovic, J., Brunner, H. I., Harris, J. G., Horton, D. B., Lovell, D. J., . . . Consolaro, A. (2019). Establishing an updated core domain set for studies in juvenile idiopathic arthritis: A report from the OMERACT 2018 JIA workshop. *Journal of Rheumatology, 46*(8), 1006–1013. https://doi.org/10.3899/jrheum.181088

Smith, C. A., Toupin April, K., Jutai, J. W., Duffy, C. M., Rahman, P., Cavallo, S., & Brosseau, L. (2015). A systematic critical appraisal of clinical practice guidelines in juvenile idiopathic arthritis using the Appraisal of Guidelines for Research and Evaluation II (AGREE II) instrument. *PLOS ONE, 10*(9), Article e0137180. https://doi.org/10.1371/journal.pone.0137180

Toupin April, K., Cavallo, S., & Feldman, D. E. (2013). Children with juvenile idiopathic arthritis: Are health outcomes better for those diagnosed younger? *Child: Care, Health and Development, 39*(3), 442–448. https://doi.org/10.1111/j.1365-2214.2012.01386.x

Musculoskeletal Conditions

Description

The musculoskeletal system is composed of all muscles, bones, joints, tendons, and connective tissues that function in the movement of body parts and organs (O'Toole, 2017). Musculoskeletal conditions include fractures, joint dislocations, ligament sprains, muscle strains, and tendon injuries to the extremities, spine, and pelvis (Porter, 2018). Musculoskeletal conditions result in the highest rate of inability to work and decline in the independent performance of activities of daily living (Roll, 2017). However, the outcome of the original trauma is influenced by personal, social, economic, and environmental factors that may not be related directly to the extent or degree of the original trauma or its source.

Cause

The most common cause of a musculoskeletal condition is trauma or an existing musculoskeletal disorder (Porter, 2018). Common sites of injuries are hand, wrist, shoulder, cervical spine, lumbar spine, and knee (Hardison & Roll, 2017). The trauma or injury may occur at home, work site, educational institution, leisure venue, or community at large. Existing disorders may include rheumatoid arthritis, osteoarthritis, fibromyalgia, psoriatic arthritis, and arthroplasty.

Evaluation/Assessment

Areas

- Activities of Daily Living/Instrumental ADL: basic ADLs, instrumental ADLs
- Education/Work: academic tasks, job/work tasks, work environment (physical and social)
- Play/Leisure: interests, frequency, location
- Rest/Sleep: sleep habits and routines
- Social Participation: type, frequency. location, with whom
- Sensorimotor: muscle strength, range of motion (flexibility), endurance/fitness, hand functions (grip, grasp, dexterity, coordination), body mechanics, and posture
- Cognitive/Perceptual: attention, memory, executive functions
- Psychosocial: depression, anxiety, sense of self-efficacy, role performance, social interaction skills
- Context/Environment: knowledge and information resources, social support, ergonomic design, assistive technology, environmental barriers
- Comorbidities: existing musculoskeletal disorders, lifestyle choices

Instruments

Instruments Developed by Occupational Therapy Personnel

- AOTA occupational profile template (AOTA, 2020)
- Canadian Occupational Performance Measure (5th ed.; COPM-5; Law et al., 2014)
- Evaluation of Daily Activity Questionnaire (EDAQ; Hammond et al., 2018, and Hammond et al., 2015, in References)
- Performance Assessment of Self-Care Skills (Version 4.1, Home Edition; PASS 4.1; Chisholm et al., 2016)
- Work Environment Impact Scale (WEIS; Moore-Corner et al., 1998)

Instruments Developed by Other Professionals and Used by Occupational Therapy Personnel

- Musculoskeletal Discomfort Questionnaire (MDQ; Wiehagen & Turin, 2004)
- Psychiatric Symptoms Index (PSI; Ilfeld, 1976)
- Rapid Upper Limb Assessment (RULA; McAtamney & Corlett, 1993)
- Work-Related Upper Extremity and Low Back Musculoskeletal Disorders Questionnaire (Kuorinka et al., 1987)

Problems/Issues

Activities of Daily Living/Instrumental ADL

- Person may be unable to perform or have difficulty performing basic ADL tasks (eating, dressing, bathing, showering, toileting, transfers).
- Person may be unable to perform or have difficulty performing IADL tasks such as meal preparation, housekeeping, laundry, driving, shopping, child care, pet care.

Education/Work

- Person may be unable to perform or have difficulty performing job/work tasks.
- Person may be absent from work due to musculoskeletal issues or may have been dismissed due to excess absence.
- Person may have difficulty meeting productivity standards (rate or pace of work).

Play/Leisure

- Person may have stopped or limited engagement in favorite leisure occupations.

Rest/Sleep

- Person may have difficulty falling asleep or staying asleep due to pain or stiffness.

Social Participation

- Person may have stopped, limited, reduced, or restricted participation in social activities.

Sensorimotor

- Person may experience decreased flexibility and range of motion.
- Person may experience loss of or decreased muscle strength.
- Person may have reduced or limited endurance and cardiovascular fitness.
- Person may have loss of or reduced hand functions (grip, grasp, dexterity, manipulation, coordination).
- Person may experience activity limitations.
- Person may experience pain and discomfort due to poor work-related posture and body mechanics (Akodu et al., 2015).

Cognitive/Perceptual

- Person may have difficulty problem solving, planning ahead, or using time scheduling effectively. (Note: Cognitive problems are not directly a result of the musculoskeletal condition, but may require consideration in intervention planning and implementation.)

Psychosocial

- Person may experience depressive symptoms.
- Person may become anxious or fearful as to what will happen in the future.
- Person may become angry or aggressive.
- Person may experience thoughts of suicide.

Context/Environment

- Person may lack knowledge or understanding of the injury or disorder.
- Person and family may lack knowledge of available resources.
- Person may be unable to take advantage of available resources due to accessibility limitations (financial, lack of transportation, physical barriers).

Intervention/Treatment

Models and programs developed by occupational therapy personnel include general occupational rehabilitation (Hardison & Roll, 2017) and recycling workers (Fisher, 2017). Models and programs developed by other professionals but used by occupational therapy personnel include comprehensive occupational rehabilitation (Hardison & Roll, 2017), Karasek's job strain model (Gilbert-Ouimet et al., 2011), motivational interviewing (Park et al., 2018), and Siegrist effort-reward imbalance (ERI) model (Gilbert-Ouimet et al., 2011). Team members include physicians, physiatrists, psychologists, nursing personnel, dieticians, case managers, vocational rehabilitation counselors, physical therapy personnel, and occupational therapy personnel. Goals are to enable client to participate and function in everyday life to the maximum degree possible, including home, work, and community, using both restorative/remedial and compensatory/adaptive approaches.

Activities of Daily Living/Instrumental ADL

- Functional mobility: provide retraining on bed mobility and safe transfers.
- ADL retraining: provide suggestions such as sitting for dressing activities, using beside commode to reduce nighttime trips to bathroom.

Education/Work

- Simulated work tasks: grade in level of difficulty, number of steps, amount of time, hand functions required, speed/rate of completion.
- Work conditioning: amount of light or noise, indoors versus outdoors, temperature control, number of fellow workers.
- Work hardening: physical requirements, time, frequency, speed.

Play/Leisure
- Not addressed directly although many of the same concepts addressed under Education/Work can be applied to leisure occupations.

Rest/Sleep
- See Sleep–Wake Disorders in Section 13: Lifestyle Conditions.

Social Participation
- Not addressed directly.

Sensorimotor
Focus on duration or length of time, number of repetitions and frequency (times per unit of time) of an activity/task/occupation.
- Range of motion/whole body flexibility: therapeutic exercises and activities focused on movement of body segments and body as a whole.
- Endurance training/cardiovascular fitness: therapeutic exercises and activities focused on increasing duration and frequency of actions.
- Muscle strengthening: therapeutic exercises and activities focused on graded resistive activities to specific muscle groups.
- Core stability exercises: therapeutic exercises and activities focused on increasing balance and trunk stabilizing.
- Pain management: activity pacing, medication scheduling.

Cognitive/Perceptual
- Assist client with problem solving, prioritizing, and time management.

Psychosocial
- Stress management: relaxation training, yoga, mindfulness.
- Anxiety/fear management: discuss with client nature of anxiety or fear and assist client to address concerns with information and action plan.
- Focus group: assist client in a group situation to identify themes and subthemes, and then set priorities for intervention individually or in group.

Context/Environment
- Client and family education: information about musculoskeletal conditions and available resources.
- Environmental accessibility: work-site modification, legal remedies.
- Employer and supervisor education: provide employer and supervisors with information about musculoskeletal conditions and ways work setting and work conditions can be changed to minimize or reduce injury or disability in the work environment.

Precautions/Safety Considerations

Person is at risk for loss of function if musculoskeletal conditions are not addressed and remediation neglected.

Prognosis and Outcome

Variable, depending on the musculoskeletal condition and client's interest and investment in occupational performance.

REFERENCES

Akodu, A., Akinefeleye, A., Atanda, L., & Giwa, S. (2015). Work-related musculoskeletal disorders of the upper extremity with reference to working posture of secretaries. *South African Journal of Occupational Therapy, 45*(3), 16–22. https://doi.org/10.17159/2310-3833/2015/v45n3/a4

Fisher, T. (2017). Role of occupational therapy in preventing work-related musculoskeletal disorders with recycling workers: A pilot study. *American Journal of Occupational Therapy, 71*(1), Article 7101190030. https://doi.org/10.5014/ajot.2017.022871

Gilbert-Ouimet, M., Brisson, C., Vézina, M., Trudel, L., Bourbonnais, R., Masse, B., Baril-Gingras, G., & Dionne, C. E. (2011). Intervention study on psychosocial work factors and mental health and musculoskeletal outcomes. *Healthcare Papers, 11*(SP), 47–66. https://doi.org/10.12927/hcpap.2011.22410

Hammond, A., Prior, Y., Horton, M. C., Tennant, A., & Tyson, S. (2018). The psychometric properties of the Evaluation of Daily Activity Questionnaire in seven musculoskeletal conditions. *Disability and Rehabilitation, 40*(17), 2070–2080. https://doi.org/10.1080/09638288.2017.1323027

Hammond, A., Prior, Y., Tennant, A., Tyson, S., & Nordenskiold, U. (2015). The content validity and acceptability of the Evaluation of Daily Activity Questionnaire in musculoskeletal conditions. *British Journal of Occupational Therapy, 78*(3), 144–157. https://doi.org/10.1177/0308022615571117

Hardison, M. E., & Roll, S. C. (2017). Factors associated with success in an occupational rehabilitation program for work-related musculoskeletal disorders. *American Journal of Occupational Therapy, 71*(1), Article 7201190040. https://doi.org/10.5014/ajot.2016.023200

O'Toole, M. T. (Ed.). (2017). *Mosby's dictionary of medicine, nursing & health professions* (10th ed.). Elsevier.

Park, J., Esmail, S., Rayani, F., Norris, C. M., & Gross, D. P. (2018). Motivational interviewing for workers with disabling musculoskeletal disorders: Results of a cluster randomized control trial. *Journal of Occupational Rehabilitation, 28*(2), 252–264. https://doi.org/10.1007/s10926-017-9712-3

Porter, R. S. (Ed.). (2018). *The Merck manual of diagnosis and therapy* (20th ed.). Merck Sharp & Dohme.

Roll, S. C. (2017). Current evidence and opportunities for expanding the role of occupational therapy for adults with musculoskeletal conditions. *American Journal of Occupational Therapy, 71*(1), Article 7101170010. https://doi.org/10.5014/ajot.2017.711002

BIBLIOGRAPHY

Amini, D., Lieberman, D., & Hunter, E. (2018). Occupational therapy interventions for adults with musculoskeletal conditions. *American Journal of Occupational Therapy, 72*(4), Article 7204380010. https://doi.org/10.5014/ajot.2018.724001

Babatunde, F., MacDermid, J., & MacIntyre, N. (2017). Characteristics of therapeutic alliance in musculoskeletal physiotherapy and occupational therapy practice: A scoping review of the literature. *BMC Health Services Research 17*, Article 375. https://doi.org/10.1186/s12913-017-2311-3

Dorsey, J., & Bradshaw, M. (2017). Effectiveness of occupational therapy interventions for lower-extremity musculoskeletal disorders: A systematic review. *American Journal of Occupational Therapy, 71*(1), Article 7101180030. https://doi.org/10.5014/ajot.2017.023028

Marik, T. L., & Roll, S. C. (2017). Effectiveness of occupational therapy interventions for musculoskeletal shoulder conditions: A systematic review. *American Journal of Occupational Therapy, 71*(1), Article 7101180020. https://doi.org/10.5014/ajot.2017.023127

Murad, M. S., O'Brien, L., Farnworth, L., & Chien, C.-W. (2013). Health status of people with work-related musculoskeletal disorders in return to work programs: A Malaysian study. *Occupational Therapy in Health Care, 27*(3), 238–255.

Smith, P., Bielecky, A., Ibrahim, S., Mustard, C., Saunders, R., Beaton, D., Koehoorn, M., McLeod, C., Scott-Marshall, H., & Hogg-Johnson, S. (2014). Impact of pre-existing chronic conditions on age differences in sickness absence after a musculoskeletal work injury: A path analysis approach. *Scandinavian Journal of Work Environment & Health, 40*(2), 167–175. https://doi.org/10.5271/sjweh.3397

Myotonic Dystrophy

*Also called DM1, myotonic muscular dystrophy,
myotonia atrophica, Steinert's disease.*

Description

Myotonic dystrophy (DM1) is a hereditary disease with multisystemic and progressive involvement (Raymond et al., 2016). Inheritance is autosomal dominant with variable degrees of penetrance; thus, signs and symptoms may vary widely from one individual to the next, even among members of the same family (Porter, 2018). Weakness usually begins distal and progresses proximally, thus weakness of the fingers, hands, and feet precedes that in the shoulders and hips (O'Toole, 2017). Myotonia refers to delayed relaxation after muscle contraction (Porter, 2018). Muscle weakness may occur in both striated and smooth muscles (Gagnon, 2015). Four forms of DM1 can be described based on age at onset, clinical symptoms, and trinucleotide (CTG) expansion: congenital, childhood, classic adult, and mild adult (Aldehag et al., 2013). This chapter focuses primarily on the adult forms, although some assessments and interventions could be applied to children and adolescents.

Cause

Unstable expansion of a trinucleotide (CTG) repeat on chromosome 19 (Aldehag et al., 2013).

Evaluation/Assessment

Areas

- Activities of Daily Living/Instrumental ADL: basic ADLs, including eating, dysphagia (swallowing), dressing, bathing/showering, toileting, grooming; IADLs, including meal preparation, housekeeping, laundry, shopping, driving
- Education/Work: academic achievement, employment history
- Play/Leisure: interests, values, frequency, location
- Rest/Sleep: sleep habits and routines, excessive daytime sleepiness
- Social Participation: types, frequency, location, with whom
- Sensorimotor: muscle strength, dexterity, coordination
- Cognitive/Perceptual: attention, memory, executive functions
- Psychosocial: apathy, level of motivation, quality of life, role performance, interpersonal relationships, stress, and coping
- Context/Environment: social support, resources, assistive devices and equipment, accessibility
- Comorbidities: cardiovascular disease, respiratory dysfunction

Instruments

Instruments Developed by Occupational Therapy Personnel

- Assessment of Motor and Process Skills (8th ed.; AMPS-8; Fisher & Bray Jones, 2016)
- Canadian Occupational Performance Measure (5th ed.; COPM-5; Law et al., 2014)
- Impact on Participation and Autonomy (IPA; Cardol et al., 1999)
- Late Life Function and Disability Instruction (Late Life FDI; Jette et al., 2002)
- Perceived Limitations in Activities and Needs Questionnaire (PLAN-Q; Pieterse et al., 2008a, 2008b)

Instruments Developed by Other Professionals and Used by Occupational Therapy Personnel

- Assessment of Life Habits, 3.1 (LIFE-H 3.1; Fourgeyrollas & Noreau, 2005)
- Muscle strength (dynamometer; JAMAR, Lafayette Instrument; Grippit sold in Europe)
- Muscular Impairment Rating Scale (MIRS; Mathieu et al., 2001)
- Purdue Pegboard Test (PPT; Tiffin, 1948)

Problems/Issues

Activities of Daily Living/Instrumental ADL
- Person may experience difficulty performing basic ADLs, including eating, dressing, bathing, showering, toileting.
- Person may experience difficulty performing IADLs, including shopping, doing household chores, driving.

Education/Work
- Person may be unable to attend educational institutions due to factors such as muscle weakness, pain, fatigue, loss of interest, absenteeism, and lack of accessibility.
- Person may be unable to continue working due to factors such as muscle weakness, pain, fatigue, excessive daytime sleepiness, absenteeism, or lack of accessibility.

Play/Leisure
- Person may be unable to engage in favorite leisure occupations due to factors such as decreased muscle strength, pain, fatigue, loss of interest, or lack of accessibility.

Rest/Sleep
- Person may experience excessive daytime sleepiness.

Social Participation
- Person may decrease or stop participation in social activities with friends or in community activities, such as singing in a choir.

Sensorimotor
- Person usually experiences muscle weakness and atrophy in the upper and lower extremities starting with hands and feet and progressing toward shoulder and hip.
- Person is at risk for falls due to muscle weakness in lower extremities.
- Person usually reports fatigue.
- Person usually experiences facial muscle weakness, including ptosis (drooping eyelids).
- Person may experience weakness in the muscles of the respiratory system.
- Person may experience cardiomyopathy including arrhythmias.
- Person may develop cataracts in the eyes.
- Person may experience pain.

Cognitive/Perceptual
- Person may have limited selective attention.
- Person usually experiences executive function impairment, especially loss of initiative.
- Person may experience executive dysfunction in making choices and participating in making decisions.
- Person may demonstrate cognitive dysfunction in memory, including loss of previously acquired or learned information or how to apply the knowledge to everyday activities.

Psychosocial
- Person may have avoidant personality traits.
- Person may stop performing or limit performance in previously held roles such as meal preparation or shopping.

Context/Environment
- Person may have lifestyle issues such as being overweight or obese, smoking, and being physically inactive.
- Person and family may have limited health literacy about the disease even though the disorder has occurred in the family for generations.
- Person and family may have limited knowledge of internet and community resources.

- Person may experience architectural and environmental barriers, including need for home modifications, resulting in decreased accessibility to home, school, employment, and community resources.
- Family or caregivers may need to assume more responsibility for role and task performance previously done by person, such as shopping for groceries.

Intervention/Treatment

Models and programs developed by occupational therapy personnel include the hand-training program (Aldehag et al., 2013). Models and programs developed by other professionals but used by occupational therapy personnel include disability creation process (Gagnon, 2015) and Stanford Chronic Disease Self-Management Program (Raymond et al., 2016). Team members include physicians, neurologists, psychologists, physical therapy personnel, speech–language pathologists, and occupational therapy personnel. Goals are to help the client improve or maintain occupational performance needed to live as independently as possible and to enable participation in occupations that give meaning and purpose to the client's life (Gagnon, 2015).

Activities of Daily Living/Instrumental ADL

- Assist client in occupational performance of daily activities (eating, dressing, grooming, bathing/showering, toileting, and general mobility) including use of adapted techniques, assistive technology, and home modification for better accessibility.
- For dysphasia, see Swallowing Disorders: Adult in Section 3: Nervous System Disorders.
- Assist client and family to determine which IADL tasks will be performed by whom, including shared tasks such as meal preparation, household tasks, yard work, driving, and shopping.
- Assist client to determine level of safe driving habits or whether driving should be discontinued.

Education/Work

- Work with educational institutions to identify ways clients can continue studies.
- Work with employers to identify ways to assist clients to continue employment in an accessible and safe environment.

Play/Leisure

- Assist client to continue enjoying leisure occupations with adaptations as needed.
- Assist client to explore new leisure occupations that are within client's level of function.

Rest/Sleep

- See Sleep–Wake Disorders in Section 13: Lifestyle Conditions.

Social Participation

- Assist client to continue participation in social activities with modifications, such as passive versus active, shorter time periods, small groups, at familiar locations, or use of communication aids and devices, including computers.

Sensorimotor

- Provide resistive exercises to maintain or increase muscle strength.
- Provide instruction in fatigue management, including energy conservation and work simplification techniques.

Cognitive/Perceptual

- Assist client to develop and follow a time-management program based on doing important tasks at time when energy level is at its best.
- Assist client to use activity pacing with cycles of work and rest.

Psychosocial

- Assist client to continue role performance including shared responsibility.

Context/Environment

- Recommend client assistive devices that may be useful, such as commode chairs, shower benches, beds and chairs that assist person to stand up, mobile arm supports, walkers, and wheelchairs.
- Recommend orthotic devices to support weak muscles including slings, splints, or braces for wrists, arms, ankles, and shoulders to improve function.
- Recommend corset or body jacket to provide better support and balance to the spine if client is at risk for scoliosis.
- Recommend home modification and assistive technology to improve quality of life.
- Recommend available internet and community resources.
- Assist client or family members to determine if outside caregiver, domestic help, or contracted services are needed to maintain person in the home and keep the home in good working order and repair.
- Assist family members or caregivers to perform roles previously performed by client.
- Collaborate with other health care professionals to create and implement program specific to the client's needs and level of function.

Precautions/Safety Considerations

Visual loss due to cataracts, increased cognitive dysfunction, falls due to muscle weakness, and loss of fine motor skills (Porter, 2018).

Prognosis and Outcome

DM1 is a chronic disorder with no known cure. Death is most commonly due to respiratory and cardiac disease. Clients who develop cardiac arrhythmias and severe muscle weakness earlier in life are at increased risk of premature death (Porter, 2018). Caregiver burden increases as disease progresses requiring caregiver to provide more directions and use more reminders to compensate for decreased initiative and lack of motivation (Cup et al., 2011). Mean age at death is 54 years (Porter, 2018).

REFERENCES

Aldehag, A., Jonsson, H., Lindblad, J., Kottorp, A., Ansved, T., & Kierkegaard, M. (2013). Effects of hand-training in persons with myotonic dystrophy type 1—A randomised controlled cross-over pilot study. *Disability and Rehabilitation, 35*(21), 1798–1807. https://doi.org/10.3109/09638288.2012.754952

Cup, E. H. C., Kinébanian, A., Satink, T., Pieterse, A. J., Hendricks, H. T., Oostendorp, R. A. B., van der Wilt, G. J., & van Engelen, B. G. M. (2011). Living with myotonic dystrophy; what can be learned from couples? A qualitative study. *BMC Neurology, 11*, Article 86. https://doi.org/10.1186/1471-2377-11-86

Gagnon, C. (2015). Occupational therapy suggestions for the management of a myotonic dystrophy patient. In *Myotonic Dystrophy Foundation toolkit* (pp. 81–90). Myotonic Dystrophy Foundation. https://www.myotonic.org/sites/default/files/pages/files/MDF-Occupational-TherapyGuidelines2_21.pdf

O'Toole, M. T. (Ed.). (2017). *Mosby's dictionary of medicine, nursing & health professions* (10th ed.). Elsevier.

Porter, R. S. (Ed.). (2018). *The Merck manual of diagnosis and therapy* (20th ed.). Merck Sharp & Dohme.

Raymond, K., Lavasseur, M., Chouinard, M.-C., Mathieu, J., & Gagnon, C. (2016). Stanford Chronic Disease Self-Management Program in myotonic dystrophy: New opportunities for occupational therapists. *Canadian Journal of Occupational Therapy, 83*(3), 166–176. https://doi.org/10.1177/0008417416646130

Osteoarthritis of the Hip and Knee

Also called OA, degenerative joint disease, osteoarthrosis, hypertrophic osteoarthritis.

Description

Osteoarthritis is a chronic joint disease (arthropathy) characterized by disruption and potential loss of joint cartilage along with other changes, including bone hypertrophy, that may occur in any joint in the body. The disease is more common in men than women beginning in the ages of 40 to 50 years (O'Toole, 2017; Porter, 2018). Major problem area is physical limitation (Klokker, Osborne, et al., 2015).

Cause

Early onset osteoarthritis is usually caused by trauma, but the cause of most osteoarthritis is unknown. Factors include chemical, mechanical, genetic, metabolic, endocrine, and emotional stress (O'Toole, 2017).

Evaluation/Assessment

Areas

- Activities of Daily Living/Instrumental ADL: self-maintenance activities, functional mobility (sit to stand, bed mobility, transfers, standing, ambulation, wheelchair or scooter mobility)
- Education/Work: work tasks, work site modification
- Play/Leisure: interests, frequency
- Rest/Sleep: sleep disturbance
- Social Participation: type, frequency, location, with whom
- Sensorimotor: muscle strength, joint range of motion, endurance and activity tolerance, balance, contractures, proprioception, pain
- Cognitive/Perceptual: not specifically involved; consider whether comorbidity of cognitive impairment exists
- Psychosocial: depression, role performance, quality of life, self-efficacy
- Context/Environment: adapted equipment, home modification, community resources
- Comorbidities: obesity, sarcopenia, cardiovascular disease

Instruments

Instruments Developed by Occupational Therapy Personnel

- Dynamic weight-bearing Assessment of Pain (DAP; Klokker, Christensen, et al., 2015, in References)
- Social Role Participation Questionnaire (SRPQ; Gignac et al., 2008)

Instruments Developed by Other Professionals and Used by Occupational Therapy Personnel

- Brief Fatigue Inventory (BFI; Mendoza et al., 1999)
- Brief Pain Inventory (BPI; Keller et al., 2004)
- Composite Indian Functional Knee Assessment Scale (CIFKAS; see Batra et al., 2010, in References)
- Western Ontario and McMaster Universities Osteoarthritis Index (WOMAC; Bellamy et al., 2010)

Problems/Issues

Activities of Daily Living/Instrumental ADL

- Person may have difficulty dressing lower extremity.
- Person may have difficulty with functional mobility (bed mobility, transfers, standing, walking, climbing stairs).

Education/Work

- Person may have difficulty getting to workstation (transportation, architectural barriers).
- Person may have difficulty performing work tasks that require standing, frequent changes from sitting to standing or sitting to walking.
- Person may have difficulty performing changes in balance and position, such as climbing stairs, climbing ladders, walking on hills, stooping, or bending over.

Play/Leisure

- Person may have difficulty playing sports or games requiring movement and agility.

Rest/Sleep

- Person may have sleep disturbances due to difficulty moving in bed or pain.

Social Participation

- Person may limit or stop participation in social activities that require movements, such as standing for long periods of time, climbing steps or hills, or walking long distances.

Sensorimotor

- Person may have limited range of motion in lower extremity.
- Person may have reduced or weak muscle strength in lower extremity.
- Person may have reduced endurance and activity tolerance.
- Person may have impaired balance reactions.
- Person may have joint stiffness.
- Person may experience difficulty changing body positions from sit to stand, stand to walk.
- Person may have soft tissue or joint contractures.
- Person may experience pain.

Cognitive/Perceptual

- Not directly affected.

Psychosocial

- Person may become depressed or withdrawn.
- Person may experience reduced quality of life.
- Person may experience changes in role functions.

Context/Environment

- Person may need adapted equipment.
- Person may need information about disease and disease progression.
- Person may lack knowledge about available community or internet resources.

Intervention/Treatment

Models and programs developed by occupational therapy personnel include cognitive-behavioral therapy (Murphy et al., 2018) and proprioceptive retraining technique (Batra et al., 2010). Models and programs developed by other professionals but used by occupational therapy personnel include aerobic exercise programs (Brosseau et al., 2017c), exercise program (Al-Khlaifat, Herrington, Hammond, et al., 2016; Al-Khlaifat, Herrington, Tyson, et al., 2016), mind–body exercise programs (Brosseau et al., 2017a), OA Go Away (Paterson et al., 2016), strengthening exercise programs (Brosseau et al., 2017b), and therapeutic exercise (Brosseau et al., 2016). Team members include general physicians, rheumatologists, psychologists, physical therapists, and occupational therapy personnel. Goals include training in safe and efficient functional mobility, maintaining muscle strength, physical endurance, and joint mobility and flexibility.

Activities of Daily Living/Instrumental ADL

- Instruction on modification of dressing techniques: sit to dress lower extremity until both feet can be used for balance (pull up pants over buttocks), lean against a wall or corner of two walls for added balance, hold onto a sturdy chair or dresser for added balance.

- Advise client on use of footwear that provides support and balance.
- Recommend use of carts for carrying loads, carrying loads close to body, carrying loads balanced on two sides of body.
- Recommend modifying kitchen so items frequently used are within reach that reduces need to bend, stoop, reach overhead, or climb.
- Instruct or review with client nutrition program including meal planning and preparation designed to control weight.

Education/Work
- Recommend modifying workstation so items frequently used are within reach that reduces need to bend, stoop, reach over head, or climb.
- Recommend modifying workplace demands to reduce need to stand for long periods of time or walk long distances (use a stool to sit, riding cart for distances).

Play/Leisure
- Consider if riding more and walking less would be helpful (playing golf, hiking).
- Consider if changing role would permit continuing participation (scorekeeper versus active player).

Rest/Sleep
- Consider whether changing bedding to silk sheets would be helpful to improve bed mobility.
- Consider whether changing mattress to a firmer or softer pile would improve sleep.

Social Participation
- Encourage social participation with modifications such as shorter outings, using a scooter for longer distances, sitting rather than standing.

Sensorimotor
- Therapeutic exercise: assist client to develop an individualized exercise program in consultation with physician and physical therapist.
- Strengthening muscles: sustained isometric exercise for both legs including quadriceps and proximal hip girdle muscles.
- Range of motion: stretching exercises/activities.
- Activity pacing: alternate cycles of rest and activity.
- Pain management programs: problem solving, coping strategies, goal setting.

Cognitive/Perceptual
- Self-management: person should learn to manage weight, nutritional needs, amount (dose) of daily physical activity.
- Assist in cognitive behavioral therapy.

Psychosocial
- Stress management: relaxation training, yoga, tai chi, mindfulness, coping strategies.

Context/Environment
- Educate client including family, partners, and caregivers about managing osteoarthritis of lower extremity and progression of disorder.
- Provide information and recommendations regarding assistive devices and walking aids.
- Provide review of home and work environments for safety (lighting, floor surfaces, stairs, railings, furniture placement).
- Provide information and recommendations for home and work modifications to reduce architectural and environmental barriers.

Precautions/Safety Considerations

Person is at risk for falls. Lifting, cumulative physical loads, full-body vibration, and kneeling/squatting/bending are risk factors for developing osteoarthritis in both men and women (Gignac et al., 2020).

Prognosis and Outcome

Condition is chronic and usually gradually gets worse. Hip or knee replacement, or both, may be needed.

REFERENCES

Al-Khlaifat, L., Herrington, L. C., Hammond, A., Tyson, S. F., & Jones, R. K. (2016). The effectiveness of an exercise programme on knee loading, muscle co-contraction, and pain in patients with medial knee osteoarthritis: A pilot study. *The Knee, 23*(1), 63–69. https://doi .org/10.1016/j.knee.2015.03.014

Al-Khlaifat, L., Herrington, L. C., Tyson, S. F., Hammond, A., & Jones, R. K. (2016). The effectiveness of an exercise programme on dynamic balance in patients with medial knee osteoarthritis: A pilot study. *The Knee, 23*(5), 849–856. https://doi.org/10.1016/j.knee.2016.05.006

Batra, V., Batra, M., Sharma, V. P., Agarwal, G. G., & Sharma, V. (2010). Context specific proprioceptive retraining technique and its implication on functional disability status in early knee osteoarthritis. *Indian Journal of Occupational Therapy, 42*(3), 13–22.

Brosseau, L., Taki, J., Desjardins, B., Thevenot, O., Fransen, M., Wells, G. A., Imoto, A. M., Toupin-April, K., Westby, M., Álvarez Gallardo, I. C., Gifford, W., Laferrière, L., Rahman, P., Loew, L., De Angelis, G., Cavallo, S., Shallwani, S. M., Aburub, A., Bennell, K. L., . . . McLean, L. (2017a). The Ottawa panel clinical practice guidelines for the management of knee osteoarthritis. Part one: Introduction, and mind–body exercise programs. *Clinical Rehabilitation, 31*(5), 582–595. https://doi.org/10.1177/0269215517691083

Brosseau, L., Taki, J., Desjardins, B., Thevenot, O., Fransen, M., Wells, G. A., Imoto, A. M., Toupin-April, K., Westby, M., Álvarez Gallardo, I. C., Gifford, W., Laferrière, L., Rahman, P., Loew, L., De Angelis, G., Cavallo, S., Shallwani, S. M., Aburub, A., Bennell, K. L., . . . McLean, L. (2017b). The Ottawa panel clinical practice guidelines for the management of knee osteoarthritis. Part two: Strengthening exercise programs. *Clinical Rehabilitation, 31*(5), 596–611. https:// doi.org/10.1177/0269215517691084

Brosseau, L., Taki, J., Desjardins, B., Thevenot, O., Fransen, M., Wells, G. A., Imoto, A. M., Toupin-April, K., Westby, M., Álvarez Gallardo, I. C., Gifford, W., Laferrière, L., Rahman, P., Loew, L., De Angelis, G., Cavallo, S., Shallwani, S. M., Aburub, A., Bennell, K. L., . . . McLean, L. (2017c). The Ottawa Panel clinical practice guidelines for the management of knee osteoarthritis. Part three: Aerobic exercise programs. *Clinical Rehabilitation, 31*(5), 612–624. https://doi .org/10.1177/0269215517691085

Brosseau, L., Wells, G. A., Pugh, A. G., Smith, C. A., Rahman, P., Alvarez Gallardo, I. C., Toupin-April, K., Loew, L., De Angelis, G., Cavallo, S., Taki, J., Marcotte, R., Fransen, M., Hernandez-Molina, G., Kenny, G. P., Regnaux, J.-P., Lefevre-Colau, M.-M., Brooks, S., Laferriere, L., . . . Longchamp, G. (2016). Ottawa panel evidence-based clinical practice guidelines for therapeutic exercise in the management of hip osteoarthritis. *Clinical Rehabilitation, 30*(10), 935–946. https://doi.org/10.1177/0269215515606198

Gignac, M. A. M., Irvin, E., Cullen, K., Van Eerd, D., Beaton, D. E., Mahood, Q., McLeod, C., & Backman, C. L. (2020). Men and women's occupational activities and the risk of developing osteoarthritis of the knee, hip, or hands: A systematic review and recommendations for future research. *Arthritis Care and Research, 72*(3), 378–396. https://doi.org/10.1002/ acr.23855

Klokker, L., Christensen, R., Osborne, R., Ginnerup E., Wæhrens, E. E., Bliddal, H., & Henriksen, M. (2015). Dynamic weight-bearing assessment of pain in knee osteoarthritis: A reliability and agreement study. *Quality of Life Research, 24*(12), 2985–2992. https://doi.org/10.1007/ s11136-015-1025-4

Klokker, L., Osborne, R., Wæhrens, E. E., Norgaard, O., Bandak, E. Bliddal, H., & Henriksen, M. (2015). The concept of physical limitations in knee osteoarthritis: As viewed by patients and health professionals. *Quality of Life Research, 24*(10), 2423–2432. https://doi.org/10.1007/s11136-015-0976-9

Murphy, S. L., Janevic, M. R., Lee, P., & Williams, D. A. (2018). Occupational therapist-delivered cognitive-behavioral therapy for knee osteoarthritis: A randomized pilot study. *American Journal of Occupational Therapy, 72*(5), Article 7205205040. https://doi.org/10.5014/ajot.2018.027870

O'Toole, M. T. (Ed.). (2017). *Mosby's dictionary of medicine, nursing & health professions* (10th ed.). Elsevier.

Paterson, G., Toupin April, K., Backman, C., & Tugwell, P. (2016). OA Go Away: Development and preliminary validation of a self-management tool to promote adherence to exercise and physical activity for people with osteoarthritis of the hip and knee. *Physiotherapy Canada, 68*(2), 124–132. https://doi.org/10.3138/ptc.2014-68

Porter, R. S. (Ed.). (2018). *The Merck manual of diagnosis and therapy* (20th ed.). Merck Sharp & Dohme.

BIBLIOGRAPHY

Backman, C. L. (2011). Enabling performance and participation for persons with rheumatic diseases. In C. H. Christiansen & K. M. Matuska (Eds.), *Ways of living* (4th ed., pp. 213–238). AOTA Press.

Beaton, D. E., Tang, K., Gignac, M. A. M., Lacaille, D., Badley, E., Anis, A. H., & Bombardier, C. (2010). Reliability, validity, and responsiveness of five at-work productivity measures in patients with rheumatoid arthritis or osteoarthritis. *Arthritis Care & Research, 62*(1), 28–37. https://doi.org/10.1002/acr.20011

Deshaies, L. (2018). Arthritis. In H. M. Pendleton & W. Schultz-Krohn (Eds.), *Pedretti's occupational therapy* (8th ed., pp. 945–971). Mosby.

Dziedzick, K., Murphy, S. L., & Myers, H. (2010). Osteoarthritis. In K. Dziedzic & A. Hammond (Eds.), *Rheumatology: Evidence-based practice for physiotherapists and occupational therapists* (pp. 235–254). Churchill Livingstone.

Fernandes, L., Hagen, K. B., Bijlsma, J. W. J., Andreassen, O., Christensen, P., Conaghan, P. G., Doherty, M., Geenen, R., Hammond, A., Kjeken, I., Lohmander, L. S., Lund, H., Mallen, C. D., Nava, T., Oliver, S., Pavelka, K., Pitsillidou, I., da Silva, J. A., de la Torre, J., Zanoli, G., & Vliet Vieland, T. P. M. (2013). EULAR recommendations for the non-pharmacological core management of hip and knee osteoarthritis. *Annals of the Rheumatic Diseases, 72*(7), 1125–1135. https://doi.org/10.1136/annrheumdis-2012-202745

Gignac, M. A. M., Backman, C. L., Davis, A. M., Lacaille, D., Cao, X., & Badley, E. M. (2013). Social role participation and the life course in healthy adults and individuals with osteoarthritis: Are we overlooking the impact on the middle-aged? *Social Science & Medicine, 81,* 87–93. https://doi.org/10.1016/j.socscimed.2012.12.013

Godziuk, K., Prado, C. M., Woodhouse, L. J., & Forhan, M. (2018). The impact of sarcopenic obesity on knee and hip osteoarthritis: A scoping review. *BMC Musculoskeletal Disorders, 2018,* 19, Article 271. https://doi.org/10.1186/s12891-018-2175-7

Hammond, A. (2014). Rheumatoid arthritis, osteoarthritis, and fibromyalgia. In M. V. Padomski & C. A. Trombly Latham (Eds.), *Occupational therapy for physical dysfunction* (7th ed., pp. 1215–1243). Wolters Kluwer.

Housman, L., Arden, N., Schnitzer, T. J., Birbara, C., Conrozier, T., Skrepnik, N., Wei, N., Bockow, B., Waddell, D., Tahir, H., Hammond, A., Goupille, P., Sanson, B.-J., Elkins, C., & Bailleul, F. (2014). Intra-articular hylastan versus steroid for knee osteoarthritis. *Knee Surgery, Sports Traumatology, Arthroscopy, 22*(7), 1684–1692. https://doi.org/10.1007/s00167-013-2438-7

Mullen, T. M. (2017). Rheumatic diseases. In B. J. Atchison & D. P. Dirette (Eds.), *Conditions in occupational therapy* (5th ed., pp. 423–446). Wolters Kluwer.

Murphy, S. L., Robinson-Lane, S. G., & Schepens Niemiec, S. L. (2016). Knee and hip osteoarthritis management: A review of current and emerging non-pharmacological approaches. *Current Treatment Options in Rheumatology*, 2, 296–311. https://doi.org/10.1007/s40674-016-0054-7

Toupin April, K., Rader, T., Hawker, G. A., Stacey, D., O'Connor, A. M., Welch, V., Lyddiatt, A., McGowan, J., Thorne, J. C., Bennett, C., Pardo Pardo, J., Wells, G. A., & Tugwell, P. (2016). Development and alpha-testing of a stepped decision aid for patients considering nonsurgical options for knee and hip osteoarthritis management. *Journal of Rheumatology*, 43(10), 1891–1896. https://doi.org/10.3899/jrheum.150736

Psoriatic Arthritis

Description

Psoriatic arthritis (PsA) is a form of chronic inflammatory arthritis associated with psoriatic lesions of the skin and nails, particularly at the distal interphalangeal joints of the fingers and toes. The main symptoms are stiffness and swelling as well as joint pain (O'Toole, 2017; Porter, 2018).

Cause

Etiology and pathophysiology are unknown (Porter, 2018).

Evaluation/Assessment

Areas

- Activities of Daily Living/Instrumental ADL: self-care, weight control, home management, shopping, driving
- Education/Work: work tasks, workstation
- Play/Leisure: types of interests, frequency, location
- Rest/Sleep: sleep disturbance
- Social Participation: type, frequency, location, with whom
- Sensorimotor: joint range of motion, joint stiffness, joint tenderness, joint swelling and edema, grip strength, dexterity, pain, skin problems, fatigue
- Cognitive/Perceptual: no information identified
- Psychosocial: anxiety, fear, stress management and coping, quality of life, sense of shame or embarrassment
- Context/Environment: assistive devices, environment modification
- Comorbidity: obesity

Instruments

Instruments Developed by Occupational Therapy Personnel

- Psoriatic Arthritis Impact of Disease (PsAID) Questionnaires 9 and 12 (Gossec et al., 2014, and Holland et al., 2018, in References)

Instruments Developed by Other Professionals and Used by Occupational Therapy Personnel

- Disease Activity Index for Reactive Arthritis (DAREA; Eberl et al., 2000; see also Nell-Duxneuner et al., 2010, in References)
- Dougados Functional Index (DFI; Dougados et al., 1988; also called the Ankylosing Spondylitis Function Index)
- Educational Needs Assessment Tool (ENAT; Hardware et al., 2004)
- Functional Assessment of Chronic Illness Therapy–Fatigue Scale (FACIT-F; Smith et al., 2010; see also Holland et al., 2018, in References)

- Health Assessment Questionnaire–Disability Index (HAQ-DI; Bruce & Fries, 2005; see also Holland et al., 2018, in References)
- pain*DETECT* Questionnaire (PD-Q; Freynhagen et al., 2006; see also Rifbjerg-Madsen et al., 2017, in References)
- Psoriasis Area and Severity Index (PASI; Fredriksson & Pettersson, 1978; see also Holland et al., 2018, in References)

Problems/Issues

Activities of Daily Living/Instrumental ADL
- Person may have difficulty performing self-care activities due to joint problems (stiffness, swelling, tenderness, pain), which may limit available range of motion.
- Person may have difficulty performing aspects of IADL tasks such as lifting, grasping, reaching.

Education/Work
- Person may have difficulty performing certain work tasks due to joint problems as noted above.

Play/Leisure
- Person may have difficulty performing certain motions or activities required to engage in specific leisure activities.

Rest/Sleep
- Person may have sleep disturbances related to positioning of body to reduce pain.

Social Participation
- Person may have reduced participation in social activities with family, friends, colleagues.

Sensorimotor
- Person usually has decreased range of motion in affected joints most commonly in the hands, wrists, feet, ankles, lower back, and neck.
- Person may have swelling in affected joints.
- Person may have tenderness in affected joints.
- Person usually has pain in affected joints.
- Person may have enthesitis: inflammation of the entheses—sites where the tendons and ligaments insert into the bone.
- Person may have dactylitis: inflammation of the digits (fingers or toes).
- Person may have reduced muscle strength related to decreased joint motion.
- Person may have reduced dexterity and manipulation skills in the hands.
- Person may experience fatigue.
- Person usually has raised red scaly patches on the skin (plaques) most commonly on the elbows, knees, and scalp.

Cognitive/Perceptual
- No information identified.

Psychosocial
- Person may express feelings of depression, anxiety, or fear related to disease progression.
- Person may experience decreased quality of life.
- Person may express feelings of shame or embarrassment due to appearance.

Context/Environment
- Person may need adapted equipment or environmental modifications.
- Person, family, coworkers may lack knowledge of the disease and methods of coping with its consequences.

Intervention/Treatment

No specific models of practice or programs are cited. The booklet published by the Psoriasis and Psoriatic Arthritis Alliance (2017) provides useful suggestions. Major issues not routinely addressed by physicians were fatigue management, adequate coping skills, and impaired social participation (Desthieux et al., 2017). Patient education needs to be more targeted to be effective (Drăgoi et al., 2013). Team members include physicians, rheumatologists, pharmacists, nursing personnel, physical therapy personnel, and occupational therapy personnel. The primary goal is to enable the person to participate in everyday life (Psoriasis and Psoriatic Arthritis Alliance, 2017).

Activities of Daily Living/Instrumental ADL
- Assist in medication management.

Education/Work
- Assist client to identify strategies that will enable client to continue to work such as pacing, pain management, adapted equipment, workplace modification.

Play/Leisure
- Assist client to modify leisure occupations, especially those involving use of hand grips.
- Assist client to explore leisure occupations that are consistent with abilities.

Rest/Sleep
- Educate client on sleep hygiene.

Social Participation
- No information identified.

Sensorimotor
- Educate client on joint protection principles.
  - ▸ Avoid griping tightly or pinching: build up handles, use palm flat, use scissor or knives to cut instead opening with fingers, use flat hand on sponge or cloth to clean surfaces, press sponge between hands to squeeze out water.
  - ▸ Use joints in neutral position.
  - ▸ Use strongest, largest, joints possible.
  - ▸ Use correct lifting and handling techniques.
  - ▸ Spread load over several joints where possible.
  - ▸ Reduce weight of objects carried.
- Provide splints to protect and support joints.
- Provide exercises to strengthen muscles and increase range of motion.
- Assist client to develop an individualized pain management program.
- Instruct person in fatigue management including activity pacing (work and rest cycles) using a timer if needed.
- Instruct person on energy conservation (motion economy) principles.
- Assist client to develop a change of position timetable to avoid staying in one position too long while doing activities such as reading, driving, watching TV, or resting.

Cognitive/Perceptual
- Assist person to problem solve difficulties with everyday tasks.

Psychosocial
- Instruct client on stress management and coping techniques such as relaxation techniques, deep breathing, imagery, yoga, mindfulness.
- Discuss with client issues that cause anxiety, fear, and depression.

Context/Environment
- Provide assistive devices to facilitate performance of everyday tasks, work, and leisure activities.

- Provide instruction of environment modification including evaluation of home furniture and objects such as height of furniture, helpful equipment such as electrical items, nonskid mats, ergonomically designed handles, use of wheeled carts, long-handled dustpans.
- Provide education to client, family, support system, and employer about psoriatic arthritis and its management.

Precautions/Safety Considerations
Monitor for side effects of medications.

Prognosis and Outcome
Condition is chronic. Management of symptoms is important to slow or prevent additional damage to joints and surrounding issue. Client/patient education and self-management are important aspects to successful outcome.

REFERENCES

Desthieux, C., Granger, B., Balanescu, A. R., Balint, P., Braun, J., Canete, J. D., Heiberg, T., Helliwell P. S., Kalyoncu, U., Kvien, T. K., Kiltz, U., Niedermayer, D., Otsa, K., Scrivo, R., Smolen, J., Stamm, T. A., Veale, D. J., de Vlam, K., de Wit, M., & Gossec, L. (2017). Determinants of patient–physician discordance in global assessment in psoriatic arthritis. A multicenter European study. *Arthritis Care and Research, 69*(10), 1606–1611. https://doi.org/10.1002/acr.23172

Drăgoi, R. G., Ndosi, M., Sadlonova, M., Hill, J., Duer, M. Graninger, W., Smolen, J., & Stamm, T. A. (2013). Patient education, disease activity and physical function: Can we be more targeted? A cross sectional study among people with rheumatoid arthritis, psoriatic arthritis and hand osteoarthritis. *Arthritis Research & Therapy, 15*, Article R156. https://doi.org/10.1186/ar4339

Gossec, L., de Wit, M., Kiltz, U., Braun, J., Kalyoncu, U., Scrivo, R., Maccarone, M., Carton, L., Otsa, K., Sooäär, I., Heiberg, T., Bertheussen, H., Cañete, J. D., Sánchez Lobarte, A., Balanescu, A., Dinte, A., de Vlam, K., Smolen, J., Stamm, T., . . . Kvien, T. K. (2014). A patient-derived and patient-reported outcome measure for assessing psoriatic arthritis: Elaboration and preliminary validation of the Psoriatic Arthritis Impact of Disease (PsAID) questionnaire, a 13-country EULAR initiative. *Annals of Rheumatic Diseases, 73*(6), 1012–1019. https://doi.org/10.1136/annrheumdis-2014-205207

Holland, R., Tillett, W., Ogdie, A., Leung, Y. Y., Gladman, D. D., Callis Duffin, K., Coates, L. C., Mease, P. J., Eder, L., Strand, V., Elmamoun, M., Højgaard, P., Chau, J., de Wit, M., Goel, N., Lindsay, C. A., FitzGerald, O., Shea, B., Beaton, D., & Orbai, A.-M. (2018). Content and face validity and feasibility of 5 candidate instruments for psoriatic arthritis randomized controlled trials: The PsA OMERACT core set workshop at the GRAPPA 2017 annual meeting. *Journal of Rheumatology Supplement, 94*, 17–25. https://doi.org/10.3899/jrheum.180142

Nell-Duxneuner, V. P., Stamm, T. A., Machold, K. P., Pflugbeil, S., Aletaha, D., & Smolen, J. S. (2010). Evaluation of the appropriateness of composite disease activity measures for assessment of psoriatic arthritis. *Annals of the Rheumatic Diseases, 69*(3), 546–549. https://doi.org/10.1136/ard.2009.117945

O'Toole, M. T. (Ed.). (2017). *Mosby's dictionary of medicine, nursing & health professions* (10th ed.). Elsevier.

Porter, R. S. (Ed.). (2018). *The Merck manual of diagnosis and therapy* (20th ed.). Merck Sharp & Dohme.

Psoriasis and Psoriatic Arthritis Alliance. (2017). *Occupational therapy & psoriatic arthritis: A positive approach to psoriasis and psoriatic arthritis.* https://www.papaa.org/shop/occupational-therapy--psoriatic-arthritis/

Rifbjerg-Madsen, S., Wæhrens, E. E., Danneskiold-Samsøe, B., & Amris, K. (2017). Psychometric properties of the painDETECT questionnaire in rheumatoid arthritis, psoriatic arthritis and spondyloarthritis: Rasch analysis and test-retest reliability. *Health and Quality of Life Outcomes*, *15*, Article 110. https://doi.org/10.1186/s12955-017-0681-1

BIBLIOGRAPHY

Jimenez-Boj, E., Stamm, T. A., Sadlonova, M., Rovensky, J., Raffayová, H., Leeb, B., Machold, K. P., Graninger, W. B., & Smolen, J. S. (2012). Rituximab in psoriatic arthritis: An exploratory evaluation. *Annals of the Rheumatic Diseases*, *71*(11), 1868–1871. https://doi.org/10.1136/annrheumdis-2012-201897

Rheumatoid Arthritis

Also called RA, inflammatory arthritis, arthritis deformans.

Description

Rheumatoid arthritis (RA) is a chronic, systemic, autoimmune disease that primarily affects the peripheral joints such as the wrists and metacarpophalangeal (MCP) joints leading to progressive destruction and sometimes deformity of articular structures. RA is characterized by symmetrical inflammation of synovial membranes and increased synovial exudate, leading to thickening of the membranes and swelling of the joints. Course of the disease is variable but is most frequently marked by periods of remission alternated by exacerbations (O'Toole, 2017; R. S. Porter, 2018). The disease process may affect the intricate balance of the hand if joint and soft tissue structures are compromised resulting in decreased function of the hand (Beasley, 2014). In addition, joints in the elbows, shoulders, jaw, hips, knees, ankles, and spine may be involved. However, the degree of involvement may be different on the two sides of the body (Deshaies, 2018). Current research is focused on targeting low-disease activity or remission management (Stoffer et al., 2016).

Cause

The precise mechanism of the disease is not known. Genetic factors are suspected, and environmental factors such as viral infections or cigarette smoking may trigger the disorder. Women are affected more than men, usually between the ages of 36 and 50 years (R. S. Porter, 2018).

Stages (Adapted from text in Beasley, 2014)

- Stage 1 (Acute stage): Client demonstrates joint swelling, inflammation, and complains of pain.
- Stage 2 (Subacute stage): Marked by decrease in symptoms, but inflammatory synovium forms a pannus (granular tissue) that extends beyond the joint cartilage and invades ligament attachments and tendons. Nodes (small round bumps) may be evident, and joint bursa (fluid filled sac) may appear, but no evidence of deformities is evident.
- Stage 3 (Destructive stage): Client may report less pain, but irreversible joint deformities are progressing.
- Stage 4 (Chronic stage, skeletal collapse): Joint deformities occur, which may result in instability, dislocation, spontaneous fusion, and bony or fibrous ankylosis (stiffening of joint).

Classification of Global Functional Status (Adapted from Hochberg et al., 1992)

- Class 1: Person is able to perform usual activities of daily living (self-care including dressing, feeding, bathing, grooming and toileting; vocational and avocational).
- Class 2: Person is able to perform usual self-care and vocational activities, but limited in avocational activities.

- Class 3: Person is able to perform usual self-care activities, but limited in vocational and avocational activities.
- Class 4: Person is limited in ability to perform usual self-care, vocational, and avocational activities.

Evaluation/Assessment
Areas
- Activities of Daily Living/Instrumental ADL: eating, dressing, grooming, bathing, toileting, general health including skin condition, weight control
- Education/Work: job satisfaction
- Play/Leisure: interests, type, frequency, location, level of satisfaction
- Rest/Sleep: sleep disturbances related to pain or medications
- Social Participation: type, frequency, location, with whom
- Sensorimotor: joint range of motion, muscle grip and pinch strength, hand functions, stage of disease process, fatigue, pain, visual functions, body image
- Cognitive/Perceptual: self-management (executive function)
- Psychosocial: coping, resilience, self-efficacy, sense of coherence, social interaction, social roles
- Context/Environment: adaptive devices, home modification
- Comorbidity: osteoporosis

Instruments
Instruments Developed by Occupational Therapy Personnel
- Arthritis Hand Function Test (AHFT; Backman et al., 1991)
- Canadian Occupational Performance Measure (5th ed.; COPM-5; Law et al., 2014)
- Ergonomic Assessment Tool for Arthritis (EATA; Backman et al., 2008)
- Evaluation of Daily Activity Questionnaire (EDAQ; Hammond et al., 2018; see Hammond et al., 2014, and Hammond et al., 2015; in References)
- Joint Protection Self-Efficacy Scale (JPSES; Niedermann, Forster, et al., 2011, in References)
- Keyboard-Personal Computer Style (K-PeCS; Baker & Redfern, 2005)
- Measure of Activity of Performance of the Hand (MAP-HAND; Paulsen et al., 2010, in References; see also Prior et al., 2018, in References)
- National Institutes of Health (NIH) Activity Record (ACTRE; Gerber & Furst, 1992)
- Nine Hole Peg Test (NHPT, 9HPT; Mathiowetz et al., 1985)
- Occupational Balance-Questionnaire (OB-Quest; Dür et al., 2014)
- Occupational Questionnaire (OQ; Smith et al., 1986)

Instruments Developed by Other Professionals and Used by Occupational Therapy Personnel
- ACR/EULAR Classification Criteria (Biliavska et al., 2013, in References)
- Arthritis Impact Measurement Scales-2 (AIMS-2; Meenan et al., 1992)
- Arthritis Self-Efficacy Scale (ASES; Lorig et al., 1989)
- Bristol Arthritis Fatigue Multi-Dimensional Questionnaire (BAFMDQ; Nicklin et al., 2010)
- Bristol Arthritis Fatigue Numeric Rating Scale (BAFNRS; Nicklin et al., 2010)
- Coping With Rheumatoid Arthritis Questionnaire (CRAQ; Englbrecht et al., 2012)
- Decision Conflict Scale (DCS; O'Connor, 1995)
- Disabilities of the Arm, Shoulder, and Hand (3rd ed.; DASH-3; Kennedy et al., 2011; see also Prodinger et al., 2019, in References)
- Disease Activity Score (DAS; van der Heijde et al., 1990)
- Educational Needs Assessment Tool (ENAT; Hardware et al., 2004)
- Effective Consumer Scale (ECS; Tugwell et al., 2005)
- Endicott Work Productivity Scale (EWPS; Endicott & Nee, 1997)
- General Self-Efficacy Scale (GES; Jerusalem & Schwarzer, 1992)
- Grip Ability Test (GAT; Dellhag & Bjelle, 1995)

- Grip strength (dynamometry; JAMAR, Lafayette Instrument; Wang et al., 2018)
- Hospital Anxiety and Depression Scale (HADS; Zigmond & Snaith, 1983)
- Jebsen-Taylor Hand Function Test (JTHFT; Jebsen et al., 1969)
- Joint Alignment and Motion Scale (JAMS; Spiegel et al., 1987)
- Joint range of motion (functional, nonpainful) goniometry or alternate (distance of finger-tips to tabletop for opening and distance of fingertips to dorsal palmar crease for closing)
- London Coping With Rheumatoid Arthritis Questionnaire (LCRAQ; Folkman & Lazarus, 1980)
- McGill Pain Questionnaire (MPQ; Melzack, 1975)
- Michigan Hand Outcomes Questionnaire (MHQ; Chung et al., 1998)
- Modified Stanford Health Assessment Questionnaire (MSHAQ; Pincus et al., 1983)
- O'Connor Finger Dexterity Test (OFDT; O'Connor, 1926)
- Pinch strength (pinch meter; B&L Engineering; Mathiowetz et al., 1985)
- Purdue Pegboard Test (PPT; Tiffin, 1948)
- Recent-Onset Arthritis Disability Index (RADI; Salaffi et al, 2005)
- Rheumatoid Arthritis Impact of Disease (RAID; Gossec et al., 2009)
- Rheumatoid Arthritis Quality of Life (RAQL; Whalley et al., 1997)
- Rheumatoid Arthritis Self-Efficacy Questionnaire (RASE; Hewlett et al., 2001)
- Score for Assessment and Quantification of Chronic Rheumatic Affections of the Hands (SACRAH; Leeb et al., 2003)
- Semmes-Weinstein monofilaments (Bell-Krotoski, 2011; Patterson Medical)
- Sequential Occupational Dexterity Assessment (SODA; van Lankveld et al., 1996)
- Short-Form 36 Health Survey (SF-36; Ware et al., 1993)
- Signals of Functional Impairment (SOFI; Eberhard et al., 1988)
- Stanford Presenteeism Scale (SPS-6; Koopman et al., 2002)
- Valued Life Activities Scale (VLAS; Katz et al., 2006)
- Volumetry (water displacement; Stern, 1991)
- Ways of Coping Inventory–Revised (WOC-R; Folkman, Lazarus et al., 1986)
- Work Experience Survey–Rheumatic Disease (WES-RD; Allaire & Keysor, 2009)
- Work Instability Scale for Rheumatoid Arthritis (RA-WIS; Gilworth et al., 2003; see also Tang et al, 2010, in References)
- Work Limitations Questionnaire (WLQ; Lerner et al., 2001)
- Workplace Activity Limitations Scale (WALS; Gignac et al., 2004)

Problems/Issues

Activities of Daily Living/Instrumental ADL
- Person may experience difficulty performing hand functions associated with ADLs such as grip and pinch strength, twisting motions of the wrist, and static positions of wrist and fingers.

Education/Work
- Person may experience difficulty performing hand functions associated with keyboarding such as moving hands to strike keys, using two or less fingers to activate keys, reducing amount of time keyboarding, using high-force keystrokes, and static holding positions involving the upper extremity, wrist, and fingers.
- Person may experience difficulty with positioning chair, monitor, mouse, and keyboard for comfort and effective use.

Play/Leisure
- Person may experience difficulty engaging in favorite leisure occupations that required grip or pinch strength, forearm supination and pronation, or static holding of upper extremity, wrist, and fingers.

Rest/Sleep
- Person may experience sleep disturbances due to pain or side effects of medication.

Social Participation

- Person may limit or withdraw from social activities where hand or leg functions are required, such as card games, needlecraft projects, bowling, running marathons, skiing, or playing golf.

Sensorimotor

- Person may experience prolonged (1–2 hours) periods of morning stiffness.
- Person may experience loss of active range of motion due to tendon rupture (most often extensor digitorum communis [EDC] at distal end of ulna or extensor pollicis longus [EPL] at Lister's tubercle (boney prominence on radius).
- Person may experience decreased grip and pinch strength.
- Person may experience flexor tendon tenosynovitis (reduces digit motion, strength).
- Person may experience trigger finger (due to nodular thickening from tenosynovitis).
- Person may experience ulnar deviation of metacarpophalangeal (MCP) joint with palmar subluxation and radial deviation of metacarpals or zigzag deformity.
- Person may experience Swan neck deformity of proximal interphalangeal (PIP) joint.
- Person may experience boutonnière deformity (PIP joint flexion and distal interphalangeal [DIP] joint hyperextension).
- Person may experience volar subluxation of wrist (carpus on radius), causing ligament laxity due to chronic synovitis.
- Person may experience instability of distal ulna dorsal subluxation, resulting in reduced pronation and supination.
- Person may experience thumb deformities such as MCP flexion and distal joint hyperextension.
- Person may have rheumatoid nodules over pressure areas such as elbows or digits.
- Person may experience episodes of fatigue and malaise.
- Person may experience pain that is symmetric and polyarticular (involves many joints).

Cognitive/Perceptual

- RA does not directly affect cognition but ability to self-manage condition is dependent on good cognitive functioning in areas of attention, memory, and problem solving.
- Person may have cognitive impairments due to other comorbidities, which must be considered in RA management program.
- Person may experience changes in visual functions.
- Person may experience changes in perception of body image.

Psychosocial

- Person may express loss of self-efficacy.
- Person may express or exhibit signs of depression.
- Person may resist changing ways task has always been performed.
- Person may express doubt and uncertainty about future occupational performance, especially "ups and downs" related to exacerbations and remissions.
- Person may express feelings of regret about loss of occupational identity.
- Person may experience changes in ability to perform socially expected role functions.
- Person may choose to be noncompliant (Ritschl et al., 2018).

Context/Environment

- Person may need to use adapted devices and equipment.
- Person may need to wear splints or orthotic devices.
- Person, family, caregivers may need information and education about RA, including community resources.

Intervention/Treatment

Models and programs developed by occupational therapy personnel: None identified. Models and programs developed by other professionals but used by occupational therapy personnel include hand exercises (Lamb et al., 2015), health education—feet (Graham et al., 2011), joint protection education program (Niedermann, de Bie, et al., 2011; Niedermann et al., 2010), Mindfulness-Based Stress Reduction (MBSR; Hawtin & Sullivan, 2011), physical activity trackers (Leese et al., 2019), Reducing Arthritis Fatigue Teams (RAFT; Hewlett et al., 2019), self-management (Hewlett et al., 2011), serial casting (Uğurlu & Özdoğan, 2016), splinting (B. J. Porter & Brittain, 2012), and team approach (O'Shaughnessy et al., 2019). Team members include physicians, nursing personnel, physical therapists, psychologists, and occupational therapy personnel. Goals are specific to client's existing deformities or potential for deformities, stage of the disease, and need or expectation to perform daily living occupations (Beasley, 2014). The general goals are to (1) reduce pain, swelling, and fatigue; (2) improve joint function while minimizing damage and deformity; (3) prevent disability and disease-related morbidity; and (4) maintain physical, social, and emotional function (Deshaies, 2018).

Activities of Daily Living/Instrumental ADL
- Explore and discuss with client whether adapted techniques and adapted equipment may decrease fatigue and increase performance of self-maintenance activities.
- Explore and discuss with client whether adapted techniques and adapted equipment may enable continued performance of housekeeping and home-management tasks such as meal preparation, light housekeeping, and doing laundry.

Education/Work
- Explore and discuss with client whether adapted techniques and adapted equipment may enable client to continue to work, including transportation, moving about the work site, organization of workstation, or modification of work schedule.

Play/Leisure
- Discuss current and past hobbies and interests to determine which ones may be continued, need modification, or should be discontinued.
- Provide opportunity to explore new interests.

Rest/Sleep
- Encourage client to keep a sleep diary to identify sleep problems.
- Reduce unnecessary stress on joints while sleeping.
- During active inflammatory stage, client should get 8 to 10 hours of sleep and ½ to 1 hour of rest during morning and afternoon (Deshaies, 2018).
- Encourage client to get rest and sleep to reduce inflammation, pain, stress, and depression.
- Assist client to rest joints with symptoms of RA by wearing a splint, avoiding or modifying activities, or positioning to prevent joint stress.

Social Participation
- Assist client to identify and plan social events that are within client's functional status and interest level, making modifications as needed such as shorter period of time, less active participation required, opportunity for rest breaks, fewer people with whom to interact, or more familiar setting.

Sensorimotor
- Energy conservation and fatigue management
  - Balance work and rest (e.g., take 5-minute break every hour; intersperse active tasks with passive or quiet ones).
  - Avoid staying in one position too long (change position every 20–30 minutes).
  - Avoid activities that cannot be stopped immediately if pain or discomfort is experienced; plan shopping around short driving or walking trips; do not do all the shopping in 1 day.
  - Use a well-planned workspace (convenient height, maintain good posture, items frequently used conveniently located, reduce clutter, store less frequently used items away from immediate workspace).

▶ Sit rather than stand when possible, using a chair, stool, or bench that is sturdy to provide good support.

- Joint protection and ergonomics
  - ▶ Purpose: decreases joint stress and damage through altered task performance.
  - ▶ Technique:
    - ○ Use each joint in its most stable anatomic and functional position.
    - ○ Avoid positions of deformity and stress.
    - ○ Use strongest joint available.
    - ○ Maintain muscle strength and joint range of motion.
- Pain management
  - ▶ Purpose: reduce and relieve pain.
  - ▶ Techniques:
    - ○ Positioning: explore with client positions in bed, sitting, standing, or moving that cause pain and approaches to reduce pain.
    - ○ Rest and relaxation: assist client to include rest and relaxation breaks in daily schedule.
    - ○ Splints: explore use of resting splints for nighttime wear.
- Physical agents
  - ▶ Purpose: relieve pain, increase circulation, reduce inflammation, or maintain and improve range of motion.
    - ○ Superficial (local or whole body) heat: pain relief, increase tissue elasticity, and blood flow; possible negative effect is increased inflammation.
    - ○ Superficial (localized) cold: reduce inflammation and decrease pain; possible negative effect is increased tissue viscosity and decreased tissue elasticity causing joint stiffness.
  - ▶ Technique:
    - ○ Heat: fluidotherapy, heat wraps, hot packs, hydrotherapy in a heated pool, paraffin, warm shower or bath.
    - ○ Cold: gel packs, ice packs.
- Splinting
  - ▶ Purpose (by stage):
    - ○ Stage 1: resting splint to decrease inflammation and pain while protecting joints against potential deformity.
    - ○ Stage 2: day splint for comfort, night splint to relive pain and protect joints; others may be used to increase range of motion.
    - ○ Stages 3 and 4: day splint to improve function by providing stability, limiting undesired motion, properly positioning joints, and reducing pain; night splint to provide comfort and positioning.
  - ▶ Types (for pictures, see Deshaies, 2018):
    - ○ Resting splint
    - ○ Swan neck deformity splint
    - ○ Thumb support
    - ○ Ulnar deviation splint (may include wrist and MCP joint or MCP joint only)
- Therapeutic activity
  - ▶ Purpose: provide physical and psychological support (see Play/Leisure, above).
  - ▶ Technique: selected activities may be graded to include range of motion and strengthening using principles of therapeutic exercise (below).
- Therapeutic exercise
  - ▶ Purpose: maintain muscle and joint function, prevent disuse atrophy, maintain or improve range of motion.
  - ▶ Technique:
    - ○ Regular aerobic and dynamic exercise for fingers, forearms and wrists, jaw, neck, shoulders, and elbows.

o Amount depends on pain tolerance; if pain lasts longer than 1 or 2 hours postexercise, amount or intensity needs to be decreased.

o Exercises for range of motion should be performed at least once daily, even during exacerbations.

o Exercises should be done slowly, smoothly, using proper technique, throughout comfortable range of motion.

o Active range of motion is preferred but therapist may provide assisted or passive range of motion if pain or muscle weakness prevents passive motion.

o Start with 5 repetitions and increase slowly to 10, one or two times daily.

Cognitive/Perceptual
- Assist client to plan, prioritize, and problem solve (PPP).
- Assist client to use diaries to track disease progress and problems.
- Assist client to use schedules to organize activities and rest breaks.

Psychosocial
- Involvement and participation in activities and exercise can reduce feelings of depression.
- Discuss with client feelings about changing role functions.

Context/Environment
- Provide client, family, and caregivers education about RA and its stages.
- Provide education and training in use of equipment including wheelchairs, walkers, splints, and assistive devices.
- Assist client, family, and caregivers to identify and use community and internet resources.
- Assistive devices
  - ► Built-up handles: eating utensils, toothbrush, pens or pencils, brush or comb, buttonhook, zipper pull, key holder
  - ► Two handles instead of one: drink cup, coffee mug
  - ► Extended handles: dressing stick, groom aids, mirrors, shoehorns, perianal hygiene aid, reacher or grabber, dustpan
  - ► Levers instead of knobs: door handles, sink handles, toilet handles
  - ► Electrical instead of manual: can opener, toothbrush
  - ► Velcro or elastic (in place of regular): shoelaces, buttons, zippers, hooks, fasteners
  - ► Suction cups: denture brush, nail clipper and brush, cutting board
  - ► Lightweight: plates, eating utensils, cups, trays
  - ► Equipment: raised toilet seat, grab bars, rolling (wheeled) cart, knob turner, speaker phone, spring-loaded scissors, jar opener

Precautions/Safety Considerations
- Monitor client for potential tendon rupture; rupture can occur with extensor pollicis longus (EPL) and extensor digitorum communis (EDC) tendons of third, fourth, and fifth digits.
- Monitor client for negative reactions to physical agent modalities (heat and cold) such as burns or pain.
- Person may be at increased risk for falls due to joint changes (dislocation, instability).
- During acute inflammatory phase (Stage 1) when joint temperatures are elevated, use of heat modalities are contraindicated because the heat may promote inflammation.
- Use of cold modalities is contraindicated if Raynaud's phenomenon (a vasospastic disorder of digits) is present.
- Strengthening program for RA hand should proceed with caution to avoid aggravation of deformities; stability should not be sacrificed for possible increase in strength, and exercises should never cause pain.
- Fingers (digits) and wrist should never be forced into an aligned position; a properly fitted orthosis should allow the joint to guide into position.

Prognosis and Outcome

Disease is progressive, and there is no cure. Disease-modifying antirheumatic drugs (DMARDs) and biologic response modifiers can slow the progression of the disease and prevent permanent damage to the joints and tissues, but cannot cure the disease. RA decreases life expectancy by 3 to 7 years, with heart disease, infection, and gastrointestinal bleeding accounting for the increased mortality (R. S. Porter, 2018).

REFERENCES

Beasley, J. (2014). Arthritis. In C. Cooper (Ed.), *Fundamentals of hand therapy* (2nd ed., pp. 457–478). Elsevier.

Biliavska, I., Stamm, T. A., Martinez-Avila, J., Huizinga, T. W., Landewé, R. B. M., Steiner, G., Aletaha, D., Smolen, J. S., & Machold, K. P. (2013). Application of the 2010 ACR/EULAR classification criteria in patients with very early inflammatory arthritis: Analysis of sensitivity, specificity and predictive values in the SAVE study cohort. *Annals of the Rheumatic Diseases*, *72*(8), 1335–1341. https://doi.org/10.1136/annrheumdis-2012-201909

Deshaies, L. (2018). Arthritis. In H. M. Pendleton & W. Schultz-Krohn (Eds.), *Pedretti's occupational therapy* (8th ed., pp. 945–971). Mosby.

Graham, A., Hammond, A., & Williams, A. (2011). Therapeutic foot health education for patients with rheumatoid arthritis: A narrative review. *Musculoskeletal Care*, *9*(3), 141–151. https://doi.org/10.1002/msc.205

Hammond, A., Tennant, A., Tyson, S. F., Nordenskiöld, U., Hawkins, R., & Prior, Y. (2015). The reliability and validity of the English version of the Evaluation of Daily Activity Questionnaire for people with rheumatoid arthritis. *Rheumatology*, *54*(9), 1605–1615. https://doi.org/10.1093/rheumatology/kev008

Hammond, A., Tyson, S., Prior, Y., Hawkins, R., Tennant, A., Nordenskiöld, U., Thyberg, I., Sandqvist, G., & Cederlund, R. (2014). Linguistic validation and cultural adaptation of an English version of the Evaluation of Daily Activity Questionnaire in rheumatoid arthritis. *Health and Quality of Life Outcomes*, *12*, Article 143. https://doi.org/10.1186/s12955-014-0143-y

Hawtin, H., & Sullivan, C. (2011). Experiences of mindfulness training in living with rheumatic disease: An interpretative phenomenological analysis. *British Journal of Occupational Therapy*, *74*(3), 137–142. https://doi.org/10.4276/030802211X12996065859283

Hewlett, S., Almeida, C., Ambler, N., Blair, P. S., Choy, E. H., Dures, E., Hammond, A., Hollingworth, W., Kadir, B., Kirwan, J. R., Plummer, Z., Rooke, C., Thorn, J., Turner, N., & Pollock, J. (2019). Reducing arthritis fatigue impact: Two-year randomised controlled trial of cognitive behavioural approaches by rheumatology teams (RAFT). *Annals of the Rheumatic Diseases*, *78*(4), 465–472. https://doi.org/10.1136/annrheumdis-2018-214469

Hewlett, S., Ambler, N., Almeida, C., Cliss, A., Hammond, A., Kitchen, K., Knops, B., Pope, D., Spears, M., Swinkels, A., & Pollock, J. (2011). Self-management of fatigue in rheumatoid arthritis: A randomised controlled trial of group cognitive-behavioural therapy. *Annals of the Rheumatic Diseases*, *70*(6), 1060–1067. https://doi.org/10.1136/ard.2010.144691

Hochberg, M. C., Chang, R. W., Dwosh, I., Lindsey, S., Pincus, T., & Wolfe, F. (1992). The American College of Rheumatology 1991 revised criteria for the classification of global functional status in rheumatoid arthritis. *Arthritis and Rheumatism*, *35*(5), 498–502. https://doi.org/10.1002/art.1780350502

Lamb, S. E., Williamson, E. M., Heine, P. J., Adams, J., Dosanjh, S., Dritsaki, M., Glover, M. J., Lord, J., McConkey, C., Nichols, V., Rahman, A., Underwood, M., & Williams, M. A. (2015). Exercises to improve function of the rheumatoid hand (SARAH): A randomised controlled trial. *Lancet*, *385*(9966), 421–429. https://doi.org/10.1016/S0140-6736(14)60998-3

Leese, J., Macdonald, G. G., Tran, B. C., Wong, R., Backman, C. L., Townsend, A. F., Davis, A. M., Jones, C. A., Gromala, D., Avina-Zubieta, J. A., Hoens, A. M., & Li, L. C. (2019). Using physical activity trackers in arthritis self-management: A qualitative study of patient and rehabilitation professional perspectives. *Arthritis Care & Research, 71*(2), 227–236. https://doi.org/10.1002/acr.23780

Niedermann, K., de Bie, R. A., Kubli, R., Ciurea, A., Steurer-Stey, C., Villiger, P. M., & Büchi, S. (2011). Effectiveness of individual resource-oriented joint protection education in people with rheumatoid arthritis: A randomized controlled trial. *Patient Education and Counseling, 82*(1), 42–48. https://doi.org/10.1016/j.pec.2010.02.014

Niedermann, K., Forster, A., Ciurea, A., Hammond, A. Uebelhart, D., & de Bie, R. (2011). Development and psychometric properties of a joint protection self-efficacy scale. *Scandinavian Journal of Occupational Therapy, 18*(2), 143–152. https://doi.org/10.3109/11038128.2010.483690

Niedermann, K., Hammond, A., Forster, A., & de Bie, R. (2010). Perceived benefits and barriers to joint protection among people with rheumatoid arthritis and occupational therapists: A mixed methods study. *Musculoskeletal Care, 8*(3), 143–156. https://doi.org/10.1002/msc.177

O'Shaughnessy, M. A., Kannas, S., Ernste, F., & Rizzo, M. (2019). Team approach: Role of medical and surgical management in rheumatoid arthritis of the hand and wrist. *Journal of Bone Joint Surgery Reviews, 7*(8), e10. https://doi.org/10.2106/JBJS.RVW.18.00196

O'Toole, M. T. (Ed.). (2017). *Mosby's dictionary of medicine, nursing & health professions* (10th ed.). Elsevier.

Paulsen, T., Grotle, M., Garratt, A., & Kjeken, I. (2010). Development and psychometric testing of the patient-reported measure of activity performance of the hand (MAP-Hand) in rheumatoid arthritis. *Journal of Rehabilitation Medicine, 42*(7), 636–644. https://doi.org/10.2340/16501977-0577

Porter, B. J., & Brittain, A. (2012). Splinting and hand exercise for three common hand deformities in rheumatoid arthritis: A clinical perspective. *Current Opinion in Rheumatology, 24*(2), 215–221. https://doi.org/10.1097/BOR.0b013e3283503361

Porter, R. S. (Ed.). (2018). *The Merck manual of diagnosis and therapy* (20th ed.). Merck Sharp & Dohme.

Prior, Y., Tennant, A., Tyson, S., Kjeken, I., & Hammond, A. (2018). Measure of activity performance of the hand (MAP-Hand) questionnaire: Linguistic validation, cultural adaptation and psychometric testing in people with rheumatoid arthritis in the UK. *BMC Musculoskeletal Disorders, 19*, Article 275. https://doi.org/10.1186/s12891-018-2177-5

Prodinger, B., Hammond, A., Tennant, A., Prior, Y., & Tyson, S. (2019). Revisiting the disabilities of the arm, shoulder and hand (DASH) and QuickDASH in rheumatoid arthritis. *BMC Musculoskeletal Disorders, 20*, Article 41. https://doi.org/10.1186/s12891-019-2414-6

Ritschl, V., Lackner, A., Boström, C., Mosor, E., Lehner, M., Omara, M., Ramos, R., Studenic, P., Smolen, J. S., & Stamm, T. A. (2018). I do not want to suppress the natural process of inflammation: New insights on factors associated with non-adherence in rheumatoid arthritis. *Arthritis Research & Therapy, 20*(1), Article 234. https://doi.org/10.1186/s13075-018-1732-7

Stoffer, M. A., Schoels, M. M., Smolen, J. S., Aletaha, D., Breedveld, F. C., Burmester, G., Bykerk, V., Dougados, M., Emery, P., Haraoui, B., Gomez-Reino, J., Kvien, T. K., Nash, P., Navarro-Compan, V., Scholte-Voshaar, M., van Vollenhoven, R., van der Heijde, D., & Stamm, T. A. (2016). Evidence for treating rheumatoid arthritis to target: Results of a systematic literature search update. *Annals of the Rheumatic Diseases, 75*(1), 16–22. https://doi.org/10.1136/annrheumdis-2015-207526

Tang, K., Beaton, D. E., Gignac, M. A. M., Lacaille, D., Zhang, W., Bombardier, C., & CANWP Group. (2010). The Work Instability Scale for Rheumatoid Arthritis predicts arthritis-related work transitions within 12 months. *Arthritis Care & Research, 62*(11), 1578–1587. https://doi.org/10.1002/acr.20272

Uğurlu, Ü., & Özdoğan, H. (2016). Effects of serial casting in the treatment of flexion contractures of proximal interphalangeal joints in patients with rheumatoid arthritis and juvenile idiopathic arthritis: A retrospective study. *Journal of Hand Therapy, 29*(1), 41–50. https://doi.org/10.1016/j.jht.2015.11.005

BIBLIOGRAPHY

Adams, J., Mullee, M., Burridge, J., Hammond, A., & Cooper, C. (2010). Responsiveness of self-report and therapist-rated upper extremity structural impairment and functional outcome measures in early rheumatoid arthritis. *Arthritis Care & Research, 62*(2), 274–278. https://doi.org/10.1002/acr.20078

Ağce, Z. B., Özkan, E., & Köse, B. (2017). Arthritis/rheumatoid arthritis. In M. Huri (Ed.), *Occupation focused holistic practice in rehabilitation* (pp. 121–147). IntechOpen. https://doi.org/10.5772/intechopen.68477

Andrade, J. A., Brandão, M. B., Pinto, M. R. C., & Lanna, C. C. D. (2016). Factors associated with activity limitations in people with rheumatoid arthritis. *American Journal of Occupational Therapy, 70*(4). Article 7004290030. https://doi.org/10.5014/ajot.2016.017467

Backman, C. L. (2011). Enabling performance and participation for persons with rheumatic diseases. In C. H. Christiansen & K. M. Matuska (Eds.), *Ways of living* (4th ed., pp. 213–238). AOTA Press.

Baker, N. A., Gustafson, N. P., & Rogers, J. (2010). The association between rheumatoid arthritis related structural changes in hands and computer keyboard operation. *Journal of Occupational Rehabilitation, 20*(1), 59–68. https://doi.org/10.1007/s10926-009-9216-x

Baker, N. A., Rubinstein, E. N., & Rogers, J. C. (2012). Problems and accommodation strategies reported by computer users with rheumatoid arthritis or fibromyalgia. *Journal of Occupational Rehabilitation, 22*(3), 353–362. https://doi.org/10.1007/s10926-012-9353-5

Barns, A., Svanholm, F., Kjellberg, A., Thyberg, I., & Falkmer, T. (2015). Living in the present: Women's everyday experiences of living with rheumatoid arthritis. *SAGE Open, 5*(4). https://doi.org/10.1177/2158244015616163

Beasley, J. (2011). Therapist's examination and conservative management of arthritis of the upper extremity. In T. M. Skirven, A. L. Osterman, J. M. Fedorczyk, & P. C. Amadio (Eds.), *Rehabilitation of the hand and upper extremity* (6th ed., pp. 1330–1343). Mosby.

Beasley, J. (2012). Osteoarthritis and rheumatoid arthritis: Conservative therapeutic management. *Journal of Hand Therapy, 25*(2), 163–172. https://doi.org/10.1016/j.jht.2011.11.001

Beaton, D. E., Tang, K., Gignac, M. A. M., Lacaille, D., Badley, E., Anis, A. H., & Bombardier, C. (2010). Reliability, validity, and responsiveness of five at-work productivity measures in patients with rheumatoid arthritis or osteoarthritis. *Arthritis Care & Research, 62*(1), 28–37. https://doi.org/10.1002/acr.20011

Carandang, K., Pyatak, E. A., & Vigen, C. L. P. (2016). Systematic review of educational interventions for rheumatoid arthritis. *American Journal of Occupational Therapy, 70*(6), Article 7006290020. https://doi.org/10.5014/ajot.2016.021386

Coenen, M., Stamm, T. A., Stucki, G., & Cieza, A. (2012). Individual interviews and focus groups in patients with rheumatoid arthritis: A comparison of two qualitative methods. *Quality of Life Research, 21*(2), 359–370. https://doi.org/10.1007/s11136-011-9943-2

College of Occupational Therapists. (2015). *Hand and wrist orthoses for adults with rheumatological conditions: Practice guideline for occupational therapists.* Author.

de Almeida, P. H. T. Q., Pontes, T. B., Matheus, J. P. C., Muniz, L. F., & da Mota, L. M. H. (2015). Occupational therapy in rheumatoid arthritis: What rheumatologists need to know? *Revista Brasileira de Reumatologia, 55*(3), 272–280. https://doi.org/10.1016/j.rbre.2014.07.008

Del Fabro Smith, L., Suto, M., Chalmers, A., & Backman, C. L. (2011). Belief in doing and knowledge in being mothers with arthritis. *OTJR: Occupation, Participation and Health, 31*(1), 40–48. https://doi.org/10.3928/15394492-20100222-01

Dür, M., Coenen, M., Stoffer, M. A., Fialka-Moser, V., Kautzky-Willer, A., Kjeken, I., Drăgoi, R. G., Mattsson, M., Boström, C., Smolen, J., & Stamm, T. A. (2015). Do patient-reported outcome measures cover personal factors important to people with rheumatoid arthritis? A mixed methods design using the International Classification of Functioning, Disability and Health as frame of reference. *Health and Quality of Life Outcomes, 13,* Article 27. https://doi .org/10.1186/s12955-015-0214-8

Dür, M., Steiner, G., Stoffer, M. A., Fialka-Moser, V., Kautzky-Willer, A., Dejaco, C., Ekmekcio-glu, C., Prodinger, B., Binder, A., Smolen, J., & Stamm, T. A. (2016). Initial evidence for the link between activities and health: Associations between a balance of activities, functioning and serum levels of cytokines and C-reactive protein. *Psychoneuroendocrinology, 65,* 138–148. https://doi.org/10.1016/j.psyneuen.2015.12.015

Dures, E., Kitchen, K., Almeida, C., Ambler, N., Cliss, A., Hammond, A., Knops, B., Morris, M., Swinkels, A., & Hewlett, S. (2012). "They didn't tell us, they made us work it out ourselves": Patient perspectives of a cognitive-behavioral program for rheumatoid arthritis fatigue. *Arthritis Care & Research, 64*(4), 494–501. https://doi.org/10.1002/acr.21562

Dziedzic, K., & Hammond, A. (2010). *Rheumatology: Evidence based practice for physiotherapists and occupational therapists.* Churchill Livingstone.

Ekelman, B. A., Hooker, L., Davis, A., Klan, J., Newburn, D., Detwiler, K., & Ricchino, N. (2014). Occupational therapy interventions for adults with rheumatoid arthritis: An appraisal of the evidence. *Occupational Therapy in Health Care, 28*(4), 347–361. https://doi.org/10.3109/07 380577.2014.919687

Forhan, M., & Backman, C. (2010). Exploring occupational balance in adults with rheumatoid arthritis. *OTJR: Occupation, Participation and Health, 30*(3), 133–141. https://doi.org/10.3928/ 15394492-20090625-01

Graham, A. S., Hammond, A., & Williams, A. E. (2012). Foot health education for people with rheumatoid arthritis: The practitioner's perspective. *Journal of Foot and Ankle Research, 5*(1), 2. https://doi.org/10.1186/1757-1146-5-2

Hammond, A. (2014). Rheumatoid arthritis, osteoarthritis, and fibromyalgia. In M. V. Radom-ski & C. A. Trombly Latham (Eds.), *Occupational therapy for physical dysfunction* (7th ed., pp. 1215–1243). Wolters Kluwer.

Hammond, A., O'Brien, R., Woodbridge, S., Bradshaw, L., Prior, Y., Radford, K., Culley, J., Whitham, D., & Pulikottil-Jacob, R. (2017). Job retention vocational rehabilitation for employed people with inflammatory arthritis (WORK-IA): A feasibility randomized controlled trial. *BMC Musculoskeletal Disorders, 18,* Article 315. https://doi.org/10.1186/s12891-017-1671-5

Hammond, A., Prior, Y., & Tyson, S. (2018). Linguistic validation, validity and reliability of the British English versions of the Disabilities of the Arm, Shoulder and Hand (DASH) questionnaire and QuickDASH in people with rheumatoid arthritis. *BMC Musculoskeletal Disorders, 19,* Article 118. https://doi.org/10.1186/s12891-018-2032-8

Li, L. C., Adam, P. M., Backman, C. L., Lineker, S., Jones, C. A., Lacaille, D., Townsend, A. F., Yacyshyn, E., Yousefi, C., Tugwell, P., Leese, J., & Stacey, D. (2014). Proof-of-concept study of a web-based methotrexate decision aid for patients with rheumatoid arthritis. *Arthritis Care & Research, 66*(10), 1472–1481. https://doi.org/10.1002/acr.22319

Li, L. C., Adam, P. M., Townsend, A. F., Lacaille, D., Yousefi, C., Stacey, D., Gromala, D., Shaw, C. D., Tugwell, P., & Backman, C. L. (2013). Usability testing of ANSWER: A web-based methotrexate decision aid for patients with rheumatoid arthritis. *BMC Medical Informatics and Decision Making, 13,* Article 131. https://doi.org/10.1186/1472-6947-13-131

Liu, C. H., Yip, K. S., & Fan, S. C. (2017). Optimal grasp distance and muscle loads for people with rheumatoid arthritis using carpometacarpal and metacarpophalangeal immobilization orthoses. *American Journal of Occupational Therapy, 71*(1), Article 7101190010. https://doi .org/10.5014/ajot.2017.017681

Lubahn, J., & Wolfe, T. L. (2011). Surgical treatment and rehabilitation of tendon ruptures and imbalances of the rheumatoid hand. In T. M. Skirven, A. L. Osterman, J. M. Fedorczyk, & P. C. Amadio (Eds.), *Rehabilitation of the hand and upper extremity* (6th ed., pp. 1399–1407). Mosby.

McDonald, H. N., Dietrich, T., Townsend, A., Li, L. C., Cox, S., & Backman, C. L. (2012). Exploring occupational disruption among women after onset of rheumatoid arthritis. *Arthritis Care & Research*, 64(2), 197–205. https://doi.org/10.1002/acr.20668

Mullen, T. M. (2017). Rheumatic diseases. In B. J. Atchison & D. P. Dirette (Eds.), *Conditions in occupational therapy* (5th ed., pp. 423–446). Wolters Kluwer.

Nicklasson, M., & Jonsson, H. (2012). Experience of participation as described by people with hand deformity caused by rheumatic disease. *British Journal of Occupational Therapy*, 75(1), 29–35. https://doi.org/10.4276/030802212X13261082051418

Packer, M., Williams, M., Samuel, D., & Adams, J. (2016). Hand impairment and functional ability: A matched case comparison study between people with rheumatoid arthritis and healthy controls. *Hand Therapy*, 21(4), 115–122. https://doi.org/10.1177/1758998316666481

Park, Y., & Chang, M. (2016). Effects of rehabilitation for pain relief in patients with rheumatoid arthritis: A systematic review. *Journal of Physical Therapy Science*, 28(1), 304–308. https://doi.org/10.1589/jpts.28.304

Poole, J.., Santhanam, D. D., & Latham, A. L. (2013). Hand impairment and activity limitations in four chronic diseases. *Journal of Hand Therapy*, 26(3), 232–237. https://doi.org/10.1016/j.jht.2013.03.002

Prior, Y., Amanna, A. E., Bodell, S. J., & Hammond, A. (2017). A qualitative evaluation of occupational therapy-led work rehabilitation for people with inflammatory arthritis: Patients' views. *British Journal of Occupational Therapy*, 80(1), 39–48. https://doi.org/10.1177/0308022616672666

Siegel, P., Tencza, M., Apodaca, B., & Poole, J. L. (2017). Effectiveness of occupational therapy interventions for adults with rheumatoid arthritis: A systematic review. *American Journal of Occupational Therapy*, 71(1), Article 7101180050. https://doi.org/10.5014/ajot.2017.023176

Smolen, J. S., Aletaha, D., Grisar, J. C. Stamm, T. A., & Sharp, J. T. (2010). Estimation of a numerical value for joint damage-related physical disability in rheumatoid arthritis clinical trials. *Annals of the Rheumatic Diseases*, 69(6), 1058–1064. https://doi.org/10.1136/ard.2009.114652

Stamm, T. A., Machold, K. P., Smolen, J., & Prodinger, B. (2010). Life stories of people with rheumatoid arthritis who retired early: How gender and other contextual factors shaped their everyday activities, including paid work. *Musculoskeletal Care*, 8(2), 78–86. https://doi.org/10.1002/msc.168

Stoffer, M. A., Smolen, J. S., Woolf, A., Ambrozic, A., Bosworth, A., Carmona, L., Fialka-Moser, V., Loza, E., Olejnik, P., Petersson I. F., Uhlig, T., Stamm, T. A., & eumusc.net-working group. (2014). Development of patient-centered standards of care for rheumatoid arthritis in Europe: The eumusc.net project. *Annals of the Rheumatic Diseases*, 73(5), 902–905. https://doi.org/10.1136/annrheumdis-2013-203743

Taylor-Gjevre, R. M., Mitchell, A., Street, M., Leswick, D. A., Stewart, S. A., & Obaid, H. (2016). The role of radiology in the quantification of digital ulnar deviation in rheumatoid arthritis patients. *Journal of Medical Imaging and Radiation Oncology*, 60(3), 323–328. https://doi.org/10.1111/1754-9485.12454

Terrono, A., Nalebuff, E. A., & Phillips, C. A. (2011). The rheumatoid thumb. In T. M. Skirven, A. L. Osterman, J. M. Fedorczyk, & P. C. Amadio (Eds.), *Rehabilitation of the hand and upper extremity* (6th ed., pp. 1344–1355). Mosby.

Tonga, E., Düger, T., & Karataş, M. (2015). Effectiveness of client-centered occupational therapy in patients with rheumatoid arthritis: Exploratory randomized controlled trail. *Archives of Rheumatology*, 31(1), 6–13. https://doi.org/10.5606/ArchRheumatol.2016.5478

Townsend, A., Backman, C. L., Adam, P., & Li, L. C. (2013). A qualitative interview study: Patient accounts of medication use in early rheumatoid arthritis from symptom onset to early post-diagnosis. *BMJ Open*, 3(2), Article e002164. https://doi.org/10.1136/bmjopen-2012-002164

Townsend, A., Backman, C. L. Adam, P., & Li, L. C. (2014). Women's accounts of help-seeking in early rheumatoid arthritis from symptom onset to diagnosis. *Chronic Illness*, 10(4), 259–272. https://doi.org/10.1177/1742395314520769

Sjögren Syndrome

Also called Sjögren's syndrome, SS.
See also Swallowing Disorders: Adult.

Description

Sjögren syndrome (SS) is a chronic autoimmune systemic, inflammatory disorder of the connective tissue characterized by dry mouth, eyes, and other mucous membranes due to deficient fluid production by the lacrimal and salivary glands. The disorder occurs most frequently among middle-aged women and may occur secondarily to other autoimmune disorders such as rheumatoid arthritis, systemic lupus erythematosus (SLE), systemic sclerosis, and mixed connective tissue disease. The disorder can lead to damage to the cornea and conjunctiva, dental disorders, and loss of taste and odor sensation (O'Toole, 2017; Porter, 2018). In addition, autonomic symptoms are common and may contribute to the overall burden of symptoms (Newton et al., 2012). Major functional impairments are associated with physical fatigue, depression, symptom burden, systemic disease activity, quality of life, mouth dryness, daytime sleepiness, and anxiety (Hackett, Newton, Frith, et al., 2012). For a comprehensive list of symptoms, see Lackner et al., 2017).

Cause

Cause is unknown. Genetic factors may contribute to the development of fatigue (Miyamoto et al., 2019). Fatigue is associated with lower levels of proinflammatory cytokines (Howard Tripp et al., 2016).

Evaluation/Assessment

Areas

- Activities of Daily Living/Instrumental ADL: dry mouth and lips, dysphagia, mouth sores (ulcers), dry skin, vaginal dryness, medication management, gastrointestinal upset
- Education/Work: absenteeism, employment history, employment status
- Play/Leisure: type, location, frequency
- Rest/Sleep: sleep disturbance, daytime sleepiness
- Social Participation: type, location, frequency, with whom
- Sensorimotor: physical fatigue, dry eyes, visual impairment, olfactory (smell), gustatory (taste), pain
- Cognitive/Perceptual: attention, memory, executive function
- Psychosocial: depression, anxiety, mental fatigue, drowsiness
- Context/Environment: knowledge of disorder, social support
- Comorbidities: anemia, celiac disease, diabetes, hypothyroidism, obesity

Instruments

Instruments Developed by Occupational Therapy Personnel

- Canadian Occupational Performance Measure (5th ed.; COPM-5; Law et al., 2014)
- Primary Sjögren's Syndrome-Quality of Life (PSS-QoL; Lackner et al., 2018, in References)

Instruments Developed by Other Professionals and Used by Occupational Therapy Personnel

- Composite Autonomic Symptom Scale (COMPASS; Suarez et al., 1999)
- Epworth Sleepiness Scale (ESS; Johns, 1991)
- European League Against Rheumatism (EULAR) Sjögren's Syndrome Disease Activity Index (ESSDAI; Seror et al., 2010; see also Lendrem et al., 2015, in References)
- European League Against Rheumatism (EULAR) Sjögren's Syndrome Patient Reported Index (ESSPRI; Seror et al., 2011; see also Lendrem et al., 2015, in References)
- European Quality of Life 5-Dimension Scale (EQ-5D; The EuroQol Group, 1990)

- Hospital Anxiety and Depression Scale (HADS; Zigmond & Snaith, 1983)
- Profile of Fatigue and Discomfort (PROFAD) Sicca Symptoms Inventory (SSI; Bowman et al., 2004)

Problems/Issues

Activities of Daily Living/Instrumental ADL

- Person usually complains of dry mouth.
- Person may report difficulty chewing due to lack of saliva.
- Person may report difficulty swallowing (dysphagia) due to lack of saliva.
- Person may report mouth sores (ulcers).
- Person may experience difficulty with speech and communication due to dry mouth.
- Person may experience increased tooth decay and loss of teeth.
- Person may experience dry eyes, including being unable to cry.
- Person may experience shortness of breath.
- Person may experience constipation.
- Person may experience vaginal dryness, which results in pain during intercourse.
- Person may have increased symptoms if taking medications that cause body to eliminate fluids (blood pressure, hypertension medications).
- Person may limit driving due to visual impairments.
- Person may have flare-up of symptoms.
- Person may restrict or stop driving due to visual impairments.

Education/Work

- Person may be unable to work or limit work due to symptoms.

Play/Leisure

- Person may be unable to engage in favorite leisure occupations due to symptoms.

Rest/Sleep (Hackett, Deary, et al., 2018; Hackett et al., 2017)

- Person may experience sleep disturbances due to pain and discomfort.
- Person may have difficulty getting to sleep.
- Person may experience frequent night awakenings.
- Person may experience excess daytime somnolence/sleepiness.
- Person may experience obstructive sleep apnea.

Social Participation

- Person may limit or restrict social activities such as going out to eat with friends.

Sensorimotor

- Person may experience decreased physical energy and increased sense of fatigue.
- Person may report muscle weakness (loss of muscle power).
- Person may experience joint pain (arthralgia).
- Person may experience decreased visual acuity due to dry eyes that may affect the cornea.
- Person may experience glare disability.
- Person may experience difficulty with visual discrimination.
- Person may experience decreased sense of smell.
- Person may experience decreased sense of taste, so food has little or no taste, regardless of flavor or added seasoning.

Cognitive/Perceptual

- Person may have difficulty concentrating and paying attention.
- Person may have difficulty with memory.
- Person may have difficulty with executive functions such as problem solving.

Psychosocial

- Person may experience decreased quality of life.

Context/Environment
- Person may lack a support group.
- Person may lack knowledge of or access to resources.
- Person may report sensitivity to cold temperatures.

Intervention/Treatment

Models and programs developed by occupational therapy personnel include occupational therapy as intervention (Hackett, Newton, & Ng, 2012). Models and programs developed by other professionals but used by occupational therapy personnel include British Society for Rheumatology Guidelines (Price et al., 2017). Team members include physicians, rheumatologists, ophthalmologists, nursing personnel, dentists, physical therapists, and occupational therapy personnel. Goals are to improve person's ability to manage symptoms, make use of available resources, and participate in everyday life occupations.

Activities of Daily Living/Instrumental ADL
- Provide activities to maintain mobility.
- Provide instruction on maintaining good nutrition and health.
- Assist client to prepare foods and meals that are easier to eat.
- Assist in reviewing medications for side effects and making adjustments to avoid aggravating symptoms.
- Review issues with driving to determine if modifications are needed.

Education/Work
- Assist client to identify changes or modifications in the workplace that would facilitate return to work or improve work environment.
- Assist client in making recommendations to employer.

Play/Leisure
- Assist client to explore whether changes or modifications would permit continued engagement in favorite activities such as cooking for others.

Rest/Sleep
- Review sleep routine and make recommendations as needed such as establishing a regular routine to "wind down" before going to bed.
- Review bedding and suggest possible changes such as different mattress, using silk or cotton flannel sheets, weighted blanket.
- Review sleep physical environment for sound (off or minimized), light (dark as possible), temperature (warm), and vibration (on or off as per choice).
- Remove all nonsleep items from the bedroom including computers, crafts, and books.
- Suggest keeping a record of sleep in a sleep diary for discussion.
- Suggest taking a "power nap" during the day for a set time period.
- Talk through thoughts or nightmares that interfere with sleep.

Social Participation
- Assist client to identify social activities that interfere less with symptoms.

Sensorimotor
- Provide a schedule of aerobic physical exercise, which is the only known effective intervention for fatigue (Miyamoto et al., 2019).
- Instruct client in fatigue management including pacing, alternate cycles of work and rest, balancing work and rest, clustering important occupations during time client has most energy.
- Instruct client in energy conservation and motion economy.
- Instruct client in pain management.

Cognitive/Perceptual
- Improve concentration through exercises and training.

- Increase client's self-management skills and sense of empowerment through increased knowledge, use of time and activity scheduling, keeping a diary of symptoms or changes in health status, and practice in problem solving.

Psychosocial
- Instruct in stress management and coping skills such as relaxation training, deep breathing exercises, mindfulness, meditation, and yoga.

Context/Environment
- Assist client to identify and participate in support group.
- Provide client with access to information and resources at local, state, or national level.
- Assist client to develop and practice explaining disorder to family, friends, and others.
- Provide client with opportunity to discuss complementary therapies and alternative remedies including aquatic therapy.
- Assist client to develop empowerment skills (Hackett, Deane, et al., 2018).

Precautions/Safety Considerations
Any changes in type of medication or frequency of taking medication should be discussed with physician.

Prognosis and Outcome
Condition is chronic. Compensatory strategies can increase person's ability to participate in everyday occupations. Clients report that fatigue is the symptom most in need of improvement, along with addressing pain, depression, and daytime sleepiness (Hackett et al., 2019).

REFERENCES
Hackett, K. L., Davies, K., Tarn, J., Bragg, R., Hargreaves, B., Miyamoto, S., McMeekin P., Mitchell, S., Bowman, S., Price, E. J., Pease, C., Emery, P., Andrews, J., Lanyon, P., Hunter, J., Gupta, M., Bombardieri, M., Sutcliffe, N., Pitzalis, C., . . . Ng, W. F. (2019). Pain and depression are associated with both physical and mental fatigue independently of comorbidities and medications in primary Sjögren's syndrome. *RMD Open, 5*(1), Article e000885. http://dx.doi.org/10.1136/rmdopen-2018-000885

Hackett, K. L., Deane, K. H. O., Newton, J. L., Deary, V., Bowman, S. J., Rapley, T., & Ng, W. F. (2018). Mixed-methods study identifying key intervention targets to improve participation in daily living activities in primary Sjögren's syndrome patients. *Arthritis Care and Research 70*(7), 1064–1073. https://doi.org/10.1002/acr.23536

Hackett, K. L., Deary, V., Deane, K. H., Newton, J. L., Ng, W. F., & Rapley, T. (2018). Experience of sleep disruption in primary Sjögren's syndrome: A focus group study. *British Journal of Occupational Therapy, 81*(4), 218–226. https://doi.org/10.1177/0308022617745006

Hackett, K. L., Gotts, Z. M., Ellis, J., Deary, V., Rapley, T., Ng, W. F., Newton, J. L., & Deane, K. H. O. (2017). An investigation into the prevalence of sleep disturbances in primary Sjögren's syndrome: A systematic review of the literature. *Rheumatology 56*(4), 570–580. https://doi.org/10.1093/rheumatology/kew443

Hackett, K. L., Newton, J. L., Frith, J., Elliott, C., Lendrem, D., Foggo, H., Edgar, S., Mitchell, S., & Ng, W.-F. (2012). Impaired functional status in primary Sjögren's syndrome. *Arthritis Care & Research, 64*(11), 1760–1764. https://doi.org/10.1002/acr.21738

Hackett, K. L., Newton, J. L., & Ng, W.-F. (2012). Occupational therapy: A potentially valuable intervention for people with primary Sjögren's syndrome. *British Journal of Occupational Therapy, 75*(5), 247–249. https://doi.org/10.4276/030802212X13361458480441

Howard Tripp, N., Tarn, J., Natasari, A., Gillespie, C., Mitchell, S., Hackett, K. L., Bowman, S. J., Price, E., Pease, C. T., Emery, P., Lanyon, P., Hunter, J., Gupta, M., Bombardieri, M., Sutcliffe, N., Pitzalis, C., McLaren, J., Cooper, A., Regan, M., . . . Ng, W. F. (2016). Fatigue in primary

Sjögren's syndrome is associated with lower levels of proinflammatory cytokines. *RMD Open, 2*(2), Article e000282. https://doi.org/10.1136/rmdopen-2016-000282

Lackner, A., Ficjan, A., Stradner, M., Hermann, J., Unger, J., Stamm, T., Stummvoll, G., Dür, M., Graninger, W. B., & Dejaco, C. (2017). It's more than dryness and fatigue: The patient perspective on health-related quality of life in primary Sjögren's syndrome—A qualitative study. *PLOS ONE, 12*(2), Article e0172056. https://doi.org/10.1371/journal.pone.0172056

Lackner, A., Stradner, M. H., Hermann, J., Unger, J., Stamm, T., Graninger, W. B., & Dejaco, C. (2018). Assessing health-related quality of life in primary Sjögren's syndrome—The PSS-QoL. *Seminars in Arthritis and Rheumatism, 48*(1), 105–110. https://doi.org/10.1016/j.semarthrit.2017.11.007

Lendrem, D., Mitchell, S., McMeekin, P., Gompels, L., Hackett, K., Bowman, S., Price, E., Pease, C. T., Emery, P., Andrews, J., Lanyon, P., Hunter, J., Gupta, M., Bombardieri, M., Sutcliffe, N., Pitzalis, C., McLaren, J., Cooper, A., Regan, M., . . . Ng, W.-F. (2015). Do the EULAR Sjögren's syndrome outcome measures correlate with health status in primary Sjögren's syndrome? *Rheumatology, 54*(4), 655–659. https://doi.org/10.1093/rheumatology/keu361

Miyamoto, S. T., Lendrem, D. W., Ng, W. F., Hackett, K. L., & Valim, V. (2019). Managing fatigue in patients with primary Sjögren's syndrome: Challenges and solutions. *Open Access Rheumatology: Research and Reviews, 11*, 77–88. https://doi.org/10.2147/OARRR.S167990

Newton, J. L., Frith, J., Powell, D., Hackett, K., Wilton, K., Bowman, S., Price, E., Pease, C., Andrews, J., Emery, P., Hunter, J., Gupta, M., Vadivelu, S., Giles, I., Isenberg, D., Lanyon, P., Jones, A., Regan, M., Cooper, A., . . . Ng, W.-F. (2012). Autonomic symptoms are common and are associated with overall symptom burden and disease activity in primary Sjögren's syndrome. *Annals of the Rheumatic Diseases, 71*(12), 1973–1979. https://doi.org/10.1136/annrheumdis-2011-201009

O'Toole, M. T. (Ed.). (2017). *Mosby's dictionary of medicine, nursing & health professions* (10th ed.). Elsevier.

Porter, R. S. (Ed.). (2018). *The Merck manual of diagnosis and therapy* (20th ed.). Merck Sharp & Dohme.

Price, E. J., Rauz, S., Tappuni, A. R., Sutcliffe, N., Hackett, K. L., Barone, F., Granata, G. Ng, W.-F., Fisher, B. A., Bombardieri, M., Astorri, E., Empson, B., Larkin, G., Crampton, B., & Bowman, S. J. (2017). The British Society for Rheumatology guideline for the management of adults with primary Sjögren's syndrome. *Rheumatology, 56*(10), e24–e48. 10.1093/rheumatology/kex375

BIBLIOGRAPHY

Hackett, K. L., Deane, K. H., Strassheim, V., Deary, V., Rapley, T., Newton, J. L., & Ng, W.-F. (2015). A systematic review of non-pharmacological interventions for primary Sjögren's syndrome. *Rheumatology, 54*(11), 2025–2032. https://doi.org/10.1093/rheumatology/kev227

Lewis, I., Hackett, K. L., Ng, W.-F., Ellis, J., & Newton, J. L. (2019). A two-phase cohort study of the sleep phenotype within primary Sjögren's syndrome and its clinical correlates. *Clinical and Experimental Rheumatology, 37*(Suppl. 118), 78–82.

Systemic Disorders

Celiac Disease

Also called celiac sprue, gluten-induced enteropathy, or nontropical sprue.

Description

Celiac disease is an immunologically mediated disease in people who are genetically suscep-tible to gluten intolerance. The disease results in mucosal inflammation and villous atrophy leading to malabsorption. Celiac disease mainly affects people of Northern European descent (Porter, 2018).

Cause

Celiac disease is a hereditary disorder caused by sensitivity to the gliadin fraction of gluten, a protein found in wheat. Similar proteins are present in rye and barley (Porter, 2018). The disease is the result of an inborn error of metabolism characterized by the inability to hydro-lyze peptides contained in gluten (O'Toole, 2017). In genetically susceptible persons, gluten-sensitive T cells are activated when gluten-derived peptide epitopes are present in the digestive system. The inflammatory response causes characteristic mucosal villous atrophy in the small bowel (Porter, 2018).

Evaluation/Assessment

Areas
- Activities of Daily Living/Instrumental ADL: dietary habits (eating wheat-based cereal), re-current abdominal pain, bloating, diarrhea or constipation, weight control
- Education/Work: academic performance, school behavior
- Play/Leisure: type, frequency, interests
- Rest/Sleep: sleep disturbance
- Social Participation: type, frequency, location, with whom
- Sensorimotor: hypotonia, muscle wasting, pallor
- Cognitive/Perceptual: attention, memory, executive functions
- Psychosocial: apathy, withdrawal, isolation, self-efficacy, quality of life
- Context/Environment: caregiver knowledge of disease and diet restrictions, social support, food availability and storage
- Comorbidities: attention-deficit/hyperactivity disorder, failure to thrive, anorexia, cancer in untreated adults

Instruments
Instruments Developed by Occupational Therapy Personnel
- Celiac Disease–Children's Activities Report (CD-Chart; Meyer & Rosenblum, 2017, in References)
- Children's Leisure Assessment Scale (CLASS; Rosenblum et al., 2010)

Instruments Developed by Other Professionals and Used by Occupational Therapy Personnel
- Celiac Disease DUX (CDDUX; van Doorn et al., 2008; see also Meyer & Rosenblum, 2016, in References)

Problems/Issues

Activities of Daily Living/Instrumental ADL
- Child may have limited food choices that are gluten free.
- Child may have to eat foods that are different from those served to other family members.

Education/Work
- Child may not be able to participate in school meals or snacks or acquire special gluten-free foods.

- Child may lack energy to focus on academic tasks if gluten-free diet is not maintained.
- Child may act out or exhibit other behavioral problems in school if gluten-free diet is not maintained.

Play/Leisure
- Child may not engage in leisure activities that involve preparing and eating foods.

Rest/Sleep
- Child may experience sleep disturbance due to body reactions to presence of gluten in the system.

Social Participation
- Child may not be able to eat at restaurants that do not have a gluten-free menu choice.
- Child may not be able to eat food served at social event (home, school, community) because there are no gluten-free options.

Sensorimotor
- Child may experience muscle weakness and pain if gluten-free diet is not maintained.

Cognitive/Perceptual
- Child may have difficulty remembering which foods are gluten free.
- Child needs to learn to read food labels for gluten-based products.

Psychosocial
- Child may resent being "different" from others, especially when food is being served.
- Child may withdraw or refuse to participate in certain activities where food is served if gluten-free options are not available.
- Child may experience apathy or decreased motivation if gluten-free diet is not maintained.
- Child may become irritable or display other behavioral problems if gluten-free diet is not maintained.

Context/Environment
- Special arrangements may be needed in the home to separate gluten-free foods from those that are not, such as separate refrigerator or pantry space.
- Family and friends may not understand the importance of maintaining a gluten-free diet.
- Family or caregivers may avoid eating out or limit eating out to only gluten-free restaurants rather than risk encountering foods that are not gluten free.
- Family or caregivers may limit travel to avoid situations where gluten-free food may not be available.

Intervention/Treatment

Models and programs developed by occupational therapy personnel: None identified. Models and programs developed by other professionals but used by occupational therapy personnel: None identified. Team members include physicians, psychologists, dieticians and nutritionists, educational personal, caregivers, and occupational therapy personnel. Goals are to enable the child to participate in everyday activities while maintaining a gluten-free diet.

Activities of Daily Living/Instrumental ADL
- Assist client and caregivers to read labels, purchase and prepare foods that are gluten free; rice and corn are good substitutes (O'Toole, 2017).
- Client and caregivers need a detailed list of foods to avoid that contain wheat, rye, or barley.
- Consider joint sessions with a dietician or nutritionist.
- Bloating, diarrhea, or constipation may be signs that compliance with gluten-free diet is not being maintained.

Education/Work
- Review with client and caregivers whether gluten-free foods are available at school or make arrangements to have child take food to school and have a place to keep it.

Play/Leisure
- Encourage engagement in play and leisure activities, but monitor those in which food may be involved to ensure compliance with gluten-free diet.

Rest/Sleep
- Sleep disturbance may be a sign that compliance to gluten-free diet is not being maintained.

Social Participation
- Encourage participation in social activities with ideas for managing eating situations.
- Encourage client to inform friends about what foods can and cannot be eaten and why it is important to adhere to the diet.

Sensorimotor
- No information identified.

Cognitive/Perceptual
- Assist client to plan ahead to anticipate whether eating is involved, such as taking gluten-free food along (a "munchy" bag) or checking to see whether gluten-free food is available at places where eating is expected to occur.
- Assist client to problem solve in unexpected situations where no gluten-free food is available or food may not be gluten free.
- Assist client to develop self-management strategies.
- Assist client to learn to read and understand food packaging labels.
- Assist client to create a list or identify a list on cell phone of allowable foods.

Psychosocial
- Encourage discussion with child or adolescent to assist in understanding why adherence to gluten-free diet is important to health and well-being, and methods of coping with temptations to "go off the diet."

Context/Environment
- Provide information on available community and internet resources.
- Encourage participation in a social support group.
- Divide refrigerator into gluten-free foods and "everything else."
- Family can practice collecting gluten-free recipes and preparing or baking gluten-free foods.

Precautions/Safety Considerations

Person must always be aware of food-related activities, roles, and strategies that support or hinder factors in everyday life (Meyer & Rosenblum, 2018). Person may also be lactose intolerant, requiring elimination of milk products. Person is at risk for cancer if gluten-free diet is not maintained throughout life.

Prognosis and Outcome

Prognosis is good if person remains on a gluten-free diet. Disease is a chronic, lifelong condition that must be managed daily.

REFERENCES

Meyer, S., & Rosenblum, S. (2016). Children with celiac disease: Health-related quality of life and leisure participation. *American Journal of Occupational Therapy, 70*(6), Article 7006220010. https://doi.org/10.5014/ajot.2016.020594

Meyer, S., & Rosenblum, S. (2017). Development and validation of the Celiac Disease-Children's Activities Report (CD-Chart) for promoting self-management among children and adolescents. *Nutrients*, 9(10), Article 1130. https://doi.org/10.3390/nu9101130

Meyer, S., & Rosenblum, S. (2018). Daily experiences and challenges among children and adolescents with celiac disease: Focus group results. *Journal of Pediatric Gastroenterology and Nutrition*, 66(1), 58–63. https://doi.org/10.1097/MPG.0000000000001635

O'Toole, M. T. (Ed.). (2017). *Mosby's dictionary of medicine, nursing & health professions* (10th ed.). Elsevier.

Porter, R. S. (Ed.). (2018). *The Merck manual of diagnosis and therapy* (20th ed.). Merck Sharp & Dohme.

BIBLIOGRAPHY

Meyer, S., & Rosenblum, S. (2017). Activities, Participation and quality of life concepts in children and adolescents with celiac disease: A scoping review. *Nutrients*, 9(9), Article 929. https://doi.org/10.3390/nu9090929

Chronic Fatigue Syndrome

Also called CFS, myalgic encephalomyelitis, ME, systemic exertion intolerance disease, SEID, neurasthenia, febricula, effort syndrome, immune dysfunction syndrome.

Description

Chronic fatigue syndrome (CFS) is a syndrome of life-altering fatigue lasting more than 6 months that is unexplained and is accompanied by various symptoms, including sleep disorders, mental cloudiness, impaired memory or concentration, fatigue, muscle pain, multijoint pain, sore throat, headache, and exacerbation of symptoms with activity (postexertional malaise). The disorder is most common in young and middle-aged women (O'Toole, 2017; Porter, 2018). Diagnostic criteria continue to be explored (Meeus et al., 2016).

Cause

Cause is unknown. No infectious, hormonal, immunologic, or psychiatric cause been established. Some genetic markers may predispose a person to CFS (Porter, 2018). Differences in autonomous response between clients and health controls has been observed (Van Cauwenbergh et al., 2014). Diagnostic criteria proposed by the Institute of Medicine (2015; now the Health and Medicine division of the National Academies of Sciences, Engineering, and Medicine) are as follows:

- Three symptoms
  - A substantial reduction or impairment in the ability to engage in pre-illness levels of occupational, educational, social, or personal activities that persists for more than 6 months and is accompanied by fatigue, which is often profound, is at new or definite onset (not lifelong), is not the result of ongoing excessive exertion, and is not substantially alleviated by rest.
  - Postexertional malaise.
  - Unrefreshing sleep.
- At least one of the following manifestations is also required:
  - Cognitive impairment.
  - Orthostatic intolerance.

Evaluation/Assessment

Areas

- Activities of Daily Living/Instrumental ADL: difficulty speaking, anomia, weight changes

- Education/Work: work experience, work tasks
- Play/Leisure: interests, values, frequency, location
- Rest/Sleep: sleep disturbance, nonrestorative sleep, nightmares
- Social Participation: types, frequency, location, with whom
- Sensorimotor: kinesiophobia, muscle weakness, endurance, fatigue, pain, headaches, seizure, numbness or tingling, balance disturbance, intolerance to bright lights, altered sense of taste, smell, or hearing (tinnitus)
- Cognitive/Perceptual: attention, memory, executive functions, blackouts, spatial relations
- Psychosocial: depression, anxiety, emotional lability (mood swings), personality changes, quality of life
- Context/Environment: knowledge of disorder, social support, resources
- Comorbidities: fibromyalgia, multiple sclerosis

Instruments

Instruments Developed by Occupational Therapy Personnel

- Canadian Occupational Performance Measure (5th ed.; COPM-5; Law et al., 2014)

Instruments Developed by Other Professionals and Used by Occupational Therapy Personnel

- Checklist Individual Strength (CIS; Vercoulen et al., 1994)
- Chronic Fatigue Syndrome-Activities and Participation Questionnaire (CFS-APQ; Nijs et al., 2002)
- Chronic Fatigue Syndrome–Symptom List (CFS-SL; De Becker et al., 2001)
- Short-Form 36 Health Survey (SF-36; Ware et al., 1993)
- Tampa Scale of Kinesiophobia–Chronic Fatigue Syndrome version (TSK-CFS; Nijs et al., 2004)

Problems/Issues

Activities of Daily Living/Instrumental ADL

- Person may frequently say the wrong word or have difficulty finding the right word.
- Person many have difficulty with calculation (doing basic math).

Education/Work

- Person may be unable to attend school or complete work tasks due to ongoing fatigue or muscle pain.

Rest/Sleep

- Person reports that sleep in not refreshing or restorative.
- Person may report feeling tired all or most of the time.
- Person may feel sleepy or drowsy all or most of the time.
- Person may report frequent or unusual nightmares.

Social Participation

- Person may restrict or stop participation in social activities.

Sensorimotor

- Person may have severe muscle weakness.
- Person may report muscle pain and headaches.
- Person many lack energy and endurance.
- Person may require prolonged rest time following physical exertion.
- Person may have difficulty with balance (disequilibrium).
- Person may have seizures.
- Person may have changes in visual acuity.
- Person may be intolerant of bright lights.
- Person may report ringing in the ears (tinnitus).
- Person may report changes or alterations of taste and smell.

Cognitive/Perceptual
- Person may have difficulty concentrating or paying attention.
- Person may have difficulty remembering.
- Person may experience spatial disorientation.
- Person may experience temporal change (Pemberton & Cox, 2014b).

Psychosocial
- Person may be depressed.
- Person may have feelings of anxiety.
- Person may exhibit emotional lability (mood swings).
- Person may exhibit personality changes or increased severity.
- Person may change amount of performance in certain roles (reduce or increase).
- Person may experience decreased sense of competency (Taylor et al., 2010).

Context/Environment
- Person may lack knowledge about chronic fatigue syndrome and its management.
- Person may lack access to community and internet resources.

Intervention/Treatment

Models and programs developed by occupational therapy personnel include Support, Empower and Employ people with ME (SEE ME; Wright & Chowdhury, 2017). Models and programs developed by other professionals but used by occupational therapy personnel include activity pacing self-management (Kos et al., 2015) and group-based self-management program (Pinxsterhuis, Hellum, et al., 2015; Pinxsterhuis et al., 2017; Pinxsterhuis, Strand, et al., 2015). Team members include physicians, psychologists, physical therapists, exercise physiologists, kinesiotherapists, and occupational therapy personnel. Goals include increasing perceived performance of and satisfaction with desired daily life activities (Kos et al., 2015).

Activities of Daily Living/Instrumental ADL
- Review daily routine focusing on meaningful occupations.

Education/Work
- Discuss with client what aspects of work are causing the most concern.
- Recommend strategies to address concerns.
- Assist client to work with employer to minimize or eliminate concerns.

Play/Leisure
- Review with client major leisure occupations and issues that may limit engagement.
- Recommend strategies to overcome limitations.
- Suggest client may want to explore new leisure occupations that are within functional limits.

Rest/Sleep
- Review sleep habits and routines for possible changes to improve quality of sleep.
- Review sleep environment (bedding, mattress, lighting, sound) for possible modifications to improve quality of sleep.

Social Participation
- Encourage participation in social activities.
- Suggest strategies that may enable participation at level client can tolerate such as having one or two friends come to the house, going for short walks, going out for 1 hour, or other limitations client can tolerate.

Sensorimotor
- Discuss with client feelings about possible dangers of movement and realistic outcomes.
- Provide a graded exercise program starting with short, easy to do, sitting down exercises and gradually increase program to standing and moving.

- Consider instruction in energy conservation and motion economy (break tasks into small units, sit rather than stand, prioritize which tasks are most important).
- Instruct in fatigue management (work and rest breaks, cluster to-do tasks during time with most energy, share tasks with other family members).
- Instruct in pain management (plan ahead, schedule rest times, perform tasks when pain is more tolerable).

Cognitive/Perceptual
- Provide exercises to increase attention and concentration.
- Provide memory training or use of memory aids.
- Provide practice in problem solving.
- Provide instruction in self-management including activity pacing.

Psychosocial
- Provide instruction and practice in coping strategies and stress reduction exercises (deep breathing, mindfulness, yoga).
- Provide activity to decrease depressive symptoms.
- Discuss issues with client that cause anxiety and possible solutions.
- Assist person to resume meaningful roles.
- Assist client to focus on believing in what can be done (positivity) instead of lamenting what cannot be done (negativity; Pemberton & Cox, 2014a).
- Assist client to develop a coherent interaction between body, occupational life, and social self (Njølstad et al., 2019).

Context/Environment
- Provide information on CFS, its management, and its impact on daily life.
- Provide information on accessing community and internet resources.

Precautions/Safety Considerations

Clients should be made aware that many sham cures that are unproven or disproven have been advertised and should be avoided; some may be harmful.

Prognosis and Outcome

Most clients improve over time, but not necessarily to their previous level of function. Functional improvement may occur over years (Porter, 2018).

REFERENCES

Institute of Medicine. (2015). *Beyond myalgic encephalomyelitis/chronic fatigue syndrome: Redefining an illness*. National Academies Press. https://doi.org/10.17226/19012

Kos, D., van Eupen, I., Meirte, J., Van Cauwenbergh, D., Moorkens, G., Meeus, M., & Nijs, J. (2015). Activity pacing self-management in chronic fatigue syndrome: A randomized controlled trial. *American Journal of Occupational Therapy, 69*(5), Article 6905290020. https://doi.org/10.5014/ajot.2015.016287

Meeus, M., Ickmans, K., Struyf, F., Kos, D., Lambrecht, L., Willekens, B., Cras, P., & Nijs, J. (2016). What is in a name? Comparing diagnostic criteria for chronic fatigue syndrome with or without fibromyalgia. *Clinical Rheumatology, 35*, 191–203. https://doi.org/10.1007/s10067-014-2793-x

Njølstad, B. W., Mengshoel, A. M., & Sveen, U. (2019). "It's like being a slave to your own body in a way": A qualitative study of adolescents with chronic fatigue syndrome. *Scandinavian Journal of Occupational Therapy, 26*(7), 505–514. https://doi.org/10.1080/11038128.2018.1455895

O'Toole, M. T. (Ed.). (2017). *Mosby's dictionary of medicine, nursing & health professions* (10th ed.). Elsevier.

Pemberton, S., & Cox, D. L. (2014a). Experiences of daily activity in chronic fatigue syndrome/myalgic encephalomyelitis (CFS/ME) and their implications for rehabilitation programmes. *Disability and Rehabilitation, 36*(21), 1790–1797. https://doi.org/10.3109/09638288.2013.874503

Pemberton, S., & Cox, D. (2014b). Perspectives of time and occupation: Experiences of people with chronic fatigue syndrome/myalgic encephalomyelitis. *Journal of Occupational Science, 21*(4), 488–503. https://doi.org/10.1080/14427591.2013.804619

Pinxsterhuis, I., Hellum, L., Aannestad, H., & Sveen, U. (2015). Development of a group-based self-management programme for individuals with chronic fatigue syndrome: A pilot study. *Scandinavian Journal of Occupational Therapy, 22*(2), 117–125. https://doi.org/10.3109/11038128.2014.985608

Pinxsterhuis, I., Sandvik, L., Strand, E. B., Bautz-Holter, E., & Sveen, U. (2017). Effectiveness of a group-based self-management program for people with chronic fatigue syndrome: A randomized controlled trial. *Clinical Rehabilitation, 31*(1), 93–103. https://doi.org/10.1177/0269215515621362

Pinxsterhuis, I., Strand, E. B., Stormorken, E., & Sveen, U. (2015). From chaos and insecurity to understanding and coping: Experienced benefits of a group-based education programme for people with chronic fatigue syndrome. *British Journal of Guidance & Counselling, 43*(4), 463–475. https://doi.org/10.1080/03069885.2014.987725

Porter, R. S. (Ed.). (2018). *The Merck manual of diagnosis and therapy* (20th ed.). Merck Sharp & Dohme.

Taylor, R., O'Brien, J., Kielhofner, G., Lee, S., Katz, B., & Mears, C. (2010). The occupational and quality of life consequences of chronic fatigue syndrome/myalgic encephalomyelitis in young people. *British Journal of Occupational Therapy, 73*(11), 524–530. https://doi.org/10.4276/030802210X12892992239233

Van Cauwenbergh, D., Nijs, J., Kos, D., Van Weijnen, L., Struyf, F., & Meeus, M. (2014). Malfunctioning of the autonomic nervous system in patients with chronic fatigue syndrome: A systematic literature review. *European Journal of Clinical Investigation, 44*(5), 516–526. https://doi.org/10.1111/eci.12256

Wright, F., & Chowdhury, S. (2017). Seeing improvements with SEE ME. *OT News, 25*(5), 15–18.

BIBLIOGRAPHY

Pinxsterhuis, J., Strand, E. B., & Sveen, U. (2015). Coping with chronic fatigue syndrome: A review and synthesis of qualitative studies. *Fatigue: Biomedicine, Health & Behavior, 3*(3), 173–188. https://doi.org/10.1080/21641846.2015.1035519

Vergauwen, K., Huijnen, I. P. J., Kos, D., Van de Velde, D., van Eupen, I., & Meeus, M. (2015). Assessment of activity limitations and participation restrictions with persons with chronic fatigue syndrome: A systematic review. *Disability and Rehabilitation, 37*(19), 1706–1716. https://doi.org/10.3109/09638288.2014.978507

Diabetes Mellitus (Type 1 and Type 2)

Note: The terms used to describe the age of onset (juvenile or adult/maturity) or type of treatment (insulin-dependent versus non-insulin-dependent) are no longer accurate because of the overlapping of age groups and interventions used to treat the disease types.

Description

Diabetes mellitus (DM) is a metabolic disorder that involves impaired insulin secretion and varying degrees of peripheral insulin resistance leading to hyperglycemia (high levels of glucose in the blood; Porter, 2018).

Cause

Type 1 diabetes mellitus is caused by a total lack of insulin, usually occurring when the body's immune system is attacked and the insulin-producing beta cells in the pancreas are unable to function or are destroyed (insulitis; Porter, 2018; *Stedman's*, 2011). Type 2 diabetes mellitus is caused by either insufficient production of insulin or the inability of the body to use insulin efficiently (*Stedman's*, 2011).

Evaluation/Assessment

Areas

- Activities of Daily Living/Instrumental ADL: nutrition and healthy eating, meal planning and preparation, diet and weight control, general fitness and wellness, medication management, glucose and lipid monitoring, mobility, dental care
- Education/Work: academic performance, work performance
- Play/Leisure: interests and values, frequency, location
- Rest/Sleep: sleep disturbance
- Social Participation: type, frequency, location, with whom
- Sensorimotor: joint range of motion, exercise program, peripheral neuropathy especially in feet, visual impairment, sensory processing
- Cognitive/Perceptual: executive functioning (problem solving, time management, and scheduling)
- Psychosocial: stress management and coping, depression, anxiety, burnout, guilt, quality of life
- Context/Environment: diabetes education, community resources, social support
- Comorbidities: obesity, arthritis, diabetic neuropathy, amputation, depression, erectile dysfunction, hypoglycemia, diabetic ketoacidosis, cardiovascular condition, coronary artery disease, hypertension, peripheral arterial disease, retinopathy, kidney failure, carpal tunnel syndrome, stiff hand syndrome, smoking or other substance abuse

Instruments

Instruments Developed by Occupational Therapy Personnel

- Adolescent/Adult Sensory Profile (AASP; Brown & Dunn, 2002)
- Arthritis Hand Function Test (AHFT; Bachman & Mackie, 1997)
- Canadian Occupational Performance Measure (5th ed.; COPM-5; Law et al., 2014)
- Community Integration Measure (CIM; McColl et al., 2001; see also Janet & LeAnne, 2016, in References)
- Hand Mobility in Scleroderma (HAMIS; Sandqvist & Eklund, 2000; see also Poole et al., 2010, in References)

Instruments Developed by Other Professionals and Used by Occupational Therapy Personnel

- Activities-Specific Balance Confidence (ABC) Scale (Powell & Myers, 1995)
- Adapted Illness Intrusiveness Ratings (AIIR; Self-Management Resource Center, 2007)
- Berg Balance Scale (BBS; Berg et al., 1989)
- Center of Epidemiologic Studies Depression Scale (CES-D; Radloff, 1977)
- Cochin Hand Function Scale (CHFS; see Hand Function Disability Scale; HFDS; see also Poole et al., 2010, in References)
- Diabetes-39 (D-39; Boyer & Earp, 1997)
- Dreiser's Functional Hand Index (DFHI; see Functional Index for Hand Osteoarthritis)
- Frenchay Activities Index (FAI; Holbrook & Skilbeck, 1983)
- Functional Index for Hand Osteoarthritis (FIHOA; Dreiser et al., 2000; see also Poole et al., 2010, in References)
- Hand Function Disability Scale (HFDS; Duruöz et al., 1996)
- Health Assessment Questionnaire (HAQ; Bruce & Fries, 2003)
- Keitel Functional Test (KFT; Holm et al., 2008; see also Poole et al., 2010, in References)

- Michigan Hand Outcomes Questionnaire (MHQ; Chung et al., 1998; see also Poole et al., 2010, in References)
- National Institutes of Health Toolbox Somatosensory Domain (Dunn et al., 2013)
- Short-Form 36 Health Survey (SF-36; Ware et al., 1993)
- Social/Role Activities Limitations Scale (S/RALS; Lorig et al., 1996)
- Stanford Diabetes Self-Efficacy Scale (SDSES; Lorig et al., 2009)
- Stanford Health Assessment Questionnaire (see Health Assessment Questionnaire)
- Summary of Diabetes Self-Care Activities (SDSCA) questionnaire (Toobert et al., 1994)
- World Health Organization Quality of Life Questionnaire BREF (WHOQOL-BREF; The WHOQOL Group, 1998)

Problems/Issues

Activities of Daily Living/Instrumental ADL
- Person may lack ability to plan and prepare nutritious, healthy meals, following a diet.
- Person may lack fitness.
- Person may have difficulty accurately measuring blood glucose level.
- Person may have difficulty managing medication schedules.
- Person may be overweight or obese or may experience loss of weight.
- Person may experience frequent urination.
- Person may experience excessive thirst or hunger.

Education/Work
- Person may be inconsistent in attending school or showing up for work.
- Person may perform poorly in the classroom or work setting.

Play/Leisure
- Person may experience limitations in ability to engage in favorite leisure activities.
- Person may feel that self-management program interferes with engagement in valued leisure activities.

Rest/Sleep
- No information identified.

Social Participation
- Person may limit participation in social activities to avoid food issues.

Sensorimotor
- Person may experience limited joint mobility and stiffness in the hands.
- Person may experience decreased grip strength.
- Person may experience loss of dexterity (Yang et al., 2015).
- Person may experience lack of energy and fatigue.
- Person may experience blurred vision or low vision (Sokol-McKay, 2010).
- Person may experience increase difficulty in processing sensory information if the glycemic level is uncontrolled in kinesthesia, tactile sensation, and stereognosis (Engel-Yeger et al., 2018; Kim et al., 2016).

Cognitive/Perceptual
- Person may not have clear goals in life, which may contribute to failing to follow self-management program (Haltiwanger, 2012b).

Psychosocial
- Person may exhibit poor self-management skills, including daily management requirements.
- Person may experience a poor quality of life related to poor management of diabetes.
- Person may deny or hide diagnosis because of social concerns about appearance of health status.
- Person may be or become depressed (Wu et al., 2018).

Context/Environment
- Person, family, or caregivers may lack access to diabetic care or refuse to fully participate in available services.
- Person may live in a stressful home situation (homelessness, violence and abuse, absent parent, foster care, substance abuse in the home).
- Community services may not be available, especially a multidisciplinary team knowledgeable about diabetes.

Intervention/Treatment

Models and programs developed by occupational therapy personnel include exercise programs (Londhe & Ferzandi, 2012), group program (Haltiwanger, 2012a), Lifestyle Redesign (Pyatak et al., 2019), managing diabetes with physical limitations (Sokol-McKay, 2013), manualized occupation-based program (Carandang & Pyatak, 2018), model of human occupation (Youngson, 2019), occupation-based activities self-management programs (Gardener et al., 2017; Piven & Duran, 2014), occupational therapy role (Sokol-McKay, 2019), strategies list (Pyatak, 2011a, 2011b), and vision rehabilitation with diabetes (Sokol-McKay, 2010). Models and programs developed by other professionals but used by occupational therapy personnel include Diabetes Empowerment Council (Weigensberg et al., 2018), group education sessions (Dahl-Popolizio et al., 2017), Let's Empower and Prepare (LEAAP; Sequeira et al., 2015), multidisciplinary diabetes self-management training class (Hreha & Noce, 2018), peer-led support group (Haltiwanger & Brutus, 2012), peer mentoring program (Lu et al., 2015), Resilient, Empowered, Active Living with Diabetes (REAL Diabetes; Pyatak et al., 2015; Pyatak, Carandang, et al., 2018), self-management (Cahill et al., 2016; Fritz, 2014; Mailoo et al., 2016; Pyatak, 2011a, 2011b), structured transition program (Pyatak et al., 2017), type 2 diabetes education program (Al-Bannay et al., 2015), and yoga/hatha yoga (Schmid et al., 2018; Van Puymbroeck et al., 2018). Team members include physicians, nursing personnel, psychologists and school counselors, physical therapists, dieticians or nutritionists, health and diabetic educators, classroom teachers, teacher's aides, social workers, and occupational therapy personnel. Goal is to "educate and train persons at risk for or who currently have diabetes to modify current habits and routines and develop new ones to promote a healthier lifestyle and minimize disease progression" (Sokol-McKay, 2011, p. 1). Intervention techniques should include self-management; leisure, social, and community activities; and fall risk management (Atler et al., 2018).

Activities of Daily Living/Instrumental ADL
- Meal management: Portions can be controlled by the Plate Method: one quarter of plate for protein (e.g., chicken), one quarter for starch (e.g., potato), and one half for nonstarchy vegetables (mixed carrots, onions, and zucchini).
- Snacks: Help person make healthy choices with ordering from a menu or picking a snack.
- Medication schedule: Suggest medications be tied to another activity that occurs regularly, such as eating meals, listening to a certain program.
- Fitness: Assist person to develop a program of physical activity that includes U.S. Department of Agriculture recommendation for 150 minutes of moderate intensity physical activity a week, preferably for 30 minutes a day.
- Habits and routines: Assist person to incorporate diabetes management program into daily activities (Pyatak, 2011a, 2011b).

Education/Work
- Assist client to locate space at school or work to perform diabetes self-management tasks.
- Assist client to develop a means to carry diabetes supplies (monitor, strips, insulin, emergency supplies).

Play/Leisure
- Assist client to find alternate leisure activities to compensate for lack of participation in activities such as ordering sugar-loaded desserts.

Rest/Sleep
- No information identified.

Social Participation
- Assist client to develop a social support group that is understanding of diabetes and self-management.

Sensorimotor
- Provide exercise program that includes both balance and resistance training exercises (Londhe & Ferzandi, 2012).
- Provide pain program focusing on upper extremities and spine.
- Provide fatigue management program.
- Provide program of information and inspection management to prevent peripheral neuropathy progression.
- Develop a strategy for inconspicuous blood checks and insulin injects if needed.

Cognitive/Perceptual
- Assist client to develop a schedule that allows time for managing diabetes at home, school, community, and travel.

Psychosocial
- Provide emotional support for depression and anxiety.
- Provide stress management and coping program: mindfulness, progressive relaxation exercises, yoga (Van Puymbroeck et al., 2018).
- Assist client to deal with stigma associated with diabetes.

Context/Environment
- Provide information and education to family and caregivers regarding diabetes as a disorder and its management long term.
- Provide skills in managing diabetes on one's own, use of monitoring devices, sports and exercise, social situations, emergencies (glucose level too high or too low), inflexible schedule management, and general management skills.
- Assist client to talk to others about being a diabetic and following a diabetic management program.

Precautions/Safety Considerations

Person is at risk for injury to feet if diabetic neuropathy, especially loss of sensation to the feet, is present. Person is at risk for injury if retinopathy is present and cannot be corrected to provide good vision; low vision techniques may be required.

Prognosis and Outcome

Diabetes, once diagnosed, is a chronic condition. Management can reduce the severity of the disorder and its effects on body systems. Poor management may result in several additional health-related problems (listed under Comorbidities, above). Treatment adherence has beneficial impact on body mass index (weight), lipid control, and glycemic control (Marinho et al., 2018). Nonadherence issues, including psychological and social stresses, should be addressed (Pyatak, Florindez, & Weigensberg, 2013; Pyatak, Sequeira, et al., 2013).

REFERENCES
Al-Bannay, H. R., Jongbloed, L. E., Jarus, T., Alabdulwahab, S. S., Khoja, T. A., & Dean, E. (2015). Outcomes of a type 2 diabetes education program adapted to the cultural contexts of Saudi women: A pilot study. *Saudi Medical Journal, 36*(7), 869–873. https://doi.org/10.15537/smj.2015.7.11681

Atler, K. E., Schmid, A. A., Klinedinst, T. C., Grimm, L. A., Marchant, T. P., Marchant, D. R., & Malcolm, M. P. (2018). The relationship between quality of life, activity and participation among people with type 2 diabetes mellitus. *Occupational Therapy in Health Care, 32*(4), 341–362. https://doi.org/10.1080/07380577.2018.1522017

Cahill, S. M., Polo, K. M., Egan, B. E., & Marasti, N. (2016). Interventions to promote diabetes self-management in children and youth: A scoping review. *American Journal of Occupational Therapy, 70*(5), Article 7005180020. https://doi.org/10.5014/ajot.2016.021618

Carandang, K. M., & Pyatak, E. A. (2018). Feasibility of a manualized occupation-based diabetes management intervention. *American Journal of Occupational Therapy, 72*(2), Article 7202345040. https://doi.org/10.5014/ajot.2018.021790

Dahl-Popolizio, S., Rogers, O., Muir, S., Carroll, J. K., & Manson, L. (2017). Interprofessional primary care: The value of occupational therapy. *Open Journal of Occupational Therapy, 5*(3), Article 11. https://doi.org/10.15453/2168-6408.1363

Engel-Yeger, B., Darawsha Najjar, S., & Darawsha, M. (2018). The relationship between health related quality of life and sensory deficits among patients with diabetes mellitus. *Disability and Rehabilitation, 40*(25), 3005–3011. https://doi.org/10.1080/09638288.2017.1365382

Fritz, H. (2014). The influence of daily routines on engaging in diabetes self-management. *Scandinavian Journal of Occupational Therapy, 21*(3), 232–240. https://doi.org/10.3109/110 38128.2013.868033

Gardener, L., Bourke-Taylor, H., & Ziviani, J. (2017). Occupational therapy: An untapped resource for children and adolescents with type 1 diabetes. *Australian Occupational Therapy Journal, 64*(1), 79–82. https://doi.org/10.1111/1440-1630.12312

Haltiwanger, E. P. (2012a). Effect of a group adherence intervention for Mexican-American older adults with type 2 diabetes. *American Journal of Occupational Therapy, 66*(4), 447–454. https://doi.org/10.5014/ajot.2012.004457

Haltiwanger, E. P. (2012b). Experience of Mexican-American elders with diabetes: A phenomenological study. *Occupational Therapy in Health Care, 26*(2-3), 150–162. https://doi.org/10 .3109/07380577.2012.694585

Haltiwanger E. P., & Brutus, H. (2012). A culturally sensitive diabetes peer support for older Mexican-Americans. *Occupational Therapy International, 19*(2), 67–75. https://doi. org/10.1002/oti.320

Hreha, K., & Noce, N. (2018). Implementation of a multidisciplinary diabetes self-management training class in acute rehabilitation. *Occupational Therapy in Health Care, 32*(4), 412–421. https://doi.org/10.1080/07380577.2018.1525509

Janet, L. P., & LeAnne, H. M. (2016). Validity of the Community Integration Questionnaire as a measure of participation in persons with diabetes mellitus. *Journal of Diabetes & Metabolism, 7*(7), Article 1000687. https://doi.org/10.4172/2155-6156.1000687

Kim, Y. J., Rogers, J. C., Kwok, G., Dunn, W., & Holm, M. B. (2016). Somatosensation differences in older adults with and without diabetes, and by age group. *Occupational Therapy in Health Care, 30*(3), 231–244. https://doi.org/10.3109/07380577.2015.1136758

Londhe, A. A., & Ferzandi, Z. D. (2012). Comparison of balance and resistive exercises versus balance exercises alone in patients with diabetic peripheral neuropathy. *Indian Journal of Occupational Therapy, 44*(2), 3–9.

Lu, Y., Pyatak, E. A., Peters, A. L., Wood, J. R., Kipke, M., Cohen, M., & Sequeira, P. A. (2015). Patient perspectives on peer mentoring: Type 1 diabetes management in adolescents and young adults. *Diabetes Educator, 41*(1), 59–68. https://doi.org/10.1177/0145721714559133

Mailoo, V. J., Best, N., Cheal, S., Kelly, F., & Turner, J. (2016). Interplay between type-1 diabetes and occupation: Results from a pilot study. *Asian Journal of Occupational Therapy, 12*(1), 1–7. https://doi.org/10.11596/asiajot.12.1

Marinho, F. S., Moram, C. B. M., Rodrigues, P. C., Leite, N. C., Salles, G. F., & Cardoso, C. R. L. (2018). Treatment adherence and its associated factors in patients with type 2 diabetes:

Results from the Rio de Janeiro type 2 diabetes cohort study. *Journal of Diabetes Research, 2018*, Article 8970196. https://doi.org/10.1155/2018/8970196

Piven, E., & Duran, R. (2014). Reduction of non-adherent behaviour in a Mexican-American adolescent with type 2 diabetes. *Occupational Therapy International, 21*(1), 42–51. https://doi.org/10.1002/oti.1363

Poole, J. L., Gonzales, I., & Tedesco, T. (2010). Self-reports of hand function in persons with diabetes. *Occupational Therapy in Health Care, 24*(3), 239–248. https://doi.org/10.3109/07380571003793957

Porter, R. S. (Ed.). (2018). *The Merck manual of diagnosis and therapy* (20th ed.). Merck Sharp & Dohme.

Pyatak, E. (2011a). Participation in occupation and diabetes self-management in emerging adulthood. *American Journal of Occupational Therapy, 65*(4), 462–469. https://doi.org/10.5014/ajot.2011.001453

Pyatak, E. A. (2011b). The role of occupational therapy in diabetes self-management interventions. *OTJR: Occupation, Participation and Health, 31*(2), 89–96. https://doi.org/10.3928/15394492-20100622-01

Pyatak, E. A., Carandang, K., & Davis, S. (2015). Developing a manualized occupational therapy diabetes management intervention: Resilient, Empowered, Active Living with Diabetes. *OTJR: Occupation, Participation and Health, 35*(3), 187–194. https://doi.org/10.1177/1539449215584310

Pyatak, E. A., Carandang, K., Vigen, C. L. P., Blanchard, J., Diaz, J., Concha-Chavez, A., Sequeira, P. A., Wood, J. R., Whittemore, R., Spruijt-Metz, D., & Peters, A. L. (2018). Occupational therapy intervention improves glycemic control and quality of life among young adults with diabetes: The Resilient, Empowered, Active Living with Diabetes (REAL Diabetes) randomized controlled trial. *Diabetes Care, 41*(4), 696–704. https://doi.org/10.2337/dc17-1634

Pyatak, E. A., Florindez, D., & Weigensberg, M. J. (2013). Adherence decision making in the everyday lives of emerging adults with type 1 diabetes. *Patient Preference and Adherence, 7*, 709–718. https://doi.org/10.2147/PPA.S47577

Pyatak, E., King, M., Vigen, C. L. P., Salazar, E., Diaz, J., Schepens Niemiec, S. L., Blanchard, J., Jordan, K., Banerjee, J., & Shukla, J. (2019). Addressing diabetes in primary care: Hybrid effectiveness-implementation study of Lifestyle Redesign occupational therapy. *American Journal of Occupational Therapy, 73*(5), Article 7305185020. https://doi.org/10.5014/ajot.2019.037317

Pyatak, E. A., Sequeira, P., Peters, A. L., Montoya, L., & Weigensberg, M. J. (2013). Disclosure of psychosocial stressors affecting diabetes care among uninsured young adults with type 1 diabetes. *Diabetic Medicine, 30*(9), 1140–1144. https://doi.org/10.1111/dme.12248

Pyatak, E. A., Sequeira, P. A., Vigen, C. L., Weigensberg, M. J., Wood, J. R., Montoya, L., Ruelas, V., & Peters, A. L. (2017). Clinical and psychosocial outcomes of a structured transition program among young adults with type 1 diabetes. *Journal of Adolescent Health, 60*(2), 212–218. https://doi.org/10.1016/j.jadohealth.2016.09.004

Schmid, A. A., Atler, K. E., Malcolm, M. P., Grimm, L. A., Klinedinst, T. C., Marchant, D. R., Marchant, T. P., & Portz, J. D. (2018). Yoga improves quality of life and fall risk-factors in a sample of people with chronic pain and type 2 diabetes. *Complementary Therapies in Clinical Practice, 31*, 369–373. https://doi.org/10.1016/j.ctcp.2018.01.003

Sequeira, P. A., Pyatak, E. A., Weigensberg, M. J., Vigen, C. P., Wood, J. R., Ruelas, V., Montoya, L., Cohen, M., Speer, H., Clark, S., & Peters, A. L. (2015). Let's Empower and Prepare (LEAP): Evaluation of a structured transition program for young adults with type 1 diabetes. *Diabetes Care, 38*(8), 1412–1419. https://doi.org/10.2337/dc14-2577

Sokol-McKay, D. A. (2010). Vision rehabilitation and the person with diabetes. *Topics in Geriatric Rehabilitation, 26*(3), 241–249. https://doi.org/10.1097/TGR.0b013e3181ef30e4

Sokol-McKay, D. A. (2011). *Fact sheet: Occupational therapy's role in diabetes self-management.* American Occupational Therapy Association.

Sokol-McKay, D. A. (2013). Managing diabetes with physical limitations. *Diabetes Self-Management, 30*(6), 8, 11–12, 14.

Sokol-McKay, D. A. (2019). Helping occupational therapy clients manage prediabetes and diabetes. *OT Practice, 24*(12), 16–19.

Stedman's medical dictionary for the health professions and nursing (7th ed.). (2011). Wolters Kluwer.

Van Puymbroeck, M., Atler, K., Portz, J. D., & Schmid, A. A. (2018). Multidimensional improvements in health following hatha yoga for individuals with diabetic peripheral neuropathy. *International Journal of Yoga Therapy, 28*(1), 71–78. https://doi.org/10.17761/2018-00027

Weigensberg, M. J., Vigen, C., Sequeira, P., Spruijt-Metz, D., Juarez, M., Florindez, D., Provisor, J., Peters, A., & Pyatak, E. A. (2018). Diabetes Empowerment Council: Integrative pilot intervention for transitioning young adults with type 1 diabetes. *Global Advances in Health and Medicine, 7.* https://doi.org/10.1177/2164956118761808

Wu, C. Y., Terhorst, L., Karp, J. F., Skidmore, E. R., & Rodakowski, J. (2018). Trajectory of disability in older adults with newly diagnosed diabetes: Role of elevated depressive symptoms. *Diabetes Care, 41*(10), 2072–2078. https://doi.org/10.2337/dc18-0007

Yang, C. J., Hsu, H. Y., Lu, C. H., Chao, Y. L., Chiu, H. Y., & Kuo, L. C. (2015). The associations among hand dexterity, functional performance, and quality of life in diabetic patients with neuropathic hand from objective- and patient-perceived measurements. *Quality of Life Research, 24,* 213–221. https://doi.org/10.1007/s11136-014-0748-y

Youngson, B. (2019). Understanding diabetes self-management using the model of human occupation. *British Journal of Occupational Therapy, 82*(5), 296–305. https://doi.org/10.1177/0308022618820010

BIBLIOGRAPHY

Dudley, B., Heiland, B., Kohler-Rausch, E., & Kovic, M. (2014). Education and technology used to improve the quality of life for people with diabetes mellitus type II. *Journal of Multidisciplinary Healthcare, 7,* 147–153. https://doi.org/10.2147/JMDH.S52681

Haltiwanger, E. P., & Galindo, D. (2013). Reduction of depressive symptoms in an elderly Mexican-American female with type 2 diabetes mellitus: A single-subject study. *Occupational Therapy International, 20*(1), 35–44. https://doi.org/10.1002/oti.1338

Malcolm, M. P., Atler, K. E., Schmid, A. A., Klinedinst, T. C., Grimm, L. A., Marchant, T. P., & Marchant, D. R. (2018). Relating activity and participation levels to glycemic control, emergency department use, and hospitalizations in individuals with type 2 diabetes. *Clinical Diabetes, 36*(3), 232–243. https://doi.org/10.2337/cd17-0118

Polo, K. M., & Cahill, S. M. (2017). Interprofessional collaboration to support children with diabetes. *Open Journal of Occupational Therapy, 5*(3), Article 3. https://doi.org/10.15453/2168-6408.1338

Poole, J. L., Cordova, J. S., Sibbitt, W. L., Jr., & Skipper, B. (2010). Quality of life in American Indian women with arthritis or diabetes. *American Journal of Occupational Therapy, 64*(3), 496–505. https://doi.org/10.5014/ajot.2010.09079

Poole, J. L., Santhanam, D. D., & Latham, A. L. (2013). Hand impairment and activity limitations in four chronic diseases. *Journal of Hand Therapy, 26*(3), 232–237. https://doi.org/10.1016/j.jht.2013.03.002

Pyatak, E. A., Florindez, D., Peters, A. L., & Weigensberg, M. J. (2014). "We are all gonna get diabetic these days": The impact of a living legacy of type 2 diabetes on Hispanic young adults' diabetes care. *Diabetes Educator, 40*(5), 648–658. https://doi.org/10.1177/0145721714535994

Pyatak, E. A., Sequeira, P. A., Whittemore, R., Vigen, C. P., Peters, A. L., & Weigensberg, M. J. (2014). Challenges contributing to disrupted transition from paediatric to adult diabetes care in young adults with type 1 diabetes. *Diabetic Medicine, 31*(12), 1615–1624. https://doi.org/10.1111/dme.12485

Ratzon, N., Futeran, R., & Isakov, E. (2010). Identifying predictors of function in people with diabetes living in the community. *British Journal of Occupational Therapy, 73*(6), 277–283. https://doi.org/10.4276/030802210X12759925469023

Thompson, M. (2014). Occupations, habits and routines: Perspectives from persons with diabetes. *Scandinavian Journal of Occupational Therapy, 21*(2), 153–160. https://doi.org/10.310 9/11038128.2013.851278

Viêro, P. B., Ponte, A. S., Pommerehn, J., & Delboni, M. C. C. (2017). Type 1 and 2 diabetes mellitus: Interference of vascular and neurological complications in occupational performance. *Cadernos de Terapia Occupacional da UFSCar São Carlos, 25*(1), 75–84. https://doi.org/ 10.4322/0104-4931.ctoAO0752

Vigen, C. L. P., Carandang, K., Blanchard, J., Sequeira, P. A., Wood, J. R., Spruijt-Metz, D., Whittemore, R., Peters, A. L., & Pyatak, E. A. (2018). Psychosocial and behavioral correlates of A1C and quality of life among young adults with diabetes. *Diabetes Educator, 44*(6), 489–500. https://doi.org/10.1177/0145721718804170

Youngson, A., Cole, F., Wilby, H., & Cox, D. (2015). The lived experience of diabetes: Conceptualisation using a metaphor. *British Journal of Occupational Therapy 78*(1), 24–32. https:// doi.org/10.1177/0308022614561240

Incontinence

Description

Incontinence is the inability to control urination or defecation (O'Toole, 2017). Urinary incontinence is a loss of bladder control. Fecal incontinence is loss of bowel control.

Cause

Causes include physiological, psychological, and pathological factors such as medication side effects, reduced or restricted mobility, stool impaction, fluid imbalance, and cognitive changes (O'Toole, 2017, Robinson et al., 2018).

Terminology (O'Toole, 2017; Porter, 2018; Robinson et al., 2018)

- *Enuresis:* Involuntary voiding during sleep as a result of dysfunctional voiding or obstructive or neurologic disease of the urinary tract (may also be called nocturnal incontinence).
- *Functional incontinence:* Caused by physical factors that prevent bathroom access in time to prevent loss of urine in other places than the toilet (issues include positioning to use the toilet, difficulty removing clothing, difficulty moving from bed or chair to toilet, or difficulty seeing in the environment).
- *Mixed incontinence:* Any combination of types. The most common combinations are urge with stress incontinence and urge or stress with functional incontinence.
- *Overflow incontinence:* Occurs when the urinary tract is obstructed, resulting in a chronically distended bladder due to intravesical pressure that exceeds the outlet resistance, permitting urine to dribble.
- *Reflex incontinence:* Occurs when there is detrusor muscle hyperreflexia and/or urethral relaxation due to neurological causes, such as spinal cord injury.
- *Stress incontinence:* Urine is lost during activities that increase abdominal press such as coughing, sneezing, straining, laughing, bending, lifting, or exercising (see also Yang et al., 2010, in References).
- *Total incontinence:* Occurs when a person loses urine in all positions and at all times. The sphincter is unable to function possibly due to surgery, nerve damage, cancer, or other causes.

- *Urge incontinence:* Strong, unexpected urge to void, followed by uncontrolled urine loss. Position and activity are not factors. Inflammation condition and neurogenic bladder disorders are factors.

Evaluation/Assessment
Areas
- Activities of Daily Living/Instrumental ADL: dressing, toileting, health expectations, functional mobility, transfers, transportation
- Education/Work: location of bathrooms to classrooms or workstation, academic performance, work performance
- Play/Leisure: interests, location, frequency
- Rest/Sleep: enuresis, sleep disturbance
- Social Participation: type, location, frequency, with whom
- Sensorimotor: sphincter control, muscle strength, coordination, pain, visual acuity
- Cognitive/Perceptual: functional cognition, cognitive impairment
- Psychosocial: depression, anxiety, embarrassment, feelings of frustration, social stigmatization, isolation, family and caregiver burden, self-image, self-esteem, role performance, quality of life
- Context/Environment: cultural factors, environmental modification, urinary tract infection
- Development (Infant, Child, Adolescent only): developmental delay
- Comorbidities: diabetes, enlarged prostate, multiple sclerosis, Parkinson's disease, poststroke, spinal cord injury

Instruments
Instruments Developed by Occupational Therapy Personnel
- Canadian Occupational Performance Measure (5th ed.; COPM-5; Law et al., 2014)

Instruments Developed by Other Professionals and Used by Occupational Therapy Personnel
- Continence Assessment Tool (CAT; Cassell, 2006)
- Incontinence Impact Questionnaire (PIIQ; Harvey et al., 2001)
- Incontinence Quality of Life (QOL) Questionnaire (Schurch et al., 2007)
- Multiple Sclerosis Quality of Life Inventory (MSQLI; Ritvo et al., 1997)
- Pelvic Floor Distress Inventory (PFDI-20; Barber et al., 2011)
- Pelvic Floor Impact Questionnaire (PFIQ-7; Barber et al., 2011)
- RAND 36 Item Health Survey (SF-36; Hays et al., 1993)
- Revised Urinary Incontinence Scale (RUIS; Sansoni et al., 2015)
- Sandvik Severity Scale (SSS; Sandvik et al., 2000)

Problems/Issues
Activities of Daily Living/Instrumental ADL
- Person may experience difficulty undressing in time to avoid dribble.
- Person may express need to watch how much liquid is consumed because of incontinence or frequently needing to void.
- Person may have difficulty getting to the toilet in time to avoid dribble.
- Person may express concerns about having sex because of incontinence.
- Person may experience symptoms while doing household chores such as cooking, laundry, or housecleaning.
- Person may experience symptoms while traveling by car or bus for more than 30 minutes.
- Person may have to press on the abdomen or vaginal area to complete urination.

Education/Work
- Person may experience embarrassment at work due to "accidents" from not getting to the bathroom on time.
- Person may have to quit work or change jobs to avoid concerns about urinary incontinence.

Play/Leisure
- Incontinence and sudden urge to go may interfere with engagement in favorite leisure occupations.
- Person may reduce or restrict engagement in leisure occupations due to concerns about being incontinent.

Rest/Sleep
- Person may experience enuresis (bed-wetting), especially at night.
- Person may express dissatisfaction with quality of sleep or rest because of having to get up to use the bathroom.

Social Participation
- Incontinence and urge to go may interfere with participation in social outings or travel.
- Person may reduce or limit participation in social activities due to concerns about being incontinent.

Sensorimotor
- Person may experience difficulty with motor coordination to get to the toilet.
- Person may have weak pelvic muscles.
- Person may experience pain or discomfort in the lower abdomen or genital region during urination.

Cognitive/Perceptual
- Person may have difficulty identifying the location of the bathroom in time to avoid dribble.
- Person can be instructed to keep a bladder diary to determine frequency and severity of symptoms (bladder retaining and fluid titration is based on findings in bladder diary).

Psychosocial
- Person may become isolated due to concerns about incontinence.
- Person may become depressed or anxious about symptoms of incontinence.
- Person may express concerns and worry about not being able to get to a toilet on time to avoid leaks.
- Person may express concerns that coughing, sneezing, bending, lifting will cause symptoms.
- Person may express concern about going to new places because the first issue is finding where the toilets are located.
- Person may have decreased sense of self-esteem and self-worth.
- Person may experience decreased sense of self-image and self-identity.
- Person may express feelings of hopelessness and helplessness due to incontinence and loss of sense of control over body functions.
- Person may express concerns about wetting self and the smell of urine, especially in public.
- Person may experience changes in role performance.
- Person may experience decreased quality of life and life satisfaction.
- Person may express feelings of being a burden on family or caregivers due to incontinence.

Context/Environment
- Person may lack knowledge about typical bladder physiology and pathology.
- Person may lack knowledge about options for intervention.
- Person may lack information about available resources.
- Person may not be familiar with environmental modifications and safety options.

Intervention/Treatment

Models and programs developed by occupational therapy personnel include case studies (Cunningham & Valasek, 2019), education program (Singh & Arya, 2010), and pelvic floor muscle rehabilitation program (Sangeetha & Rao, 2010). Models and programs developed by other professionals but used by occupational therapy personnel include bladder buzz (Mathis et al., 2013). Team members include physicians, nursing personnel, psychologists, physical therapy personnel, family members and other caregivers, and occupational therapy personnel. Goals are reduced incidence of urinary incontinence and improving client's quality of life.

Activities of Daily Living/Instrumental ADL
- Food and fluid management.
- Dressing/undressing: Discuss clothing options to make dressing and undressing lower extremities easier, such as elastic waistband.
- Skin inspection: Assist client to develop a habit and routine for inspecting skin during toileting and bathing/showering to check for skin redness or breakdown.
- Transfers: Assist client to transfer from bed to toilet.
- Bladder training: Timing voiding (every 2 to 3 hours) while awake.

Education/Work
- Workplace modification: Explore with client whether modifications in the work environment would reduce concerns at work, such as moving workstation closer to a bathroom.
- Change of location (consider whether person could work at home).

Play/Leisure
- Assist person to review leisure occupations for possible changes, such as taking more frequent "potty" breaks during a sports activity such as bowling or playing tennis or during a trip to the zoo or museum.
- Explore with client whether there are new leisure occupations that are of interest, which allow flexibility for "potty" breaks.

Rest/Sleep
- See Sleep–Wake Disorders in Section 13: Lifestyle Conditions.

Social Participation
- Assist person to review social activities to determine whether modifications can be made to permit closer access to bathrooms and/or more frequent breaks to use the bathroom.
- Explore with person whether new social activities would permit participation within the person's need for access to bathrooms.

Sensorimotor
- Pelvic floor exercises (Kegel exercises): Client contracts the pelvic muscles (pubococcygeus and paravaginal), not the thigh, abdominal, or buttock muscles. Muscles are contracted for 10 seconds then relaxed for 10 seconds, 10 to 15 times.
- Pelvic floor electrical stimulation: Automated version of Kegel exercise; uses electrical current to inhibit detrusor overactivity and contract pelvic muscles.
- Biofeedback: Provides visual or audio responses when muscle contraction or relaxation has occurred.
- Pain: If pain is experienced, client should be referred to a physician for further examination.

Cognitive/Perceptual
- Scheduling: Client creates a reminder to void at specific times, such as every 3 hours.

Psychosocial
- Relaxation training: Standing in place or sitting down (rather than rushing to the toilet) and tightening pelvic floor muscles.
- Stress management: Mindfulness, increased awareness of pelvic floor and urinary function.

Context/Environment
- Consider whether a bedside commode would be useful for person with reduced mobility.

- Assist client in proper use of mobility aids (canes, walkers, wheelchairs) so that adapted devices do not interfere with access to the bathroom.
- Assist in environmental modification.
  - ▶ Placing bed as close to the bathroom as possible and removing furniture or other objects that might reduce access or act as barriers to bathroom.
  - ▶ Improving lighting, such as a bedside lamp or reflector lights in wall sockets or reflective tape on doorway.
  - ▶ Reduce conditions that might make floor surface a tripping hazard (throw rugs, glazed floor title, uneven surface).
  - ▶ If a wheelchair is involved, determine whether wheelchair can pass through the bathroom doorframe or if a commode will be needed.
  - ▶ Consider whether signage may be helpful to direct person with cognitive impairment to the bathroom.

Precautions/Safety Considerations

Person who wears disposable undergarments should be educated to self-examine for skin rash or skin breakdown. Persons who are bedridden are at risk for pressure sores.

Prognosis and Outcome

Urinary incontinence may be acute due to a side effect of medication that can be resolved by changing or discontinuing the medication; more often, it is a chronic condition that should be managed, as may occur following a stroke (White et al., 2014).

REFERENCES

Cunningham, R., & Valasek, S. (2019). Occupational therapy interventions for urinary dysfunction in primary care: A case series. *American Journal of Occupational Therapy, 73*(5), Article 7305185040. https://doi.org/10.5014/ajot.2019.038356

Mathis, S., Ehlman, K., Dugger, B. R., Harrawood, A., & Kraft, C. M. (2013). Bladder buzz: The effect of a 6-week evidence-based staff education program on knowledge and attitudes regarding urinary incontinence in a nursing home. *Journal of Continuing Education in Nursing, 44*(11), 498–506. https://doi.org/10.3928/00220124-20130903-78

O'Toole, M. T. (Ed.). (2017). *Mosby's dictionary of medicine, nursing & health professions* (10th ed.). Elsevier.

Porter, R. S. (Ed.). (2018). *The Merck manual of diagnosis and therapy* (20th ed.). Merck Sharp & Dohme.

Robinson, M. R., Kemple, C., & Smith-Gabai, H. (2018). Gastrointestinal system. In H. Smith-Gabai & S. E. Holm (Eds.), *Occupational therapy in acute care* (2nd ed., pp. 407–440). AOTA Press.

Sangeetha, J. M., & Rao, S. (2010). The efficacy of a comprehensive pelvic floor muscle rehabilitation program of stress urinary incontinence in women. *Indian Journal of Occupational Therapy, 42*(1), 3–6.

Singh, N., & Arya, K. N. (2010). Controlled trial of occupational therapy based education program in the management of stress urinary incontinence (SUI) in women. *Indian Journal of Occupational Therapy, 42*(2), 10–14.

White, J. H., Patterson, K., Jordan, L. A., Magin, P., Attia, J., & Sturm, J. W. (2014). The experience of urinary incontinence in stroke survivors: A follow-up qualitative study. *Canadian Journal of Occupational Therapy, 81*(2), 124–134. https://doi.org/10.1177/0008417414527257

Yang, J.-M., Yang, S.-H., Yang, S.-Y., Yang, E., Huang, W.-C., & Tzeng, C.-R. (2010). Clinical and pathophysiological correlates of the symptom severity of stress urinary incontinence. *International Urogynecology Journal, 21*(6), 637–643.

Scleroderma

Also called systemic sclerosis.

Description

Scleroderma is a chronic disease characterized by diffuse fibrosis, degenerative changes, and vascular abnormalities in the skin, joints, and internal organs, especially the esophagus, lower gastrointestinal tract, lungs, heart, and kidneys (Porter, 2018). There are two types: diffuse and limited. Diffuse scleroderma (dSSc) is characterized by symmetrical and generalized thickening of the skin of the trunk, face, and extremities, and, in addition, early involvement of the internal organs, which may result in pulmonary, renal, and gastrointestinal complications, cardiac fibrosis, and interstitial lung disease. Disability occurs early in the progression of the disease, and mortality is high. Limited cutaneous scleroderma (lcSSc) skin thickening is generally restricted to the face and hands initially, with involvement of internal organs occurring later. Although the progression of the disease is slower, vascular involvement can lead to digital ulcers, esophageal disease, and pulmonary arterial hypertension. Disability may occur later in the progression of the disease (Mendelson et al., 2013).

Cause

Etiology is unknown, but factors such as immunologic mechanisms and heredity are thought to be involved. The disorder is four times more common in women than in men (Porter, 2018).

Associated Hand Conditions (Melvin, 2011; Young et al., 2016)

- *Calcium deposits:* Accumulation of calcium salts under the skin; their hardness makes the skin and tissue over them sensitive to pressure.
- *Claw hand deformity:* Severe contractures including hyperextension of metacarpophalangeal (MCP) joints, flexion contractures of proximal interphalangeal (PIP) and distal interphalangeal (DIP) joints.
- *Digital ischemic ulcers:* There are three typical forms of presentation: (1) small ulcers over the fingertips or palmar surface, which are often very painful; (2) ulcers that occur over the dorsum of the PIP joints, which result in pressure from PIP joint flexion contractures; and (3) ulcer that occurs on the sides of hand or ends of the fingers that can progress to gangrene.
- *Raynaud's phenomenon:* An episodic ischemia characterized by blanching (vasospasm) cyanosis and suffusion or erythema as the blood returns to the hands; occurs in 90% of people with scleroderma.
- *Resorption:* The distal tuft of the distal phalanx as resorption occurs, resulting in a shortening of the digit and a rounded tip as the soft tissue contracts.
- *Telangiectasias:* Lesions formed by dilated capillaries that appear as dark red spots in the skin or just below the surface.
- *Tendon friction rubs:* A form of crepitation, the rubs are the result of thickened tendons rubbing against other structures during motion and are common in the diffuse cutaneous form of scleroderma.

Evaluation/Assessment

Areas

- Activities of Daily Living/Instrumental ADL: eating (chewing, swallowing)
- Education/Work: computer keyboards
- Play/Leisure: types, frequency, location
- Rest/Sleep: sleep disturbance
- Social Participation: types, frequency, location, with whom

- Sensorimotor: hand functions (grasp, dexterity), grip and pinch strength, contractures, ulceration of fingertips, fatigue, pain, edema, vasospasms, tenosynovitis, nerve entrapment, ischemia; lower extremity range of motion, muscle strength, and mobility should also be included
- Cognitive/Perceptual: self-management
- Psychosocial: depression, self-efficacy
- Context/Environment: environmental modification, adapted equipment
- Comorbidities: carpal tunnel syndrome, Raynaud's phenomenon, rheumatoid arthritis, organ dysfunction and failure

Instruments

(Note: Thirty-five instruments are listed in Mattsson et al., 2015.)

Instruments Developed by Occupational Therapy Personnel

- Arthritis Hand Function Test (AHFT; Backman et al., 1991)
- Canadian Occupational Performance Measure (5th ed.; COPM-5; Law et al., 2014)
- Computer Problems Survey (ComPS; Baker et al., 2009)
- Delta Finger-to-Palm (Delta FTP; Torok et al., 2010, in References)
- Hand Mobility in Scleroderma (HAMIS; Sandqvist & Eklund, 2000)

Instruments Developed by Other Professionals and Used by Occupational Therapy Personnel

- Arthritis Self-Efficacy Scale (ASES; Lorig et al., 1989)
- Center for Epidemiologic Studies Depression Scale (CES-D; Radloff, 1977)
- Duruöz Hand Function Scale (see Hand Function Disability Scale)
- Grip strength (dynamometer; JAMAR, Lafayette Instrument; Grippit, Vigrometer; Wang et al., 2018)
- Grooved Pegboard Test (GPT; Trites, 2002)
- Hand Function Disability Scale (HFDS; Duruöz et al., 1996)
- Health Assessment Questionnaire (HAQ; Bruce & Fries, 2005)
- Joint range of motion (goniometry; Shurtleff & Kaskutas, 2018)
- Keitel Functional Test (KFT; Holm et al., 2008; see also Poole et al., 2018, in References)
- Multidimensional Assessment of Fatigue (MAF; Belza, 1995)
- Pinch meter (pinch strength; B&E Engineering; Mathiowetz et al., 1985)
- RAND 36 Item Health Survey (SF-36; Hays et al., 1993)
- Rheumatoid and Arthritis Outcome Scale (RAOS; Bremander et al., 2003)
- Rheumatoid Hand Function Disability Scale (RHFDS; see Hand Function Disability Scale)
- Scleroderma Functional Assessment Questionnaire (SFAQ; Silman et al., 1998)
- Work Experience Survey (WES; Roessler & Gottcent, 1994)

Problems/Issues

Activities of Daily Living/Instrumental ADL

- Person may have difficulty performing self-care tasks that require fine motor coordination (such as buttoning or zipping) or gross motor tasks (such as getting in and out of the tub or shower).
- Person may have difficulty performing oral hygiene due to decreased oral aperture (microstomia), loss of tongue mobility, and dry mouth (xerostomia).
- Person may experience increased periodontal disease; decayed, missing and filled teeth; and mandibular bone resorption and erosion (Poole et al., 2010).
- Person may have difficulty performing homemaking tasks that require fine motor skills, such as turning a key in a lock, opening a jar, handwriting a shopping list.
- Person may experience difficulty with functional mobility.
- Person may experience difficulty swallowing during meals.
- Person may experience difficulty with transportation especially in cold weather.
- Person may report difficulty with child care activities related to pain and fatigue.

Education/Work

- Person may have difficulty performing certain work tasks such as keyboarding, lifting, sitting, standing up.
- Person may have difficulty maintaining a regular work schedule due to fatigue or amount of physical demands.
- Person may have difficulty with physical aspects of work environment such as comfortable chairs, heavy or hard to open doors, or turning doorknobs, handles, or levers.
- Person may complain about working in cold temperatures.
- Person may have difficulty travelling to and from work.
- Person may have difficulty getting around the work site.

Play/Leisure

- Person may be unable to engage in favorite leisure occupations.

Rest/Sleep

- Person may experience sleep disturbance.

Social Participation

- Person may withdraw from participation in social activities due higher level of disability, depression, or severity of disease symptoms (Poole et al., 2015).

Sensorimotor

- Person usually has tightening of skin.
- Person usually has shortening of tendons.
- Person usually has decreased muscle strength.
- Person usually has decreased joint range of motion, especially in the hands, specifically loss of flexion at the metacarpophalangeal (MCP) joints, extension of the proximal interphalangeal (PIP) joints, and decreased thumb movements (Poole, Santhanam, & Latham, 2013).
- Person usually experiences decreased hand functions such as decreased grip strength, grasp and pinch strength, decreased coordination and dexterity of the fingers and thumb, and inability to place the hand flat (full extension) on a surface.
- Person usually experiences pain in legs and hands.
- Person usually experiences fatigue.
- Person usually experiences Raynaud's phenomenon, especially in cold temperatures.
- Person may experience swelling, especially in legs.
- Person may develop contractures.
- Person may develop skin ulcers, especially on the fingers.
- Person may lack joint range of motion, muscle strength, and mobility in the lower extremities (Poole & Brandenstein, 2016).

Cognitive/Perceptual

- Person may choose to hide disease and disability from others.

Psychosocial

- Person may experience depression, anxiety, and fear about condition.
- Person may express feelings of loss, dependence, helplessness, guilt, shame, sadness, insecurity.
- Person may express feelings of frustration, annoyance.
- Person may express feelings of general emotional distress.
- Person may develop a negative self-image.
- Person may experience difficulty maintaining role performance.
- Person may experience decreased sense of self-efficacy (Buck et al., 2010).

Context/Environment

- Person may need adapted devices and equipment.

- Person may need environmental modification (modifications to personal transportation might include automatic car starters, car seat warmers, access to covered parking, and assignment to handicapped parking spaces).
- Person, family, colleagues, coworkers may have little knowledge about the disease and its effect on occupational performance.

Intervention/Treatment

Models and programs developed by occupational therapy personnel include environmental and ergonomic accommodations (Baker et al., 2012), intervention suggestions (Hays-Elliott, 2011), and upper extremity treatment protocol (Murphy et al., 2018). Models and programs developed by other professionals but used by occupational therapy personnel include case study (Poole, MacIntyre, & deBoer, 2013), oral hygiene (Poole et al., 2010), orofacial exercises (Yuen et al., 2012), and self-administered stretching program (Stefanantoni et al., 2016). Team members include physicians, psychologists, dentists, nursing personnel, physical therapy personnel, and occupational therapy personnel. The goal of intervention is to allow the person to regain and maintain the ability to perform daily tasks (Poole, MacIntyre, & deBoer, 2013).

Activities of Daily Living/Instrumental ADL

- Assist client to select or modify clothing to facilitate fastening (buttoning and zipping), such as using a buttonhook, changing buttons to Velcro, putting a large ring on the zipper pull.
- Assist client to develop and implement an oral hygiene program (Yuen et al., 2012).
- Encourage eating a healthy diet through meal planning and shopping.

Education/Work

- Assist client to try out different work equipment such as ergonomically designed keyboard and adjustable workstation heights.
- Assist client to obtain job accommodations.
- Assist client to determine whether workstation redesign may be helpful.

Play/Leisure

- Assist client in adapting current leisure activities and exploring new ones if previous interests are no longer feasible.

Rest/Sleep

- Provide information on good sleep hygiene.
- Assist client to modify sleeping quarters.

Social Participation

- Encourage client to continue participation in social activities with modifications as needed.

Sensorimotor

- Educate client in energy conservation (motion economy) techniques.
- Assist client to create a priority schedule that maximizes highest energy level with tasks that most need to be accomplished.
- Educate client in activity pacing (rest and work cycles).
- Education client in joint protection protocol such as carrying objects close to the body trunk and using the elbow/forearm to carry handles/straps rather than fingers or hand.
- Assist client to identify pain and discomfort and to stop activities in which pain occurs.
- Instruct client in using good body mechanics.
- Provide exercises to keep joints moving and skin as elastic as possible.
- Instruct client in skin protection such as wearing mittens in cold weather or using battery operated warming gloves.
- During therapy session use of lukewarm water as a warm-up strategy prior to scheduled therapy may be as effective as use of paraffin (Kristensen et al., 2019).

Cognitive/Perceptual
- Assist client to plan activity schedule to maximize use of energy resources and avoid stressful situations.

Psychosocial
- Assist client to learn stress management techniques such as imagery and deep-breathing techniques to facilitate relaxation to reduce anxiety and fears.

Context/Environment
- With client, determine which adapted devices or equipment would facilitate function, especially those that assist with hand function.
- With client, determine which environmental modifications to home or work situations would reduce barriers to function, such as grab bars in tub/shower or work chairs with adjustable levels for height and back tilt and support, ergonomic keyboard and mouse.
- Provide information on available community or internet resources.
- Provide information about legal requirements, such as those covered in the Americans With Disabilities Act.

Precautions/Safety Considerations

Protect skin from additional damage.

Prognosis and Outcome

Life expectancy is around 10 years, but persons with mild form may live 30 to 50 years (O'Toole, 2017; Porter, 2018). Death is usually caused by heart failure, kidney insufficiency, or visceral complications (Porter, 2018).

REFERENCES

Baker, N. A., Aufman, E. L., & Poole, J. L. (2012). Computer use problems and accommodation strategies at work and home for people with systemic sclerosis: A needs assessment. *American Journal of Occupational Therapy, 66*(3), 368–375. https://doi.org/10.5014/ajot.2012.003467

Buck, U., Poole, J., & Mendelson, C. (2010). Factors related to self-efficacy in persons with scleroderma. *Musculoskeletal Care, 8*(4), 197–203. https://doi.org/10.1002/msc.181

Hays-Elliott, C. (2011, Spring). Occupational therapy and scleroderma: Providing a bridge to function. *Voice Magazine*.

Kristensen, L. Q., Oestergaard, L. G., Bovbjerg, K., Rolving, N., & Søndergaard, K. (2019). Use of paraffin instead of lukewarm water prior to hand exercises had no additional effect on hand mobility in patients with systemic sclerosis: A randomized clinical trial. *Hand Therapy, 24*(1), 13–21. https://doi.org/10.1177/1758998318824346

Mattsson, M., Boström, C., Mihai, C., Stöcker, J., Geyh, S., Stummvoll, G., Gard, G., Möller, B., Hesselstrand, R., Sandqvist, G., Draghicescu, O., Gherghe, A. M., Voicu, M. Distler, O., Smolen, J. S., & Stamm, T. A. (2015). Personal factors in systemic sclerosis and their coverage by patient-reported outcome measures. *European Journal of Physical and Rehabilitation Medicine, 51*(4), 405–421.

Melvin, J. L. (2011). Scleroderma (Systemic sclerosis): Treatment of the hand. In T. M. Skirven, A. L. Osterman, J. M. Fedorczyk, & P. C. Amadio (Eds.), *Rehabilitation of the hand and upper extremity* (6th ed., pp. 1434–1448). Mosby.

Mendelson, C., Poole, J. L., & Allaire, S. (2013). Experiencing work as a daily challenge: The case of scleroderma. *Work, 44*(4), 405–413. https://doi.org/10.3233/WOR-2012-1420

Murphy, S. L., Barber, M. W., Homer, K., Dodge, C., Cutter, G. R., & Khanna, D. (2018). Occupational therapy treatment to improve upper extremity function in individuals with early systemic sclerosis: A pilot study. *Arthritis Care & Research, 70*(11), 1653–1660. https://doi.org/10.1002/acr.23522

O'Toole, M. T. (Ed.). (2017). *Mosby's dictionary of medicine, nursing & health professions* (10th ed.). Elsevier.

Poole, J. L., & Brandenstein, J. (2016). Difficulty with daily activities involving the lower extremities in people with systemic sclerosis. *Clinical Rheumatology, 35*(2), 483–488. https://doi.org/10.1007/s10067-015-3137-1

Poole, J. L., Chandrasekaran, A., Hildebrand, K., & Skipper, B. (2015). Participation in life situations by persons with systemic sclerosis. *Disability and Rehabilitation, 37*(10), 842–845. https://doi.org/10.3109/09638288.2014.944624

Poole, J., Conte, C., Brewer, C., Good, C. C., Perella, D., Rossie, K. M., & Steen, V. (2010). Oral hygiene in scleroderma: The effectiveness of a multi-disciplinary intervention program *Disability and Rehabilitation, 32*(5), 379–384. https://doi.org/10.3109/09638280903171527

Poole, J. L., MacIntyre, N. J., & deBoer, H. N. (2013). Evidence-based management of hand and mouth disability in a woman living with diffuse systemic sclerosis (scleroderma). *Physiotherapy Canada, 65*(4), 317–320. https://doi.org/10.3138/ptc.2012-40

Poole, J. L., New, A., & Garcia, C. (2018). A comparison of performance on the Keitel Functional Test by persons with systemic sclerosis and rheumatoid arthritis. *Disability and Rehabilitation, 40*(21), 2505–2508. https://doi.org/10.1080/09638288.2017.1337240

Poole, J. L., Santhanam, D. D., & Latham, A. L. (2013). Hand impairment and activity limitations in four chronic diseases. *Journal of Hand Therapy, 26*(3), 232–237. https://doi.org/10.1016/j.jht.2013.03.002

Porter, R. S. (Ed.). (2018). *The Merck manual of diagnosis and therapy* (20th ed.). Merck Sharp & Dohme.

Stefanantoni, K., Sciarra, I., Iannace, N., Vasile, M., Caucci, M., Scavalli, A. S., Massimiani, M. P., Passi, L., Maset, L., & Riccieri, V. (2016). Occupational therapy integrated with a self-administered stretching program on systemic sclerosis patients with hand involvement. *Clinical and Experimental Rheumatology, 34*(5), 157–161.

Torok, K. S., Baker, N. A., Lucas, M., Domsic, R. T., Boudreau, R., & Medsger, T. A., Jr. (2010). Reliability and validity of the delta finger-to-palm (FTP), a new measure of finger range of motion in systemic sclerosis. *Clinical and Experimental Rheumatology, 28*(2, Suppl. 58), S28–S36.

Young, A., Namas, R., Dodge, C., & Khanna, D. (2016). Hand impairment in systemic sclerosis: Various manifestations and currently available treatment. *Current Treatment Options in Rheumatology, 2*(3), 252–269. https://doi.org/10.1007/s40674-016-0052-9

Yuen, H. K., Marlow, N. M., Reed, S. G., Mahoney, S., Summerlin, L. M., Leite, R., Slate, E., & Silver, R. M. (2012). Effect of orofacial exercises on oral aperture in adults with systemic sclerosis. *Disability and Rehabilitation, 34*(1), 84–89. https://doi.org/10.3109/09638288.2011.587589

BIBLIOGRAPHY

DeLea, S. L., Chavez-Chiang, N. R., Poole, J. L., Norton, H. E., Sibbitt, W. L., Jr., & Bankhurst, A. D. (2011). Sonographically guided hydrodissection and corticosteroid injection for scleroderma hand. *Clinical Rheumatology, 30*(6), 805–813. https://doi.org/10.1007/s10067-010-1653-6

Moran, M. E. (2014). Scleroderma and evidence based non-pharmaceutical treatment modalities for digital ulcers: A systematic review. *Journal of Wound Care, 23*(10), 510–516. https://doi.org/10.12968/jowc.2014.23.10.510

Poole, J., Hare, K., Turner-Montez, S., Mendelson, C., & Skipper, B. (2014). Mothers with chronic disease: A comparison of parenting in mothers with systemic sclerosis and systemic lupus erythematosus. *OTJR: Occupation, Participation and Health, 34*(1), 12–19. https://doi.org/10.3928/15394492-20131029-06

Poole, J. L., Anwar, S., Mendelson, C., & Allaire, S. (2016). Workplace barriers encountered by employed persons with systemic sclerosis. *Work, 55*(4), 923–929. https://doi.org/10.3233/WOR-162448

Poole, J. L., Willer, K., Mendelson, C., Sanders, M., & Skipper, B. (2011). Perceived parenting ability and systemic sclerosis. *Musculoskeletal Care, 9*(1), 32–40. https://doi.org/10.1002/msc.197

Thombs, B. D., Jewett, L. R., Assassi, S., Baron, M., Bartlett, S. J., Maia, A. C., El-Baalbaki, G., Furst, D. E., Gottesman, K., Haythornthwaite, J. A., Hudson, M., Impens, A., Korner, A., Leite, C., Mayes, M. D., Malcarne, V. L., Motivala, S, J., Mouthon, L., Nielson, W. R., . . . Khanna, D. (2012). New directions for patient-centred care in scleroderma: The Scleroderma Patient-Centred Intervention Network (SPIN). *Clinical and Experimental Rheumatology, 30*(2, Suppl. 71), S23–S29.

Sickle Cell Disease

Also called sickle cell anemia, crescent cell anemia.

Description

Sickle cell disease causes a chronic hemolytic anemia occurring mostly in Black individuals. Sickle-shaped red blood cells cause vaso-occlusion and are prone to hemolysis, leading to severe pain crises, organ ischemia, and other systemic complications such as leg ulcers and bone deformities (Porter, 2018; *Stedman's*, 2011). Sickle cell disease (SCD) is a group of chronic genetic disorders involving the red blood cells characterized by the production of abnormal hemoglobin (HbS, Berg et al., 2012). The anemia is characterized by crises of joint pain, thrombosis, and fever and by chronic anemia, with splenomegaly, lethargy, and weakness (O'Toole, 2017).

Cause

Sickle cell disease is caused by homozygous inheritance of the hemoglobin S. Sickle cell disease is an autosomal dominant disorder.

Evaluation/Assessment

Areas

- Activities of Daily Living/Instrumental ADL: independent living, home management, managing clothing (laundry), money management, medication management, health-care skills (including seeking emergency care and number of hospitalizations), nutrition, sexual development, driver training
- Education/Work: absenteeism, academic achievement, work-related interests and skills, employment history and status, volunteering
- Play/Leisure: interests, play skills, values, frequency, location
- Rest/Sleep: sleep disturbance
- Social Participation: frequency, type, location, with whom
- Sensorimotor: pain, fatigue, temperature
- Cognitive/Perceptual: attention, memory (working memory), executive functions (planning, initiating, organizing, monitoring, completing, terminating), general intelligence, processing speed (of information), auditory processing
- Psychosocial: social skills, social roles, sense of autonomy, perceived competence, self-efficacy, quality of life, goal setting
- Context/Environment: social support, qualifications for special education (Individualized Education Program [IEP], 504 program, transitional program), knowledge and information about sickle cell disease management, government assistance programs
- Development (Infant, Child, Adolescent only): developmental delay
- Comorbidities and Complications: cerebrovascular accident (silent or overt stroke), anemia, blood transfusions, acute chest syndrome, substance abuse

Instruments

Instruments Developed by Occupational Therapy Personnel

- Assessment of Motor and Process Skills (8th ed.; AMPS-8; Fisher & Bray Jones, 2016)
- Children's Kitchen Task Assessment (CKTA; Rocke et al., 2008; see also Berg et al., 2012, in References)
- Role Checklist Version 3: Participation and Satisfaction (RCv3; Scott, 2019; Scott et al., 2017)

Instruments Developed by Other Professionals and Used by Occupational Therapy Personnel

- Adolescent Autonomy Checklist (AAC; Goodwyn, 1990)
- Bayley Scales of Infant and Toddler Development (4th ed.; Bayley-4; Bayley & Aylward, 2019)
- Behavior Rating Inventory of Executive Function (BRIEF: Parent and Teacher forms; Gioia et al., 2015; first three subscales also called the Behavioral Regulation Index [BRI]; last five subscales form the Metacognition Index [MI])
- Delis-Kaplan Executive Function System (D-KEFS) Color Word Interferences Test (Delis et al., 2001)
- Delis-Kaplan Executive Function System (D-KEFS) Sorting Test (Delis et al., 2001)
- Goal Attainment Scaling (GAS; Kiresuk et al., 1994)
- Home Observation for Measurement of the Environment (HOME; Caldwell & Bradley, 2003)
- Norbeck Social Support Questionnaire (NSSQ; Norbeck et al., 1981)
- Sickle Cell Self-Efficacy Scale (SCSES; Edwards et al., 2000)

Problems/Issues

Activities of Daily Living/Instrumental ADL

- Child/person may reach adulthood without having been educated or trained in independent living skills including home management, money management, medication management, clothing management, or health-care skills.
- Child/person may experience a stroke (silent or overt) caused by sickle cell disease.
- Parent or caregiver may lack knowledge and types of play activities designed to promote language development (receptive and expressive).

Education/Work

- Child may miss school due to pain or intravenous treatment related to sickle cell disease.
- Person may need practice in work-related skills such as writing a resume or completing an application.

Play/Leisure

- Child may be unable to engage in play or leisure activities due to pain or lack of energy related to sickle cell disease.

Rest/Sleep

- Child/person may experience sleep disturbance due to pain related to sickle cell disease.

Social Participation

- Child/person may be unable to participate in certain social activities due to pain or fatigue.

Sensorimotor

- Child/person usually experiences pain related to sickle cell disease.
- Child/person may experience motor or sensory loss related to stroke.
- Child/person may be hypersensitive to changes in temperature such as air conditioner or heating system coming on, or going from inside to outside on a very cold day.

Cognitive/Perceptual

- Child/person may have loss of general intelligence related to sickle cell disease.
- Child/person may have decreased cognitive functional ability, including use of some executive functions such as needing additional cues to initiate (start) a task and to state when the task is completed.

- Child/person may have difficulty remembering rules or steps to complete a task without reminders (verbal, written directions).
- Child/person may have difficulty with time management to initiate, monitor, or complete a task within a given time period.
- Child/person may have difficulty organizing and maintaining the work space in a manner that optimizes task performance.
- Child/person may have decreased ability to use metacognition.
- Parent or caregiver may lack knowledge, toys, and other learning materials to promote cognitive skills.

Psychosocial
- Child/person may lack social skills due to restricted opportunity to practice related to pain crisis, fatigue, medical crises, and hospitalization.
- Child may have fewer reciprocal friendships that typically developing children.
- Child/person may restrict or be limited in role performance (da Silva Cunha et al., 2018).

Context/Environment
- Family or caregivers may lack knowledge about typical development of skills in gross and fine motor, cognitive, and receptive and expressive language.
- Family or caregivers may lack knowledge about parenting skills, including how to play with a child and provide appropriate discipline to promote cognitive skills and expressive language (Fields et al., 2016).
- Child's living environment may contain few toys, books, or other learning materials.
- Child, family, or caregivers may not be familiar with special education qualifications and availability of programs.
- Child, family, or caregivers may live in an area that does not provide special education programs, such as transitional program.
- Child, family, or caregivers may be unfamiliar with available resources in the community.
- Educators and caregivers may be unfamiliar with sickle cell disease, its problems, and management.
- Child/person may lack a consistent social support system.

Intervention/Treatment

Models and programs developed by occupational therapy personnel include the CO-OP model (Dawson et al., 2017). Models and programs developed by other professionals but used by occupational therapy personnel include the home-based education model (Drazen et al., 2014) and parents as teachers (PAT; Drazen et al., 2014; Fields et al., 2016). Approaches may include coaching, direct service, or consultation to address issues such as activity modification, developmental progress, environmental modification, learning needs, parenting skills, psychosocial barriers, and transitioning (Hoyt, 2011). Team members include physicians (hematologist), nursing personnel, respiratory or inhalation therapists, psychologists, social workers, and occupational therapy personnel. The goal is to develop life skills that target cognitive, emotional, and social skills needed for self-management into adulthood (Raines et al., 2019).

Activities of Daily Living/Instrumental ADL
- Provide programs in independent living, including home management.
- Provide life-skills-based programming such as making phone calls, scheduling and attending appointments, budgeting, medication management.
- Provide practice in symptom management of sickle cell disease.

Education/Work
- Assist educators in management issues in schools such as
  - ▶ alerting educators that more frequent bathroom breaks may be needed because a child with SCD may not concentrate urine as well as typically developing children,

> ▸ identifying developmental delays that may result in need for remedial education or repeating a certain academic task to achieve proficiency, and
>
> ▸ identifying and suggesting strategies for behavior management issues that may disturb classroom activity.

- Provide opportunity to explore career choices.
- Provide practice in writing a resume and completing a work application.

Play/Leisure

- Provide opportunity to explore leisure activities.

Rest/Sleep

- No information identified.

Social Participation

- No information identified.

Sensorimotor

- Provide examples of toys and play materials to promote gross and fine motor skills.

Cognitive/Perceptual

- Assist parents and caregivers to use toys and play materials to promote cognitive skills in attention, memory, and executive functioning.
- Assist client to develop goals and plan to achieve goals.
- Assist client to develop adaptive and compensatory techniques to optimize following rules and directions such as self-talk to repeat directions to self, rereading the written directions, replaying auditory directions.

Psychosocial

- Assist client to become an advocate for self-identified needs, such as insurance coverage.

Context/Environment

- Assist client, family, caregivers, and educators to increase health literacy about sickle cell disease.
- Assist client, family, and caregivers to access community resources.

Precautions/Safety Considerations

Monitor for increased chest pain, signs of infection, and difficulty breathing (Porter, 2018).

Prognosis and Outcome

Sickle cell disease is a chronic lifelong condition requiring transition to adult health care and medical management and to independent living (Abel et al., 2015; Berg et al., 2018).

REFERENCES

Abel, R. A., Cho, E., Chadwick-Mansker, K. R., D'Souza, N., Housten, A. J., & King, A. A. (2015). Transition needs of adolescents with sickle cell disease. *American Journal of Occupational Therapy, 69*(2), Article 6902350030. https://doi.org/10.5014/ajot.2015.013730

Berg, C., Edwards, D. F., & King, A. (2012). Executive function performance on the Children's Kitchen Task Assessment with children with sickle cell disease and matched controls. *Child Neuropsychology, 18*(5), 432–448. https://doi.org/10.1080/09297049.2011.613813

Berg, C., King, A., & Edwards, D. F. (2018). Mentoring program for young adults with sickle cell disease. *Occupational Therapy in Health Care, 32*(2), 124–136. https://doi.org/10.1080/07380577.2018.1443363

da Silva Cunha, J. H., Montero, C. F., Ferreira, L. A., Cordeiro, J., R., & de Paula Souza, L. M. (2018). Occupational roles of individuals with sickle cell anemia. *Revista de Terapia Ocupacional da Universidade de São Paulo, 28*(2), 230–238. https://doi.org/10.11606/issn.2238-6149.v28i2p230-238

Dawson, D. R., McEwen, S. E., & Polatajko, H. J. (Eds.). (2017). *Cognitive orientation to daily occupational performance in occupational therapy*. AOTA Press.

Drazen, C. H., Abel, R., Lindsey, T., & King, A. A. (2014). Development and feasibility of a home-based education model for families of children with sickle cell disease. *BMC Public Health, 14*, Article 116. https://doi.org/10.1186/1471-2458-14-116

Fields, M. E., Hoyt-Drazen, C., Abel, R., Rodeghier, M. J., Yarboi, J. M., Compas, B. E., & King, A. A. (2016). A pilot study of parent education intervention improves early childhood development among toddlers with sickle cell disease. *Pediatric Blood & Cancer, 63*(12), 2131–2138. https://doi.org/10.1002/pbc.26164

Hoyt, C. (2011). Branching out: Occupational therapy and children with sickle cell disease. *OT Practice, 16*(4), 24–25.

O'Toole, M. T. (Ed.). (2017). *Mosby's dictionary of medicine, nursing & health professions* (10th ed.). Elsevier.

Porter, R. S. (Ed.). (2018). *The Merck manual of diagnosis and therapy* (20th ed.). Merck Sharp & Dohme.

Raines, G. M., Stasher-Booker, B., & Stapleton, D. H. (2019). Promoting mental health and wellness for adolescents living with sickle cell disease. *SIS Quarterly Practice Connections, 4*(4), 19–22.

Stedman's medical dictionary for the health professions and nursing (7th ed.). (2011). Wolters Kluwer.

BIBLIOGRAPHY

Drazen, C. H., Abel, R., Gabir, M., Farmer, G., & King, A. A. (2016). Prevalence of developmental delay and contributing factors among children with sickle cell disease. *Pediatric Blood & Cancer, 63*(3), 504–510. https://doi.org/10.1002/pbc.25838

Systemic Lupus Erythematosus

Also called SLE, disseminated lupus erythematosus.

Description

Systemic lupus erythematosus is a chronic, multisystem, inflammatory disorder of the autoimmune system occurring primarily in young women. Common manifestations include arthralgia and arthritis, severe vasculitis, lesions of the skin (rashes), pleuritis or pericarditis, renal or central nervous system involvement. A common rash is a "butterfly shaped" rash across the nose the checks under the eyes (O'Toole, 2017; Porter, 2018).

Cause

Etiology is an autoimmune reaction in the connective tissues that may have genetic origins that are triggered by immune system dysfunction or by unknown environmental factors such as virus infections or adverse reactions to certain drugs (O'Toole, 2017; Porter, 2018).

Classification (Porter, 2018)

- Mild: Includes fever, arthritis, pleurisy, pericarditis, headache, and rash.
- Severe: Includes hemolytic anemia, thrombocytopenic, purpura, massive pleural and pericardial involvement, significant renal damage, acute vasculitis of the extremities or gastrointestinal tract, and florid central nervous system involvement.

Evaluation/Assessment

Areas

- Activities of Daily Living/Instrumental ADL: basic ADLs (eating, dressing, grooming, bathing/showering, brushing teeth, transfers); IADLs (meal preparation/cooking, house cleaning,

laundry and clothes care, child care, shopping, household and yard maintenance), functional mobility (indoors, outdoors), functional communication
- Education/Work: physical requirements (crouching, bending, kneeling, lifting, carrying, reaching), job duties (pace, schedule), mobility requirements (at work, getting to and from work), transportation needs
- Play/Leisure: hobbies, interests, recreational activities, frequency, type
- Rest/Sleep: sleep disturbance
- Social Participation: frequency, type, location, with whom
- Sensorimotor: range of motion, joint stiffness, fatigue, pain (resting, moving)
- Cognitive/Perceptual: attention and concentration
- Psychosocial: anxiety, depression, quality of life, role performance, self-efficacy
- Context/Environment: adapted devices, patient education, social support, community resources
- Comorbidities: glomerulonephritis, pleuritis, pericarditis, peritonitis, neuritis, anemia, renal failure (Porter, 2018)

Instruments

Instruments Developed by Occupational Therapy Personnel
- Energy Conservation Strategies Survey (ECSS; Mallik et al., 2005)
- Evaluation of Daily Activity Questionnaire (EDAQ; Hammond et al., 2018; see also Hammond et al., 2018, in References)

Instruments Developed by Other Professionals and Used by Occupational Therapy Personnel
- Fatigue Impact Scale (FIS; Fisk et al., 1994)
- Fatigue Severity Scale (FSS; Krupp et al., 1989)
- Frenchay Activities Index (FAI; Holbrook & Skilbeck, 1983)
- Health Assessment Questionnaire (HAQ; Bruce & Fries, 2005)
- Hospital Anxiety and Depression Scale (HADS; Zigmond & Snaith, 1983)
- Job Content Questionnaire (JCQ; Karasek et al., 1998)
- Lupus Quality of Life Questionnaire (LupusQoL; McElhone et al., 2007)
- Multidimensional Assessment of Fatigue (MAF; Belza, 1995)
- Pain Catastrophizing Scale (PCS; Sullivan et al., 1995)
- Parenting Disability Index (PDI; Katz et al., 2003)
- Profile of Mood States–Fatigue Subscale (POMS; McNair et al., 1971)
- Self-Administered Comorbidity Questionnaire (SACQ; Sangha et al., 2003)
- Self-Efficacy for Performing Energy Conservation Strategies Assessment (SEPECSA; Swain, 2000)
- Short-Form 36 Health Survey (SF-36; Ware et al., 1996)
- Systemic Lupus Activity Questionnaire (SLAQ; Karlson et al., 2003)
- Visual analogue scale (VAS-pain)
- Workplace Activity Limitations Scale (WALS; Gignac et al., 2004)

Problems/Issues

Activities of Daily Living/Instrumental ADL
- Person may experience difficulty performing basic ADLs during early stage of disease.
- Person is likely to experience difficulty performing household chores including preparing meals, cleaning, shopping, laundry, child care, and gardening/lawn maintenance (Poole et al., 2012).

Education/Work (Al Dhanhani et al., 2014)
- Person may experience difficulty performing physical demands involving crouching, bending, kneeling, lifting, carrying, reaching, moving items, or working in awkward positions.
- Person may experience difficulty attending to or concentrating on task.

- Person may experience difficulty keeping up with the pace or scheduling of work demands.
- Person may experience difficulty sitting or standing for long periods of time.
- Person may experience difficulty moving about work setting or getting in and from work place.
- Person may experience difficulty performing tasks that require hand dexterity or manipulation.

Play/Leisure

- Person may be unable due to level of fatigue to continue engaging in leisure activities with high physical energy demands, such as cycling, swimming, playing badminton, or other high energy demand sports or activities.

Rest/Sleep

- Person may experience pain that interferes with sleep.
- Person may continue to feel fatigued even after a period of rest or sleep.

Social Participation

- Person may be unable to continue participation in social activities that require higher energy level.

Sensorimotor

- Person usually experiences feelings of fatigue that decreases physical functioning; nature of fatigue may be intermittent or persistent; fatigue increases following stress, physical activity, and joint pain (Connolly et al., 2014).
- Person usually experiences intermittent or acute polyarthritis arthralgia (joint pain).
- Person usually experiences skin lesions (rash) on the face.
- Person may experience neurologic symptoms including headaches, ischemic stroke, subarachnoid hemorrhage, seizures, organic brain syndrome, aseptic meningitis, peripheral and cranial neuropathies, transverse myelitis, or cerebellar dysfunction (Porter, 2018).
- Person may experience deformities of the metacarpophalangeal (MCP) and interphalangeal (IP) joints.
- Person may experience abdominal pain resulting from nausea, vomiting, bowel formation, pseudo-obstruction, and serositis (inflammation of tissue lining internal organs).
- Person may experience skin lesions on the neck, upper chest, and elbows.
- Person may experience cardiopulmonary manifestations, including pleurisy and pulmonary hypertension.

Cognitive/Perceptual

- Person may experience difficulty attending to or concentrating on task due to fatigue, pain, or both.

Psychosocial

- Person may experience personality changes.
- Person may experience episodes of psychosis, including changes in mood from depression to happiness.
- Person may be unable to continue performing certain roles or role functions, such as homemaking or child care.

Context/Environment

- Person may lack social support.
- Person may lack knowledge of available community and internet resources.
- Person may need access to adapted devices.

Intervention/Treatment

Models and programs developed by occupational therapy personnel include fatigue and activity management education (FAME; O'Riordan et al., 2017) and Wii Fit (Yuen et al., 2011).

Models and programs developed by other professionals but used by occupational therapy personnel include optimal management of fatigue (Yuen & Cunningham, 2014). Team members include physicians, nursing personnel, physical therapists, psychologists, and occupational therapy personnel. Goals are to retain functional and occupational performance and remain an active participant in home and community activities.

Activities of Daily Living/Instrumental ADL
- Assist client to prioritize, organize, and schedule ADLs and IADLs to maximize functional performance.

Education/Work
- Client may need to consider working part-time, flextime, or working from home.
- Client may need to consider selecting or changing to an occupation and job setting with less physical demands.
- Client may need to organize and schedule work activities to be more efficient in use of physical demands.
- Client may need to change job demands or reschedule tasks to time when fatigue is less a factor, such as in the morning.

Play/Leisure
- Client may need to stop engaging in physically demanding leisure pursuits or alter them to accommodate fatigue.
- Client may need to explore and develop new leisure activities that are within person's level of energy.

Rest/Sleep
- Assist client to determine if changes or modifications in bedding or environment (lighting, noise) may facilitate better sleep.
- Assist client to determine whether rest breaks are more effective based on length of time, timing with daily schedule, or location (easy chair, bed, lounge chair).

Social Participation
- Assist client to evaluate which social activities are most important and what modifications may enable continued participation.
- Assist client to explore new social activities with demands that accommodate client's level of energy.

Sensorimotor
- Instruct person in fatigue management techniques including exercises to reduce joint stiffness, if present.
- Explore with person what energy conservation or work simplification strategies may be useful.
- Consider if activity pacing (alternative cycles of work and rest) may be useful.
- Consider if rescheduling or reorganizing tasks within the day may facilitate performance.

Cognitive/Perceptual
- Encourage client to focus on planning ahead and being flexible.
- Assist client to develop self-management strategies.

Psychosocial
- Encourage person to engage in stress reduction activities such as deep-breathing exercises, yoga, mindfulness, massage, Pilates, meditation.
- Assist person to change or modify roles and role functions especially mothering role (Poole et al., 2012).
- Assist person to consider maximizing abilities rather than focusing on limitations.

Context/Environment
- Engage person to make use of social supports to perform selected activities.

- Provide adapted devices as useful (may be temporary).
- Provide access to community and internet resources.

Precautions/Safety Considerations

Major issue is management of fatigue.

Prognosis and Outcome

Disease is marked by chronic remission and exacerbation, which results in both uncertainty and opportunities (Mattsson et al., 2012; O'Toole, 2017). However, the long-term prognosis is usually good, including the 10-year survival rate if initial acute phase is controlled (Porter, 2018). However, if end-stage renal failure occurs, dialysis or kidney transplant may be needed.

REFERENCES

Al Dhanhani, A. M., Gignac, M. A. M., Beaton, D. E., Su, J., & Fortin, P. R. (2014). Work factors are associated with workplace activity limitations in systemic lupus erythematosus. *Rheumatology, 53*(11), 2044–2052. https://doi.org/10.1093/rheumatology/keu242

Connolly, D., McNally, A., Moran, D., & Ryan, M. (2014). Fatigue in systemic lupus erythematosus: Impact on occupational participation and reported management strategies. *British Journal of Occupational Therapy, 77*(7), 373–380. https://doi.org/10.4276/030802214X14044755581862

Hammond, A., Prior, Y., Horton, M. C., Tennant, A., & Tyson, S. (2018). The psychometric properties of the Evaluation of Daily Activity Questionnaire in seven musculoskeletal conditions. *Disability and Rehabilitation, 40*(17), 2070–2080. https://doi.org/10.1080/09638288.2017.1323027

Mattsson, M., Möller, B., Stamm, T., Gard, G., & Boström, C. (2012). Uncertainty and opportunities in patients with established systemic lupus erythematosus: A qualitative study. *Musculoskeletal Care, 10*(1), 1–12. https://doi.org/10.1002/msc.220

O'Riordan, R., Doran, M., & Connolly, D. (2017). Fatigue and activity management education for individuals with systemic lupus erythematosus. *Occupational Therapy International, 2017,* Article 4530104. https://doi.org/10.1155/2017/4530104

O'Toole, M. T. (Ed.). (2017). *Mosby's dictionary of medicine, nursing & health professions* (10th ed.). Elsevier.

Poole, J., Rymek-Gmytrasiewicz, M., Mendelson, C., Sanders, M., & Skipper, B. (2012). Parenting: The forgotten role of women living with systemic lupus erythematosus. *Clinical Rheumatology, 31*(6), 995–1000. https://doi.org/10.1007/s10067-011-1929-5

Porter, R. S. (Ed.). (2018). *The Merck manual of diagnosis and therapy* (20th ed.). Merck Sharp & Dohme.

Yuen, H. K., & Cunningham, M. A. (2014). Optimal management of fatigue in patients with systemic lupus erythematosus: A systematic review. *Therapeutics and Clinical Risk Management, 2014*(10), 775–786. https://doi.org/10.2147/TCRM.S56063

Yuen, H. K., Holthaus, K., Kamen, D. L., Sword, D. O., & Breland, H. L. (2011). Using Wii Fit to reduce fatigue among African American women with systemic lupus erythematosus: A pilot Study. *Lupus, 20*(12), 1293–1299. https://doi.org/10.1177/0961203311412098

BIBLIOGRAPHY

Poole, J. L., Hare, K. S., Turner-Montez, S., Mendelson, C., & Skipper, B. (2014). Mothers with chronic disease: A comparison of parenting in mothers with systemic sclerosis and systemic lupus erythematosus. *OTJR: Occupation, Participation and Health, 34*(1), 12–19. https://doi.org/10.3928/15394492-20131029-06

Immunologic and Infection Diseases

Breast Cancer

See also Cancer: Adult, Cancer: Childhood and Adolescent, Cancer Survivor, Lymphedema.

Description

Cancer in the breast tissue. Breast cancer most often involves glandular breast cells in the ducts or lobules. The most frequent postsurgery complications are pain, scaring, altered sensitivity, range of motion limitation, lymphedema, and seroma (mass or lump; Dias et al., 2017).

Cause

Genetic (*BRCA1, BRCA2, HER2* genes), hormone-based tumors (estrogen, progesterone), or unknown (Porter, 2018).

Evaluation/Assessment

Areas

- Activities of Daily Living/Instrumental ADL: basic ADLs (eating, dressing, grooming, bathing, functional mobility), medication management, meal preparation, homemaking, shopping, driving, caring for children or pets, sexual activity
- Education/Work: work skills (paid or volunteer) performance, retirement planning
- Play/Leisure: interests, frequency, location
- Rest/Sleep: sleep disturbances due to medications or pain
- Social Participation: type, frequency, with whom
- Sensorimotor: joint range of motion, muscle weakness, fatigue and tiredness, pain, posture, edema and lymphedema, sensation (nerve damage), scar management
- Cognitive/Perceptual: attention and concentration, memory, executive functions, body image
- Psychosocial: depression, anxiety, role performance, quality of life
- Context/Environment: home and community modification, adaptive devices
- Comorbidity: osteoporosis

Instruments

Instruments Developed by Occupational Therapy Personnel

- Activity Card Sort (2nd ed.; ACS-2; Baum & Edwards, 2008)
- Canadian Occupational Performance Measure (5th ed.; COPM-5; Law et al., 2014)
- Carolina Frailty Index (CFI; Guerard et al., 2017)
- Engagement in Meaningful Activities Survey (EMAS; Eakman et al., 2010)
- Occupational Performance History Interview (Version 2.1; OPHI-II; Kielhofner et al., 2004)
- Worker Role Interview (Version 10.0; WRI 10.0; Braveman et al., 2005)

Instruments Developed by Other Professionals and Used by Occupational Therapy Personnel

- Arm circumference (cloth tape measure)
- Beck Depression Inventory (2nd ed.; BDI-II; Beck et al., 1996)
- Blessed Orientation Memory and Concentration (BOMC; Kawas et al., 1995)
- Cancer Fatigue Scale (CRS; Okuyama et al., 2000)
- Cognitive Symptom Checklist W21 (CSC-W21; Ottati & Feuerstein, 2013)
- Dynamometer (measure grip strength; JAMAR Dynamometer, Lafayette Instrument)
- Goniometer (measure joint range of motion; multiple sources)
- Hospital Anxiety and Depression Scale (HADS; Zigmond & Snaith, 1983)
- Karnofsky Performance Status (KPS; Karnofsky & Burchenal, 1949)
- Kwan's Arm Problem Scale (KAPS; Kwan et al., 2002)
- Patient-Specific Functional Scale (PSFS; Strafford et al., 1995)
- Quality of Life Questionnaire-C30 (QLQ-30; European Organization for Research and Treatment of Cancer; Aaronson et al., 1993)

- Supportive Care Needs Survey (SCNS-SF34; Bonevski et al., 2000)
- Volumetry (measure edema or lymphedema)
- Wingate Functional Evaluation of the Ipsilateral Shoulder questionnaire (WFEISQ; Wingate et al., 1989)
- Work Limitations Questionnaire (WLQ; Lerner et al., 2001)

Problems/Issues

Activities of Daily Living/Instrumental ADL

- Person may experience difficulty completing basic ADLs, such as dressing self, due to decreased joint range of motion of the upper extremity shoulder.
- Person may experience hair loss due to side effects of medication.
- Person may experience difficulty performing IADLs tasks, such as housekeeping, due to fatigue and lack of endurance.
- Person may experience difficulty caring for children and maintaining good relationships with them.
- Person may experience difficulty driving due to decreased ability to attend and concentrate related to side effects of medication.

Education/Work

- Person may be unable to continue working due to fatigue, lack of endurance, depression, or cognitive impairments due to side effects of medication.

Play/Leisure

- Person may discontinue engagement in meaningful leisure activities.

Rest/Sleep

- Person may experience sleep disturbances due to pain or side effects of medication.
- Person may have difficulty getting adequate sleep (i.e., fall asleep and stay asleep).

Social Participation

- Person may limit or cease participation in social activities due to fatigue, concern about body image, or cognitive impairments.

Sensorimotor

- Person usually experiences fatigue and sense of tiredness.
- Person usually experiences decreased muscle strength.
- Person usually experiences decreased endurance and activity tolerance.
- Person may experience decreased joint range of motion.
- Person may experience edema and lymphedema.

Cognitive/Perceptual

- Person may experience decreased ability to attend and concentrate.
- Person may experience memory loss.
- Person may experience executive dysfunction, such decreased problem-solving skills.
- Person may experience negative changes in body image.

Psychosocial

- Person may experience depression and anxiety.
- Person may feel increased sense of stress and decreased ability to cope.

Context/Environment

- Person, family, relatives, friends may lack information about cancer and its management and rehabilitation approaches.
- Person may lack knowledge about community resources.

Intervention/Treatment

Models and programs developed and implemented by occupational therapy personnel include community-based occupational therapy program (Petruseviciene et al., 2018), early detection program (Thomas et al., 2019), intervention approaches (Deluliis & Hughes, 2012), occupation-based problem-solving strategies (OB-PSS; Şahin & Uyanik, 2019), occupational project (Moreno-Chaparro et al., 2018), Pilates exercise program (Gajbhiye & Deshpande, 2013), Perceive, Recall, Plan, and Perform (PRPP) System (Lewis et al., 2016), return-to-work program (Désiron, 2010; Désiron et al., 2016; Désiron et al., 2015; Désiron et al., 2013), Take Action program (Newman, 2013), upper extremity screening program (Thomas et al., 2019), and tailored occupational therapy approach (Ryan et al., 2011). Models and programs developed by other professionals but implemented by occupational therapy personnel include empowerment (Fisher & Howell, 2010), integrated rehabilitation (Cheville et al., 2019), multidisciplinary preoperative teaching session (Ibrahim et al., 2018; Loh & Musa, 2015), practice recommendations (Lattanzi et al., 2010), problem-solving treatment program (Hegel et al., 2011; Lyons et al., 2012; Lyons, Hull, et al., 2015; Lyons, Svensborn, et al., 2015), and self-management intervention program (Loh et al., 2010). Team members include physicians, plastic surgeons, nursing personnel, physical therapists, certified lymphedema specialists, dietitians or nutritionists, and occupational therapy personnel. The goal is to adapt existing occupations to facilitate performance, find new meaningful occupations, learn to plan and prioritize which occupations to do when, improve role performance, and to gather information about resources or options (Keesing et al., 2018; Lyons et al., 2012).

Activities of Daily Living/Instrumental ADL
- Suggest compensatory techniques for meal preparation, such as one-skillet meals or sharing meal preparation with other family members.
- Assist person to develop a diet that provides adequate nutrition.
- Assist person in selecting hair pieces, wigs, hat, cap, or alternate hairstyle if hair loss has occurred.
- Assist client to develop a child care program (or parent care program) that accounts for limitations such as increased external daycare time.
- Discuss with client strategies to resume safe and comfortable sexual activity.

Education/Work
- Assist client in identifying job duties and suggest modifications to those that are problematic or difficult to perform.
- Assist client in terminating if a change of job is desirable or retirement planning is an option.

Play/Leisure
- Encourage person to reengage in meaningful leisure occupations, with modifications if necessary.
- Support development of new leisure occupations, especially if previously enjoyed occupations must be curtailed.
- Note: Person may prefer to engage in "needed" or "necessary" occupations initially before engaging in leisure occupations (Fleischer & Howell, 2017).

Rest/Sleep
- Review sleep habits and routines and recommend changes as needed.
- Suggest modifications such as adding pillows under affected arm.
- Review postsurgery precautions such as protective instructions, which may include avoiding sleeping on the affected arm and side of body for about 2 weeks.
- Review bed mobility issues, including rolling over, getting out of bed, using silk sheets to reduce friction, monitoring room temperature.

Social Participation

- Encourage participation in social activities with modifications as needed such as shorter time periods, less strenuous physical demands, more relaxed environments.
- Encourage participation in support group for breast cancer survivors.

Sensorimotor

- Provide instruction in energy conservation (motion economy).
- Provide instruction in fatigue management.
- Instruct client in protective use of affected arm following surgery.
  - ▶ Avoid overuse of arm to reduce pain and edema.
  - ▶ Avoid lifting more than 5 pounds.
  - ▶ Avoid lifting arm above 90 degrees of shoulder motion (reaching above shoulder height).
  - ▶ Instruction in use of one-handed techniques may be helpful postsurgery.
- Provide an aerobic exercise program to increase overall strength and endurance and reduce edema and lymphedema.
- Provide instructions to reduce edema and lymphedema such as avoiding long periods of dependent positions of affected upper extremity (see Lymphedema chapter).
- Instruct client in pain self-management program.
  - ▶ Recommend observing and adjusting medication peak with activity and exercise.
  - ▶ Instruct client in maintaining good posture during activities.
  - ▶ Teach relaxation.
  - ▶ Use pillows for postural support.

Cognitive/Perceptual

- Provide instruction in self-care management such as skin care, infection prevention, and adapted clothing.
- Assist in developing interventions to improve health body image.

Psychosocial

- Assist person to tailor role performance to allow participation as parent, homemaker, and worker.
- Provide stress management and coping skills approaches such as relaxation training, deep-breathing exercises, imagery, yoga.
- Encourage and support self-efficacy and empowerment to increase participation in daily activities.

Context/Environment

- Recommend and/or provide adaptive devices and equipment as needed.
- Instruct use of pillows to relax arm and shoulder during sitting or lying down.
- Provide information on community and internet resources.
- Provide information to family or caregivers regarding postoperative activity limitations and precautions.

Precautions/Safety Considerations

Impairment in upper extremity function may persist for many years following surgical intervention (Fisher & Howell, 2010).

Prognosis and Outcome

Variable. Intervention for early stage diagnosis and intervention is good, but poor for late stage diagnosis. Persons from Latina backgrounds may require additional information and assistance to overcome participation restrictions including language barriers and lack of general health knowledge (Sleight et al., 2018). Quality of life may continue to be an ongoing issue for various survivors (Sleight et al., 2019; Williams et al., 2019).

REFERENCES

Cheville, A. L., McLaughlin, S. A., Haddad, T. C., Lyons, K. D., Newman, R., & Ruddy, K. J. (2019). Integrated rehabilitation for breast cancer survivors. *American Journal of Physical Medicine & Rehabilitation, 98*(2), 154–164. https://doi.org/10.1097/PHM.0000000000001017

Deluliis, E. D., & Hughes, J. K. (2012). *Fact sheet: Occupational therapy's role in breast cancer rehabilitation.* American Occupational Therapy Association.

Désiron, H. A. M. (2010). Occupational therapy and return to work for breast cancer survivors. *World Federation of Occupational Therapists Bulletin, 61*(1), 45–51. https://doi.org/10.1179/otb.2010.61.1.013

Désiron, H. A. M., Crutzen, R., Godderis, L., Van Hoof, E., & de Rijk, A. (2016). Bridging health care and the workplace: Formulation of a return-to-work intervention for breast cancer patients using an intervention mapping approach. *Journal of Occupational Rehabilitation, 26*(3), 350–365. https://doi.org/10.1007/s10926-015-9620-3

Désiron, H. A. M., Donceel, P., Godderis, L., Van Hoof, E., & de Rijk, A. (2015). What is the value of occupational therapy in return to work for breast cancer patients? A qualitative inquiry among experts. *European Journal of Cancer Care, 24*(2), 267–280. https://doi.org/10.1111/ecc.12209

Désiron, H. A. M., Donceel, P., de Rijk, A., & Van Hoof, E. (2013). A conceptual-practice model for occupational therapy to facilitate return to work in breast cancer patients. *Journal of Occupational Rehabilitation, 23*, 516–526. https://doi.org/10.1007/s10926-013-9427-z

Dias, M., Zomkowski, A., Michels, F. A. S., & Sperandio, F. F. (2017). Breast cancer surgery effect over professional activities. *Cadernos Brasileiros de Terapia Ocupacional São Carlos, 25*(2), 325–332.

Fisher, M. I., & Howell, D. (2010). The power of empowerment: An ICF-based model to improve self-efficacy and upper extremity function of survivors of breast cancer. *Rehabilitation Oncology, 28*(3), 19–25. https://doi.org/10.1097/01893697-201028030-00003

Fleischer, A., & Howell, D. (2017). The experience of breast cancer survivors' participation in important activities during and after treatments. *British Journal of Occupational Therapy, 80*(8), 470–478. https://doi.org/10.1177/0308022617700652

Gajbhiye, P. P., & Deshpande, L. (2013). To compare the effects of Pilates exercises and conventional therapy on upper extremity function and quality of life in women with breast cancer. *Indian Journal of Occupational Therapy, 45*(1), 3–9.

Hegel, M. T., Lyons, K. D., Hull, J. G., Kaufman, P., Urquhart, L., Li, Z., & Ahles, T. A. (2011). Feasibility study of a randomized controlled trial of a telephone-delivered problem-solving–occupational therapy intervention to reduce participation restrictions in rural breast cancer survivors undergoing chemotherapy. *Psycho-Oncology, 20*(10), 1092–1101. https://doi.org/10.1002/pon.1830

Ibrahim, M., Lau, G. J., Smirnow, N., Buono, A. T., Cooke, A., Gartshore, K., Loiselle, C. G., & Johnson, K. (2018). A multidisciplinary preoperative teaching session for women awaiting breast cancer surgery: A quality improvement initiative. *Rehabilitation Process and Outcome, 7*. https://doi.org/10.1177/1179572718790937

Keesing, S., Rosenwax, L., & McNamara, B. (2018). Identifying the contribution of occupational therapy in meeting the needs of women survivors of breast cancer. *British Journal of Occupational Therapy, 81*(7), 402–412. https://doi.org/10.1177/0308022618762080

Lattanzi, J. B., Giuliano, S., Meehan, C., Sander, B., Wootten, R., & Zimmerman, A. (2010). Recommendations for physical and occupational therapy practice from the perspective of clients undergoing therapy for breast cancer-related impairments. *Journal of Allied Health, 39*(4), 257–264.

Lewis, J., Chapparo, C., Mackenzie, L., & Ranka, J. (2016). Work after breast cancer: Identification of cognitive difficulties using the Perceive, Recall, Plan, and Perform (PRPP) system of task analysis. *British Journal of Occupational Therapy, 79*(5), 323–332. https://doi.org/10.1177/0308022616639983

Loh, S. Y., & Musa, A. N. (2015). Methods to improve rehabilitation of patients following breast cancer surgery: A review of systematic reviews. *Breast Cancer: Targets and Therapy, 7,* 81–98. https://doi.org/10.2147/BCTT.S47012

Loh, S. Y., Packer, T., Passmore, A., Yip, C. H., Tan, F. L., & Xavier, M. (2010). Psychological distress of women newly diagnosed with breast cancer: Relationship with a self-management intervention program. *Asian Journal of Occupational Therapy, 8*(1), 5–11. https://doi.org/10.11596/ASIAJOT.8.5

Lyons, K. D., Erickson, K. S., & Hegel, M. T. (2012). Problem-solving strategies of women undergoing chemotherapy for breast cancer. *Canadian Journal of Occupational Therapy, 79*(1), 33–40. https://doi.org/10.2182/cjot.2012.79.1.5

Lyons, K. D., Hull, J. G., Kaufman, P. A., Li, Z., Seville, J. L., Ahles, T. A., Kornblith, A. B., & Hegel, M. T. (2015). Development and initial evaluation of a telephone-delivered, behavioral activation and problem-solving treatment program to address functional goals of breast cancer survivors. *Journal of Psychosocial Oncology, 33*(2), 199–218. https://doi.org/10.1080/07347 332.2014.1002659

Lyons, K. D., Svensborn, I. A., Kornblith, A. B., & Hegel, M. T. (2015). A content analysis of functional recovery strategies of breast cancer survivors. *OTJR: Occupation, Participation and Health 35*(2), 73–80. https://doi.org/10.1177/1539449214567306

Moreno-Chaparro, J., Jaramillo-Corredor, C., & Faustino, Y. (2018). Breaking paradigms, new breast cancer rehabilitation methods from occupational therapy: Case report. *Case Reports, 4*(2), 78–90. https://doi.org/10.15446/cr.v4n2.69693

Newman, R. M. (2013). Re-defining one's occupational self 2 years after breast cancer: A case study. *Work, 46*(4), 439–444. https://doi.org/10.3233/WOR-131679

Petruseviciene, D., Surmaitiene, D., Baltaduoniene, D., & Lendraitiene, E. (2018). Effect of community-based occupational therapy on health-related quality of life and engagement in meaningful activities of women with breast cancer. *Occupational Therapy International, 2018,* Article 6798697. https://doi.org/10.1155/2018/6798697

Porter, R. S. (Ed.). (2018). *The Merck manual of diagnosis and therapy* (20th ed.). Merck Sharp & Dohme.

Ryan, E. L., Miskovitz, G., Sutton, D., & Ahles, T. (2011). A tailored occupational therapy approach to cognitive rehabilitation of chemotherapy-related cognitive side effects in breast cancer survivors: Two case studies of premenopausally affected women. *Psicooncología, 8*(2-3), 315–342. https://doi.org/10.5209/rev_PSIC.2011.v8.n2-3.37884

Şahin, S., & Uyanik, M. (2019). The impact of occupation-based problem-solving strategies training in women with breast cancer. *Health and Quality of Life Outcomes, 17,* Article 104. https://doi.org/10.1186/s12955-019-1170-5

Sleight, A. G., Lyons, K. D., Vigen, C., Macdonald, H., & Clark, F. (2019). The association of health-related quality of life with unmet supportive care needs and sociodemographic factors in low-income Latina breast cancer survivors: A single-centre pilot study. *Disability and Rehabilitation, 41*(26), 3151–3156. https://doi.org/10.1080/09638288.2018.1485179

Sleight, A. G., Lyons, K. D., Vigen, C., Macdonald, H., & Clark, F. (2018). Supportive care priorities of low-income Latina breast cancer survivors. *Supportive Care in Cancer, 26*(11), 3851–3859. https://doi.org/10.1007/s00520-018-4253-7

Thomas, E., Polo, K. M., Blackham, K., & Gill, J. (2019). An early detection program for performance deficit in patients receiving breast cancer-related surgical intervention. *Special Interest Section Quarterly Practice Connections, 4*(1), 27–29.

Williams, G. R., Deal, A. M., Sanoff, H. K., Nyrop, K. A., Guerard, E., Pergolotti, M., Shachar, S. S., Reeve, B. B., Bensen, J. T., Choi, S. K., & Muss, H. B. (2019). Frailty and health-related quality of life in older women with breast cancer. *Supportive Care in Cancer, 27*(7), 2693–2698. https://doi.org/10.1007/s00520-018-4558-6

BIBLIOGRAPHY

Cheng, A. S. K., Lau, L. O. C., Ma, Y. N. H., Ngai, R. H., & Fong, S. S. L. (2016). Impact of cognitive and psychological symptoms on work productivity and quality of life among breast cancer survivors in Hong Kong. *Hong Kong Journal of Occupational Therapy, 28*(1), 15–23. https://doi.org/10.1016/j.hkjot.2016.11.002

Jakobsen, K., Magnus, E., Lundgren, S., & Reidunsdatter, R. J. (2018). Everyday life in breast cancer survivors experiencing challenges: A qualitative study. *Scandinavian Journal of Occupational Therapy, 25*(4), 298–307. https://doi.org/10.1080/11038128.2017.1335777

Lin, Y., & Pan, P. J. (2012). The use of rehabilitation among patients with breast cancer: A retrospective longitudinal cohort study. *BMC Health Services Research, 12*, Article 282. https://doi.org/10.1186/1472-6963-12-282

Palmadottir, G. (2010). The role of occupational participation and environment among Icelandic women with breast cancer: A qualitative study. *Scandinavian Journal of Occupational Therapy, 17*(4), 299–307. https://doi.org/10.3109/11038120903302874

Player, L., Mackenzie, L., Willis, K., & Loh, S. Y. (2014). Women's experiences of cognitive changes or "chemobrain" following treatment for breast cancer: A role for occupational therapy? *Australian Occupational Therapy Journal, 61*(4), 230–240. https://doi.org/10.1111/1440-1630.12113

Sleight, A. G. (2017). Occupational engagement in low-income Latina breast cancer survivors. *American Journal of Occupational Therapy, 71*(2), Article 67102100020. https://doi.org/10.5014/ajot.2017.023739

Cancer: Adult

See also Breast Cancer; Cancer: Child and Adolescent; Cancer Survivor; Lymphedema; Terminal Illness, End of Life, Palliative Care, and Hospice.

Description

Cancer is the unregulated proliferation of cells. The important property is a lack of differentiation of cells, local invasion of adjoining tissues, and, often, metastasis (spread to distant sites through the bloodstream or the lymphatic system). The majority of cancers are now curable, particularly if detected at an early state, and long-term remission is often possible in those detected at later stages (Porter, 2018). Cancer is a general term for malignant neoplasms—carcinoma or sarcoma. Medical interventions may include surgery, chemotherapy, radiation, and stem cell transplant. Cancers may be categorized in four stages in which Stage 1 is most curable and Stage IV is most life threatening. The specific descriptions of the categories depend on whether the type of cancer is considered a "solid organ" (lung, breast) type or "liquid" (blood, lymphatic) type. This chapter focuses more on the acute or hospital management of cancer. The chapter on Cancer Survivor focuses more on posthospitalization and home care.

Cause

Immunodeficiency states are associated with an increased incidence of various kinds of cancer, particularly those associated with viral infection, and tumors arising in the lymphatic system and the skin (Porter, 2018).

Evaluation/Assessment

Areas

- Activities of Daily Living/Instrumental ADL: basic ADL skills (eating, dressing, toileting, bathing/showering, grooming), shopping, finances, meal preparation, medication management, home management, driving, caring for others, caring for pets, sexual relations

- Education/Work: academic performance if enrolled in an educational setting, work skill (paid or volunteer) requirements, retirement status
- Play/Leisure: interests, type, frequency
- Rest/Sleep: sleep disturbance, insomnia
- Social Participation: type, frequency, location
- Sensorimotor: gross motor, fine motor, balance and coordination (falls), joint range of motion, muscle strength, endurance, shortness of breath, posture, pain (central, headache, muscle and joint), fatigue and tiredness, scar tissue management, edema (swelling, lymphedema), peripheral neuropathy (numbness and tingling), pressure sores
- Cognitive/Perceptual: attention and concentration, memory, executive functions, body image
- Psychosocial: depression, anxiety, interpersonal relations, role performance, quality of life
- Context/Environment: home modification, adapted equipment
- Comorbidities: arthritis, lung or gastrointestinal disorders, diabetes, depression

Instruments

Instruments Developed by Occupational Therapy Personnel

- Activities of Daily Living Questionnaire (ADLQ; Waehrens et al., 2012)
- Activity Measure for Post-Acute Care (AM-PAC; Jette et al., 2015)
- Arnadottir OT-ADL Neurobehavioral Evaluation (A-One; Arnadottir, 1990)
- Canadian Occupational Performance Measure (5th ed., COPM-5; Law et al., 2014)
- Carolina Frailty Index (CFI; Guerard et al., 2017, in References)
- Executive Function Performance Test (EFPT; Baum & Wolf, 2013)
- Kettle Test (KT; Harman-Maeir et al., 2009)
- Manual Ability Measure (MAM-16, MAM-20, or MAM-36; Chen et al., 2005; Chen & Bode, 2010; Chen & Bode, 2011; see also Hill & Chen, 2012, in References)
- Mental Health Index-13 (MHI-13; Pergolotti, Langer, et al., 2019, in References)
- Model of Human Occupation Screening Tool (MHOST; Parkinson et al., 2006)
- Possibilities for Activity Scale (PActS; Pergolotti & Cutchin, 2015, and Pergolotti et al., 2015, in References)
- Possibilities for Activity Scale for Women (PActS-W; Pergolotti, Doll, et al., 2019, in References)
- Valued Activity Inventory for Adults with Cancer (VAI-AC; Lyons et al., 2012, in References)
- Worker Role Inventory (Version 10.0; WRI 10.0; Braveman et al., 2005)

Instruments Developed by Other Professionals and Used by Occupational Therapy Personnel

- Brief Fatigue Inventory (BFI; Mendoza et al., 1999)
- Coping thermometer (visual analogue scale using an 11-point scale ranging from 0 [*I have no difficulty coping*] to 10 [*I have great difficulty coping*])
- Core Quality of Life Questionnaire C30 (QLQ-C30; European Organization for Research and Treatment of Cancer [EORTC], 1995)
- Distress thermometer (visual analogue scale using an 11-point scale ranging from 0 [*no distress*] to 10 [*extreme distress*])
- Eastern Cooperative Oncology Group Performance Status (ECOG Performance Status; Oken et al., 1982)
- Edmonton Symptom Assessment System (ESAS; Bruera et al., 1991; see also Cheifetz et al., 2014, in References)
- Edmonton Symptom Assessment System-r (ESAS-r; Nekolaichuk et al., 2018)
- Five-Meter Walk Test (no source found)
- Functional Assessment of Cancer Therapy (FACT; Cella et al., 1993)
- Karnofsky Performance Status (KPS; Karnofsky & Burchenal, 1949)
- Katz Activities of Daily Living Index (Katz ADL Index; see Index of Activities of Daily Living, Katz et al., 1970)

- Lee Fatigue Scale (LFS; Lee et al., 1991; see also Lerdal et al., 2016, in References)
- Montreal Cognitive Assessment (MoCA; Nasreddine et al., 2005; see also Arcuri et al., 2015, in References)
- Multidimensional Fatigue Inventory (MFI; Smets et al., 1995)
- Multiple Errands Test (MET; Shallice & Burgess, 1991)
- Patient-Generated Subjective Global Assessment (PGSGA) of nutritional status (Ottery, 1996)
- Rivermead Behavioural Memory Test (3rd ed.; RBMT-3; Wilson et al., 2008)
- Sheffield Profile for Assessment and Referral for Care questionnaire (SPARC; Hughes et al., 2015)
- Short-Form 36 Health Survey (SF-36; Ware et al., 1993)
- Six-Minute Walk Test (6MWT; American Thoracic Society, 2002)
- World Health Organization Quality of Life–BREF (WHOQOL-BREF; The WHOQOL Group, 1998)
- Wong-Baker FACES Pain Rating Scale (FACES; Wong & Baker, 1998)

Problems/Issues

Activities of Daily Living/Instrumental ADL
(Note: See Lindahl-Jacobsen et al., 2015, for a full list of problems in ADLs and IADLs.)

- Person may experience difficulty eating and swallowing depending on the type of cancer and side effects of chemotherapy or radiation.
- Person may experience nausea and loss of appetite.
- Person may experience weight loss and have difficulty maintaining normal weight for age and sex.
- Person may experience difficulty with bathing or showering.
- Person may experience difficulty getting dressed and undressed.
- Person may be experience difficulty with mobility including difficulty with transfers, difficulty walking more than short distances and climbing stairs.
- Person may experience changes in sexual habits and concepts of sexuality.
- Person may be unable to prepare meals or need assistance.
- Person may have difficulty performing housekeeping activities including cleaning and doing laundry.
- Person may be unable to shop for groceries and other household needs.
- Person may be unable to drive or take public transportation.
- Person may be able to perform many of the ADL and IADL tasks but require extra time to complete.

Education/Work
- Person may be unable to participate in classroom activities.
- Person may be unable to perform required work tasks (paid or volunteer) at expected level of performance.
- Person may express feelings of inadequacy in performing worker role.

Play/Leisure
- Person may be unable to engage in favorite leisure activities.

Rest/Sleep
- Person may experience changes in sleep routines due to effects of chemotherapy or pain.
- Person may experience episodes of drowsiness during the day regardless of quality of nighttime sleep. Drowsiness may be a side effect of medication.
- Person may experience sleep disturbances such as night sweats.

Social Participation

- Person may withdraw from participation in social activities.

Sensorimotor

- Person usually experiences decreased endurance and increased symptoms of cancer-related fatigue, including shortness of breath.
- Person may experience decreased range of motion.
- Person may experience decreased muscle strength.
- Person may experience pain.
- Person may experience swelling.
- Person may have changes in posture.
- Person may experience neuropathy or neuropathies.

Cognitive/Perceptual

- Person may experience changes in cognitive functions due to the side effects of chemotherapy.
- Person may have difficulty with goal setting and problem solving.
- Person may experience changes in perception, especially vision, due to side effects of chemotherapy.
- Person may experience changes in body image, especially in head and neck cancer (Teo et al., 2016).

Psychosocial

- Person may experience depression, distress, and anxiety.
- Person may experience a decreased quality of life.
- Person may experience changes in role performance.
- Person may experience changes in interpersonal relationships with family, friends, and colleagues.

Context/Environment

- Lack of information about community or national resources.
- Person may lack information about adapted devices and equipment.

Intervention/Treatment

Models of practice and programs developed by occupational therapy personnel include activity-based program (Maher & Mendonca, 2018), AOTA Practice Guidelines (Braveman & Hunter, 2017), case studies (Braveman et al., 2017; Coss, 2019), Cancer-Related Fatigue Intervention Trial (CAN-FIT; Purcell et al., 2010), clinical case (Braveman et al., 2017), Canadian model of occupational performance (Shipp et al., 2015), goal attainment (Lyons et al., 2018), knowledge translation model (Caldwell et al., 2011), Occupational Therapy Cognitive Behavioral Stress Management (OT-CBSM; Huri et al., 2015), occupation-based intervention (Sagari et al., 2018), occupational therapy role (American Occupational Therapy Association, 2011; Lemoignan et al., 2010; Taylor, 2018), person-environment-occupation-performance model (Hammill et al., 2019), and storytelling (la Cour et al., 2016). Models of practice and programs developed by other professionals but used by occupational therapy personnel include cancer home-life intervention (Brandt et al., 2016), cancer screening (Rockson et al., 2016), ENABLE (Educate, Nurture, Advise, Before Life End; Dionne-Odom et al., 2016), fatigue management (Harris & Belancic, 2018), family member occupational performance patterns (Minami et al., 2013; Minami & Kobayashi, 2016), goal attainment (Lyons et al., 2018), interdisciplinary nutrition program (Gagnon et al., 2013; Lemoignan et al., 2010), mindfulness (Black et al., 2017), residential cancer rehabilitation course (la Cour et al., 2015), psychosocial rehabilitation intervention program (Ledderer et al., 2014; Ledderer et al., 2013), and surveillance model (Alfano & Pergolotti, 2018). Team members include physicians (plastic surgeons, orthopedists), nursing personnel, psychologists, social workers, physical therapists, dieticians or nutritionists, speech–language pathologists, and occupational therapy personnel. The goal includes use of both remedial and compensatory occupation-based approaches to set client-centered goals with the aim of maintaining dignity and enabling improved quality of life by maximizing function, promoting independence, facilitating engagement in meaningful occupations, and assisting in adaptation as needed while also addressing physical, social, emotional, and spiritual needs (Aslam, 2017; Bentley et al., 2013; Occupational Therapy Australia, 2015).

Activities of Daily Living/Instrumental ADL

- Aim to optimize independence in ADLs and IADLs by maintaining functional performance and use of adapted devices and assistive technology as needed.
- Monitor for signs of symptoms of lymphedema or issues such as graph versus host disease in stem cell transplants.
- Discuss issues of sexual health and sexuality or arrange for referral.

Education/Work

- Support engagement in valued vocational interests.
- Provide a return-to-work program or refer client to an existing program in the community.
- Review existing or prospective work environment for possible modifications such as organizing workspace to reduce need to reach overhead or use a cart rather than carry items.

Play/Leisure

- Encourage person to engage or reengage in favorite and valued leisure activities; modifications may be necessary such as gardening in pots on a raised platform instead of gardening at ground level in the backyard.

Rest/Sleep

- Sleep habits and routines: Explore with client whether changes in sleep habits or routines would provide better sleep and rest periods.
- Sleep environment: Explore with client if changes in sleep environment would improve quality of sleep such as a different mattress, silk sheets to improve bed mobility, decreasing light and noise, using essential oils such as lavender, changing room temperature.

Social Participation

- Encourage person to continue participation or reestablish participation in social activities starting with more passive activities, such going to movies or concerts, and increasing toward more active involvement such as eating out with friends.

Sensorimotor

- Joint range of motion and stretching exercises.
- Energy conservation strategies (motion economy) including planning/scheduling, pacing work and rest periods, and prioritizing.
- Work simplification: Cutting out unnecessary steps or substituting one approach for another that is less complicated.
- Pain management program: Adjusting medication effectiveness to coincide with peak activity or energy expenditure.
- Fatigue management program including keeping a daily fatigue journal noting which activities produced the most fatigue symptoms, keeping a weekly calendar of activities, scheduling rest breaks, and prioritizing most valued occupations.

Cognitive/Perceptual

- Negotiate individualized, meaningful goals with the person and the social support group (family, friends, caregivers, colleagues).
- Problem solving: Assisting clients to use problem-solving strategies to address everyday activities.
- Self-management: Encouraging client to develop and implement approaches to manage daily activities using prioritizing activities, scheduling important activities when medication is most effective.

- Body image: Encourage client to identify makeup and clothing that looks best on the individual.

Psychosocial

- Provide stress management training such as relaxation, deep-breathing exercise, yoga, mindfulness, expressive writing, aromatherapy (essential oils), and visual imagery to reduce anxiety, distress, and depression. Family members and caregivers may benefit from the training as well as the client.
- Promote autonomy of decision making and participation in care planning and choices.
- Consider what tasks could be delegated to others short term and long term.

Context/Environment

- Refer client to other professional such as psychologist.
- Provide instruction and training to family and caregivers regarding managing client especially in advanced (Stage IV) cancer.
- Use of adaptive or assistive devices should consider if the devices will address fatigue and pain issues as well as provide additional functional performance.
- Provide information and advice on environmental modifications to make the home, yard, and community more accessible.
- Include social support group (circle of support) as part of the intervention planning team.
- Respect and consider cultural language and spiritual needs in developing care plans.
- Provide access to community and internet resources.

Precautions/Safety Considerations

Blood cell counts: red blood cell count, white blood cell count, hemoglobin, and hematocrit may affect performance. Coagulation panels: prothrombin time, international normalized ration, and partial thromboplastin time. Basic metabolic panels: blood sugar, calcium, creatinine, potassium, blood urea nitrogen. Increased fall risk due to decreased balance and coordination. Increased burn or injury risk due to peripheral neuropathy.

Prognosis and Outcome

Variable. Good outcome expected if cancer is identified and treated in Stage 1. Outcome is less successful when cancer is identified as Stage 4 or has progressed to Stage 4. High level of motor ability to perform ADLs is associated with a higher quality of life (Brekke et al., 2019). Poorer quality of life is associated with high comorbidity, decreased ability to participate in daily activities, and older Black adults with cancer (Pergolotti et al., 2017). Risk of functional decline is a major reason for referral to occupational therapy services (Pergolotti et al., 2016).

REFERENCES

Alfano, C. M., & Pergolotti, M. (2018). Next-generation cancer rehabilitation: A giant step forward for patient care. *Rehabilitation Nursing, 43*(4), 186–194. https://doi.org/10.1097/rnj.0000000000000174

American Occupational Therapy Association. (2011). *Fact sheet: The role of occupational therapy in oncology.* Author.

Arcuri, G. G., Palladini, L., Dumas, G., Lemoignan, J., & Gagnon, B. (2015). Exploring the measurement properties of the Montreal Cognitive Assessment in a population of people with cancer. *Supportive Care in Cancer, 23*(9), 2779–2787. https://doi.org/10.1007/s00520-015-2643-7

Aslam, A. (2017). Working with complex cancer patients. *OT News, 25*(2), 36–38.

Bentley, R., Hussain, A., Maddocks, M., & Wilcock, A. (2013). Occupational therapy needs of patients with thoracic cancer at the time of diagnosis: Findings of a dedicated rehabilitation service. *Supportive Care in Cancer, 21,* 1519–1524. https://doi.org/10.1007/s00520-012-1687-1

Black, D. S., Peng, C., Sleight, A. G., Nguyen, N., Lenz, H. J., & Figueiredo, J. C. (2017). Mindfulness practice reduces cortisol blunting during chemotherapy: A randomized controlled study of colorectal cancer patients. *Cancer, 123*(16), 3088–3096. https://doi.org/10.1002/cncr.30698

Brandt, Å., Pilegaard, M. S., Oestergaard, L. G., Lindahl-Jacobsen, L., Sørensen, J., Johnsen, A. T., & la Cour, K. (2016). Effectiveness of the "Cancer Home-Life Intervention" on everyday activities and quality of life in people with advanced cancer living at home: A randomised controlled trial and an economic evaluation. *BMC Palliative Care, 15,* Article 10. https://doi.org/10.1186/s12904-016-0084-9

Braveman, B., & Hunter, E. G. (2017). *Occupational therapy practice guidelines for cancer rehabilitation with adults.* AOTA Press.

Braveman, B., Hunter, E. G., Nicholson, J., Arbesman, M., & Lieberman, D. (2017). Occupational therapy interventions for adults with cancer. *American Journal of Occupational Therapy, 71*(5), Article 7105395010. https://doi.org/10.5014/ajot.2017.715003

Brekke, M. F., la Cour, K., Brandt, Å., Peoples, H., & Wæhrens, E. E. (2019). The association between ADL ability and quality of life among people with advanced cancer. *Occupational Therapy International, 2019,* Article 2629673. https://doi.org/10.1155/2019/2629673

Caldwell, E., Fleming, J., Purcell, A., Whitehead, M., & Cox, R. (2011). Knowledge translation in cancer services: Implementing the research and evidence in practice model. *British Journal of Occupational Therapy, 74*(11), 535–539. https://doi.org/10.4276/030802211X13204135680947

Cheifetz, O., Packham, T. L., & MacDermid, J. C. (2014). Rasch analysis of the Edmonton Symptom Assessment System and research implications. *Current Oncology, 21*(2), e186–e194. https://doi.org/10.3747/co.21.1735

Coss, D. (2019). Occupational therapy interventions in cancer care. *OT Practice, 24*(7), 10–14.

Dionne-Odom, J. N., Lyons, K. D., Akyar, I., & Bakitas, M. A. (2016). Coaching family caregivers to become better problem solvers when caring for persons with advanced cancer. *Journal of Social Work in End-of-Life & Palliative Care. 12*(1-2), 63–81. https://doi.org/10.1080/15524256.2016.1156607

Gagnon, B., Murphy, J., Eades, M., Lemoignan, J., Jelowicki, M., Carney, S., Amdouni, S., Di Dio, P., Chasen, M., & MacDonald, N. (2013). A prospective evaluation of an interdisciplinary nutrition-rehabilitation program for patients with advanced cancer. *Current Oncology, 20*(6), 310–318. https://doi.org/10.3747/co.20.1612

Guerard, E. J., Deal, A. M., Chang, Y., Williams, G. R., Nyrop, K. A., Pergolotti, M., Muss, H. B., Sanoff, H. K., & Lund, J. L. (2017). Frailty index developed from a cancer-specific geriatric assessment and the association with mortality among older adults with cancer. *Journal of the National Comprehensive Cancer Network, 15*(7), 894–902. https://doi.org/10.6004/jnccn.2017.0122

Hammill, K., Stewart, C. G., Kosic, N., Bellamy, L. Irvine, H., Hutley, D., & Arblaster, K. (2019). Exploring the impact of brain cancer on people and their participation. *British Journal of Occupational Therapy, 82*(3), 162–169. https://doi.org/10.1177/0308022618800186

Harris, I., & Belancic, M. (2018). Stepping out of the bubble. *OT News, 26*(7), 42–44.

Hill, A. E., & Chen, C. (2012). The Manual Ability Measure in oncology: An occupation-based hand assessment. *OT Practice, 17*(11), CE-1–CE-8.

Huri, M., Huri, E., Kayihan, H., & Altuntas, O. (2015). Effects of occupational therapy on quality of life of patients with metastatic prostate cancer: A randomized controlled study. *Saudi Medical Journal, 36*(8), 954–961.

la Cour, K., Ledderer, L., & Hansen, H. P. (2015). "An arena for sharing": Exploring the joint involvement of patients and their relatives in a cancer rehabilitation intervention study. *Cancer Nursing, 38*(2), E1–E9. https://doi.org/10.1097/NCC.0000000000000149

la Cour, K., Ledderer, L., & Hansen, H. P. (2016). Storytelling as part of cancer rehabilitation to support cancer patients and their relatives. *Journal of Psychosocial Oncology, 34*(6), 460–475. https://doi.org/10.1080/07347332.2016.1217964

Ledderer, L., la Cour, K., & Hansen, H. P. (2014). Outcome of supportive talks in a hospital setting: Insights from cancer patients and their relatives. *Patient, 7*(2), 219–229. https://doi.org/10.1007/s40271-014-0047-2

Ledderer, L., la Cour, K., Mogensen, O., Jakobsen, E., Depont Christensen, R., Kragstrup, J., & Hansen, H. P. (2013). Feasibility of a psychosocial rehabilitation intervention to enhance the involvement of relatives in cancer rehabilitation: Pilot study for a randomized controlled trial. *Patient, 6*(3), 201–212. https://doi.org/10.1007/s40271-013-0019-y

Lemoignan, J., Chasen, M., & Bhargava, R. (2010). A retrospective study of the role of an occupational therapist in the cancer nutrition rehabilitation program. *Supportive Care in Cancer, 18,* 1589–1596. https://doi.org/10.1007/s00520-009-0782-4

Lerdal, A., Kottorp, A., Gay, C., Aouizerat, B. E., Lee, K. A., & Miaskowski, C. (2016). A Rasch analysis of assessments of morning and evening fatigue in oncology patients using the Lee Fatigue Scale. *Journal of Pain and Symptom Management, 51*(6), 1002–1012. https://doi.org/10.1016/j.jpainsymman.2015.12.331

Lindahl-Jacobsen, L., Hansen, D. G., Wæhrens, E. E., la Cour, K., & Søndergaard, J. (2015). Performance of activities of daily living among hospitalized cancer patients. *Scandinavian Journal of Occupational Therapy, 22*(2), 137–146. https://doi.org/10.3109/11038128.2014.985253

Lyons, K. D., Hegel, M. T., Hull, J. G., Li, Z., Balan, S., & Bartels, S. (2012). Reliability and validity of the Valued Activity Inventory for Adults with Cancer (VAI-AC). *OTJR: Occupation, Participation and Health, 32*(1), 238–245. https://doi.org/10.3928/15394492-20110623-02 (Form included)

Lyons, K. D., Newman, R. M., Kaufman, P. A., Bruce, M. L., Stearns, D. M., Lansigan, F., Chamberlin, M., Bartels, S. J., Whipple, J., & Hegel, M. T. (2018). Goal attainment and goal adjustment of older adults during person-directed cancer rehabilitation. *American Journal of Occupational Therapy, 72*(2), Article 7202205110. https://doi.org/10.5014/ajot.2018.023648

Maher, C., & Mendonca, R. J. (2018). Impact of an activity-based program on health, quality of life, and occupational performance of women diagnosed with cancer. *American Journal of Occupational Therapy, 72*(2), Article 7202205040. https://doi.org/10.5014/ajot.2018.023663

Minami, S., & Kobayashi, R. (2016). An occupational performance patterns of family members of terminal cancer patients: Typology of family palliative caregivers and occupation performance patterns. *Asian Journal of Occupational Therapy, 12*(1), 29–36.

Minami, S., Kobayashi, R., Kyougoku, M., & Matuda, I. (2013). Occupational experiences of and psychological adjustment by family members of cancer patients. *Hong Kong Journal of Occupational Therapy, 23*(1), 32–38. https://doi.org/10.1016/j.hkjot.2013.06.002

Occupational Therapy Australia. (2015). *Position paper: Occupational therapy in oncology.*

Pergolotti, M., & Cutchin, M. P. (2015). The Possibilities for Activity Scale (PActS): Development, validity, and reliability. *Canadian Journal of Occupational Therapy, 82*(2), 85–92. https://doi.org/10.1177/0008417414561493

Pergolotti, M., Cutchin, M. P., & Muss, H. B. (2015). Predicting participation in meaningful activity for older adults with cancer. *Quality of Life Research, 24*(5), 1217–1222. https://doi.org/10.1007/s11136-014-0849-7

Pergolotti, M., Deal, A. M., Williams, G. R., Bryant, A. L., Bensen, J. T., Muss, H. B., & Reeve, B. B. (2017). Activities, function, and health-related quality of life (HRQOL) of older adults with cancer. *Journal of Geriatric Oncology, 8*(4), 249–254. https://doi.org/10.1016/j.jgo.2017.02.009

Pergolotti, M., Doll, K. M., Fawaz, E. O., & Reeve, B. B. (2019). Adaptation of the Possibilities for Activity Scale for women encountering cancer (PActS-W). *Australian Occupational Therapy Journal, 66*(2), 154–163. https://doi.org/10.1111/1440-1630.12520 (Form included)

Pergolotti, M., Langer, M. M., Deal, A. M., Muss, H. B., Nyrop, K., & Williams, G. (2019). Mental status evaluation in older adults with cancer: Development of the Mental Health Index-13. *Journal of Geriatric Oncology, 10*(2), 241–245. https://doi.org/10.1016/j.jgo.2018.08.009

Pergolotti, M., Williams, G. R., Campbell, C., Munoz, L. A., & Muss, H. B. (2016). Occupational therapy for adults with cancer: Why it matters. *Oncologist, 21*(3), 314–319. https://doi.org/10.1634/theoncologist.2015-0335

Porter, R. S. (Ed.). (2018). *The Merck manual of diagnosis and therapy* (20th ed.). Merck Sharp & Dohme.

Purcell, A., Fleming, J., Bennett, S., & Haines, T. (2010). Development of an educational intervention for cancer-related fatigue. *British Journal of Occupational Therapy, 73*(7), 327–333. https://doi.org/10.4276/030802210X12759925544425

Rockson, L. E., Swarbrick, M. A., & Pratt, C. (2016). Cancer screening among peer-led community wellness center enrollees. *Journal of Psychosocial Nursing and Mental Health Services, 54*(3), 36–40. https://doi.org/10.3928/02793695-20160219-06

Sagari, A., Ikio, Y., Imamura, N., Deguchi, K., Sakai, T., Tabira, T., & Higashi, T. (2018). Effect of occupation-based interventions in patients with haematopoietic malignancies undergoing chemotherapy: A pilot randomised controlled trial. *Hong Kong Journal of Occupational Therapy, 31*(2), 97–105. https://doi.org/10.1177/1569186118818680

Shipp, S., McKinstry, C., & Pearson, E. (2015). The impact of colorectal cancer on leisure participation: A narrative study. *British Journal of Occupational Therapy, 78*(5), 311–319. https://doi.org/10.1177/0308022614562794

Taylor, S. F. (2018). Occupational therapy and the cancer care continuum: Adjusting treatment focuses. *OT Practice 23*(16), CE-1–CE-12.

Teo, I., Fronczyk, K. M., Guindani, M., Vannucci, M., Ulfers, S. S., Hanasono, M. M., & Fingeret, M. C. (2016). Salient body image concerns of patients with cancer undergoing head and neck reconstruction. *Head & Neck, 38*(7), 1035–1042. https://doi.org/10.1002/hed.24415

BIBLIOGRAPHY

Braveman, B., Munoz, L. A., Hughes, J. K., & Nicholson, J. (2018). Cancer and oncology rehabilitation. In H. M. Pendleton & W. Schultz-Krohn (Eds.), *Pedretti's occupational therapy: Practice skills for physical dysfunction* (8th ed., pp. 1134–1141). Elsevier.

Burkhardt, A., & Schultz-Krohn, W. (2013). Oncology. In H. M. Pendleton & W. Schultz-Krohn (Eds.), *Pedretti's occupational therapy: Practice skills for physical dysfunction* (7th ed., pp. 1215–1227). Mosby.

Capozzi, L. C., Dolgoy, N. D., & McNeely, M. L. (2018). Physical rehabilitation and occupational therapy. *Oral and Maxillofacial Surgery Clinics of North America, 30*(4), 471–486. https://doi.org/10.1016/j.coms.2018.06.008

Fieldson, H. (2018). Adopting enhanced recovery principles with cancer treatment. *OT News, 26*(12), 44–45.

Funch, A., Kruse, N. B., la Cour K., Peoples, H. Wæhrens, E. E., & Brandt, Å. (2019). The association between having assistive devices and activities of daily living ability and health-related quality of life: An exploratory cross-section study among people with advanced cancer. *European Journal of Cancer Care, 28*(3), Article e13002. https://doi.org/10.1111/ecc.13002

Hunter, E. G., Gibson, R. W., Arbesman, M., & D'Amico, M. (2017). Systematic review of occupational therapy and adult cancer rehabilitation: Part 1. Impact of physical activity and symptom management interventions. *American Journal of Occupational Therapy, 71*(2), Article 7102100030. https://doi.org/10.5014/ajot.2017.023564

Hunter, E. G., Gibson, R. W., Arbesman, M., & D'Amico, M. (2017). Systematic review of occupational therapy and adult cancer rehabilitation: Part 2. Impact of multidisciplinary rehabilitation and psychosocial, sexuality, and return-to-work interventions. *American Journal of Occupational Therapy, 71*(2), Article 7102100040. https://doi.org/10.5014/ajot.2017.023572

Leak Bryant, A., Walton, A. L., Pergolotti, M., Phillips, B., Bailey, C., Mayer, D. K., & Battaglini, C. (2017). Perceived benefits and barriers to exercise for recently treated adults with acute leukemia. *Oncology Nursing Forum, 44*(4), 413–420. https://doi.org/10.1188/17.ONF.413-420

Lyons, K. D., Radomski, M. V., Alfano, C. M., Finkelstein, M., Sleight, A. G., Marshall, T. F., McKenna, R., & Fu, J. B. (2017). Delphi study to determine rehabilitation research priorities for older adults with cancer. *Archives of Physical Medicine and Rehabilitation, 98*(5), 904–914. https://doi.org/10.1016/j.apmr.2016.11.015

Park, P., & Hashmi, M. (2018). Occupational therapy for the head and neck cancer patient. *Cancer Treatment and Research, 174,* 225–235. https://doi.org/10.1007/978-3-319-65421-8_13

Pergolotti, M., Cutchin, M. P., Weinberger, M., & Meyer, A. M. (2014). Occupational therapy use by older adults with cancer. *American Journal of Occupational Therapy, 68*(5), 597–607. https://doi.org/10.5014/ajot.2014.011791

Pergolotti, M., Deal, A. M., Lavery, J., Reeve, B., & Muss, H. B. (2015). The prevalence of potentially modifiable functional deficits and the subsequent use of occupational and physical therapy by older adults with cancer. *Journal of Geriatric Oncology, 6*(3), 194–201. https://doi.org/10.1016/j.jgo.2015.01.004

Pergolotti, M., Lyons, K. D., & Williams, G. R. (2018). Moving beyond symptom management towards cancer rehabilitation for older adults: Answering the 5W's. *Journal of Geriatric Oncology, 9*(6), 543–549. https://doi.org/10.1016/j.jgo.2017.11.009

Radomski, M. V., Anheluk, M., Gabe, K., Hopkins, S. E., & Zola, J. (2014). Cancer. In M. V. Radomski & C. A. T. Latham (Eds.), *Occupational therapy for physical dysfunction* (7th ed., pp. 1368–1387). Lippincott Williams & Wilkins.

Rijpkema, C., Van Hartingsveldt, M., & Stuiver, M. M. (2018). Editorial: Occupational therapy in cancer rehabilitation: Going beyond physical function to enabling activity and participation. *Expert Review of Quality of Life in Cancer Care, 3*(1), 1–3. https://doi.org/10.1080/23809000.2018.1438844

Smith-Gabai, H. (2011). Oncology. In H. Smith-Gabai (Ed.), *Occupational therapy in acute care* (pp. 407–442). AOTA Press.

Stein Duker, L. I., & Sleight, A. G. (2019). Occupational therapy practice in oncology care: Results from a survey. *Nursing and Health Sciences, 21*(2), 164–170. https://doi.org/10.1111/nhs.12576

Taylor, S. F. (2017). Cancer. In B. J. Atchison & D. P. Dirette (Eds.), *Conditions in occupational therapy* (5th ed., pp. 513–539). Wolters Kluwer.

Williams, G. R., Deal, A. M., Muss, H. B., Weinberg, M. S., Sanoff, H. K., Guerard, E. J., Nyrop, K. A., Pergolotti, M., & Shachar, S. S. (2018). Frailty and skeletal muscle in older adults with cancer. *Journal of Geriatric Oncology, 9*(1), 68–73. https://doi.org/10.1016/j.jgo.2017.08.002

Wilson, C. M., Colombo, R., & Hakmeh, B. (2018). New Horizons in oncology rehabilitation. *Oncology Issues, 33*(1), 28–35. https://doi.org/10.1080/10453356.2018.1400871

Cancer: Childhood and Adolescent

Description

A diagnosis of cancer occurring in persons ages 0 to 18. Leukemia is the most common type overall. Brain tumors are the most common solid cancer in children under 15 years old and are the second leading cause of death due to cancer (Porter, 2018). Types of tumors include astrocytomas, medulloblastoma, ependymomas, neuroblastoma, retinoblastoma, rhabdomyosarcoma, and Wilms tumor, also called nephroblastoma. Other types of childhood cancer include lymphomas, osteosarcoma, and Ewing sarcoma (Porter, 2018).

Cause

The cause of most childhood brain tumors is unknown, but two risk factors are ionizing radiation and specific genetic syndromes such as neurofibromatosis (Porter, 2018).

Evaluation/Assessment

Areas

- Activities of Daily Living/Instrumental ADL: basic ADLs (eating, dressing, toileting, mobility, communication)
- Education/Work: academic performance and participation in school activities
- Play/Leisure: play skills, leisure interests, frequency of engagement
- Rest/Sleep: sleep habits, sleep environment
- Social Participation: type, frequency, with whom
- Sensorimotor: gross and fine motor development, balance and coordination, fatigue, sensory responsiveness, visuomotor skills, bilateral integration, pain and discomfort
- Cognitive/Perceptual: attention, orientation, memory, executive function, visual perceptual skills
- Psychosocial: anxiety, quality of life
- Context/Environment: adapted equipment, modifications to home or school
- Development (Infant, Child, Adolescent only): developmental milestones, regression to previous levels of development, endocrine function

Instruments

Instruments Developed by Occupational Therapy Personnel

- Assessment of Motor Process Skills (8th ed.; AMPS-8; Fisher & Bray Jones, 2016)
- Children's Assessment of Participation and Enjoyment and Preferences for Activities of Children (CAPE/PAC; King et al., 2004)
- Loewenstein Occupational Therapy Cognitive Assessment (2nd ed.; see Dynamic Loewenstein Occupational Therapy Cognitive Assessment, Katz et al., 2012)
- Observation Protocol (Miralles et al., 2016, in References)
- Play History (PH; Takata, 1969)

Instruments Developed by Other Professionals and Used by Occupational Therapy Personnel

- Bruininks-Oseretsky Test of Motor Proficiency (2nd ed., Brief Form; BOT-2 Brief; Bruininks & Bruininks, 2010)
- Children's Memory Scale (CMS; Cohen, 1997)
- Movement Assessment Battery for Children (2nd ed.; M-ABC-2; Henderson et al., 2007)
- Rehabilitation service: OT/PT Screen 12-36 Months (Miale et al., 2013, in References)
- Rivermead Behavioural Memory Test (3rd ed.; RBMT-3; Wilson et al., 2008)
- Rivermead Behavioural Memory Test for Children (RBMT-C; Wilson et al., 1991)
- Short-Form Health Survey (SF-12; Ware et al., 1996)
- Test of Everyday Attention for Children (2nd ed.; TEA-Ch2; Manley et al., 2016)
- Wong-Baker FACES Pain Rating Scale (FACES; Wong & Baker, 1998)

Problems/Issues

Activities of Daily Living/Instrumental ADL

- Child or adolescent may have decreased ability to perform basic ADLs.
- Child or adolescent may have difficulty participating in routine activities.
- Child or adolescent may experience diminished functional mobility including loss of previously learned motor skills.

Education/Work
- Child or adolescent may have difficulty completing academic assignments.
- Child or adolescent may have difficulty participating in school activities due to hospitalization or home treatment program.
- Child or adolescent may have difficulty with handwriting.

Play/Leisure
- Child may fail to develop or lose development skills in play.
- Child or adolescent may discontinue or decrease engagement in leisure activities.

Rest/Sleep
- Child or adolescent may experience sleep disturbances.

Social Participation
- Child or adolescent may limit or discontinue participating in social activities.

Sensorimotor
- Child or adolescent may have decreased muscle strength.
- Child or adolescent may have impaired balance and coordination.
- Child or adolescent may experience difficulties with manual dexterity.
- Child or adolescent may have decreased endurance.
- Child or adolescent may experience decreased activity tolerance.
- Child or adolescent may have decreased level of physical fitness.
- Child or adolescent may experience peripheral neuropathy.

Cognitive/Perceptual
- Child or adolescent may experience cognitive deficits.

Psychosocial
- Child or adolescent may have decreased motivation.
- Child or adolescent may have decreased self-esteem.
- Child or adolescent may experience decreased peer interaction.
- Child or adolescent may experience diminished quality of life.
- Child or adolescent may experience decreased emotional stability.

Context/Environment
- Child or adolescent may experience decreased ability to keep up with peers.
- Child and family may lack knowledge about childhood cancer, especially Hispanic populations (Sleight et al., 2019).
- Child and caregivers may lack knowledge about available resources.

Intervention/Treatment

Models and programs developed by occupational therapy personnel include play-based occupational therapy (Mohammadi et al., 2017). Models and programs developed by other professionals but used by occupational therapy personnel include self-rehabilitation (Nicholson, 2018). Team members include physicians (surgeons, oncologists, pathologists, nursing personnel, psychologists, social workers, physical therapists, speech–language pathologists, dieticians and nutritionists, educators, family, volunteers, and occupational therapy personnel. The goal is to improve the quality of life of children through rehabilitation, prevention of sequelae, maintenance of activities approach to age group, and to develop or redevelop abilities and skills (Joaquim et al., 2017). The goal is to maintain, stimulate, and rehabilitate components of occupational, sensory motor, cognitive, and psychosocial performance, preventing disability and promoting the functionality of children.

Activities of Daily Living/Instrumental ADL
- Assist child to perform age-appropriate basic ADLs as needed.
- Assist child to perform functional mobility.
- Assist adolescents to develop independent living skills.

Education/Work
- Assist in maintaining active participation in academics and classroom activities.

Play/Leisure
- Promote development of play skills in young clients.
- Encourage engagement in favorite and meaningful leisure activities for children and adolescents.

Rest/Sleep
- See Sleep–Wake Disorders in Section 13: Lifestyle Conditions.

Social Participation
- Encourage age-appropriate participation is social activities (passive and active).

Sensorimotor
- Provide opportunity to practice gross motor skills.
- Provide opportunity to improve fine motor skills.
- Provide instruction in energy conservation.
- Assist in development of a pain management program.
- Prevent disabilities and deformities in muscles, joints, and tendons.
- Promote function and activity tolerance.
- Promote activities to increase muscle strength and maintain range of motion.
- Promote use of sensory skills such as registration and discrimination.

Cognitive/Perceptual
- Promotor development of cognitive skills including attention, awareness, memory, and executive skills.
- Promote development of visual perceptual skills.

Psychosocial
- Facilitate motivation for play.
- Promote behavior and emotional regulation.
- Encourage development of friendships and social interaction skills.

Context/Environment
- Provide assistive technology as needed to perform tasks such as ADL tasks or schoolwork.
- Provide information about childhood cancer and its rehabilitation.
- Assist child and family to identify and use community and internet resources.
- Assist family or teachers to make modifications to home or school environment.

Precautions/Safety Considerations

The condition of children with cancer is a dynamic and changing one that requires monitoring over time. Impairment may be global and may result in failure to develop skills that should have been acquired at an earlier age (Adcock & Burke, 2014). The result may mean the child does not have the judgment of safety that another child of similar age has acquired.

Prognosis and Outcome

Variable, depending in part on the type of cancer and on responsiveness to treatment. Performance deficits in motor and process skills may remain after active medical intervention has ceased (Demers et al., 2016). Chemotherapy may cause peripheral neuropathy resulting in decreased fine motor abilities (Sabarre et al., 2014).

REFERENCES

Adcock, F., & Burke, G. A. (2014). Children with brain tumours: A critical reflection on a specialist coordinated assessment. *British Journal of Occupational Therapy, 77*(8), 429–433. https://doi.org/10.4276/030802214X14071472109950

Demers, C., Gélinas, I., & Carret, A.-S. (2016). Activities of daily living in survivors of childhood brain tumor. *American Journal of Occupational Therapy, 70*(1), Article 700122004. https://doi.org/10.5014/ajot.2016.014993

Joaquim, R. H. V. T., Soares, F. B., Figueiredo, M. O., & Brito, C. M. D. (2017). Occupational therapy and pediatric oncology: Characterization of professionals from reference health centers in the state of São Paulo. *Revista de Terapia Ocupacional da Universidade de São Paulo, 28*(1), 36–45. https://doi.org/10.11606/issn2238-6149.v28i1p36-45

Miale, S., Stimler, L., & Riedel, E. R. (2013). Using a simple screening tool to enhance awareness and utilization of rehabilitation services for pediatric oncology patients in the acute care setting. *Rehabilitation Oncology, 31*(2), 6–10. https://doi.org/10.1097/01893697-201331020-00003

Miralles, P. M., Ramón, N. C., & Valero, S. A. (2016). Adolescents with cancer and occupational deprivation in hospital settings: A qualitative study. *Hong Kong Journal of Occupational Therapy, 27*(1), 26–34. https://doi.org/10.1016/j.hkjot.2016.05.001

Mohammadi, A., Mehraban, A. H., & Damavandi, S. A. (2017). Effect of play-based occupational therapy on symptoms of hospitalized children with cancer: A single-subject study. *Asia-Pacific Journal of Oncology Nursing, 4*(2), 168–172. https://doi.org/10.4103/apjon.apjon_13_17

Nicholson, A. (2018). Promoting self-rehabilitation through purposeful activities. *OT News, 26*(2), 27.

Porter, R. S. (Ed.). (2018). *The Merck manual of diagnosis and therapy* (20th ed.). Merck Sharp & Dohme.

Sabarre, C. L., Rassekh, S. R., & Zwicker, J. G. (2014). Vincristine and fine motor function of children with acute lymphoblastic leukemia. *Canadian Journal of Occupational Therapy, 81*(4), 256–264. https://doi.org/10.1177/0008417414539926

Sleight, A. G., Ramirez, C. N., Miller, K. A., & Milam, J. E. (2019). Hispanic orientation and cancer-related knowledge in childhood cancer survivors. *Journal of Adolescent and Young Adult Oncology, 8*(3), 363–367. https://doi.org/10.1089/jayao.2018.0099

BIBLIOGRAPHY

O'Toole, M. T. (Ed.). (2017). *Mosby's dictionary of medicine, nursing & health professions* (10th ed.). Elsevier.

Cancer Survivor

See also Breast Cancer; Cancer: Adult; Cancer: Child and Adolescent; Lymphedema; Terminal Illness, End of Life, Palliative Care, and Hospice.

Description

"A cancer survivor is a person diagnosed with cancer, from the time of diagnosis throughout their lifespan" (Centers for Disease Control and Prevention, 2021, para. 2). However, this chapter focuses on studies documenting problems after the initial treatment period and when the cancer diagnosis has become a chronic condition. Survivors may have residual physical, cognitive, emotional, and social problems that prevent or inhibit them from participating in everyday meaningful occupations and may reduce their quality of life. Survivors have functional deficit scores in occupational therapy categories of areas of occupation, body function, performance skills, and psychosocial well-being (Hwang et al., 2015).

Cause

A cancer diagnosis is the cause for which a person is labeled a cancer survivor.

Evaluation/Assessment

Areas

- Activities of Daily Living/Instrumental ADL: basic ADLs (eating, dressing, bathing, toileting) home management, meal preparation
- Education/Work: return to work
- Play/Leisure: interests, frequency
- Rest/Sleep: sleep habits and routines
- Social Participation: type, frequency, with whom
- Sensorimotor: endurance, fatigue, activity tolerance
- Cognitive/Perceptual: attention and concentration, memory, executive functions
- Psychosocial: depression, anxiety, stress, emotional stability, role performance, quality of life
- Context/Environment: home and environmental modification, adapted devices and equipment, caregiver education, community resources
- Comorbidities: osteoporosis, smoking, alcohol abuse, stress

Instruments

Instruments Developed by Occupational Therapy Personnel

- Canadian Occupational Performance Measure (5th ed.; COPM-5; Law et al., 2014)
- Nottingham Extended Activities of Daily Living (NEADL; Nouri & Lincoln, 1987)
- Possibilities for Activity Scale (PActS; Pergolotti & Cutchin, 2015)

Instruments Developed by Other Professionals and Used by Occupational Therapy Personnel

- Berg Balance Scale (BBS; Berg et al., 1989)
- Disabilities of the Arm, Shoulder, and Hand (3rd ed.; DASH-3; Kennedy et al., 2011)
- Montreal Cognitive Assessment (MoCA; Nasreddine et al., 2005)
- Patient-Reported Outcomes Measurement Information System (PROMIS; Hahn et al., 2014)
- Visual analogue scale (VAS; pain scale: scored 0 = *no pain*, 10 = *worst pain ever*)

Problems/Issues

Activities of Daily Living/Instrumental ADL

- Person may experience difficulty performance basic ADLs such as getting dressed or undressed, getting in or out of the tub, safely showering while standing.
- Person may experience urinary incontinence.
- Person may be unable to drive or require retraining to drive safely.
- Person may experience sexual dysfunction.

Education/Work

- Person may be unable to work or need work site modification.
- Person may need to consider changing type or line of work activity.

Play/Leisure

- Person may be unable to engage in favorite leisure occupations unless modified.
- Person may need to find alternative leisure occupations.

Rest/Sleep

- Person may experience sleep disturbances due to pain or medications.

Social Participation
- Person may be unable to participate or experience difficulty in participating in preferred social occupations.

Sensorimotor
- Person may have muscle weakness.
- Person may experience loss of hand function including reduced grip strength.
- Person may have reduced range of motion.
- Person may experience fatigue, especially older adults (Lyons et al., 2013).
- Person may have lymphedema.
- Person may have hyper- or hyposensitivity in one or more sensory systems.
- Person may experience pain.
- Person may have scars due to surgery.

Cognitive/Perceptual
- Person may have difficulty paying attention or concentrating.
- Person may experience difficulty with working memory.
- Person may experience executive dysfunction.
- Person may lack self-awareness, insight, and self-acceptance.

Psychosocial
- Person may experience stress and anxiety.
- Person may become depressed.
- Person may express feelings of loss of self-efficacy and self-worth.
- Person may experience loss of self-confidence.
- Person may experience loss of roles and role performance.
- Person may become emotionally labile and experience difficulty with emotional stabilization.

Context/Environment
- Person may experience breakdown of family and partnerships and loss of social support.
- Person may lack access to community resources.
- Community resources may be lacking.
- Cultural beliefs about cancer may interfere with intervention programs.

Intervention/Treatment

Models and programs developed by occupational therapy personnel include cancer home-life intervention (Pilegaard, la Cour, et al., 2018; Pilegaard, Oestergaard, et al., 2020), case study—lung cancer (White, 2016), in-home occupational therapy (Imanishi et al., 2015), and workbook (Taylor & Jones, 2017). Models and programs developed by other professionals but used by occupational therapy personnel include cancer rehabilitation (Lyons et al., 2019; Silver & Gilchrist, 2011), cognitive rehabilitation (Sleight, 2016), health promotion model (Liaset & Kvam, 2018), interdisciplinary nutrition program (Eades et al., 2013), OptiMal (Boland et al., 2019), return-to-work planning tool (Amin et al., 2017), spinal cord compression care (Warnock et al., 2014), and work readiness (Stergiou-Kita et al., 2016). Team members include physicians, oncologists, surgeons, nursing personnel, psychologists, physical therapy personnel, vocational rehabilitation specialists, and occupational therapy personnel. Goals are to address the residual physical and psychosocial complications that prevent a person from fully engaging in everyday life and compromise quality of life (Baxter et al., 2017).

Activities of Daily Living/Instrumental ADL
- See Cancer: Adult; and Cancer: Childhood and Adolescent chapters.

Education/Work
- Assist client with recommendations for work site modification.
- Assist client with transportation to and from work and on-site navigation.

- Assist client to determine what amount/percentage of work time is feasible.
- Assist client to evaluate work and job performance skills and capacity.

Play/Leisure
- Assist client to modify leisure occupations to account for reduced physical fitness and energy level.
- Assist client to explore new leisure occupations that are more congruent with level of physical fitness and energy level.

Rest/Sleep
- Assist client to address sleep disturbances, including habits, routines, medications, and pain management.

Social Participation
- Encourage client to participate in social activities with modifications if needed.

Sensorimotor
- Provide information and practice on using energy conservation and work simplification techniques.
- Provide information and practice in managing fatigue.
- Monitor for signs and symptoms of lymphedema (see Lymphedema chapter, this section).

Cognitive/Perceptual
- Assist client to evaluate cognitive skills including attending behavior, concentration, memory, planning, and problem solving, and self-awareness.

Psychosocial
- Provide strategies for stress reduction: deep breathing, yoga, mindfulness.
- Assist client to develop confidence in abilities and reduce feelings of inadequacy.

Context/Environment
- Provide assistive devices as useful to facilitate functional performance.
- Provide information on home modification to promote safety and energy conservation, such as having laundry room on same floor as clothes closets.
- Provide information on community and internet resources such as cancer survivor groups.
- Provide home exercise program including range of motion, stretching, and postural exercises.
- Assist family and caregivers to provide social support.

Precautions/Safety Considerations

Client should know signs to observe for return of same cancer or evidence of other cancers.

Prognosis and Outcome

Early diagnosis and Stage 1 tumor have better prognosis than later diagnosis and Stage 4 tumor (has metastasized to other parts of the body). Supporting people with advanced cancer to remain in their home doing familiar occupations and occupational performance assists person to maintain sense of self and reduces loss of identity (Maersk et al., 2018; Maersk et al., 2019; Minami & Kobayashi, 2016; Peoples et al., 2017).

REFERENCES

Amin, L., Stergiou-Kita, M., & Jones, J. M. (2017). Development of a return-to-work planning tool for cancer survivors. *Canadian Journal of Occupational Therapy, 84*(4-5), 223–228. https://doi.org/10.1177/0008417417700916

Baxter, M. F., Newman, R., Longpré, S. M., & Polo, K. M. (2017). Occupational therapy's role in cancer survivorship as a chronic condition. *American Journal of Occupational Therapy, 71*(3), Article 7103090010. https://doi.org/10.5014/ajot.2017.713001

Boland, L., Bennett, K., Cuffe, S., Gleeson, N., Grant, C., Kennedy, J., & Connolly, D. (2019). Cancer survivors' experience of OptiMal, a 6-week, occupation-based, self-management intervention. *British Journal of Occupational Therapy, 82*(2), 90–100. https://doi.org/10.1177/0308022618804704

Centers for Disease Control and Prevention. (2021). *Supporting cancer survivors and caregivers.* https://www.cdc.gov/cancer/ncccp/priorities/cancer-survivor-caregiver.htm

Eades, M., Murphy, J., Carney, S., Amdouni, S. Lemoignan, J., Jelowicki, M., Nadler, M., Chasen, M., & Gagnon, B. (2013). Effect of an interdisciplinary rehabilitation program on quality of life in patients with head and neck cancer: Review of clinical experience. *Head & Neck, 35*(3), 343–349. https://doi.org/10.1002/hed.22972

Hwang, E. J., Lokietz, N. C., Lozano, R. L., & Parke, M. A. (2015). Functional deficits and quality of life among cancer survivors: Implications for occupational therapy in cancer survivorship care. *American Journal of Occupational Therapy, 69*(6), Article 6906290010. https://doi.org/10.5014/ajot.2015.015974

Imanishi, M., Tomohisa, H., & Higaki, K. (2015). In-home occupational therapy for a patient with stage IV lung cancer: Changes in quality of life and analysis of causes. *SpringerPlus, 4,* Article 157. https://doi.org/10.1186/s40064-015-0931-9

Liaset, I. F., & Kvam, L. (2018). Experiences of returning to work after brain tumor treatment. *Work, 60*(4), 603–612. https://doi.org/10.3233/WOR-182768

Lyons, K. D., Lambert, L. A., Balan, S., Hegel, M. T., & Bartels, S. (2013). Changes in activity levels of older adult cancer survivors. *OTJR: Occupation, Participation and Health, 33*(1), 31–39. https://doi.org/10.3928/15394492-20120607-02

Lyons, K. D., Padgett, L. S., Marshall, T. F., Greer, J. A., Silver, J. K., Raj, V. S., Zucker, D. S., Fu, J. B., Pergolotti, M., Sleight, A. G., & Alfano, C. M. (2019). Follow the trail: Using insights from the growth of palliative care to propose a roadmap for cancer rehabilitation. *CA: A Cancer Journal for Clinicians, 69*(2), 113–126. https://doi.org/10.3322/caac.21549

Maersk, J. L., Cutchin, M. P., & la Cour, K. (2018). Identity and home: Understanding the experience of people with advanced cancer. *Health & Place, 51,* 11–18. https://doi.org/10.1016/j.healthplace.2018.02.003

Maersk, J. L., Johannessen, H., & la Cour, K. (2019). Occupation as marker of self: Occupation in relation to self among people with advanced cancer. *Scandinavian Journal of Occupational Therapy, 26*(1), 9–18. https://doi.org/10.1080/11038128.2017.1378366

Minami, S., & Kobayashi, R. (2016). An occupational performance patterns of family members of terminal cancer patients: Typology of family palliative caregivers and occupation performance patterns. *Asian Journal of Occupational Therapy, 12*(1), 29–36.

Peoples, H., Brandt, Å., Wæhrens, E. E., & la Cour, K. (2017). Managing occupations in everyday life for people with advanced cancer living at home. *Scandinavian Journal of Occupational Therapy, 24*(1), 57–64. https://doi.org/10.1080/11038128.2016.1225815

Pilegaard, M. S., la Cour, K., Oestergaard, L.G., Johnsen, A. T., Lindahl-Jacobsen, L., Højris, I., & Brandt, Å. (2018). The "Cancer Home-Life Intervention": A randomised controlled trial evaluating the efficacy of an occupational therapy-based intervention in people with advanced cancer. *Palliative Medicine, 32*(4), 744–756. https://doi.org/10.1177/0269216317747199

Pilegaard, M. S., Oestergaard, L. G., la Cour, K., Johnsen, A. T., & Brandt, Å. (2020). Subgroup effects of occupational therapy-based intervention for people with advanced cancer. *Scandinavian Journal of Occupational Therapy, 27*(7), 517–523. https://doi.org/10.1080/11038128.2018.1455897

Silver, J. K., & Gilchrist, L. S. (2011). Cancer rehabilitation with a focus on evidence-based outpatient physical and occupational therapy interventions. *American Journal of Physical Medicine & Rehabilitation, 90*(5, Suppl. 1), S5–S15. https://doi.org/10.1097/PHM.0b013e31820be4ae

Sleight, A. (2016). Coping with cancer-related cognitive dysfunction: A scoping review of the literature. *Disability and Rehabilitation, 38*(4), 400–408. https://doi.org/10.3109/09638288.2015.1038364

Stergiou-Kita, M., Pritlove, C., Holness, D. L., Kirsh, B., van Eerd, D., Duncan, A., & Jones, J. (2016). Am I ready to return to work? Assisting cancer survivors to determine work readiness. *Journal of Cancer Survivorship, 10*, 699–710. https://doi.org/10.1007/s11764-016-0516-9

Taylor, J., & Jones, V. (2017). The development of a workbook to explore meaningful occupations after life-changing events. *British Journal of Occupational Therapy, 80*(7), 440–447. https://doi.org/10.1177/0308022617698168

Warnock, C., Hodson, S., Tod, A., Mills, R., Crowther, L., Buchanan, J., & Foran, B. (2014). Improving care of patients with metastatic spinal cord compression. *British Journal of Nursing, 23*(4, Suppl.), S14–S18. https://doi.org/10.12968/bjon.2014.23.Sup2.S14

White, K. M. (2016). The role of the occupational therapist in the care of people living with lung cancer. *Translational Lung Cancer Research, 5*(3), 244–246. https://doi.org/10.21037/tlcr.2016.05.02

BIBLIOGRAPHY

Buckland, N., & Mackenzie, L. (2017). Exploring the role of occupational therapy in caring for cancer survivors in Australia: A cross sectional study. *Australian Occupational Therapy Journal, 64*(5), 358–368. https://doi.org/10.1111/1440-1630.12386

Cedar, S. H., White, M., & Atwal, A. (2018). The efficacy of complementary therapy for patients receiving palliative cancer care. *International Journal of Palliative Nursing, 24*(3), 146–151. https://doi.org/10.12968/ijpn.2018.24.3.146

Dionne-Odom, J. N., Hull, J. G., Martin, M. Y., Lyons, K. D., Prescott, A. T., Tosteson, T., Li, Z., Akyar, I., Raju, D., & Bakitas, M. A. (2016). Associations between advanced cancer patients' survival and family caregiver presence and burden. *Cancer Medicine 5*(5), 853–862. https://doi.org/10.1002/cam4.653

la Cour, K., & Hansen, H. P. (2012). Aesthetic engagements: "Being" in everyday life with advanced cancer. *American Journal of Hospice and Palliative Care, 29*(2), 126–133. https://doi.org/10.1177/1049909111413117

Polo, K. M., & Smith, C. (2017). Taking our seat at the table: Community cancer survivorship. *American Journal of Occupational Therapy, 71*(2), Article 7102100010. https://doi.org/10.5014/ajot.2017.020693

Şahin, S., Akel, S., & Zarif, M. (2017). Occupational therapy in oncology and palliative care. In M. Huri (Ed.), *Occupational therapy: Occupation focused holistic practice in rehabilitation* (pp. 207–221). InTech.

Sakellariou, D., Anstey, S., Polack, S., Rotarou, E. S., Warren, N., Gaze, S., & Courtenay, M. (2020). Pathways of disability-based discrimination in cancer care. *Critical Public Health, 30*(5), 533–543. https://doi.org/10.1080/09581596.2019.1648762

Sleight, A. G., & Clark, F. (2015). Unlocking the core self: Mindful occupation for cancer survivorship. *Journal of Occupational Science, 22*(4), 477–487. https://doi.org/10.1080/14427591.2015.1008025

Sleight, A. G., & Stein Duker, L. I. (2016). Toward a broader role for occupational therapy in supportive oncology care. *American Journal of Occupational Therapy, 70*(4), Article 7004360030. https://doi.org/10.5014/ajot.2016.018101

Stergiou-Kita, M., Grigorovich, A., Tseung, V., Milosevic, E., Hebert, D., Phan, S., & Jones, J. (2014). Qualitative meta-synthesis of survivors' work experiences and the development of strategies to facilitate return to work. *Journal of Cancer Survivorship, 8*, 657–670. https://doi.org/10.1007/s11764-014-0377-z

Stergiou-Kita, M., Qie, X., Yau, H. K., & Lindsay, S. (2017). Stigma and work discrimination among cancer survivors: A scoping review and recommendations. *Canadian Journal of Occupational Therapy, 84*(3), 178–188. https://doi.org/10.1177/0008417417701229

Stergiou-Kita, M., Pritlove, C., & Kirsh, B. (2016). The "Big C"—Stigma, cancer, and workplace discrimination. *Journal of Cancer Survivorship, 10*, 1035–1050. https://doi.org/10.1007/s11764-016-0547-2

Stergiou-Kita, M., Pritlove, C., van Eerd, D., Holness, L. D., Kirsh, B., Duncan, A., & Jones, J. (2016). The provision of workplace accommodations following cancer: Survivor, provider, and employer perspectives. *Journal of Cancer Survivors, 10*(3), 489–504. https://doi.org/10.1007/s11764-015-0492-5

Williams, G. R., Dunham, L., Chang, Y., Deal, A. M., Pergolotti, M., Lund, J. L. Guerard, E., Kenzik, K., Muss, H. B., & Sanoff, H. K. (2019). Geriatric assessment predicts hospitalization frequency and long-term care use in older adult cancer survivors. *Journal of Oncology Practice, 15*(5), e399-e409. https://doi.org/10.1200/JOP.18.00368

Williams, G. R., Deal, A. M., Lund, J. L., Chang, Y., Muss, H. B., Pergolotti, M., Guerard, E. J., Shachar, S. S., Wang, Y., Kenzik, K., & Sanoff, H. K. (2018). Patient-reported comorbidity and survival in older adults with cancer. *The Oncologist, 23*(4), 433–439. https://doi.org/10.1634/theoncologist.2017-0404

HIV and AIDS

Description

The human immunodeficiency virus (HIV) infection destroys CD4-positive helper T lymphocytes and impairs cell-mediated immunity, increasing risk of certain infections and cancers. HIV can damage the brain, gonads, kidneys, and heart, causing cognitive impairment including acquired immunodeficiency syndrome (AIDS) dementia complex, hypogonadism, renal insufficiency, and cardiomyopathy (Porter, 2018). At-risk populations are gay and bisexual men, male-to-male sexual contact, injection drug use, and heterosexual contact.

Cause

The HIV infection is caused by one of two similar retroviruses (HIV-1 and HIV-2). In the United States, the HIV-1 is more common (Porter, 2018). HIV is transmitted through contact with an infected individual's blood, semen, breast milk, cervical secretions, cerebrospinal fluid, or synovial fluid (O'Toole, 2017). Although HIV/AIDS infection is now considered a chronic disorder, the episodic cycle of wellness and illness may restrict the person's ability to participate in meaningful occupations and present a number of occupational challenges (Lapointe et al., 2013).

Classification
- By CD4 (CD4 positive) cell count persons 6 years or older (Selik et al., 2014)
  - ▶ Stage 1: cell count of 500 or more CD4+ cells per microliter of blood
  - ▶ Stage 2: cell counts from 200 to 499 CD4+
  - ▶ Stage 3: cell count below 200 CD4+
- By stages of disease (Centers for Disease Control and Prevention, n.d.)
  - ▶ Stage 1: Acute HIV Infection
    - ○ People have a large amount of HIV in their blood; they are very contagious.
    - ○ Some people have flu-like symptoms; this is the body's natural response to infection.
    - ○ Some people may not feel sick right away or at all.
    - ○ If a person has flu-like symptoms and may have been exposed to HIV, the person should seek medical care and ask for a test to diagnose acute infection (wording modified to third person).
    - ○ Only antigen/antibody tests or nucleic acid tests (NATs) can diagnose acute infection.
  - ▶ Stage 2: Chronic HIV Infection
    - ○ This stage is also called asymptomatic HIV infection or clinical latency.
    - ○ HIV is still active but reproduces at very low levels.
    - ○ Person may not have any symptoms or get sick during this phase.
    - ○ Without taking HIV medicine, this period may last a decade or longer, but some people may progress faster.

○ People can transmit HIV in this phase.

○ At the end of this phase, amount of HIV in the blood (called viral load) goes up and the CD4 cell count goes down; the person may have symptoms as the virus levels increase in the body, and the person moves into Stage 3.

○ People who take HIV medicine as prescribed may never move into Stage 3.

▶ Stage 3: Acquired Immunodeficiency Syndrome (AIDS)

○ The most severe phase of HIV infection.

○ People with AIDS have such a badly damaged immune system that they get an increasing number of severe illnesses, called opportunistic infections.

○ People receive an AIDS diagnosis when the CD4 cell count drops below 200 cells/mm, or if they develop certain opportunistic infections.

○ People with AIDS can have a high viral load and be very infectious.

○ Without treatment, people with AIDS typically survive about 3 years.

Evaluation/Assessment

Areas

- Activities of Daily Living/Instrumental ADL: medical management and side effects, weight control, functional oral and written communication, cooking and meal preparation, housekeeping, driving, shopping
- Education/Work: job performance
- Play/Leisure: leisure interests, type and frequency in adults, play skills in children
- Rest/Sleep: sleep disturbances
- Social Participation: type, frequency, with whom
- Sensorimotor: fine and gross motor skills, balance and falls, pain such as burning sensations, peripheral neuropathy, muscle weakness, fatigue and reduced endurance, shortness of breath, activity tolerance
- Cognitive/Perceptual: memory and concentration, visual spatial relations
- Psychosocial: anger, fear, depression, irritability, self-awareness, role performance, withdrawal from others, level of motivation, quality of life
- Context/Environment: social support, community resources, social sigma, living environment such as large city or farming community
- Comorbidities and risk factors: opportunistic infections (candidiasis, pneumonia, tuberculosis), cancers such as Kaposi's sarcoma, depression, renal failure, diabetes, cardiovascular disease

Instruments

Instruments Developed by Occupational Therapy Personnel

- Assessment of Motor and Process Skills (8th ed.; AMPS-8; Fisher & Bray Jones, 2016; see also Merritt et al., 2013, in References)
- Communicating Cognitive Concerns Questionnaire (CeQ-60; Askari et al., 2018, in References)
- Lee Visual Analogue Fatigue Scale–Short Version (LVAFS-SV; Lerdal et al., 2013b, in References)
- Patient-Reported Outcomes Quality of Life–HIV (PROQOL-HIV; Askari et al., 2018, in References)
- Pizzi Assessment of Productive Living for Adults with HIV Infection and AIDS (PAPL; Pizzi, 1991; see form in Pizzi & Teaford, 2018, pp. 1177–1180, in References)
- Positive Outlook Self-Efficacy Scale (POSE; Millard et al., 2016, in References)
- Test of Playfulness (Version 4.2; ToP 4.2; Bundy, 2010)

Instruments Developed by Other Professionals and Used by Occupational Therapy Personnel

- Center for Epidemiologic Studies Depression Scale (CES-D; Radloff, 1977; see also Gay et al., 2016, in References)

- Depression Anxiety and Stress Scale-21 (DASS-21; Lovibond & Lovibond, 1995a, 1995b)
- Dix-Hallpike maneuver (DH; Dix & Hallpike, 1952)
- Duke Social Support Index (DSSI; Goodger et al., 1999)
- Fatigue Severity Scale (FSS; Krupp et al., 1989; see also Johansson et al., 2014, and Lerdal et al., 2011, in References)
- Head Thrust Test (HTT; Halmagyi & Curthoys, 1988)
- Health Education Impact Questionnaire (heiQ; Osborne et al., 2007)
- Lee Fatigue Scale (LFS; Lee et al., 1991; see also Lerdal et al., 2013a, 2013b, in References)
- Lee Fatigue and Energy Scales (see Lee Fatigue Scale)
- Mental Adjustment to HIV Scale (MAH-HIV; Ross et al., 1994)
- Patient Reported Outcomes Quality of Life–HIV (PROQOL-HIV; Duracinsky et al., 2012)
- Patient's Assessment of Own Functioning Inventory (PAOFI; Richardson-Vejlgaard et al., 2009)
- Romberg Balance test (RBT; Cohen et al., 1993)

Problems/Issues

Activities of Daily Living/Instrumental ADL
- Person may forget to take medications due to cognitive impairment.
- Person may have difficulty with handwriting due to fine motor deficit.
- Person may have difficulty with communication such as finding words or expressing ideas.
- Person may have difficulty with financial issues such as balancing a checkbook.

Education/Work
- Person may be unable or have difficulty completing academic assignments due to cognitive impairment.
- Person may be unable to perform or have difficulty performing work tasks due to cognitive or motor deficits.

Play/Leisure
- Person may limit engagement or stop engaging in leisure activities due to cognitive or motor deficits.

Rest/Sleep
- Person may experience sleep disturbances including night sweats, chills, and fever.

Social Participation
- Person may limit or stop participation in social activities.

Sensorimotor
- Person may have difficulty with fine motor activities such as handwriting.
- Person may experience difficulty with balance.
- Person may experience muscle weakness in upper or lower extremities.
- Person may experience increased episodes of breathlessness (dyspnea).
- Person may experience fatigue, feelings of tiredness, lethargy.
- Person may experience neuropathic pain such as a burning sensation in the extremities.
- Person may experience general sense of malaise.
- Person may have skin rash or lesions.

Cognitive/Perceptual
- Person may experience decreased ability to concentrate and focus attention such as reading a magazine or watching a movie or television program.
- Person may demonstrate decreased information processing speed.
- Person may experience changes in executive-functioning such as being organized, calculating tips, making everyday decisions.

- Person may have memory impairment such as forgetting appointments (episodic memory).
- Person may lack self-awareness of impaired cognitive functions (Juengst et al., 2012).
- Person may demonstrate deficits in visuospatial relations.

Psychosocial

- Person may express anger, depression, anxiety, and irritability.
- Person may become withdrawn from others including family and friends.
- Person may lack initiation and reduced motivation to start new occupations.
- Person may experience occupational deprivation and occupational imbalance.
- Person may lack awareness of disability and limitations.
- Person may experience changes (reductions, reversals) in role performance.
- Person may experience reduced or unsatisfactory quality of life.
- Person may be afraid (risk adverse) to leave the house for fear of falling.

Context/Environment

- Person may lack a social support system due to stigma about HIV/AIDS.
- Person, family, and caregivers may lack knowledge and information about community resources.

Intervention/Treatment

Models and programs developed by occupational therapy personnel include case studies (Misko et al., 2015; Sherry & Martin, 2010), play-informed, caregiver-implemented, home-based program (Ramugondo et al., 2018), PRPP System of Task Analysis (Ranka & Chapparo, 2010), and regaining productive occupations (Ledgister & Fleming-Castaldy, 2017). Models and programs developed by other professionals but used by occupational therapy personnel include episodic disability framework (Hawkins & Eva, 2014), grounded theory of social participation (Siemon et al., 2013), Nine Circles Community Health Centre (Lapointe et al., 2013), online self-management program (Millard et al., 2014; Millard et al., 2015), positive outlook program (Millard et al., 2016), and self-management programs (Bernardin et al., 2013; Millard et al., 2013; Millard et al., 2014). Team members include physicians, nursing personnel, physical therapists, social workers, health educators, pharmacists, dieticians, and mental health therapists. The goal is to enable the person to live a meaningful and productive life (Lapointe et al., 2013).

Activities of Daily Living/Instrumental ADL

- Provide opportunity to practice preparing and eating healthy meals.
- Provide opportunity to explore and practice moving about the community.

Education/Work

- Review work setting for energy conservation and work simplification techniques.
- Review education or work setting for safety issues and recommend modifications.
- Encourage person to continue education or work with modifications as needed.

Play/Leisure

- Encourage client to engage in enjoyable and meaningful leisure interests and occupations.

Rest/Sleep

- Review sleep habits and routines.
- Discuss and check bedding, sleep posture, auditory and visual disrupters.

Social Participation

- Encourage person to continue participation in social activities modifying duration (amount of time), complexity (type of event, number of persons expected, role of client), and distance and transportation needs (walking distance, short ride, requires changing types of transportation).

Sensorimotor
- Instruct client in energy conservation (motion economy) techniques.
- Instruct client in work simplification techniques.
- Develop a fatigue management program such as pacing, alternate rest and activity cycles.

Cognitive/Perceptual
- Discuss and recommend use of external memory devices.
- Provide opportunity to problem solve and make decisions.

Psychosocial
- Provide information and instruction on stress management techniques such as relaxation training, deep-breathing exercises, yoga.
- Discuss copies strategies.
- Explore approaches to increase self-esteem and feelings of empowerment.
- Develop a self-management program.

Context/Environment
- Suggest use of adaptive devices and equipment.
- Instruct family and caregivers about changes that occur in functional status as the disease process progresses.
- Provide instruction on prevention of injury and falls.
- Discuss and recommend safety adaptations to the home such as grab bars, railings.

Precautions/Safety Considerations

Person is at risk for falls and should be monitored for dizziness and imbalance symptoms (Erlandson et al., 2016).

Prognosis and Outcome

HIV and AIDS infections are chronic conditions. Episodes of wellness alternating with episodes of illness are common (Hawkins & Eva, 2014). Women ageing with HIV need access to peer support groups, community social support services, and ongoing education regarding managing their health for themselves and their families (Akhtar et al., 2017).

REFERENCES

Akhtar, N. F., Garcha, R. K., & Solomon, P. (2017). Experiences of women aging with the human immunodeficiency virus: A qualitative study. *Canadian Journal of Occupational Therapy*, *84*(4-5), 253–261. https://doi.org/10.1177/0008417417722574

Askari, S., Fellows, L., Brouillette, M. J., Moriello, C., Duracinsky, M., & Mayo, N. E. (2018). Development of an item pool reflecting cognitive concerns expressed by people with HIV. *American Journal of Occupational Therapy*, *72*(2), Article 7202205070. https://doi.org/10.5014/ajot.2018.023945

Bernardin, K. N., Toews, D. N., Restall, G. J., & Vuongphan, L. (2013). Self-management interventions for people living with human immunodeficiency virus: A scoping review. *Canadian Journal of Occupational Therapy*, *80*(5), 314–327. https://doi.org/10.1177/0008417413512792

Centers for Disease Control and Prevention. (n.d.) *About HIV*. Retrieved April 4, 2022, from https://www.cdc.gov/hiv/basics/whatishiv.html

Erlandson, K. M., Plankey, M. W., Springer, G., Cohen, H. S., Cox, C., Hoffman, H. J., Yin, M. T., & Brown, T. T. (2016). Fall frequency and associated factors among men and women with or at risk for HIV infection. *HIV Medicine*, *17*(10), 740–748. https://doi.org/10.1111/hiv.12378

Gay, C. L., Kottorp, A., Lerdal, A., & Lee, K. A. (2016). Psychometric limitations of the Center for Epidemiologic Studies-Depression Scale for assessing depressive symptoms among adults with HIV/AIDS: A Rasch analysis. *Depression, Research and Treatment,* 2016, Article 2824595. https://doi.org/10.1155/2016/2824595

Hawkins, C., & Eva, G. (2014). Understanding HIV management. *OT News, 22*(12), 44–45.

Johansson, S., Kottorp, A., Lee, K. A., Gay, C. L., & Lerdal, A. (2014). Can the Fatigue Severity Scale 7-item version be used across different patient populations as a generic fatigue measure—A comparative study using a Rasch model approach. *Health and Quality of Life Outcomes, 12,* Article 24. https://doi.org/10.1186/1477-7525-12-24

Juengst, S., Skidmore, E., Pramuka, M., McCue, M., & Becker, J. (2012). Factors contributing to impaired self-awareness of cognitive functioning in an HIV positive and at-risk population. *Disability and Rehabilitation, 34*(1), 19–25. https://doi.org/10.3109/09638288.2011.587088

Lapointe, J., James, D., & Craik, J. (2013). Occupational therapy services for people living with HIV: A case of service delivery in a primary health care setting. *Occupational Therapy Now, 15*(5), 22–24.

Ledgister, K., & Fleming-Castaldy, R. P. (2017). The perceptions of persons living with human immunodeficiency virus/acquired immune deficiency syndrome about their experiences in regaining productive occupations: A Delphi study. *Occupational Therapy in Mental Health, 33*(3), 235–258. https://doi.org/10.1080/0164212X.2017.1311241

Lerdal, A., Kottorp, A., Gay, C., Aouizerat, B. E., Portillo, C. J., & Lee, K. A. (2011). A 7-item version of the fatigue severity scale has better psychometric properties among HIV-infected adults: An application of a Racsh model. *Quality of Life Research, 20*(9), 1447–1456. https://doi.org/10.1007/s11136-011-9877-8

Lerdal, A., Kottorp, A., Gay, C. L., & Lee, K. A. (2013a). Development of a short version of the Lee Visual Analogue Fatigue Scale in a sample of women with HIV/AIDS: A Rasch analysis application. *Quality of Life Research, 22*(6), 1467–1472. https://doi.org/10.1007/s11136-012-0279-3

Lerdal, A., Kottorp, A., Gay, C. L., & Lee, K. A. (2013b). Lee Fatigue and Energy Scales: Exploring aspects of validity in a sample of women with HIV using an application of a Rasch model. *Psychiatry Research, 205*(3), 241–246. https://doi.org/10.1016/j.psychres.2012.08.031

Merritt, B., Gahagan, J., & Kottorp, A. (2013). HIV and disability: A pilot study exploring the use of the Assessment of Motor and Process Skills to measure daily life performance. *Journal of the International AIDS Society, 16*(1), Article 17339. https://doi.org/10.7448/IAS.16.1.17339

Millard, T., Agius, P. A., McDonald, K., Slavin, S., Girdler, S., & Elliott, J. H. (2016). The positive outlook study: A randomised controlled trial evaluating online self-management for HIV positive gay men. *AIDS and Behavior, 20,* 1907–1918. https://doi.org/10.1007/s10461-016-1301-5

Millard, T., Elliott, J., & Girdler, S. (2013). Self-management education programs for people living with HIV/AIDS: A systematic review. *AIDS Patient Care and STDs, 27*(2), 103–113. https://doi.org/10.1089/apc.2012.0294

Millard, T., McDonald, K., Elliott, J., Slavin, S., Rowell, S., & Girdler, S. (2014). Informing the development of an online self-management program for men living with HIV: A needs assessment. *BMC Public Health 14,* Article 1209. https://doi.org/10.1186/1471-2458-14-1209

Millard, T., McDonald, K., Girdler, S., Slavin, S., & Elliot, J. (2015). Online self-management for gay men living with HIV: A pilot study. *Sexual Health, 12*(4), 308–314. https://doi.org/10.1071/SH15064

Misko, A. N., Nelson, D. L., & Duggan, J. M. (2015). Three case studies of community occupational therapy for individuals with human immunodeficiency virus. *Occupational Therapy in Health Care, 29*(1), 11–26. https://doi.org/10.3109/07380577.2014.941452

O'Toole, M. T. (Ed.). (2017). *Mosby's dictionary of medicine, nursing & health professions* (10th ed.). Elsevier.

Pizzi, M., & Teaford, G. (2018). HIV infection and AIDS. In H. M. Pendleton & W. Schultz-Krohn (Eds.), *Pedretti's occupational therapy* (8th ed., pp. 1167–1183). Elsevier.

Porter, R. S. (Ed.). (2018). *The Merck manual of diagnosis and therapy* (20th ed.). Merck Sharp & Dohme

Ramugondo, E., Ferreira, A., Chung, D., & Cordier, R. (2018). A feasibility RCT evaluating a play-informed, caregiver-implemented, home-based intervention to improve the play of children who are HIV positive. *Occupational Therapy International, 2018,* Article 3652529. https://doi.org/10.1155/2018/3652529

Ranka, J. L., & Chapparo, C. J. (2010). Assessment of productivity performance in men with HIV Associated Neurocognitive Disorder (HAND). *Work, 36*(2), 193–206. https://doi.org/10.3233/WOR-2010-1020

Selik, R. M., Mokotoff, E. D., Branson, B., Owen, S. M., Whitmore, S., & Hall, H. I. (2014, April 11). Revised surveillance case definition for HIV infection—United States, 2014. *Morbidity and Mortality Weekly Report: Recommendations and Reports, 63,* 1–10.

Sherry, K., & Martin, I. Z. (2010). HIV, occupational performance and the role of occupational therapy. In V. Alvers & R. Couch (Eds.), *Occupational therapy: An African perspective* (pp. 232–251).

Siemon, J. S., Blenkhorn, L., Wilkins, S., O'Brien, K. K., & Solomon, P. E. (2013). A grounded theory of social participation among older women living with HIV. *Canadian Journal of Occupational Therapy, 80*(4), 241–250. https://doi.org/10.1177/0008417413501153

BIBLIOGRAPHY

Cohen, H. S., Cox, C., Springer, G., Hoffman, H. J., Young, M. A., Margolick, J. B., & Plankey, M. W. (2012). Prevalence of abnormalities in vestibular function and balance among HIV-seropositive and HIV-seronegative women and men. *PLOS ONE, 7*(5), Article e38419. https://doi.org/10.1371/journal.pone.0038419

Corvinelli, A. (2012). Boredom in recovery from adult substance users with HIV/AIDS attending an urban day treatment program. *Occupational Therapy in Mental Health, 28*(3), 201–319. https://doi.org/10.1080/0164212X.2012.708643

Leidel, S., Leslie, G., Boldy, D., & Girdler, S. (2017). A comprehensive theoretical framework for the implementation and evaluation of opt-out HIV testing. *Journal of Evaluation in Clinical Practice, 23*(2), 301–307. https://doi.org/10.1111/jep.12602

Leidel, S., Leslie, G., Boldy, D., Davies, A., & Girdler, S. (2017). "We didn't have to dance around it": Opt-out HIV testing among homeless and marginalised patients. *Australian Journal of Primary Health, 23*(3), 278–283. https://doi.org/10.1071/PY16120

Leidel, S., McConigley, R., Boldy, D., Wilson, S., & Girdler, S. (2015). Australian health care providers' views on opt-out HIV testing. *BMC Public Health, 15*(1), Article 888. https://doi.org/10.1186/s12889-015-2229-9

Leidel, S., Wilson, S., McConigley, R., Boldy, D., & Girdler, S. (2015). Health-care providers' experiences with opt-out HIV testing: A systematic review. *AIDS Care, 27*(12), 1455–1467. https://doi.org/10.1080/09540121.2015.1058895

Matovu, S. N., la Cour, K., & Hemmingsson, H. (2012). Narratives of Ugandan women adhering to HIV/AIDS medication. *Occupational Therapy International, 19*(4), 176–184. https://doi.org/10.1002/oti.1330

Opacich, K. J. (2014). Human immunodeficiency virus. In M. V. Radomski & C. A. Trombly Latham (Eds.), *Occupational therapy for physical dysfunction* (7th ed., pp. 1352–1367). Wolters Kluwer.

Restall, G. J., Carnochan, T. N., Roger, K. S., Sullivan, T. M., Etcheverry, E. J., & Roddy, P. (2016). Collaborative priority setting for human immunodeficiency virus rehabilitation research: A case report. *Canadian Journal of Occupational Therapy, 83*(1), 7–13. https://doi.org/10.1177/0008417415577423

Lymphedema

See also Breast Cancer; Cancer: Adult, Cancer: Childhood and Adolescent;
Terminal Illness, End of Life, Palliative Care, and Hospice.

Description

Lymphedema is edema (swelling) of a limb characterized by an accumulation of lymph in soft tissue and the resultant swelling caused by inflammation, obstruction, or removal of lymph channels (O'Toole, 2017). Breast-cancer-related lymphedema (BCRL) is a blockage in the one-way lymphatic transport system from physical trauma to the affected area caused by surgery or radiation (McClure et al., 2010).

Cause

Primary cause is due to lymphatic hypoplasia, which is usually an inherited condition, such as Milroy disease, Meige disease, or lymphedema tarda. Secondary cause is due to obstruction or disruption of lymphatic vessels resulting from conditions such as surgery, radiation therapy, trauma, tumor obstruction, or lymphatic filariasis (Porter, 2018).

Stages
- Stage 1: The edema is pitting, and the affected area often returns to normal by morning.
- Stage 2: The edema is nonpitting, and chronic soft-tissue inflammation causes early fibrosis.
- Stage 3: The edema is brawny and irreversible, largely because of soft-tissue fibrosis (Porter, 2018).

Evaluation/Assessment

Areas
- Activities of Daily Living/Instrumental ADL: basic ADLs (dressing, grooming, bathing, mobility), don and doff compression garments or self-bandaging
- Education/Work: work requirements (positions, frequency of repeated tasks)
- Play/Leisure: interests, values, frequency, location
- Rest/Sleep: sleep habits, sleep disturbance
- Social Participation: type, frequency, with whom
- Sensorimotor: joint range of motion, muscle strength, dexterity, swelling, pain, skin care, wound care
- Cognitive/Perceptual: cognitive impairment (chemo brain)
- Psychosocial: depression, anxiety, role performance, quality of life, sense of independence
- Context/Environment: pressure garments, home modifications
- Comorbidities: cancer metastases, infection

Instruments
Instruments Developed by Occupational Therapy Personnel
- Assessment of Lymphedema of the Head and Neck (ALOHA; Purcell et al., 2016, in References)

Instruments Developed by Other Professionals and Used by Occupational Therapy Personnel
- Beck Depression Inventory (2nd ed.; BDI-II; Beck et al., 1996)
- Circumference measurement/limb girth circumference (tape measure)
- Disabilities of the Arm, Shoulder, and Hand (3rd ed.; DASH-3; Kennedy et al., 2011)
- ImpediMed (Bioelectrical Impedance Analysis System; commercial product)
- Joint range of motion (goniometry; Shurtleff & Kaskutas, 2018)
- M. D. Anderson Head and Neck Lymphedema Rating Scale (Smith & Lewin, 2010)
- MositureMeterD (MMD; commercial product)

- Short-Form 36 Health Survey (SF-36; Ware, 1993)
- Skin or soft-tissue tonometry (pressure measurement; commercial product)
- Truncated Cone Volume Measurement (TCVM; Latchford & Casley-Smith, 1997)
- Volumetery (measuring water volume displaced by the submerged limb; Stern, 1991)

Problems/Issues

Activities of Daily Living/Instrumental ADL

- Person may have difficulty performing basic ADLs such as dressing, grooming, and bathing due to limited range of motion related to edema.
- Person may find that certain clothing cannot be worn because the sleeves are too tight or small to accommodate the swelling.
- Person may have difficulty performing any task that is usually performed by or with the affected extremity, such as meal preparation, housecleaning, vacuuming, doing laundry.

Education/Work

- Person may have difficulty performing work tasks that require body positions that tend to increased edema.

Play/Leisure

- Person may be unable to or have difficulty engaging in favorite and meaningful leisure activities.

Rest/Sleep

- Person may experience sleep disturbance.

Social Participation

- Person may limit or discontinue participation in social activities.

Sensorimotor

- Person may have current symptoms of lymphedema such as swelling (edema).
- Person may have loss of limb flexibility including joint range of motion.
- Person may experience decreased muscle strength especially in the hand.
- Person may have tissue fibrosis.
- Person may experience discomfort and pain related to the swelling.

Cognitive/Perceptual

- Not discussed in relation to lymphedema management, but may be present due to management of breast cancer.

Psychosocial

- Person may have symptoms of depression, anxiety, frustration, and distress.
- Person may experience decreased quality of life due to activity limitations as a result of the lymphedema and its management requirements.
- Person may experience changes in role performance.

Context/Environment

- Provide education on monitoring for signs and symptoms of infection.
- Provide instruction on donning and doffing fitted graduated compression garments.

Intervention/Treatment

Models and programs developed by occupational therapy personnel include self-management (Pigott et al., 2018). Models and programs developed by other professionals but used by occupational therapy personnel include breast cancer recovery program (BCRP; McClure et al., 2010), decongestive lymphatic therapy (DLT; King et al., 2012), Kinesio Taping and manual edema mobilization (Miller et al., 2017), and smart pressure monitored suits (Feng et al., 2013).

Team members include surgeons, oncologists, nursing personnel, lymphedema specialists, physical therapists, psychologists, dieticians or nutritionists, and occupational therapy personnel. The goal is to enable occupation by decreasing barriers to and increased participation in occupational performance (Shier, 2012).

Activities of Daily Living/Instrumental ADL
- Assist client to modify as needed performance requirements related to dressing (including putting on compression garments or bandaging), grooming, bathing.

Education/Work
- Assist client to modify work requirements if needed.
- Assist client to plan for retirement if continuing to work is not possible.

Play/Leisure
- Encourage client to continue engagement in favorite leisure activities.
- Assist client to explore new leisure interests, especially if previous interests cannot be continued.

Rest/Sleep
- Assist client in determining what modifications are need in technology, sensory experiences, environmental controls (heat, light, noise) to facilitate sleep.

Social Participation
- Encourage client to continue participation in social activities.
- Assist client to modify participation as needed such as less travel time, shorter outings, or other accommodations.

Sensorimotor
- Assist client in learning manual lymphatic drainage techniques.
- Assist client in managing gradient pressure bandages or sleeves.
- Assist client to learn limb exercises such as gravity-resistive arm movements using concentric muscle-shortening motions out away from the body.
- Promote arm motions that promote shoulder flexion (SF), abduction (AB), and external rotation along with inhaling breath.
- Management may include limb massage including intermittent pneumatic compression.
- Provide instruction in managing skin care.

Cognitive/Perceptual
- No information identified.

Psychosocial
- Encourage use of stress reduction techniques such as deep diaphragmatic breathing.

Context/Environment
- Provide client education on how to prevent lymphedema.
- Provide information on different types of pressure garments such as compression stocking, smart pressure monitored suits (Feng et al., 2013).

Precautions/Safety Considerations

Client is at increased risk for skin infection and monitoring procedures should be observed. Client may be at increased risk for injury to affected arm due to decreased sensation.

Prognosis and Outcome

Cure is unusual once lymphedema occurs. Treatment and preventive measures can lessen symptoms, slow, or halt disease progression, and prevent complications (Porter, 2018). The most widely used modalities were self-massage, compression garments, therapist-delivered manual lymphatic drainage, and exercise (Sierla et al., 2013).

Cost Effectiveness

Health-care costs between lymphedema group and nonlymphedema group ranged from $14,877 to $23,167. A prospective surveillance model (lymphedema education and arm measurements) has been an effective method of preventing lymphedema and showed a cost saving (Dominick et al., 2014).

REFERENCES

Dominick, S. A., Natarajan, L., Pierce, J. P., Madanat, H., & Madlensky, L. (2014). Patient compliance with a health care provider referral for an occupational therapy lymphedema consult. *Supportive Care in Cancer, 22*, 1781–1787. https://doi.org/10.1007/s00520-014-2145-z

Feng, B., Pao, W. Y., Wu, A., Li, H. C. K., & Li-Tsang, C. W. P. (2013). Are "smart pressure monitored suits" "smarter" than conventional garments in clinical applications? *Hong Kong Journal of Occupational Therapy, 23*(2), 82–88. https://doi.org/10.1016/j.hkjot.2013.11.002

King, M., Deveaux, A., White, H., & Rayson, D. (2012). Compression garments versus compression bandaging in decongestive lymphatic therapy for breast cancer-related lymphedema: A randomized controlled trial. *Supportive Care in Cancer, 20*(5), 1031–1036. https://doi.org/10.1007/s00520-011-1178-9

McClure, M. K., McClure, R. J., Day, R., & Brufsky, A. M. (2010). Randomized controlled trial of the Breast Cancer Recovery Program for women with breast cancer-related lymphedema. *American Journal of Occupational Therapy, 64*(1), 59–72. https://doi.org/10.5014/ajot.64.1.59

Miller, L. K., Jerosch-Herold, C., & Shepstone, L. (2017). Effectiveness of edema management techniques for subacute hand edema: A systematic review. *Journal of Hand Therapy, 30*(4), 432–446. https://doi.org/10.1016/j.jht.2017.05.011

O'Toole, M. T. (Ed.). (2017). *Mosby's dictionary of medicine, nursing & health professions* (10th ed.). Elsevier.

Pigott, A., Nixon, J., Fleming, J., & Porceddu, S. (2018). Head and neck lymphedema management: Evaluation of a therapy program. *Head & Neck, 40*(6), 1131–1137. https://doi.org/10.1002/hed.25086

Porter, R. S. (Ed.). (2018). *The Merck manual of diagnosis and therapy* (20th ed.). Merck Sharp & Dohme.

Purcell, A., Nixon, J., Fleming, J., McCann, A., & Porceddu, S. (2016). Measuring head and neck lymphedema: The "ALOHA" trial. *Head & Neck, 38*(1), 79–84. https://doi.org/10.1002/hed.23853

Shier, B. (2012). The occupational therapist's role in lymphedema self-management. *Occupational Therapy Now, 14*(3), 19–21.

Sierla, R., Lee, T. S. M., Black, D., & Kilbreath, S. L. (2013). Lymphedema following breast cancer: Regions affected, severity of symptoms, and benefits of treatment from the patients' perspective. *Clinical Journal of Oncology Nursing, 17*(3), 325–331. https://doi.org/10.1188/13.CJON.325-331

Skin Disorders

Burn Scars

Description

Burn scars can be described as the "laying down of disorganized connective tissue in the newly forming scar" tissue (Agency for Clinical Innovation, 2017, p. 2). Burn scars can be described by 10 characteristics: color, fragility, hardness, hydration, raised, scar sensitivity, scar surface appearance, stretchability, surface area, and thickness (Simons et al., 2018). The term *hypertrophic scarring* refers to skin tissue that is "raised, fibrous (firm, tight) erythematous (red) dry, painful and pruritic (itchy)" (Agency for Clinical Innovation, 2017, p. 2). Hypertrophic scarring and contracture adversely affect flexor surfaces of joints, mobile skin area such as the face, and concave areas (axilla, web-spaces between fingers and thumb) and are most active during the first 4–6 months after healing (Kurakazu & Hirai, 2018).

Cause

Burn scars occur when skin in the dermal layer is damaged or lost. Superficial burns that heal within 2 weeks usually do not form scars (Kurakazu & Hirai, 2018). The original cause of the burn injury may have been flame, steam, hot liquids, hot surfaces, dry ice, frost, or radiation.

Evaluation/Assessment

Areas

- Activities of Daily Living/Instrumental ADL: eating, dressing, mobility, daily routine
- Education/Work: education, work history, job duties, hand dominance
- Play/Leisure: interests and avocations, frequency, location
- Rest/Sleep: no information identified
- Social Participation: frequency, type, with whom
- Sensorimotor: gross and fine motor skills, joint range of motion, muscle strength, pain, itching, endurance and deconditioning, changes in sensation
- Cognitive/Perceptual: no information identified
- Psychosocial: body image, resilience, motivation
- Context/Environment: family and social support
- Development (Infant, Child, Adolescent only): expected growth of body, especially in infants and toddlers
- Comorbidities: check for diabetes, fractures, or other musculoskeletal injuries

Instruments

(See Tyack et al., 2012, for review of burn scar rating scales and Tyack et al., 2013, for guide to choosing a rating scale.)

Instruments Developed by Occupational Therapy Personnel

- Brisbane Burn Scar Impact Profile (BBSIP; Tyack et al., 2015, in References; see also Simons et al., 2019a, 2019b, in References)
  - BBSIP for Adults (Version 1.0; Queensland Health, 2013)
  - BBSIP for Children aged 8 to 18 years (Queensland Health, 2013)
  - BBSIP for Caregivers of Children aged 8 to 18 years (Queensland Health, 2013)
  - BBSIP for Caregivers of Children aged less than 8 years (Queensland Health, 2013)
- Burn Scar Contracture Severity Scale (BSCSS; Niedzielski & Chapman, 2015, in References)

Instruments Developed by Other Professionals and Used by Occupational Therapy Personnel

- Cutometer (measures pliability; MPA 580; Courage + Khazaka Electronic GmbH, Koln, Germany)
- DermaScan C (ultrasound scanner; Cortex Technology, Handsund, Denmark)
- Derriford Appearance Scale (DAS-59; Carr et al., 2000)

- Disabilities of the Arm, Shoulder, and Hand (3rd ed.; DASH-3; Kennedy et al., 2011)
- Grip strength (dynamometer; JAMAR Dynamometer, Lafayette Instrument; Wang et al., 2018)
- Injury Severity Score (ISS; Baker et al., 1974)
- Joint range of motion (goniometry; Shurtleff & Kaskutas, 2018)
- Manchester Scar Scale (MSS; Beausang et al., 1998)
- Manual Muscle Test (MMT; Kaskutas, 2018)
- Matching Assessment of Scars and Photographs (MAPS; Masters et al., 2005)
- Mexameter (measures erythema and pigmentation of scars; MX18; Courage + Khazaka Electronic GmbH, Koln, Germany)
- Modified Vancouver Scar Scale (MVSS; Baryza & Baryza, 1995)
- Patient and Observer Scar Assessment Scale (POSAS; Draaijers et al., 2004)
- Photography (see Simons & Tyack, 2011, and Simons et al., 2013, in References)
- Pliance X (measures pressure; see Wiseman et al., 2018, in References)
- Ultrasound (measures scar height; see Simons et al., 2017, in References)
- Vancouver Scar Scale (VSS; Sullivan et al., 1990)

Problems/Issues

Activities of Daily Living/Instrumental ADL

- Person may have difficulty performing tasks required within the ADL—for example, person has difficulty grasping buttons, zippers, or snaps because scar tissue has formed and contracted skin tissue on dorsum of hand, limiting finger flexion and thumb opposition (webspace inability) of index and thumb.
- Person may have difficulty performing tasks required with IADL—for example, person has difficulty turning the steering wheel in the truck due to scarring and contractures in both axillas, which limit forward flexion and abduction of the shoulders necessary to grasp the steering wheel and turn it clockwise or counterclockwise to turn the truck left or right.

Education/Work

- Person may be unable to perform required academic tasks, such as keyboarding, due to lack of finger flexion.
- Person may have difficulty performing tasks required on the job such as lifting, stooping, pushing, pulling, handling and manipulating objects.

Play/Leisure

- Person may limit or stop engagement in favorite leisure activities because scar tissue and contractures have made movement difficult.

Rest/Sleep

- Not discussed (see Sleep–Wake Disorders in Section 13: Lifestyle Conditions).

Social Participation

- Person may restrict participation in social activities because of concerns about appearance.

Sensorimotor

- Person usually experiences contractures that can limit movement and mobility, increase pain, and slow wound healing.
- Person may experience pain related to scarring, contractures, and associated interventions.
- Person may experience reduced activity tolerance and endurance, limiting tolerance to movement needed to increase joint mobility.
- Person may have reduced joint range of motion due to burn scars, contractures, and immobility while burns are healing.
- Person may have reduced muscle strength and deconditioning due to loss of movement and activity.

Cognitive/Perceptual
- Not discussed.

Psychosocial
- Person may experience changes in body image, depending on location and extent of scar tissue.
- Person may lack motivation to participate in scar management program.
- Person may express feelings of anger and show signs of depression related to both burn injury and resulting scars.
- Person may have difficulty accepting the "new me," including the scarring and contractures.

Context/Environment
- Person may lack social support system to facilitate and follow scar management program.
- Person may need assistive devices to facilitate certain activities.

Developmental
- Child may experience restricted growth in areas of body with scar tissue.

Intervention/Treatment

Models and programs developed by occupational therapy personnel: None identified. Models and programs developed by other professionals but used by occupational therapy personnel include the conceptual model (Simons et al., 2016), massage (Nedelec et al., 2019), mechanical stretch (Zhang et al., 2017), and pressure therapy (Sharp, 2014). Team members include physicians, nursing personnel, physical therapists, psychologists, social workers, and occupational therapy personnel. Goal should be to enable the person to return to work or school, engage in activities such as sports, and participate in premorbid routine as soon as possible by increasing independence, reinforcing need for active movement, and providing information and education on managing postburn activities to reduce impact of scarring and contractures on everyday life (Kurakazu & Hirai, 2018).

Activities of Daily Living/Instrumental ADL
- Encourage independence and self-management as early as possible.
- Daily routine and exercise program should be integrated.
- Clients with facial burns may benefit from using camouflage makeup for special occasions.
- Client with severe burns may require a fitness to drive assessment.

Education/Work
- Client may require a work evaluation to determine if job duties can be performed.
- Client may require workplace accommodation.

Play/Leisure
- Encourage client to resume leisure activities.

Rest/Sleep
- No information identified.

Social Participation
- Encourage client to participate in previously enjoyed social activities.

Sensorimotor
- Compression garments
  - ▶ Rationale: Compression is assumed to reduce the excessive blood flow that delivers scarring mediators.
  - ▶ Types of materials include flexible bandage, tubular elastic stocking, bandaging, and pressure garments (customized or off the shelf), Coban or Co-Flex (for small hands and fingers).

- ► Type depends on wound health, area of body affected, time in healing process, and individual client needs (young children may require several types).
- ► Pressure garments are worn at all times, except for bathing or showering, massage, or moisturizing skin.
- ► Two sets are needed: One is being worn and the other is being washed.
- ► Typically, compression garments are worn by adults for 12 to 18 months but may require a longer period in children.
- ► Typically, compression garments must be replaced every 3 to 5 months because material loses tension for compression.
- ► Compression garments may need to be suspended if skin deteriorated, infection occurred, deep venous thrombosis occurs, excesses swelling occurs, or surgery is scheduled.
- • Contracture management: see sections on exercise, pressure garments, and splinting.
- • Edema management (may include any or all of the following items):
  - ► Positioning: see section below on positioning.
  - ► Elevation to facilitate postural drainage.
  - ► Splinting: see section on splinting.
  - ► Pressure garments: see section on pressure garments.
  - ► Exercise, active and passive to facilitate circulation.
  - ► Massage to promote drainage.
  - ► Participation in activities of daily living as part of the daily routine.
  - ► Avoid as much as possible limb dependency, lack of movement and mobility, inappropriate compression or bandaging.
- • Exercise
  - ► Commence exercise program as early as possible, especially to face, mouth, neck, axilla, elbows, hand, wrists, knees, ankles, and feet.
  - ► Active range of motion should be encouraged as soon as possible, but active-assist and passive are useful adjuncts.
  - ► Use range of motion activities to affected areas: ambulation if possible, performing any activity of daily living when possible.
  - ► Exercise program will be needed until scar maturation has occurred.
  - ► Pay extra attention to burns over or adjacent to joints to maintain joint range of motion.
  - ► Stretching exercises should be low in repetitions but long in duration (sustained stretch).
  - ► Use stretching exercise in lines of tension, not necessarily in the anatomical plane.
  - ► Where possible, combine stretching over multiple joints.
  - ► Stretching exercises should be done without dressing or pressure garments in place to identify and optimize lengthening.
  - ► Aerobic exercise may include walking, cycling, or jogging.
  - ► The actual exercise prescription must be individualized in frequency, intensity, amount of time, type, pain tolerance, and motivation.
- • Massage
  - ► Massage is used to break down the collagen bundles that form the scar tissue.
  - ► Most effective during the early weeks of treatment to increase skin elasticity and reduce scar thickness (Nedelec et al., 2019).
  - ► Young children and adults may need assistance with massage to areas that are hard to reach.
  - ► Use of a moisturizer along with the massage is recommended if skin is dry.
  - ► Massage with firm pressure so skin blanches a light color or white.
  - ► Use a slow circular motion with a flat hand and fingers; if scar is very thick, use a pinch and roll technique.
  - ► Massage should be continued until the scar is mature.
  - ► Monitor for irritation from moisturizing product, fragile skin breakdown, excessive discomfort and pain.
- • Pain management

- ► Work with team members to determine pharmacological treatment and monitor side effects.
- ► Work with physical therapist to determine whether transcutaneous electrical nerve stimulation might be helpful.
- ► Consider whether cognitive behavior therapy might be effective.
- ► Consider whether sensory modification could be used.
- ► Work to minimize pain, such as providing adequate pressure support before having client with burns on lower extremities stand, transfer, or walk.
- ► Assist client to determine amount of time to spend on pain management to encourage client to take control.
- Positioning: Recommended positioning is neck extension or hyperextension, shoulder 90 to 160 degrees of abduction (maintain stretch on axilla) and external rotation, elbow extension, forearm supination, wrist neutral and digits extended. Trunk in straight alignment. Lower extremities abducted 20-degree separation, no hip external rotation or flexion, knees extended, with ankle dorsiflexion (Agency for Clinical Innovation, 2017).
- Pressure
  - ► Most effective to decrease hypertrophic scar height and erythema (Sharp, 2014). Not recommended to decrease abnormal scar pigmentation or hasten rate or time to scar maturation.
  - ► For garment pressure see compression garments above.
  - ► Orthotic mask (transparent rigid plastic or fabric device) may be used on face to provide pressure on scars to face, nose, and lips and on the hand (especially dorsal aspect) using a casting system or computer program to design.
  - ► All pressure systems must be inspected frequently and adjustments made to continue the pressure.
- Reconstructive therapy
  - ► Indications are functional restrictions due to contractures, growth in children, tissue loss, or cosmetic enhancement.
  - ► Types of surgery include excision of scar tissue and grating, Z-plasty, full thickness grafting, and skin and muscle flaps.
- Silicone and scar softening
  - ► Use medical grade silicone products to soften red, raised, or thickened (hypertrophic) scars.
  - ► Silicone is available in gel sheet, liquid, and putty forms.
  - ► Silicone can be used on conjunction with pressure garments and splints.
  - ► Skin should be fully healed, clean, and dry before application of silicone.
  - ► Silicone should be removed before water-based activities, heavy exercise, and not be worn for 24 hours per day to allow the skin to breathe.
  - ► Silicone can be applied until scar is mature.
  - ► Silicone should be discontinued if wound develops, skin breakdown occurs, red rash occurs, or skin become itchy where silicone is to be applied.
  - ► Monitoring should occur for young children or for persons with cognitive impairment.
- Skin care
  - ► Skin should be monitored regularly for signs of breakdown, infection, or wound development.
- Splinting
  - ► Splinting should be applied to maximize the lengthening of the skin of affected area to minimize contractures and scarring.
  - ► When possible, splint the joint or joints at end of range to maximize stretch of burn scars or pull on burn area to prevent contractures.
  - ► Note that splints used for burn injuries may not be a "functional" position as usually recommended for other types of injuries, diseases, or disorders.
  - ► Splints are most often applied to high-risk areas such as face, mouth, neck (collar), wrists, hands, palms, hips, knees, and toes.

- ► Types of splinting materials include thermoplastics, plaster of Paris, and negative pressure wound management dressing.
- ► Serial casting may be used if a joint is losing range.
- ► Position of safe immobilization of the hand is wrist extension 10–45 degrees, metacarpophalangeal (MCP) flexion 60–80 degrees, and proximal interphalangeal (PIP) and distal interphalangeal (DIP) in full extension.
- ► Splints should be removed during exercises.
- ► Splints may have to be adjusted to account for child's growth.
- ► Splints are worn at night until scar is mature, but daytime schedule is balanced against daily activities program.
- ► Splints should be checked regularly for changes in edema, fragile skin, circulation, range of motion, client's weight, or sweating.
- ► To prevent brachial plexus injury, ensure sufficient forward flexion of the shoulder.
- • Specialized treatments
  - ► Some clients may benefit from corticosteroid injection, dry needling, or laser therapy.

Cognitive/Perceptual

- • Assist client to set goals within rehabilitation program to encourage participation and monitor progress.

Psychosocial

- • Provide stress management and coping strategies such as relaxation techniques, breathing exercises, guided imagery, aromatherapy, use of music.

Context/Environment

- • Provide education to client, family, and caregivers regarding the importance of scar management and detailed instructions of what needs to be done.
- • Use adapted devices for early success, but discontinue as soon as person can perform activity without assistance.

Precautions/Safety Considerations

- • Burned skin and active scars contract within hours, rather than over days or weeks; active scar management must be initiated as soon as possible.
- • Aerobic exercises may be restricted for a person with inhalation injury and possible scarring of lung tissue.
- • Always monitor carefully any exercise or activity following skin grafting, which may require a period of immobilization to allow for healing.
- • Donor sites for grafting may be painful but are not usually a contraindication to exercise.
- • Special precautions should be considered if any of the following are present: exposed tendons, flaps, reconstruction areas, regrafting, k-wires, or medical conditions such as low blood pressure, infections, graft fragility, heterotopic ossification, peripheral neuropathy, and wound breakdown.

Prognosis and Outcome

Outcome depends in part on the severity of burn area, intervention program developed, and compliance by client and social support system. Clients can resume participation in school, work, homelife, and community.

REFERENCES

Agency for Clinical Innovation. (2017). *Clinical guideline: Burn physiotherapy and occupational therapy guidelines.* https://aci.health.nsw.gov.au/__data/assets/pdf_file/0018/236151/Burns-PT-OT-Guidelines.pdf

Kurakazu, D., & Hirai, A. H. (2018). Burns and burn rehabilitation. In H. H. Pendleton & W. Schultz-Krohn (Eds.), *Pedretti's occupational therapy* (8th ed., pp. 1048–1082). Elsevier.

Nedelec, B., Couture, M. A., Calva, V., Poulin, C., Chouinard, A., Shashoua, D., Gauthier, N., Correa, J. A., de Oliveira, A., Mazer, B., & LaSalle, L. (2019). Randomized controlled trial of the immediate and long-term effect of massage on adult postburn scar. *Burns, 45*(1), 128–139. https://doi.org/10.1016/j.burns.2018.08.018

Niedzielski, L. S., & Chapman, M. T. (2015). Changes in burn scar contracture: Utilization of a severity scale and predictor of return to duty for service members. *Journal of Burn Care & Research, 36*(3), e212–e219. https://doi.org/10.1097/BCR.0000000000000148

Sharp, P. (2014). *Use of pressure therapy for management of hypertrophic scarring.* Cincinnati Children's Hospital Medical Center.

Simons, M., Kee, E. G., Kimble, R., & Tyack, Z. (2017). Ultrasound is a reproducible and valid tool for measuring scar height in children with burn scars: A cross-sectional study of the psychometric properties and utility of the ultrasound and 3D camera. *Burns, 43*(5), 993–1001. https://doi.org/10.1016/j.burns.2017.01.034

Simons, M., Kimble, R., McPhail, S., & Tyack, Z. (2019a). The Brisbane Burn Scar Impact Profile (child and young person version) for measuring health-related quality of life in children with burn scars: A longitudinal cohort study of reliability, validity and responsiveness. *Burns, 45*(7), 1537–1552. https://doi.org/10.1016/j.burns.2019.07.012

Simons, M., Kimble, R., McPhail, S., & Tyack, Z. (2019b). The longitudinal validity reproducibility and responsiveness of the Brisbane Burn Scar Impact Profile (caregiver report for young children version) for measuring health-related quality of life in children with burn scars. *Burns, 45*(8), 1792–1809. https://doi.org/10.1016/j.burns.2019.04.015

Simons, M., Lim, P. C. C., Kimble, R. M., & Tyack, Z. (2018). Towards a clinical and empirical definition of burn scarring: A template analysis using qualitative data, *Burns, 44*(7), 1811–1819. https://doi.org/10.1016/j.burns.2018.04.006

Simons, M., Price, N., Kimble, R., & Tyack, Z. (2016). Patient experiences of burn scars in adults and children and development of a health-related quality of life conceptual model: A qualitative study. *Burns, 42*(3), 620–632. https://doi.org/10.1016/j.burns.2015.11.012

Simons, M., & Tyack, Z. (2011). Health professionals' and consumers' opinion: What is considered important when rating burn scars from photographs? *Journal of Burn Care & Research, 32*(2), 275–285. https://doi.org/10.1097/BCR.0b013e31820aaf09

Simons, M., Ziviani, J., Thorley, M., McNee, J., & Tyack, Z. (2013). Exploring reliability of scar rating scales using photographs of burns from children aged up to 15 years. *Journal of Burn Care & Research, 34*(4), 427–438. https://doi.org/10.1097/BCR.0b013e3182700054

Tyack, Z., Simons, M., Spinks, A., & Wasiak, J. (2012). A systematic review of the quality of burn scar rating scales for clinical and research use. *Burns, 38*(1), 6–18. https://doi.org/10.1016/j.burns.2011.09.021

Tyack, Z., Wasiak, J., Spinks, A., Kimble, R., & Simons, M. (2013). A guide to choosing a burn scar rating scale for clinical or research use. *Burns, 39*(7), 1341–1350. https://doi.org/10.1016/j.burns.2013.04.021

Tyack, Z., Ziviani, J., Kimble, R., Plaza, A., Jones, A., Cuttle, L., & Simons, M. (2015). Measuring the impact of burn scarring on health-related quality of life: Development and preliminary content validation of the Brisbane Burn Scar Impact Profile (BBSIP) for children and adults. *Burns, 41*(7), 1405–1419. https://doi.org/10.1016/j.burns.2015.05.021

Wiseman, J., Simons, M., Kimble, R., & Tyack, Z. (2018). Reliability and clinical utility of the Pliance X for measuring pressure at the interface of pressure garments and burn scars in children. *Burns, 44*(7), 1820–1828. https://doi.org/10.1016/j.burns.2018.05.002

Zhang, Y.-T., Li-Tsang, C. W. P., & Au, R. K. C. (2017). A systematic review on the effect of mechanical stretch on hypertrophic scars after burn injuries. *Hong Kong Journal of Occupational Therapy, 29*(1), 1–9. https://doi.org/10.1016/j.hkjot.2016.11.001

BIBLIOGRAPHY

Burn Therapy Standards Working Group. (2017). *Standards of physiotherapy ad occupational therapy practice in the management of burn injured adults and children*. British Burn Association.

Nedelec, B., Correa, J. A., de Oliveira, A., LaSalle, L., & Perrault, I. (2014). Longitudinal burn scar quantification. *Burns, 40*(8), 1504–1512. https://doi.org/10.1016/j.burns.2014.03.002

Parry, I., Walker, K., Niszczak, J., Palmieri, T., & Greenhalgh, D. (2010). Methods and tools used for the measurement of burn scar contracture. *Journal of Burn Care & Research, 31*(6), 888–903. https://doi.org/10.1097/BCR.0b013e3181f9354f

Slocombe, P. D., Simons, M. A., & Kimble, R. M. (2011). A modification of the Hynes procedure—A surgical innovation in the treatment of mature hypertrophic scars in children. *Burns, 37*(7), 1265–1267. https://doi.org/10.1016/j.burns.2011.04.012

Tyack, Z., Kimble, R., McPhail, S., Plaza, A., & Simons, M. (2017). Psychometric properties of the Brisbane Burn Scar Impact Profile in adults with burn scars. *PLOS ONE, 12*(9), Article e0184452. https://doi.org/10.1371/journal.pone.0184452

Wiseman, J., Simons, M., Kimble, R., & Tyack, Z. (2019). Variability of pressure at the pressure garment-scar interface in children after burn: A pilot longitudinal cohort study. *Burns, 45*(1), 103–113. https://doi.org/10.1016/j.burns.2018.08.029

Burns: Adults

Description

A burn is any injury to tissues of the body caused by hot objects or flames, electricity, chemicals, radiation, or gases (O'Toole, 2017). Frostbite, although not technically a burn by definition, is included because the condition is treated in a similar matter (Bearden, 2017). The extent of the injury is described by the nature of the burn agent, the length of time the person's tissue was exposed, body parts involved, and depth of burn into the tissue.

Cause

Burns are caused by thermal, electrical, chemical, radiation, gases, or frostbite. Motivation may be as an assault, self-inflicted, failure to understand level of danger, unintentional, or careless (Bearden, 2017; O'Toole, 2017).

Definitions (O'Toole, 2017)

- *First-degree burn* (superficial epidermal): Involves only a superficial layer of epidermal (skin) cells.
- *Second-degree burn* (superficial dermal burn, superficial partial-thickness): Involves superficial partial-thickness and deep partial-thickness, but damage to skin is not sufficient to prevent skin regeneration.
- *Third-degree burn* (deep dermal or deep partial-thickness): Extends through the entire thickness of the epidermis and dermis.
- *Fourth-degree burn* (full thickness): All epidermis and dermis are lost and burn has penetrated the subcutaneous tissue, muscle, and periosteum or bone.
- *Zone of coagulation*: Usually found in or near the center of the burn and characterized as the part of the burn with maximum damage; tissue in this zone may be permanently damaged.
- *Zone of stasis*: Tissue surrounding the zone of coagulation that has decreased perfusion. The zone of stasis may convert to the zone of coagulation but usually the tissue can be salvaged if treated properly. Avoid occlusive dressing, splints, edema, and inadequate fluid resuscitation.
- *Zone of hyperemia*: Outermost area of the burn area that is characterized by increased tissue perfusion and viable tissue; tissue in this zone should recover unless complications occur (Bearden, 2017).

Evaluation/Assessment
Areas
- Activities of Daily Living/Instrumental ADL: eating (mouth opening if facial burns are involved), dressing, body weight, and nutritional status
- Education/Work: vocation, return to work, or continue education
- Play/Leisure: not discussed
- Rest/Sleep: sleep disturbance
- Social Participation: previous social activities
- Sensorimotor: depth of burn, areas of body burned, percentage of body burned, joints affected and range of motion, skin fragility for friction and shearing forces, muscle strength, hand functions (grasp and release, fine motor control, web-space between thumb and index finger), edema, pain, body temperature
- Cognitive/Perceptual: not discussed
- Psychosocial: client compliance, stress and coping, body image, depression, anxiety, quality of life
- Context/Environment: splinting, pressure garments, community resources
- Comorbidities: infection, pruritus, shock, pressure sores (decubitus ulcers), acute stress disorder (ASD), posttraumatic stress disorder (PTSD), self-inflected burn injury, assault by burn

Instruments
Instruments Developed by Occupational Therapy Personnel
- Australian Therapy Outcome Measures (3rd ed.; AusTOMS-3; Unsworth & Duncombe, 2014)
- Mouth Impairment and Disability Assessment (MIDA; Couture et al., 2018, in References)
- Posttraumatic Growth Inventory (PTGI; Martin et al., 2016, in References)
- Upper Extremity Performance Evaluation Test for the Elderly (TEMPA; see Upper Extremity Performance Test for the Elderly; Desrosiers et al., 1995)

Instruments Developed by Other Professionals and Used by Occupational Therapy Personnel
- Burn Specific Health Scale–Brief (BSHS-B; Kildal et al., 2001)
- Circumferential measurement (tape measure)
- Disabilities of the Arm, Shoulder, and Hand (3rd ed.; DASH-3; Kennedy et al., 2011)
- Dynamometry (grip strength; JAMAR Dynamometer, Lafayette Instrument)
- Functional Assessment for Burns (FAB; Smailes et al., 2013)
- Functional Independence Measure (FIM; Uniform Data System for Medical Rehabilitation, 1997)
- Get Up and Go test (GUG test; Mathias et al., 1986)
- Goniometry (joint range of motion)
- Jepsen-Taylor Hand Function Test (JTHFT; Jepsen et al., 1969)
- McGill Pain Questionnaire (MPQ; Melzack, 1975)
- Michigan Hand Outcomes Questionnaire (MHQ; Chung et al., 1998)
- Modified Barthel Index (MBI; Shah et al., 1989)
- Pittsburgh Sleep Quality Index (PSQI; Buysse et al.,1989)
- Self-Rating Anxiety Scale (SRAS; Zung, 1965)
- Self-Rating Depression Scale (SRDS; Zung, 1965)
- Sollerman Hand Function Test (SHFT; Sollerman & Ejeskär, 1995)
- Volumetry (water displacement)
- World Health Organization Quality of Life–BREF (WHOQOL-BREF; WHOQOL Group, 1998)

Problems/Issues
Activities of Daily Living/Instrumental ADL
- Person may experience loss of ability to perform self-maintenance activities such eating, brushing teeth, and grooming if face is involved.

- Person may experience loss of ability to perform self-maintenance activities such as dressing and toileting if one or both upper extremities are involved.
- Person may experience loss of mobility if lower extremities are involved.
- Person may experience decreased function in independent living skills depending on areas of burn such as meal preparation and cleanup, homemaking (laundry, vacuuming, dusting), shopping, banking, and driving or taking public transportation.

Education/Work
- Person may have difficulty continuing education depending on area(s) of burn.
- Person may be unable to perform work tasks depending on area(s) of burn.

Play/Leisure
- No information identified.

Rest/Sleep
- Person may experience sleep disturbances.

Social Participation
- Person may be unable or unwilling to participate in social activities.

Sensorimotor
- Person may experience loss of range of motion in the mouth, neck, axilla, elbow, wrist, hand, knee, or ankle.
- Person may experience decreased cardiovascular fitness due to prolonged immobilization.
- Person may experience hypersensitivity as the skin tissue heals.
- Person may experience loss of sensation in the area of burn related to tactile, temperature, and pressure.
- Person may experience contractures if corrective splinting and positioning is not applied to affected area such as the mouth, neck, axilla, elbow, wrist, hand, knee, or ankle.
- Person may experience heterotopic ossification.
- Person may experience graft failure if protective guidelines are not followed.
- Person may experience damage to the extensor tendons if the dorsum of the hand is involved.
- Person may experience chronic itch.

Cognitive/Perceptual
- No information identified.

Psychosocial
- Person may become depressed.
- Person may experience difficulty coping with treatment program.
- Person may experience changes in body image, including identifiable disfigurement.
- Person may experience decreased quality of life.

Context/Environment
- Person and family may need information on burn management program during hospitalization, including the use of specialized equipment and related supplies such as IVs for fluid management, tracheotomy for breathing, pressure garments to manage scars, specific positioning to manage edema, wound management dressings, splints to reduce contractures, and dressings to protect graft areas.
- Person and family may need information on home management programs upon discharge.

Intervention/Treatment

Models and programs developed by occupational therapy personnel include burn contracture management (Adsule et al., 2011; Adsule & Desai, 2012), mind–body interventions (Anderson et al., 2019), occupational therapy for burned hands (Aghajanzade et al., 2019), occupational therapy for upper extremities (T. Williams & Berenz, 2017), orthotics (splints and casts; Parry et al., 2020; Procter, 2010), and serial splintage (Puri et al., 2013). Models and programs developed by other professionals but used by occupational therapy personnel include case studies (Nedelec, Calva, et al., 2016); contracture positioning (Procter, 2010); edema (Burn Therapy Standards Working Group, 2017); Grading of Recommendations, Assessment, Development and Evaluation (GRADE) classification (Goutos et al., 2010); guidelines for cardiovascular fitness (Nedelec, Parry, et al., 2016); guidelines for ambulation (Nedelec et al., 2012); guidelines for gel (Nedelec et al., 2015); guidelines for vocational evaluation (Stergiou-Kita et al., 2014); inpatient rehabilitation (Schneider et al., 2012); knowledge translation (Lamble et al., 2019); leap motion control (Wu et al., 2019); pain and sensation (Burn Therapy Standards Working Group, 2017); pressure garment therapy (Pillay et al., 2016); range of motion and strength (Burn Therapy Standards Working Group, 2017); and work reintegration (Nguyen et al., 2016). Team members include physicians (plastic surgeons), nursing personnel, psychologists, physical therapists, dieticians and nutritionists, and occupational therapy personnel. Goals are focused on minimizing the adverse effects caused by the injury (joint range of motion, contracture, and scaring), maximizing functional ability, psychological well-being, and social integration with the aim of resuming independence in self-care, leisure, and work activities to regain quality of life (Agency for Clinical Innovation, 2017; Procter, 2010). For practitioner competency skills, see Parry et al. (2017).

Activities of Daily Living/Instrumental ADL
- Provide retraining in eating, dressing, toileting.
- Assist team to maintain balance of body fluids and electrolytes.
- Work with dietician or nutritionist to maintain or increase body weight and improve nutritional status.
- Assist in providing corrective cosmetics for facial burns.
- Provide retraining in communication skills such as writing or keyboarding.
- Assist in providing driver training or retraining.

Education/Work
- Assist in educational activities, including getting a GED or participating in continuing education.
- Assist in return-to-work program.

Play/Leisure
- No information identified.

Rest/Sleep
- See Sleep–Wake Disorders in Section 13: Lifestyle Conditions.

Social Participation
- Assist person to resume participation in social activities.

Sensorimotor
- Position body to prevent pressure sores from developing, including schedule to change body position.
- Positioning to support joints in best alignment possible in relation to burn rehabilitation.
- Assist in managing edema (swelling) through:
  - ► Applying compression using bandages or garments.
  - ► Supporting and elevating swollen limbs.
  - ► Maintaining joint range of motion as much as possible.
- Facilitate normal joint and muscle movement to perform everyday activities.
- Provide scar management program.
  - ► Apply compression bandages or garments.
  - ► Apply silicone products (gel sheets, liquid or putty).
  - ► Demonstrate to family and professionals appropriate scare massage.

- Address functional upper limb.
  - ▶ Maintain or improve joint range of motion.
  - ▶ Maintain or improve muscle strength.
  - ▶ Maintain or improve sensation in skin receptors (touch, temperature, pressure).
  - ▶ Increase fine motor control including grasp and release and object manipulation.
- Provide assistance in reducing burn skin hypersensitivity.
- Provide home program of active range of motion (AROM) and passive range of motion (PROM) exercises upon discharge.
- Provide home program of scar management and use of pressure garments, if needed, upon discharge.

Cognitive/Perceptual
- No information identified.

Psychosocial
- Provide stress management and coping strategies such as relaxation training, deep-breathing exercises, mediation, mindfulness, positive thinking, yoga.
- Assist person to resume social roles.

Context/Environment
- Provide splints to secure newly grafted skin in place.
- Provide splints to maintain good body alignment and prevent contractures depending on the area of burn: mouth, neck, axilla, elbow, wrist, hand, knee, or ankle (Bearden, 2017).
- Provide education about the importance of skin care to overall health, sun protection, protective clothing, and footwear.
- Provide assistive devices where necessary, such as adapted eating devices for a client with burns to the hands.
- Recommend home modifications for safety and independence such as grab bars, bannisters, ramps, rearrangement of furniture, removal of rugs.
- Provide information to client and family about other resources available in the community.

Precautions/Safety Considerations
- Maintain aseptic (sterile) conditions to prevent infection. Monitor client for shock reactions.
- Monitor client for changes in skin conditions, especially if grafts have been applied.
- Monitor client for respiratory distress if inhalation injury may have occurred. In hand injuries, monitor first web-space contractures, which can limit recovery (Ghalayini et al., 2019).

Prognosis and Outcome
The earlier burn injuries are treated with proper protocols, the better the outcome including a lower risk of functional deficits (Bearden, 2017). Recovery for isolated hand burns is good (N. Williams et al., 2012).

REFERENCES
Adsule, P. R., Borkar, R., & Desai, S. P. (2011). Effectiveness of pre operative splints and conventional occupational therapy in reduction of the area required for skin grafting in cases of elbow post burn contracture. *Indian Journal of Occupational Therapy, 43*(3), 23–29.

Adsule, P. R., & Desai, S. P. (2012). To study the effectiveness of pre operative splints and conventional occupational therapy in moderate and severe contracture of the hand. *Indian Journal of Occupational Therapy, 44*(1), 13–18.

Agency for Clinical Innovation. (2017). *Clinical Guideline: Burn physiotherapy and occupational therapy guidelines.* https://aci.health.nsw.gov.au/__data/assets/pdf_file/0018/236151/Burns-PT-OT-Guidelines.pdf

Aghajanzade, M., Momeni, M., Niazi, M., Ghorbani, H., Saberi, M., Kheirkhah, R., Rahbar, H., & Karimi, H. (2019). Effectiveness of incorporating occupational therapy in rehabilitation of hand burn patients. *Annals of Burns and Fire Disasters, 32*(2), 147–152.

Anderson, A. K., Hoffman, A. L., Atler, K., Yuma, P., Hill, H., Pauley, J., & Schmid, A. A. (2019). Mind over matter: An exploratory case study of mind–body interventions in the burn unit. *Journal of Acute Care Occupational Therapy, 2*(3), 1–27.

Bearden, M. D. (2017). Burns. In H. Smith-Gabai & S. E. Holm (Eds.), *Occupational therapy in acute care* (2nd ed., pp. 571–581). AOTA Press.

Burn Therapy Standards Working Group. (2017). *Standards of physiotherapy and occupational therapy practice in the management of burn injured adults and children*. British Burn Association.

Couture, M. A., Calva, V., de Oliveira, A., LaSalle, L., Forget, N., & Nedelec, B. (2018). Development and clinimetric evaluation of the mouth impairment and disability assessment (MIDA). *Burns, 44*(4), 980–994. https://doi.org/10.1016/j.burns.2017.10.024

Ghalayini, G., O'Brien, L., & Bourke-Taylor, H. M. (2019). Recovery in the first six months after hand and upper limb burns: A prospective cohort study. *Australian Occupational Therapy Journal, 66*(2), 201–209. https://doi.org/10.1111/1440-1630.12538

Goutos, I., Clarke, M., Upson, C., Richardson, P. M., & Ghosh, S. J. (2010). Review of therapeutic agents for burns pruritus and protocols for management in adult and paediatric patients using the GRADE classification. *Indian Journal of Plastic Surgery, 43*(Suppl. 1), S51–S62. https://doi.org/10.4103/0970-0358.70721

Lamble, M., Seto, V., Ye, Z., Couture, C., de Oliveira, A., Calva, V., Couture, M.-A., Poulin, C., LaSalle, L., & Nedelec, B. (2019). Perceived value of a knowledge translation intervention designed to facilitate burn survivors' work reintegration. *Journal of Burn Care & Research, 40*(6), 846–856. https://doi.org/10.1093/jbcr/irz100

Martin, L., Byrnes, M., McGarry, S., Rea, S., & Wood, F. (2016). Evaluation of the posttraumatic growth inventory after severe burn injury in Western Australia: Clinical implications for use. *Disability and Rehabilitation, 38*(24), 2398–2405. https://doi.org/10.3109/09638288.2015.1129448

Nedelec, B., Carter, A., Forbes, L., Hsu, S.-C. C., McMahon, M., Parry, I., Ryan, C. M., Serghiou, M. A., Schneider, J. C., Sharp, P. A., de Oliveira, A., & Boruff, J. (2015). Practice guidelines for the application of nonsilicone or silicone gels and gel sheets after burn injury. *Journal of Burn Care & Research, 36*(3), 345–374. https://doi.org/10.1097/BCR.0000000000000124

Nedelec, B., Calva, V., Chouinard, A., Couture, M.A., Godbout, E., de Oliveira, A., & LaSalle, L. (2016). Somatosensory rehabilitation for neuropathic pain in burn survivors: A case series. *Journal of Burn Care & Research, 37*(1), e37–e46. https://doi.org/10.1097/BCR.0000000000000321

Nedelec, B., Parry, I., Acharya, H., Benavides, L., Bills, S., Bucher, J. L., Cheal, J., Chouinard, A, Crump, D., Duch, S., Godleski, M., Guenther, J., Knox, C., LaBonte, E., Lorello, D., Lucio, J. X., Macdonald, L. E., Kemp-Offenberg, J., Osborne, C., Pontius, K., Yelvington, M., de Olveira, A., & Kloda, L. A. (2016). Practice guidelines for cardiovascular fitness and strengthening exercise prescription after burn injury. *Journal of Burn Care & Research 37*(6), e539–e558. https://doi.org/10.1097/BCR.0000000000000282

Nedelec, B., Serghiou, M. A., Niszczak, J., McMahon, M., & Healey, T. (2012). Practice guidelines of early ambulation for burn survivors after lower extremity grafts. *Journal of Burn Care & Research, 33*(3), 319–329. https://doi.org/10.1097/BCR.0b013e31823359d9

Nguyen, N. T., Lorrain, M., Pognon-Hanna, J. N., Elfassy, C., Calva, V., de Oliveira, A., & Nedelec, B. (2016). Barriers and facilitators to work reintegration and burn survivors' perspectives on educating work colleagues. *Burns, 42*(7), 1477–1486. https://doi.org/10.1016/j.burns.2016.05.014

O'Toole, M. T. (Ed.). (2017). *Mosby's dictionary of medicine, nursing & health professions* (10th ed.). Elsevier.

Parry, I., Forbes, L., Lorello, D., Benavides, L., Calvert, C., Hsu, S.-C., Chouinard, A., Godleski, M., Helm, P., Holavanahalli, R. K., Kemp-Offenberg, J., Ruiz, C. E., Shon, R., Schneider, J. C., Shetler, M., Suman, O. E., & Nedelec, B. (2017). Burn Rehabilitation Therapists Competency Tool–Version 2: An expansion to include long-term rehabilitation and outpatient care. *Journal of Burn Care & Research, 38*(1), e261–e268. https://doi.org/ 10.1097/BCR.0000000000 000364

Parry, I. S., Schneider, J. C., Yelvington, M., Sharp, P., Serghiou, M., Ryan, C. M., Richardson, E., Pontius, K., Niszczak, J., McMahon, M., MacDonald, L. E., Lorello, D., Kehrer, C. K., Godleski, M., Forbes, L., Duch, S., Crump, D., Chouinard, A., Calva, V., Bills, S., Benavides, L., Acharya, H. J., de Oliveira, A., Boruff, J., & Nedelec, B. (2020). Systematic review and expert consensus on the use of orthoses (splints and casts) with adults and children after burn injury to determine practice guidelines. *Journal of Burn Care & Research, 41*(3), 503–534. https://doi.org/10.1093/ jbcr/irz150

Pillay, R., Visagie, S., & Mji, G. (2016). An exploration of burn survivors' experiences of pressure garment therapy at a tertiary hospital in South Africa. *South African Journal of Occupational Therapy, 46*(3), 73–79. https://doi.org/10.17159/2310-3833/2016/v46n3a12

Procter, F. (2010). Rehabilitation of the burn patient. *Indian Journal of Plastic Surgery, 43*(Suppl. 1), S101–S113. https://doi.org/10.4103/0970-0358.70730

Puri, V., Khare, N., Venkateshwaran, N., Bharadwaj, S., Choudhary, S., Deshpande, O., & Borkar, R. (2013). Serial splintage: Preoperative treatment of upper limb contracture. *Burns, 39*(6), 1096–1100. https://doi.org/10.1016/j.burns.2013.01.010

Schneider, J. C., Qu, H. D., Lowry, J., Walker, J., Vitale, E., & Zona, M. (2012). Efficacy of inpatient burn rehabilitation: A prospective pilot study examining range of motion, hand function and balance. *Burns, 38*(2), 164–171. https://doi.org/10.1016/j.burns.2011.11.002

Stergiou-Kita, M., Grigorovich, A., & Gomez, M. (2014). Development of an inter-professional clinical practice guideline for vocational evaluation following severe burn. *Burns, 40*(6), 1149–1163. https://doi.org/10.1016/j.burns.2014.01.001

Williams, N., Stiller, K., Greenwood, J., Calvert, P., Masters, M., & Kavanagh, S. (2012). Physical and quality of life outcomes of patients with isolated hand burns—A prospective audit. *Journal of Burn Care & Research, 33*(2), 188–198. https://doi.org/10.1097/BCR.0b013e318242eeef

Williams, T., & Berenz, T. (2017). Postburn upper extremity occupational therapy. *Hand Clinics, 33*(2), 293–304. https://doi.org/10.1016/j.hcl.2016.12.015

Wu, Y. T., Chen, K. H., Ban, S. L., Tung, K. Y., & Chen, L. R. (2019). Evaluation of leap motion control for hand rehabilitation in burn patients: An experience in the dust explosion disaster in Formosa Fun Coast. *Burns, 45*(1), 157–164. https://doi.org/10.1016/j.burns.2018.08.001

BIBLIOGRAPHY

Ablort-Morgan, C., Allorto, N. L., & Rode, H. (2016). Rehabilitation of a bilateral upper limb amputee in a resource restricted burn service. *Burns, 42*(5), e81–e85. https://doi.org/10.1016/ j.burns.2016.01.027

Deshaies, L. (2014). Burns. In C. Cooper (Ed.), *Fundamentals of hand therapy* (2nd ed., pp. 479–490). Elsevier.

Holavanahalli, R. K., Helm, P. A., Parry, I. S., Dolezal, C. A., & Greenhalgh, D. G. (2011). Select practices in management and rehabilitation of burns: A survey report. *Journal of Burn Care & Research, 32*(2), 210–223. https://doi.org/10.1097/BCR.0b013e31820aadd5

Knight, A., Wasiak, J., Salway, J., & O'Brien, L. (2017). Factors predicting health status and recovery of hand function after hand burns in the second year after hospital discharge. *Burns, 43*(1), 100–106. https://doi.org/10.1016/j.burns.2016.07.025

Kurakazu, D., & Hirai, A. H. (2018). Burns and burn rehabilitation. In H. H. Pendleton & W. Schultz-Krohn (Eds.), *Pedretti's occupational therapy* (8th ed., pp. 1048–1082). Elsevier.

Lin, S.-Y., Chang, J.-K., Chen, P.-C., & Mao, H.-F. (2013). Hand function measures for burn patients: A literature review. *Burns, 39*(1), 16–23. https://doi.org/10.1016/j.burns.2012.08.020

Nedelec, B., & Carrougher, G. J. (2017). Pain and pruritus postburn injury. *Journal of Burn Care & Research, 38*(3), 142–145. https://doi.org/10.1097/BCR.0000000000000534

Nedelec, B., de Oliveira, A., Calva, V., Couture, M. A., Poulin, C., LaSalle, L., & Correa, J. A. (2020). Longitudinal evaluation of pressure applied by custom fabricated garments worn by adult burn survivors. *Journal of Burn Care & Research, 41*(2), 254–262. https://doi.org/10.1093/jbcr/irz154

Nedelec, B., Forget, N. J., Hurtubise, T., Cimino S., de Muszka, F., Legault, A., Liu, W. L., de Oliveira, A., Calva, V., & Correa, J. A. (2016). Skin characteristics: Normative data for elasticity, erythema, melanin, and thickness at 16 different anatomical locations. *Skin Research and Technology, 22*(3), 263–275. https://doi.org/10.1111/srt.12256

Nedelec, B., & LaSalle, L. (2018). Postburn itch: A review of the literature. *Wounds: A Compendium of Clinical Research and Practice, 30*(1), e118–e124.

Ozelie, R. (2017). Burns. In B. J. Atchison & D. P. Dirette (Eds.), *Conditions in occupational therapy* (5th ed., pp. 387–401). Wolters Kluwer.

Parnell, L. K. S., Nedelec, B., Rachelska, G., & LaSalle, L. (2012). Assessment of pruritus characteristics and impact on burn survivors. *Journal of Burn Care & Research, 33*(3), 407–418. https://doi.org/10.1097/BCR.0b013e318239d206

Pressina, M. A., & Orroth, A. C. (2014). Burn injuries. In M. V. Radomski & C. A. Trombly Latham (Eds.), *Occupational therapy for physical dysfunction* (7th ed., pp. 1244–1265). Wolters Kluwer.

Prochazka, M., Thornton, S., & Dodd, H. S. (2011). Enabling life roles after severe burns. In C. H. Christiansen & K. M. Matuska (Eds.), *Ways of living* (4th ed., pp. 349–378). AOTA Press.

Stergiou-Kita, M., Mansfield, E., Bayley, M., Cassidy, J. D., Colantonio, A., Gomez, M., Jeschke, M., Kirsh, B., Kristman, V., Moody, J., & Vartanian, O. (2014). Returning to work after electrical injuries: Workers' perspectives and advice to others. *Journal of Burn Care & Research, 35*(6), 498–507. https://doi.org/10.1097/BCR.0000000000000041

Tang, D., Li-Tsang, C. W. P., Au, R. K. C., Li, K.-C., Yi, X.-F., Liao, L.-R., Cao, J.-Y., Feng, Y.-N., & Liu, C.-S. (2015). Functional outcomes of burn patients with or without rehabilitation in mainland China. *Hong Kong Journal of Occupational Therapy, 26*(1), 15–23. https://doi.org/10.1016/j.hkjot.2015.08.003

Burns: Child and Adolescent

Description

Burns are injuries to the skin and other tissue. Burns are classified by tissue depth (superficial and deep partial-thickness, and full-thickness) and percentage of total body surface area (TBSA) involved (Porter, 2018). In children, the area of the head includes a larger percentage of TBSA and the lower extremities a lesser percentage. The percentages shift as the child grows older. In children, both sides of the trunk account for 26%, whereas in adults both sides account for 36%. Wound healing of burns is described in three phases: inflammatory phase (vascular and cellular response, 3–10 days), proliferation phase (revascularization, reepithelialization and contraction of wound, approximately 10–21 days), and maturation phrase (collagen remodeling, 3 weeks to 2 years).

Cause

Burns are caused by thermal, radiation, chemical, or electrical contact. Thermal burns may result from flame, hot liquids, hot solid objects, steam, or toxic smoke inhalation. Radiation burns usually occur as a result of exposure to solar ultraviolet radiation (sunburn), from ultraviolet radiation (tanning beds), sources of X-ray, or other nonsolar radiation. Chemical burns may be caused by strong acids, strong alkalis (lye, cement), phenols, cresols, mustard gas, phosphorus, and certain petroleum products (gasoline, paint thinner). Electrical burns are the result of heat generation and electroporation of cell membranes caused by contact with a massive current of electrons, which can cause extensive damage to electrically conductive tissues such as muscles, nerves, and blood vessels (Porter, 2018).

Evaluation/Assessment

Areas

- Activities of Daily Living/Instrumental ADL: eating, dressing, grooming, writing, mobility
- Education/Work: academic level, keyboarding, return-to-school plan
- Play/Leisure: play skills, interests (hobbies, sports), frequency of involvement
- Rest/Sleep: sleep pattern, sleep disturbance
- Social Participation: frequency, type (formal, informal), location
- Sensorimotor: depth and location of burn area, joint range of motion, fine motor skills, pain, itch, skin fragility, touch sensation
- Cognitive/Perceptual: age-appropriate attention, memory, executive functions, and self-awareness
- Psychosocial: depression, anxiety, stress and coping mechanisms, quality of life, motivation, compliance, grief or loss, body image, self-concept, social roles, guilt on the part of parents
- Context/Environment: home life or child protective services, peer and social support, adapted devices, information and education to family and caregivers, community resources
- Development (Infant, Child, Adolescent only): developmental level
- Comorbidity: ventilator dependence if inhalation injury has occurred

Instruments

Instruments Developed by Occupational Therapy Personnel

- Brisbane Burn Scar Impact Profile (BBSIP; Tyack et al., 2015)
- Children's Assessment of Participation and Enjoyment and Preferences for Activities of Children (CAPE/PAC; King et al., 2004).
- Rainbow Pain Scale (RPS; Mahon et al., 2015)

Instruments Developed by Other Professionals and Used by Occupational Therapy Personnel

- Circumferential measurements (tape measure)
- Dynamometer (muscle strength; JAMAR Dynamometer, Lafayette Instrument)
- Goniometer (joint range of motion; Shurtleff & Kaskutas, 2018)
- Itch Man Scale (IMS; Blakeney & Marvin, 2000; see also Blankers et al., 2019, in References)
- Jepsen-Taylor Hand Function Test (JPHFT; Jepsen et al., 1969)
- Modified Lund and Browder Chart (determine burn size area; Murari, 2017)
- Pediatric Quality of Life (PedsQL; Varni et al., 2001)
- Photography of burn areas
- Toronto Pediatric Itch Scale (TPIS; Everett et al., 2015)
- Vancouver Scar Scale (VSS; Sullivan et al., 1990)
- Visual Analogue Scale (VAS) Numeric Pain Rating Scale (NPRS; 0 = *no pain* to 10 = *worst pain ever*)
- Volumeter (water displacement measure of edema; Stern, 1991)

Problems/Issues

Activities of Daily Living/Instrumental ADL

- Child may have difficulty eating if the face is burned.
- Child may have difficulty performing self-maintenance skills, especially if upper extremities and hands are involved, such as dressing and grooming.

- Child may experience difficulty with mobility if lower extremities are involved.
- Child may be restricted in ability to perform ADLs or IADLs due to positioning or bandaging applied during the acute phase of burn care.

Education/Work
- Child may not be able to attend school physically or may participate in a hospital or home-based program until medical management is stable.

Play/Leisure
- Child may be restricted in ability to engage in play or leisure activities, especially if upper extremities and hands are involved.

Rest/Sleep
- Child may experience difficulty sleeping.

Social Participation
- Child may reduce or eliminate participation in formal social activities, preferring informal instead.

Sensorimotor
- Child usually experiences pain.
- Child may experience itching (pruritus).
- Child may experience loss of joint range of motion in joints where burn injury has occurred or in joints that must be positioned to decrease incidence of contractures.
- Child may experience loss of muscle strength due to injury to muscles directly or general deconditioning related to medical management program.
- Child may experience loss of endurance and cardiovascular fitness.
- Child may lose gross motor abilities.
- Child may experience loss of hand function including fine motor skills if burns involve the hands.
- Child may experience loss of sensation (touch, temperature, pressure, proprioception, stereognosis).

Cognitive/Perceptual
- Child may regress in level of cognitive function.
- Child may experience hypersensitivity of skin.
- Child may lose perceptual functions if hands are burned.

Psychosocial
- Child may be difficult to motivate due to pain.

Context/Environment
- Child and family may need access to community and internet resources.
- Child and family may need information about burn management and rehabilitation.
- Child and family may need information about assistive technology.

Intervention/Treatment

Models and programs developed by occupational therapy personnel include alternate splint (Sudhakar & Le Blanc, 2011), Oculus Rift Virtual Reality goggles (Hoffman et al., 2014), orthotics (splints and casts; Parry et al., 2020), pain management (Kipping & Miller, 2017), and purposeful activity-based play (Omar et al., 2012). Models and programs developed by other professionals but used by occupational therapy personnel include burn guidelines (Agency for Clinical Innovation, 2017), Ditto program (Brown et al., 2015; Brown et al., 2014), multimodal distraction (Miller et al., 2010; Miller et al., 2011), and standards of practice (Burn Therapy Standards Working Group, 2017). Team members include physicians (plastic surgeons), nursing personnel, physical therapists, social workers, psychologists, educators, and occupational therapy personnel. Goals are to improve the quality of life and optimize the outcomes in both the short and long term, including managing debilitating scarring, controlling pain, improving functional recovery, and increasing activity and occupational participation (Atiyeh & Janom, 2014; Grice et al., 2015).

Activities of Daily Living/Instrumental ADL

- Consider use of compensatory techniques to facilitate self-maintenance and basic self-care activities, including use of assistive devices for eating, dressing, bathing/showering, toileting, mobility, and communication.

Education/Work

- Assist educators to facilitate participation in educational activities, making modifications as needed within medical management program.

Play/Leisure

- Provide opportunity to play or engage in leisure activities within limits of burn-management protocol.

Rest/Sleep

- Assist in developing a sleep routine and make adjustments as burn injuries heal.

Social Participation

- Encourage child to participate in formal and informal social activities.

Sensorimotor

- Edema management
  - ▶ Purpose: Reduce limitations to wound health, joint movement, and function
  - ▶ Techniques
    - ○ Apply compression using bandages or garments.
    - ○ Support or elevate swollen limbs.
    - ○ Encourage normal movements in daily tasks and occupations.
- Exercise (passive and active)
  - ▶ Purpose: Maintain joint mobility, sensation, and strength
  - ▶ Techniques/considerations
    - ○ Focus on grasp and release, fine motor control, and object manipulation.
    - ○ Use daily activities (eating, dressing, writing, coloring).
    - ○ Provide assistive devices where necessary.
    - ○ Stretches should address lines of tension and may not necessarily be in anatomical plane.
    - ○ Stretching should be observed and performed without dressing or garments to observe effect directly.
- Joint protection
  - ▶ Purpose: Maintain joint alignment and mobility
  - ▶ Techniques
    - ○ Support joints in best possible position given burn area.
    - ○ Manage edema.
    - ○ Facilitate normal movement for daily tasks and occupations.
- Massage
  - ▶ Purpose: Break up collagen bundles that form scar tissue and assist with desensitization
  - ▶ Techniques
    - ○ Massage scar area with moisturizer several times per day.
    - ○ Massage with firm pressure so skin blanches.
    - ○ Massage in slow circular motions using flat hand and fingers.
- Pain management (see also Pain and Chronic Pain in Section 2: Sensory Disorders)
  - ▶ Purpose: Control pain to extent possible

- ► Techniques
  - ○ Virtual reality may be used as a distractor (Miller et al., 2010).
  - ○ Positioning to reduce contractures.
  - ○ Active and passive exercises.
  - ○ Engaging in everyday activities.
- Positioning
  - ► Purpose: Reduce flexion contractures and prevent pressure injury development
  - ► Recommended position (Note: splinting may require changes)
    - ○ Neck: extension/hyperextension.
    - ○ Arms abducted, externally rotated with 90 degrees from arm to trunk.
    - ○ Forearm: supinated.
    - ○ Trunk: supine in straight alignment.
    - ○ Hips: neutral, no external rotation or flexion.
    - ○ Legs: extended/straight about 20 degrees apart.
    - ○ Feet: dorsiflexed.
- Pressure/compression garments
  - ► Purpose: Garments are worn at all times except for showering/bathing, massage, or moisturizing to reduce scarring
  - ► Techniques/considerations
    - ○ Young children may require new garments every 3 months due to growth and fabric fatigue.
    - ○ To aid dressing and undressing, zippers may be added to arm, hand, and leg garments.
    - ○ Vests should have back closures to prevent child from removing vest.
    - ○ Velcro closures allow for weight fluctuations.
    - ○ Suspenders on pants are important for children up to age 10.
- Sensory retraining: See Sensory Processing Disorders: Child in Section 2: Sensory Disorders.
- Skin care
  - ► Purpose: Compensate for decreased ability of skin to perform normal functions
  - ► Techniques/considerations
    - ○ Daily washing or showering to cleanse skin and add moisturizer.
    - ○ Control environmental temperature to compensate for decreased ability of skin to sweat or heat up.
    - ○ Avoid ultraviolet light that may increase risk of skin cancer.
    - ○ Sun exposure may increase risk of skin discoloration.
- Silicone sheet products
  - ► Purpose: Reduce scarring
  - ► Techniques/considerations
    - ○ For school-age children products are usually worn at night because activities tend to build up heat and become uncomfortable.
    - ○ Younger children that are less active may wear product during day hours.
- Splinting
  - ► Purpose
    - ○ Maintain full range of motion and prevent contractures.
    - ○ Prevent newly grafted skin from moving.
  - ► Type
    - ○ Mouth: Mouth exerciser and splint.
    - ○ Hand, general: Wrist extension 10–45 degrees, metacarpophalangeal (MCP) flexion 60–80 degrees, proximal interphalangeal (PIP) and distal interphalangeal (DIP) in full extension.
    - ○ Burns in hands require MCP or thumb extension and neutral wrist position.
    - ○ Axilla: Shoulder is abducted overhead to about 160 degrees with forward flexion to prevent brachial plexus injury; elbow may be extended or flexed.

▶ Considerations
  ○ Splinting in pediatric population differs from adults: Is generally done more frequently, for longer periods within 24-hour period, and for longer course of time for scar management.
  ○ Splint position is at end of range or as close as possible.
  ○ Splints are worn 24 hours per day and removed only for exercises, dressing changes, and participation in daily activities (eating, bathing, swimming).
  ○ Splints should be checked for changes in edema, breakdown, fragile skins, changes in range of motion, hot weather, or maceration.
  ○ Splints must be checked frequently to ensure proper fit as child grows.

Cognitive/Perceptual
- Maintain cognitive functions to age-appropriate level.
- Be prepared to repeat information and instructions frequently to compensate for sleep deprivation, pain, medications, and stress.

Psychosocial
- Assist in providing stress management and coping techniques (deep breathing, mindfulness, yoga).
- Discuss with child or adolescent what is bothering him or her and provide answers at age-appropriate level of understanding.

Context/Environment
- Provide adaptive devices as needed and instructions in their use.
- Provide information to family and caregivers regarding burn treatment protocol.
- Provide access to community and online resources such as the burn support network or local camps for burn survivors.

Precautions/Safety Considerations

If inhalation injury has occurred, be aware of signs of allergies or respiratory distress. Watch for signs of infection or wound separation (dehiscence) and report immediately to medical management team.

Prognosis and Outcome

Recovery depends in part on severity of burn injury, intervention program, social support, and compliance (Kurakazu & Hirai, 2018). Teenagers with burn injuries are 3 times more likely than typical peers of having mental health problems, including mood and anxiety disorders and substance abuse (Duke et al., 2018). Scar maturation typically occurs between 12 and 18 months depending on individual variation (Agency for Clinical Innovation, 2017). Mental health support is an ongoing need through childhood and adulthood (Duke et al., 2018).

REFERENCES

Agency for Clinical Innovation. (2017). *Clinical guidelines: Burn physiotherapy and occupational therapy guidelines.*

Atiyeh, B., & Janom, H. H. (2014). Physical rehabilitation of pediatric burns. *Annals of Burns and Fire Disasters, 27*(1), 37–43.

Blankers, K., Dankerlui, N., van Loey, N., Pursad, M., Rode, H., & van Dijk, M. (2019). Cross-cultural validation of the Itch Man Scale in pediatric burn survivors in a South African setting. *Burns, 45*(3), 725–731. https://doi.org/10.1016/j.burns.2018.09.027

Brown, N. J., David, M., Cuttle, L., Kimble, R. M., Rodger, S., & Higashi, H. (2015). Cost-effectiveness of a nonpharmacological intervention in pediatric burn care. *Value in Health, 18*(5), 631–637. https://doi.org/10.1016/j.jval.2015.04.011

Brown, N. J., Kimble, R. M., Rodger, S., Ware, R. S., & Cuttle, L. (2014). Play and heal: Randomized controlled trial of Ditto intervention efficacy on improving re-epithelialization in pediatric burns. *Burns, 40*(2), 204–213. https://doi.org/10.1016/j.burns.2013.11.024

Burn Therapy Standards Working Group. (2017). *Standards of physiotherapy and occupational therapy practice in the management of burn injured adults and children.* British Burn Association.

Duke, J. M., Randall, S. M., Vetrichevvel, T. P., McGarry, S., Boyd, J. H., Rea, S., & Wood, F. M. (2018). Long-term mental health outcomes after unintentional burns sustained during childhood: A retrospective cohort study. *Burns & Trauma, 6,* 32. https://doi.org/10.1186/s41038-018-0134-z

Grice, K. O., Barnes, K. J., & Vogel, K. A. (2015). Influence of burn injury on activity participation of children. *Journal of Burn Care & Research, 36*(3), 414–420. https://doi.org/10.1097/BCR.0000000000000105

Hoffman, H. G., Meyer, W. J., III, Ramirez, M., Roberts, L., Seibel, E. J., Atzori, B., Sharar, S. R., & Patterson, D. R. (2014). Feasibility of articulated arm mounted Oculus Rift virtual reality goggles for adjunctive pain control during occupational therapy in pediatric burn patients. *Cyberpsychology, Behavior, and Social Networking, 17*(6), 397–401. https://doi.org/10.1089/cyber.2014.0058

Kipping, B., & Miller, K. (2017). Occupational therapists' role in facilitating pain management in children with burn injuries. *Australian Occupational Therapy Journal, 64*(Suppl. S1), 35–38. https://doi.org/10.1111/1440-1630.12378

Kurakazu, D., & Hirai, A. H. (2018). Burns and burn rehabilitation. In H. H. Pendleton & W. Schultz-Krohn (Eds.), *Pedretti's occupational therapy* (8th ed., pp. 1048–1082). Elsevier.

Miller, K., Rodger, S., Bucolo, S., Greer, R., & Kimble, R. M. (2010). Multi-modal distraction: Using technology to combat pain in young children with burn injuries. *Burns, 36*(5), 647–658. https://doi.org/10.1016/j.burns.2009.06.199

Miller, K., Rodger, S., Kipping, B., & Kimble, R. M. (2011). A novel technology approach to pain management in children with burns: A prospective randomized controlled trial. *Burns, 37*(3), 395–405. https://doi.org/10.1016/j.burns.2010.12.008

Omar, M. T. A., Hegazy, F. A., & Mokashi, S. P. (2012). Influences of purposeful activity versus rote exercise on improving pain and hand function in pediatric burn. *Burns, 38*(2), 261–268. https://doi.org/10.1016/j.burns.2011.08.004

Parry, I. S., Schneider, J. C., Yelvington, M., Sharp, P., Serghiou, M., Ryan, C. M., Richardson, E., Pontius, K., Niszczak, J., McMahon, M., MacDonald, L. E., Lorello, D., Kehrer, C. K., Godleski, M., Forbes, L., Duch, S., Crump, D., Chouinard, A., Calva, V., Bills, S., Benavides, L., Acharya, H. J., de Oliveira, A., Boruff, J., & Nedelec, B. (2020). Systematic review and expert consensus on the use of orthoses (splints and casts) with adults and children after burn injury to determine practice guidelines. *Journal of Burn Care & Research, 41*(3), 503–534. https://doi.org/10.1093/jbcr/irz150

Porter, R. S. (Ed.). (2018). *The Merck manual of diagnosis and therapy* (20th ed.). Merck Sharp & Dohme.

Sudhakar, G., & Le Blanc, M. (2011). Alternate splint for flexion contracture in children with burns. *Journal of Hand Therapy, 24*(3), 277–279. https://doi.org/10.1016/j.jht.2010.10.008

BIBLIOGRAPHY

Brown, N. J., Kimble, R. M., Gramotnev, G., Rodger, S., & Cuttle, L. (2014). Predictors of re-epithelialization in pediatric burn. *Burns, 40*(4), 751–758. https://doi.org/10.1016/j.burns.2013.09.027

Brown, N. J., Kimble, R. M., Rodger, S., Ware, R. S., McWhinney, B. C., Ungerer, J. P., & Cuttle, L. (2014). Biological markers of stress in pediatric acute burn injury. *Burns, 40*(5), 887–895. https://doi.org/10.1016/j.burns.2013.12.001

Goutos, I., Clarke, M., Upson, C., Richardson, P. M., & Ghosh, S. J. (2010). Review of therapeutic agents for burns pruritus and protocols for management in adult and paediatric patients using the GRADE classification. *Indian Journal of Plastic Surgery* 43(Suppl. 1), S51–S62. https://doi.org/10.4103/0970-0358.70721

Heath, K., Timbrell, V., Calvert, P., & Stiller, K. (2011). Outcome measurement tools currently used to assess pediatric burn patients: An occupational therapy and physiotherapy perspective. *Journal of Burn Care & Research, 32*(6), 600–607. https://doi.org/10.1097/BCR .0b013e31822dc450

Kipping, B., Rodger, S., Miller, K., & Kimble, R. M. (2012). Virtual reality for acute pain reduction in adolescents undergoing burn wound care: A prospective randomized controlled trial. *Burns, 38*(5), 650–657. https://doi.org/10.1016/j.burns.2011.11.010

McGarry, S., Elliott, C., McDonald, A., Valentine, J., Wood, F., & Girdler, S. (2015). "This is not just a little accident": A qualitative understanding of paediatric burns from the perspective of parents. *Disability and Rehabilitation, 37*(1), 41–50. https://doi.org/10.3109/09638288.2 014.892640

McGarry, S., Elliott, C., McDonald, A., Valentine, J., Wood, F., & Girdler, S. (2014). Paediatric burns: From the voice of the child. *Burns, 40*(4), 606–615. https://doi.org/10.1016/j .burns.2013.08.031

McGarry, S., Girdler, S., McDonald, A., Valentine, J., Wood, F., & Elliott, C. (2013). Paediatric medical trauma: The impact on parents of burn survivors. *Burns, 39*(6), 1114–1121. https:// doi.org/10.1016/j.burns.2013.01.009

Ohgi, S., & Gu, S. (2013). Pediatric burn rehabilitation: Philosophy and strategies. *Burns & Trauma, 1*(2), 73–79. https://doi.org/10.4103/2321-3868.118930

Pressina, M. A., & Orroth, A. C. (2014). Burn injuries. In M. V. Radomski & C. A. Trombly Latham (Eds.), *Occupational therapy for physical dysfunction* (7th ed., pp. 1244–1265). Wolters Kluwer.

Simons, M. A., Ziviani, J., & Copley, J. (2010). Predicting functional outcome for children on admission after burn injury: Do parents hold the key? *Journal of Burn Care & Research, 31*(5), 750–765. https://doi.org/10.1097/BCR.0b013e3181eebe88

Pressure Ulcers

Also called pressure sores, pressure injuries, decubitus ulcers, bedsores, skin breakdown.

Description

Pressure ulcers (PUs) are areas of necrosis and ulceration in the skin tissues that have been compressed between bony prominences and hard surfaces in the environment such as a bed or chair (Porter, 2018). Pressure ulcers can be life threatening since they can become infected, but most are preventable with proper care, including weight shifts, pressure redistribution, skin inspection, routine turning and repositioning, keeping skin clean and dry, maintaining adequate nutrition and hydration, and wearing properly fitting clothing and shoes. Specialized mattress and wheelchair seat cushions, proper transfer technique, and protection of bony prominences with various types of padding are also important. Major issues leading to pressure ulcers may be person's lack of rudimentary knowledge pertaining to wound care, unavailable or nonuse of equipment and supply, comorbidities, person's nonadherence to prescribed bed rest, inactivity, and circumstances beyond caregiver/therapist's reach (Floríndez et al., 2020). Spasticity and dementia may increase risk of developing pressure ulcers (Jaul et al., 2019).

Cause

Pressure ulcers are lesions or injuries to the skin or underlying tissue that are caused by a loss of blood flow to the area. The mechanical and fluid dynamic causes of the lesions or injuries are the result of a combination of pressure, friction, shearing forces, trauma to the skin (cuts, burns, bumps), and moisture on the skin tissues. Risk factors include age 65 or older, loss of sensation or feeling, impaired circulation, immobilization such as lying or sitting in one position without moving for several hours, undernutrition, and incontinence, which causes a skin irritant (Porter, 2018). Pressure ulcers occur most frequently on the bony prominences over the sacrum ischium, trochanters, heels, and elbows but can occur elsewhere on the body.

Stages
- Suspected deep tissue injury: Purple or maroon localized area of discolored skin or blood-filled blister.
- Stage 1: Intact skin with nonblanchable redness of a localized area, usually over a bony prominence.
- Stage 2: Partial thickness loss of dermis presenting as a shallow open ulcer with red/pink wound bed, without slough.
- Stage 3: Full thickness tissue loss. Subcutaneous fat may be visible, but bone, tendon, or muscle is not exposed. Slough may be present. May include undermining and tunneling.
- Stage 4: Full thickness tissue loss with exposed bone, tendon, or muscle. Slough or eschar may be present on some parts of the wound bed. Often includes undermining and tunneling.
- Unstageable: Full thickness loss with the base of the ulcer covered by slough and/or eschar in the wound bed (Spencer et al., 2012).

Evaluation/Assessment

Areas
- Activities of Daily Living/Instrumental ADL: skin inspection
- Education/Work: potential workplace hazards (cuts, bruises, scratches) or routines (long periods of time in one position)
- Play/Leisure: potential hazards or routines, interests, frequency, location
- Rest/Sleep: potential hazards (scratchy bedding or bed clothes, sweat or moisture) or routines (sleeping in one position for long periods of time)
- Social Participation: potential hazards or routines, frequency, location, with whom
- Sensorimotor: muscle weakness, joint range of motion, positioning, fatigue, pain, sensation loss
- Cognitive/Perceptual: awareness, memory, executive functioning, time management, and scheduling
- Psychosocial: motivation, depression, anxiety, quality of life, life habits, sense of self-efficacy, role performance, emotional control
- Context/Environment: patient and caregiver education, wheelchair or scooter cushions, bed and mattress, adapted devices, social support, community and internet resources
- Comorbidities: level of spinal cord injury, diabetes, spasticity, dementia, brain injury, decreased sensory acuity due to aging

Instruments
Instruments Developed by Occupational Therapy Personnel:
- Questionnaire (Mathew et al., 2013, in References)

Instruments Developed by Other Professionals and Used by Occupational Therapy Personnel
- Braden Scale (BS; Bergstrom et al., 1987)
- "Pressure Zone Mapping" (instrumentation; McCarthy, 2011, and Mendes et al., 2016, in References)
- Spinal Cord Injury Pressure Ulcer Scale (SCIPUS; Salzberg et al., 1996; see also Krishnan et al., 2016, in References)

Problems/Issues

Activities of Daily Living/Instrumental ADL

- Person may be limited in ability to perform self-care tasks due to restricted positions required to permit pressure ulcer to heal, such as bathing or showering.
- Person may experience difficulty maintaining nutritional status, including food and liquid intake necessary to promote healing.
- Person may experience difficulty avoiding moisture build-up on ulcerated skin from urine and sweat, which may reduce healing process.
- Person may be limited in mobility depending on location of pressure ulcer (bed mobility, use of wheelchair, walking).
- Person may need to limit friction and shear forces to avoid damaging skin as it heals.
- Person may be limited or unable to perform independent living skills such as driving, shopping, or housekeeping tasks.

Education/Work

- Person may be limited or unable to attend educational classes while pressure ulcer heals, requiring remote learning.
- Person may be limited or unable to perform work tasks that require physical mobility such as lifting, bending, stooping, climbing, reaching, or carrying.

Play/Leisure

- Person may be limited or unable to engage in leisure occupations that require physical mobility until pressure ulcer heals.

Rest/Sleep

- Person may be limited in body positions that can be assumed depending on location of pressure ulcer.

Social Participation

- Person may be limited or be unable to participate in social activities due to restricted physical mobility.

Sensorimotor

- Person may lose physical fitness due to restricted positions imposed while healing occurs.
- Person may lose joint range of motion due to restricted movement imposed while healing occurs.
- Person may experience spasticity or contractures due to limited mobility.
- Person may experience impaired sensation to touch or pressure in area of skin where pressure ulcer has occurred, especially if the ulcer involves all layers of skin; during healing process skin sensation may be hypersensitive.
- Person may experience pain caused by the pressure ulcer and skin healing process.
- Person may experience discomfort related to restricted movement.

Cognitive/Perceptual

- Not directly involved but person may report reduced ability to attend due to pain and discomfort.

Psychosocial

- Person may report reduced quality of life.
- Person may be unable to perform or be limited in performance of role functions.
- Person may report feelings of depression and anxiety due to restricted mobility.
- Person may report loss of sense of self-efficacy and self-worth.
- Person's preinjury habits may determine ability to adhere to intervention program or risk of potential noncompliance (Fogelberg et al., 2016).

Context/Environment

- Person may be restricted to home or health facility while healing occurs.
- Person may require assistance from family, caregivers, or healthcare workers to provide for physical care while healing occurs, including assistance in changing positions every 2 to 4 hours.

Intervention/Treatment

Models and programs developed by occupational therapy personnel include lifestyle intervention (Ghaisas et al., 2015), manualization of occupational therapy program (Blanche et al., 2011; Vaishampayan et al., 2011), occupational therapy role (Evers et al., 2015; Macens et al., 2011), and posture control and cushion air management (Park & Lee, 2019). Models and programs developed by other professionals but used by occupational therapy personnel include clinical practice guidelines (Robertson & Stern, 2012), electrical stimulation therapy (Lala et al., 2016), National Institute for Health and Care Excellence (NICE) Guidelines (Stuart, 2014), pressure injury prevention best practices (Scovil et al., 2019), Pressure Ulcer Prevention Initiative (Cobb et al., 2014), pressure ulcer prevention program (Carlson et al., 2019; Martin et al., 2017; Sleight et al., 2019), seating guidelines (Stephens & Barley, 2018), and skin-care internet intervention (Hilgart et al., 2014). Team members include physicians, nursing personnel, dietitians and nutritionists, pharmacists, physical therapists, and occupational therapy personnel. Goal is to maintain skin integrity and prevent skin breakdown.

Activities of Daily Living/Instrumental ADL

- Daily inspection of skin for signs of pressure ulcers needs to be added to daily bathing or showering routine for older individuals or for those at risk.
- Reestablish routines such as wiping wetness form vulnerable areas, using padded surfaces, changing out of sweaty clothes, setting reminders to change positions.
- Assist client to establish and maintain healthy eating habits high in protein for good nutrition and healthy skin.

Education/Work

- Assist client to plan for paid or unpaid work or volunteering.
- Asist client to establish a work/rest routine.

Play/Leisure

- Assist client to identify meaningful leisure occupations.
- Assist client to reconnect with established leisure occupations and explore new ones.

Rest/Sleep

- Assist client to determine whether pressure relief devices can be static (low tech: foam or gel mattress) or dynamic (high tech: mechanical).
- Factor to consider is amount of independence with bed mobility including ability to turn over or move from back to side.

Social Participation

- Assist client to identify meaningful social occupations.
- Assist client to modify existing social occupations to meet current level of function and explore new ones.

Sensorimotor

- Reduce pressure: practice weight shifts including shifting weight side to side or front to back or lifting buttocks off seat with upper extremities (alternate: power chair with tilt-in-space or can recline).
- Avoid friction.
- Avoid shearing force.

- Provide wound care.
- Skin grafts or myocutaneous flaps may be needed in late-stage ulcer.

Cognitive/Perceptual

- Establish a pressure relief schedule: 2 minutes of relief for every hour of sitting; in bed position should be changed every 2 hours.
- Assist person to identify cause of pressure ulcer, including actions or activities that contributed, if one has occurred; start prevention process to avoid repeated occurrence.
- Assist person to learn to watch for potential hazards (rough surfaces, sharp edges) and harmful routines (sitting too long in one position).

Psychosocial

- Assist person to identify how pressure ulcer may limit participation in day-to-day living and quality of life.

Context/Environment

- Provide instruction and training on examination of skin using adaptive equipment, such as a mirror, if needed to examine buttocks, heels, and elbows.
- Provide assistance and recommendations in selection of appropriate equipment such as seating systems, mattresses, bedding, cushions, or padded shower chairs.
- Instruct family and caregivers to watch for signs of developing problems.
- Recommend use of technology such as smartphone apps to act as reminders.
- If adapted devices such as hand splints or body jackets are used, additional inspection sites must be included in daily inspection routine.
- Assist in identification and use of equipment including cushions, mattress, wedges or heel boot, and household tools such as handheld mirror to inspect skin, or timer to remind client or caregiver to reposition or shift weight.

Precautions/Safety Considerations

Moisture increases risk of additional skin breakdown. Area around ulcer site should remain dry. Inadequate nutrition adds to length of time for healing process to occur. Monitor any out-of-bed mobility for risk of falls. Monitor in-bed mobility to reduce friction and shear forces, which can increase ulceration or damage new skin formation.

Prognosis and Outcome

Prognosis is excellent if ulcer is treated in an early stage. Late-stage ulcers are at risk of becoming infected and may be difficult to heal.

Cost

The cost in the United Kingdom of treating pressure ulcers has been estimated at £1.7 billion annually (Stinson et al., 2013).

REFERENCES

Blanche, E. I., Fogelberg, D., Diaz, J., Carlson, M., & Clark, F. (2011). Manualization of occupational therapy interventions: Illustrations from the pressure ulcer prevention research program. *American Journal of Occupational Therapy, 65*(6), 711–719. https://doi.org/10.5014/ajot.2011.001172

Carlson, M., Vigen, C. L. P., Rubayi, S., Blanche, E. I., Blanchard, J., Atkins, M., Bates-Jensen, B., Garber, S. L., Pyatak, E. A., Diaz, J., Florindez, L. I., Hay, J. W., Mallinson, T., Unger, J. B., Azen, S. P., Scott, M., Cogan, A., & Clark, F. (2019). Lifestyle intervention for adults with spinal cord injury: Results of the USC-RLANRC pressure ulcer prevention study. *Journal of Spinal Cord Medicine, 42*(1), 2–19. https://doi.org/10.1080/10790268.2017.1313931

Cobb, J. E., Bélanger, L. M., Park, S. E., Shen, T., Rivers, C. S., Dvorak, M. F., Street, J. T., & Noonan, V. K. (2014). Evaluation of a pilot Pressure Ulcer Prevention Initiative (PUPI) for patients with traumatic spinal cord injury. *Journal of Wound Care, 23*(5), 211–226. https://doi.org/10.12968/jowc.2014.23.5.211

Evers, S., Anderson, K., & Pagel, L. (2015). Occupational therapy's role in pressure. *OT Practice, 20*(2), 13–15.

Floríndez, L. I., Carlson, M. E., Pyatak, E., Blanchard, J., Cogan, A. M., Sleight, A. G., Hill, V., Diaz, J., Blanche, E., Garber, S. L., & Clark, F. (2020). A qualitative analysis of pressure injury development among medically underserved adults with spinal cord injury. *Disability and Rehabilitation, 42*(15), 2093–2099. https://doi.org/10.1080/09638288.2018.1552328

Fogelberg, D. J., Powell, J. M., & Clark, F. A. (2016). The role of habit in recurrent pressure ulcers following spinal cord injury. *Scandinavian Journal of Occupational Therapy, 23*(6), 467–476. https://doi.org/ 10.3109/11038128.2015.1130170

Ghaisas, S., Pyatak, E. A., Blanche, E., Blanchard, J., Clark, F., & PUPS II Study Group. (2015). Lifestyle changes and pressure ulcer prevention in adults with spinal cord injury in the pressure ulcer prevention study lifestyle intervention. *American Journal of Occupational Therapy, 69*(1), Article 6901290020. https://doi.org/10.5014/ajot.2015.012021

Hilgart, M., Ritterband, L., Baxter, K., Alfano, A., Ratliff, C., Kinzie, M., Cohn, W., Whaley, D., Lord, H., & Garber, S. (2014). Development and perceived utility and impact of a skin care internet intervention. *Internet Interventions, 1*(3), 149–157. https://doi.org/10.1016/j.invent.2014.07.003

Jaul, E., Factor, H., Karni, S., Schiffmiller, T., & Meiron, O. (2019). Spasticity and dementia increase the risk of pressure ulcers. *International Wound Journal, 16*(3), 847–851. https://doi.org/10.1111/iwj.13110

Krishnan, S., Brick, R. S., Karg, P. E., Tzen, Y.-T., Garber, S. L., Sowa, G. A., & Brienza, D. M. (2016). Predictive validity of the Spinal Cord Injury Pressure Ulcer Scale (SCIPUS) in acute care and inpatient rehabilitation in individuals with traumatic spinal cord injury. *Neuro-Rehabilitation, 38*(4), 401–409. https://doi.org/10.3233/NRE-161331

Lala, D., Spaulding, S. J., Burke, S. M., & Houghton, P. E. (2016). Electrical stimulation therapy for the treatment of pressure ulcers in individuals with spinal cord injury: A systematic review and meta-analysis. *International Wound Journal, 13*(5), 1214–1226. https://doi.org/10.1111/iwj.12446

Macens, K., Rose, A., & Mackenzie, L. (2011). Pressure care practice and occupational therapy: Findings of an exploratory study. *Australian Occupational Therapy Journal, 58*(5), 346–354. https://doi.org/ 10.1111/j.1440-1630.2011.00962.x

Martin, D., Albensi, L., Van Haute, S., Froese, M., Montgomery, M., Lam, M., Gierys, K., Lajeunesse, R., Guse, L., & Basova, N. (2017). Healthy skin wins: A glowing pressure ulcer prevention program that can guide evidence-based practice. *Worldviews on Evidence-Based Nursing, 14*(6), 473–483. https://doi.org/10.1111/wvn.12242

Mathew, A., Samuelkamaleshkumar, S., Radhika, S., & Elango, A. (2013). Engagement in occupational activities and pressure ulcer development in rehabilitated South Indian persons with spinal cord injury. *Spinal Cord, 51*, 150–155. https://doi.org/10.1038/sc.2012.112

McCarthy, S. (2011). Low pressure zone. *Rehab Management, 24*(9), 10, 12–14.

Mendes, P. V. B., Paulisso, D. C., Caro, C. C., & Cruz, D. M. C. (2016). Comparison of wheelchair cushion calibration by users with spinal cord injury and by occupational therapists, using a pressure mapping system. *European International Journal of Science and Technology, 5*(6), 77–85.

Park, M. O., & Lee, S. H. (2019). Effects of seating education and cushion management for adaptive sitting posture in spinal cord injury: Two case reports. *Medicine, 98*(4), Article e14231. https://doi.org/10.1097/MD.0000000000014231

Porter, R. S. (Ed.). (2018). *The Merck manual of diagnosis and therapy* (20th ed.). Merck Sharp & Dohme.

Robertson, J., & Stern, M. (2012). *Pressure ulcer prevention and treatment: Clinical practice guideline*. Winnipeg Regional Health Authority.

Scovil, C. Y., Delparte, J. J., Walia, S., Flett, H. M., Guy, S. D., Wallace, M., Burns, A. S., & Wolfe, D. L. (2019). Implementation of pressure injury prevention best practices across 6 Canadian rehabilitation sites: Results from the spinal cord injury knowledge mobilization network. *Archives of Physical Medicine and Rehabilitation, 100*(2), 327–335. https://doi.org/10.1016/j .apmr.2018.07.444

Sleight, A. G., Cogan, A. M., Hill, V. A., Pyatak, E. A., Díaz, J., Floríndez, L. I., Blanchard, J., Vigen, C., Garber, S. L., & Clark, F. A. (2019). Factors protecting against pressure injuries in medically underserved adults with spinal cord injury: A qualitative study. *Topics in Spinal Cord Injury Rehabilitation, 25*(1), 31–40. https://doi.org/10.1310/sci2501-31

Spencer, M., Bogosian, C., & Campbell, S. (2012). Overcoming pressure. *Rehab Management, 25*(9), 16, 18, 20–21.

Stephens, M., & Bartley, C. A. (2018). Understanding the association between pressure ulcers and sitting in adults what does it mean for me and my carers? Seating guidelines for people, carers and health & social care professionals. *Journal of Tissue Viability, 27*(1), 59–73. https:// doi.org/10.1016/j.jtv.2017.09.004

Stinson, M., Gillan, C., & Porter-Armstrong, A. (2013). A literature review of pressure ulcer prevention: Weight shift activity, cost of pressure care and role of the occupational therapists. *British Journal of Occupational Therapy, 76*(4), 169–178. https://doi.org/10.4276/0308022 13X13651610908371

Stuart, L. (2014). Relieve the pressure. *OT News, 22*(8), 38–39.

Vaishampayan, A., Clark, F., Carlson, P., & Blanche, E. I. (2011). Preventing pressure ulcers in people with spinal cord injury: Targeting risky life circumstances through a community-based intervention for people with spinal cord injury. *Advances in Skin and Wound Care, 24*(6), 275–284. https://doi.org/10.1097/01.ASW.0000398663.66530.46

BIBLIOGRAPHY

American Occupational Therapy Association. (2013). The role of occupational therapy in wound management. *American Journal of Occupational Therapy, 67*(Suppl. 6), S60–S68. https://doi.org/10.5014/ajot.2013.67S60

Brienza, D., Kelsey, S., Karg, P., Allegretti, A., Olson, M., Schmeler, M., Zanca, J., Geyer, M. J., Kusturiss, M., & Holm, M. (2010). A randomized clinical trial on preventing pressure ulcers with wheelchair seat cushions. *Journal of the American Geriatrics Society, 58*(12), 2308–2314. https://doi.org/10.1111/j.1532-5415.2010.03168.x

Brienza, D., Krishnan, S., Karg, P., Sowa, G., & Allegretti, A. L. (2018). Predictors of pressure ulcer incidence following traumatic spinal cord injury: A secondary analysis of a prospective longitudinal study. *Spinal Cord, 56*(1), 28–34. https://doi.org/10.1038/sc.2017.96

Cogan, A. M., Blanchard, J., Garber, S. L., Vigen, C. L. P., Carlson, M., & Clark, F. A. (2017). Systematic review of behavioral and educational interventions to prevent pressure ulcers in adults with spinal cord injury. *Clinical Rehabilitation, 31*(7), 871–880. https://doi .org/10.1177/0269215516660855

Folan, A., Downie, S., & Bond, A. (2015). Systematic review: Is prescription of pressure-relieving air cushions justified in acute and subacute settings? *Hong Kong Journal of Occupational Therapy, 26*(1), 25–32. https://doi.org/10.1016/j.hkjot.2015.12.002

Jackson, J., Carlson, M., Rubayi, S., Scott, M. D., Atkins, M. S., Blanche, E. I., Saunders-Newton, C., Mielke, S., Wolfe, M. K., & Clark, F. A. (2010). Qualitative study of principles pertaining to lifestyle and pressure ulcer risk in adults with spinal cord injury. *Disability and Rehabilitation, 32*(7), 567–578. https://doi.org/10.3109/09638280903183829

Lee, S.-H., Park, J.-S., Jung, B.-K., & Lee, S.-A. (2016). Effects of different seat cushions on interface pressure distribution: A pilot study. *Journal of Physical Therapy Science, 28*, 227–230.

Mortenson, W. B., Thompson, S. C., Wright, A. L., Boily, J., Waldorf, K., & Leznoff, S. (2018). A survey of Canadian occupational therapy practices to prevent pressure injuries among wheelchair users via weight shifting. *Journal of Wound, Ostomy and Continence Nursing, 45*(3), 213–220. https://doi.org/10.1097/WON.0000000000000428

Rae, K. E., Isbel, S., & Upton, D. (2018). Support surfaces for the treatment and prevention of pressure ulcers: A systematic literature review. *Journal of Wound Care, 27*(8), 467–474. https://doi.org/ 10.12968/jowc.2018.27.8.467

Rose, A., & Mackenzie, L. (2010). "Beyond the cushion": A study of occupational therapists' perceptions of their role and clinical decisions in pressure care. *Disability and Rehabilitation, 32*(13), 1099–1108. https://doi.org/10.3109/09638280903410748

Taule, T., Bergfjord, K., Holsvik, E. E., Lunde, T., Stokke, B. H., Storlid, H., Sørheim, M. V., & Rekand, T. (2013). Factors influencing optimal seating pressure after spinal cord injury. *Spinal Cord, 51*(4), 273–277. https://doi.org/10.1038/sc.2012.163

Trewartha, M., & Stiller, K. (2011). Comparison of the pressure redistribution qualities of two air-filled wheelchair cushions for people with spinal cord injuries. *Australian Occupational Therapy Journal, 58*(4), 287–292. https://doi.org/10.1111/j.1440-1630.2011.00932.x

Webb, J., Twiste, M., Walton, L. A., & Hogg, P. (2018). The impact of hoist sling fabrics on interface pressure whilst sitting in healthy volunteers and wheelchair users: A comparative study. *Journal of Tissue Viability, 27*(2), 90–94. https://doi.org/10.1016/j.jtv.2017.12.001

Worsley, P. R., Clarkson, P., Bader, D. L., & Schoonhoven, L. (2017). Identifying barriers and facilitators to participation in pressure ulcer prevention in allied healthcare professionals: A mixed methods evaluation. *Physiotherapy, 103*(3), 304–310. https://doi.org/10.1016/j .physio.2016.02.005

Wu, G. A., Garber, S. L., & Bogie, K. M. (2016). Utilization and user satisfaction with alternating pressure air cushions: A pilot study of at-risk individuals with spinal cord injury. *Disability and Rehabilitation Assistive Technology, 11*(7), 599–603. https://doi.org/10.3109/17483107 .2015.1027303

Cognitive-Perceptual Disorders

Alzheimer's Disease

Also called Alzheimer disease.

See also Cognitive Impairment, Dementia, Executive Dysfunction, Memory Impairment.

Description

Alzheimer's disease is a neurocognitive disorder and is the most common cause of dementia accounting for 60% to 80% of the dementias in the elderly. The disease is twice as common among women as among men. Alzheimer's disease causes progressive cognitive deterioration and is characterized by beta-amyloid deposits and neurofibrillary tangles in the cerebral cortex and subcortical gray matter (Porter, 2018). Progressive cognitive deterioration is manifested by loss of memory, decreased ability to calculate, problems with visual-spatial orientation, confusion, and disorientation (*Stedman's*, 2011).

Probable Alzheimer's disease might be considered if either of the following is present:

- Evidence of a causative Alzheimer's disease genetic mutation from family history or genetic testing.
- All of the following conditions are present:
  ▶ Clear evidence of decline in memory and learning and at least one other cognitive domain.
  ▶ Steadily progressive, gradual decline in cognition, without extended plateaus.
  ▶ No evidence of mixed etiology.

Possible Alzheimer's disease might be considered if there is no evidence of a causative Alzheimer's disease genetic mutation from either family history or genetic testing, but all three of the conditions are present (American Psychiatric Association, 2013).

Cause

Most cases are sporadic with late onset at or after 65 years of age. However, about 5% to 15% of cases are familial with about half of the familial cases having a presenile onset before age 65 (Porter, 2018).

Stages (Adapted from Arrighi et al., 2013; Glogoski & Schultz-Krohn, 2018)

- Stage I: Very Mild to Mild Cognitive Decline (mild problems with memory, less initiative, difficulty with word finding and attention/concentration, repetition may be needed, decline in job performance, conversation more superficial, minimal changes in social and physical ability).
- Stage II: Mild to Moderate Decline in Cognition (mood and behavior changes more noticeable, memory loss noticeable in current events, tendency to lose or misplace objects, difficulty learning new information, visuospatial deficits more apparent, moves more slowly, has more difficulty with instrumental activities of daily living and social interactions, unable to work, does not engage in favorite leisure activities, cannot live independently, difficulty paying bills, difficulty following medication schedule).
- Stage III: Moderate to Moderately Severe Decline in Cognition (behavior changes occur more frequently with antisocial behavior present, unaware of most current events although past history may be mostly intact, disoriented to place and time, slow response, unable to perform ADLs as well as IADLs, wandering behavior occurs).
- Stage IV: Severe Cognitive Decline and Moderate to Severe Physical Decline (memory impairment severe including lack of recognition of family members, gait and balance disturbances present, severe psychomotor retardation, unable to communicate with language other than single words or grunts, incontinence, difficulty eating or requires feeding tube, requires full-time care. Additional problems may include seizures, contractures, pressure ulcers, urinary tract infections, and pneumonia).

Evaluation/Assessment
Areas

- Activities of Daily Living/Instrumental ADL: self-maintenance skills, aphasia (expressive and receptive language), anomia (difficulty with word finding), circumlocution (talking around the intended word), finances, mobility, transfers, community activities
- Education/Work: work performance
- Play/Leisure: interests, frequency of engagement
- Rest/Sleep: sleep disturbances
- Social Participation: frequency, type, with whom
- Sensorimotor: balance, endurance, gait, joint mobility, body mechanics, muscle strength, posture, range of motion, sensory awareness
- Cognitive/Perceptual: arousal, attention (sustained, divided, shifting, concentrated, distractibility), memory (orientation to person, place, and date/time; topographical orientation, working memory; short-term or recent memory, long-term or remote memory, personal episodic memory, sematic memory), learning and retention of new materials/routines, executive functions (planning, decision making, responding to feedback/error correction, mental flexibility, judgment, insight, visual field, spatial relations)
- Psychosocial: anxiety, depression, sense of control, quality of life, antisocial behavior, psychosis
- Context/Environment: adapted devices, assistive/positioning equipment, mobility aids
- Comorbidities: depression, anxiety, suicide

Instruments

Instruments Developed by Occupational Therapy Personnel

- Allen Cognitive Level Screen (5th ed.; ACLS-5) and Large Allen Cognitive Level Screen (5th ed.; LACLS-5; Allen et al., 2007)
- Allen Diagnostic Module (2nd ed.; ADM-2; Earhart, 2006)
- Assessment of Motor and Process Skills (8th ed.; AMPS-8; Fisher & Bray Jones, 2016)
- Disability Assessment for Dementia (DAD; Gélinas et al., 1999)
- Dynamic Loewenstein Occupational Therapy Cognitive Assessment–Geriatric (DLOTCA-G; Katz et al., 2012)
- Everyday Technology Use Questionnaire (ETUQ; Rosenberg et al., 2009; see Nygård et al., 2012, in References)
- Management of Everyday Technology Assessment (META; Malinowsky et al., 2011)
- Occupational Therapy–Driver Off-Road Assessment Battery (OT-DORA Battery; Unsworth et al., 2012)
- Perceive, Recall, Plan, Perform (PRPP) System of Task Analysis (Chapparo & Ranka, 2006)
- Performance Assessment of Self-Care Skills (Version 4.1; PASS 4.1; Chisholm et al., 2016)
- Routine Task Inventory–Expanded (RTI-E; Katz, 2006)
- Safety Assessment of Function and the Environment for Rehabilitation–Health Outcome Measurement and Evaluation (3rd ed.; SAFER-HOME 3; Chiu & Oliver, 2006)
- Short Form-Everyday Technology Use Questionnaire (S-ETUQ; Kottorp & Nygård, 2011, in References)

Instruments Developed by Other Professionals and Used by Occupational Therapy Personnel

- Alzheimer's Disease Assessment Scale (ADAS; Mohs & Cohen, 1988)
- Alzheimer's Disease Cooperative Study/Activities of Daily Living (ADCS-ADL; Galasko et al., 1997)
- Barthel Index (BI; Mahoney & Barthel, 1965)
- Behavioural Assessment of the Dysexecutive Syndrome (BADS; Wilson et al., 1996)
- Berg Balance Scale (BBS; Berg et al., 1989)
- Borg Rating of Perceived Exertion Scale (BRPES; Borg, 1982)
- Clinical Dementia Rating (CDR; Morris, 1997)

- Cohen-Mansfield Agitation Inventory (CMAI; Cohen-Mansfield, 1986)
- Frenchay Activities Index (FAI) and Self-Report Frenchay Activities Index (SR-FAI; see Fujita et al., 2018, in References)
- Functional Assessment Staging (FAST) scale (FAST; Reisberg, 1988)
- Functional Independence Measure (FIM; Uniform Data System for Medical Rehabilitation, 1997)
- Functional Reach Test (FRT; Duncan et al., 1990)
- Geriatric Depression Scale (GDS; Yesavage et al., 1982)
- Instrumental Activities of Daily Living Scale (IADL; Lawton & Brody, 1969)
- Interview for Deterioration in Daily Living Activities in Dementia (IDDD; Teunisse & Derix, 1997)
- Joint range of motion (goniometry; Shurtleff & Kaskutas, 2018)
- Manual Muscle Test (MMT; Kaskutas, 2018)
- Mini-Mental State Examination (MMSE; Folstein et al., 1975)
- Neurobehavioral Cognitive Status Examination (NCSE, Cognistat; Kiernan et al., 1987)
- Perceived Quality of Life Scale (PQLS; Patrick et al., 1988)
- Problems in Everyday Living (PEDL; Leckey & Beatty, 2002)
- Quality of Life in Alzheimer's Disease (QOL-AD; Logsdon et al., 2007)
- Revised Cambridge Examination for Mental Disorders of the Elderly (CAMDEX-R; Roth et al., 1999)
- Short Physical Performance Battery (SPPB; Guralnik et al., 1994)
- Short Portable Sarcopenia Measure (SPSM; Miller et al., 2009)
- Timed Up and Go test (TUG; Podsiadlo & Richardson, 1991)
- Verbal Fluency Test (VFT; Benton et al., 1994)

Problems/Issues
Activities of Daily Living/Instrumental ADL
- Person will lose ability to perform self-maintenance activities as the disease progresses.
- Person may experience communication disorders such as aphasia, anomia, and circumlocution.
- Person may need mobility assistance including a wheelchair in later stage.

Education/Work
- Person may be terminated from employment because he or she is unable to perform work tasks.

Play/Leisure
- Person may reduce or stop engagement in favorite leisure activities.

Rest/Sleep
- Person may experience sleep disturbances.

Social Participation
- Person may reduce or stop participation in social activities because of symptoms and disregard following social rules of behavior.
- Person may experience increased social isolation because friends are unable or unwilling to deal with changes in person's cognition and behavior.

Sensorimotor
- Person usually experiences loss of strength.
- Person usually experiences loss of joint range of motion.
- Person usually experiences loss of endurance.
- Person usually loses postural control, which leads to being bedbound in later stage.
- Person may experience fatigue.
- Person may experience apraxia (difficulty with motor planning).

- Person may wander (walk away from location) if not monitored closely.
- Person may have sensory loss or sensitivities.
- Person may demonstrate agnosia (difficulty recognizing objects or persons).
- Person may have difficulty with constructional activities, such as finding the armholes and leg holes of garments.
- Person may be unable to judge distance and depth.
- Person may have difficulty differentiating foreground and background.

Cognitive/Perceptual

- Person usually has impaired attention skills, which increases in severity as the disease progresses.
- Person usually has impaired memory, which increases in severity as the disease progresses.
- Person usually has impaired executive function skills, which increases in severity.
- Person usually has perceptual dysfunction, which increases in severity.
- Person may be unable to concentrate and pay attention for more than seconds.
- Person may be become disoriented as to person, place (topographical orientation), time, and date.
- Person may have impaired personal episodic memory (time-related information about one's self and one's activities).
- Person may have impaired semantic memory (remembering the names of common objects and general knowledge).
- Person may have difficulty problem solving and making decisions.
- Person may have poor judgment of safety and ability to weigh consequences of actions.
- Person may have difficulty considering alternative solutions to a problem.
- In severe stage person may be unable to engage in purposeful, goal-directed occupation.

Psychosocial

- Person usually loses ability to perform roles such as spouse, parent, grandparent, friend, colleague.
- Person may become rigid in following a set routine and become upset if routine is varied.
- Person may have impaired self-awareness of disability.
- Person may become agitated or restless.
- Person may become depressed.
- Person may become aggressive, hostile, or violent.
- Person may express paranoid or delusional behavior.
- Person may be suspicious of others' behavior.
- Person may confabulate (make up stories that are not true).
- Person may experience sundown syndrome (behavior changes and mental status declines in the evening).

Context/Environment

- Person usually requires monitoring of activities by family and caregivers.
- Person's behavior, such as wandering, may require home modification.

Intervention/Treatment

Models and programs developed by occupational therapy personnel include the AOTA Practice Guidelines (Schaber, 2010), AOTA Guideline Summary (Piersol & Jensen, 2017), assistive technology (Collins, 2018; Lindqvist et al., 2013), case study (Piersol et al., 2018), computer-assisted errorless learning program (CELP; Lee et al., 2013), functional task-based exercise program (Law et al., 2013, 2014), home-based occupational therapy intervention (Ávila et al., 2018; Schmid et al., 2015), home modifications (Struckmeyer & Pickens, 2016), music to reduce agitation (Cox et al., 2011), and small-scale shared housing arrangements (Bortnick, 2017). Models and programs developed by other professionals but used by occupational therapy personnel include cognitive rehabilitation (Kim, 2015). Team members may include geriatricians, gerontologists, nursing personnel, psychologists, speech–language pathologists, dieticians, physical therapists, social workers, family members, paid or volunteer caregivers, and occupational therapy personnel. Goals include adapting the environment and focusing on what the person can do (functional capacity) to maximize engagement in occupation, supporting emotional regulation and behavior, adapting and modifying the environment, promoting safety, and enhancing, quality of life (American Occupational Therapy Association, 2011; Bernardo, 2018; Bernardo & Raymundo, 2018; Wiemer & Slowman, 2016).

Activities of Daily Living/Instrumental ADL
- Have client complete functional skills during time of day client is least symptomatic.
- Dressing may be facilitated by laying items out in the order they are to be put on (use of procedural memory, which tends to remain intact until severe stage).
- Pictures or photography may be useful to provide instructions in order they are to be performed.
- Use of step-by-step instructions for simple tasks (such as using the microwave or getting dressed) can be helpful in early stages when physical skills are still relatively intact.
- Verbal instructions may need to be repeated several times.
- Move from verbal to gestures to physical assistance as disorder progresses.
- Supervise person or have person act as a helper in the kitchen when preparing meals.
- Encourage participation in familiar household activities.
- Consider use of critical incident approach for independent living tasks such as grocery shopping (Brorsson et al., 2013).
- Performance of IADL tasks involves consideration of both cognitive and physical functions (Fujita et al., 2018; Unsworth & Chan, 2016).

Education/Work
- Assist person in changing status from worker to retiree.

Play/Leisure
- Maintain interests through sharing of photos or scrapbooks.
- Assist person to engage in favorite leisure activities, providing adaptations as needed.

Rest/Sleep
- Review sleep routine and provide recommendations as needed (see Sleep–Wake Disorders in Section 13: Lifestyle Conditions).

Social Participation
- Engage person to participate in social activities.
- Make recommendations for adaptations or modifications to facilitate participation such as shorter visits, going to familiar places, fewer people.

Sensorimotor
- Assist in providing exercise programs (with physical therapist, if needed) to maintain range of motion to maintain mobility and prevent contractures.
- Assist in providing resistive exercises to maintain muscle strength for as long as possible.
- Assist in providing an activity program to promote endurance.

Cognitive/Perceptual
- Use large, clearly written letters, words, and signs when giving directions.
- When working with the client, always introduce self at the beginning of each session and wear a name tag.
- Limit choices to two items when possible.
- Reduce distractions and keep only necessary items in view (visual field).
- Use client's previous interests when possible in current activities.
- When routine must be changed, provide explanation and warning.

Psychosocial

- Assist in providing reality orientation and reminiscence tasks.
- Provide reassurance as client is performing tasks.
- Assist in planning and implementing a predictable routine.
- Familiar music and songs may be useful to maintain calm behavior and avoid disruptive behavior (anger, aggression, hostility, irritability).

Context/Environment

- Assistive devices may be useful to the client in early stage of the disease (but not in later stages) to compensate for decreased cognitive abilities.
- Assist family and caregivers to identify assistive devices and equipment that will make caregiving tasks easier and safer.
- Assist family and caregivers to promote safety by removing access to dangerous items such as sharps, flammable liquids, stove knobs, and other items that may be hazardous.
- Assist family and caregivers to modify living environment to prevent falls such as installing grab bars, removing throw rugs, reducing clutter, clearing pathways, providing adequate light in bathroom and hallways, installing adjustable shower head, providing a shower bench or chair.
- Assist family and caregivers to reduce wandering behavior such as putting "Stop" signs on doors leading to the outside, installing deadbolt locks on doors and windows, installing motion sensors and nightlights, having person wear a global positioning system (GPS) locator or carry a smartphone (Note: devices may reduce ability to wander, but do not reduce urge to wander).
- Provide information to the family and caregivers about the progression of the disorder.

Precautions/Safety Considerations

Person is at risk for falls (Stark et al., 2013). Person is at risk for wandering away without telling anyone. Person is at risk for pressure sores due to immobility.

Prognosis and Outcome

There is no known cure. Cognitive decline is inevitable, although rate of progression varies. Average survival rate from time of diagnosis is 4–8 years. Average survival rate from time person can no longer walk is about 6 months (Porter, 2018). Death is usually the result of an infection such as pneumonia, or body system failure such as heart failure.

Cost Effectiveness

Callahan et al. (2017) did not find benefit for a home-based occupational therapy program; a 2-year study did not show the program slowed the progress of the disease. Voigt-Radloff et al. (2011) found that 10 home visits were not better than one in changing the performance of clients. Corvol et al. (2018) suggested that measuring cost-effective intervention in working with clients with Alzheimer's disease deviates from the evidence-based model focused on functional improvement.

REFERENCES

American Occupational Therapy Association. (2011). *Tips for living life to its fullest: Living with Alzheimer's disease.*

American Psychiatric Association. (2013). *Diagnostic and statistical manual of mental disorders* (5th ed.). https://doi.org/10.1176/appi.books.9780890425596

Arrighi, H. M., Gélinas, I., McLaughlin, T. P., Buchanan, J., & Gauthier, S. (2013). Longitudinal changes in functional disability in Alzheimer's disease patients. *International Psychogeriatrics,* 25(6), 929–937. https://doi.org/10.1017/S1041610212002360

Ávila, A., De-Rosende-Celeiro, I., Torres, G., Vizcaíno, M., Peralbo, M., & Durán, M. (2018). Promoting functional independence in people with Alzheimer's disease: Outcomes of a home-based occupational therapy intervention in Spain. *Health and Social Care in the Community, 26*(5), 734–743.

Bernardo, L. D. (2018). Older adults with Alzheimer's disease: A systematic review about the occupational therapy intervention in changes of performance skills. *Cadernos Brasileiros Terapia Ocupacional São Carlos, 26*(4), 926–942. https://doi.org/10.4322/2526-8910.ctoAR1066

Bernardo, L. D., & Raymundo, T. M. (2018). Physical and social environment in the occupational therapeutic intervention process for elderly with Alzheimer's disease and their caregivers: A systematic review of the literature. *Cadernos Brasileiros Terapia Ocupacional São Carlos, 26*(2), 460–477. https://doi.org/10.4322/2526-8910.ctoAO1064

Bortnick, K. N. (2017). An ecological framework to support small-scale shared housing for persons with neurocognitive disorders of the Alzheimer's and related types: A literature review. *Hong Kong Journal of Occupational Therapy, 29*(1), 26–38. https://doi.org/10.1016/j.hkjot.2017.03.001

Brorsson, A., Öhman, A., Cutchin, M., & Nygård, L. (2013). Managing critical incidents in grocery shopping by community-living people with Alzheimer's disease. *Scandinavian Journal of Occupational Therapy, 20*(4), 292–301. https://doi.org/10.3109/11038128.2012.752031

Callahan, C. M., Boustani, M. A., Schmid, A. A., LaMantia, M. A., Austrom, M. G., Miller, D. K., Gao, S., Ferguson, D. Y., Lane, K. A., & Hendrie, H. C. (2017). Targeting functional decline in Alzheimer disease: A randomized trial. *Annals of Internal Medicine, 166*(3), 164–171. https://doi.org/10.7326/M16-0830

Collins, M. E. (2018). Occupational therapists' experience with assistive technology in provision of service to clients with Alzheimer's disease and related dementias. *Physical & Occupational Therapy in Geriatrics, 36*(2-3), 179–188. https://doi.org/10.1080/02703181.2018.1458770

Corvol, A., Netter, A., Campeon, A., & Somme, D. (2018). Implementation of an occupational therapy program for Alzheimer's disease patients in France: Patients' and caregivers' perspectives. *Journal of Alzheimer's Disease, 62*(1), 157–164. https://doi.org/10.3233/JAD-170765

Cox, E., Nowak, M., & Buettner, P. (2011). Managing agitated behavior in people with Alzheimer's disease: The role of live music. *British Journal of Occupational Therapy, 74*(11), 517–524. https://doi.org/10.4276/030802211X13204135680866

Fujita, T., Notoya, M., Sunahara, N., Nakatani, K., & Kimura, D. (2018). Risk factors for impaired instrumental activities of daily living in Alzheimer's disease. *Asian Journal of Occupational Therapy, 14*(1), 9–16. https://doi.org/10.11596/asiajot.14.9

Glogoski, C., & Schultz-Krohn, S. (2018). Alzheimer's disease. In H. M. Pendleton & W. Schultz-Krohn (Eds.), *Pedretti's occupational therapy* (8th ed., pp. 878–885). Elsevier.

Kim, S. (2015). Cognitive rehabilitation for elderly people with early-stage Alzheimer's disease. *Journal of Physical Therapy Science, 27*(2), 543–546. https://doi.org/10.1589/jpts.27.543

Kottorp, A., & Nygård, L. (2011). Development of a short-form assessment for detection of subtle activity limitations: Can use of everyday technology distinguish between MCI and Alzheimer's disease? *Expert Review of Neurotherapeutics, 11*(5), 647–655. https://doi.org/10.1586/ern.11.55

Law, L. L. F., Barnett, F., Yau, M. K., & Gray, M. A. (2013). Development and initial testing of functional task exercise on older adults with cognitive impairment at risk of Alzheimer's disease—FcTSim programme—A feasibility study. *Occupational Therapy International 20*(4), 185–197. https://doi.org/10.1002/oti.1355

Law, L. L. F., Barnett, F., Yau, M. K., & Gray, M. A. (2014). Effects of functional tasks exercise on older adults with cognitive impairment at risk of Alzheimer's disease: A randomised controlled trial. *Age and Ageing, 43*(6), 813–820. https://doi.org/10.1093/ageing/afu055

Lee, G. Y., Yip, C. C. K., Yu, E. C. S., & Man, D. W. K. (2013). Evaluation of a computer-assisted errorless learning-based memory training program for patients with early Alzheimer's disease in Hong Kong: A pilot study. *Clinical Interventions in Aging, 8,* 623–633. https://doi .org/10.2147/CIA.S45726

Lindqvist, E., Nygård, L., & Borell, L. (2013). Significant junctures on the way towards becoming a user of assistive technology in Alzheimer's disease. *Scandinavian Journal of Occupational Therapy, 20*(5), 386–396. https://doi.org/10.3109/11038128.2013.766761

Nygård, L., Pantzar, M., Uppgard, B., & Kottorp, A. (2012). Detection of activity limitations in older adults with MCI or Alzheimer's disease through evaluation of perceived difficulty in use of everyday technology: A replication study. *Aging & Mental Health, 16*(3), 361–371. https://doi.org/10.1080/13607863.2011.605055

Piersol, C. V., & Jensen, L. (2017). *Guideline summary: Occupational therapy practice guidelines for adults with Alzheimer's disease and related major neurocognitive disorders.* AOTA Press. https:// doi.org/10.7139/2017.978-1-56900-408-1

Piersol, C. V., Jensen, L., Lieberman, D., & Arbesman, M. (2018). Evidence connection—Occupational therapy interventions for people with Alzheimer's disease. *American Journal of Occupational Therapy, 72*(1), Article 7201390010. https://doi.org/10.5014/ajot.2018.721001

Porter, R. S. (Ed.). (2018). *The Merck manual of diagnosis and therapy* (20th ed.). Merck Sharp & Dohme.

Schaber, P. (2010). *Occupational therapy practice guidelines for adults with Alzheimer's disease and related disorders.* AOTA Press.

Schmid, A. A., Spangler-Morris, C., Beauchamp, R. C., Wellington, M. C., Hayden, W. M., Porterfield, H. S., Ferguson, D., & Callahan, C. M. (2015). The home-based occupational therapy intervention in the Alzheimer's disease multiple intervention trial (ADMIT). *Occupational Therapy in Mental Health, 31*(1), 19–34. https://doi.org/10.1080/0164212X.2014.1002963

Stark, S. L., Roe, C. M., Grant, E. A., Hollingsworth, H., Benzinger, T. L., Fagan, A. M., Buckles, V. D., & Morris, J. C. (2013). Preclinical Alzheimer disease and risk of falls. *Neurology, 81*(5), 437–443. https://doi.org/10.1212/WNL.0b013e31829d8599

Stedman's medical dictionary for the health professions and nursing (7th ed.). (2011). Wolters Kluwer.

Struckmeyer, L. R., & Pickens, N. D. (2016). Home modifications for people with Alzheimer's disease: A scoping review. *American Journal of Occupational Therapy, 70*(1), Article 7001270020. https://doi.org/10.5014/ajot.2015.016089

Unsworth, C., & Chan, S.-P. (2016). Determining fitness to drive among drivers with Alzheimer's disease or cognitive decline. *British Journal of Occupational Therapy, 79*(2), 102–110. https:// doi.org/10.1177/0308022615604645

Voigt-Radloff, S., Graff, M., Leonhart, R., Schornstein, K., Jessen, F., Bohlken, J., Metz, B., Fellgiebel, A., Dodel, R., Eschweiler, G., Vernooij-Dassen, M., Rikkert, M. O., & Hüll, M. (2011). A multicentre RCT on community occupational therapy in Alzheimer's disease: 10 sessions are not better than one consultation. *BMJ Open, 1*(1), Article e000096. https://doi.org/10.1136/ bmjopen-2011-000096

Wiemer, H., & Slowman, L. S. (2016). *Clinical review: Alzheimer's disease: Occupational therapy.* CINAHL Information Systems.

BIBLIOGRAPHY

Bernard, B. L., Bracey, L. E., Lane, K. A., Ferguson, D. Y., LaMantia, M. A., Gao, S., Miller, D. K., & Callahan, C. M. (2016). Correlation between caregiver reports of physical function and performance-based measures in a cohort of older adults with Alzheimer Disease. *Alzheimer Disease and Associated Disorders, 30*(2), 169–174. https://doi.org/10.1097/WAD.0000000000 000101

Fraker, J., & Yatczak, J. (2017). Neurocognitive disorders. In B. J. Atchison & D. P. Dirette (Eds.), *Conditions in occupational therapy* (5th ed., pp. 165–192). Wolters Kluwer.

Jensen, L., & Padilla, R. (2017). Effectiveness of environment-based interventions that address behavior, perception, and falls in people with Alzheimer's disease and related major neurocognitive disorders: A systematic review. *American Journal of Occupational Therapy, 71*(5), Article 7105180030. https://doi.org/10.5014/ajot.2017.027409

Jensen, L. E., & Padilla, R. (2011). Effectiveness of interventions to prevent falls in people with Alzheimer's disease and related dementias. *American Journal of Occupational Therapy, 65*(5), 532–540. https://doi.org/10.5014/ajot.2011.002626

Letts, L., Edwards, M., Berenyi, J., Moros, K., O'Neill, C., O'Toole, C., & McGrath, C. (2011). Using occupations to improve quality of life, health and wellness, and client and caregiver satisfaction for people with Alzheimer's disease and related dementias. *American Journal of Occupational Therapy, 65*(5), 497–504. https://doi.org/10.5014/ajot.2011.002584

Letts, L., Minezes, J., Edwards, M., Berenyi, J., Moros, K., O'Neill, C., & O'Toole, C. (2011). Effectiveness of interventions designed to modify and maintain perceptual abilities in people with Alzheimer's disease and related dementias. *American Journal of Occupational Therapy, 65*(5), 505–513. https://doi.org/10.5014/ajot.2011.002592

Padilla, R. (2011a). Effectiveness of environment-based interventions for people with Alzheimer's disease and related dementias. *American Journal of Occupational Therapy, 65*(5), 514–522. https://doi.org/10.5014/ajot.2011.002600

Padilla, R. (2011b). Effectiveness of interventions designed to modify the activity demands of the occupations of self-care and leisure for people with Alzheimer's disease and related dementias. *American Journal of Occupational Therapy, 65*(5), 523–531. https://doi.org/10.5014/ajot.2011.002618

Piersol, C. V., Canton, K., Connor, S. E., Giller, I., Lipman, S., & Sager, S. (2017). Effectiveness of interventions for caregivers of people with Alzheimer's disease and related major neurocognitive disorders: A systematic review. *American Journal of Occupational Therapy, 71*(5), Article 7095189920. https://doi.org/10.5014/ajot.2017.027581

Rao, A. K., Chou, A., Bursley, B., Smulofsky, J., & Jezequel, J. (2014). Systematic review of the effects of exercise on activities of daily living in people with Alzheimer's disease. *American Journal of Occupational Therapy, 68*(1), 50–56. https://doi.org/10.5014/ajot.2014.009035

Robert, A., Gélinas, I., & Mazer, B. (2010). Occupational therapists use of cognitive interventions for clients with Alzheimer's disease. *Occupational Therapy International, 17*(1), 10–19. https://doi.org/10.1002/oti.283

Rosenberg, L., & Nygård, L. (2014). Learning and using technology in intertwined processes: A study of people with mild cognitive impairment or Alzheimer's disease. *Dementia, 13*(5), 662–677. https://doi.org/10.1177/1471301213481224

Ryd, C., Nygård, L., Malinowsky, C., Öhman, A., & Kottorp, A. (2015). Associations between performance of activities of daily living and everyday technology use among older adults with mild stage Alzheimer's disease or mild cognitive impairment. *Scandinavian Journal of Occupational Therapy, 22*(1), 33–42. https://doi.org/10.3109/11038128.2014.964307

Schaber, P., Blair, K., Jost, E., Schaffer, M., & Thurner, E. (2016). Understanding family interaction patterns in families with Alzheimer's disease. *OTJR: Occupation, Participation and Health, 36*(1), 25–33. https://doi.org/10.1177/1539449215610566

Smallfield, S., & Heckenlaible, C. (2017). Effectiveness of occupational therapy interventions to enhance occupational performance for adults with Alzheimer's disease and related major neurocognitive disorders: A systematic review. *American Journal of Occupational Therapy, 71*(5), Article 7105189910. https://doi.org/10.5014/ajot.2017.024752

Vermeersch, S., Gorus, E., Cornelis, E., & De Vriendt, P. (2015). An explorative study of the relationship between functional and cognitive decline in older persons with mild cognitive impairment and Alzheimer's disease. *British Journal of Occupational Therapy, 78*(3), 166–174. https://doi.org/10.1177/0308022614565114

Apraxia

*See also Cognitive-Perceptual Disorders; Dyspraxia and Developmental Dyspraxia,
a condition associated with sensory processing disorders in children;
Executive Dysfunction; Memory Impairment.*

Description

Praxis is the ability to organize and skillfully execute purposeful movements (Giles, 2014).
Apraxia is the inability to execute purposeful, previously learned motor tasks, despite physical ability and willingness or impaired ability to do previously learned motor activities despite intact motor function (Porter, 2018). Apraxia is a cognitive impairment in the ability
to perform purposeful acts or to manipulate objects without any loss of muscle strength, abnormal tone, hand coordination, sensory loss, incomprehension, inattention, or noncoopera-
tion (Giles, 2014; O'Toole, 2017). Diagnosis is based on exclusion as opposed to inclusion
of symptoms. Two major types of apraxia are recognized in adults: ideational and ideomotor.
Ideational apraxia occurs when the cognitive conceptual process is lost and the individual is
unable to formulate a plan of movement or does not know the proper use of an object due of
lack of perception of its purpose (O'Toole, 2017). *Ideomotor apraxia* is the inability to translate
an idea into motion, resulting from some interference with the transmission of the appropriate impulses from the brain to the motor centers. There is no loss of the ability to perform the
action automatically, but the action cannot be performed upon request or verbal command
(e.g., person can tie shoelaces automatically as part of putting on socks and shoes but cannot
tie the shoelaces if asked to demonstrate the task by a therapist, although the person can name
and describe the action steps). Ideational apraxia is also called conceptual, dissociation, or
conduction apraxia. Ideomotor apraxia is also called ideokinetic apraxia, limb kinetic apraxia,
or transcortical apraxia. A third type of apraxia is called *oral apraxia*, which is related to difficulty initiating chewing and swallowing (Giles, 2014). Arntzen and Elstad (2013) identified
five types of altered bodily intentionality in persons with apraxia, including a gap between
intention and bodily action, fragmented awareness of action or intention, peculiar action and
odd body parts (person unable to identify action or why body part was needed), intentionality
on the loose (action appeared unconnected to intended target), and fighting against tools (difficulty using tools for intended or designed purpose). Poole et al. (2011) reported that poorer
ipsilesional motor performance was associated with longer completion time in clients with
right hemisphere damage, and poorer contralesional motor performance and greater aphasia
were associated with less independence in clients with left hemisphere damage.

Cause

Brain damage such as by infarct, tumor, trauma, or degeneration, usually in the parietal lobes
or their connections, which retain memories of learned movement patterns. Less common
cause is damage to the premotor cortex or other parts of the frontal lobe, corpus callosum, or
diffuse damage related to degenerative dementias (Porter, 2018). Impaired anticipatory control
for familiar objects may be due to damage to the inferior parietal and superior and middle
temporal lobes (Dawson et al., 2010). Ideomotor apraxia (IMA) is a common disorder after
a left hemisphere stroke. Apraxia has been reported and observed as a symptom in diseases
and disorders such as stroke, parkinsonism, dementia including Alzheimer's disease, multiple
sclerosis, posterior cortical atrophy, and corticobasal degeneration syndrome (Porter, 2018).

Evaluation/Assessment

Areas

- Activities of Daily Living/Instrumental ADL: basic ADLs (bathing, dressing, grooming, toileting, brushing teeth); IADLs (meal planning, paying bills, doing laundry, driving a car,
  checking a bus schedule)

- Education/Work: work skills involving thinking conceptually (ideational) or motor performance (ideomotor)
- Play/Leisure: leisure occupations involving thinking conceptually (ideational) or motor performance (ideomotor)
- Rest/Sleep: may not be able to describe sleep routine (ideational) or demonstrate (ideomotor)
- Social Participation: social activities involving thinking conceptually or motor performance
- Sensorimotor: tasks involving motor planning and executive functioning, motor performance on command, gesture imitation, pantomiming, object use
- Cognitive/Perceptual: awareness, memory, executive functions: goal selection, initiate and execute a planned action, anticipate results, problem solving, self-awareness of deficits
- Psychosocial: anxiety, role performance
- Context/Environment: habits, rituals, or routines associated with cultural activities
- Comorbidities: stroke, parkinsonism, dementia, multiple sclerosis, posterior cortical atrophy, and corticobasal degeneration syndrome

Instruments

(Note: No single test captures all types of apraxia possibility because apraxia is a heterogeneous group of disorders; Giles, 2014.)

Instruments Developed by Occupational Therapy Personnel

- Canadian Occupational Performance Measure (5th ed.; COPM-5; Law et al., 2014)
- Nottingham Stroke Dressing Assessment (NSDA; Fletcher-Smith et al., 2010, in References; see also Walker et al., 2012, in References)

Instruments Developed by Other Professionals and Used by Occupational Therapy Personnel

- Apraxia Screen of TULIA (AST; Vanbellingen & Bohlhalter, 2009)
- Arm Motor Ability Test (AMAT; Kopp et al., 1997)
- Assessment of Apraxia (AoA; Heugten & Kinebanian (1999)
- Assessment of Disabilities in Stroke Patients with Apraxia (ADSPA; see Assessment of Apraxia)
- Florida Apraxia Battery–Extended and Revised Sydney (FABERS; Power et al., 2010)
- Florida Apraxia Screening Test–Revised (FAST-R; Rothi et al., 1991)
- Fugl-Meyer Assessment (FMA; Fugl-Meyer et al., 1975)
- Functional Independence Measure (FIM; Uniform Data System for Medical Rehabilitation, 1997)
- Gesture Imitation (GI; Kimura & Archibald, 1974)
- Screening for Apraxia (SFA; Almeida et al., 2002)
- Test for Upper Limb Apraxia (TULIA; Vanbellingen et al., 2010)

Problems/Issues

Activities of Daily Living/Instrumental ADL

- Person may have difficulty in organizing and selecting eating utensils.
- Person may have difficulty moving food to mouth.
- Person may have difficulty initiating chewing or moving food to back of mouth to initiate swallowing (oral apraxia; Note: difficulty not related to loss of motor actions).
- Person may have difficulty selecting correct garment if asked to identify which type of coat to wear if the weather forecast is for rain.
- Person may have difficulty with meal preparation (planning, initiation, carrying out).
- Person may have difficulty driving a vehicle (putting foot on correct pedal, initiating a turn) leading to unsafe driving.

Education/Work

- Person (as a result of apraxia) may have difficulty completing work tasks due to failure to initiate a task, failure to complete a task, using wrong tools, using tool inappropriately, omitting required steps, using body part when a tool is usually required, repeating steps already completed, not able to self-monitor actions to correct errors and account for safety (Note: problems are not due to lack of motor ability or cognitive knowledge and learning).

Play/Leisure

- Person (as a result of apraxia) may have difficulty engaging in leisure occupations successfully due to failure to initiate a task, failure to complete a task, using wrong tools or objects, using tool or object inappropriately, omitting required steps, using body part instead of recommended tool or object, repeating steps already completed, not able to self-monitor actions to correct errors and account for safety (Note: problems might be due to lack of motor ability or cognitive knowledge and learning).

Rest/Sleep

- Person (as a result of apraxia) may experience disturbances in sleep habits and routines.

Social Participation

- Person (as a result of apraxia) may have difficulty engaging in social activities successfully due to failure to initiate a task, failure to complete a task, using wrong tools or objects, using tool or object inappropriately, omitting required steps, using body part instead of recommended tool or object, repeating steps already completed, not able to self-monitor actions to correct errors and account for safety (Note: problems might be due to lack of motor ability or cognitive knowledge and learning).
- Person (unintentionally) violates expected social norms.

Sensorimotor

- Note: Person should be evaluated to determine whether there is identifiable motor or sensory losses or impairments.
- Note: Person should be evaluated to determine whether there is identifiable loss of motor skill or evidence of never having achieved basic mastery of the motor skill.

Cognitive/Perceptual

- Note: Person should be evaluated to determine whether there is lack of knowledge about a task and that the person has previously learned how to perform the task or tasks being presented.
- Person may use object incorrectly such as shaving beard with toothbrush (incorrect tool use).
- Person may use extended index finger to brush teeth, to spread butter on toast, or stir coffee (called body part as object or tool omission).
- Person may target wrong part of body with a tool, such as using shaver designed to shave beard but instead places shaver on hair (wrong target).
- Person may use wrong hand function, such as attempting to pick up and hold a comb using a full hand grasp instead of pincer grasp (wrong hand grasp).
- Person attempts to pick up object by wrong part, such as attempting to pick up coffee pot by the lid instead of the handle (wrong orientation).
- Person may substitute one object for another, such as putting jar of instant coffee on burner instead of the coffee pot (substitution).
- Person may be unable to initiate symbolic or expressive gestures, such as waving good-bye, making the OK sign, stop/cut the action, make hitchhiking sign, or initiate any other gesture upon command (Note: motor ability is intact).
- Person may be unable to pantomime how to use scissors to cut paper, use a hammer to hammer a nail, use a comb to comb hair, use a salt shaker to salt food, use a spoon to stir coffee (Note: motor ability is intact).
- Person may be unable to imitate directional gestures made by therapist such as touching the top of head or wiping (dust) off the shoulder (motor ability is intact).
- Person may be unable to initiate an action such as stirring a powdered drink into a cup of hot water.

- Person may be unaware that any type of error has been made, whether the error is classified as omission, substitution, addition, perseveration, inappropriate, unsafe, inexact, too many, too few, wrong answer, or other error classification.

Psychosocial

- Person (as a result of apraxia) may have difficulty performing expected role behaviors successfully due to failure to initiate a task, failure to complete a task, using wrong tools or objects, using tool or object inappropriately, omitting required steps, using body part instead of recommended tool or object, repeating steps already completed, not able to self-monitor actions to correct errors and account for safety (Note: Problems might be due to lack of motor ability or cognitive knowledge and learning).
- Person may express anxiety or frustration.

Context/Environment

- Family members and caregivers may become frustrated with person due to lack of understanding of the apraxia disorder.
- Family members and caregivers may lack knowledge of how to manage person with apraxia.
- Community and internet resources may be lacking or unavailable to assist person and family.

Intervention/Treatment

Models and programs developed by occupational therapy personnel include strategy training (Lindsten-McQueen et al., 2014). Models and programs developed by other professionals but used by occupational therapy personnel include combined physical and mental practice (Wu et al., 2011) and summary of interventions (Tempest, 2017). Team members include physicians, psychologists, and occupational therapy personnel. Goal is to enable person to participate in all desired life tasks.

Activities of Daily Living/Instrumental ADL

- Picture sequences, video recordings, or audio instructions may provide assistance to perform problem tasks (eating, shaving, dressing, combing hair) correctly or to initiate sequence of action steps.
- Ask the person to conceptualize (rehearse) the selected goal, how to initiate and execute required movements, and anticipate results before starting the task.
- Standby assistance may be required to compensate when client is unable to initiate, continue, or terminate actions.
- Strategy training: Focus on teaching client intrinsic strategies (mental practice approaches) or providing extrinsic strategies such as providing instruction, physical assistance, and feedback.

Education/Work

- Not discussed. See concepts under ADL/IADH.

Play/Leisure

- Not discussed. See concepts under ADL/IADL.

Rest/Sleep

- Not discussed. See concepts under ADL/IADL. See also Sleep–Wake Disorders in Section 13: Lifestyle Conditions.

Social Participation

- Not discussed. See concepts under ADL/IADL.

Sensorimotor

- Gentle hand-over-hand tactile cues may promote initiation of tasks and allow client's motor memory to be activated sufficiently to perform the task correctly.
- Use pantomime to aid performance if ideomotor apraxia is present.

- Use gestures.
  - ▶ Transitive: Tool based (e.g., Hold comb in hand and comb hair. Instruct client to do same action).
  - ▶ Intransitive-symbolic: Symbols based but no tools used (e.g., waving good-bye or thumbs-up sign).
  - ▶ Intransitive-nonsymbolic: Action based without tools (e.g., flying, walking like a dog or four-footed animal).

Cognitive/Perceptual
- Give concrete and contextual directions to improve performance.
- Have client repeat movement and activity to promote motor learning.
- Provide practice sessions of task such as reaching using actual objects.
- Provide guided mental practice using audiotape for instruction.
- Errorless learning approach may be useful in providing support and cueing critical stages in training.

Psychosocial
- Not discussed. See concepts under ADL/IADL.

Context/Environment
- Set up task with commonly used items in sight to reduce symptoms of apraxia or decreased attention skills and promote correct response to natural environmental cues.
- Remove objects from the environment not needed, including unnecessary tools/equipment/items for an ADL task.
- Consider removing objects that may be used in an unsafe manner such as sharp knives, razor blades, or pointed scissors.

Precautions/Safety Considerations

Watch for correct and safe use of eating utensils, toothbrush, kitchen utensils used to prepare a meal; use of a hammer, screwdriver, or scissors; unsafe driving.

Prognosis and Outcome

Client may become dependent, requiring help with ADLs, and require some degree of supervision. Clients whose apraxia is associated with a stroke may have a stable course and even improve somewhat (Porter, 2018). Recording errors in context (perseveration, related, non-related), spatial (amplitude, internal and external configuration, body part as tool, movement error), timing (sequencing, occurrences), and other (no response, unrecognizable) can be used to report progress. Clients with apraxia upon admission are less likely to be independent upon discharge (Wu et al., 2014).

REFERENCES

Arntzen, C., & Elstad, I. (2013). The bodily experience of apraxia in everyday activities: A phenomenological study. *Disability and Rehabilitation, 35*(1), 63–72. https://doi.org/10.3109/09638288.2012.687032

Dawson, A. M., Buxbaum, L. J., & Duff, S. V. (2010). The impact of left hemisphere stroke on force control with familiar and novel objects: Neuroanatomic substrates and relationship to apraxia. *Brain Research, 1317*, 124–136. https://doi.org/10.1016/j.brainres.2009.11.034

Fletcher-Smith, J., Walker, M., Sunderland, A., Garvey, K., Wan, A., & Turner, H. (2010). An inter-rater reliability study of the Nottingham Stroke Dressing Assessment. *British Journal of Occupational Therapy, 73*(12), 570–578. https://doi.org/10.4276/030802210X12918167234127

Giles, G. M. (2014). Cognition and cognitive rehabilitation in neurocognitive disorders—Apraxia. In M. A. Corcoran (Ed.), *Neurocognitive disorders (NCD): Interventions to support occupational performance* (pp. 90–93). AOTA Press.

Lindsten-McQueen, K., Weiner, N. W., Wang, H. Y., Josman, N., & Connor, L. T. (2014). Systematic review of apraxia treatments to improve occupational performance outcomes. *OTJR: Occupation, Participation and Health, 34*(4), 183–192. https://doi.org/10.3928/15394492-20141006-02

O'Toole, M. T. (Ed.). (2017). *Mosby's dictionary of medicine, nursing & health professions* (10th ed.). Elsevier.

Poole, J. L., Sadek, J., & Haaland, K. Y. (2011). Meal preparation abilities after left or right hemisphere stroke. *Archives of Physical Medicine and Rehabilitation, 92*(4), 590–596. https://doi.org/10.1016/j.apmr.2010.11.021

Porter, R. S. (Ed.). (2018). *The Merck manual of diagnosis and therapy* (20th ed.). Merck Sharp & Dohme.

Tempest, S. (2017). Purposeful movement and apraxia. In L. Maskill & S. Tempest (Eds.), *Neuropsychology for occupational therapists: Cognition in occupational performance* (4th ed., pp. 149–163). Wiley.

Walker, M. F., Sunderland, A., Fletcher-Smith, J., Drummond, A., Logan, P., Edmans, J. A., Garvey, K., Dineen, R. A., Ince, P., Horne, J., Fisher, R. J., & Taylor, J. L. (2012). The DRESS trial: A feasibility randomized controlled trial of a neuropsychological approach to dressing therapy for stroke inpatients. *Clinical Rehabilitation, 26*(8), 675–685. https://doi.org/10.1177/0269215511431089

Wu, A. J., Burgard, E., & Radel, J. (2014). Inpatient rehabilitation outcomes of patients with apraxia after stroke. *Topics in Stroke Rehabilitation, 21*(3), 211–219. https://doi.org/10.1310/tsr2103-211

Wu, A. J., Radel, J., & Hanna-Pladdy, B. (2011). Improved function after combined physical and mental practice after stroke: A case of hemiparesis and apraxia. *American Journal of Occupational Therapy, 65*(2), 161–168. https://doi.org/10.5014/ajot.2011.000786

Cognitive Impairment

Also called cognitive deficit, cognitive defect, cognitive disability, cognitive dysfunction, mild cognitive impairment, early stage cognitive decline.

See also Alzheimer's Disease, Anxiety and General Anxiety Disorder, Autism Spectrum Disorder: Adolescent and Adult, Bipolar Disorders, Brain Injuries: Adult, Brain Injuries: Child and Adolescent, Concussion and Post-Concussion, Delirium, Dementia, Depression and Depressive Disorders, Driving Cessation and Driving Retirement, Driving Fitness, Executive Dysfunction, Fetal Alcohol Spectrum Disorder, Huntington's Disease, Intellectual Disability, Memory Impairment, Parkinson's Disease, Multiple Sclerosis, Schizophrenia, Stroke: Acute, Stroke: Chronic, Substance-Related and Addictive Disorders.

Description

Cognition refers to the information processing functions carried out by the brain, including attention, memory, executive functions, comprehension, formation of speech, calculation ability, visual perception, and praxis skills (American Occupational Therapy Association, 2013). *Cognitive impairment* is present when a person has trouble remembering, learning new things, concentrating, or making decisions that affect their everyday life (American Occupational Therapy Association, 2013; Centers for Disease Control, 2011). Two subtypes are recognized: amnestic cognitive impairment involves primarily memory loss, whereas nonamnestic cognitive impairment involves other domains such as language, visual-spatial relations, or executive functions.

Related terms include the following: A *cognitive deficit* is a cognitive performance (e.g., in memory tasks) "as measured by individually administered standardized assessments that is . . . substantially below that expected given the individual's chronological age and formal education" (VandenBos, 2015, p. 203). A *cognitive disability* includes physiologic or biochemical impairment in information-processing capacities, which produces observable and measurable limitations in routine task behavior (Jacobs & Simon, 2015). *Cognitive dysfunction* is "any disruption in mental activities associated with thinking, knowing, and remembering" (VandenBos, 2015, p. 204). A *cognitive disorder* is "any disorder that involves impairment of the executive functions, such as organization, regulation, and perception" (VandenBos, 2015, p. 203). *Functional cognition* is defined as the ability to use and integrate thinking and performance skills to accomplish complex everyday activities. *Functional cognition* influences how an individual uses and integrates "thinking and processing skills to accomplish everyday activities in clinical and community living environments" (American Occupational Therapy Association, 2021, para. 4; Giles et al., 2017). *Cognitive rehabilitation* is a general term used to refer to the therapeutic intervention designed to improve cognitive functioning and participation in activities that may be affected by difficulties in one or more cognitive domains (American Occupational Therapy Association, 2013).

Cause

Any disorder that involves the brain and central nervous system may produce signs and symptoms of cognitive impairment. Four categories can be described: human genetics and development; neurologic disease, injuries, and disorders; mental illness; and transient or continuing life stresses (Giles, 2017). Some examples are stroke, traumatic brain injury, Alzheimer's disease, Parkinson's, multiple sclerosis, Huntington's disease, concussion, autism spectrum disorder, fetal alcohol spectrum, intellectual disability, delirium, dementia, brain tumors, schizophrenia, bipolar disorder, depression, anxiety disorders, posttraumatic stress disorder, pain syndromes, cardiac diseases, and others. The normal process of aging may result in cognitive decline, but not always. In addition, pharmaceuticals that act on the central nervous system may produce cognitive impairment.

Evaluation/Assessment

Areas

- Activities of Daily Living/Instrumental ADL: self-maintenance and basic ADL activities; independent living: meal preparation, housekeeping, driving, shopping, child care
- Education/Work: academic performance, work performance
- Play/Leisure: interests, values, frequency, type, location, level of satisfaction
- Rest/Sleep: sleep disturbances, daytime sleepiness
- Social Participation: frequency, type, location, with whom
- Sensorimotor: psychomotor retardation, sensory processing, visual-spatial relations
- Cognitive/Perceptual: arousal, attention, memory, executive functions, processing speed
- Psychosocial: anxiety, depression, self-awareness, behavioral changes, role performance, quality of life, life satisfaction, self-efficacy
- Context/Environment: adapted devices, environmental modifications, education of family and caregivers
- Comorbidities: diabetes, hypertension, obesity, cerebral hypoxia, heart failure, neurological disorder, mental or behavioral disorder

Instruments

Instruments Developed by Occupational Therapy Personnel

- Activity Card Sort (2nd ed.; ACS-2; Baum & Edwards, 2008)
- Allen Cognitive Levels Screen (5th ed.; ACLS-5; Allen et al., 2007)
- Allen Diagnostic Module (2nd ed.; ADM-2; Earhart, 2006)
- Assessment of Awareness of Disability (AAD; Tham et al., 1999)
- Assessment of Motor and Process Skills (8th ed.; AMPS-8; Fisher & Bray Jones, 2016)

- Children's Kitchen Task Assessment (CKTA; Rocke et al., 2008; see also Reifenberg et al., 2018, in References)
- Computer Adaptive Measure of Functional Cognition for TBI (CAMFC-TBI; Donovan et al., 2011, in References)
- Everyday Technology Use Questionnaire (ETUQ; Rosenberg et al., 2009)
- Executive Function Performance Test (EFPT; Baum & Wolf, 2013)
- Instrumental Activities of Daily Living Profile (IADL Profile; Bottari et al., 2009)
- Kohlman Evaluation of Living Skills, (4th ed.; KELS-4; Kohlman-Thomson & Robnett, 2016)
- Large Allen Cognitive Level Screen (5th ed.; LACLS-5; Allen et al., 2007)
- Performance Assessment of Self-Care Skills (PASS 4.1; Chisholm et al., 2016)
- Routine Task Inventory–Expanded (RTI-E; Katz, 2006)
- Weekly Calendar Planning Activity (WCPA; Toglia, 2015)

Instruments Development by Other Professionals and Used by Occupational Therapy Personnel
- Alzheimer's Disease Cooperative Study/Activities of Daily Living (ADCS-ADL; Galasko et al., 1997)
- Assessment of Capacity for Everyday Decision Making (ACED; Lai et al., 2008)
- Birmingham Cognitive Screen (BCoS; Bickerton et al., 2012; see also Bisiker & Bickerton, 2013, in References)
- Brief Cognitive Assessment Tool (BCAT; Mansbach et al., 2012)
- Clock Drawing Test (CDT; Agrell & Dehun, 1998)
- Disability Assessment in Dementia-6 (DAD-6; de Rotrou et al., 2012)
- Everyday Cognition Battery Memory Test (ECB; Allaire et al., 2009)
- Everyday Problems Test (EPT; Burton et al., 2006)
- Everyday Problems for Cognitively Challenged Elderly (EPCCE; Allaire & Willis, 2006)
- Executive Function Route-Finding Task (EFRFT; Boyd & Sautter, 1993; see also Kizony et al., 2011, in References)
- Functional Activities Questionnaire (FAQ; Pfeffer et al., 1982)
- Montreal Cognitive Assessment (MoCA; Nasreddine et al., 2005; see also van der Wijst et al., 2014, in References)
- Quick Mild Cognitive Impairment screen (QMCI; Lee et al., 2018, in References)
- Repeatable Battery for the Assessment of Neuropsychological Status (RBANS; Randolph et al., 1998)

Problems/Issues
Activities of Daily Living/Instrumental ADL
- Person may require more time to complete ADL or IADL tasks due to slower processing speed.
- Person may forget to complete ADL, IADL, or health maintenance tasks due to memory impairment such as buying certain items during a shopping trip or taking medications.
- Person may make poor decisions regarding finances such as difficulty managing bank account, or making unwise financial decisions.
- Person may experience difficulty driving or have license suspended, which may affect ability to get to work or shop for groceries and other supplies.
- Person may experience language and communication problems including difficulty thinking of common words (anomia), errors in speaking (misusing common words), or errors in writing (misspelling common words).

Education/Work
- Person may have difficulty initiating, planning, and executing a work task or job without structure or guidance.

- Person may have difficulty remembering to follow-up or follow through with a task such as returning a phone call or returning a cart to its assigned storage area.
- Person may have difficulty following instructions or applying the instructions to similar tasks.

Play/Leisure

- Person may reduce or stop engagement in favorite leisure occupations due to decreased ability to perform tasks required in the activity.
- Person may have lost interest in leisure occupations.

Rest/Sleep

- Person may have difficulty falling asleep or remaining asleep: Note that lack of sleep may result in more errors and fatigue.
- Person may not maintain a sleeping (going to bed) routine.

Social Participation

- Person may reduce or stop participation in social activities due to decreased ability to perform tasks expected in social activity.

Sensorimotor

- Person may have visual-spatial impairments that result in misunderstanding written instructions or overlooking items needed to complete a task (visual-spatial neglect).
- Person may experience auditory processing impairment, especially in noisy environments.

Cognitive/Perceptual

- Person may have decreased ability to attend and concentrate (focus) attention on a task.
- Person may be easily distracted by environmental factors.
- Person may have difficulty understanding instructions.
- Person may have difficulty acquiring or remembering new information such as asking repetitive questions, frequently misplacing objects, or forgetting appointments.
- Person may have difficulty doing more than one thing at a time resulting in tasks started but not completed.
- Person may have difficulty remembering to do or how to do tasks (see Memory Impairment).
- Person may demonstrate slow processing speed (see Memory Impairment).
- Person may have difficulty with tasks requiring reasoning and quick decision making, such as driving in traffic.
- Person may have difficulty performing complex tasks, such as preparing several different foods for a meal.
- Person may have difficulty problem solving without supervision or guidance (see Executive Dysfunction).
- Person may have difficulty planning and prioritizing (see Executive Dysfunction).
- Person may have difficulty with time management (see Executive Dysfunction).
- Person may perform tasks in an unsafe manner or place self in danger of injury due to deficits in judgment.

Psychosocial

- Person may become anxious and depressed due to awareness that his or her ability to function is decreasing.
- Person may become irritable with others.
- Person may have difficulty performing expected role responsibilities, such as paying bills.
- Person may express feelings of worthlessness or loss of self-efficacy.

Context/Environment

- Person may get lost in environments (local community) once familiar and easily traversed.
- Person, family, or caregivers may not understand or have knowledge about cognitive impairment.
- Person, family, or caregivers may lack access to resources about cognitive impairment.

Intervention/Treatment

Giles (2017) suggested five general categories of intervention without regard to which profession developed the approach: (1) global strategy learning and awareness, (2) domain-specific strategy training, (3) cognitive retaining embedded in functional activity, (4) specific functional skills training, and (5) environmental modification and use of assistive technology. Toglia et al. (2012) suggested intervention strategies can be grouped into three general categories: modality-specific, mental or self-verbalization, and task specification/modification. An additional general category is client/family/caregiver education (Karmali et al., 2018). Models and programs developed by occupational therapy personnel include case studies (Bottari et al., 2017), Cognitive Orientation to daily Occupation Performance (CO-OP; Jackman et al., 2018), medication management (Lui et al., 2012), multifaceted cognitive training program (Lim et al., 2012), neurofunctional approach (Clark-Wilson et al., 2014), occupation-centered cognitive rehabilitation program (Kim & Cho, 2018; Park et al., 2015), occupational therapy intervention program (Peralta et al., 2017), occupational therapy role in return to work (Purdy, 2012), and occupational therapy task-oriented approach (Preissner, 2010). Models and programs developed by other professionals but used by occupational therapy personnel include attention training (Yoshida et al., 2014), cognitive behavior therapy (Arundine et al., 2012), education program for caregivers (Harada & Yamane, 2016), eHEALTH (Jakobsson et al., 2019), FcTSim Programme (Law et al., 2013, 2014), functional tasks exercise (Law et al., 2014; Law et al., 2018; Law et al., 2019), rehabilitation living lab in the mall (Auger et al., 2014), and transcranial direct-current stimulation (Gonzalez et al., 2018). Team members include physicians, psychologists, sports medicine personnel, and occupational therapy personnel. Goal is to use daily function tasks that are innately cognitively demanding and involve components of an exercise program that are meaningful and practical for the client (Law et al., 2013).

Activities of Daily Living/Instrumental ADL
- Assist client to complete basic ADLs using visual and/or auditory memory aids.
- Assist client in developing a financial management program such as teaching or reviewing basic monetary skills, teaching or reviewing basic calculations, maintaining and balancing a checkbook, basic banking tasks, paying bills (written or electronic), developing and following a budget plan, monitoring and regulating spending, shifting responsibility for finances to another family member, and understanding financial terminology and concepts (Engel et al., 2016; Koller et al., 2016).
- Evaluate driving ability and examine if other modes of transportation are suitable and acceptable to the person. See also chapters in Section 13, Driving Fitness and Driving Cessation.
- Assist person in developing a shopping management program such using a list, shopping at times when fewer customers are present, shopping online using pickup at store or home delivery program.

Education/Work
- Assist client to analyze workplace and worker roles to make recommendations to client and supervisor that will allow the client to be successful and continue employment. Examples: memory aids, energy conservation, work simplification, more frequent rest breaks, environmental modification to light, noise, clutter, and temperature.

Play/Leisure
- Explore if leisure activities can be adapted or modified to allow client to continue engagement.
- Provide opportunity to develop new leisure activities that are within client's ability level and interest.

Rest/Sleep
- Assist client (family, caregivers) to develop a sleep schedule and routine.
- Suggest adding stress reduction techniques before going to bed.

Social Participation
- Encourage person to continue participation in social activities with modifications as useful (less time, fewer people, less cognitively demanding, limit to familiar places).

Sensorimotor
- Assist person with visual rehabilitation such as scanning techniques, use of magnification on computer screen (see chapter in Section 2, Visual Impairments Due to Neurologic Conditions.
- Assist person with auditory processing impairment such as providing written, electronic or pictorial instructions in addition to verbal instructions, give instructions in a quiet area.

Cognitive/Perceptual
- Assist person to develop goals and steps to achieve the goals such as increasing attention span, memory training, reality orientation, solving problems, sequencing tasks.
- Assist client to use memory aids: create checklists, a memory book, or use of other external aids such as smartphone to assist with organizing daily activities.

Psychosocial
- Listen to person express anxiety or feelings of depression and address concerns.
- Teach stress management techniques: mindfulness, yoga, relaxation training, deep-breathing exercises.
- Promote self-efficacy by helping person learn to cope using environmental modifications or adapted devices.

Context/Environment
- Reduce distractions: clutter, noise, visually "busy" environments, glare, slippery surfaces, rough or sharp edges, heavy loads.
- Increase lighting in dark or dim areas, use of good contrasts between light and dark materials, noise cancelling equipment
- Provide education to client, family, and caregivers about cognitive impairment and its management.
- Provide information to client, family, and caregivers about available resources in the community or on the internet to learn more about cognitive impairment and strategies to compensate for decrease cognitive functions (Poulin et al., 2019).

Precautions/Safety Considerations

Person is at increased risk of unintended self-injury due to failure to self-monitor to detect and recognize actual danger or potentially dangerous situations, such as potential for burns, cuts, or falls.

Prognosis and Outcome

Prognosis and outcome depend in part on cause of cognitive impairment and in part on response of client to intervention. Cognitive impairment due to neurodegenerative disorders is likely to get worse over time. Cognitive impairment due to conditions that can be treated successfully may improve. Clients who are able to participate actively in intervention may be able to compensate for deficits in cognitive functioning.

REFERENCES

American Occupational Therapy Association. (2013). Cognition, cognitive rehabilitation, and occupational performance. *American Journal of Occupational Therapy, 67*(Suppl.), S9–S31. https://doi.org/10.5014/ajot.2013.67S9

American Occupational Therapy Association. (2021). *Role of OT in assessing functional cognition.* https://www.aota.org/Advocacy-Policy/Federal-Reg-Affairs/Medicare/Guidance/role-OT -assessing-functional-cognition.aspx

Arundine, A., Bradbury, C. L., Dupuis, K., Dawson, D. R., Ruttan, L. A., & Green, R. E. A. (2012). Cognitive behavior therapy after acquired brain injury: Maintenance of therapeutic benefits at 6 months posttreatment. *Journal of Head Trauma Rehabilitation, 27*(2), 104–112. https://doi.org/10.1097/HTR.0b013e3182125591

Auger, C., Leduc, E., Labbé, D., Guay, C., Fillion, B., Bottari, C., & Swaine, B. (2014). Mobile applications for participation at the shopping mall: Content analysis and usability for persons with physical disabilities and communication or cognitive limitations. *International Journal of Environmental Research and Public Health, 11*(12), 12777–12794. https://doi.org/10.3390/ijerph111212777

Bisiker, J., & Bickerton, W. L. (2013). Using a comprehensive and standardized cognitive screen to guide cognitive rehabilitation in stroke. *British Journal of Occupational Therapy, 76*(3), 151–156. https://doi.org/10.4276/030802213X13627524435261

Bottari, C., Gosselin, N., Chen, J. K., & Ptito, A. (2017). The impact of symptomatic mild traumatic brain injury on complex everyday activities and the link with alterations in cerebral functioning: Exploratory case studies. *Neuropsychological Rehabilitation, 27*(5), 871–890. https://doi.org/10.1080/09602011.2015.1110528

Centers for Disease Control. (2011). *Cognitive impairment: A call for action now!* https://www.cdc.gov/aging/pdf/cognitive_impairment/cogimp_poilicy_final.pdf

Clark-Wilson, J., Giles, G. M., & Baxter, D. (2014). Revisiting the neurofunctional approach: Conceptualizing the core components for the rehabilitation of everyday living skills. *Brain Injury, 28*(13-14), 1646–1656. https://doi.org/10.3109/02699052.2014.946449

Donovan, N. J., Heaton, S. C., Kimberg, C. I., Wen, P. S., Waid-Ebbs, J. K., Coster, W., Singletary, F., & Velozo, C. A. (2011). Conceptualizing functional cognition in traumatic brain injury rehabilitation. *Brain Injury, 25*(4), 348–364. https://doi.org/10.3109/02699052.2011.556105

Engel, L., Bar, Y., Beaton, D. E., Green, R. E., & Dawson, D. R. (2016). Identifying instruments to quantify financial management skills in adults with acquired cognitive impairments. *Journal of Clinical and Experimental Neuropsychology, 38*(1), 76–95. https://doi.org/10.1080/13803395.2015.1087468

Giles, G. M. (2017). *Fact sheet: Occupational therapy's role in adult cognitive disorders.* American Occupational Therapy Association.

Giles, G. M., Edwards, D. F., Morrison, M. T., Baum, C., & Wolf, T. J. (2017). Screening for functional cognition in postacute care and the Improving Medicare Post-Acute Care Transformation (IMPACT) act of 2014. *American Journal of Occupational Therapy, 71*(5), Article 7105090010. https://doi.org/10.5014/ajot.2017.715001

Gonzalez, P. C., Fong, K. N. K., Chung, R. C. K., Ting, K. H., Law, L. L. F., & Brown, T. (2018). Can transcranial direct-current stimulation alone or combined with cognitive training be used as a clinical intervention to improve cognitive functioning in persons with mild cognitive impairment and dementia? A systematic review and meta-analysis. *Frontiers in Human Neuroscience, 12*, Article 416. https://doi.org/10.3389/fnhum.2018.00416

Harada, S., & Yamane, H. (2016). Effect of education programs for caregivers with the provision of the elderly with mental and cognitive impairments. *Asian Journal of Occupational Therapy, 11*(1), 9–17.

Jackman, M., Novak, I., Lannin, N. Froude, E., Miller, L., & Galea, C. (2018). Effectiveness of Cognitive Orientation to daily Occupational Performance over and above functional hand splints for children with cerebral palsy or brain injury: A randomized controlled trial. *BMC Pediatrics, 18*, Article 248. https://doi.org/10.1186/s12887-018-1213-9

Jacobs, K., & Simon, L. (Eds.). (2015). *Quick reference dictionary for occupational therapy* (6th ed.). Slack.

Jakobsson, E., Nygård, L., Kottorp, A., & Malinowsky, C. (2019). Experiences from using eHealth in contact with health care among older adults with cognitive impairment. *Scandinavian Journal of Caring Sciences, 33*(2), 380–389. https://doi.org/10.1111/scs.12634

Karmali, S., Hagstrom, L., Mah, K., Mishima, G., & Seminary, J. (2018). Functional cognitive assessment and intervention in acute care. *SIS Quarterly Practice Connections Productive Aging, 3*(3), 21–23.

Kim, K. S., & Cho, Y. S. (2018). The effects of an occupation-centered cognitive rehabilitation program on elderly individuals with mild cognitive impairment. *Journal of Physical Therapy Science, 30*(2), 332–334.

Kizony, R., Demayo-Dayan, T., Sinoff, G., & Josman, N. (2011). Validation of the Executive Function Route-Finding Task (EFRT) in people with mild cognitive impairment. *OTJR, Occupation, Participation and Health, 31*(1 Suppl.), S47–S52. https://doi.org/10.3928/15394492-20101108-08

Koller, K., Woods, L., Engel, L., Bottari, C., Dawson, D. R., & Nalder, E. (2016). Loss of financial management independence after brain injury: Survivors' experiences. *American Journal of Occupational Therapy, 70*(3), Article 7003180070. https://doi.org/10.5014/ajot.2016.020198

Law, L. L. F., Barnett, F., Yau, M. K., & Gray, M. A. (2013). Development and initial testing of functional task exercise on older adults with cognitive impairment at risk of Alzheimer's disease—FcTSim Programme—A feasibility study. *Occupational Therapy International, 20*, 185–197. https://doi.org/10.1002/oti.1355

Law, L. L. F., Barnett, F., Yau, M. K., & Gray, M. A. (2014). Effects of functional tasks exercise on older adults with cognitive impairment at risk of Alzheimer's disease: A randomised controlled trial. *Age and Ageing, 43*(6), 813–820. https://doi.org/10.1093/ageing/afu055

Law, L. L. F., Fong, K. N. K., & Yau, M. M. K. (2018). Can functional task exercise improve executive function and contribute to functional balance in older adults with mild cognitive impairment? A pilot study. *British Journal of Occupational Therapy, 81*(9), 495–502. https://doi.org/10.1177/0308022618763492

Law, L. L. F., Mok, V. C. T., & Yau, M. M. K. (2019). Effects of functional tasks exercise on cognitive functions of older adults with mild cognitive impairment: A randomized controlled pilot trial. *Alzheimer's Research & Therapy, 11*, Article 98. https://doi.org/10.1186/s13195-019-0548-2

Lee, M.-T., Chang, W.-Y., & Jang, Y. (2018). Psychometric and diagnostic properties of the Taiwan version of the Quick Mild Cognitive Impairment screen. *PLOS ONE, 13*(12), Article e0207851. https://doi.org/10.1371/journal.pone.0207851

Lim, M. H. X., Liu, K. P. Y., Cheung, G. S. F., Kuo, M. C. C., Li, R., & Tong, C. Y. (2012). Effectiveness of a multifaceted cognitive training programme for people with mild cognitive impairment: A one-group pre- and posttest design. *Hong Kong Journal of Occupational Therapy, 22*(1), 3–8. https://doi.org/10.1016/j.hkjot.2012.04.002

Lui, V. W.-C., Lam, L. C.-W., Chau, R. C.-M., Fung, A. W.-T., Wong, B. M.-L., Leung, G. T.-Y., Leung, K.-F., Chiu, H. F.-K., Karlawish, J. H. T., & Appelbaum, P. S. (2012). Capacity to make decisions on medication management in Chinese older persons with mild cognitive impairment and mild Alzheimer's disease. *International Psychogeriatrics, 24*(7), 1103–1111. https://doi.org/10.1017/S1041610212000129

Maskill, L., & Tempest, S. (2017). Intervention for cognitive impairments and evaluating outcomes. In L. Maskill & S. Tempest (Eds.), *Neuropsychology for occupational therapists* (4th ed., pp. 33–49). Wiley Blackstone.

Park, H. Y., Maitra, K., & Martinez, K. M. (2015). The effect of occupation-based cognitive rehabilitation for traumatic brain injury: A meta-analysis of randomized controlled trials. *Occupational Therapy International, 22*, 104–116. https://doi.org/10.1002/oti.1389

Peralta, P., Gascón, A., & Latorre, E. (2017). Occupational therapy prevents cognitive impairment on long-term care residents. *Physical & Occupational Therapy in Geriatrics, 35*(3-4), 119–131. https://doi.org/10.1080/02703181.2017.1339757

Poulin, V., Dawson, D. R., Bottari, C., Verreault, C., Turcotte, S., & Jean, A. (2019). Managing cognitive difficulties after traumatic brain injury: A review of online resources for families.

Disability and Rehabilitation, 41(16), 1955–1965. https://doi.org/10.1080/09638288.2018.1451560

Preissner, K. (2010). Use of the Occupational Therapy Task-Oriented Approach to optimize the motor performance of a client with cognitive limitations. *American Journal of Occupational Therapy, 64*(5), 727–734. https://doi.org/10.5014/ajot.2010.08026

Purdy, S. (2012). *Fact sheet: Returning to work with cognitive impairments.* American Occupational Therapy Association.

Reifenberg, G., Kiger, M. A., & Cronin, A. (2018). Using the Children's Kitchen Task Assessment to measure functional cognition in children with developmental disabilities. *SIS Quarterly Practice Connections, 3*(4), 5–7.

Toglia, J. P., Rodger, S. A., & Polatajko, H. J. (2012). Anatomy of cognitive strategies: A therapist's primer for enabling occupational performance. *Canadian Journal of Occupational Therapy, 79*(4), 225–236. https://doi.org/10.2182/cjot.2012.79.4.4

van der Wijst, E., Wright, J., & Steultjens, E. (2014). The suitability of the Montreal Cognitive Assessment as a screening tool to identify people with dysfunction in occupational performance after mild stroke. *British Journal of Occupational Therapy, 77*(10), 526–532. https://doi.org/10.4276/030802214X14122630932511

VandenBos, G. (Ed.). (2015). *APA dictionary of psychology* (2nd ed.). American Psychological Association.

Yoshida, K., Sawamura, D., Ogawa, K., Ikoma, K., Asakawa, K., Yamauchi, T., & Sakai, S. (2014). Flow experience during attentional training improves cognitive functions in patients with traumatic brain injury: An exploratory case study. *Hong Kong Journal of Occupational Therapy, 24*(2), 81–87. https://doi.org/10.1016/j.hkjot.2015.01.001

BIBLIOGRAPHY

Adolfsson, P., Lindstedt, H., & Janeslätt, G. (2015). How people with cognitive disabilities experience electronic planning devices. *NeuroRehabilitation, 37*(3), 379–392. https://doi.org/10.3233/NRE-151268

Adolfsson, P., Lindstedt, H., Pettersson, I., Hermansson, L. N., & Janeslätt, G. (2016). Perception of the influence of environmental factors in the use of electronic planning devices in adults with cognitive disabilities. *Disability and Rehabilitation: Assistive Technology, 11*(6), 493–500. https://doi.org/10.3109/17483107.2014.989418

Andersen, J., Kot, N., Ennis, N., Colantonio, A., Ouchterlony, D., Cusimano, M. D., & Topolovec-Vranic, J. (2014). Traumatic brain injury and cognitive impairment in men who are homeless. *Disability and Rehabilitation, 36*(26), 2210–2215. https://doi.org/10.3109/09638288.2014.895870

Baum, C. (2017). Editorial: Functional cognition: the occupational therapist's expertise. *Revista de Terapia Ocupacional de Galicia, 14*(25), 10–13.

Baker, N., Barbour, K. E., Helmick, C. G., Zack, M., & Al Snih, S. (2017). Arthritis and cognitive impairment in older adults. *Rheumatology International, 37*(6), 955–961. https://doi.org/10.1007/s00296-017-3698-1

Belchior, P., Holmes, M., Bier, N., Bottari, C., Mazer, B., Robert, A., & Kaur, N. (2015). Performance-based tools for assessing functional performance in individuals with mild cognitive impairment. *Open Journal of Occupational Therapy, 3*(3), Article 3. https://doi.org/10.15453/2168-6408.1173

Belchior, P., Korner-Bitensky, N., Holmes, M., & Robert, A. (2015). Identification and assessment of functional performance in mild cognitive impairment: A survey of occupational therapy practices. *Australian Occupational Therapy Journal, 62*(3), 187–196. https://doi.org/10.1111/1440-1630.12201

Earl, R., Falkmer, T., Girdler, S., Morris, S. L., & Falkmer, M. (2018). Viewpoints of pedestrians with and without cognitive impairment on shared zones and zebra crossings. *PLOS ONE*, *13*(9), Article e0203765. https://doi.org/10.1371/journal.pone.0203765

Fang, M. L., Coatta, K., Badger, M., Wu, S., Easton, M., Nygård, L., Astell, A., & Sixsmith, A. (2017). Informing understandings of mild cognitive impairment for older adults: Implications from a scoping review. *Journal of Applied Gerontology*, *36*(7), 808–839. https://doi.org/10.1177/0733464815589987

Gillen, G. (2018). Evaluation and treatment of limited occupational performance secondary to cognitive dysfunction. In H. M. Pendleton & W. Schultz-Kohn (Eds.), *Pedretti's occupational therapy* (8th ed., pp. 646–668). Elsevier.

Gillen, G., Nilsen, D. M., Attridge, J., Banakos, E., Morgan, M., Winterbottom, L., & York, W. (2015). Effectiveness of interventions to improve occupational performance of people with cognitive impairments after stroke: An evidence-based review. *American Journal of Occupational Therapy*, *69*(1), Article 6902280040, Supplemental Table 1-4. https://doi.org/10.5014/ajot.2015.012138

Hedman, A., Kottorp, A., Almkvist, O., & Nygård, L. (2018). Challenge levels of everyday technologies as perceived over five years by older adults with mild cognitive impairment. *International Psychogeriatrics*, *30*(10), 1447–1454. https://doi.org/10.1017/S1041610218000285

Hedman, A., Kottorp, A., & Nygård, L. (2018). Patterns of everyday technology use and activity involvement in mild cognitive impairment: A five-year follow-up study. *Aging & Mental Health*, *22*(5), 603–610. https://doi.org/10.1080/13607863.2017.1297361

Hedman, A., Lindqvist, E., & Nygård, L. (2016). How older adults with mild cognitive impairment relate to technology as part of present and future everyday life: A qualitative study. *BMC Geriatrics*, *16*, Article 73. https://doi.org/10.1186/s12877-016-0245-y

Hedman, A., Nygård, L., Almkvist, O., & Kottorp, A. (2013). Patterns of functioning in older adults with mild cognitive impairment: A two-year study focusing on everyday technology use. *Aging & Mental Health*, *17*(6), 679–688. https://doi.org/10.1080/13607863.2013.777396

Hedman, A., Nygård, L., Almkvist, O., & Kottorp, A. (2015). Amount and type of everyday technology use over time in older adults with cognitive impairment. *Scandinavian Journal of Occupational Therapy*, *22*(3), 196–206. https://doi.org/10.3109/11038128.2014.982172

Hedman, A., Nygård, L., & Kottorp, A. (2017). Everyday technology use related to activity involvement among people in cognitive decline. *American Journal of Occupational Therapy*, *71*(5), Article 710519040. https://doi.org/10.5014/ajot.2017.027003

Hoffmann, T., Bennett, S., Koh, C. L., & McKenna, K. (2010). A systematic review of cognitive interventions to improve functional ability in people who have cognitive impairment following stroke. *Topics in Stroke Rehabilitation*, *17*(2), 99–107. https://doi.org/10.1310/tsr1702-99

Hoffmann, T., Bennett, S., Koh, C. L., & McKenna, K. T. (2010). Occupational therapy for cognitive impairment in stroke patients. *Cochrane Database of Systematic Reviews*, *9*, Article CD006430. https://doi.org/10.1002/14651858.CD006430.pub2

Holmqvist, K., Ivarsson, A. B., & Holmefur, M. (2014). Occupational therapist practice patterns in relation to clients with cognitive impairment following acquired brain injury. *Brain Injury*, *28*(11), 1365–1373. https://doi.org/10.3109/02699052.2014.919529

Kaur, N., Belchior, P., Gélinas, I., & Bier, N. (2016). Critical appraisal of questionnaires to assess functional impairment in individuals with mild cognitive impairment. *International Psychogeriatrics*, *28*(9), 1425–1439. https://doi.org/10.1017/S104161021600017X

Katz, N., & Toglia, J. (Eds.). *Cognition, occupation, and participation across the lifespan* (4th ed.). AOTA Press.

Korner-Bitensky, N., Barrett-Bernstein, S., Bibas, G., & Poulin, V. (2011). National survey of Canadian occupational therapists' assessment and treatment of cognitive impairment post-stroke. *Australian Occupational Therapy Journal*, *58*(4), 241–250. https://doi.org/10.1111/j.1440-1630.2011.00943.x

Kringle, E. A., Terhorst L., Butters, M. A., & Skidmore, E. R. (2018). Clinical predictors of engagement in inpatient rehabilitation among stroke survivors with cognitive deficits: An exploratory study. *Journal of the International Neuropsychological Society, 24*(6), 572–583. https://doi.org/10.1017/S1355617718000085

Law, L. L. F., Barnett, F., Yau, M. K., & Gray, M. A. (2012). Measures of everyday competence in older adults with cognitive impairment: A systematic review. *Age and Ageing, 41*(1), 9–16. https://doi.org/10.1093/ageing/afr104

Lindqvist, E., PerssonVasiliou, A., Hwang, A. S., Mihailidis, A., Astelle, A., Sixsmith, A., & Nygård, L. (2018). The contrasting role of technology as both supportive and hindering in the everyday lives of people with mild cognitive deficits: A focus group study. *BMC Geriatrics, 18,* Article 185. https://doi.org/10.1186/s12877-018-0879-z

Maskill, L., & Tempest, S. (2017). Assessment and measuring change. In L. Maskill & S. Tempest (Eds.), *Neuropsychology for occupational therapists* (4th ed., pp. 17–31). Wiley Blackstone.

Norris, J. (2018). Cognitive function in cardiac patients: Exploring the occupational therapy role in lifestyle medicine. *American Journal of Lifestyle Medicine, 14*(1), 61–70. https://doi.org/10.1177/1559827618757189

Nygård, L., Pantzar, M., Uppgard, B., & Kottorp, A. (2012). Detection of activity limitations in older adults with MCI or Alzheimer's disease through evaluation of perceived difficulty in use of everyday technology: A replication study. *Aging & Mental Health, 16*(3), 361–371. https://doi.org/10.1080/13607863.2011.605055

Öhman, A., Nygård, L., & Kottorp, A. (2011). Occupational performance and awareness of disability in mild cognitive impairment or dementia. *Scandinavian Journal of Occupational Therapy, 18*(2), 133–142. https://doi.org/10.3109/11038121003645993

Radomski, M. V., Anheluk, M., Bartzen, M. P., & Zola, J. (2016). Effectiveness of interventions to address cognitive impairments and improve occupational performance after traumatic brain injury: A systematic review. *American Journal of Occupational Therapy, 70*(3), 7003180050. https://doi.org/10.5014/ajot.2016.020776

Radomski, M. V., & Giles, G. M. (2014). Optimizing cognitive performance. In M. V. Radomski & C. A. Trombly Latham (Eds.), *Occupational therapy for physical dysfunction* (7th ed., pp. 725–752). Wolters Kluwer.

Radomski, M. V., & Morrison, M. T. (2014). Assessing abilities and capacities: Cognition. In M. V. Radomski & C. A. Trombly Latham (Eds.), *Occupational therapy for physical dysfunction* (7th ed., pp. 121–143). Wolters Kluwer.

Rodakowski, J., Saghafi, E., Butters, M. A., & Skidmore, E. R. (2015). Non-pharmacological interventions for adults with mild cognitive impairment and early stage dementia: An updated scoping review. *Molecular Aspects of Medicine, 43-44,* 38–53. https://doi.org/10.1016/j.mam.2015.06.003

Rodakowski, J., Skidmore, E. R., Reynolds, C. F., III, Dew, M. A., Butters, M. A., Holm, M. B., Lopez, O. L., & Rogers, J. C. (2014). Can performance on daily activities discriminate between older adults with normal cognitive function and those with mild cognitive impairment? *Journal of the American Geriatrics Society, 62*(7), 1347–1352. https://doi.org/10.1111/jgs.12878

Ryd, C., Nygård, L., Malinowsky, C., Öhman, A., & Kottorp, A. (2015). Associations between performance of activities of daily living and everyday technology use among older adults with mild stage Alzheimer's disease or mild cognitive impairment. *Scandinavian Journal of Caring Sciences, 22*(1), 33–42. https://doi.org/10.3109/11038128.2014.964307

Ryd, C., Nygård, L., Malinowsky, C., Öhman, A., & Kottorp, A. (2017). Can the everyday technology use questionnaire predict overall functional level among older adults with mild cognitive impairment or mild-stage Alzheimer's disease?—A pilot study. *Scandinavian Journal of Occupational Therapy, 31*(1), 201–209. https://doi.org/10.1111/scs.12330

Sansonetti, D., & Hoffmann, T. (2013). Cognitive assessment across the continuum of care: The importance of occupational performance-based assessment for individuals post-stroke and traumatic brain injury. *Australian Occupational Therapy Journal, 60*(5), 334–342. https://doi .org/1111/1440-1630.12069

Scanlan, J. N., & Still, M. (2013). Functional profile of mental health consumers assessed by occupational therapists: Level of independence and associations with functional cognition. *Psychiatry Research, 208*(10), 29–32. https://doi.org/10.1016/j.psychres.2013.02.032

Sinnott, C., Foley, T., Forsyth, J., McLoughlin, K., Horgan, L., & Bradley, C. P. (2018). Consultations on driving in people with cognitive impairment in primary care: A scoping review of the evidence. *PLOS ONE, 13*(1), Article e0205580. https://doi.org/10.1371/journal.pone.0205580

Sinnott, C., Foley, T., Horgan, L., McLoughlin, K., Sheehan, C., & Bradley, C. (2019). Shifting gears versus sudden stops: Qualitative study of consultations about driving in patients with cognitive impairment. *BMJ Open, 9*(8), Article e024452. https://doi.org/10.1136/bm jopen-2018-024452

Sirois, K., Tousignant, B., Boucher, N., Achim, A. M., Beauchamp, M. H., Bedell, G., Massicotte, E., Vera-Estay, E., & Jackson, P. L. (2019). The contribution of social cognition in predicting social participation following moderate and severe TBI in youth. *Neuropsychological Rehabilitation, 29*(9), 1383–1398. https://doi.org/10.1080/09602011.2017.1413987

Sleight, A. (2016). Coping with cancer-related cognitive dysfunction: A scoping review of the literature. *Disability and Rehabilitation, 38*(4), 400–408. https://doi.org/10.3109/09638288.20 15.1038364

Spitzer, J., Tse, T., Baum, C. M., & Carey, L. M. (2011). Mild impairment of cognition impacts on activity participation after stroke in a community-dwelling Australian cohort. *OTJR: Occupation, Participation and Health, 31*(1 Suppl.), S8–S15. https://doi.org/10.3928/15394492-20101108-03

Steel, E. J., & Janeslätt, G. (2017). Drafting standards on cognitive accessibility: A global collaboration. *Disability and Rehabilitation: Assistive Technology, 12*(4), 385–389. https://doi.org/ 10.1080/17483107.2016.1176260

Stephens, J. A., Williamson, K. N., & Berryhill, M. E. (2015). Cognitive rehabilitation after traumatic brain injury: A reference for occupational therapists. *OTJR: Occupation, Participation and Health, 35*(1), 5–22.

Tempest, S., & Maskill, L. (2017). Occupation and cognitive rehabilitation. In L. Maskill & S. Tempest (Eds.), *Neuropsychology for occupational therapists* (4th ed., pp. 3–16). Wiley Blackstone.

Thorton, J., & Velez-Spina, M. (2016). OT's role in functional cognition rehabilitation. *Rehab Care,* (April 22), 1–2.

Tulsky, D. S., Holdnack, J. A., Cohen, M. L., Heaton, R. K., Carlozzi, N. E., Wong, A. W. K., Boulton, A. J., & Heinemann, A. W. (2017). Factor structure of the NIH Toolbox Cognitive Battery in individuals with acquired brain injury. *Rehabilitation Psychology, 62*(4), 435–442. https://doi.org/10.1037/rep0000183

Walsh, R., Leggett, C., & Lee, J. (2019). Everyday technology use, occupation-based assessment, and functional cognition in older adults post-stroke. *OT Practice, 24*(6), 20–23.

Wesson, J., Clemson, L., Brodaty, H., & Reppermund, S. (2016). Estimating functional cognition in older adults using observational assessments of task performance in complex everyday activities: A systematic review and evaluation of measurement properties. *Neuroscience & Biobehavioral Reviews, 68,* 335–360. https://doi.org/10.1016/j.neubiorev.2016.05.024

Wesson, J., Clemson, L., Crawford, J. D., Kochan, N. A., Brodaty, H., & Reppermund, S. (2017). Measurement of functional cognition and complex everyday activities in older adults with mild cognitive impairment and mild dementia: Validity of the Large Allen's Cognitive Level Screen. *American Journal of Geriatric Psychiatry, 25*(5), 471–482. https://doi.org/10.1016/j.ja gp.2016.11.021

White, A., Hocking, C., & Reid, H. (2014). How occupational therapists engage adults with cognitive impairments in assessments. *British Journal of Occupational Therapy, 77*(1), 2–9. https://doi.org/10.4276/030802214X13887685335427

Wolf, T. J., Barco, P. P., & Giles, G. M. (2019). Functional cognition: Understanding the importance to occupational therapy. *OT Practice, 24*(12), 12–15.

Wolf, T. J., Edwards, D. F., & Giles, G. M. (2019). *Functional cognition and occupational therapy: A practical approach to treating individuals with cognitive loss.* AOTA Press.

Wong, G. K. C., Wong, R., & Poon, W. S. (2011). Cognitive outcomes and activity of daily living for neurosurgical patients with intrinsic brain lesions: A 1-year prevalence study. *Hong Kong Journal of Occupational Therapy, 21*(1), 27–32.

APPENDIX A: COGNITIVE STRATEGIES TO TEACH THE CLIENT

Modality-Specific Strategies

- Auditory (hearing): sounds, songs, singing, tones, tunes, rhythms, instruments (solo, band, orchestra), verbal prompts
- Gustatory (tasting): sweet, sour, salty, bitter
- Kinesthetic (muscle movement): gestures, pantomime
- Olfactory (smell): flowery, rancid, fruity
- Proprioception (joint movement): static or dynamic postures
- Tactile (touch): light touch, deep pressure, static, dynamic/moving
- Vision (seeing): pictures, signs, symbols, colors, visual prompts (pointing, gesturing), reading, written instructions

Mental or Self-Verbalization Strategies

- Anticipation (mental, verbal): Thinking, imagining, or verbalizing in advance about challenges, obstacles, or scenarios that might occur to prepare for a task such as going shopping, dealing with crowds, noisy situations, or flashing lights.
- Association: Linking similar information (ideas, concepts) together based on previous experiences, knowledge of categories, or physical similarities.
- Chunking: Grouping information together into manageable combinations to aid memory and recall such as remembering phone numbers in groups of 3 (area code), 3 (first 3 numbers), 4 (last 4 numbers).
- Elaboration (mental, verbal): Expand or add to information such as adding new words, sentences, images, symbols, or actions and relate new information to previously learned/known information.
- Imagery: Transformation of physical objects, events, actions, or experiences into mental images, symbols, or representations using vision, smell, textures, sounds, or movements.
- Knowledge: Identifying, verbalizing, or thinking about what is known (facts, information) about a task before initiating, starting, or beginning to do the task.
- Mnemonic technique (mental, verbal, visual, auditory): Forming associations between words, sets of words, pictures, or images to cue actions or recall.
- Reconstruction (mental, verbal): Thinking back to previous occurrences by replaying, imagining, or verbalizing a previous activity, experience, or context to assist or guide performance in a new or potentially occurring situation.
- Rehearsal: Repeating or practicing information mentally or verbally such as key words, rules, procedures, actions steps, or facts to enhance retention (memorization) of information or procedures in lieu of actual performance.
- Rote scripts: Repeating information that has been coded or abbreviated to guide a sequence of action steps or enhance recall of information.
- Self-coaching: Positive self-talk, thinking, and encouragement to increase persistence or to help regulate and control emotions, such as "You can do this, stay calm."

- Self-guidance: Person provides self with instructions, self-cues, or reminders to prepare or guide the individual through a task (self-instruction, self-talk, talk aloud).
- Self-questioning: Person asks himself or herself key questions related to the task to be performed.
- Translation: Changing the format of information such as changing written instruction, procedures, or actions into images, phrases, or more manageable chunks of information.

Task Specific/Modification Strategies

- Attention to doing: Identifying key cues or features to focus attention during a performance.
- Finger pointing: Point to relevant task stimuli to enhance attention to details or to pace timing within a task.
- Lists (checklists): Creating or using a written, pictorial, audiotaped list of steps to guide performance or cue actions.
- Organization (association, categorization): Grouping task materials or steps so that similar items or steps are together or in a particular order.
- Pacing strategies: Actions that assist with the timing of activities such as taking breaks, spreading activities throughout the day, completing partial tasks and then taking a break before completing the rest of the tasks. Other actions may include humming tone, singing a song, moving to a rhythm, or counting to oneself or out loud, tapping one's foot to a rhythm to assist with the timing of actions including getting started.
- Stimuli reduction: Decreasing the amount of information, decluttering, or reducing the number of items presented at any one time. Also covering or removing part of task stimuli from view at a given time.
- Task simplification: Breaking a task apart into steps or reducing the number of steps or activity into more manageable parts.
- Task specification: Identifying specific relevant features or components of a task prior to an activity that require careful consideration, planning, or attention.
- Work simplification: Identifying if a task or steps in a task can be done using less energy, time, and/or more safely by modifying elements in the environment such as using wheeled equipment, sliding instead of lifting, using shoulder bags instead of handbags to carry items.

Adapted and expanded from Toglia et al. (2012).

APPENDIX B: THERAPY TECHNIQUES IN REHABILITATION
Behavioral Methods

Changing behavior(s) through positive reinforcement using verbal praise for appropriate behavior or tangible rewards for achieving goals that are meaningful to the client. Clients with executive dysfunction should participate in setting the goal(s) and determining the type of reward (verbal, tangible) to be used toward achieving the goal. Clients with severe cognitive impairment or dementia usually need assistance in setting goals and determining the type of reward system to be used.

Chaining

The chosen task is first broken or separated into steps or stages. In forward chaining, the client completes the steps or stages in sequence beginning with the first item and the therapist completes the rest. After the client masters the first item, the client performs the first and second items and the therapist completes the rest. After the client masters the first two items, the third is added and the therapist completes the rest. The process is continued until all items are performed in order by the client. In backwards or reverse chaining, the therapist completes all but the last item, which the client performs until mastered. Then the therapist completes all but the last two items, which the client performs until mastered. Next the therapist leaves the last three items for the client to perform and so forth until all items are performed by the client in a forward chained process.

Cueing

The process of guiding and directing performance through prompts. Cues can be verbal (spoken or written), gesture (pointing or demonstration), physical (guiding or placing a body part), or environmental (color coding, symbols, items to be used). Cueing can be adjusted in form, frequency, and content depending of the level of the client's functional cognition.

Environmental Modification/Manipulation

Clients may be able to perform better if the environment is adjusted to remove or reduce distractions (noise, sounds, clutter, glare, people, animals) or by adding selected items such as light, contrast between background and foreground, safety bars, chairs with arms, built-up handles.

Errorless or Error-Free Learning

Setting up performance tasks so that only correct responses are made without any mistakes. Approach is useful in teaching or reteaching client rote tasks that do not require problem solving, decision making, transfer of training, or generalization to a different environment or setting.

Feedback and Knowledge of Results

Intrinsic feedback occurs through the senses and external feedback occurs through the actions of others (such as therapist response) regarding the effectiveness or efficiency of the client's actions or performance. Feedback is an essential element in learning or relearning a task or occupation. Feedback can be positive or negative, given immediately, delayed or at intervals during the process, or as a summary at completion.

Grading Intervention

Grading involves setting the time, complexity, and therapeutic use of self as parameters in the therapeutic process. The "how," "when," "what," and "how much" depend on the client's needs and progression toward goals and outcomes.

Practice Patterns

Issues are random versus blocked, top-down versus bottom-up, and remedial versus compensatory/adaptive. Clients with higher levels of cognitive dysfunction primarily in the areas of executive function can benefit from random, top-down, and remedial practice approaches. Clients with severe cognitive dysfunction are more likely to benefit from blocked, bottom-up, and compensatory/adaptive approaches. Some clients will need a combination of both as their condition improves or declines.

Shaping

Shaping involves rewarding behavior that approximates the desired behavior. Next, behavior is only rewarded when it more closely resembles the actual behavior desired, and finally, only the desired behavior is rewarded. The approach can be used when various behaviors are involved, including both desirable and undesirable behaviors. Desirable behaviors are rewarded while undesirable behaviors are not, so that the person learns which behaviors are more desirable.

Strategy Training

Technique is used to assist a client to identify his or her own difficulties, then solve problems and implement and evaluate task-specific cognitive strategies to overcome the difficulties.

Adapted from Maskill and Tempest (2017).

Delirium

Also called acute confusional state, toxic encephalopathy, metabolic encephalopathy, substance intoxication delirium, substance withdrawal delirium.

Description

Delirium is "an acute, transient, usually reversible, fluctuating disturbance in attention, cognition, and consciousness level" (Porter, 2018, p. 1871). In contrast, dementia affects mainly memory caused by anatomic changes in the brain, has a slower onset, and generally is not reversible. Delirium is an altered state of consciousness, consisting of confusion, distractibility, disorientation, disordered thinking and memory, defective perception (illusions and hallucinations), prominent hyperactivity, agitation, and autonomic nervous system overactivity. (*Stedman's*, 2011).

- Delirium is a disturbance in attention (i.e., reduced ability to direct, focus, sustain, and shift attention) and awareness (reduced orientation to the environment)
- The disturbance develops over a short period of time (usually hours to a few days), represents a change from baseline attention and awareness, and tends to fluctuate in severity during the course of a day
- An additional disturbance in cognition (e.g., memory deficit, disorientation, language, visuo-spatial ability or perception) is present (American Psychiatric Association, 2013)

Cause

Causes include most disorders and drugs. Delirium may occur at any age but is more common among the elderly. Examples of causes include a recent illness or injury such as a broken hip, an infection in the lung or bladder, new medications, side effects of medications, wrong dose of medication, dehydration, withdrawal from alcohol or drugs, pain, and changes in vision or hearing among others (The Ottawa Hospital, 2016). Multiple causes can occur. Identifying the cause or causes is important in planning and implementing an effective intervention program.

Evaluation/Assessment

Areas
- Activities of Daily Living/Instrumental ADL: self-maintenance
- Education/Work: academic or job performance (paid or volunteer)
- Play/Leisure: type, frequency, location
- Rest/Sleep: sleep disturbance
- Social Participation: frequency, type, location, with whom
- Sensorimotor: changes in motor skills, changes in sensory function
- Cognitive/Perceptual: attention, memory (recent, working), executive functions, agnosia, daytime versus nighttime performance
- Psychosocial: life history, self-awareness, agitation, aggression, restlessness
- Context/Environment: changes in environment
- Comorbidities: substance abuse, infections, injuries, surgery

Instruments
Instruments Developed by Occupational Therapy Personnel
- None identified

Instruments Developed by Other Professionals and Used by Occupational Therapy Personnel
- Confusion Assessment Method (CAM; Inouye et al., 1990)
- Delirium Rating Scale–Revised–98 (DRS-R-98; Trzepacz et al., 2001)
- Glasgow Coma Scale (GCS; Teasdale & Jennett, 1974; also see https://www.glasgowcomascale.org/)
- Intensive Care Delirium Screening Checklist (ICDSC; Bergeron et al., 2001)

- JFK Coma Recovery Scale–R (CRS-R; Giacino et al., 2004)
- Richmond Agitation–Sedation Scale (RASS; Sessler et al, 2002)

Problems/Issues

Activities of Daily Living/Instrumental ADL
- Person may display impairment in performance of daily life activities, which is usually temporary and reversible.
- Person may have difficulty following a conversation.

Education/Work
- Person may display impairment in performance of academic or work tasks, which is usually temporary and reversible.

Play/Leisure
- No information identified.

Rest/Sleep
- Person may experience sleep/wake disturbances.
- Person may drift between being asleep and awake.
- Person may sleep during the day and be awake and restless at night.

Social Participation
- Person may display impairment in ability to participate in social activities, which is usually temporary and reversible.

Sensorimotor
- Person may be hyperactive-agitated or experience hypoactive-psychomotor retardation or shift from one to the other motor action.
- Person may experience edema due to poor positioning, which may decrease mobility.
- Person may experience sensory disturbances (visual, hearing).

Cognitive/Perceptual
- Person may have attention deficit (difficulty paying attention, focusing, or concentrating attention on a task).
- Person may experience periods of amnesia (loss of memory of certain events).
- Person may be forgetful.
- Person may be very worried and upset.
- Person may have disorganized thoughts.
- Person may experience disorientation (person, place, time).
- Person may mix up names, dates, times, and events.
- Person may experience altered state of consciousness.
- Person may have memory deficit (but not permanent memory loss as in dementia).
- Person may demonstrate poor judgment of safety.
- Person may experience perceptual disturbances.
- Person may not recognize family members.
- Person's symptoms may be worse at night than during the day.

Psychosocial
- Person may experience illusions, delusions, or hallucinations.
- Person may experience loss of sense of self.
- Person may experience loss of continuity with life history (dates, events, significant people).
- Person may display behavioral disturbances such as agitation or aggression.
- Person may be uncooperative and unwilling to follow directions.
- Person may wander without apparent sense of purpose.
- Person may display mood swings fluctuating from elation, crying, fearful, or other emotion.

- Person's behavior may be worse (more challenging) at night than during the day.
- Person may be restless (try to climb out of bed at night, pick at blankets or tubes).

Context/Environment

- Person's symptoms or severity of symptoms may change throughout the day.
- Person's symptoms may change depending on the environment (physical, social) or environmental demands.

Intervention/Treatment

Models and programs developed by occupational therapy personnel include delirium management (Morrow & Laxton, 2019), guide for caregivers (The Ottawa Hospital, 2016), delirium prevention (Tobar et al., 2017), occupational therapy enhanced programs (Álvarez et al., 2017a, 2017b; Pozzi et al, 2017), prevention and management program (Amadi, 2013), and sensory approach (Perryman & Smith, 2018). Models and programs developed by other professionals or multidisciplinary teams include the D.E.L.I.R.I.U.M (Rains & Chee, 2017) and nonpharmacological intervention (Oh-Park et al., 2018). The goal is to minimize effects of delirium.

Activities of Daily Living/Instrumental ADL

- Maintain or promote routine performance of basic ADL tasks (eating, dressing, grooming, bathing, toileting).
- Encourage independence by using as few cues as necessary to accomplish performance.
- Be sure to maintain hydration level (drinking fluids or checking to make sure tubes are clear and working properly).

Education/Work

- Usually not possible during episodes of delirium.

Play/Leisure

- Familiar card, board, or computer games may be used to promote awareness and alertness, and visual perception.
- Puzzles (flat or 3D) may facilitate problem solving.

Rest/Sleep

- Adjust lights and sounds to decrease effects at night or during rest periods, and increase during the day or activity periods.

Social Participation

- Engage contact with family and friends. May need to keep visits short or limit number of people visiting at one time.

Sensorimotor

- Polysensory or multisensory stimulation using different sensory inputs may be useful to increase level of alertness (auditory, music, pressure/mechanical, tactile, visual).
- Use stretching or other mild exercises of the upper extremities to maintain functional range of motion and strength.
- Monitor client for signs of fatigue. Shorter more frequent sessions may be necessary.

Cognitive/Perceptual

- Keep instructions simple. One step at a time. Picture or printed instructions may help.
- Reorient person frequently to names, date, place, time of day.
- Create a reminiscence box of objects (obsolete or historical items, familiar songs, childhood games or toys) that can be used to provide conversation in group.
- Provide copies of current newspapers and magazines to read or to provide topics for discussion.
- Cognitive exercises such as word or number puzzles may provide mental stimulation.
- Promote visual perception through activities such as card and computer games.

Psychosocial
- Avoid arguing with person or asking why the person did or did not do a particular action.

Context/Environment
- Be sure person has glasses or hearing aids available (check that they are in good condition).
- Suggest family or caregiver bring items from home that are familiar to the person such as pictures, blanket, music, reading material, photo albums, scrapbooks.
- Provide education to family, caregivers, hospital staff about delirium assessment and management.

Precautions/Safety Considerations
Maintain safety protocols. Client's judgment of safety may be compromised.

Prognosis and Outcome
Delirium usually is self-limiting, lasting a few days. Person should improve over time.

REFERENCES
Álvarez, E., Garrido, M. A., Tobar, E. A., Prieto, S. A., Vergara, S. O., Briceño, C. D., & González, F. J. U. (2017a). Occupational therapy for delirium management in elderly patients without mechanical ventilation in an intensive care unit: A pilot randomized clinical trial. *Journal of Critical Care, 37,* 85–90. https://doi.org/10.1016/j.jcrc.2016.09.002

Álvarez, E., Garrido, M. A., Tobar, E. A., Prieto, S. A., Vergara, S. O., Briceño, C. D., & González, F. J. (2017b). Occupational therapy for delirium management in elderly patients without mechanical ventilation in an intensive care unit: A pilot randomized clinical trial: Dear editor. *Journal of Critical Care, 40,* 265. https://doi.org/10.1016/j.jcrc.2017.03.016

Amadi, A. (2013). The prevention and management of delirium: A student OT's perspective. *OT News, 21*(1), 37.

American Psychiatric Association. (2013). *Diagnostic and statistical manual of mental disorders* (5th ed.). https://doi.org/10.1176/appi.books.9780890425596

Morrow, M., & Laxton, L. (2019). *Delirium management in the ICU: The role of occupational therapy.* AOTA Press.

Oh-Park, M., Chen, P., Romel-Nichols, V., Hreha, K., Boukrina, O., & Barrett, A. M. (2018). Delirium screening and management in inpatient rehabilitation facilities. *American Journal of Physical Medicine & Rehabilitation, 97*(10), 754–762. https://doi.org/10.1097/PHM.0000000000000962

The Ottawa Hospital. (2016). *Delirium: A guide for caregivers.*

Perryman, M., & Smith C. (2018). The green team: Finding occupation in delirium. *OT News, 26*(12), 46–47.

Porter, R. S. (Ed.). (2018). *The Merck manual of diagnosis and therapy* (20th ed.). Merck Sharp & Dohme.

Pozzi, C., Lucchi, E., Lanzoni, A., Gentile, S., Trabucchi, M., Bellelli, G., & Morandi, A. (2017). Preliminary evidence of a positive effect of occupational therapy in patients with delirium superimposed on dementia. *Journal of the American Medical Directors Association, 18*(12), 1091–1092. https://doi.org/10.1016/j.jamda.2017.09.005

Rains, J., & Chee, N. (2017). The role of occupational and physiotherapy in multi-modal approach to tackling delirium in the intensive care. *Journal of the Intensive Care Society, 18*(4), 318–322. https://doi.org/10.1177/1751143717720589

Stedman's medical dictionary for the health professions and nursing (7th ed.). (2011). Wolters Kluwer.

Tobar, E., Alvarez, E., & Garrido, M. (2017). Cognitive stimulation and occupational therapy for delirium prevention. *Revista Brasileira de Terapia Intensiva, 29*(2), 248–252. https://doi.org/10.5935/0103-507X.20170034

BIBLIOGRAPHY

Needham, D. M., Korupolu, R., Zanni, J. M., Pradhan, P., Colantuoni, E., Palmer, J. B., Brower, R. G., & Fan, E. (2010). Early physical medicine and rehabilitation for patients with acute respiratory failure: A quality improvement project. *Archives of Physical Medicine and Rehabilitation, 91*(4), 536–542. https://doi.org/10.1016/j.apmr.2010.01.002

Pozzi, C., Tatzer, V. C., Álvarez, E. A., Lanzoni, A., & Graff, M. J. L. (2020). The applicability and feasibility of occupational therapy in delirium care. *European Geriatric Medicine, 11*, 209–216. https://doi.org/10.1007/s41999-020-00308-z

Dementia

Also called neurocognitive disorders.

See also Memory Impairment, Executive Dysfunction, Alzheimer's Disease, Frontotemporal Dementia, Huntington's Disease, Parkinson's Disease, Stroke: Chronic.

Description

Dementia is "chronic, global, usually irreversible deterioration of cognition" (Porter, 2018, p. 1874). The loss, usually progressive, of cognitive and intellectual functions occurs without impairment of perception or consciousness. Dementia is a progressive organic mental disorder characterized by chronic personality disintegration, confusion, disorientation, stupor, deterioration of intellectual capacity and function, and impairment of control of memory, judgment, and impulses (O'Toole, 2017). The most common types of dementia are the following:

- Alzheimer's disease. See Alzheimer's Disease in Section 11: Cognitive-Perceptual Disorders).
- Frontotemporal dementia: cognitive disorder affecting the frontal and temporal lobes; includes Pick disease (Porter, 2018). See Frontotemporal Dementia in Section 11: Cognitive-Perceptual Disorders.
- HIV-associated dementia: chronic cognitive deterioration due to brain infections by HIV (Porter, 2018). See HIV and AIDS in Section 9: Immunologic and Infection Diseases.
- Lewy body dementia: chronic cognitive deterioration characterized by cellular inclusions called Lewy bodies in the cytoplasm of cortical neurons; often in Parkinson's disease (Porter, 2018).
- Vascular dementia: acute or chronic cognitive deterioration due to diffuse or focal cerebral infarction that is most often related to cerebrovascular disease (Porter, 2018).

Cause

Dementia may result from primary diseases of the brain such as beta-amyloid deposits and neurofibrillary tangles, alpha-syndrome abnormalities, Huntington gene mutation, cerebrovascular disease, ingestion of drugs or toxin, infections, prion disorders, structural brain disorder, depression, hypothyroidism, and vitamin B12 deficiency (Porter, 2018). Dementia also occurs in disorders such as Parkinson's disease, Huntington's disease, Creutzfeldt-Jakob disease, Gerstmann-Sträussler-Scheinker syndrome, and neurosyphilis.

Stages of Dementia (Adapted from Reisberg et al., 1982, Global Deterioration Scale; Levy, 2018)

- No cognitive decline/absence of functional-cognitive disability: Person reports no subjective complaints or there is no evidence on interview or assessment; person is able to retrieve information from memory to be activated and used purposefully to carry out complex occupations with accuracy and safety; person can inhibit automatic responses appropriately.

- Very mild subjective cognitive decline (age-associated memory impairment)/no equivalent in Levy.
  - ► Person complains of memory deficits such as
    - ○ Forgetting where familiar objects have been placed.
    - ○ Forgetting names of familiar, well-known people.
  - ► No objective deficits are present on testing.
  - ► No identifiable deficits are reported from employer or others in social situations.
- Mild cognitive and functional decline (mild cognitive impairment, mental age equivalent 12+)/mild functional decline: Earliest clear-cut deficits.
  - ► Person gets lost when traveling to unfamiliar locations.
  - ► Coworkers are aware of person's relatively poor performance.
  - ► Word and name finding deficit becomes evident to family and close associates.
  - ► Person retains relatively little material from reading.
  - ► Person does not remember names upon introduction to new people.
  - ► Person may lose or misplace object of value.
  - ► Person may demonstrate attention/concentration deficit during testing.
  - ► Person demonstrates decreased performance in demanding employment and social settings.
  - ► Inhibitory processes weaken, such as ability to inhibit autonomic responses and irrelevant cues.
  - ► Information processing slows.
  - ► Episodic memory impairment becomes apparent.
  - ► Semantic memory impairment beings.
  - ► Deficits in executive functioning emerge (planning ahead, problem solving, judgment, multitasking).
  - ► Person has difficulty learning new material.
  - ► Complex IADLs are performed with less efficiency and more errors.
  - ► Person may become impulsive, distractible and less able to anticipate consequences before acting.
  - ► Person may begin to deny loss of cognitive functions.
  - ► Person is still capable of independent living but some help with IADLs may be needed.
  - ► Person can perform basic ADLs without assistance.
- Moderate cognitive decline (mild dementia, mental age equivalent 8–12 years)/moderate decline: Clear-cut deficits.
  - ► Person demonstrates decreased knowledge of current and recent events.
  - ► Person is less able to maintain attention when distractions occur.
  - ► Person is less able to use abstract reasoning and relies more on concrete thinking.
  - ► Person may exhibit some deficit in memory of personal history.
  - ► Person demonstrates concentration deficit elicited on serial subtractions (or similar task).
  - ► Person demonstrates decreased ability to travel, handle finances, and other IADLs.
  - ► Person demonstrates decreased ability to perform complex tasks.
  - ► Person uses denial as the dominant defense mechanism.
  - ► Person frequently withdraws from challenging situations.
  - ► Deficits in executive functioning increase (planning ahead, problem solving, judgment, multitasking).
  - ► Problem solving based on visual information is severely impaired.
  - ► New learning becomes more difficult.
  - ► Processing speed of information slows.
  - ► Person increasingly relies on procedural actions triggered by established memories retrieved from environmentally recognized cues.
  - ► Inhibitory processes markedly decline.

- ▶ Person may not demonstrate any deficits in the following areas:
  - ○ Orientation to time and place.
  - ○ Recognition of familiar persons and faces.
  - ○ Ability to travel in familiar locations.
  - ○ Ability to perform basic ADLs but may require verbal cueing to initiate from a caregiver.
- • Moderately severe cognitive decline (moderate dementia, mental age equivalent 5–7 years)/ no equivalent in Levy.
  - ▶ Person can no longer survive without assistance from a caregiver 24 hours per day.
  - ▶ Person is unable to recall major relevant aspects of his or her current life, such as address, telephone number, names of family members, names of high school or college from which he or she graduated.
  - ▶ Person frequently is disoriented in time (date, day of week, season) or to place.
  - ▶ Person may have difficulty counting backwards from 40 by fours or from 20 by twos.
  - ▶ Person may require assistance in choosing proper clothing to wear.
  - ▶ Person may not demonstrate any deficits in the following areas:
    - ○ Knows own name and those of spouse and children.
    - ○ Person retains knowledge of many major facts about self and others.
    - ○ Person does not require assistance with eating or toileting.
- • Severe cognitive decline (moderately severe dementia, mental age equivalent 2–4 years)/ severe functional decline.
  - ▶ Person may occasionally forget the name of the spouse or caregiver upon whom he or she is totally dependent for survival.
  - ▶ Person is generally unaware of all recent events and experiences in his or her life.
  - ▶ Person may retain some knowledge of life history but details are very sketchy.
  - ▶ Person is generally unaware of surroundings, the year, or the seasons.
  - ▶ Person loses awareness of conventional goals and outcomes in everyday life such as relationship of grocery shopping, meal preparation, eating, and health status.
  - ▶ Person may have difficulty counting backwards from 10 and sometime forwards.
  - ▶ Person's actions may be limited to tactile exploration of objects in the environment.
  - ▶ Actions may be repeated many times to verify that similar results occur.
  - ▶ Person's environment needs to be simplified, and safety proofed.
  - ▶ Person requires one-on-one assistance with all basic ADLs.
  - ▶ Person requires travel assistance but may be able to travel to familiar locations.
  - ▶ Person may experience disturbance of diurnal rhythm (day and night).
  - ▶ A variety of personality and emotional changes occur, such as the following:
    - ○ Delusional behavior such as accusing spouse of being an imposter, talking to imaginary figures in the environment, or talking to own reflection in the mirror.
    - ○ Obsessive symptoms such as continually repeating simple cleaning activities.
    - ○ Anxiety symptoms, agitation, and sometimes violent behavior.
    - ○ Loss of willpower (cognitive abulia) because person cannot carry a thought long enough to determine a purposeful course of action.
  - ▶ Person usually does recall his or her own name.
- • Very severe cognitive decline (severe dementia, mental age equivalent 0–1 year)/very severe functional decline.
  - ▶ Person's attention is focused on internal cues from body movements and touch.
  - ▶ Person loses verbal abilities except from some utterances or a particular word or phrase.
  - ▶ Person is incontinent.
  - ▶ Person requires assistance in feeding.
  - ▶ Behavioral actions are limited to spontaneous and imitated gross motor actions.
  - ▶ Basic psychomotor skills such as ability to walk, sit up, or smile are increasingly lost.
  - ▶ Generalized rigidity and developmental neurologic reflexes are frequently present.
  - ▶ Person responds to pain and sensory inputs only.

  ▶ Person is not capable of setting goals or performing purposeful actions based on external cues.
  ▶ Person requires palliative care (see Terminal Illness, End of Life, Palliative Care, and Hospice in Section 13: Lifestyle Conditions).

Evaluation/Assessment

Areas

- Activities of Daily Living/Instrumental ADL: eating, continence, dressing, hygiene, meal preparation, finances, shopping, communication, telephoning, housekeeping, medications, driving
- Education/Work: work status, job requirements
- Play/Leisure: interests, types of hobbies, frequency, location
- Rest/Sleep: sleep disturbance
- Social Participation: types of activities, frequency, location, with whom
- Sensorimotor: visuospatial orientation, praxis (motor planning), visuoconstructional ability
- Cognitive/Perceptual: attention and concentration, memory and learning, executive functions
- Psychosocial: self-awareness, depression, anxiety, aggression, agitation, delusions, hallucinations, apathy, disinhibition
- Context/Environment: home and environmental modification, safety check, caregiver education
- Comorbidities: older adult, genetic disorders, neurological disorders

Instruments

Instruments Developed by Occupational Therapy Personnel

- Assessment of Awareness of Disability (AAD; Tham et al., 1999; Kottorp, 2006)
- Assessment of Motor and Process Skills (8th ed.; AMPS-8; Fisher & Bray Jones, 2016)
- Disability Assessment for Dementia (DAD; Gélinas & Gauthier, 1994; Gélinas et al., 1999)
- Instrumental Activities of Daily Living Profile (IADL Profile; Bottari et al., 2009; see also Bier et al., 2016, in References)
- Participation in Activities and Places Outside Home Questionnaire (ACT-OUT; Margot-Cattin et al., 2019, in References; see also Gaber et al., 2019, in References)
- Perceive, Recall, Plan, Perform (PRPP) System of Task Analysis (Chapparo & Ranka, 2014; see also Steultjens et al., 2012, in References)
- Pool Activity Level (PAL) Instrument for Occupational Profiling (4th ed.; Pool, 2012; see also Dudzinski, 2016, in References)
- Residential Environment Impact Scale (REIS; Fisher et al., 2014)

Instruments Developed by Other Professionals and Used by Occupational Therapy Personnel

- Advanced Activities of Daily Living (A-ADL; De Vriendt et al., 2013)
- Cornell Scale for Depression in Dementia (CSDD; Alexopoulos et al., 1988)
- Dementia Care Mapping (DCM; Bradford Dementia Group, 1997; see also du Toit & Surr, 2012, in References)
- Geriatric Depression Scale (GDS; Yesavage et al., 1982–1983)
- Global Deterioration Scale (GDS; Reisberg et al., 1982)
- Index of Activities of Daily Living (Index of IADL; Katz et al., 1963)
- Instrumental Activities of Daily Living Scale (IADL or LIADL; Lawton & Brody, 1969)
- Interview for Deterioration in Daily Living Activities in Dementia (IDDD; Teunisse & Derix, 1997)
- Mini-Mental Status Examination (MMSE; Folstein et al., 1975)
- Multidimensional Observation for Elderly Subjects (MOSES; Heimes et al., 1987)
- Neuropsychiatric Inventory Questionnaire (NPI-Q; Cummings et al., 1994)
- Quality of Life in Alzheimer's Disease (QOL-AD; Logsdon et al., 2007)
- Rowland Universal Dementia Assessment Scale (RUDAS; Storey et al., 2004; see also Joliffe et al., 2015, in References)

- Vitality Index (VI; Toba et al., 2002)
- Zarit Burden Interview (ZARIT-BI; Zarit et al., 1980)

Problems/Issues

Activities of Daily Living/Instrumental ADL

- Person may experience difficulty with daily activities related to difficulty planning, organizing, and sequencing tasks.
- Person may experience language disturbance (expressive and receptive aphasia, word finding/anomia).

Education/Work

- Person usually is unable to continue paid or volunteer work activities unless directly supervised during repetitive tasks.

Play/Leisure

- Person may not initiate or engage in favorite leisure activities.

Rest/Sleep

- Person may have sleep/wake disturbances.

Social Participation

- Person may become socially withdrawn.
- Person may discontinue participating in familiar social activities.

Sensorimotor

- Person may experience apraxia (difficulty with motor planning).
- Person may experience altered sensory perception (vision, hearing).

Cognitive/Perceptual

- Person may have attention deficit (short attention span, difficulty concentrating or focusing attention on task).
- Person usually has memory loss, beginning with short-term and working memory.
- Person may have disorganized thoughts.
- Person may become disoriented (person, place, and time including day, month, year, season).
- Person may have disturbances in executive functioning (planning sequencing, organizing, abstracting).
- Person may have difficulty identifying objects (agnosia).

Psychosocial

- Person may experience hallucinations.
- Person gradually experiences loss of sense of self.
- Person gradually experiences loss of continuity with life history (facts, dates, and events).
- Person may experience behavioral changes such as agitation and aggression.
- Person may wander without apparent sense of direction.
- Person may experience mood swings (affective lability).

Context/Environment

- Person may be unable to navigate environment without getting lost.
- Environmental modification may be needed to ensure safety and protect again injury or wandering behavior.
- Assistive technology may be needed to assist client and caregivers to perform everyday tasks.

Intervention/Treatment

Models of practice and programs developed by occupational therapy personnel include the cognitive disabilities model (Levy, 2018), Community Occupational Therapy in Dementia (COTiD;

Döpp et al., 2015; Hynes et al., 2016; Van't Leven et al., 2012), environment design (Clarke, 2015), home support program (HoSt-D; Clarkson et al., 2017), home visit program (Bennett et al., 2019; Nishida et al., 2017), Interdisciplinary Home-bAsed Reablement (I-HARP; Jeon et al., 2019), Kawa model (du Toit & Surr, 2012), lifestyle matters (Andrew, 2014), multicomponent rehabilitation program (Cornelis et al., 2018), occupational adaptation model (McKay, 2019), parametric speaker and music program (Nishiura et al., 2018), personalized email support intervention (Chiu et al., 2010), self-management program (Coe et al., 2019), stages of dementia (Sarsak, 2018), and Stepping Stones (Han & Brown, 2018). Models and programs developed by other professionals but used by occupational therapy personnel include ambient assisted living (Hwang et al., 2017; Hwang et al., 2015); assistive technology (Kenigsberg et al., 2019); Care of People with dementia in their Environments (COPE; Clemson et al., 2018); cognitive stimulation therapy (Yuill & Hollis, 2011); cooking task (Bier et al., 2013; Bier et al., 2011); Describe, Investigate, Create and Evaluate (DICE) approach (Fraker et al., 2014); memory clinic (Kumar et al., 2013); person-centered care model (du Toit & Surr, 2012); photo documentation (Brorsson et al., 2020; Brorsson et al., 2016); reminiscence program (Nakamae et al., 2014); remotivation process (Raber et al., 2016); Tailored Activity Program, (TAP-VA; Gitlin et al, 2018; Gitlin et al., 2010; Gitlin et al., 2017; Marx et al., 2019); and videophone (Boman, Lundberg, et al., 2014; Boman, Nygård, & Rosenberg, 2014). Team members may include physicians, nursing personnel, social workers, physical therapists, and occupational therapy personnel. Goals include "maintenance or remediation of cognitive function, compensation for deficits, reduction of be havioral symptoms and facilitation of supportive social and care giving relationships" (Yuill & Hollis, 2011, p. 165).

Activities of Daily Living/Instrumental ADL
- Assist in monitoring and modifying as needed ADLs such as dressing, toileting, feeding, and functional mobility.
- Assist person and family in determining when driving and unsupervised travel, including shopping, should stop.

Education/Work
- Assist person in planning for retirement from paid work.
- Person may be able to continue repetitive tasks in highly structured environment.

Play/Leisure
- Provide vintage (old time) objects familiar to client(s) when younger.
- Explore interests previously known to client but may have been neglected for many years.

Rest/Sleep
- See Sleep–Wake Disorders in Section 13: Lifestyle Conditions.

Social Participation
- Modify social activities from active participation to passive observer as dementia symptoms progress.

Sensorimotor
- Enhance contrast sensitivity of light and dark to aid identification and location.
- Use of color to personalize and aid identification.
- Use sensory cues to clue motor behavior (running water to promote bathing, lay out clothes to promote dressing).

Cognitive/Perceptual
- Use scheduling (time management) to provide predictability in routine.
- Repeat orienting information frequently.
- Order use of cues from verbal to gestures to physical assistance as dementia progresses.

Psychosocial
- Use sensory stimulation or sensory dampening to facilitate control of behavior.
- Use reminiscence group approaches to support memory of life history and past events.

Context/Environment
- Assist in modifying environment to aid in orientation, ensure safety from injury (falls, cuts from sharps, burns) or wandering behavior.
- Assist in selection and use of assistive technology to facilitate care (assistive technology is more useful to caregivers than to client).
- Assist family or caregivers to adjust daily routine to accommodate change in person's ability to function independently, including the need for role performance reversal and increased caregiving responsibilities.
- Provide information and resources to family or caregivers regarding progression of symptoms and management of dementia in the home or care facility.

Precautions/Safety Considerations
- Person is at risk for seizures in all stages of dementia due to changes in brain anatomy and physiology.
- Person is at risk for wandering away from home (or any living situation) and getting lost; precautions are needed to ensure physical safety.
- Person is at risk for falls; evaluate environment to reduce fall risk.
- Person is at risk for injury from sharps or excessive heat; remove or lock up sharp knives and scissors, unplug or remove knobs from stove, reduce temperature of hot water.

Prognosis and Outcome

Dementia is progressive and permanent, but the rate of progression varies widely and depends on the cause. Dementia shortens life expectancy, but survival rates vary (Porter, 2018). Admission criteria for dementia care units includes "lack of socially inappropriate behaviors, dependency in activities of daily living, and inability to participate in dementia care activities" (Mortenson & Bishop, 2016).

Cost Effectiveness

A study by Gitlin et al. (2010) identified a cost saving to caregivers of 1 extra hour per day doing things for the client at a cost of $2.37 per day, and 1 extra hour per day of being on duty to care for client at a cost of $1.10 per day.

REFERENCES

Andrew, C. (2014). Lifestyle matters for people with dementia. *OT News, 22*(3), 36–37.

Bennett, S., Laver, K., Voigt-Radloff, S., Letts, L., Clemson, L., Graff, M., Wiseman, J., & Gitlin, L. (2019). Occupational therapy for people with dementia and their family carers provided at home: A systematic review and meta-analysis. *BMJ Open, 9*(11), Article e026308. https://doi.org/10.1136/bmjopen-2018-026308

Bier, N., Belchior, P. D. C., Paquette, G., Beauchemin, É., Lacasse-Champagne, A., Messier, C., Pellerin, M.-L., Petit, M., Mioshi, E., & Bottari, C. (2016). The Instrumental Activity of Daily Living Profile in Aging: A feasibility study. *Journal of Alzheimer's Disease, 52*(4), 1361–1371. https://doi.org/10.3233/JAD-150957

Bier, N., Bottari, C., Hudon, C., Joubert, S., Paquette, G., & Macoir, J. (2013). The impact of semantic dementia on everyday actions: Evidence from an ecological study. *Journal of the International Neuropsychological Society, 19*(2), 162–172. https://doi.org/10.1017/S1355617712001105

Bier, N., Macoir, J., Joubert, S., Bottari, C., Chayer, C., Pigot, H., Giroux, S., & SemAssist Team. (2011). Cooking "shrimp à la Créole": A plot study of an ecological rehabilitation in semantic dementia. *Neuropsychological Rehabilitation, 21*(4), 455–483. https://doi.org/10.1080/0960 2011.2011.580614

Boman, I. L., Lundberg, S., Starkhammar, S., & Nygård, L. (2014). Exploring the usability of a videophone mock-up for persons with dementia and their significant others. *BMC Geriatrics, 14*, Article 49. https://doi.org/10.1186/1471-2318-14-49

Boman, I. L., Nygård, L., & Rosenberg, L. (2014). Users' and professionals' contributions in the process of designing an easy-to-use videophone for people with dementia. *Disability and Rehabilitation Assistive Technology, 9*(2), 164–172. https://doi.org/10.3109/17483107.2013.769124

Brorsson, A., Öhman, A., Lundberg, S., Cutchin, M. P., & Nygård, L. (2020). How accessible are grocery shops for people with dementia? A qualitative study using photo documentation and focus group interviews. *Dementia, 19*(6), 1872–1888. https://doi.org/10.1177/1471301218 808591

Brorsson, A., Öhman, A., Lundberg, S., & Nygård, L. (2016). Being a pedestrian with dementia: A qualitative study using photo documentation and focus group interviews. *Dementia, 15*(5), 1124–1140. https://doi.org/10.1177/1471301214555406

Chiu, T. M. L., Marziali, E., Tang, M., Colantonio, A., & Carswell, A. (2010). Client-centred concepts in a personalized e-mail support intervention designed for Chinese caregivers of family members with dementia: A qualitative study. *Hong Kong Journal of Occupational Therapy, 20*(2), 87–93. https://doi.org/10.1016/S1569-18611170008-0

Clarke, V. (2015). Environmental design in dementia care. *OT News, 23*(9), 28–29.

Clarkson, P., Davies, L., Jasper, R., Loynes, N. Challis D., & Home Support in Dementia (HoSt-D) Programme Management Group. (2017). A systematic review of the economic evidence for home support interventions in dementia. *Value in Health, 20*(8), 1198–1209. https://doi .org/10.1016/j.jval.2017.04.004

Clemson, L., Laver, K., Jeon, Y.-H., Comans, T. A., Scanlan, J., Rahja, M., Culph, J., Low, L.-F., Day, S., Cations, M., Crotty, M., Kurrle, S., Piersol, C., & Gitlin, L. N. (2018). Implementation of an evidence-based intervention to improve the wellbeing of people with dementia and their carers: Study protocol for "Care of People with dementia in their Environments (COPE)" in the Australian context. *BMC Geriatrics, 18*, Article 108. https://doi.org/10.1186/s12877-018-0790-7

Coe, Á., Martin, M., & Stapleton, T. (2019). Effects of an occupational therapy memory strategy education group intervention on Irish older adults' self-management of everyday memory difficulties. *Occupational Therapy in Health Care, 33*(1), 37–63. https://doi.org/10.1080/0738 0577.2018.1543911

Cornelis, E., Gorus, E., Beyer, I., Van Puyvelde, K., Lieten, S., Versijpt, J., Vande Walle, N., Aerts, G., De Roover, K., & De Vriendt, P. (2018). A retrospective study of a multicomponent rehabilitation programme for community-dwelling persons with dementia and their caregivers. *British Journal of Occupational Therapy, 81*(1), 5–14. https://doi.org/10.1177/0308022617728680

Döpp, C. M. E., Graff, M. J. L., Teerenstra, S., Olde Rikkert, M. G. M., Nijhuis-van der Sanden, M. W. G., & Vernooij-Dassen, M. J. F. J. (2015). Effectiveness of a training package for implementing a community-based occupational therapy program in dementia: A cluster randomized controlled trial. *Clinical Rehabilitation, 29*(10), 974–986. https://doi.org/10.1177/0269 215514564699

du Toit, S. H. J., & Surr, C. (2012). Opinion piece: The potential of Dementia Care Mapping as a practice development tool for occupational therapists in South Africa. *South African Journal of Occupational Therapy, 42*(3), 32–39.

Dudzinski, E. (2016). Using the Pool Activity Level instrument to support meaningful activity for a person with dementia: A case study. *British Journal of Occupational Therapy, 79*(2), 65–68. https://doi.org/10.1177/0308022615600182

Fraker, J., Kales, H. C., Blazek, M., Kavanagh, J., & Gitlin, L. N. (2014). The role of the occupational therapist in the management of neuropsychiatric symptoms of dementia in clinical settings. *Occupational Therapy in Health Care, 28*(1), 4–20. https://doi.org/10.3109/073805 77.2013.867468

Gaber, S. N., Nygård, L., Brorsson, A., Kottorp, A., & Malinowsky, C. (2019). Everyday technologies and public space participation among people with and without dementia. *Canadian Journal of Occupational Therapy, 86*(5), 400–411. https://doi.org/10.1177/0008417419837764

Gitlin, L. N., Arthur, P., Piersol, C., Hessels, V., Wu, S. S., Dai, Y., & Mann, W. C. (2018). Targeting behavioral symptoms and functional decline in dementia: A randomized clinical trial. *Journal of the American Geriatrics Society, 66*(2), 339–345. https://doi.org/10.1111/jgs.15194

Gitlin, L. N., Hodgson, N., Jutkowitz, E., & Pizzi, L. (2010). The cost-effectiveness of a nonpharmacologic intervention for individuals with dementia and family caregivers: The tailored activity program. *American Journal of Geriatric Psychiatry, 18*(6), 510–519. https://doi.org/10.1097/JGP.0b013e3181c37d13

Gitlin, L. N., Marx, K. A., Alonzi, D., Kvedar, T., Moody, J., Trahan, M., & Van Haitsma, K. (2017). Feasibility of the tailored activity program for hospitalized (TAP-H) patients with behavioral symptoms. *The Gerontologist, 57*(3), 575–584. https://doi.org/10.1093/geront/gnw052

Han, A., & Brown, D. (2018). Perspectives of caregivers and volunteers on *Stepping Stones* for people with dementia. *Hong Kong Journal of Occupational Therapy, 31*(2), 86–96. https://doi.org/10.1177/1569186118812948

Hwang, A. S., Rosenberg, L., Kontos, P., Cameron, J. I. O., Mihailidis, A., & Nygård, L. (2017). Sustaining care for a parent with dementia: An indefinite and intertwined process. *International Journal of Qualitative Studies on Health and Well-being, 12*(1), Article 1389578. https://doi.org/10.1080/17482631.2017.1389578

Hwang, A. S., Truong, K. N., Cameron, J. I., Lindqvist, E., Nygård, L., & Mihailidis, A. (2015). Co-designing ambient assisted living (AAL) environments: Unraveling the situated context of informal dementia care. *BioMed Research International, 2015*, Article 720483. https://doi.org/10.1155/2015/720483

Hynes, S. M., Field, B., Ledgerd, R., Swinson, T., Wenborn, J., di Bona, L., Moniz-Cook, E., Poland, F., & Orrell, M. (2016). Exploring the need for a new UK occupational therapy intervention for people with dementia and family carers: Community Occupational Therapy in Dementia (COTiD): A focus group study. *Aging & Mental Health, 20*(7), 762–769. https://doi.org/10.1080/13607863.2015.1037243

Jeon, Y., Simpson, J., Low, L., Woods, R., Norman, R., Mowszowski, L., Clemson, L., Naismith, S. L., Brodaty, H., Hilmer, S., Amberber, A. M., Gitlin, L., & Szanton, S. (2019). A pragmatic randomised controlled trial (RCT) and realist evaluation of the Interdisciplinary Home-bAsed Reablement program (I-HARP) for improving functional independence of community dwelling older people with dementia: An effectiveness-implementation hybrid design. *BMC Geriatrics, 19*(1), Article 199. https://doi.org/10.1186/s12877-019-1216-x

Joliffe, L., Brown, T., & Fielding, L. (2015). Are clients' performances on the Rowland Universal Dementia Assessment Scale associated with their functional performance? A preliminary investigation. *British Journal of Occupational Therapy, 78*(1), 16–23. https://doi.org/10.1177/0308022614561236

Kenigsberg, P. A., Aquino, J. P., Bérard, A., Brémond, F., Charras, K., Dening, T., Droës, R.-M., Gzil, F., Hicks, B., Innes, A., Nguyen, S.-M., Nygård, L., Pino, M., Sacco, G., Salmon, E., van der Roest, H., Villet, H., Villez, M., Robert, P., & Manera, V. (2019). Assistive technologies to address capabilities of people with dementia: From research to practice. *Dementia, 18*(4), 1568–1595. https://doi.org/10.1177/1471301217714093

Kumar, P., Tiwari, S. C., Vishnubhatla, S., Kumar, N., Tripathi, R. K., & Dey, A. B. (2013). Profile of older adults in memory outpatients' clinic setting and effectiveness of novel occupational therapy intervention in patients with mild to moderate dementia. *Indian Journal of Physiotherapy and Occupational Therapy, 7*(3), 297–302. https://doi.org/10.5958/j.0973-5674.7.3.111

Levy, L. L. (2018). Neurocognition and function: Intervention in dementia based on cognitive disabilities model. In N. Katz & J. Toglia (Eds.), *Cognition, occupation, and participation across the life span* (4th ed., pp. 499–522). AOTA Press.

Margot-Cattin, I., Kuhne, N., Kottorp, A., Cutchin, M., Öhman, A., & Nygård, L. (2019). Development of a questionnaire to evaluate out-of-home participation for people with dementia. *American Journal of Occupational Therapy, 73*(1), Article 7301205030. https://doi.org/10.5014/ajot.2019.027144

Marx, K. A., Scott, J. B., Piersol, C. V., & Gitlin, L. N. (2019). Tailored activities to reduce neuropsychiatric behaviors in persons with dementia: Case report. *American Journal of Occupational Therapy, 73*(2), Article 730295160. https://doi.org/10.5014/ajot.2019.029546

McKay, H. (2019). The role of occupational therapy in consultation with dementia care teams: An occupational adaptation-based approach. *SIS Quarterly Practice Connections, 4*(3), 22–25.

Mortenson, W. B., & Bishop, A. M. (2016). Discharge criteria and follow-up support for dementia care units. *Journal of Applied Gerontology, 35*(3), 321–330. https://doi.org/10.1177/0733464815577140

Nakamae, T., Yotsumoto, K., Tatsumi, E., & Hashimoto, T. (2014). Effects of productive activities with reminiscence in occupational therapy for people with dementia: A pilot randomized controlled study. *Hong Kong Journal of Occupational Therapy, 24*(1), 13–19. https://doi.org/10.1016/j.hkjot.2014.01.003

Nishida, S., Kondo, S., Takagi, M., Buthod, T., Yamanishi, Y., Koyama, C., & Kamijo, K. (2017). Effectiveness of an occupation-based home-visit program for clients with dementia and caregivers: A pilot study. *Asian Journal of Occupational Therapy, 13*(1), 7–12.

Nishiura, Y., Hoshiyama, M., & Konagaya, Y. (2018). Use of parametric speaker for older people with dementia in a residential care setting: A preliminary study of two cases. *Hong Kong Journal of Occupational Therapy, 31*(1), 30–35. https://doi.org/10.1177/1569186118759611

O'Toole, M. T. (Ed.). (2017). *Mosby's dictionary of medicine, nursing & health professions* (10th ed.). Elsevier.

Porter, R. S. (Ed.). (2018). *The Merck manual of diagnosis and therapy* (20th ed.). Merck Sharp & Dohme.

Raber, C., Purdin, S., Hupp, A., & Stephenson, B. (2016). Occupational therapists' perspectives on using the remotivation process with clients experiencing dementia. *British Journal of Occupational Therapy, 79*(2), 92–101. https://doi.org/10.1177/0308022615615892

Reisberg, B., Ferris, S. H., de Leon, M. J., & Crook, T. (1982). The Global Deterioration Scale for assessment of primary degenerative dementia. *American Journal of Psychiatry, 139*(9), 1136–1139. https://doi.org/10.1176/ajp.139.9.1136

Sarsak, H. (2018). Overview: Dementia and the role of occupational therapy practitioner. *MOJ Yoga & Physical Therapy, 3*(5), 98–100. https://doi.org/10.15406/mojypt.2018.03.00053

Steultjens, E. M., Voigt-Radloff, S., Leonhart, R., & Graff, M. J. L. (2012). Reliability of the Perceive, Recall, Plan, and Perform (PRPP) assessment in community-dwelling dementia patients: Test consistency and inter-rater agreement. *International Psychogeriatrics, 24*(4), 659–665. https://doi.org/10.1017/S1041610211002249

Van't Leven, N., Graff, M. J. L., Kaijen, M., de Swart, B. J. M., Olde Rikkert, M. G. M., & Vernooij-Dassen, M. J. M. (2012). Barriers to and facilitators for the use of an evidence-based occupational therapy guideline for older people with dementia and their carers. *International Journal of Geriatric Psychiatry, 27*(7), 742–748. https://doi.org/10.1002/gps.2782

Yuill, N., & Hollis, V. (2011). A systematic review of cognitive stimulation therapy for older adults with mild to moderate dementia: An occupational therapy perspective. *Occupational Therapy International, 18*(4), 163–186.

BIBLIOGRAPHY

du Toit, S., & van der Merwe, R. (2013). Scientific letter: Promoting person-centred care for people with advanced dementia through environmental adaptation. *South African Journal of Occupational Therapy, 43*(2), 2–4.

Gitlin, L. N., & Piersol, C. V. (2014). *A caregiver's guide to dementia: Using activities and other strategies to prevent, reduce and manage behavioral symptoms.* Camino Books.

Haigh, J., & Mytton, C. (2016). Sensory interventions to support the wellbeing of people with dementia: A critical review. *British Journal of Occupational Therapy, 79*(2), 120–126. https://doi.org/10.1177/0308022615598996

Hall, L., & Skelton, D. A. (2012). Occupational therapy for caregivers of people with dementia: A review of the United Kingdom literature. *British Journal of Occupational Therapy, 75*(6), 281–288. https://doi.org/10.4276/030802212X13383757345184

Iverson, D. J., Gronseth, G. S., Reger, M. A., Classen, S., Dubinsky, R. M., & Rizzo, M. (2010). Practice parameter update: Evaluation and management of driving risk in dementia. *Neurology, 74*(16), 1316–1324.

Jarvis, F., Clemson, L. M., & Mackenzie L. (2017). Technology for dementia: Attitudes and practices of occupational therapists in providing assistive technology for way finding. *Disability and Rehabilitation: Assistive Technology, 12*(4), 373–377. https://doi.org/10.3109/17483107.2016.1173729

Jeon, Y., Clemson, L., Naismith, S., Mowszowski, L., McDonagh, N., Mackenzie, M., Dawes, C., Krein, L., & Szanton, S. (2018). Improving the social health of community dwelling older people living with dementia through a reablement program. *International Psychogeriatrics, 30*(6), 915–920. https://doi.org/10.1017/S1041610217001533

Kim, S.-Y., Yoo, E.-Y., Jung, M.-Y., Park, S.-H., & Park, J.-H. (2012). A systematic review of the effects of occupational therapy for persons with dementia: A meta-analysis of randomized controlled trials. *NeuroRehabilitation, 31*(2), 107–115. https://doi.org/10.3233/NRE-2012-0779

Laver, K., Clemson, L., Bennett, S., Lannin, N. A., & Brodaty, H. (2014). Unpacking the evidence: Interventions for reducing behavioral and psychological symptoms in people with dementia. *Physical & Occupational Therapy in Geriatrics, 32*(4), 294–309.

Laver, K., Dyer, S., Whitehead, C., Clemson, L., & Crotty, M. (2016). Interventions to delay functional decline in people with dementia: A systematic review of systematic reviews. *BMJ Open, 6*(4), Article 1013. https://doi.org/10.1136/bmjopen-2015-010767

Lu, K., Wang, H. K., Yeh, C. C., Huang, C. Y., Sung, P. S., Wang, L. C., Muo, C. H., Sung, F. C., Chen, H. J., Li, Y. C., Chang, L. C., & Tsai, K. J. (2014). Association between autoimmune rheumatic diseases and the risk of dementia. *BioMed Research International, 2014,* Article 861812. https://doi.org/10.1155/2014/861812

Malinowsky, C., Almkvist, O., Kottorp, A., & Nygård, L. (2010). Ability to manage everyday technology: A comparison of persons with dementia or mild cognitive impairment and older adults without cognitive impairment. *Disability and Rehabilitation Assistive Technology, 5*(6), 462–469. https://doi.org/10.3109/17483107.2010.496098

Malinowsky, C., Rosenberg, L., & Nygård, L. (2014). An approach to facilitate healthcare professionals' readiness to support technology use in everyday life for persons with dementia. *Scandinavian Journal of Occupational Therapy, 21*(3), 199–209. https://doi.org/10.3109/11038128.2013.847119

McLaren, A. N., LaMantia, M. A., & Callahan, C. M. (2013). Systematic review of non-pharmacologic interventions to delay functional decline in community-dwelling patients with dementia. *Aging & Mental Health, 17*(6), 655–666. https://doi.org/10.1080/13607863.2013.781121

Monnat, M. L. (2011). Incorporating occupational therapy to decrease agitation in nursing home residents with dementia. *Journal of the American Geriatrics Society, 59*(3), 556–557. https://doi.org/10.1111/j.1532-5415.2010.03297.x

Nickel, F., Barth, J., & Kolominsky-Rabas, P. L. (2018). Health economic evaluations of non-pharmacological interventions for persons with dementia and their informal caregivers: A systematic review. *BMC Geriatrics, 18,* Article 69. https://doi.org/10.1186/s12877-018-0751-1

Ogawa, M., Nishida, S., & Shirai, H. (2017). A qualitative study to explore ways to observe results of engaging activities in clients with dementia. *Occupational Therapy International, 2017,* Article 7513875. https://doi.org/10.1155/2017/7513875

Öhman, A., Nygård, L., & Kottorp, A. (2011). Occupational performance and awareness of disability in mild cognitive impairment or dementia. *Scandinavian Journal of Occupational Therapy*, 18(2), 133–142. https://doi.org/10.3109/11038121003645993

Ojagbemi, A., & Owolabi, M. (2017). Do occupational therapy interventions improve quality of life in persons with dementia? A meta-analysis with implications for future directions. *Psychogeriatrics*, 17(2), 133–141. https://doi.org/10.1111/psyg.12201

Rahja, M., Comans, T., Clemson, L., Crotty, M., & Laver, K. (2018). Are there missed opportunities for occupational therapy for people with dementia? An audit of practice in Australia. *Australian Occupational Therapy Journal*, 65(6), 565–574. https://doi.org/10.1111/1440-1630.12514

Rodakowski, J., Saghafi, E., Butters, M. A., & Skidmore, E. R. (2015). Non-pharmacological interventions for adults with mild cognitive impairment and early stage dementia: An updated scoping review. *Molecular Aspects of Medicine*, 43-44, 38–53. https://doi.org/10.1016/j.mam.2015.06.003

Rosenberg, L., Kottorp, A., & Nygård, L. (2012). Readiness for technology use with people with dementia: The perspectives of significant others. *Journal of Applied Gerontology*, 31(4), 510–530. https://doi.org/10.1177/0733464810396873

Schaber, P. (2019). Neurocognitive disorders (dementia). In C. Brown, V. C. Stoffel, & J. P. Muñoz (Eds.), *Occupational therapy in mental health* (2nd ed., pp. 250–263). F.A. Davis.

Schulte, O. J., Stephens, J., & Ann, J. (2013). Aging, dementia and disorders of cognition. In D. A. Umphred, G. U. Burton, R. T. Lazaro, & M. L. Roller (Eds.), *Umphred's neurological rehabilitation* (6th ed., pp. 835–862). Elsevier.

Simpson, C., Statton, L., & Spencer, S. (2018). Environmental design and dementia. *OT News*, 26(12), 32–33.

Tatzer, V. E. (2019). Narratives-in-action in people with moderate to severe dementia in long-term care: Understanding the link between occupation and identity. *Journal of Occupational Science*, 26(2), 245–257. https://doi.org/10.1080/14427591.2019.1600159

Thinnes, A., & Padilla, R. (2011). Effect of educational and supportive strategies on the ability of caregivers of people with dementia to maintain participation in that role. *American Journal of Occupational Therapy*, 65(5), 541–549. https://doi.org/10.5014/ajot.2011.002634

Voigt-Radloff, S., Leonhart, R., Schützwohl, M., Jurjanz, L., Reuster, T., Gerner, A., Marschner, K., van Nes, F., Graff, M., Vernooij-Dassen, M., Olde Rikkert, M., Holthoff, V., & Hüll, M. (2012). Interview for deterioration in daily living activities in dementia: Construct and concurrent validity in patients with mild to moderate dementia. *International Psychogeriatrics*, 24(3), 382–390. https://doi.org10.1017/S1041610211001785

Wong, C., & Leland, N. E. (2016). Non-pharmacological approaches to reducing negative behavioral symptoms: A scoping review. *OTJR: Occupation, Participation and Health*, 36(1), 34–41. https://doi.org/10.1177/1539449215627278

Executive Dysfunction

Also called disturbance in executive functioning, dysexecutive syndrome.

See also Cognitive Impairment, Memory Impairment, Alzheimer's Disease, Attention-Deficit/Hyperactivity Disorder, Dementia, Down Syndrome.

Description

Executive functions are higher level cognitive processes of planning, decision-making, problem-solving, action sequencing, task assignment and organization effortful and persistent goal pursuit, inhibition of competing impulses, flexibility in goal selection, and goal-conflict resolution. A cognitive disorder that involves impairment of the executive functions may affect such functions as organization, regulation, and perception. Impairments in these fundamental processes can affect performance in many cognitive areas, including processing speed, reasoning, emotional engagement and regulation, perseveration, impulse control, awareness, attention, language, learning, memory, and timing (VandenBos, 2015).

Executive functions often involve the use of language, judgment, abstraction and concept formation, and logic and reasoning (VandenBos, 2015). Executive functions act as an integrated process allowing people to perform complex, novel, and dynamic occupations.

Executive functioning is an umbrella term that includes an interrelated set of abilities that direct and coordinate cognitive control and goal-directed actions (Toglia & Katz, 2018, p. 129). Executive functioning is a construct that involves complex, high-order or high-level abilities, processes, capacities, or functions that draw on, manage, or supervise low-level, primary, or basic elements of metacognition or cognition (Cramm et al., 2016).

Dysexecutive syndrome includes impaired judgment, impulsiveness, apathy, poor insight, and lack of organization, planning, and decision-making, in addition to behavioral disinhibition and impaired intellectual disabilities (Gillen, 2018)

Executive dysfunction is defined as impairment in the ability to think abstractly, plan, solve problems, and synthesize information or start, continue, and stop complex behavior. Executive dysfunction is related especially to disorders of the frontal lobe or associated subcortical pathways. Deficits in executive functioning are seen in various disorders, including Alzheimer's disease and schizophrenia (VandenBos, 2015).

Cause

Multiple causes are involved including human genetics and development, neurologic disease, injuries and disorders, mental illness, and transient or continuing life stresses. Deficits in executive functioning are frequently associated with changes in the neural networks that include the frontal lobe, particularly the prefrontal cortex (VandenBos, 2015).

Evaluation/Assessment

Areas
- Activities of Daily Living/Instrumental ADL: cooking/meal preparation, shopping
- Education/Work: academic performance, work task performance
- Play/Leisure: interests, values, frequency, location
- Rest/Sleep: sleep disorders
- Social Participation: type, frequency, location, with whom
- Sensorimotor: sensory processing
- Cognitive/Perceptual: attention, memory, specific executive function skills listed below:
  - ▶ Ability to orient self to place (topographical orientation) and time (temporal orientation)
  - ▶ Ability to set goals and plan ahead into the future
  - ▶ Ability to organize and prioritize tasks (what to do first)
  - ▶ Ability to make decisions (choose between two or more choices)
  - ▶ Ability to plan how, where, and when to do a task
  - ▶ Ability to organize the set of steps or sequence to complete a task
  - ▶ Ability to initiate/start/begin a task
  - ▶ Ability to anticipate consequence of actions in advance of initiation
  - ▶ Ability to monitor how the task is progressing (self-monitoring)
  - ▶ Ability to problem solve (identify a problem, examine alternative solutions, select best alternative, put solution into action)
  - ▶ Ability to identify and correct errors
  - ▶ Ability to switch gears/look for or consider alternatives (mental flexibility)
  - ▶ Ability to deal with novelty or creativity (new or different situations or scenarios)
  - ▶ Ability to follow the rules (legal laws and regulations, policies and procedures, written and unwritten, social mores and manners)

► Ability to pay/focus/maintain/concentrate attention including start, stop, and restart
► Ability to evaluate the task and performance upon completion to avoid errors (error correction) next time.
► Ability to multitask (do more than one thing at a time)
► Ability to integrate learned information into future tasks (generalization)
► Ability to adjust the speed of processing information (thought to action; Toglia et al., 2012; VandenBos, 2015)

- Psychosocial: emotional self-regulation/self-control/self-monitoring, impulse control/inhibition, self-awareness, motivation, flexibility
- Context/Environment: familiar or unfamiliar (novel, new)
- Development (Infant, Child, Adolescent only): cognitive development, executive function development
- Comorbidities: Alzheimer's disease, attention-deficit/hyperactivity disorder, autism spectrum disorder, cognitive disabilities, dementia, epilepsy, fetal alcohol spectrum disorder, heart failure, multiple sclerosis, neurofibromatosis type 1, Parkinson's disease, schizophrenia, stroke, Tourette's syndrome, traumatic brain injury

Instruments

Instruments Developed by Occupational Therapy Personnel

(Note: Tests with an asterisk have components of executive function but include other functions.)

- Adapted Four-Item Shopping Task (AFIST; Nir-Hadad et al., 2017, in References)
- ADL Profile (Activities of Daily Living Profile; Dutil et al., 1990)
- Assessment of Motor and Process Skills (8th ed.; AMPS-8; Fisher & Bray Jones, 2016)*
- Assessment of Sensory Processing and Executive Functions in Childhood (EPYFEI; Romero-Ayuso et al., 2018, in References)
- Assessment of Time Management Skills (ATMS; White et al., 2013; see also Janeslätt et al., 2018, in References)
- Baycrest Multiple Errands Test (BMET-R; Clark et al., 2017, in References)
- Charge of Quarters (CQ) Duty Task (for servicemembers; Smith et al., 2014, in References)
- Children's Cooking Task (CCT; Chevignard et al., 2010, in References)
- Children's Kitchen Task Assessment (CKTA; Rocke et al., 2008; see also Berg et al., 2012, in References)
- Clinical Reasoning Tool (CRT; Toglia et al., 2012, in References)
- Complex Task Performance Assessment (CTPA; Wolf et al., 2008; see also Wolf et al., 2017, in References)
- Cooking Task (CT; Poncet et al., 2015, in References)
- Do-Eat (D-E; Josman et al., 2010)
- Execution of a Cooking Test (ECT; Chevignard et al., 2000, adult version)
- Executive Function Performance Test (EFPT; Baum & Wolf, 2013; see also Baum et al., 2017; Cederfeldt et al., 2015; Cederfeldt et al., 2011; Conti & Dozzi Brucki, 2018; Hahn et al., 2014; Kim et al., 2017; Rand et al., 2018; Raphael-Greenfield, 2012; Voelbel et al., 2011; and Wolf et al., 2010, in References)
- Instrumental Activities of Daily Living Profile (IADL Profile; Bottari et al., 2009)
- Kettle Test (Hartman Maeir et al., 2005; Hartman-Maeir et al., 2009)*
- Meal Preparation Scale (MPS; Jongbloed et al., 1988)
- Multiple Errands Test–Revised (MET-R; Morrison et al., 2013, in References)
- Performance-Based Measure of Executive Functions (PEF; Chiu et al., 2015, in References)
- Pictorial Interview of Children's Metacognition and Executive Functions (PIC-ME; see Bar-Ilan et al., 2018, in References)
- Rabideau Kitchen Evaluation–Revised (RKE-R; Neistadt, 1992, 1994)
- Rivermead Activities of Daily Living Assessment (R-ADL; Whiting & Lincoln, 1980)
- School Function Assessment (SFA; Coster et al., 1998)

- Virtual Multiple Errands Test (VMET; Rand et al., 2009)
- Weekly Calendar Planning Activity (WCPA; Toglia, 2015, in References; see also Goverover et al., 2020; and Weiner et al., 2012, in References)

Instruments Developed by Other Professionals and Used by Occupational Therapy Personnel

- Behavior Rating Inventory of Executive Function (2nd ed.; BRIEF-2; Gioia et al., 2015; see also Linder et al., 2010, in References)
- Behavioural Assessment of the Dysexecutive Syndrome (BADS; Wilson et al., 1996)
- Behavioural Assessment of the Dysexecutive Syndrome in Children (BADS-C; Emslie et al., 2003)
- Brixton Spatial Anticipation Test (BSAT; Burgess & Shallice, 1997)
- Childhood Executive Functioning Inventory (CHEXI; Thorell & Nyberg, 2008)
- Delis-Kaplan Executive Function System (D-KEFS; Delis et al., 2001)
- Dysexecutive Questionnaire (DQ; part of the Behavioural Assessment of the Dysexecutive Syndrome [BADS]; Wilson et al., 1996)
- Executive Function Route-Finding Task (EFRFT; Boyd & Sautter, 1993; see also Kizony et al., 2011, in References)
- Executive Interview-25 (EXIT-25) and Quick EXIT (Royall et al., 1992)
- Executive Secretarial Task (EST; Lamberts et al., 2010)
- Frontal Assessment Battery (FAB; Dubois et al., 2001)
- Hayling Sentence Completion Test (HSCT; subtest of Hayling and Brixton Tests; Burgess & Shalice, 1997)
- Montreal Cognitive Assessment (MoCA; Nasreddine et al., 2005)
- Multi-Level Action Test (MLAT; Buxbaum, 1998)
- Multiple Errands Test (MET; Shallice & Burgess, 1991; see also Maeir et al., 2011; and Nalder et al., 2017, in References)
- Naturalistic Action Test (NAT; Schwartz et al., 2001)
- Observed Tasks of Daily Living–Revised (OTDL-R; Diehl et al., 2005)
- Preschool Executive Task Assessment (PETA; Downes et al., 2018)
- Ruff Neurobehavioral Inventory (RNI; Ruff & Hibbard, 2003)
- Stroop Color and Word Test (Stroop Test, SCWT; Golden & Freshwater, 2002)
- Tinker Toy Test (TTT; Lezak, 1982)
- Tower of London (ToL; Shallice, 1982)
- Trail Making Test A and B (TMT-A, TMT-B; Bowie & Harvey, 2006; Reitan & Wolfson, 1995)
- Virtual Action Planning Supermarket (VAP-S; Klinger et al., 2004, 2006)
- Wechsler Abbreviated Scale of Intelligence (2nd ed.; WASI-II; Wechsler, 2011)
- Wisconsin Card Sorting Test (WCST; Heaton et al., 1993)

Problems/Issues

Activities of Daily Living/Instrumental ADL

- Person may have difficulty cooking or preparing a meal.
- Person may have difficulty maintaining finances such as paying bills, budgeting.
- Person may have difficulty shopping such as making decisions on what and how much to buy, considering alternatives if desired objects are not available.

Education/Work

- Person may be unable to perform work tasks due to loss of executive function skills.
- Person may make errors while performing work tasks.

Play/Leisure

- Person may discontinue engaging in favorite leisure activities.

Rest/Sleep

- Not discussed.

Social Participation
- Person may withdraw from social activities.

Sensorimotor
- Person may perseverate (repeat the same action many times without purpose).

Cognitive/Perceptual
- Person usually is forgetful (forgetting appointments, forgetting to buy needed items).
- Person may have difficulty with time management (keeping a schedule, getting to appointments on time).
- Person may be disorganized (misplacing items, creating clutter).
- Person may be unable to plan ahead or present a poorly organized plan.
- Person may have difficulty starting/commencing tasks.
- Person may have difficulty completing task, leaving a task half done.
- Person may have difficulty correctly sequencing the steps in a task (steps out of order, deleted, or unnecessary steps added).
- Person may be easily distracted from what he or she was doing.
- Person may demonstrate poor time management skills (allowing too much time or not enough).
- Person may be able to verbally explain what he or she is going to do, but does not complete the action plan.
- Person may have difficulty with abstract thinking.
- Person may confabulate (make up facts or incidents when unable to remember actual information).
- Person may have difficulty dealing with new situations or new information.

Psychosocial
- Person may lack self-awareness of deficits.
- Person may be apathetic and lack motivation.
- Person may be impulsive (buying unneeded items, making hasty decisions).
- Person may demonstrate lack of concern for others.
- Person may have difficulty inhibiting behavior or inappropriate responses.
- Person may disobey social rules of conduct without awareness or remorse.

Context/Environment
- Problems reported by person may differ significantly from those reported by family, friends, or caregivers. Clients may report difficulty with abstract thinking, impulsivity, poor temporal sequencing, and variable motivation. Caregivers are more likely to report person's lack of concern for social rules, lack of concern for others, lack of planning behavior, and euphoria.

Intervention/Treatment

Models and programs developed by occupational therapy personnel include Cognitive Orientation to daily Occupational Performance (CO-OP; Dawson et al., 2014; Ng et al., 2013; Poulin et al., 2017), frontal/executive program (Miyajima et al., 2018), mindfulness parenting program (Mollo et al., 2018), multicontextual approach (Toglia et al., 2011), multidisciplinary rehabilitation program (Poncet et al., 2018), person–environment–occupational performance (Matheson et al., 2011), VMALL (virtual supermarket; Erez et al., 2013), and Weekly Calendar Planning Activity (WCPA; Toglia, 2015; Toglia et al., 2017). Models and programs developed by other personnel include cognitive rehabilitation therapy (CRT; Jones, 2017), computer-based EF Training (COMPUTER; Poulin et al., 2017), exergaming (Hilton et al., 2014), goal management training (Gillen, 2018), metacognitive training (Gillen, 2018), problem-solving training (Gillen, 2018), and Short-Term Executive Plus (STEP; Hildebrandt, 2017). The goal of intervention varies with type of executive dysfunction.

Activities of Daily Living/Instrumental ADL

- Provide step-by-step instructions for simple tasks using visuals and/or audio supports, depending on which sensory input system is most successful for the individual client.
- Have client perform tasks in a familiar environment (unfamiliar environment such as a clinic adversely affects performance, especially in older adults).

Education/Work

- Start with simple and/or familiar tasks using visuals and/or audio supports depending on client preference and response.
- Using a variety of learning strategies such as reinforcement, modeling, shaping, prompting, fading, and chaining to support skill acquisition (e.g., use problem-solving approach from CO-OP model: "Goal, Plan, Do, Check").
- Provide structured situation (coaching, on-site supervision, work hardening) to practice skills needed to perform work task.
- Consider whether modifications to workstation or work environment may facilitate better performance (light, noise, heat, clutter, number of coworkers, height of workstation or monitor, etc.).

Play/Leisure

- Assist client to select one leisure occupation to initiate or reinitiate within current level of executive functioning.
- Select which sensory input system and learning strategy or strategies are most successful for client.
- Provide opportunity to engage in leisure occupation.
- Consider whether modifications of the environment or context may improve performance.

Rest/Sleep

- See Sleep–Wake Disorders in Section 13: Lifestyle Conditions.

Social Participation

- Assist client to select a social activity within the client's current executive functioning.
- Select which sensory input system or systems and learning strategy or strategies are most successful for the client.
- Facilitate opportunity to participate in social occupation.
- Consider whether environmental modifications or adaptations may improve performance.

Sensorimotor

- If motor dysfunction is also present, consider techniques for improving gross or fine motor skills or compensating for dysfunction.
- If sensory dysfunction is also present, consider techniques for improving sensory function or compensating for dysfunction.

Cognitive/Perceptual

- Establish structure (person, place, and time) with the client in his or her daily routine.
- Use step-by-step instructions for simple tasks.
- Use external cue devices (checklists, smartphones, home security systems).
- Use a cueing system (modified from Seo, 2018).
  - ▶ 0 = No cue required. Task performed independently.
  - ▶ 1 = General verbal guidance. Therapist gives direct instructions and answers general questions.
  - ▶ 2 = Gesture guidance. Therapist demonstrates the motions needed to complete the task or shows body motions to reengage the client.
  - ▶ 3 = Direct verbal assistance. Therapist tells client what to do, where to start.
  - ▶ 4 = Physical assistance. Therapist helps the client perform the task.

▶ 5 = Doing for the client. Therapist helps throughout the entire process of performing the task.
- Assist client to develop routines, including modifying and simplifying tasks.
- Use Goal Management Training (GMT).
  - ▶ Stop and ask "What am I doing?"
  - ▶ Define the main goal or task at hand.
  - ▶ List steps to complete task.
  - ▶ Learn the steps, check and ask "Am I doing what I planned to do?"

Psychosocial
- Assist client to develop or increase self-awareness.
- Assist client to develop or improve self-control and regulation skills such as self-instruction, learning problem-solving techniques, and training in goal management.

Context/Environment
- Educate client, family, and caregivers regarding executive dysfunction and effect on daily life functions.
- Assist person to develop a support system.
- Plan the environment in advance (antecedent control) to include only what is needed and eliminate all extraneous items and people.
- Organize living environment (and work environment if still working) for efficiency (keep what is needed and get rid of anything not needed, things needed most within arm's reach).

Precautions/Safety Considerations

Person is at risk for injury including falls due to decreased or loss of judgment of distance and depth and/or impulsive behavior.

Prognosis and Outcome

Variable depending on the underlying cause of the dysfunction. In traumatic brain injury, schizophrenia, or stroke, some remediation may be possible. In conditions with dementia, prognosis is poor.

REFERENCES

Bar-Ilan, R. T., Cohen, N., & Maeir, A. (2018). Comparison of children with and without ADHD on a new pictorial self-assessment of executive functions. *American Journal of Occupational Therapy, 72*(3), Article 7203205040. https://doi.org/10.5014/ajot.2018.021485

Baum, C. M., Wolf, T. J., Wong, A. W. K., Chen, C. H., Walker, K., Young, A. C., Carlozzi, N. E., Tulsky, D. S., Heaton, R. K., & Heinemann, A. W. (2017). Validation and clinical utility of the Executive Function Performance Test in persons with traumatic brain injury. *Neuropsychological Rehabilitation, 27*(5), 603–617. https://doi.org/10.1080/09602011.2016.1176934

Berg, C., Edwards, D. F., & King, A. (2012). Executive function performance on the Children's Kitchen Task Assessment with children with sickle cell disease and matched controls. *Child Neuropsychology, 18*(5), 432–448. https://doi.org/10.1080/09297049.2011.613813

Cederfeldt, M., Carlsson, G., Dahlin-Ivanoff, S., & Gosman-Hedstrom, G. (2015). Inter-rater reliability and face validity of the Executive Function Performance Test (EFPT). *British Journal of Occupational Therapy, 78*(9), 563–569. https://doi.org/10.1177/0308022615575744

Cederfeldt, M., Widell, Y., Elgmark Andersson, E., Dahlin-Ivanoff, S., & Gosman-Hedström, G. (2011). Concurrent validity of the Executive Function Performance Test in people with mild stroke. *British Journal of Occupational Therapy, 74*(9), 443–449. https://doi.org/10.4276/030802211X13153015305673

Chevignard, M. P., Catroppa, C., Galvin, J., & Anderson, V. (2010). Development and evaluation of an ecological task to assess executive functioning post childhood TBI: The Children's Cooking Task. *Brain Impairment*, *11*(2), 125–143. https://doi.org/10.1375/brim.11.2.125 (Scoring included)

Chiu, E. C., Lee, S. C., Kuo, C. J., Lung, F. W., Hsueh, I.-P., & Hsieh, C. L. (2015). Development of a performance-based measure of executive functions in patients with schizophrenia. *PLOS ONE*, *10*(11), Article e0142790. https://doi.org/10.1371/journal.pone.0142790

Clark, A. J., Anderson, N. D., Nalder, E., Arshad, S., & Dawson, D. R. (2017). Reliability and construct validity of a revised Baycrest Multiple Errands Test. *Neuropsychological Rehabilitation*, *27*(5), 667–684. https://doi.org/10.1080/09602011.2015.1117981 (Form in Appendix A)

Conti, J., & Dozzi Brucki, S. M. (2018). Executive Function Performance Test: Transcultural adaptation, evaluation of psychometric properties in Brazil. *Arquivos de Neuro-Psiqulatria*, *76*(11), 767–774. https://doi.org/10.1590/0004-282X20180127

Cramm, H., Krupa, T., Missiuna, C., Lysaght, R., & Parker, K. (2016). The expanding relevance of executive functioning in occupational therapy: Is it on your radar? *Australian Occupational Therapy Journal*, *63*(3), 214–217. https://doi.org/10.1111/1440-1630.12244

Dawson, D., Richardson, J., Troyer, A., Binns, M., Clark, A., Polatajko, H., Winocur, G., Hunt, A., & Bar, Y. (2014). An occupation-based strategy training approach to managing age-related executive changes: A pilot randomized controlled trial. *Clinical Rehabilitation*, *28*(2), 118–127. https://doi.org/10.1177/0269215513492541

Erez, N., Weiss, P. L., Kizony, R., & Rand, D. (2013). Comparing performance within a virtual supermarket of children with traumatic brain injury to typically developing children: A pilot study. *OTJR: Occupation, Participation and Health*, *33*(4), 218–227. https://doi.org/10.3928/15394492-20130912-04

Gillen, G. (2018). Evaluation and treatment of limited occupational performance secondary to cognitive dysfunction. In H. M. Pendleton & W. Schultz-Kohn (Eds.), *Pedretti's occupational therapy* (8th ed., pp. 646–668). Elsevier.

Goverover, Y., Toglia, J., & DeLuca, J. (2020). The weekly calendar planning activity in multiple sclerosis: A top-down assessment of executive functions. *Neuropsychological Rehabilitation*, *30*(7), 1372–1387. https://doi.org/10.1080/09602011.2019.1584573

Hahn, B., Baum, C., Moore, J., Ehrlich-Jones, L., Spoeri, S., Doherty, M., & Wolf, T. J. (2014). Development of additional tasks for the Executive Function Performance Test. *American Journal of Occupational Therapy*, *68*(6), e241–e246. https://doi.org/10.5014/ajot.2014.008565

Hildebrandt, S. (2017). Executive functions. In L. Maskill & S. Tempest (Eds.), *Neuropsychology for occupational therapists* (4th ed., pp. 165–176). Wiley.

Hilton, C. L., Cumpata, K., Klohr, C., Gaetke, S., Artner, A., Johnson, H., & Dobbs, S. (2014). Effects of exergaming on executive function and motor skills in children with autism spectrum disorder: A pilot study. *American Journal of Occupational Therapy*, *68*(1), 57–65. https://doi.org/10.5014/ajot.2014.008664

Janeslätt, G. K., Holmqvist, K. L., White, S., & Holmefur, M. (2018). Assessment of time management skills: Psychometric properties of the Swedish version. *Scandinavian Journal of Occupational Therapy*, *25*(3) 153–161. https://doi.org/10.1080/11038128.2017.1375009

Jones, C. (2017). Brain boot camp: Helping Canadian armed forces members with executive cognitive dysfunction. *Occupational Therapy Now*, *19*(3), 15–17.

Kim, H., Lee, Y. N., Jo, E. M., & Lee, E. Y. (2017). Reliability and validity of culturally adapted Executive Function Performance Test for Koreans with stroke. *Journal of Stroke and Cerebrovascular Diseases*, *26*(5), 1033–1040. https://doi.org/10.1016/j.jstrokecerebrovasdis.2016.12.013

Kizony, R., Demayo-Dayan, T., Sinoff, G., & Josman, N. (2011). Validation of the Executive Function Route-Finding Task (EFRT) in people with mild cognitive impairment. *OTJR: Occupation, Participation and Health*, *31*(1, Suppl.), S47–S52. https://doi.org/10.3928/15394492-20101108-08

Linder, N., Kroyzer, N., Maeir, A., Wertman-Elad, R., & Pollak, Y. (2010). Do ADHD and executive dysfunctions, measured by the Hebrew version of Behavior Rating Inventory of Executive

Functions (BRIEF), completely overlap? *Child Neuropsychology, 16*(5), 494–502. https://doi.org/10.1080/09297041003781884

Maeir, A., Krauss, S., & Katz, N. (2011). Ecological validity of the Multiple Errands Test (MET) on discharge from neurorehabilitation hospital. *OTJR: Occupation, Participation and Health, 31*(1, Suppl.), S38–S46. https://doi.org/10.3928/15394492-20101108-07

Matheson, L. N., Dodson, M. B., & Wolf, T. J. (2011). Executive dysfunction and work: Tying it all together. *Work & Industry Special Interest Section Quarterly, 25*(1), 1–4.

Miyajima, M., Omiya, H., Yamashita, K., Yambe, K., Matsui, M., & Denda, K. (2018). Therapeutic responses to a frontal/executive programme in autism spectrum disorder: Comparison with schizophrenia. *Hong Kong Journal of Occupational Therapy, 31*(2), 69–75. https://doi.org/10.1177/1569186118808217

Mollo, K. S., Merizalde, B. A., & Lape, J. (2018). Increasing competency for parents of adolescents with executive functioning deficits: Enhancing occupational performance with mindfulness. *Open Journal of Occupational Therapy, 6*(3) Article 9. https://doi.org/10.15453/2168-6408.1445

Morrison, M. T., Giles, G. M., Ryan, J. D., Baum, C. M., Dromerick, A. W., Polatajko, H. J., & Edwards, D. F. (2013). Multiple Errands Test-Revised (MET-R): A performance-based measure of executive function in people with mild cerebrovascular accident. *American Journal of Occupational Therapy, 67*(4), 460–468. https://doi.org/10.5014/ajot.2013.007880

Nalder, E. J., Clark, A. J., Anderson, N. D., & Dawson, D. R. (2017). Clinicians' perceptions of the clinical utility of the Multiple Errands Test for adults with neurological conditions. *Neuropsychological Rehabilitation, 27*(5), 685–706. https://doi.org/10.1080/09602011.2015.1067628

Ng, E. M. W., Polatajko, H. J., Marziali, E., Hunt, A., & Dawson, D. R. (2013). Telerehabilitation for addressing executive dysfunction after traumatic brain injury. *Brain Injury, 27*(5), 548–564. https://doi.org/10.3109/02699052.2013.766927

Nir-Hadad, S. Y., Weiss, P. L., Waizman, A., Schwartz, N., & Kizony, R. (2017). A virtual shopping task for the assessment of executive functions: Validity for people with stroke. *Neuropsychological Rehabilitation, 27*(5), 808–833. https://doi.org/10.1080/09602011.2015.1109523

Poncet, F., Swaine, B., Migeot, H., Lamoureux, J., Picq, C., & Pradat, P. (2018). Effectiveness of a multidisciplinary rehabilitation program for persons with acquired brain injury and executive dysfunction. *Disability and Rehabilitation, 40*(13), 1569–1583. https://doi.org/10.1080/09638288.2017.1300945

Poncet, F., Swaine, B., Taillefer, C., Lamoureux, J., Pradat-Diehl, P., & Chevignard, M. (2015). Reliability of the cooking task in adults with acquired brain injury. *Neuropsychological Rehabilitation, 25*(2), 298–317. https://doi.org/10.1080/09602011.2014.971819

Poulin, V., Korner-Bitensky, N., Bherer, L., Lussier, M., & Dawson, D. R. (2017). Comparison of two cognitive interventions for adults experiencing executive dysfunction post-stroke: A pilot study. *Disability and Rehabilitation, 39*(1), 1–13. https://doi.org/10.3109/09638288.2015.1123303

Rand, D., Ben-Haim, K. L., Malka, R., & Portnoy, S. (2018). Development of internet-based tasks for the Executive Function Performance Test. *American Journal of Occupational Therapy, 72*(2), Article 7202205060. https://doi.org/10.5014/ajot.2018.023598

Raphael-Greenfield, E. (2012). Assessing executive and community functioning among homeless persons with substance use disorders using the Executive Function Performance Test. *Occupational Therapy International, 19*(3), 135–143. https://doi.org/10.1002/oti.1328

Romero-Ayuso, D., Jorquera-Cabrera, S., Segura-Fragoso, A., Toledano-González, A., Rodriguez-Martinez, M. C., & Triviño-Juárez, J. M. (2018). Assessment of sensory processing and executive functions in childhood: Development, reliability, and validity of the EPYFEI. *Frontiers in Pediatrics, 6*, Article 71. https://doi.org/10.3389/fped.2018.00071

Seo, S. M. (2018). The impact of group occupational therapy using a cueing system on executive function of preschool-aged children with brain lesions. *Journal of Physical Therapy Science, 30*(2), 339–342. https://doi.org/10.1589/jpts.30.339

Smith, L. B., Radomski, M. V., Davidson, L. F., Finkelstein, M., Weightman, M. M., McCulloch, K. L., & Scherer, M. R. (2014). Development and preliminary reliability of a multitasking assessment for executive functioning after concussion. *American Journal of Occupational Therapy, 68*(4), 439–443. https://doi.org/10.5014/ajot.2014.012393

Toglia, J. (2015). *Weekly Calendar Planning Activity (WCPA): A performance test for executive function.* AOTA Press.

Toglia, J., Goverover, Y., Johnston, M. V., & Dain, B. (2011). Application of the multicontextual approach in promoting learning and transfer of strategy use in an individual with TBI and executive dysfunction. *OTJR: Occupation, Participation and Health, 31*(1, Suppl.), S53–S60. https://doi.org/10.3928/15394492-20101108-09

Toglia, J., & Katz, N. (2018). Executive functioning: Prevention and health promotion for at-risk population and those with chronic disease. In N. Katz & J. Toglia (Eds.), *Cognition, occupation, and participation across the lifespan* (4th ed., pp.129–142). AOTA Press.

Toglia, J., Lahav, O., Ben Ari, E., & Kizony, R. (2017). Adult age and cultural differences in performance on the Weekly Calendar Planning Activity (WCPA). *American Journal of Occupational Therapy, 71*(5), Article 7105270010. https://doi.org/10.5014/ajot.2016.020073

Toglia, J., Rodger, S. A., & Polatajko, H. J. (2012). Anatomy of cognitive strategies: A therapist's primer for enabling occupational performance. *Canadian Journal of Occupational Therapy, 79*(4), 225–236. https://doi.org/10.2182/cjot.2012.79.4.4

VandenBos, G. (Ed.). (2015). *APA dictionary of psychology* (2nd ed.). American Psychological Association.

Voelbel, G. T., Goverover, Y., Gaudino, E. A., Moore, N. B., Chiaravalloti, N., & DeLuca, J. (2011). The relationship between neurocognitive behavior of executive functions and the EFPT in individuals with multiple sclerosis. *OTJR: Occupation, Participation and Health 31*(1, Suppl.), S30–S37. https://doi.org/10.3928/15394492-20101108-06

Weiner, N. W., Toglia, J., & Berg, C. (2012). Weekly Calendar Planning Activity (WCPA): A performance-based assessment of executive function piloted with at-risk adolescents. *American Journal of Occupational Therapy, 66*(6), 699–708. https://doi.org/10.5014/ajot.2012.004754

Wolf, T. J., Dahl, A., Auen, C., & Doherty, M. (2017). The reliability and validity of the Complex Task Performance Assessment: A performance-based assessment of executive function. *Neuropsychological Rehabilitation, 27*(5), 707–721. https://doi.org/10.1080/09602011.2015.1037771

Wolf, T. J., Stift, S., Connor, L. T., Baum, C., & the Cognitive Rehabilitation Research Group. (2010). Feasibility of using the EFPT to detect executive function deficits at the acute stage of stroke. *Work, 36*(4), 405–412. https://doi.org/10.3233/WOR-2010-1045

BIBLIOGRAPHY

Akyurek, G. (2018). Executive functions and neurology in children and adolescents. In M. Huri (Ed.). *Occupational Therapy: Therapeutic and creative use of activity* (pp. 29–49). IntechOpen. https://doi.org/10.5772/intechopen.78312

Bottari, C., & Dawson, D. R. (2011). Executive functions and real-world performance: How good are we at distinguishing people with acquired brain injury from healthy controls? *OTJR: Occupation, Participation and Health. 31*(1, Suppl.), S61–S68. https://doi.org/10.3928/153944 92-20101108-10

Cermak, S., & Toglia, J. (2018). Cognitive development across the lifespan: Development of cognition and executive functioning in children and adolescents. In N. Katz & J. Toglia (Eds.), *Cognition, occupation, and participation across the lifespan* (4th ed., pp. 9–28). AOTA Press.

Chaimaha, N., Sriphetcharawut, S., Lersilp, S., & Chinchai, S. (2017). Effectiveness of therapeutic programs for students with ADHD with executive function deficits. *Journal of Occupational Therapy, Schools, & Early Intervention, 10*(4), 436–456. https://doi.org/10.1080/19411243.20 17.1359131

Connor, L. T., & Maeir, A. (2011). Putting executive performance in a theoretical context. *OTJR: Occupational, Participation and Health 31*(1, Suppl.), S3–S7. https://doi.org/10.3928/153944 92-20101108-02

Cramm, H., Krupa, T., Missiuna, C., Lysaght, R. M., & Parker, K. C. H. (2013a). Broadening the occupational therapy toolkit: An executive functioning lens for occupational therapy with children and youth. *American Journal of Occupational Therapy, 67*(6), e139–e147. https://doi .org/10.5014/ajot.2013.008607

Cramm, H., Krupa, T., Missiuna, C., Lysaght, R. M., & Parker, K. H. (2013b). Executive functioning: A scoping review of the occupational therapy literature. *Canadian Journal of Occupational Therapy, 80*(3), 131–140. https://doi.org/10.1177/0008417413496060

Daunhauer, L. A., Fidler, D. J., Hahn, L., Will, E., Lee, N. R., & Hepburn. S. (2014). Profiles of everyday executive functioning in young children with Down syndrome. *American Journal on Intellectual and Developmental Disabilities, 119*(4), 303–318. https://doi.org/10.1352/1944-7558-119.4.303

Daunhauer, L. A., Gerlach-McDonald, B., Will, E., & Fidler, D. J. (2017). Performance and ratings based measures of executive function in school-aged children with Down syndrome. *Developmental Neuropsychology, 42*(6), 351–368. https://doi.org/10.1080/87565641.2017.1360303

Driscoll, J. (2014). Executive function and occupational therapy: Lessons drawn from the literature and lived experience with 22q11.2 deletion syndrome. *Occupational Therapy Now, 16*(6), 17–19.

Erez, A. B., Rothschild, E., Katz, N., Tuchner, M., & Hartman-Maeir, A. (2009). Executive functioning, awareness, and participation in daily life after mild traumatic brain injury: A preliminary study. *American Journal of Occupational Therapy, 63*(5), 634–640. https://doi.org/10.5014/ ajot.63.5.634

Foster, E. R., Cunnane, K. B., Edwards, D. F., Morrison, M. T., Ewald, G., Geltman, E. M., & Zazulia, A. R. (2011). Executive dysfunction and depressive symptoms associated with reduced participation of people with severe congestive heart failure. *American Journal of Occupational Therapy, 65*(3), 306–313. https://doi.org/10.5014/ajot.2011.000588

Foster, E. R., & Hershey, T. (2011). Everyday executive function is associated with activity participation in Parkinson disease without dementia. *OTJR: Occupation, Participation and Health, 31*(1, Suppl.), S16–S22. https://doi.org/10.3928/15394492-20101108-04

Gilboa, Y., Rosenblum, S., Fattal-Valevski, A., Toledano-Alhadef, H., & Josman, N. (2014). Is there a relationship between executive functions and academic success in children with neurofibromatosis type 1? *Neuropsychological Rehabilitation, 24*(6), 918–935. https://doi.org/10.1080/09 602011.2014.920262

Hellinger, N., Lipskaya-Velikovsky, L., Weizman, A., & Ratzon, N. Z. (2019). Comparing executive functioning and clinical and sociodemographic characteristics of people with schizophrenia who hold a driver's license to those who do not. *Canadian Journal of Occupational Therapy, 86*(1), 70–80. https://doi.org/10.1177/0008417419831399

Hunt, A. W., Turner, G. R., Polatajko, H., Bottari, C., & Dawson, D. R. (2013). Executive function, self-regulation and attribution in acquired brain injury: A scoping review. *Neuropsychological Rehabilitation, 23*(6), 914–932. https://doi.org/10.1080/09602011.2013.835739

Josman, N., & Meyer, S. (2019). Conceptualisation and use of executive functions in paediatrics: A scoping review of occupational therapy literature. *Australian Occupational Therapy Journal, 66*(1), 77–90. https://doi.org/10.1111/1440-1630.12525

Lee, N. R., Anand, P., Will, E., Adeyemi, E. I., Clasen, L. S. Blumenthal, J. D., Giedd, J. N., Daunhauer, L. A., Fidler, D. J., & Edgin, J. O. (2015). Everyday executive functions in Down syndrome from early childhood to young adulthood: Evidence for both unique and shared characteristics compared to youth with sex chromosome trisomy (XXX and XXY). *Frontiers in Behavioral Neuroscience, 9*, Article 264. https://doi.org/10.3389/fnbeh.2015.00264

Lee, N. R., Fidler, D. J., Blakeley-Smith, A., Daunhauer, L., Robinson, C., & Hepburn, S. L. (2011). Caregiver report of executive functioning in a population-based sample of young children with Down syndrome. *American Journal on Intellectual & Developmental Disabilities, 116*(4), 290–304. https://doi.org/10.1352/1944-7558-116.4.290

Mazor-Karsenty, T., Parush, S., Bonneh, Y., & Shalev, L. (2015). Comparing the executive attention of adult females with ADHD to that of females with sensory modulation disorder

(SMD) under aversive and non-aversive auditory conditions. *Research in Developmental Disabilities, 37*(1), 17–30. https://doi.org/10.1016/j.ridd.2014.10.041

Obermeyer, I. (2018). Executive function for school-age students. *SIS Quarterly Practice Connection, 3*(4), 2–5.

Poncet, F., Swaine, B., Dutil, E., Chevignard, M., & Pradat-Diehl, P. (2017). How do assessments of activities of daily living address executive functions: A scoping review. *Neuropsychological Rehabilitation, 27*(5), 618–666. https://doi.org/10.1080/09602011.2016.1268171

Poulin, V., Korner-Bitensky, N., & Dawson, D. R. (2013). Stroke-specific executive function assessment: A literature review of performance-based tools. *Australian Occupational Therapy Journal, 60*(1), 3–19. https://doi.org/10.1111/1440-1630.12024

Poulin, V., Korner-Bitensky, N., Dawson, D. R., & Bherer, L. (2012). Efficacy of executive function interventions after stroke: A systematic review. *Topics in Stroke Rehabilitation, 19*(2), 158–171. https://doi.org/10.1310/tsr1902-158

Preston, J., Ballinger, C., & Gallagher, H. (2014). Understanding the lived experience of people with multiple sclerosis and dysexecutive syndrome. *British Journal of Occupational Therapy, 77*(10), 484–490. https://doi.org/10.4276/030802214X14122630932313

Preston, J., Hammersley, R., & Gallagher, H. (2013). The executive dysfunctions most commonly associated with multiple sclerosis and their impact on occupational performance. *British Journal of Occupational Therapy, 76*(5), 225–233. https://doi.org/10.4276/030802213X136792 75042726

Provencher, V., Demers, L., Gagnon, L., & Gélinas, I. (2012). Impact of familiar and unfamiliar settings on cooking task assessments in frail older adults with poor and preserved executive functions. *International Psychogeriatrics, 24*(5), 775–783. https://doi.org/10.1017/S1041610 21100216X

Schultz-Kohn, W. (2019). Best practices in cognition and executive functioning to enhance participation. In G. F. Clark, J. E. Rioux, & B. E. Chandler (Eds.), *Best practices for occupational therapy in schools* (2nd ed., pp. 457–463). AOTA Press.

Schworer, E., Fidler, D. J., Lunkenheimer, E., & Daunhauer, L. A. (2019). Parenting behaviour and executive function in children with Down syndrome. *Journal of Intellectual Disability Research, 63*(4), 298–312. https://doi.org/10.1111/jir.12575

Shimoni, M., Engel-Yeger, B., & Tirosh, E. (2012). Executive dysfunctions among boys with attention deficit hyperactivity disorder (ADHD): Performance-based test and parents report. *Research in Developmental Disabilities, 33*(3), 858–865. https://doi.org/10.1016/j.ridd.2011.12.014

Stern, A., & Maeir, A. (2014). Validating the measurement of executive functions in an occupational context for adults with attention deficit hyperactivity disorder. *American Journal of Occupational Therapy, 68*(6), 719–728. https://doi.org/10.5014/ajot.2014.012419

Toglia, J., & Berg, C. (2013). Performance-based measure of executive function: Comparison of community and at-risk youth. *American Journal of Occupational Therapy, 67*(5), 515–523. https://doi.org/10.5014/ajot.2013.008482

Waldman-Levi, A., & Obermeyer, I. S. (2018). Addressing executive function in schools. In N. Katz & J. Toglia (Eds.), *Cognition, occupation, and participation across the lifespan* (4th ed., pp. 259–272). AOTA Press.

Wasmuth, S. L., Outcalt, J., Buck, K., Leonhardt, B. L., Vohs, J., & Lysaker, P. H. (2015). Metacognition in persons with substance abuse: Findings and implications for occupational therapists. *Canadian Journal of Occupational Therapy, 82*(3), 150–159. https://doi.org/10.1177/000 8417414564865

Wheeler, S. (2014). Approaches to managing executive cognitive functioning impairment following TBI: A focus on facilitating community participation. In F. Sadaka (Ed.), *Traumatic brain injury.* IntechOpen. https://doi.org/10.5772/57395

Will, E., Fidler, D. J., Daunhauer, L., & Gerlach-McDonald, B. (2017). Executive function and academic achievement in primary-grade students with Down syndrome. *Journal of Intellectual Disability Research, 61*(2), 181–195. https://doi.org/10.1111/jir.12313

Wolf, T. J. (2010). Participation in work: The necessity of addressing executive function deficits. *Work, 36*(4), 459–463. https://doi.org/10.3233/WOR-2010-1049

Wolf, T. J., Barbee, A. R., & White, D. (2011). Executive dysfunction immediately after mild stroke. *OTJR: Occupation, Participation and Health 31*(1, Suppl.), S23–S29. https://doi.org/10.3928/15394492-20101108-05

Zlotnik, S., Schiff, A., Ravid, S., Shahar, E., & Toglia, J. (2020). A new approach for assessing executive functions in everyday life, among adolescents with genetic generalised epilepsies. *Neuropsychological Rehabilitation, 30*(2), 333–345. https://doi.org/10.1080/09602011.2018.1468272

Frontotemporal Dementia

Also called frontal-temporal dementia,
major or mild frontotemporal neurocognitive disorder.

Description

Frontotemporal dementia (FTD) refers to disorders that affect the frontal and temporal lobes of the brain. The dementia is chronic, global, and usually irreversible deterioration of cognition. FTD accounts for about 10% of dementias. Age of onset is usually younger (age 55 to 65) than in Alzheimer's disease, but affects men and woman about equally (Porter, 2018). Note that there is no definitive laboratory or observation diagnostic test for FTD. Diagnosis is based on clinical criteria that are not yet consistent. Classification varies depending on resources consulted. The National Institute on Aging (2019) classification of frontotemporal disorders and the current criteria for diagnosing a major form of frontotemporal dementia are listed below. Most articles in which occupational therapy services are provided focus on the behavior and personality problems.

Cause

Approximately half of FTD cases are inherited. The others involve mutations of chromosome 17q21-22 and result in abnormalities of the microtubule-binding tau protein (Porter, 2018).

Types (National Institute on Aging, 2019)

- Progressive behavior/personality decline
  - ▶ Behavioral variant FTD (bvFTD): Characterized by behavior and personality change assumed to have started in the frontal lobe or evident on magnetic resonance imagery.
  - ▶ Temporal/frontal variant FTD (tvFTD, fbFTD): Characterized by behavior, personality change, or language disorders assumed to have started in the temporal lobe and then to the frontal lobe.
  - ▶ Pick's disease: Term used to describe pathological changes in FTD including severe atrophy, neuronal loss, gliosis, and presence of abnormal neurons (Porter, 2018).
- Progressive language decline
  - ▶ Primary progressive aphasia FTD (PPA, ppaFTD): Characterized by language function deterioration (finding the right words while speaking, hesitation and/or pauses in speech).
  - ▶ Progressive nonfluent aphasia (agrammatic primary progressive aphasia): Characterized by omitting words that link nouns and verbs together, such as *as to*, *from*, or *the*.
  - ▶ Sematic dementia FTD (sdFTD): Characterized by difficulty with word comprehension and understanding language.
- Corticobasal syndrome (CBS): Muscle rigidity, difficulty with fine motor skills and swallowing, language, or spatial orientation problems.
- Progressive supranuclear palsy (PSP): Progressive problems with balance and walking, slow movement, falling, body stiffness, and restricted eye movements.

- FTD with parkinsonism: Movement problems similar to Parkinson's disease, such as slowed movement and stiffness and changes in behavior or language.
- FTD with amyotrophic lateral sclerosis (FTD-ALS): Changes in behavior and/or language, muscle weakness and loss, fine jerks in muscles.

Evaluation/Assessment
Areas
- Activities of Daily Living/Instrumental ADL: basic—changes in eating habits and dietary preferences, hyperorality, communication and language (syntax and fluency), dressing and undressing, bathing/showering, grooming, toileting; independent living—finances, medication management, driving
- Education/Work: work history, work performance
- Play/Leisure: type, level of interest, frequency, location
- Rest/Sleep: habits, routines
- Social Participation: level of interest, frequency, location, with whom
- Sensorimotor: dystonia, gait disorder, tremor, clumsiness, apraxia, neuromuscular weakness
- Cognitive/Perceptual: attention (maintaining and shifting), executive functions (abstract thinking, sequencing tasks, judgment of safety; Note: memory and learning are less affected than in Alzheimer's disease, and visuospatial and constructional tasks are usually preserved)
- Psychosocial: apathy (lack of drive or initiative), emotional regulation (disinhibition), social interaction skills (disinhibition), role performance (decreased), emotional blunting (apathy, empathy, affection), personal safety (wandering away from home), quality of life
- Context/Environment: stress on caregivers, home safety and modification, community services, joint services with speech–language pathologist
- Comorbidities: Alzheimer's disease, motor neuron disease, parkinsonism

Instruments
Instruments Developed by Occupational Therapy Personnel
- Cambridge Behavioural Inventory Revised (CBI-R; Wear et al., 2008)
- Frontotemporal Dementia Rating Scale (FTD-FRS; Mioshi et al., 2010 in References; see also Lima-Silva et al., 2018, in References)
- Mini-Addenbrooke's Cognitive Examination (M-ACE; Hsieh et al., 2015, in References)

Instruments Developed by Other Professionals and Used by Occupational Therapy Personnel
- Addenbrooke's Cognitive Examination III (ACE-III; Hsieh et al., 2013, in References)
- Clinical Dementia Rating (CDR; Morris, 1997)
- Clinical Dementia Rating–Frontotemporal Lobar Degeneration (CDR-FTLD; Knopman et al., 2008)
- Intimate Bond Measure (IBM; Wilhelm & Parker, 1988)
- Social Network Index (SNI; Cohen et al., 1997)
- Zarit Burden Interview–Abridged (ZBI-A; O'Rourke & Tuokko, 2003)

Criteria for Behavioral Variant Frontotemporal Dementia (bvFTD; Adapted from Piguet et al., 2011; Rascovsky et al., 2011)

I. Neurodegenerative disease: Patient must show progressive deterioration of behavior and/or cognition by observation or history

II. Possible bvFTD
- Early (3 years) behavior disinhibition
- Early (3 years) apathy or inertia
- Early (3 years) loss of sympathy or empathy
- Early (3 years) perseveration, stereotyped or compulsive/ritualistic behavior

- Hyperorality and dietary changes
- Neuropsychological profile of executive/generation deficits with relative sparing of memory and visuospatial functions

III. Probable bvFTD: All of the following symptoms must be present to meet criteria
- Meets criteria for possible bvFTD
- Exhibits significant functional decline (by caregiver report or functional scales)
- Imaging results consistent with bvFTD (i.e., frontal and/or anterior temporal atrophy on CT or MRI or frontal hypoperfusion or hypometabolism on SPECT or PET)

IV. bvFTD with defined frontotemporal lobar degeneration (FTLD) pathology: Criterion A and either Criterion B or C must be present
- Meets criteria for possible or probably bvFTD
- Histopathological evidence of FTLD
- Presence of known pathogenic mutation

V. Exclusionary criteria for bvFTD
- Criteria A and B must be answered negatively for any bvFTD diagnosis
- Criterion C can be positive for possible bvFTD but must be negative for probably bvFTD

VI. Additional features
- Presence of motor neuron findings suggestive of motor neuron disease
- Motor symptoms and signs similar to corticobasal degeneration and progressive supranuclear palsy
- Impaired word and object knowledge
- Motor speech deficits
- Substantial grammatical deficits

Problems/Issues
Activities of Daily Living/Instrumental ADL
- Person may develop cravings for sweets or carbohydrates.
- Person may restrict food intake to a few types of food such as cake and ice cream.
- Person may take food from others plates without asking or understanding the social reactions.
- Person may binge eat, especially breads or sweets.
- Person may refuse to eat or forget to eat.
- Person may eat items that are not food substances (pica).
- Person may refuse to get dressed or undressed.
- Person may want to keep same clothes on or not want to wear any clothes.
- Person may have incontinence (have accidents getting to toilet in time).
- Person may refuse to bathe or shower (task too complex, requires undressing, water temperature is too hot or too cold).
- Person may have difficulty with word finding.
- Person may have difficulty with language comprehension including loss of meaning of written words.
- Person may have dysarthria or difficulty with speech production.
- Person may speak fluently, but much of what is said makes little sense within the immediate situation.
- Person may refuse to take medications.
- Person may reduce initiation of sexual activity and responsiveness or engage in hypersexual behavior, increased interest in sex (Ahmed et al., 2015).

- Person may exhibit unsafe driving behaviors (impulsive, poor judgment of safety).
- Person may become excessively religious.

Education/Work

- Person may become argumentative with coworkers or supervisors.
- Person may refuse to change method of performing tasks or adapt to changes in task performance.

Play/Leisure

- Person may lose interest in engaging in favorite occupations.

Rest/Sleep

- Person may have difficulty getting to sleep or staying asleep.
- Person may wander in home or to outside.

Social Participation

- Person may lose interest in participating in social activities.
- Person's behavior may be socially unacceptable (due to disinhibition) such as saying inappropriate remarks, "stealing" food off other people's plates, wandering instead of sitting, not participating in topic of conversation or group task.

Sensorimotor

- In bvFTD, generally no measurable change in sensorimotor functions is observed until severe stage of disorder; any change is age related and not out of norm for age and sex.
- In CBS, PSP, parkinsonism, or ALS types, changes in sensorimotor function may include decreased movement fluency, shuffling gait, falling, muscle stiffness, loss of hand dexterity, and decreased muscle strength.

Cognitive/Perceptual

- Person may have difficulty with sustained and changing focus of (maintain and shifting) attention.
- Person may have difficulty with episodic memory but other types of memory are usually intact.
- Person usually has difficulty with executive functions especially doing sequential tasks, making decisions, exercising good judgment of safety, use of insight into the meaning or significance of one's actions on others, prioritizing, multitasking, self-monitoring.
- Person may experience prosopagnosia or inability to recognize familiar faces.
- Person may experience topographic disorientation and get lost even in familiar environments.

Psychosocial

- Person usually demonstrates apathy, lack of motivation, boredom, listlessness.
- Person may demonstrate lack of emotional regulation (act out, speak out of turn, say socially unacceptable words, perform socially unacceptable acts).
- Person may lack impulsive control without regard for consequences of his or her actions, including lack of social tactfulness.
- Person may become agitated and impatient.
- Person may perseverate (repeating the same word[s] or action[s] over and over even when the word[s] or action[s] no longer makes sense).
- Person may become aggressive if demands are denied or not quickly granted.
- Person may exhibit compulsive behaviors and hoarding of self-selected objects.
- Person may demonstrate emotional blunting (lack of empathy, does not show affection even to loved ones and family members).
- Person may fail to perform expected tasks of social roles (spouse, parent, friend, colleague).
- Person may express delusions comprised of persecutory, somatic, jealous, or grandiose features.
- Person may have visual or tactile hallucinations.

Context/Environment

- Home and neighborhood may be unsafe for person with FTD.
- Caregivers may not know how to manage person with FTD.
- Caregivers may be experiencing increased stress and fatigue greater than in other forms of dementia (Mioshi, Foxe, et al., 2013).
- Community and internet resources may be limited or unavailable.
- Access to other professionals such as speech–language pathologist may be limited.
- Misdiagnosis is common including schizophrenia, motor neuron disease, Alzheimer's disease, delirium, other types of dementia.

Intervention/Treatment

Models and programs developed by occupational therapy personnel include case study (Association for Frontotemporal Degeneration, 2016; Guilmette & Hoffman, 2014). Models and programs developed by other professionals but used by occupational therapy personnel include caregivers program (Mioshi, McKinnon, et al., 2013) and tailored activity program (O'Connor et al., 2019; O'Connor et al., 2013). Team members include physicians, nurses, psychologists, social workers, and speech–language-pathologists. Goals are to modify the environment to support memory, orientation, and promote safety. For example, environment should be bright, cheerful, and familiar (photos, favorite objects) and should reinforce orientation to time and place (clocks, calendars), and include safety features such as a signal monitoring system for clients who wander (Porter, 2018).

Activities of Daily Living/Instrumental ADL

- Eating/diet
  - ▶ Alter how food is served: vegetables can be offered with dip, sauce, or gravy; serve carrot cake, peaches, and ice cream.
  - ▶ Serve food with high calories (more gravy) if weight loss occurs, or add calorie drinks.
  - ▶ Create a visual meal schedule to remind person when food is being served.
  - ▶ Popsicles and soups may facilitate increasing fluid intake.
- Dressing/undressing
  - ▶ Consider buying larger-sized clothing that is easier to put on.
  - ▶ Buy clothing with elastic waistbands that are easy to get off and pull up after toileting.
  - ▶ Get slip-on shoes (sandals, loafers) or shoes with Velcro fasteners.
  - ▶ If undressing at inappropriate times is an issue, jumpsuits with zipper in back may solve problem.
  - ▶ If changing clothes is a problem, tie changing clothes to toileting or bathing.
- Bathing/showering
  - ▶ Consider whether changing time of day may make bathing or showering easier.
  - ▶ Consider changing from tub or shower to sponge bathing.
  - ▶ Consider sponge bathing upper half today and lower half tomorrow.
  - ▶ Provide a reward for completing bathing/showering task.
- Grooming
  - ▶ Consider a shorter haircut that is easier to style and care for.
  - ▶ Consider an electric shaver instead of a razor to increase safety.
- Brushing teeth
  - ▶ A children's toothpaste with increased sweetness may be more acceptable.
  - ▶ Try different mouth rinses.
- Toileting
  - ▶ Consider creating a toileting schedule.
  - ▶ Consider placing a commode next to the bed at night or near where person sits during the day (a curtain for privacy may help).

- ▶ Adding a bell to the bathroom door may alert caregiver when person uses toilet at night.
- ▶ Reduce fluid intake at 6 p.m. and avoid caffeine to decrease chance of bed-wetting.
- Communication
  - ▶ Talk in a slow, calm tone.
  - ▶ Reduce distractions such as background sounds or sights.
  - ▶ Communicate at eye level.
  - ▶ Avoid open-ended questions.
- Finances
  - ▶ Review with family current spending habits.
  - ▶ Consider whether changes in spending habits (use of credit or debit cards, writing checks) should be changed.
- Medications
  - ▶ Provide information on rationale for medications.
  - ▶ Set up a medication schedule such as taking pill(s) before meals or before bedtime.
- Driving
  - ▶ Review driving habits and consider whether driving should be revoked.
  - ▶ Arrange alternate forms of transportation.

Education/Work

- Retirement or phased retirement appears to be the best approach because the disorder is progressive.
- Work-task modification (work simplification) or workplace modification (reduce distractions, change location of workstation) may help in the short term.

Play/Leisure

- Encourage engagement in leisure occupations; modify existing occupations by simplifying.
- Encourage exploration of new leisure occupations that are within client's functional ability level.

Rest/Sleep

- Decrease caffeine intake and screen time (TV, computer) close to set bedtime schedule.
- Encourage activity during the day.
- Set a scheduled time for starting bedtime routine and going to bed.
- Use of aroma therapy or essential oils such as lavender may help.

Social Participation

- Encourage participation in social activities; modification may be necessary such as limiting amount of time, travel distance, number of other participants, educating family and friends regarding the disorder and its associated behavior and personality changes.

Sensorimotor

- Not usually a major issue in bvFTD.

Cognitive/Perceptual

- Attention
  - ▶ Organize participation into short time periods based on individual performance.
  - ▶ Control environment to decrease distractions.
- Memory
  - ▶ Use activities in the "here and now."
  - ▶ Reminiscent activities may not be useful because of decreased episodic memory.
- Executive functions
  - ▶ Limit choices to two items (beef or chicken, carrots or beans, potatoes or rice).
  - ▶ Pictures may facilitate sequential task performance and setting a daily schedule.
  - ▶ Safety may require alarms on doors or painting doors and walls the same color so as to make doors less obvious.

➤ Avoid arguing with client (change the activity or subject) or expecting client to self-monitor behavior (therapist or caregiver must monitor).

Psychosocial

- Avoid arguing or reasoning with client about behavioral issues because client cannot control behavior or have insight that behavior is unusual or upsetting to others.
- Attempt to control environment (social and physical) in advance to reduce incident of unwanted behavior occurring (e.g., if client tends to lick and mouth small figurine objects sitting on the mantle, remove the figurines to storage or place in a locked cabinet).
- Maintaining a consistent schedule can help manage behavior.

Context/Environment

- Provide caregiver(s) with information about symptoms and assist in developing management strategies.
- Provide information on available community and internet resources.

Precautions/Safety Considerations

Client may wander away from home; safety alarms on doors, notification of police of condition may be useful. Client may be taking medications for conditions the client does not have due to misdiagnosis. Side effects from those medications may be masking or exaggerating symptoms associated with FTD. Review of existing medications and reasons for prescribing the medication may be useful in developing an effective plan of care.

Prognosis and Outcome

FTD is a progressive disorder and there is no known effective cure. Treatment is supportive based on symptoms. In severe stage, client is bedridden.

REFERENCES

Ahmed, R. M., Kaizik, C., Irish, M., Mioshi, E., Dermody, N., Kiernan, M. C., Piguet, O., & Hodges, J. R. (2015). Characterizing sexual behavior in frontotemporal dementia. *Journal of Alzheimer's Disease, 46*(3), 677–686. https://doi.org/10.3233/JAD-150034

Association for Frontotemporal Degeneration. (2016). Think like an occupational therapist: The importance of individual activities in FTD care. *Partners in FTD Care*. https://www.theaftd .org/issue-19-the-importance-of-individualized-activities-in-ftd-care/

Guilmette, J., & Hoffman, P. (2014). Fronto-temporal dementia. *OT Practice, 19*(3), 13–17.

Hsieh, S., McGrory, S., Leslie, F., Dawson, K., Ahmed, S., Butler, C. R., Rowe, J. B., Mioshi, E., & Hodges, J. R. (2015). The Mini-Addenbrooke's Cognitive Examination: A new assessment tool for dementia. *Dementia and Geriatric Cognitive Disorders, 39*, 1–11. https://doi.org/10.1159/00 0366040

Hsieh, S., Schubert, S., Hoon, C., Mioshi, E., & Hodges, J. R. (2013). Validation of the Addenbrooke's Cognitive Examination III in frontotemporal dementia and Alzheimer's disease. *Dementia and Geriatric Cognitive Disorders, 36*(3-4), 242–250. https://doi.org/10.1159/ 000351671

Lima-Silva, T. B., Bahia, V. S., Cecchini, M., Cassimiro, L., Guimarães, H. C., Gambogi, L. B., Caramelli, P., Balthazar, M., Damasceno, B., Brucki, S. M. D., de Souza, L. C., Nitrini, R., Mioshi, E., & Yassuda, M. S. (2018). Validity and reliability of the Frontotemporal Dementia Rating Scale (FTD-FRS) for the progression and staging of dementia in Brazilian patients. *Alzheimer Disease and Associated Disorders, 32*(3), 220–225. https://doi.org/10.1097/WAD.0000000000000246

Mioshi, E., Foxe, D., Leslie, F., Savage, S., Hsieh, S., Miller, L., Hodges, J. R., & Piguet, O. (2013). The impact of dementia severity on caregiver burden in frontotemporal dementia and Alzheimer disease. *Alzheimer Disease and Associated Disorders, 27*(1), 68–73. https://doi.org/10.1097/ WAD.0b013e318247a0bc

Mioshi, E., Hsieh, S., Savage, S., Hornberger, M., & Hodges, J. R. (2010). Clinical staging and disease progression in frontotemporal dementia. *Neurology, 74*(20), 1591–1597. https://doi.org/10.1212/WNL.0b013e3181e04070

Mioshi, E., McKinnon, C., Savage, S., O'Connor, C. M., & Hodges, J. R. (2013). Improving burden and coping skills in frontotemporal dementia caregivers: A pilot study. *Alzheimer Disease and Associated Disorders, 27*(1), 84–86.

National Institute on Aging. (2019). *What are frontotemporal disorders? Causes, symptoms, and treatment.* https://www.nia.nih.gov/health/what-are-frontotemporal-disorders

O'Connor, C., Clemson, L., Brodaty, H., Low, L., Jeon, Y., Gitlin, L., Piguet, O., & Mioshi, E. (2019). The tailored activity program (TAP) to address behavioral disturbances in frontotemporal dementia: A feasibility and pilot study. *Disability and Rehabilitation, 41*(3), 299–310. https://doi.org/10.1080/09638288.2017.1387614

O'Connor, C., Clemson, L., da Silva, T. B. L., Piguet, O., Hodges, J. R., & Mioshi, E. (2013). Enhancement of carer skills and patient function in the non-pharmacological management of frontotemporal dementia (FTD): A call for randomised controlled studies. *Dementia & Neuropsychologia, 7*(2), 143–150. https://doi.org/10.1590/S1980-57642013DN70200002

Piguet, O., Hornberger, M., Mioshi, E., & Hodges, J. R. (2011). Behavioural-variant frontotemporal dementia: Diagnosis, clinical staging, and management. *Lancet Neurology, 10*(2), 162–172. https://doi.org/10.1016/S1474-4422(10)70299-4

Porter, R. S. (Ed.). (2018). *The Merck manual of diagnosis and therapy* (20th ed.). Merck Sharp & Dohme.

Rascovsky, K., Hodges, J. R., Knopman, D., Mendez, M. F., Kramer, J. H., Neuhaus, J., van Swieten, J. C., Seelaar, H., Dopper, E. G. P., Onyike, C. U., Hillis, A. E., Josephs, K. A., Boeve, B. F., Kertesz, A., Seeley, W. W., Rankin, K. P., Johnson, J. K., Gorno-Tempini, M.-L., Rosen, H., . . . Miller, B. L. (2011). Sensitivity of revised diagnostic criteria for the behavioural variant of frontotemporal dementia. *Brain, 134*(9), 2456–2477. https://doi.org/10.1093/brain/awr179

BIBLIOGRAPHY

Devenney, E. M., Landin-Romero, R., Irish, M., Hornberger, M., Mioshi, E., Halliday, G. M., Kiernan, M. C., & Hodges, J. R. (2017). The neural correlates and clinical characteristics of psychosis in the frontotemporal dementia continuum and the C9orf72 expansion. *NeuroImage: Clinical, 13*, 439–445. https://doi.org/10.1016/j.nicl.2016.11.028

Hornberger, M., Savage, S., Hsieh, S., Mioshi, E., Piguet, O., & Hodges, J. R. (2010). Orbitofrontal dysfunction discriminates behavioral variant frontotemporal dementia from Alzheimer's disease. *Dementia and Geriatric Cognitive Disorders, 30*(6), 547–552. https://doi.org/10.1159/000321670

Kaizik, C., Caga, J., Camino, J., O'Connor, C. M., McKinnon, C., Oyebode, J. R., Piguet, O., Hodges, J. R., & Mioshi, E. (2017). Factors underpinning caregiver burden in frontotemporal dementia differ in spouses and their children. *Journal of Alzheimer's Disease, 56*(3), 1109–1117. https://doi.org/10.3233/JAD-160852

Mekala, S., Alladi, S., Chandrasekar, K., Fathima, S., O'Connor, C. M., McKinnon, C., Hornberger, M., Piguet, O., Hodges, J. R., & Mioshi, E. (2013). Cultural differences are reflected in variables associated with carer burden in FTD: A comparison study between India and Australia. *Dementia & Neuropsychologia, 7*(1), 104–109. https://doi.org/10.1590/S1980-57642013DN70100016

Mioshi, E., Flanagan, E., & Knopman, D. (2017). Detecting clinical change with the CDR-FTLD: Differences between FTLD and AD dementia. *International Journal of Geriatric Psychiatry, 32*(9), 977–982. https://doi.org/10.1002/gps.4556

Mioshi, E., Hodges, J. R., & Hornberger, M. (2013). Neural correlates of activities of daily living in frontotemporal dementia. *Journal of Geriatric Psychiatry and Neurology, 26*(1), 51–57. https://doi.org/10.1177/0891988713477474

O'Connor, C., Clemson, L., Brodaty, H., Gitlin, L., Piguet, O., & Mioshi, E. (2016). Enhancing caregivers' understanding of dementia and tailoring activities in frontotemporal dementia: Two case studies. *Disability and Rehabilitation, 38*(7), 704–714. https://doi.org/10.3109/0963 8288.2015.1055375

O'Connor, C., Clemson, L., Hornberger, M., Leyton, C., Hodges, J., Piguet, O., & Mioshi, E. (2016). Longitudinal change in everyday function and behavioral symptoms in frontotemporal dementia. *Neurology: Clinical Practice, 6*(5), 419–428. https://doi.org/10.1212/CPJ.00 00000000000264

O'Connor, C., Landin-Romero, R., Clemson, L., Kaizik, C., Daveson, N., Hodges, J., Hsieh, S., Piguet, O., & Mioshi, E. (2017). Behavioral-variant frontotemporal dementia: Distinct phenotypes with unique functional profiles. *Neurology, 89*(6), 570–577. https://doi.org/10.1212/ WNL.0000000000004215

Yassuda, M., Lima da Silva, T. B., O'Connor, C. M., Mekala, S., Alladi, S., Bahia, V. S., Amaral-Carvalho, V., Guimaraes, H. C., Caramelli, P., Balthazar, M. L. F., Damasceno, B., Brucki, S. M. D., Nitrini, R., Hodges J. R., Piguet, O., & Mioshi, E. (2018). Apathy and functional disability in behavioral variant frontotemporal dementia. *Neurology: Clinical Practice, 8*(2) 120–128. https://doi.org/10.1212/CPJ.0000000000000429

Impaired Self-Awareness

Also called anosognosia (neurologic conditions literature), impaired insight, lack of insight (psychiatric literature), impaired self-understanding, unawareness, inability to self-reflect (psychological literature).

See also Cognitive Impairment, Executive Dysfunction, Memory Impairment, other specific diagnoses.

Description

Self-awareness is described as a person's understanding of their own strengths and weaknesses, including attitudes, motives, reactions, and defenses. Self-awareness may also be described as the ability to objectively perceive oneself while maintaining a sense of subjectivity (Schmidt et al., 2012). Self-awareness involves "the conscious knowledge of one's abilities and impact of those abilities on daily functioning" (Dirette, 2010, p. 310). Self-awareness may include the metacognitive abilities of self-monitoring and self-regulation (Toglia & Maier, 2018). Three domains are recognized: awareness or knowledge of the existence of health conditions and impairments, awareness or knowledge of ability to function, and awareness of task specific performance (Toglia, & Maier, 2018).

Impaired self-awareness manifests itself when the person has difficulty recognizing that impairment exists, has difficulty understanding the implications of the impairment, and has difficulty setting realistic goals for the future (Doig et al., 2014). Impaired self-awareness may impact the person's recovery during the treatment process and impair the person's ability to return to all areas of occupation performance (Dirette, 2010). Persons with impaired self-awareness may overestimate or overstate their ability to perform a task, may engage in occupations that exceed their capabilities, may set unrealistic performance goals, and are less likely to use adaptive compensatory strategies (Anderson et al., 2010).

Cause

Most common cause is an acquired brain injury which affects areas of the brain responsible for attention, memory, and executive function (Anderson et al., 2010). Examples of acquired brain injury include hematoma, hemorrhage, contusion, viral encephalitis, closed head injury, tumor, lobectomy, and anoxia (Anderson et al., 2010). Other causes include attention-deficit/hyperactivity disorder, schizophrenia, stroke, and older adults with mild cognitive impairment or dementia (Toglia & Maeir, 2018). Impaired self-awareness can affect people of all ages, gender, education levels, and socioeconomic status (Dirette, 2010).

Terminology (Rotenberg-Shpigelman et al., 2014)

- *Anticipatory awareness:* "A person's expectations regarding task outcomes that depend on appraisal of the task and/or the situation and interaction with previous self-knowledge" (Rotenberg-Shpigelman et al., 2014, p. 48).
- *Emergent awareness:* "A person's ability to recognize errors in performance due to a discrepancy between expected outcomes and what actually occurs, or due to changes in task demands and/or context" (Rotenberg-Shpigelman et al., 2014, p. 48).
- *Metacognition:* Knowledge a person "holds regarding task characteristics, cognitive strategies, and functional demands as well as self-awareness, concerning ones capacities and limitations" (Rotenberg-Shpigelman et al., 2014, p. 48). Also called intellectual awareness. Metacognition is considered to be a fairly stable or unchanging concept.
- *Online awareness:* "Dynamic ongoing process of self-monitoring and self-regulation of performance, activated within the context of a specific task and situation" (Rotenberg-Shpigelman et al., 2014, p. 48). Online awareness is considered to be a very unstable concept that changes with task performed and the situation (context, environment) in which the performance occurs.
- *Self-regulation:* Internal processes involved in "the ability to adjust performance and shift set or plan as needed, depending on accurate monitoring that detect errors" (Rotenberg-Shpigelman et al., 2014, p. 48).

Evaluation/Assessment

Areas

- Activities of Daily Living/Instrumental ADL: basic ADLs (eating, dressing, grooming, toileting, transfers), independent living skills (meal preparation, housekeeping, financial management, medication management, doing laundry, shopping, driving or use of public transportation)
- Education/Work: educational attainment, work history including paid and unpaid job skills
- Play/Leisure: interests, frequency, location
- Rest/Sleep: not discussed
- Social Participation: type, frequency, location, with whom
- Sensorimotor: gross and fine motor skills, speed, accuracy, dexterity, history of falls, sensory awareness and registration
- Cognitive/Perceptual: memory, executive functioning (problem solving, planning, setting goals, judgment of safety, time management, metacognition)
- Psychosocial: self-image, self-efficacy, self-confidence, emotional regulation, social relations, role performance, quality of life
- Context/Environment: cultural values and beliefs, social support, community and internet resources
- Comorbidities: acquired or traumatic brain injury, Alzheimer's disease, attention-deficit/hyperactivity disorder, dementia, mild cognitive impairment (MCI), mood disorders, stroke

Instruments

Instruments Developed by Occupational Therapy Personnel

- Assessment of Awareness of Ability (A3; new name for the Assessment of Awareness of Disability; Kottorp et al., 2013)
- Assessment of Awareness of Disability (AAD; Tham et al., 1999; see also Anderson et al., 2010; Asaba et al., 2012, in References)

- Assessment of Motor and Process Skills (8th ed.; AMPS-8; Fisher & Bray Jones, 2016)
- Brain Injury Driving Self-Awareness Measure (BIDSAM; Gooden et al., 2017, in References)
- Canadian Occupational Performance Measure (5th ed.; COPM-5; Law et al., 2014)
- Client-Centredness of Goal Setting (C-COgS) scale (Doig et al., 2015)
- Driving Awareness Questionnaire (Drive-Aware; Kay et al., 2009)
- Meal Independence Rating Scale (MIRS; Schmidt et al., 2015, in References)
- Paediatric Awareness Questionnaire (PAQ; Lloyd et al., 2018, in References)
- Self-Awareness of Deficits Interview (SADI; Fleming et al., 1996)
- Self-Awareness of Falls Risk Measure (SAFR; Mihaljcic et al., 2014, in References)
- Self-Perceptions in Rehabilitation Questionnaire (SPIRQ; Ownsworth et al., 2013, in References)

Instruments Developed by Other Professionals and Used by Occupational Therapy Personnel
- Anosognosia Questionnaire-Dementia (AQ-D; Migliorelli et al., 1995)
- AwareCare (AC; Clare et al., 2012)
- Awareness Interview (AI; Anderson & Tranel, 1989)
- Awareness Questionnaire (AQ; Sherer et al., 1998; see also Ownsworth et al., 2019, in References)
- Denial of Disability (DD) scale (Prigatano & Klonoff, 1998)
- Depression Anxiety Stress Scale-21 (DASS-21; Lovibond & Lovibond, 1995a, 1995b)
- Functional Independence Measure (FIM; Uniform Data System for Medical Rehabilitation, 1997)
- Goal Attainment Scaling (GAS; Kiresuk & Sherman, 1968; Kiresuk et al., 1994)
- Indiana Psychiatric Illness Interview (IPII; Lysaker et al., 2002)
- Insight Interview (II; Malouf et al., 2014)
- ISA and Denial of Disability Clinician's Rating Scale (ISA-DDCRS; Prigatano & Klonoff, 1998)
- Knowledge of Injury Checklist (KIC; Beardmore et al., 1999)
- Mayo-Portland Adaptability Index (MPAI-4; Malec & Lezak, 2008)
- Memory Awareness Rating Scale (MARS; Clare et al., 2002)
- Patient Competency Rating Scale (PCRS; Prigatano & Fordyce, 1986)
- Patient Competency Rating Scale for Neuro-Rehabilitation (PCRSNR; Borgaro & Prigatano, 2003)
- Patient Distress Scale (PDS; Borgaro et al., 2003)
- Questionnaire of Executive Functioning (QEF; Geurten et al., 2016)
- Scale to Assess Unawareness of Mental Disorders (SUMD; Amador et al., 1991)
- Self-Regulation Skills Interview (SRSI; Ownsworth et al., 2000)
- Structured Clinical Interview for Insight and Judgment in Dementia (SIJID; Parrao et al., 2017)
- Sydney Psychosocial Reintegration Scale (Version 2; SPRS-2; Tate, 2011)

Problems/Issues
Activities of Daily Living/Instrumental ADL
(Note: The following are examples; individuals may exhibit none or all of the examples.)

- Person may fail to perform critical step in a task (puts on shirt but does not button the buttons).
- Person may fail to perform a critical task (put on deodorant).
- Person may fail to recognize a dangerous situation (water on the floor, food burning on the stove, smoke coming from the oven, broken glass, too heavy a load to carry, etc.).
- Person may fail to recognize limits such as credit card limit and overspends 4 months in a row.
- Person may have difficulty balancing the checkbook manually or online.
- Person may get lost while walking in the neighborhood.
- Person may be driving too slow or too fast for weather conditions or posted speed limits.

Education/Work
- Person may sign up for too many college courses or ones for which the person does not have prerequisite knowledge or interest.
- Person may attempt to return to work but perform some tasks poorly or fail to perform other required tasks.

Play/Leisure
- Person may attempt to engage in a leisure occupation previously known such as a card game, but not be able to follow the rules or makes poor choices that usually result in losing the game.
- Person overestimates or is overly optimistic about performance in a leisure occupation such as stating he or she can bowl a perfect game (300) but actually unable to bowl a single strike.

Rest/Sleep
- No information identified.

Social Participation
- Person is confident he or she can join friends who usually order steak for dinner when individual has difficulty using hands in a coordinated manner.

Sensorimotor
- Person may attempt to walk across on open space when balance is poor and an adaptive device (cane, walker, scooter, wheelchair) is usually needed.

Cognitive/Perceptual
- Person may make decisions without thinking through the consequences such as driving at night in a rural area without checking to see if the tank is full of gas.
- Person may decide to cross a busy street in the middle of the street because he or she sees something of interest in a store window without regard for traffic.

Psychosocial
- Person may be overly confident in ability or capacity to perform a task or totally lack confidence.
- Person may be motivated to "try anything" or unwilling to try any task.
- Person may experience more anxiety and stress if better self-awareness is present (Geytenbeek et al., 2017).

Context/Environment
- Person may come from a culture where admitting weakness or limitations is not acceptable, especially for males.
- Person, family, caregivers, peers, or employer may not know that certain cognitive dysfunctions are common in the disorder or diagnosis the individual has been given.
- Person or family may not know about available community or internet resources.

Intervention/Treatment

Models and programs created by occupational therapy personnel include the awareness intervention (Miyahara et al., 2018), goal-planning procedure (Doig et al., 2014), Self-Awareness Enhancement through Learning and Function (SELF; (Dirette, 2010), awareness intervention protocol (Miyahara et al., 2018), goal setting (Prescott et al., 2019), online awareness and error behavior (Doig, Fleming, & Lin, 2017; Doig, Fleming, Ownsworth, Fletcher, 2017), verbal feedback (Fleming et al., 2020), and Weekly Calendar Planning Activity (WCPA; Zlotnik & Toglia, 2018). Models and programs created by other professionals but used by occupational therapy personnel include strategy training (Kersey et al., 2019; Skidmore et al., 2018) and video feedback (Schmidt et al., 2013, 2015). Team members include psychiatrists, psychologists, social workers, and occupational therapy personnel. Goal is to enable the person to achieve conscious awareness of functional status and the ability to self-interpret and set personal goals, which lead to mastery and the individual's evaluation of personal performance after a response is generated (Dirette, 2010).

Activities of Daily Living/Instrumental ADL
- Select basic ADL or independent living tasks or occupations can be performed and evaluated using one or more of the approaches listed under Cognitive/Perceptual, Psychosocial, or Context/Environment sections.

Education/Work
- Selected academic or work-related tasks or occupations can be performed and evaluated using one or more of the approaches listed under Cognitive/Perceptual, Psychosocial, or Context/Environmental sections.

Play/Leisure
- Selected play activities for children or leisure occupations for older children, adolescents, and adults can be performed and evaluated using one or more of the approaches listed under Cognitive/Perceptual, Psychosocial, or Context/Environment sections.

Rest/Sleep
- No information identified.

Social Participation
- Selected social or cultural activities can be performed and evaluated using one or more of the approaches listed under Cognitive/Perceptual, Psychosocial, or Context/Environment sections.

Sensorimotor
- Section motor or sensory tasks can be performed and evaluated using one or more of the approaches listed under Cognitive/Perceptual, Psychosocial, or Context/Environment sections.

Cognitive/Perceptual
- Awareness protocol (three steps; adapted from Miyahara et al., 2018)
  - Step 1: Before starting the occupation: (a) explain the procedure for the occupation, (b) have subject anticipate difficulties and strategies by him- or herself, and (c) if the client has difficulty with describing the strategy, the therapist proposes them.
  - Step 2: Client performs the occupation: (a) if the strategy is not used, the therapist indicates it should be, and (b) therapist provides assistance if difficulties arise.
  - Step 3: After the occupation is performed: (a) client self-assesses mistakes and strategies, and (b) client completes the Self-Regulation Skills Interview.
- General cognitive deterioration (dementia, schizophrenia, or severe emotional defense mechanisms)
  - Use adaptive or compensatory approaches.
  - Do not confront person with deficits or attempt to use remedial approaches.
  - Therapeutic technique: Listen-Empathize-Agree-Partner (partner compensates for unawareness and focuses on collaborating around functional interests and getting tasks done the best way possible).
- Self-awareness
  - Focus on increasing self-knowledge (intellectual awareness) or increasing self-monitoring skills (online awareness) or combination.
  - Assist person to better understand individual strengths, abilities, and challenges.
  - Assist person to advocate for self when help is needed to facilitate occupational performance.
- Metacognition approaches
  - Identify tasks that may be easy or hard.
  - Before beginning a task, self-predict whether it will be easy or hard to do.

- After performing a task, self-check whether the task was easy or hard and whether it was done correctly and if errors occurred (corrected or uncorrected).
- Assist client by asking questions to facilitate reflection such as the following: Were you able to complete the task as you predicted? Did any problems or errors occur? Were you able to correct the problems or fix the errors? What about (situation where problem or error occurred)?
- Video feedback
  - Video feedback can help the client observe and recognize his or her own errors in the playback of performance.
  - Video feedback can facilitate discussion of what actually happened when the person performed a task or engaged in an interaction with other people.
  - Video feedback may reduce the "not me" or the "I would never do that" denial of that behavior.
  - Video feedback can be played back repeatedly and can be used to compare one performance to another to show improvement in task or interaction performance.
  - Video feedback can be used for self-checking and self-appraisal with or without the assistance of a therapist.
- Errorless learning
  - Errorless learning focuses on teaching steps in a task or behavior so that each step is performed successfully (to an expected standard) without any errors occurring.
  - Errorless learning requires that the teaching situation be totally under the control of the instructor (therapist, caregiver) so that all possible sources of errors can be avoided.
  - Errorless learning is useful for persons with mild cognitive dysfunction and impaired self-awareness who might not recognize errors if they occurred or be able to make corrections. The task and associated behavior are only done one way—the correct way—for the person, environment, and occupation.
  - Errorless learning works best in stable or consistent environment where little or no deviations or unexpected changes occur in task performance expectations. (Positive example: Morning routine in a nursing home. Negative example: Driving protocol in a large metropolitan community.)

Psychosocial

- Group programs
  - Activities that encourage reflection on the person's life narrative and life history presented to others focused on strengths (I'm good at ____; I'm not so good at ____) and limitations (I know how to ____; I don't know how to ____).
  - Activities that provide opportunity to describe abilities, challenges, interests, goals, or aspirations through photo collages, digital stories, videos, or PowerPoint presentations.
  - Opportunities to reflect and focus on strengths that can be used to overcome challenges.

Context/Environment

- Caregiver or family member intervention.
  - Teach caregiver to increase observation skills to watch for and recognize signs of impairment and lack of awareness.
  - Provide caregiver with techniques to adapt situations to facilitate performance such as using environmental cues (smell the coffee, hear the running water for a shower, see food contrasted from plate or bowl, use lavender scents to calm a person, play favorite type of music, view favorite TV or movie programs).

Precautions/Safety Considerations

Person may tend to overestimate ability or skills in situations, which may result in harm to the person and/or others. Monitor regularly for safety and dangerous situations.

Prognosis and Outcome

Person's self-awareness may improve over time. Therapy intervention during the first year following diagnosis appears to be helpful. However, if cognitive decline is expected, self-awareness is less likely to improve and may deteriorate.

REFERENCES

Anderson, R. L., Doble, S. E., Merritt, B. K., & Kottorp, A. (2010). Assessment of awareness of disability measures among persons with acquired brain injury. *Canadian Journal of Occupational Therapy, 77*(1), 22–29. https://doi.org/10.2182/cjot.2010.77.1.4

Asaba, E., Petersson, I, Bontje, P., & Kottorp, A. (2012). The Assessment of Awareness of Ability (A3) in a Japanese context: A Rasch model application. *Scandinavian Journal of Occupational Therapy, 19*(4), 370–376. https://doi.org/10.3109/11038128.2011.614277

Dirette, D. (2010). Self-awareness enhancement through learning and function (SELF): A theoretically based guideline for practice. *British Journal of Occupational Therapy, 73*(7), 309–318. https://doi.org/10.4276/030802210X12759925544344

Doig, E., Fleming, J., & Lin, B. (2017). Comparison of online awareness and error behaviour during occupational performance by two individuals with traumatic brain injury and matched controls. *NeuroRehabilitation, 40*(4), 519–529. https://doi.org/10.3233/NRE-171439

Doig, E., Fleming, J, Ownsworth, T., & Fletcher, S. (2017). An occupation-based metacognitive approach to assessing error performance and online awareness. *Australian Occupational Therapy Journal, 64*(2), 137–148. https://doi.org/10.1111/1440-1630.12322

Doig, E., Kuipers, P., Prescott, S., Cornwell, P., & Fleming, J. (2014). Development of self-awareness after severe traumatic brain injury through participation in occupation-based rehabilitation: Mixed-methods analysis of a case series. *American Journal of Occupational Therapy, 68*(5), 578–588. https://doi.org/10.5014/ajot.2014.010785

Fleming, J., Tsi Hui Goh, A., Lannin, N. A., Ownsworth, T., & Schmidt, J. (2020). An exploratory study of verbal feedback on occupational performance for improving self-awareness in people with traumatic brain injury. *Australian Occupational Therapy Journal, 67*(2), 142–152. https://doi.org/10.1111/1440-1630.12632

Geytenbeek, M., Fleming, J., Doig, E., & Ownsworth, T. (2017). The occurrence of early impaired self-awareness after traumatic brain injury and its relationship with emotional distress and psychosocial functioning. *Brain Injury, 31*(13-14), 1791–1798. https://doi.org/10.1080/02699052.2017.1346297

Gooden, J. R., Ponsford, J. L., Charlton, J. L., Ross, P. E., Marshall, S., Gagnon, S., Bédard, M., & Stolwyk, R. J. (2017). The development and initial validation of a new tool to measure self-awareness of driving ability after brain injury. *Australian Occupational Therapy Journal, 64*(1), 33–40. https://doi.org/10.1111/1440-1630.12306

Kersey, J., Juengst, S. B., & Skidmore, E. (2019). Effect of strategy training on self-awareness of deficits after stroke. *American Journal of Occupational Therapy, 73*(3), Article 7303345020. https://doi.org/10.5014/ajot.2019.031450

Lloyd, O., Ownsworth, T., Fleming, J., & Zimmer-Gembeck, M. J. (2018). Development and preliminary validation of the Paediatric Awareness Questionnaire for children and adolescents with traumatic brain injury. *Child Neuropsychology, 24*(5), 702–722. https://doi.org/10.1080/09297049.2017.1332173

Mihaljcic, T., Haines, T. P., Ponsford, J. L., & Stolwyk, R. J. (2014). Development of a new self-awareness of falls risk measure (SAFRM). *Archives of Gerontology and Geriatrics, 59*(2), 249–256. https://doi.org/10.1016/j.archger.2014.06.001

Miyahara, T., Shimizu, H., Yamane, S., & Hanaoka, H. (2018). Occupation-based intervention to improve self-awareness in persons with acquired brain injury: A single-case experimental design. *Asian Journal of Occupational Therapy, 14*(1), 33–41.

Ownsworth, T., Fleming, J., Doig, E., Shum, D. H. K., & Swan, S. (2019). Concordance between the Awareness Questionnaire and Self-Awareness of Deficits Interview for identifying impaired self-awareness in individuals with traumatic brain injury in the community. *Journal of Rehabilitation Medicine, 51*(5), 376–379. https://doi.org/10.2340/16501977-2537

Ownsworth, T., Stewart, E., Fleming, J., Griffin, J., Collier, A. M., & Schmidt, J. (2013). Development and preliminary psychometric evaluation of the Self-Perceptions in Rehabilitation Questionnaire (SPIRQ) for brain injury rehabilitation. *American Journal of Occupational Therapy, 67*(3), 336–344. https://doi.org/10.5014/ajot.2013.007625

Prescott, S., Fleming, J., & Doig, E. (2019). Effect of self-awareness on goal engagement and outcomes after acquired brain injury. *British Journal of Occupational Therapy, 82*(12), 726–731. https://doi.org/10.1177/0308022619851434

Rotenberg-Shpigelman, S., Rosen-Shilo, L., & Maeir, A. (2014). Online awareness of functional tasks following ABI: The effect of task experience and associations with underlying mechanisms. *NeuroRehabilitation, 35*(1), 47–56. https://doi.org/10.3233/NRE-141101

Schmidt, J., Fleming, J., Ownsworth, T., & Lannin, N. A. (2013). Video feedback on functional task performance improves self-awareness after traumatic brain injury: A randomized controlled trial. *Neurorehabilitation and Neural Repair, 27*(4), 316–324. https://doi.org/10.1177/1545968312469838

Schmidt, J., Fleming, J., Ownsworth, T., & Lannin, N. A. (2015). An occupation-based video feedback intervention for improving self-awareness: Protocol and rationale. *Canadian Journal of Occupational Therapy, 82*(1), 54–63. https://doi.org/10.1177/0008417414550999

Schmidt, J., Fleming, J., Ownsworth, T., Lannin, N., & Khan, A. (2012). Feedback interventions for improving self-awareness after brain injury: A protocol for a pragmatic randomised controlled trial. *Australian Occupational Therapy Journal, 59*(2), 138–146. https://doi.org/10.1111/j.1440-1630.2012.00998.x

Skidmore, E. R., Swafford, M., Juengst, S. B., & Terhorst, L. (2018). Self-awareness and recovery of independence with strategy training. *American Journal of Occupational Therapy, 72*(1), Article 7201345010. https://doi.org/10.5014/ajot.2018.023556

Toglia, J., & Maeir, A. (2018). Self-awareness and metacognition: Affect on occupational performance and outcome across the lifespan. In N. Katz & J. Toglia (Eds.), *Cognition, occupation, and participation across the lifespan* (4th ed., pp. 143–163). AOTA Press.

Zlotnik, S., & Toglia, J. (2018). Measuring adolescent self-awareness and accuracy using a performance-based assessment and parental report. *Frontiers in Public Health, 6*, Article 15. https://doi.org/ 10.3389/fpubh.2018.00015

BIBLIOGRAPHY

Engel, L., Chui, A., Goverover, Y., & Dawson, D. R. (2019). Optimising activity and participation outcomes for people with self-awareness impairments related to acquired brain injury: An interventions systematic review. *Neuropsychological Rehabilitation, 29*(2), 163–198. https://doi.org/10.1080/09602011.2017.1292923

Goverover, Y., & Chiaravalloti, N. (2014). The impact of self-awareness and depression on subjective reports of memory, quality-of-life and satisfaction with life following TBI. *Brain Injury, 28*(2), 174–180. https://doi.org/10.3109/02699052.2013.860474

Juengst, S., Skidmore, E., Pramuka, M., McCue, M., & Becker, J. (2012). Factors contributing to impaired self-awareness of cognitive functioning in an HIV positive and at-risk population. *Disability and Rehabilitation, 34*(1), 19–25. https://doi.org/10.3109/09638288.2011.587088

Leung, D. P., & Liu, K. P. (2011). Review of self-awareness and its clinical application in stroke rehabilitation. *International Journal of Rehabilitation Research, 34*(3), 187–195. https://doi.org/10.1097/MRR.0b013e3283487f31

Mahoney, D., Gutman, S. A., & Gillen, G. (2019). A scoping review of self-awareness instruments for acquired brain injury. *Open Journal of Occupational Therapy, 7*(2) Article 3. https://doi.org/10.15453/2168-6408.1529

Ohman, A., Nygård, L., & Kottorp, A. (2011). Occupational performance and awareness of disability in mild cognitive impairment or dementia. *Scandinavian Journal of Occupational Therapy, 18*(2), 133–142. https://doi.org/10.3109/11038121003645993

Schmidt, J., Lannin, N., Fleming, J., & Ownsworth, T. (2011). Feedback interventions for impaired self-awareness following brain injury: A systematic review. *Journal of Rehabilitation Medicine, 43*(8), 673–680. https://doi.org/10.2340/16501977-0846

Stapleton, T., Connolly, D., & O'Neill, D. (2012). Exploring the relationship between self-awareness of driving efficacy and that of a proxy when determining fitness to drive after stroke. *Australian Occupational Therapy Journal, 59*(1), 63–70. https://doi.org/10.1111/j.1440-1630.2011.00980.x

Wales, L., Hawley, C., & Sidebotham, P. (2013). How an occupational therapist should conceptualise self-awareness following traumatic brain injury in childhood—A literature review. *British Journal of Occupational Therapy, 76*(7), 325–332. https://doi.org/10.4276/030802213X13729279115013

Memory Impairment

See also Cognitive Impairment, Dementia, Executive Dysfunction, Impaired Self-Awareness.

Description

Difficulty of a person to register, retrieve, manipulate (apply), retain, and recall or recognize information needed to perform everyday occupations over time. Note that memory impairment is not the same as memory loss, in which memory processes cease to function, as occurs in dementia or Alzheimer's disease. Memory impairment involves difficulty using memory processes effectively and efficiently (Baird & Maskill, 2017).

Cause

Dysfunction of the nervous system, especially conditions that affect the frontal lobes directly or interfere with access to frontal lobes such as traumatic brain injury, stroke, dementia, attention-deficit/hyperactivity disorder, Parkinson's disease, multiple sclerosis, schizophrenia, bipolar disorder, psychosis, and side effects of some medications used to treat conditions such as cancer (Baird & Maskill, 2017). Major brain areas involved in memory are the diencephalon, medial temporal lobe, and frontal lobe (Baird & Maskill, 2017).

Types of Memory (Adapted from Baird & Maskill, 2017)

- Declarative (Explicit, Nonprocedural): Knowledge of people, objects, places, and events through conscious recall or recognition.
- Episodic: Knowledge of facts and events in context of time (recent or remote) and place.
- Long term: Retention of information over long periods of time.
- Metamemory: Ability to self-assess that information has been learned and can be used in the future.
- Procedural (Implicit, Nondeclarative): Retrieval of information through performance (doing, action) rather than through conscious recall or recognition. Two subtypes are time-based procedural memory (TBPM; performance is based on the time, such as a morning routine) and event-based procedural memory (EBPM; performance is based on a specific event, such as eating dinner or going to a sporting event; see Korman et al., 2017; Pavol et al., 2018).

- Prospective: Remembering to do things in the future, recalling decisions and plans in order to carry them through and act (see Au et al., 2014; Au et al., 2017; Hogan et al., 2016).
- Semantic: Memory of vocabulary, concepts, and associations, knowledge of the world in general (see Bier et al., 2013; Bier et al., 2011).
- Short term: Retention of small amounts of information over a few seconds; includes verbal (auditory) information and/or visual information.
- Working (bench): Temporary storage and manipulation of information necessary for such complex cognitive tasks as language comprehension, learning, and reasoning; sources of working memory are incoming sensory input and/or long-term memory storage (see Chehreh-Negar et al., 2012; Coe et al., 2019; Green et al., 2018, Johansson & Tornmalm, 2012; Leung et al., 2016; Stephens & Berryhill, 2016).

Types of Remedial Memory Strategies (Nadar & McDowd, 2010)

- Chunking: Related items of information are grouped together into small units, such as three or four items. Examples: Phone number is grouped into three, three, four numbers (123-456-7891); Social Security number is grouped into three, two, four (123-45-6789).
- Errorless learning: Focus on one cognitive domain and a single component of behavior creating step-by-step learning (brushing teeth).
- Mnemonics—Loci: Items to be memorized are paired or associated with a known list. Example: familiar places such as rooms in a house (kitchen, dining room, bathroom) or parts of a room (bed, closet, door, table, chair).
- Mnemonics—Pegword: Association using a rhyming system (1 = bun, 2 = shoe, 3 = tree, 4 = door, 5 = hive) or a phrase (spell the word arithmetic: "a rat in the house may eat the ice cream"; remember the names and order of the 12 cranial nerves: "On old Olympus towering tops, A Finn and German viewed some hops").
- Rehearsal—Maintenance: Repeat some information several times.
- Rehearsal—Elaborative: Actively reorganizing and associating to-be-learned material to other information already in long-term memory.

Types of Compensatory Memory Strategies

- Time dependent
  - ▶ Calendars (weekly, monthly, yearly; paper, computer)
  - ▶ Daily (hourly, 1/2 hour, 1/4 hour) schedules (paper, sticky notes, pager, phone, computer)
- Event dependent
  - ▶ Eating dinner
  - ▶ Going for a walk outside
  - ▶ Driving to an appointment
- Sensory based
  - ▶ Voice/sound reminders (phone, pager, computer software program)
  - ▶ Visual reminders (arrows, red lines, pictures, photos)
  - ▶ Tactile (raised dots, different textures, surface treads)
- Action based
  - ▶ Pantomime
  - ▶ Gestures
  - ▶ Hand over hand (therapist guided)

Evaluation/Assessment

Areas

- Activities of Daily Living/Instrumental ADL: self-maintenance activities, time management, financial management,
- Education/Work: academic achievement, work performance
- Play/Leisure: interests, values, frequency, location

- Rest/Sleep: sleep disturbances
- Social Participation: type, frequency, with whom
- Sensorimotor: sensory awareness, sensory registration
- Cognitive/Perceptual: short-term memory, long-term memory, working memory, declarative memory, procedural memory, episodic, semantic
- Psychosocial: self-awareness
- Context/Environment: home, community, treatment center or clinic
- Development (Infant, Child, Adolescent only): developmental milestones in cognition
- Comorbidities: sensory loss (hearing, vision, smell, taste, touch, proprioception), perceptual dysfunction

Instruments

Instruments Developed by Occupational Therapy Personnel

- Addenbrooke's Cognitive Examination Revised (ACE-R; Mioshi et al., 2006, screen for dementia)
- Canadian Occupational Performance Measure (5th ed.; COPM-5; Law et al., 2014)
- Instrumental Activities of Daily Living Profile (IADL Profile; Bottari et al., 2009)

Instruments Developed by Other Professionals and Used by Occupational Therapy Personnel

- Cambridge Prospective Memory Test (CPMT; Wilson et al., 2005; see also Au et al., 2014, in References)
- Doors and People (DAP; Baddeley et al., 2006)
- Everyday Memory Questionnaire–Revised (EMQ-R; Royle & Lincoln, 2008)
- Memory Self Efficacy Scale (MSES; Berry & West, 1993)
- Mini-Mental State Examination (MMSE; Folstein et al., 1975)
- Prospective and Retrospective Memory Questionnaire (PRMQ; Smith et al., 2000)
- Rivermead Behavioural Memory Test-3 (RBMT-3; Wilson et al., 2008)
- Visual analogue scale (quality of life satisfaction)
- Wechsler Memory Scale (4th ed.; WMS-IV; Wechsler, 2009)

Problems/Issues

Activities of Daily Living/Instrumental ADL

- Person may not perform tasks in daily routine, such as taking medications or bathing/showering, without reminders.
- Person may have difficulty initiating a task, such as brushing teeth or combing hair, but can perform a task once first step is started.

Education/Work

- Person may not complete school assignments as per instructions.
- Person may not perform work tasks as stated in job description.
- Person may make errors in performing routine work task.

Play/Leisure

- Person may have discontinued engaging in favorite leisure activities.

Rest/Sleep

- Person may have sleep disturbances.

Social Participation

- Person may withdraw from participation in social activities with family, friends, colleagues.

Sensorimotor

- Person may have difficulty with visual perception.

Cognitive/Perceptual

- Person may be confused about how to perform a familiar task.

Psychosocial

- Person may lack awareness that errors in performance have occurred.
- Person may or may not be aware that performance level has changed.
- Person may report increased sense of stress related to memory impairment.

Context/Environment

- Person may have difficulty performing routine activities in a clinic or hospital environment that are performed in the home living environment.
- Person may report getting lost in a community that is known to the individual.

Intervention/Treatment

Models and programs developed by occupational therapy personnel include electronic memory aids (Boman et al., 2010), Memory Strategy Education Group (MSEG; Coe et al., 2019), and Cogmed QM (Johansson & Tornmalm, 2012). Models and programs developed by other professionals include the Modified Approach to Stroke Rehabilitation (MAStR; Pavol et al., 2018). Team members include physicians, neurologists, nursing personnel, psychologists, caregivers, and occupational therapy personnel. Goal is to assist client to learn and apply compensatory approaches for memory limitation to improve the level of functional performance and to increase participation and life satisfaction in everyday occupations (Baird & Maskill, 2017).

Activities of Daily Living/Instrumental ADL

- Determine which ADL and IADL tasks are most important to the person, family, or caregivers.

Education/Work

- Determine whether time-based or event-based procedural memory approach may be helpful.

Play/Leisure

- Use cognitive stimulation to keep memory processes active such as reminiscence groups, memory games, making family photo albums, doing puzzles, music activities, and familiar activities such as baking cookies or making pizza.

Rest/Sleep

- See Sleep–Wake Disorders in Section 13: Lifestyle Conditions.

Social Participation

- Encourage participation in social activities. Modifications may include smaller number of individuals, shorter time frame, or reduce demand on client to perform certain tasks.

Sensorimotor

- See Visual Impairment Due to Neurologic Conditions in Section 2: Sensory Disorders.

Cognitive/Perceptual

- Focus on client's goals rather than on specific memory remediation tasks such as paper-and-pencil exercises or reciting the alphabet backwards.
- Use preserved abilities (what person can do with assistance as needed) rather than trying to remediate dysfunction (what person cannot do or can only do with maximum assistance).
- Use event-based procedural memory to initiate task: turn water on for shower, use smell of coffee to facilitate eating breakfast, lay out clothes in order to be donned; also called maximizing antecedent events in the environment.
- Use time-based procedural memory to facilitate tasks such as determining when person is most able to performance task (see example in Korman et al., 2017).
- Give brief instruction summary of task, such as, "I want to see if you can get from the bed to the chair. Can you repeat that (sentence) back to me?"
- Give detailed, step-by-step verbal instructions, such as "To do this safely, you need to (1) move your body forward to the edge of bed, (2) check that your feet are on the floor, (3) bring

your shoulders forward so you can reach for the chair arm, (4) stand up, (5) pivot your body to the chair, (6) grab the chair arms with both hands, (7) sit down."

- Before client initiates task, have client repeat the instructions.
- Allow time for person to respond (slow processing speed) before repeating instructions.
- Keep choices simple (e.g., Coffee or tea? Eggs scrambled or sunny-side up? Red socks or blue socks?). Avoid open-ended questions when possible, such as "What do you want to eat?"
- Have client state each step before performing each step of the task.
- For retention, have person repeat summary of task: (1) Move to edge of bed, (2) check that feet are on the floor, (3) reach for chair, (4) stand up, (5) pivot to chair, (6) grab chair arms, (7) sit down.
- To check for retrieval, have person repeat the instructions at the next session before initiating the task again.

Psychosocial
- No information identified.

Context/Environment
- Educate client, family, friends, caregivers about memory impairment and how it affects everyday life.
- Recommend and provide training as needed in use of memory aids: checklists, notebooks, picture/photo instructions, whiteboards, smartphone reminder apps, environmental control devices.
- If client is not in home living (natural) environment, try to simulate environment as close to natural environment as possible.
- Labeling objects in the home can facilitate memory.
- Organizing items in drawers and closets can facilitate memory.
- Keep items stored where they belong when not in use (a place for everything and everything in its place).
- Remove items not needed (declutter) from the environment.

Precautions/Safety Considerations

Person may get lost easily even in a familiar environment. Monitor client. Be sure client has global positioning system (GPS) on cell phone. Monitor environment for safety consideration: lights, fall hazards, sharps, clutter, signage, labels, organization of drawers and closets.

Prognosis and Outcome

Memory impairment due to cognitive diseases or disorders with a cognitive impairment is progressive and not reversible. Exception might be a reaction to a medication in which memory functions may improve when medication is stopped or dose adjusted.

REFERENCES

Au, R. W. C., Man, D., Shum, D., Lee, E., Xiang, Y. T., Ungvari, G. S., & Tang, W. K. (2014). Assessment of prospective memory in schizophrenia using the Chinese version of the Cambridge Prospective Memory Test: A controlled study. *Asia-Pacific Psychiatry*, 6(1), 54–61. https://doi.org/10.1111/j.1758-5872.2012.00217.x

Au, R. W. C., Xiang, Y. T., Ungvari, G. S., Lee, E., Shum, D. H. K., Man, D., & Tang, W. K. (2017). Prospective memory performance in persons with schizophrenia and bipolar disorder and healthy persons. *Perspectives in Psychiatric Care*, 53(4), 266–274. https://doi.org/10.1111/ppc.12172

Baird, T., & Maskill, L. (2017). Memory. In L. Maskill & S. Tempest (Eds.), *Neuropsychology for occupational therapy* (4th ed., pp. 123–148). Wiley/Blackwell.

Bier, N., Bottari, C., Hudon, C., Joubert, S., Paquette, G., & Macoir, J. (2013). The impact of semantic dementia on everyday actions: Evidence from an ecological study. *Journal of the*

International Neuropsychological Society, 19(2), 162–172. https://doi.org/10.1017/S1355617
712001105

Bier, N., Macoir, J., Joubert, S., Bottari, C., Chayer, C., Pigot, H., Giroux, S., & SemAssist Team.
(2011). Cooking "shrimp à la Créole": A pilot study of an ecological rehabilitation in semantic dementia. *Neuropsychological Rehabilitation, 21*(4), 455–483. https://doi.org/10.1080/096
02011.2011.580614

Boman, I. L., Bartfai, A., Borell, L., Tham, K., & Hemmingsson, H. (2010). Support in everyday
activities with a home-based electronic memory aid for persons with memory impairments.
Disability and Rehabilitation: Assistive Technology, 5(5), 339–350. https://doi.org/10.3109/1748
3100903131777

Chehreh-Negar, N., Shams, F., Zarshenas, S., & Nikseresht, A. R. (2012). Correlation between
working memory and quality of life in multiple sclerosis patients. *Feyt, Journal of Kashan
University of Medical Sciences, 16*(4), 337–345. (Abstract in English, article in Arabic)

Coe, Á., Martin, M., & Stapleton, T. (2019). Effects of an occupational therapy memory strategy
education group intervention on Irish older adults' self-management of everyday memory
difficulties. *Occupational Therapy in Health Care, 33*(1), 37–63. https://doi.org/10.1080/07
380577.2018.1543911

Green, S. L., Keightley, M. L., Lobaugh, N. J., Dawson, D. R., & Mihailidis, A. (2018). Changes in
working memory performance in youth following concussion. *Brain Injury, 32*(2), 182–190.
https://doi.org/10.1080/02699052.2017.1358396

Hogan, C., Fleming, J., Cornwell, P., & Shum, D. (2016). Prospective memory after stroke: A
scoping review. *Brain Impairment, 17*(2), 123–142. https://doi.org/10.1017/BrImp.2016.12

Johansson, B., & Tornmalm, M. (2012). Working memory training for patients with acquired
brain injury: Effects in daily life. *Scandinavian Journal of Occupational Therapy, 19*(2), 176–183.
https://doi.org/10.3109/11038128.2011.603352

Korman, M., Levy, I., & Karni, A. (2017). Procedural memory consolidation in attention-deficit/
hyperactivity disorder is promoted by scheduling of practice to evening hours. *Frontiers in
Psychiatry, 8*, Article 140. https://doi.org/10.3389/fpsyt.2017.00140

Leung, A. W., Barrett, L. M., Butterworth, D., Werther, K., Dawson, D. R., & Brintnell, E. S.
(2016). Neural plastic effects of working memory training influenced by self-perceived stress
in stroke: A case illustration. *Frontiers in Psychology, 7*, Article 1266. https://doi.org/10.3389/
fpsyg.2016.01266

Nadar, M. S., & McDowd, J. (2010). Comparison of remedial and compensatory approaches
in memory dysfunction: A comprehensive literature review. *Occupational Therapy in Health
Care, 24*(3), 274–289. https://doi.org/10.3109/07380577.2010.483269

Pavol, M. A., Bassile, C. C., Lehman, J. R., Harmon, E., Ferreira, N., Shinn, B., St. James, N.,
Callender, J., & Stein, J. (2018). Modified Approach to Stroke Rehabilitation (MAStR): Feasibility study of a method to apply procedural memory concepts to transfer training. *Topics
in Stroke Rehabilitation, 25*(5), 351–358. https://doi.org/10.1080/10749357.2018.1458462

Stephens, J. A., & Berryhill, M. E. (2016). Older adults improve on everyday tasks after working memory training and neurostimulation. *Brain Stimulation, 9*(4), 553–559. https://doi.org/
10.1016/j.brs.2016.04.001

BIBLIOGRAPHY

Brown, C. (2019). Cognition. In C. Brown, V. C. Stoffel, & J. P. Muñoz (Eds.), *Occupational
therapy in mental health* (2nd ed., pp. 281–300). F.A. Davis.

Gillen, G. (2018). Evaluation and treatment of limited occupational performance secondary to
cognitive dysfunction. In H. M. Pendleton & W. Schultz-Kohn (Eds.), *Pedretti's occupational
therapy* (8th ed., pp. 646–668). Elsevier.

Judge, K. S., & Dawson, N. T. (2018). Cognitive function. In B. Bonder & V. D. Bell-Haas (Eds.),
Functional performance in older adults (4th ed., pp. 93–108). F.A. Davis.

Levy, L. L. (2018). Cognitive aging: Considerations for adults and older adults. In N. Katz & J. Toglia (Eds.), *Cognition, occupation, and participation across the lifespan* (4th ed., pp. 29–49). AOTA Press.

Toglia, J. P., Golisz, K. M., & Goverover, Y. (2019). Cognition, perception and occupational performance. In B. A. Boyt Schell & G. Gillen (Eds.), *Willard and Spackman's occupational therapy* (13th ed., pp. 901–941). Wolters Kluwer.

Unilateral Spatial Neglect

Also called unilateral neglect, spatial neglect, hemispatial neglect, hemispatial inattention, visuospatial neglect, visual neglect, poststroke neglect, hypokinesia.

Description

Unilateral spatial neglect (USN) is a disorder of attention, perception, processing of, and responding to stimuli in contralesional personal, peripersonal, or extrapersonal space (Hreha, Chaudhari, et al., 2018; Shah et al., 2013). The disorder is characterized by a failure or slowness to respond, orient, or initiate action toward contralesional stimuli. USN can affect how an individual perceives his or her personal, near extrapersonal, and far extrapersonal space (Petzold et al., 2012). In addition, the disorder is considered to be a debilitating neurocognitive disorder associated with prolonged hospitalization, poor rehabilitation outcomes in stroke survivors, increased risk of falls, and unsafe navigation while walking and using a wheelchair, thus resulting in a functional disability (P. Chen et al., 2012). Although neglect may occur on either side of the body, more commonly neglect involves the left side of body and the left side of the environment as oriented by the person. However, aphasia may be a clue for neglect in left hemisphere strokes (Hreha et al., 2017).

Cause

The majority of cases of neglect are seen in people with right parietal lobe damage, but cases of neglect to the left parietal lobe have been reported, as has damage to the premotor area (Tempest & Maskill, 2017, p. 117). The most common cause is a stroke involving the middle cerebral artery. However, spatial neglect has been reported in traumatic brain injury (P. Chen et al., 2016), and hemispatial inattention has been reported in patients with schizophrenia (Liu et al., 2011).

Types and Terminology

- *Allocentric neglect or object-centered neglect:* Person neglects one side of an object or person, such as food on the left side of the plate, shaving the right side of the face but not the left, or dressing the right side of body but not the left (P. Chen et al., 2017).
- *Anticipatory anosognosia for spatial neglect (anticipatory ASN):* Person is aware that spatial difficulties are likely to occur in an upcoming task (P. Chen & Toglia, 2019).
- *Egocentric neglect or viewer-centered neglect:* Person neglects one side of the environment, such as objects or people in the left viewing area of the environment (P. Chen et al., 2017).
- *Offline anosognosia for spatial neglect (offline ASN):* Person is unaware of having experienced spatial deficits (P. Chen & Toglia, 2019).
- *Online anosognosia for spatial neglect (online ASN):* Person is aware of deficit of underestimating spatial difficulties (P. Chen & Toglia, 2019).
- *Stimulus-centered deficits:* Person cannot distinguish correct stimulus from incorrect stimulus (e.g., cancellation test includes forward- or right-facing letter "C"s and backward- or left-facing letter "C"s. Person is unable to cancel left-facing "C"s as incorrect stimulus; P. Chen et al., 2017).

Evaluation/Assessment
Areas
- Activities of Daily Living/Instrumental ADL: eating, hair combing, brushing teeth, dressing, grooming, counting money, clock (analogue) reading, cleaning up after a meal, telephone number dialing, address copying, filling out a form, locating common objects such as glasses, handbag, toothbrush, cell phone, clothing, greeting cards, navigation
- Education/Work: work performance, work tasks
- Play/Leisure: interests, values, frequency, location
- Rest/Sleep: sleep behavior
- Social Participation: type, frequency, location, with whom
- Sensorimotor: gaze orientation, auditory attention
- Cognitive/Perceptual: object cancellation, clock drawing, figure copying, text reading, star cancellation, line bisection, visual searches
- Psychosocial: awareness or lack of awareness of neglect, awareness of difficulty with spatial relations
- Context/Environment: observation of occupational performance in environmental situations
- Comorbidities: stroke, tumor, traumatic brain injury, schizophrenia

Instruments
(Note: Brown & Powell, 2017, and Grattan & Woodbury, 2017, recommend use of multiple assessments when evaluating unilateral spatial neglect including ones that assess everyday tasks and environments.)

Instruments Developed by Occupational Therapy Personnel
- 3s Spreadsheet Test (3S Test; P. Chen et al., 2017, in References)
- Catherine Bergego Scale (CBS; Azouvi, 1996; see P. Chen et al., 2012, for form and instructions in English. Also included in the KF-NAP below.)
- Kessler Foundation Neglect Assessment Process (KF-NAP; P. Chen et al., 2014, and P. Chen et al., 2015, in References)

Instruments Developed by Other Professionals and Used by Occupational Therapy Personnel
- Action Research Arm Test (ARAT; Lyle, 1981)
- Apples Test (AT; Humphreys et al., 2012)
- Barthel Index (BI; Mahoney & Barthel, 1965)
- Behavioral Inattention Test (BIT; Wilson et al., 1987)
- Bells Test (BT; Gauthier et al., 1989)
- Cancellation Test (CT; Weintraub & Mesulam, 1988)
- Circle Discriminative Cancellation Test (CDCT; Ota et al., 2001)
- Eschenbeck Activities of Daily Living (ADL) Scale (EADLS; Eschenbeck et al., 2010)
- Florida Mental Status Examination (FMSE; Doty et al., 1990)
- Gap Detection Test (GDT; Ota et al., 2001)
- Life Space Questionnaire (LSQ; Stalvey et al., 1999)
- Line Cancellation Test (LCT; also called Line Crossing Test; Albert, 1973)
- One-Word Reading Test (OWRT; Hillis et al., 2005)
- Repeatable Battery for the Assessment of Neuropsychological Status (RBANS; Randolph et al., 1998)
- "Trees & House" Figure Copying Test (Gainotti et al., 1972)

Problems/Issues
Activities of Daily Living/Instrumental ADL
- Person may not eat food or drink liquids on the left side (or contralesional side) of the plate or complain that only part of the food or liquids is being provided because some items are on the left side.

- Person may only dress the right side (or contralesional side) of the body.
- Person may only comb the right side (or contralesional) of his or her hair.
- Person may only brush the right side of his or her teeth or only wash the right side of the face.
- Person may only complete the right side of a food menu or only read the right side of greeting card or newspaper.
- Person may use only one upper extremity, such as right, to complete daily living activities (in other words, act as though he or she is one-handed).

Education/Work
- Person may be unable to locate doors on the left side of room.
- Person may be unable to locate desk items on the left side such as a telephone.

Play/Leisure
- Person may be unable to engage in leisure activities because of the left side neglect.

Rest/Sleep
- Person may feel he or she is all alone if bed is oriented so right-side gaze faces a wall or window.

Social Participation
- Person may neglect or fail to respond to people on his or her left side, but people may feel they are being purposely ignored.

Sensorimotor
- Person may have asymmetric strength in the lower extremities, specifically left weaker than right.
- Person may walk into objects or walls on the left side or bump into walls with a wheelchair.
- Person may have bruises or other injuries on the left side of body and be unaware of the skin damage.
- Person may fall due to muscle weakness or neglect of objects or dangers in the left side of the environment.
- Person may have no sensation on the left side of the body.

Cognitive/Perceptual
- Person may have no perceptual awareness of the left side of the body.
- Person may state he or she has no left side or that the body parts on the left side do not belong to him or her.
- Person may draw a clock with all 12 numbers located on the right half of the circle.
- Person may draw only the right side of familiar objects such as a house, cat, or flower.
- Person may circle only the right-side words of meal item. Example "fresh vegetables" is circled for a menu item reading "meat and fresh vegetables."
- Person may be concerned that his or her occupational therapist is a rapist because he or she is reading only the last six letters, which spell "rapist."

Psychosocial
- Person may not interact with people on his or her left side at the party or other social situation.
- Person may demonstrate signs of depression because he or she reports "always losing things" on the left side.

Context/Environment
- Person may be hospitalized longer or remain in rehabilitation program longer.
- Person may have lower initial scores on the Functional Independence Measure on both the motor and cognitive sections and recover more slowly with lower discharge scores.

Intervention/Treatment

Successful intervention for unilateral spatial neglect (USN) requires an understanding that neglect appears to have two manifestations: spatial representation (perception of whole of space) and motor exploration guided by visual searching (oculomotor scanning). The amount or degree of dysfunction between the two manifestations appears to vary from client to client making a "gold standard" of intervention difficult to describe. Of 28 known techniques, the following were cited most often by experts: For spatial perception—prism lenses glasses, space remapping training, sustained attention training, visual scanning, and visuomotor imagery training. For motor exploration—active limb activities, passive limb activation, and trunk rotation (P. Chen et al., 2018). Models and programs developed by occupational therapy personnel: None identified. Models and programs developed by other professionals but used by occupational therapy personnel include case study (Shah et al., 2013), constraint-induced therapy and eye patching (Wu et al., 2013), listening to classical music program (M. C. Chen et al., 2013; Tsai et al., 2013), prisms (Champod et al., 2018), repetitive task-specific practice program (Grattan et al., 2016), sensory cueing (Fong et al., 2013), and vibration (Kamada et al., 2011). Team members may include physiatrists, neurologists, nursing personnel, psychologists or neuropsychologists, physical therapists, speech–language pathologists, and occupational therapy personnel. The goal is to improve functional training and abilities to perform specific tasks and activities in everyday life (P. Chen et al., 2018).

Activities of Daily Living/Instrumental ADL
- Approaches listed under Sensorimotor or Cognitive/Perceptual can be adapted for self-maintenance activities.

Education/Work
- Approaches listed under Sensorimotor or Cognitive/Perceptual can be adapted for paid or unpaid work tasks.

Play/Leisure
- Approaches listed under Sensorimotor or Cognitive/Perceptual can be adapted for engagement in favorite leisure occupations.

Rest/Sleep
- No information identified.

Social Participation
- Approaches listed under Sensorimotor or Cognitive/Perceptual can be adapted for participation in social occupations.

Sensorimotor
- Active limb activation: Client is asked to initiate spontaneous movement of the contralateral upper limb in the contralesional space (left side of body for lesion in right hemisphere).
- Passive limb activation: Client's contralesional upper limb is moved passively in the contralesional space (Yoshihiro & Ito, 2017).
- Trunk rotation: Client's trunk is rotated toward the contralesional side while the head faces straight forward.
- Prism adaptation: Client perform goal-direct movements while wearing prism lenses that shift the entire visual field horizontally toward the ipsilesional space (Hreha, Gillen, et al., 2018; Oh et al., 2015; Turton et al., 2010).
- Space remapping training: Client performs goal-directed movements in a simulated environment (virtual reality), which dissociates visual feedback from the actual movement.
- Sustained attention training: Client is trained to maintain a high level of alertness such as "get ready to" do the next task.
- Visuomotor imagery training: Client uses imagery training following detailed verbal descriptions of spatial layout (visual imagery) and verbal or figural instructions of body postures (movement imagery).
- Visual scanning: Client is trained to initiate a visual scanning pattern starting from the contralesional space (see Visual anchors and Visual guides).

- Visual anchors: Anchors are targets to visually orient person to the left side. Examples are bright colored lines drawn down the left side a paper or menu, use of bright colored Post-it notes stuck on the left side of a computer screen, colored strips of tape placed on edges of tables, walls, or doorframes to orient person to the environment. The person is taught to return the eyes to the anchor or to scan for the anchor.
- Visual guides: Guides are objects used to direct the person's eyes toward the information that needs to be processed. Examples including using a finger to help scan text, using a piece of paper or template to mark the line of text to be read, or notecards and flashcards to identify important words or pictures of important objects to be located in the environment (Note: textual cues start with large lettering using plain font style with no serifs and good contrast between foreground and background).

Cognitive/Perceptual

- Verbal or written commands: Commands are reminders to perform a certain action, such as "Turn to the left" or "Find the red line" on the left side. The purpose is to counteract the tendency of the person to turn toward the right.
- Combined approach: Anchors, guides, and commands can be used in any combination. Example: The client enters the room, pausing at the doorway to anchor the visual attention to the left wall, scans the room using the right hand as a guide, and turns to left to locate the cue card labeled "Closet."
- Self-cuing: Initially, the cues are given verbally by the therapist or caregiver; the objective is to have the client self-direct.

Psychosocial

- No information identified.

Context/Environment

- Provide information to client and family about USN and related conditions such as impaired self-awareness (anosognosia), and the effect on the performance of everyday activities.
- Recommend environment modifications such as having the bed positioned so the person's right side is facing the door.

Precautions/Safety Considerations

Person should be monitored carefully when moving in the environment to avoid injury to self or others. Moving to the left usually requires the most monitoring. Person is at increased risk of falling.

Prognosis and Outcome

Intervention may or may not be effective (Fong et al., 2013). Condition may be self-limiting or become chronic.

REFERENCES

Brown, E. V. D., & Powell, J. M. (2017). Assessment of unilateral neglect in stroke: Simplification and structuring of test items. *British Journal of Occupational Therapy, 80*(7), 448–452. https://doi.org/10.1177/0308022616685582

Champod, A. S., Frank, R. C., Taylor, K., & Eskes, G. A. (2018). The effects of prism adaptation on daily life activities in patients with visuospatial neglect: A systematic review. *Neuropsychological Rehabilitation, 28*(4), 491–514. https://doi.org/10.1080/09602011.2016.1182032

Chen, M.-C., Tsai, P.-L., Huang, Y.-T., & Lin, K.-C. (2013). Pleasant music improves visual attention in patients with unilateral neglect after stroke. *Brain Injury, 27*(1), 75–82. https://doi.org/10.3109/02699052.2012.722255

Chen, P., Caulfield, M. D., Hartman, A. J., O'Rourke, J., & Toglia, J. (2017). Assessing viewer-centered and stimulus-centered spatial bias: The 3s spreadsheet test version 1. *Applied Neuropsychology: Adult, 24*(6), 532–539. https://doi.org/10.1080/23279095.2016.1220382

Chen, P., Chen, C. C., Hreha, K., Goedert, K. M., & Barrett, A. M. (2015). Kessler Foundation Neglect Assessment Process uniquely measures spatial neglect during activities of daily living. *Archives of Physical Medicine and Rehabilitation, 96*(5), 869–876. https://doi.org/10.1016/j.apmr.2014.10.023

Chen, P., Hreha, K., Fortis, P., Goedert, K. M., & Barrett, A. M. (2012). Functional assessment of spatial neglect: A review of the Catherine Bergego Scale and an introduction of the Kessler Foundation Neglect Assessment Process. *Topics in Stroke Rehabilitation, 19*(5), 423–435. https://doi.org/10.1310/tsr1905-423

Chen, P., Hreha, K., & Pitteri, M. (2014). *Kessler Foundation Neglect Assessment Process: KF-NAP 2014 manual.* Kessler Foundation.

Chen, P., Pitteri, M., Gillen, G., & Ayyala, H. (2018). Ask the experts how to treat individuals with spatial neglect: A survey study. *Disability and Rehabilitation, 40*(22), 2677–2691. https://doi.org/10.1080/09638288.2017.1347720

Chen, P., & Toglia, J. (2019). Online and offline awareness deficits: Anosognosia for spatial neglect. *Rehabilitation Psychology, 64*(1), 50–64. https://doi.org/10.1037/rep0000207

Chen, P., Ward, I., Khan, U., Liu, Y., & Hreha, K. (2016). Spatial neglect hinders success of inpatient rehabilitation in individuals with traumatic brain injury: A retrospective study. *Neurorehabilitation and Neural Repair, 30*(5), 451–460. https://doi.org/10.1177/1545968315604397

Fong, K. N. K., Yang, N. Y. H., Chan, M. K. L., Chan, D. Y. L., Lau, A. F. C., Chan, D. Y. W., Cheung, J. T. Y., Cheung, H. K. Y., Chung, R. C. K., & Chan, C. C. H. (2013). Combined effects of sensory cueing and limb activation on unilateral neglect in subacute left hemiplegic stroke patients: A randomized controlled pilot study. *Clinical Rehabilitation, 27*(7), 628–637. https://doi.org/10.1177/0269215512471959

Grattan, E. S., Lang, C. E., Birkenmeier, R., Holm, M., Rubinstein, E., Van Swearingen, J., & Skidmore, E. R. (2016). Examining the feasibility, tolerability, and preliminary efficacy of repetitive task-specific practice for people with unilateral spatial neglect. *American Journal of Occupational Therapy, 70*(4), Article 7004290020. https://doi.org/10.5014/ajot.2016.019471

Grattan, E. S., & Woodbury, M. L. (2017). Do neglect assessments detect neglect differently? *American Journal of Occupational Therapy, 71*(3), Article 7103190050. https://doi.org/10.5014/ajot.2017.025015

Hreha, K., Chaudhari, A., Kong, Y., Maduri, P., & Barrett, A. M. (2018). Illustrating where spatial perception versus memory-based representation: Spatial neglect in a distinguished artist; a case report. *Neurocase, 24*(3), 151–155. https://doi.org/10.1080/13554794.2018.1495741

Hreha, K., Gillen, G., Noce, N., & Nilsen, D. (2018). The feasibility and effectiveness of using prism adaptation to treat motor and spatial dysfunction in stroke survivors with multiple incidents of stroke. *Topics in Stroke Rehabilitation, 25*(4), 305–311. https://doi.org/10.1080/10749357.2018.1437937

Hreha, K., Mulry, C., Gross, M., Jedziniak, T., Gramas, N., Ohevshalom, L., Sheridan, A., Szabo, G., Davison, C., & Barrett, A. M. (2017). Assessing chronic stroke survivors with aphasia sheds light on prevalence of spatial neglect. *Topics in Stroke Rehabilitation, 24*(2), 91–98. https://doi.org/10.1080/10749357.2016.1196906

Kamada, K., Shimodozono, M., Hamada, H., & Kawahira, K. (2011). Effects of 5 minutes of neck-muscle vibration immediately before occupational therapy on unilateral spatial neglect. *Disability and Rehabilitation, 33*(23-24), 2322–2328. https://doi.org/10.3109/09638288.2011.570411

Liu, Y.-C., Chen, K.-C., Yang, Y. K., Chen, Y.-L., & Lin, K.-C. (2011). Relationship between hemispatial inattention and performance of activities of daily living in patients with schizophrenia. *Perceptual and Motor Skills, 112*(3), 703–710. https://doi.org/10.2466/02.09.13.PMS.112.3.703-710

Oh, S.-I., Kim, J.-K., & Park, S.-Y. (2015). The effects of prism glasses and intensive upper limb exercise on hemineglect, upper limb function, and activities of daily living in stroke patients: A case series. *Journal of Physical Therapy Science, 27*(12), 3941–3943. https://doi.org/10.1589/jpts.27.3941

Petzold, A., Korner-Bitensky, N., Salbach, N. M., Ahmed, S., Menon, A., & Ogourtsova, T. (2012). Increasing knowledge of best practices for occupational therapists treating post-stroke unilateral spatial neglect: Results of a knowledge-translation intervention study. *Journal of Rehabilitation Medicine, 44*(2), 118–124. https://doi.org/10.2340/16501977-0910

Shah, P. P., Spaldo, N., Barrett, A. M., & Chen, P. (2013). Assessment and functional impact of allocentric neglect: A reminder from a case study. *Clinical Neuropsychologist, 27*(5), 840–863. https://doi.org/10.1080/13854046.2013.783120

Tempest, S., & Maskill, L. (2017). Complex perceptual functions: Body scheme and agnosia, constructional skills and neglect. In L. Maskill & S. Tempest (Eds.), *Neuropsychology for occupational therapists* (4th ed., pp. 113–122). Wiley Blackwell.

Tsai, P.-L., Chen, M.-C., Huang, Y.-T., Lin, K.-C., Chen, K.-L., & Hsu, Y.-W. (2013). Listening to classical music ameliorates unilateral neglect after stroke. *American Journal of Occupational Therapy, 67*(3), 328–335. https://doi.org/10.5014/ajot.2013.006312

Turton, A. J., O'Leary, K., Gabb, J., Woodward, R., & Gilchrist, I. D. (2010). A single blinded randomised controlled pilot trial of prism adaptation for improving self-care in stroke patients with neglect. *Neuropsychological Rehabilitation, 20*(2), 180–196. https://doi.org/10.1080/0960 2010903040683

Wu, C.-Y., Wang, T.-N., Chen, Y. T., Lin, K. C., Chen, Y. A., Li, H.-T., & Tsai, P.-L. (2013). Effects of constraint-induced therapy combined with eye patching on functional outcomes and movement kinematics in poststroke neglect. *American Journal of Occupational Therapy, 67*(2), 236–245. https://doi.org/10.5014/ajot.2013.006486

Yoshihiro, N., & Ito, E. (2017). Effect of passive limb activation by functional electrical stimulation on wheelchair driving in patients with unilateral spatial neglect: A case study. *Hong Kong Journal of Occupational Therapy, 30*(1), 14–21. https://doi.org/10.1016/j.hkjot.2017.10.003

BIBLIOGRAPHY

Chen, P., Hreha, K., Kong, Y., & Barrett, A. M. (2015). Impact of spatial neglect on stroke rehabilitation: Evidence from the setting of an inpatient rehabilitation facility. *Archives of Physical Medicine and Rehabilitation, 96*(8), 1458–1466. https://doi.org/10.1016/j.apmr.2015.03.019

Grattan, E. S., Skidmore, E. R., & Woodbury, M. L. (2018). Examining anosognosia of neglect. *OTJR: Occupation, Participation and Health, 38*(2), 113–120. https://doi.org/10.1177/15394 49217747586

Kwon, J. S. (2018). Therapeutic intervention for visuo-spatial neglect after stroke: A meta-analysis of randomized controlled trials. *Osong Public Health and Research Perspectives, 9*(2), 59–65. https://doi.org/10.24171/j.phrp.2018.9.2.04

Liu, K. P. Y., Hanly, J., Fahey P., Fong, S. S. M., & Bye, R. (2019). A systematic review and meta-analysis of rehabilitative interventions for unilateral spatial neglect and hemianopia poststroke from 2006 through 2016. *Archives of Physical Medicine and Rehabilitation, 100*(5), 956–979. https://doi.org/10.1016/j.apmr.2018.05.037

Toglia, J. P., Golisz, K. M., & Goverover, Y. (2019). Cognition, perception and occupational performance. In B. A. Boyt Schell & G. Gillen (Eds.), *Willard and Spackman's occupational therapy* (13th ed., pp. 901–941). Wolters Kluwer.

Wagener, S. G., Anheluk, M., Arulanantham, C., & Scheiman, M. (2014). Vision assessment and intervention. In M. Weightman, M. V. Radomski, P. A. Mashima, & C. R. Roth (Eds.), *Mild traumatic brain injury rehabilitation toolkit* (pp. 97–146). Borden Institute.

Yang, N. Y. H., Zhou, D., Chung, R. C. K., Li-Tsang, C. W. P., & Fong, K. N. K. (2013). Rehabilitation interventions for unilateral neglect after stroke: A systematic review from 1997 through 2012. *Frontiers in Human Neuroscience, 7,* Article 187. https://doi.org/10.3389/fnhum.2013.00187

Vegetative and Minimally Conscious States

Also called unresponsive wakefulness syndrome (UWS) and disorders of consciousness (DOC). UWS is offered as a new name for the vegetative state to counter the negative connotation of the term "vegetative," but the term "vegetative state" still appears more frequently in the literature and diagnostic terms.

Description

In a vegetative state (VS) the person is unresponsive and unaware of self, other people, or the environment due to significant dysfunction of the cerebral hemispheres, but with sufficient sparing of the diencephalon and brain stem to preserve autonomic and motor reflexes and sleep–wake cycles (Porter, 2018). Typical responses are eye opening, reactive pupils, oculocephalic reflex, and a sleep–wake cycle that is not related to a specific circadian (day–night) rhythm. More complex brain stem reflexes such as yawning, chewing, swallowing, guttural vocalizations, cry or smile for no apparent reason, reaction to loud sounds (startle reflex) or blinking in response to bright lights may be present (Porter, 2018). A permanent or persistent vegetative state is one that lasts longer than 6 months for anoxic or other metabolic brain injury and 12 months for those with a traumatic brain injury (TBI; Dhamapurkar et al., 2018). Corresponds to Rancho Levels of Cognitive Functioning (Hagen, 1998).

A minimally conscious state (MCS) is characterized by some evidence of awareness of self and the environment (Porter, 2018). Person may establish eye contact, may purposefully grasp objects, may respond to commands in a stereotypical manner, and may answer commands with single words. However, responses may be inconsistent. Two subcategories are recognized on the Wessex Head Injury Matrix: MCS-Minus and MCS-Plus. MCS-Minus is described as a minimal level of behavioral interaction characterized by the presence of very basic nonreflex movements such as orientation to noxious stimuli or pursuit of eye movements that occur appropriately in relation to relevant environmental stimuli. MCS-Plus is described as the presence of overt command following, intelligible verbalization, reproducible gestures, or verbal "yes" or "no" responses (Gilutz et al., 2015). Permanent MCS is assumed if the condition lasts 5 years or more (Dhamapurkar et al., 2018).

Emergence from an MCS (emerging MCS) is defined by overt functional communication or functional use of objects (Gilutz et al., 2015; corresponds to Rancho Scale (1998). Minimally Conscious State-Plus (MCS-Plus) is able to follow commands, has intelligible verbalization, or gestural or verbal yes/no intentional communication. Minimally Conscious State-Minus (MCS-Minus) has automatic motor behaviors (e.g., nose scratching); demonstrates object manipulation (e.g., grasping and holding a cup); can localize objects in space (e.g., reach and grasp examiner's hand); can localize noxious stimuli (e.g., rubbing an area that has just been pinched); demonstrates visual pursuit and visual fixation; does not demonstrate receptive or expressive language function (Giacino et al., 2014).

Prolonged disorder of consciousness (PDOC) is a disordered state of consciousness that lasts more than 4 weeks (Dhamapurkar et al., 2017).

Cause

Injury to brain tissue due to trauma (traumatic brain injury), anoxia or hypoxia (oxygen deprivation due to stroke, TBI, cardiac or pulmonary arrest, hanging, drowning, suicide attempt from carbon monoxide poisoning, embolism, drug overdose), metabolic event (severe hypoglycemia), infection (encephalitis), advanced dementia, or other neurodegenerative disease (Wilson et al., 2016).

Evaluation/Assessment

Areas

- Activities of Daily Living/Instrumental ADL: functional movement, functional communication, transfers, bladder and bowel management, oral hygiene

- Education/Work: none
- Play/Leisure: interests, values, frequency, location
- Rest/Sleep: sleep–wake cycle, daytime sleepiness
- Social Participation: type, frequency, location, with whom
- Sensorimotor: brain steam reflexes, voluntary responses, joint movement and range of motion, vision (eyes open, object recognition, fixation, pursuit/tracking eye movements), reproducible gestures (nonverbal, verbal), object manipulation, deep pressure response, oral reflexes (clamping, tongue movement), chewing, sitting (with support, independent), muscle tone, pain (often due to tight muscles)
- Cognitive/Perceptual: state or level of arousal/awareness, attention span and concentration, memory, orientation to noxious stimuli, following overt commands
- Psychosocial: irritability, agitation
- Context/Environment: adaptive technology, family support including information and care instructions, splinting and instructions for use and care
- Comorbidities: hydrocephalus, osteoporosis, pressure sores, contractures

Instruments

Instruments Developed by Occupational Therapy Personnel

- Sensory Modality Assessment and Rehabilitation Technique (SMART; Gill-Thwaites & Munday, 2004)

Instruments Developed by Other Professionals and Used by Occupational Therapy Personnel

- Coma Recovery Scale-Revised (see JFK Coma Recovery Scale–Revised)
- Glasgow Outcome Scale (GOS; Jennett & Bond, 1975)
- JFK Coma Recovery Scale–Revised (CRS-R; Giacino et al., 2004, in References; see also Tamashiro et al., 2014, in References)
- Neurobehavioural Rating Scale (NRS; Levin et al., 1987)
- Rancho Los Amigos Cognitive Scale–Revised (Rancho Scale–Revised, Rancho Levels of Cognitive Functioning; Hagen, 1998, in References)
- Reuth DOC Response Assessment (RDOC-RA; Gilutz et al., 2015, in References)
- Wessex Head Injury Matrix (WHIM; Shiel et al., 2000; see also Dhamapurkar et al., 2018, in References)

Problems/Issues

Activities of Daily Living/Instrumental ADL

- Person is usually unable to perform basic self-maintenance activities independently.
- Person usually requires maximum assistance to perform any transfer.
- Person is unable to respond to verbal commands.

Education/Work

- Not discussed.

Play/Leisure

- Not discussed.

Rest/Sleep

- Person usually experiences difficulty with sleep–wake cycles.

Social Participation

- Not discussed.

Sensorimotor

- Person usually is unable to move voluntarily although some reflex movements may be possible.
- Person may have limited joint range of motion including possible contracture.
- Person may have reduced use of sensory systems including auditory, smell, taste, tactile, and vision.

Cognitive/Perceptual
- Person may have difficulty maintaining state of consciousness, including alertness.
- Person may have difficulty maintaining level of arousal.
- Person may have difficulty maintaining attention and concentration.
- Person may have impaired memory.

Psychosocial
- Person may become irritable or agitated.
- Person usually is unable to interact with others, including family and friends.

Context/Environment
- Family may have limited knowledge about altered states of consciousness.
- Person may need adapted devices including mobility and transfer equipment.

Intervention/Treatment

Models and programs developed by occupational therapy personnel include case study (Dhamapurkar et al., 2016; Wilson et al., 2016) and SMART (da Conceição Teixeira et al., 2018; Morrissey et al., 2018; Tennant & Gill-Thwaites, 2017). Models and programs developed by other professionals but used by occupational therapy personnel include positioning (Wilson et al., 2013), Reuth DOC Periodic Intervention Model (RDOC-PIM; Gilutz et al., 2015), sensory stimulation (Padilla & Domina, 2016), and specialized early treatment (Seel et al., 2013). Team members include physicians, nursing personnel, psychologists, physical therapists, speech–language pathologists, speech therapists, and occupational therapy personnel. Goals include enabling person to attain functional communication or functional use of objects (Gilutz et al., 2015). Some clients may continue to recover and be able to participate in the everyday occupations of self-maintenance including self-care, enjoy leisure occupations, engage in paid or unpaid work, attend school, and participate in social activities.

Activities of Daily Living/Instrumental ADL
- Maintain routine as much as possible. Perform ADLs at normal scheduled time such as bathing in the morning.
- Assist with bowel and bladder relief using catheter or diapers.

Education/Work
- Not discussed.

Play/Leisure
- Not discussed.

Rest/Sleep
- Maintain normal day–night schedule—lights on during day, off at night.

Social Participation
- Always speak to client before beginning an intervention even if client gives no indication of response.
- Provide family and friends with guidelines for interacting with client based on level of consciousness.

Sensorimotor
- Positioning: Be sure client is turned in bed on a schedule to prevent pressure sores.
- Recommend special bedding to help prevent pressure sores if not already in use.
- As feasible, increase client's position to sitting supported in bed, sitting assisted (two persons) on side of bed, sitting supported in a chair with armrests, sitting without support, standing supported. Record position and amount of time in specific position. (Note: Responses to testing may improve as more upright position is obtained. Record position when reporting evaluation results.)

- Use passive range of motion to maintain joint mobility and decrease contractures.
- Consider splinting to decrease contractures.
- Reduce extraneous noise as much as possible to avoid overstimulation. Generally no TV, radio, and mute sound of machines (monitors) as much as possible.
- Increase response reaction to sensory stimulation, such as grasping a cold washcloth.
- Increase visual skills (look at a family member for more than 10 seconds).
- Increase auditory skills (turns head toward person speaking when greeted).
- Improve fine motor skills (grasp objects full hand, then fingers and thumb).

Cognitive/Perceptual
- Use of bimodal or multimodal sensory stimulation (combinations of auditory, gustatory, olfactory, tactile/kinesthetic, and visual input) may increase level of arousal and alertness (Padilla & Domina, 2016).
  - Auditory: music, voices of loved ones, loud clapping, tuning forks, bells, singing.
  - Gustatory: tastes of sour, salty, sweet, mouthwash on mouth swab.
  - Olfactory: scents of perfume, vinegar, lemon, vanilla, coffee.
  - Tactile/kinesthetic: massage, touch, temperature, noxious stimuli, pressure, range of motion exercises.
  - Visual: colored paper, light pens, pictures and photos of family members or favorite items.
- Use hand-over-hand technique with verbal directions to facilitate basic activities (washing, eating).
- Increase response time to verbal stimulation (eyes open, eyes focus).
- Increase ability to follow verbal directions to make motor responses (squeeze my hand, wave hand, move leg).
- Increase ability to follow verbal commands (wash face, say your name, turn head five times).
- Increase attention span (follow two or more commands).

Psychosocial
- Observe client for signs of irritability (increased respiration, heart rate, closing eyes).

Context/Environment
- Provide family and caregivers with information about disorders of consciousness.
- Provide family and caregivers with instructions for use and care of adapted equipment such as wheelchair.
- Provide nursing staff with information and care if splints are used to maintain positioning and for prevention of contractures.

Precautions/Safety Considerations

Clients are at increased risk of infection; behavioral changes or cognitive deterioration may be first indicator. Monitor feeding tube, especially if repositioning client. Monitor client for breathing difficulties, including suctioning and care of a tracheostomy tube if present. Monitor client for signs of seizures.

Prognosis and Outcome

Prognosis of clients with persistent deficits is typically poor. Clients with minimally conscious state tend to improve (Porter, 2018).

REFERENCES

da Conceição Teixeira, L., Gill-Thwaites, H., Reynolds, F., & Duport, S. (2018). Can behavioural observations made during the SMART assessment detect the potential for later emergence from vegetative state? *Neuropsychological Rehabilitation, 28*(8), 1340–1349. https://doi.org/10.1080/09602011.2016.1243482

Dhamapurkar, S. K., Rose, A., Florschutz, G., & Wilson, B. A. (2016). The natural history of continuing improvement in an individual after a long period of impaired consciousness: The story of I.J. *Brain Injury, 30*(2), 230–236. https://doi.org/10.3109/02699052.2015.1094132

Dhamapurkar, S. K., Wilson, B. A., Rose, A., Florschutz, G., Watson, P., & Shiel, A. (2018). Does a regular Wessex Head Injury Matrix assessment identify early signs of infections in people with prolonged disorders of consciousness? *Brain Injury, 32*(9), 1103–1109. https://doi.org/10.1080/02699052.2018.1484165

Dhamapurkar, S. K., Wilson, B. A., Rose, A., Watson, P., & Shiel, A. (2017). Does Modafinil improve the level of consciousness for people with a prolonged disorder of consciousness? A retrospective pilot study. *Disability and Rehabilitation, 39*(26), 2633–2639. https://doi.org/10.1080/09638288.2016.1236414

Giacino, J. T., Kalmar, K., & Whyte, J. (2004). The JFK Coma Recovery Scale–Revised: Measurement characteristics and diagnostic utility. *Archives of Physical Medicine and Rehabilitation, 85*(12), 2020–2029. https://doi.org/10.1016/j.apmr.2004.02.033

Gilutz, Y., Lazary, A., Karpin, H., Vatine, J.-J., Misha, T., Fortinsky, H., & Sharon, H. (2015). Detailed behavioral assessment promotes accurate diagnosis in patients with disorders of consciousness. *Frontiers in Human Neuroscience, 9*, Article 87. https://doi.org/10.3389/fnhum.2015.00087

Hagen, C. (1998). *Rancho levels of cognitive functioning* (3rd ed.). Rancho Los Amigo Medical Center.

Morrissey, A. M., Gill-Thwaites, H., Wilson, B., Leonard, R., McLellan, L., Pundole, A., & Shiel, A. (2018). The role of the SMART and WHIM in behavioural assessment of disorders of consciousness: Clinical utility and scope for a symbiotic relationship. *Neuropsychological Rehabilitation, 28*(8), 1254–1265. https://doi.org/10.1080/09602011.2017.1354769

Padilla, R., & Domina, A. (2016). Effectiveness of sensory stimulation to improve arousal and alertness of people in a coma or persistent vegetative state after traumatic brain injury: A systematic review. *American Journal of Occupational Therapy, 70*(3), Article 7003180030. https://doi.org/10.5014/ajot.2016.021022

Porter, R. S. (Ed.). (2018). *The Merck manual of diagnosis and therapy* (20th ed.). Merck Sharp & Dohme.

Seel, R. T., Douglas, J., Dennison, A. C., Heaner, S., Farris, K., & Rogers, C. (2013). Specialized early treatment for persons with disorders of consciousness: Program components and outcomes. *Archives of Physical Medicine and Rehabilitation, 94*(10), 1908–1923. https://doi.org/10.1016/j.apmr.2012.11.052

Tamashiro, M., Rivas, M. E., Ron, M., Salierno, F., Dalera, M., & Olmos, L. (2014). A Spanish validation of the Coma Recovery Scale-Revised (CRS-R). *Brain Injury, 28*(13-14), 1744–1747. https://doi.org/10.3109/02699052.2014.947621

Tennant, A., & Gill-Thwaites, H. (2017). A study of the internal construct and predictive validity of the SMART assessment for emergence from vegetative state. *Brain Injury, 31*(2), 185–192. https://doi.org/10.1080/02699052.2016.1225983

Wilson, B. A., Dhamapurkar, S., & Rose, A. (2016). Assessment and treatment of people with a disorder of consciousness: An account of some recent studies. *Psychology & Neuroscience, 9*(2), 221–229. https://doi.org/10.1037/pne0000053

Wilson, B. A., Dhamapurkar, S., Tunnard, C., Watson, P., & Florschutz, G. (2013). The effect of positioning on the level of arousal and awareness in patients in the vegetative state or the minimally conscious state: A replication an extension of a previous finding. *Brain Impairment, 14*(3), 475–479. https://doi.org/10.1017/Brimp.2013.34

BIBLIOGRAPHY

Hamby, J. R. (2018). The nervous system. In H. Smith-Gabai & S. E. Holm (Eds.), *Occupational therapy in acute care* (2nd ed., pp. 293–391). AOTA Press.

Klingshirn, H., Grill, E., Bender, A., Strobl, R., Mittrach, R., Braitmayer, K., & Müller, M. (2015). Quality of evidence of rehabilitation interventions in long-term care for people with severe disorders of consciousness after brain injury: A systematic review. *Journal of Rehabilitation Medicine, 47*(7), 577–585. https://doi.org/10.2340/16501977-1983

Wilson, B. A., Dhamapurkar, S. K., & Rose, A. (2016). *Surviving brain damage after assault: From vegetative state to meaningful life.* Routledge.

Mental and Behavioral Disorders

Anxiety and General Anxiety Disorder

Description

"Anxiety is a distressing, unpleasant emotional state of nervousness and uneasiness" and "is often accompanied by physical changes and behaviors similar to those caused by fear" (Porter, 2018, p. 1741). Anxiety is defined as apprehension of danger and dread accompanied by restlessness, tension, tachycardia, and dyspnea unattached to a clearly identifiable stimulus (*Stedman's*, 2011). Kinds of anxiety include castration anxiety, free-floating anxiety, generalized anxiety disorder, separation anxiety, situational anxiety, and panic disorder (O'Toole, 2017). The impact of anxiety on a person's everyday living may result in significant functional decline and may affect all aspects of occupational performance, including self-care, parenting, leisure, social life, and work (Cara, 2013). Bodily functions may be involved including autonomic, cardiovascular, gastrointestinal, genital, muscular, respiratory, and urinary (Cara, 2013).

General anxiety disorder (GAD) "is characterized by excessive anxiety and worry about a number of activities or events" that is present for 6 months or longer (Porter, 2018, p. 1742). People with GAD have difficulty controlling the worries, which may be associated with three or more of the following symptoms: restlessness, easily fatigability, difficulty concentrating, irritability, muscle tension, and disturbed sleep (Porter, 2018).

The *Diagnostic and Statistical Manual of Mental Disorders* (5th ed.; *DSM-5*; American Psychiatric Association, 2013) lists, in addition to the general anxiety disorder, eight other anxiety conditions: agoraphobia, panic disorder, selective mutism, separation anxiety disorder, specific phobia, social anxiety disorder (social phobia), substance/medication-induced anxiety disorder, and anxiety disorder due to another medical condition, such as Parkinson's disease. Formal criteria for a diagnosis of anxiety are listed in the *DSM-5* (American Psychiatric Association, 2013).

Cause

The cause of anxiety is not fully known but is associated with both psychiatric and general medical factors. The cause of GAD is unknown, but commonly exists in people who have alcohol abuse, major depression, or panic disorder (Porter, 2018). For theories about the causation of overresponsivity see Green and Ben-Sasson (2010).

Evaluation/Assessment

Areas

- Activities of Daily Living/Instrumental ADL: self-care, meal preparation, shopping, driving
- Education/Work: academic or work performance
- Play/Leisure: interests, values, frequency, location
- Rest/Sleep: sleep habits, sleep disturbance
- Social Participation: type, frequency, location, with whom
- Sensorimotor: muscle tension, restlessness, physical fitness, sensory processing
- Cognitive/Perceptual: concentration, mental fatigue
- Psychosocial: worry, fear, irritability, feelings of vulnerability, role performance, quality of life
- Context/Environment: home, family, community, natural and built environments
- Comorbidities: autism spectrum disorder, bipolar disorder, dementia, depression, obsessive-compulsive disorder, Parkinson's disease, posttraumatic stress disorder, sensory processing disorder, substance abuse

Instruments
Instruments Developed by Occupational Therapy Personnel
- Adolescent/Adult Sensory Profile (AASP; Brown & Dunn, 2002)
- Role Checklist (RC; Oakley et al., 1986)
- Role Checklist Version 3: Participation and Satisfaction (RCv3; Scott, 2019)
- Self-Assessment of Activities (SAA; Cara, 2013, in References)

Instruments Developed by Other Professionals and Used by Occupational Therapy Personnel
- Agitated Behavior Scale (ABS; Corrigan, 1989)
- Beck Anxiety Inventory (BAI; Beck & Steer, 1993)
- Beck Depression Inventory (2nd ed.; BDI-II; Beck et al., 1996)
- Function Questionnaire (FQ; Taylor & Arrow, 1988; see also Cara, 2013, in References)
- Maslach Burnout Inventory (3rd ed.; MBI-3; Maslach et al., 1997)
- Observed Emotion Rating Scale (OERS; Lawton et al., 1999; original name: Philadelphia Geriatric Center Affect Rating Scale, 1996)
- Return-to-Work Self-Efficacy Scale (RWEFS; Lagerveld et al., 2010)
- Rosenberg Self-Esteem as a Worker Scale (RSEWS; Corbière et al., 2009)
- Work Role Functioning Questionnaire (WRFQ; Durand et al., 2004)

Problems/Issues

Activities of Daily Living/Instrumental ADL
- Person may stop communicating with others such as turning off the phone and refusing to answer the doorbell.
- Person may report doing only survival skills, including reducing the amount of food eaten.

Education/Work
- Person may worry about ability to perform job requirements.

Play/Leisure
- Person may stop engaging in fun or favorite leisure occupations.
- Person may engage in passive activities only such as watching television.

Rest/Sleep
- Person often experiences sleep disturbances: inability to fall asleep or stay asleep.
- Person may report nightmares or night terrors.

Social Participation
- Person may stop participating in social activities.

Sensorimotor
- Person may be overresponsive to certain stimuli.

Cognitive/Perceptual
- Person may lack understanding of the consequences of acting or not acting in specific situations such as the effects on the physical body or mental health.

Psychosocial
- Person may worry about the consequences of real or imagined physical condition.
- Person may be fearful about engaging in activities.
- Person may lack self-confidence and belief in the self because of some prior experience.
- Person may worry about having a panic attack.
- Person may refuse to interact with others and disconnect interpersonal relations.
- Person may report that once enjoyable activities are no longer enjoyed.
- Person may report feelings of being uneasy or off balance.
- Person may report feelings of being overwhelmed.
- Person may report feelings of impending doom.
- Person may report feelings of helplessness and out of control.
- Person may report feelings of "going insane."
- Person may report feelings of depersonalization (having feelings of unreality, as if in a dream state).
- Person may report feelings of detachment from environment and personal surroundings.

Context/Environment
- Person may experience anxiety in contexts, environments, or situations that are similar, in the person's mind, to those that triggered original anxiety.

Intervention/Treatment

Models of practice developed by occupational therapists include case study (Cara, 2013), model of human occupation (Lalande et al., 2017), Redesigning Daily Occupations (ReDO) program (Eklund, 2013), sensory modulation (Cara, 2013), tree theme method (Gunnarsson et al., 2018), and weighted blanket approach (Chen et al., 2013). Models developed by other professionals include Acceptance and Commitment Therapy (ACT; Hayes et al., 2012), cognitive behavioral therapy (CBT; Lalande et al., 2017), integrative group therapy model (Söchting et al., 2013), coping/stress management techniques (autogenic training, breathing exercises, progressive muscle relaxation, relaxation training, visualization; Cara, 2013), craft and art activities (Cara, 2013), education and lifestyle alterations (Cara, 2013), functional behavioral training (Cara, 2013), journal and diary writing (Cara, 2013), levels of intervention (American Occupational Therapy Association, 2012), rational-cognitive approaches (Cara, 2013), time management (Cara, 2013), virtual nature experience (Reynolds et al., 2018), and social skills training (Cara, 2013). For children, the children's group therapy program (Tokolahi et al., 2013). For adults, the focus is on using narrative and meaningful occupation to connect the person to individual sense of self and to appreciate personal experience to cope with mental health difficulties (Mulholland & Jackson, 2018). For children, the aim was to use developmentally appropriate occupations to teach cognitive, behavioral, and functional skills through participation as a means for managing anxiety (Tokolahi et al., 2013).

Activities of Daily Living/Instrumental ADL
- Encourage person to perform self-care activities.
- Encourage person to perform instrumental ADLs, such as doing household chores and caring for the pet.

Education/Work
- Return-to-work program (Lalande et al., 2017).
  - ► Activity 1: Individual occupational therapy meetings and follow-up adapted to the needs of each client.
  - ► Activity 2: A physical conditioning program offered in collaboration with kinesiologists.
  - ► Activity 3: Group intervention sessions (topics included energy management, occupational balance, values and beliefs associated with work, resistance to change, interpersonal relationships in the workplace, mindfulness meditation and its everyday use, prevention of relapse, stigma associated with work, sick leave, cognitive skills, and return to work).

Play/Leisure
- Encourage engagement in leisure activities.

Rest/Sleep
- See Sleep–Wake Disorders in Section 13: Lifestyle Conditions.

Social Participation
- Encourage person to remain engaged in social activities.
- Encourage person to reestablish contacts with friends.

Sensorimotor
- Encourage person to remain physically active.

Cognitive/Perceptual
- Assist person to maintain habits, routines, and conscious structuring (time management) of daily activities.
- Tokolahi et al. (2013) provides a nine-step program for working with children.

Psychosocial

- Assist person to develop and maintain a positive state of mind focusing on what can be done versus what cannot be done from the individual's perspective and situation.
- Encourage person to maintain roles and roles performance.

Context/Environment

- Encourage person to engage in activities in the natural environment: walks, hikes, bird watching.

Precautions/Safety Considerations

Anxiety can be very distressing (potential suicide or suicidal behavior). Anxiety can interfere with occupational performance and everyday functioning.

Prognosis and Outcome

Anxiety may be transient and focused on a particular event or situation, which can be addressed through management of specific symptoms. Anxiety can become a chronic condition that reoccurs throughout the person's life. Different approaches may be needed to manage symptoms depending on what event(s) or situation(s) are most distressing to the person at a particular time (American Psychiatric Association, 2013).

REFERENCES

American Occupational Therapy Association. (2012). Anxiety disorders. In *School mental health toolkit.* https://www.aota.org/-/media/Corporate/Files/Practice/Children/SchoolMHToolkit/Anxiety%20Disorders%20Info%20Sheet.pdf

American Psychiatric Association. (2013). *Diagnostic and statistical manual of mental disorders* (5th ed.). https://doi.org/10.1176/appi.books.9780890425596

Cara, E. (2013). Anxiety disorders. In E. Cara & A. MacRae (Eds.), *Psychosocial occupational therapy: An evolving practice* (3rd ed., pp. 258–307). Delmar Cengage Learning.

Chen, H. Y., Yang, H., Chi, H. Y., & Chen, H. M. (2013). Physiological effects of deep touch pressure on anxiety alleviation: The weighted blanket approach. *Journal of Medical and Biological Engineering, 33*(5), 463–470.

Eklund, M. (2013). Anxiety, depression, and stress among women in work rehabilitation for stress-related disorders. *International Journal of Mental Health, 42*(4), 34–47. https://doi.org/10.2753/IMH0020-7411420402

Green, S. A., & Ben-Sasson, A. (2010). Anxiety disorders and sensory over-responsivity in children with autism spectrum disorders: Is there a causal relationship? *Journal of Autism and Developmental Disorders, 40*(12), 1495–1504. https://doi.org/10.1007/s10803-010-1007-x

Gunnarsson, A. B., Wagman, P., Hedin, K., & Håkansson, C. (2018). Treatment of depression and/or anxiety—Outcomes of a randomised controlled trial of the tree theme method versus regular occupational therapy. *BMC Psychology, 6,* Article 25. https://doi.org/10.1186/s40359-018-0237-0

Hayes, S. C., Strosahl, K. D., & Wilson, K. G. (2012). *Acceptance and commitment therapy* (2nd ed.). Guildford Press.

Lalande, M., Vachon, B., Hogue-Harwood, M., & Rivard, S. (2017). Promoting recovery for people with workplace absence issues attributed to anxiety or mood disorders. *Occupational Therapy Now, 19*(6), 11–13.

Mulholland, E., & Jackson, J. (2018). The experience of older adults with anxiety and depression living in the community: Aging, occupation and mental wellbeing. *British Journal of Occupational Therapy, 81*(11), 657–666. https://doi.org/10.1177/0308022618777200

O'Toole, M. T. (Ed.). (2017). *Mosby's dictionary of medicine, nursing & health professions* (10th ed.). Elsevier.

Porter, R. S. (Ed.). (2018). *The Merck manual of diagnosis and therapy* (20th ed.). Merck Sharp & Dohme.

Reynolds, L., Rodiek, S., Lininger, M., & McCulley, M. A. (2018). Can a virtual nature experience reduce anxiety and agitation in people with dementia. *Journal of Housing for the Elderly, 32*(2), 176–193. https://doi.org/10.1080/02763893.2018.1431583

Söchting, I., O'Neal, E., Third, B., Rogers, J., & Ogrodniczuk, J. S. (2013). An integrative group therapy model for depression and anxiety in later life. *International Journal of Group Psychotherapy, 63*(4), 502–523. https://doi.org/10.1521/ijgp.2013.63.4.502

Stedman's medical dictionary for the health professions and nursing (7th ed.). (2011). Wolters Kluwer.

Tokolahi, E., Em-Chhour, C., Barkwill, L., & Stanley, S. (2013). An occupation-based group for children with anxiety. *British Journal of Occupational Therapy, 76*(1), 31–36. https://doi.org/10.4276/030802213X13576469254694

BIBLIOGRAPHY

Davis, J., & Noves, S. (2019). Anxiety, obsessive-compulsive and related disorders. In C. Brown, V. C. Stoffel, & J. P. Muñoz (Eds.), *Occupational therapy in mental health: A vision for participation* (2nd ed., pp. 197–210). F.A. Davis.

Fox, J., Erlandsson, L. K., & Shiel, A. (2019). A systemic review and narrative synthesis of occupational therapy-led interventions for individuals with anxiety and stress-related disorders. *Occupational Therapy in Mental Health, 35*(2), 179–204. https://doi.org/10.1080/0164212X.2018.1516172

Green, S. A., Ben-Sasson, A., Soto, T. W., & Carter, A. S. (2012). Anxiety and sensory over-responsivity in toddlers with autism spectrum disorders: Bidirectional effects across time. *Journal of Autism and Developmental Disorders, 42*(6), 1112–1119. https://doi.org/10.1007/s10803-011-1361-3

Lovegrove, C., Bannigan, K., Cheeseman, D., & Latour, J. M. (2017). The involvement of people with Parkinson's in designing a study of the lived experience of anxiety. *British Journal of Occupational Therapy, 80*(8), 494–501. https://doi.org/10.1177/0308022617700654

Lutz, S. G., Holmes, J. D., Ready, E. A., Jenkins, M. E., & Johnson, A. M. (2016). Clinical presentation of anxiety in Parkinson's disease: A scoping review. *OTJR: Occupation, Participation and Health, 36*(3), 134–147. https://doi.org/10.1177/1539449216661714

Roush, S., Monica, C., Carpenter-Song, E., & Drake, R. E. (2015). First-person perspectives on dual diagnosis anonymous (DDA): A qualitative study. *Journal of Dual Diagnosis, 11*(2), 136–141. https://doi.org/10.1080/15504263.2015.1025215

Serafini, G., Engel-Yeger, B., Vazquez, G. H., Pompili, M., & Amore, M. (2017). Sensory processing disorders are associated with duration of current episode and severity of side effects. *Psychiatry Investigation, 14*(1), 51–57. https://doi.org/10.4306/pi.2017.14.1.51

Urish, C. K. (2017). Anxiety disorders. In B. J. Atchison & D. P. Dirette (Eds.), *Conditions in occupational therapy* (5th ed., pp. 147–164). Wolters Kluwer.

Bipolar Disorders

Also called manic depressive disorders, affective disorders, mood disorders.

Description

Bipolar disorders are characterized by episodes of manic and depression behaviors that may alternate, although many people have a predominance of one or the other. Bipolar disorders usually begin during the teenage or early adult years. Lifetime prevalence is about 4%. Rates of Bipolar I disorder are about equal for men and women (R. S. Porter, 2018).

Cause

The exact cause is unknown, but heredity, changes in the level of brain neurotransmitters, and psychosocial factors may be involved. Drugs such as sympathomimetics, alcohol, and certain antidepressants may trigger exacerbations in some people with bipolar disorders (R. S. Porter, 2018).

Bipolar disorders are classified as Bipolar I (mania with or without major depressive episode), Bipolar II (major depressive episode with a hypomanic episode), and unspecified bipolar disorder (bipolar features, but do not meet criteria for other classification (American Psychiatric Association, 2013). Formal criteria for a diagnosis of bipolar disorders are listed in the *Diagnostic and Statistical Manual of Mental Disorders* (5th ed.; *DSM-5*; American Psychiatric Association, 2013).

Evaluation/Assessment

Areas

- Activities of Daily Living/Instrumental ADL: cooking, dieting, housekeeping, laundry, shopping, financial planning and budgeting, driving
- Education/Work: work performance
- Play/Leisure: interests, values, frequency, location
- Rest/Sleep: sleep disturbance
- Social Participation: type, frequency, location, with whom
- Sensorimotor: exercise, energy level, fatigue
- Cognitive/Perceptual: prospective memory, executive functions
- Psychosocial: mindfulness, mood, self-awareness,
- Context/Environment: knowledge of illness by person, family, and others; knowledge of resources, emergency plan for relapse, social support system
- Comorbidities: substance abuse, anxiety (Roush et al., 2015), pneumonia (Yang et al., 2013)

Instruments

Instruments Developed by Occupational Therapy Personnel

- Adolescent/Adult Sensory Profile (AASP; Brown & Dunn, 2002)
- Assessment of Motor and Process Skills (8th ed.; AMPS-8; Fisher & Bray Jones, 2010)
- Functional Needs Assessment (FNA; Dombrowski, 1990)
- Occupational Self-Assessment (Version 2.2; OSA 2.2; Baron et al., 2006)

Instruments Developed by Other Professionals and Used by Occupational Therapy Personnel

- Beck Depression Inventory (2nd ed.; BDI-II; Beck et al., 1996)
- Beck Hopelessness Scale (BHS; Beck, 1993)
- Beck Scale for Suicide Ideation (BSS; Beck, 1991)
- Cambridge Prospective Memory Test (CAMPROMPT; Wilson et al., 2005)
- Cognitive Complaints in Bipolar Disorder Rating Assessment (COBRA; Rosa et al., 2013)
- European Quality of Life 5-Dimension Scale (EuroQol 5 Dimension; EQ-5D; EuroQol Group, 1990)
- Hamilton Rating Scale for Depression (HRSD; Hamilton, 1959)
- Manchester Short Assessment of Quality of Life (MANSA; Priebe et al., 1999)
- Mini-International Neuropsychiatric Interview (MINI; Sheehan et al., 1998)
- Mini-Mental State Examination (MMSE; Folstein et al., 1975)
- Multidimensional Scale of Independent Functioning (MSIF; Jaeger et al., 2003)
- Pearlin Self-Mastery Scale (PSMS; Pearlin & Schooler, 1978; also called Pearlin Mastery Scale)
- Positive and Negative Syndrome Scale (PANSS; Kay et al., 1987)
- Quality of Life Enjoyment and Satisfaction Questionnaire (QLESQ; Endicott et al., 1993)
- Rivermead Behavioural Memory Test (3rd ed.; RBMT-3; Wilson et al., 1991)
- Social Adjustment Scale (SAS; Weissman & Bothwell, 1976)
- Social Support Questionnaire–Short Form (SSQ-SF; Sarason et al., 1987)
- Stroop Color and Word Test (SCWT; Golden & Freshwater, 2002)

- Temperament Evaluation of Memphis (TEM) Pisa, Paris and San Diego (TEMPS-A; Akiskal & Akiskal, 2005)
- Test of Nonverbal Intelligence (4th ed.; TONI-4; Brown et al., 2010)
- Toronto Alexithymia Scale (TAS-20; Bagby et al., 1994)
- World Health Organization Quality of Life–BREF (WHOQOL-BREF; The WHOQOL Group, 1998)
- Young Mania Rating Scale (YMRS; Young et al., 1978)

Problems/Issues

Activities of Daily Living/Instrumental ADL
- Person may experience loss of appetite (both manic and depressive).
- Person may have difficulty with cooking, meal preparation, cleanup.
- Person may have difficulty with planning and completing shopping trips.
- Person may have difficulty with housekeeping chores including dusting and vacuuming.
- Person may have difficulty washing clothes (during laundry) and maintaining clothes in good repair.
- Person may have difficulty driving safely including speeding, making poor decisions, and not feeling in control of the vehicle (McNamara & Buckley, 2015).
- Person may have difficulty with communication tasks, such as reading and handwriting.
- Person may experience change in sexual desire (manic: increased sexual preoccupation; depressive: loss of sexual desire).

Education/Work
- Person may lack confidence to return to work after a relapse.
- Person may have been terminated due to excessive absenteeism, overuse of sick leave time, or poor job performance rating.

Play/Leisure
- Person may have few or no leisure interests.
- Person may have stopped or discontinued engagement in favorite leisure activities.

Rest/Sleep
- Person may have no regular sleep pattern.
- Person may report sleep disturbances.
- Person may be staying awake for days at time (manic) or sleeping for days at time (depressive).
- Sensory hypersensitivity may contribute to reduced sleep quality (Engel-Yeger et al., 2017).

Social Participation
- Person may be "out on the town" all the time or home alone all the time.

Sensorimotor
- Person may have a deficit in sensory gating, the ability to filter out redundant sensory stimuli or attenuation of neural response to the second identical stimulus (Cheng et al., 2016).
- Person may perform tasks in a manner that appears clumsy or uncoordinated (Decker et al., 2017).
- Person may perform tasks using more effort and energy that appears necessary to accomplish the task (Decker, et al., 2017).
- Person with bipolar disorder may have a lower registration of sensory input and a higher tendency for sensory sensitivity/avoidance (Serafini et al., 2017; Serafini et al., 2016).
- Person with unipolar disorder may have a greater registration of sensory input and lower avoidance (Serafini et al., 2017; Serafini et al., 2016).
- During periods of hypomania or depression, person may experience lower registration of sensory input and sensory sensitivity (Engel-Yeger et al., 2018).

Cognitive/Perceptual

- Person may have deficits in phases of prospective memory (encoding, retention, retrieval, execution, and evaluation) related to event planning and time planning (Note: related to dysfunction of the prefrontal and parietal lobes; Au et al., 2013; Au et al., 2017; Lee et al., 2010; Xiang et al., 2014; Zhou et al., 2013).
- Person may appear disorganized in the use of time, space, or objects (Decker et al., 2017).
- Person may perform tasks in a manner that is unsafe (Decker et al, 2017).
- Person may have deficits in attending behavior (Moore et al., 2010).
- Person may demonstrate reduced information processing speed (Gildengers et al., 2012; Träger et al., 2017).

Psychosocial

- Person may experience changes in self-concept (manic: inflated sense of worth and power; depressive: sense of worthlessness or guilt).
- Person may experience changes in level of motivation (manic: increased energy, agitation, distraction, low frustration tolerance; depressive: decreased energy, paralysis of will and initiation, avoidance or escapist wishes).
- Person may experience changes in type of emotions (manic: euphoric mood and grandiosity; depressive: depleted mood, sense of hopelessness, decrease sense of humor, and lack of pleasure in occupations).
- Person may experience decreased quality of life, especially when correlated with low sensory registration, sensory sensitivity, and sensation avoidance (Engel-Yeger et al., 2016).
- Person may demonstrate limited coping strategies.
- Person may overstate competence level compared to actually observed performance (e.g., driving ability; McNamara & Buckley, 2015).

Context/Environment

- Person, family, friends, and work colleagues may have minimal knowledge and little understanding of the disorder.

Intervention/Treatment

Models and programs developed by occupational therapy personnel include case studies (Cara, 2013; Chapleau & Harrison, 2017; Tse & Spangler, 2019), empowerment (Johanson & Bejerholm, 2017), occupational lifestyle redesign (Chan, 2014), quality of life enhancement program (Chen et al., 2015), and self-management (Hale, 2011). Models and programs developed by other professionals but used by occupational therapy personnel include day hospital program (Lambert-Comeau et al., 2018), illness management and recovery program (Chan, 2014), and recovery model (Chan, 2014). Team members include psychiatrists, physicians, psychologists, nursing personnel, social workers, and occupational therapy personnel. Goal of intervention is on improving ability to perform instrumental activities of daily living, addressing cognitive issues, and increasing self-management skills (Hale, 2011).

Activities of Daily Living/Instrumental ADL

- Assist person to develop and maintain a healthy diet including cooking, meal planning, meal preparation, and cleanup.
- Initiate groups to address life skills management (housekeeping, budgeting, shopping).
- Assist person to evaluate driving participation and safety during periods of relapse.
- Assist person to take public transportation.

Education/Work

- Provide supported employment to rebuild client's confidence (Johanson et al., 2019; S. Porter et al., 2018).
- Help client identify personal determinants that facilitate or hinder work adaption.

- Help client improve personal determinants that can facilitate work adaption.
- Help client clarify personal values, interests, routines, and perceptions concerning work.
- Help client reinitiate and reintegrate a satisfactory work schedule.
- Help client develop performance capacities needed to perform work including physical, cognitive, emotional, and social factors.
- Help client put into place the environment conditions at home and at work that promote work adaptation (Lalande et al., 2017).

Play/Leisure
- Help person identify leisure activities such as drawing, painting, or sculpting as a means of structure attention.

Rest/Sleep
- Assist person to develop and maintain a regular sleep pattern.

Social Participation
- Maintain time management schedule to avoid overscheduling parties, outings, etc. (Michalak et al., 2016).

Sensorimotor
- Assist person to develop and maintain a regular exercise program.

Cognitive/Perceptual
- Assist person to develop and maintain time management/scheduling skills to focus attention on tasks to be performed but not overschedule; include time for rest and relaxation (Michalak et al., 2016).
- Assist person to learn self-management skills including how to identify changes in sleep patterns, mood, or energy level as possible risk factors and triggers for relapse (Murray et al., 2011).
- Person may attend to tasks better if environmental distractions are reduced (Moore et al., 2010).
- Help person learn to set realistic expectations and reduce tendency toward perfection in all activities (Michalak et al., 2016).

Psychosocial
- Help person learn effective coping skills that may include meditation, increased self-awareness, yoga, tai chi.
- Address anxieties by using distractions such as electronic devices (Nayler, 2010).
- Quality of life and life satisfaction may be improved by addressing depression symptoms; therapist can encourage client to report symptoms or, if in immediate contact with a physician, report symptoms directly.
- A focus on maintaining hope is important in addressing symptoms of depression (Michalak et al., 2016).

Context/Environment
- Increase person's knowledge of the illness.
- Help person educate family, friends, work colleagues about the illness.
- Help person develop a support system that includes names and contact information to assist in monitoring and taking actions to act if relapse may be occurring (Hale, 2011).

Precautions/Safety Considerations

Person is at risk for suicide and suicidal thoughts and behaviors, especially if person is feeling anxious or fearful of a relapse (Cara, 2013). Persons treated for bipolar disorders may be at higher risk of being diagnosed with cancer (Hung et al., 2014). Persons with bipolar disorders may have atypical reactions to medications (R. S. Porter, 2018).

Prognosis and Outcome

Condition is chronic but many cases can be managed with a combination of self-management and medication compliance.

Cost Effectiveness

The individual enabling and support (IES) model was cost effective in comparison to traditional vocational rehabilitation (Saha et al., 2018).

REFERENCES

American Psychiatric Association. (2013). *Diagnostic and statistical manual of mental disorders* (5th ed.). https://doi.org/10.1176/appi.books.9780890425596

Au, R. W., Ungvari, G. S., Lee, E., Man, D., Shum, D. H., Xiang, Y. T., & Tang, W. K. (2013). Prospective memory impairment and its implications for community living skills in bipolar disorder. *Bipolar Disorders, 15*(8), 885–892. https://doi.org/10.1111/bdi.12122

Au, R. W. C., Xiang, Y. T., Ungvari, G. S., Lee, E., Shum, D. H. K., Man, D., & Tang, W. K. (2017). Prospective memory performance in persons with schizophrenia and bipolar disorder and healthy persons. *Perspectives in Psychiatric Care, 53*(4), 266–274. https://doi.org/10.1111/ppc.12172

Cara, E. (2013). Mood disorders. In E. Cara & A. MacRae (Eds.), *Psychosocial occupational therapy: An evolving practice* (3rd ed., pp. 221–257). Delmar Cengage Learning.

Chan, I. W. M. (2014). My recovery journey—Service uses experience of occupational therapy. Recovery Oriented Practice in Hong Kong. *World Federation of Occupational Therapists Bulletin, 70*(1), 36–38. https://doi.org/10.1179/otb.2014.70.1.010

Chapleau, A., & Harrison, J. (2017). Mood disorders. In B. J. Atchison & D. P. Dirette (Eds.), *Conditions in occupational therapy* (5th ed., 119–132). Wolters Kluwer.

Chen, Y.-L., Pan, A.-W., Hsiung, P.-C., & Chung, L. (2015). Quality of life enhancement programme for individuals with mood disorder: A randomized controlled pilot study. *Hong Kong Journal of Occupational Therapy, 25*(1), 23–31. https://doi.org/10.1016/j.hkjot.2015.04.001

Cheng, C.-H., Chan, P.-Y. S., Liu, C.-Y., & Hsu, S.-C. (2016). Auditory sensory gating in patients with bipolar disorders: A meta-analysis. *Journal of Affective Disorders, 203*, 199–203. https://doi.org/10.1016/j.jad.2016.06.010

Decker, L., Träger, C., Miskowiak, K., Wæhrens, E. E., & Vinberg, M. (2017). Ability to perform activities of daily living among patients with bipolar disorder in remission. *Edorium Journal of Disability and Rehabilitation, 3*, 69–79. https://doi.org/10.5348/D05-2017-33-OA-9

Engel-Yeger, B., Gonda, X., Canepa, G., Pompili, M., Rihmer, Z., Amore, M., & Serafini, G. (2018). Sensory profiles as potential mediators of the association between hypomania and hopelessness in 488 major affective outpatients. *Journal of Affective Disorders, 225*, 466–473. https://doi.org/10.1016/j.jad.2017.08.036

Engel-Yeger, B., Gonda, X., Muzio, C., Rinosi, G., Pompili, M., Amore, M., & Serafini, G. (2016). Sensory processing patterns, coping strategies, and quality of life among patients with unipolar and bipolar disorders. *Revista Brasileira de Psiquiatria, 38*(3), 207–215. https://doi.org/10.1590/1516-4446-2015-1785

Engel-Yeger, B., Gonda, X., Walker, M., Rihmer, Z., Pompili, M., Amore, M., & Serafini, G. (2017). Sensory hypersensitivity predicts reduced sleeping quality in patients with major affective disorders. *Journal of Psychiatric Practice, 23*(1), 11–24. https://doi.org/10.1097/PRA.0000000000000210

Gildengers, A. G., Butters, M. A., Chisholm, D., Anderson, S. J., Begley, A., Holm, M., Rogers, J. C., Reynolds, C. F., III, & Mulsant, B. H. (2012). Cognition in older adults with bipolar disorder versus major depressive disorder. *Bipolar Disorders, 14*(2), 198–205. https://doi.org/10.1111/j.1399-5618.2012.00995.x

Hale, S. (2011). Listening to clients: Self-management strategies to stay well with bipolar disorder. *Occupational Therapy Now, 13*(5), 18–19.

Hung, Y.-N., Yang, S.-Y., Huang, M.-C., Lung, F.-W., Lin, S.-K., Chen, K.-Y., Kuo, C.-J., & Chen, Y.-Y. (2014). Cancer incidence in people with affective disorder: Nationwide cohort study in Taiwan, 1997–2010. *British Journal of Psychiatry, 205*(3), 183–188. https://doi.org/10.1192/bjp.bp.114.144741

Johanson, S., & Bejerholm, U. (2017). The role of empowerment and quality of life in depression severity among unemployed people with affective disorders receiving mental healthcare. *Disability and Rehabilitation, 39*(18), 1807–1813. https://doi.org/10.1080/09638288.2016.1211758

Johanson, S., Markström, U., & Bejerholm, U. (2019). Enabling the return-to-work process among people with affective disorders: A multiple-case study. *Scandinavian Journal of Occupational Therapy, 26*(3), 205–218. https://doi.org/10.1080/11038128.2017.1396356

Lalande, M., Vachon, B. N., Hogue-Harwood, M., & Rivard, S. (2017). Promoting recovery for people with workplace absence issues attributed to anxiety or mood disorders. *Occupational Therapy Now, 19*(6), 11–13.

Lambert-Comeau, P., Cossette-Lavallée, M., Sirois-Giguère, G., Pham, K., Gaudet, V. C., & Larivière, N. (2018). Progress of clients with mood and anxiety disorders in a day hospital program: Examination of clinical, functional and recovery outcomes. *Journal of Psychosocial Rehabilitation and Mental Health, 5*(1), 5–16. https://doi.org/10.1007/s40737-018-0104-6

Lee, E., Xiang, Y. T., Man, D., Au, R. W., Shum, D., Tang, W. K., Chiu, H. F. K., Wong, P., & Ungvari, G. S. (2010). Prospective memory deficits in patients with bipolar disorder: A preliminary study. *Archives of Clinical Neuropsychology, 25*(7), 640–647. https://doi.org/10.1093/arclin/acq061

McNamara, C., & Buckley, S. E. (2015). The road to recovery: Experiences of driving with bipolar disorder. *British Journal of Occupational Therapy, 78*(6), 356–363. https://doi.org/10.1177/0308022614562581

Michalak, E. E., Suto, M. J., Barnes, S. J., Hou, S., Lapsley, S., Scott, M. W., Murray, G., Austin, J., Elliott, N. B., Berk, L., & CREST.BD. (2016). Effective self-management strategies for bipolar disorder: A community-engaged Delphi Consensus Consultation study. *Journal of Affective Disorders, 206,* 77–86. https://doi.org/10.1016/j.jad.2016.06.057

Moore, K., Merritt, B., & Doble, S. E. (2010). ADL skill profiles across three psychiatric diagnoses. *Scandinavian Journal of Occupational Therapy, 17*(1), 77–85. https://doi.org/10.3109/11038120903165115

Murray, G., Suto, M., Hole, R., Hale, S., Amari, E., & Michalak, E. E. (2011). Self-management strategies used by 'high functioning' individuals with bipolar disorder: From research to clinical practice. *Clinical Psychology and Psychotherapy, 18*(2), 95–109. https://doi.org/10.1002/cpp.710

Nayler, S. (2010). How my occupational therapist helped me. *Mental Health Occupational Therapy, 15*(3), 76.

Porter, R. S. (Ed.). (2018). *The Merck manual of diagnosis and therapy* (20th ed.). Merck Sharp & Dohme.

Porter, S., Lexén, A., Johanson, S., & Bejerholm, U. (2018). Critical factors for the return-to-work process among people with affective disorders: Voices from two vocational approaches. *Work, 60*(2), 221–234. https://doi.org/10.3233/WOR-182737

Roush, S., Monica, C., Carpenter-Song, E., & Drake, R. E. (2015). First-person perspectives on dual diagnosis anonymous (DDA): A qualitative study. *Journal of Dual Diagnosis, 11*(2), 136–141. https://doi.org/10.1080/15504263.2015.1025215

Saha, S., Bejerholm, U., Gerdtham, U. G., & Jarl, J. (2018). Cost-effectiveness of supported employment adapted for people with affective disorders. *Nordic Journal of Psychiatry, 72*(3), 236–239. https://doi.org/10.1080/08039488.2017.1422801

Serafini, G., Engel-Yeger, B., Vazquez, G. H., Pompili, M., & Amore, M. (2017). Sensory processing disorders are associated with duration of current episode and severity of side effects.
Psychiatry Investigation, 14(1), 51–57. https://doi.org/10.4306/pi.2017.14.1.51

Serafini, G., Gonda, X., Pompili, M., Rihmer, Z., Amore, M., & Engel-Yeger, B. (2016). The relationship between sensory processing patterns, alexithymia, traumatic childhood experiences,
and quality of life among patients with unipolar and bipolar disorders. *Child Abuse & Neglect, 62*, 39–50. https://doi.org/10.1016/j.chiabu.2016.09.013

Träger, C., Decker, L., Wæhrens, E. E., Knorr, U., Miskowiak, K., & Vinberg, M. (2017). Influences of patient informed cognitive complaints on activities of daily living in patients with
bipolar disorder. An exploratory cross-sectional study. *Psychiatry Research, 249*, 268–274.
https://doi.org/10.1016/j.psychres.2016.12.058

Tse, S., & Spangler, N. W. (2019). Mood disorders. In C. Brown, V. C. Stoffel, & J. P. Muñoz
(Eds.), *Occupational therapy in mental health: A vision for participation* (2nd ed., pp. 182–196).
F.A. Davis.

Xiang, Y.-T., Li, L.-J., Zhou, J.-J., Wang, C.-Y., Dixon, L. B., Dickerson, F., Zhou, F.-C., Ungvari, G. S.,
Zhang, X.-Y., Shum, D. H. K., Au, R. W. C., Tang, W.-K., Man, D., & Chiu, H. F. K. (2014). Quality of life of patients with euthymic bipolar disorder and its associations with demographic
and clinical characteristics, psychopathology, and cognitive deficits. *Perspectives in Psychiatric
Care, 50*(1), 44–50. https://doi.org/10.1111/ppc.12024

Yang, S.-Y., Liao, Y.-T., Liu, H.-C., Chen, W. J., Chen, C.-C., & Kuo, C.-J. (2013). Antipsychotic
drugs, mood stabilizers, and risk of pneumonia in bipolar disorder: A nationwide case-
control study. *Journal of Clinical Psychiatry, 74*(1), e79–e86. https://doi.org/10.4088/JCP.12
m07938

Zhou, J.-J., Xiang, Y.-T., Wang, C.-Y., Zhou, F.-C., Ungvari, G. S., Dickerson, F., Chiu, H. F. K.,
Lai, K. Y. C., Shum, D. H. K., Lee, E., Au, R. W. C., Tang, W.-K., & Man, D. (2013). Prospec-
tive memory deficits in euthymic bipolar disorder patients: A preliminary study. *Asia-Pacific
Psychiatry, 5*(3), 183–190. https://doi.org/10.1111/appy.12019

BIBLIOGRAPHY

Birken, M., & Harper, S. (2017). Experiences of people with a personality disorder or mood disorder regarding carrying out daily activities following discharge from hospital. *British Journal
of Occupational Therapy, 80*(7), 409–416. https://doi.org/10.1177/0308022617697995

Duncan, M., & Prowse, C. (2014). Occupational therapy with mood disorders. In R. Crouch & V.
Alers (Eds.), *Occupational therapy in psychiatry and mental health* (5th ed., pp. 389–407). Wiley.

Engel-Yeger, B., Bloch, B., Gonda, X., Canepa, G., Pompili, M., Sher, L., Rihmer, Z., Amore, M.,
& Serafini, G. (2018). Sensory profiles in unipolar and bipolar affective disorders: Possible
predictors of response to antidepressant medications? A prospective follow-up study. *Journal
of Affective Disorders, 240*, 237–246. https://doi.org/10.1016/j.jad.2018.07.032

Engel-Yeger, B., Muzio, C., Rinosi, G., Solano, P., Geoffroy, P. A., Pompili, M., Amore, M., & Serafini, G. (2016). Extreme sensory processing patterns and their relation with clinical conditions among individuals with major affective disorders. *Psychiatry Research, 236*, 112–118.
https://doi.org/10.1016/j.psychres.2015.12.022

Lalande, M., Vachon, B., Hogue-Harwood, M., & Rivard, S. (2017). Promoting recovery for
people with workplace absence issues attributed to anxiety or mood disorders. *Occupational
Therapy Now, 19*(6), 11–13.

Porter, S., & Bejerholm, U. (2018). The effect of individual enabling and support on empowerment and depression severity in persons with affective disorders: Outcome of a randomized
control trial. *Nordic Journal of Psychiatry, 72*(4), 259–267. https://doi.org/10.1080/080394
88.2018.1432685

Borderline Personality Disorder and Type B Personality Disorders

Also called emotionally unstable personality disorder.

Description

Borderline personality disorder (BPD) is characterized by a pervasive pattern of instability and hypersensitivity in interpersonal relationships, instability in self-image, extreme mood fluctuations, and impulsivity. Persons with borderline personality disorder have an intolerance of being alone; they make frantic efforts to avoid abandonment and generate crises, such as making suicidal gestures in a way that invites rescue and caregiving by others. Patients often have a number of comorbidities particularly depression, anxiety disorders (e.g., panic disorder), and posttraumatic stress disorder as well as eating disorders and substance use disorders (Porter, 2018).

Persons with borderline personality disorders have persistent patterns of behavior. Some of those identified as potential criteria for a diagnosis of borderline personality disorder according to the American Psychiatric Association (2013) can be described as follows:

- Chronic feelings of emptiness
- Desperate or frantic efforts to avoid actual or imagined abandonment
- Disturbance marked by unstable self-image or sense of self
- Impulsivity that could result in self-harm, such as unsafe sex, binge eating, substance abuse, or reckless driving
- Inappropriate intense anger or problems controlling anger, such as seen in frequent displays of temper, constant anger, or recurrent physical fights
- Rapid changes in affect or mood, lasting usually only a few hours
- Repeated or recurrent suicidal behavior or gestures or threats to self-mutilate
- Temporary or transient paranoid thoughts or severe dissociative symptoms triggered by stress
- Unstable intense relationships that alternate between idealizing and devaluing the other person (American Psychiatric Association, 2013; Porter, 2018)

Cause

Stresses during early childhood may contribute to the development of borderline personality disorder. A childhood history of physical and sexual abuse, neglect, separation for caregivers, and/or loss of a parent, is common among patients with borderline personality disorder (Porter, 2018).

Certain people may have a genetic tendency to have pathologic responses to environment life stressors, and borderline personality disorder appears to have a heritable component.

Evaluation/Assessment

Areas

- Activities of Daily Living/Instrumental ADL: basic ADLs (medication management); independent living (meal planning, cooking, shopping)
- Education/Work: employment status, academic status
- Play/Leisure: interests, frequency, location
- Rest and Sleep: sleep disturbance
- Social Participation: type, location, frequency, with whom
- Sensorimotor: no specific issue; general fitness
- Cognitive/Perceptual: executive functions (problem solving, goal setting, scheduling, time management)

- Psychosocial: depression, anxiety, suicide behavior, interpersonal relations, social isolation, stigma, motivation, self-discipline, role performance
- Context/Environment: family relations, social support, community resources, effect of repeated hospitalization
- Comorbidities: anxiety, bipolar or mood disorder, depression, eating disorder, posttraumatic stress disorder, substance abuse

Instruments

Instruments Developed by Occupational Therapy Personnel

- Life Balance Inventory (LBI; Matuska, 2012a, 2012b)
- Model of Human Occupation Screening Tool (Version 2.0; MOHOST 2.0; Parkinson et al., 2006)
- Occupational Circumstances Assessment-Interview and Rating Scale (Version 4.0; OCAIRS; Forsyth et al., 2005)
- Occupational Questionnaire (OQ; Smith et al., 1986)

Instruments Developed by Other Professionals and Used by Occupational Therapy Personnel

- Assessment of Life Habits (LIFE-H 3.1; Fourgeyrollas & Noreau, 2005)
- Depression Anxiety and Stress Scale-21 (DASS-21; Lovibond & Lovibond, 1995a, 1995b)
- Life Habits Scale 3.1 (see Assessment of Life Habits)
- Quality of Life Index (QLI; Ferrans & Powers, 1985)
- Rosenberg Self-Esteem Scale (RSES; Rosenberg, 1965)
- Symptom Checklist-90-Revised (SCL-90-R; Derogatis, 1994)

Problems/Issues

Activities of Daily Living/Instrumental ADL

- Person may restrict food intake or use diet as a means of controlling body sensations as a means of controlling "something" in life (Potvin et al., 2019).
- Person may view certain self-care (e.g., bathing) and repetitive instrumental tasks (e.g., meal preparation) as tedious chores, boring, frustrating, or meaningless occupations.
- Person may have difficulty with money management related to job instability or impulsive spending.

Education/Work

- Person may have a history of failing to complete academic studies that is not due to limited intelligence or cognitive dysfunction.
- Person may have a history of job instability or multiple career changes (paid or unpaid).
- Person may exceed allowed sick leave (absenteeism) and be terminated.
- Person may be unemployed and not seeking employment.
- Person may lack work skills needed for employment.
- Person may need on-the-job work training, such as supported employment.
- Person may have a history of conflicts/interpersonal issues with employer, supervisor, or fellow employees.

Play/Leisure

- Person may have limited or no active leisure activities.
- Person may have passive leisure activities only, such as watching TV.

Rest and Sleep

- Person usually has sleep disturbances.
- Person may use sleep as an escape to numb emotional pain and find shelter (Potvin et al., 2019).

Social Participation

- Person may have difficulty participating in social activities (exhibits unacceptable behavior for given setting or situation).
- Person may engage in a socially accepted occupation to an extreme that is beyond social standards (text repeatedly and intrusively on cell phone, spend days at the movies or in bed, binge watch TV programs).
- Person may prefer virtual life (on cell phone) to face-to-face contact.

Sensorimotor

- Person may engage in movement and action to point of physical harm (work too many hours per week, hike to point of exhaustion).

Cognitive/Perceptual

- Person may be oversensitive to criticism.
- Person may avoid certain situations/tasks or procrastinate.
- Person may have poor problem-solving skills.
- Person may have poor time management/life balance skills (too much work, not enough leisure).

Psychosocial

- Person usually has poor emotional regulation, such as impulsivity, unpredictability, inappropriate or uncontrolled anger, identity disturbance, rapid shifts of mood, suicidal thoughts or acts, self-mutilations, chronic feelings of emptiness, paranoid ideation, or boredom.
- Person may express feelings of anxiety and depression.
- Person usually has poor interpersonal skills, including intolerance of being alone, unstable interpersonal relationships, martial instability, conflicts with work supervisor/employer, few or no friends, limited social network.
- Person usually has a history of suicide attempts or threats.
- Person usually has poor coping skills.
- Person may have poor or limited self-awareness.
- Person may have poor or limited self-image.
- Person may have a negative body image and limited sense of talents and capacities.
- Person may have low and fragile self-esteem or self-worth.
- Person may demonstrate active passivity (tendency to approach problems passively and helplessly instead of actively and with determination; Falklöf & Haglund, 2010).
- Person may demonstrate apparent competence (tendency to appear competent and able to cope) sometimes and at other times appear incompetent (Falklöf & Haglund, 2010).
- Person may be ambivalent to change, including avoiding attending inpatient intervention sessions and terminating attendance early to outpatient programs (Larivière et al., 2010).

Context/Environment

- Person may have difficulty identifying and coordinating services needed to cope with disorder.
- Person may engage in socially disapproved occupations (substance abuse, gaming, smoking) as a means of attaining a group identity (Potvin et al., 2019).
- Person may have limited or absent social support from family or friends.
- Person may actively engage in occupations that offer an escape from a distressing or alienating reality (substance abuse, gaming).

Intervention/Treatment

Models and programs developed by occupational therapy personnel include case study (Cara, 2013), model of human occupation (MOHO; Falklöf & Haglund, 2010; Lee & Harris, 2010), person-environment-occupation (Larivière et al., 2015), and redesigning daily occupations

(ReDo; Dahl et al., 2017). Models and programs developed by other professionals but used by occupational therapy personnel include dialectical behavior therapy (Falklöf & Haglund, 2010; Lee & Harris, 2010), constructivist grounded theory (Desrosiers et al., 2015), and psychiatric day hospital program (Larivière et al., 2010). Team members include psychiatrists, psychologists, social workers, and occupational therapy personnel. Goals include a focus on recovery, which includes letting go of the past (person), having healthy relationships (environment), and being involved in meaningful activities (occupation).

Activities of Daily Living/Instrumental ADL
- Skills classes in instrumental ADLs, such a preparing healthy meals.

Education/Work
- Assist person in participation in a work or volunteer program.
- Person may benefit from work accommodations such as the following:
  - ▶ clarity and stability in the structure, conditions, and expectations of the workplace;
  - ▶ flexible work schedule;
  - ▶ support from supervisor and coworkers;
  - ▶ ability to change job tasks or department;
  - ▶ training and coaching; and
  - ▶ progressive return to work program (Dahl et al., 2017).

Play/Leisure
- Assist client to explore leisure interests and abilities.
- Provide opportunity to try out different leisure activities.
- Encourage integration of leisure activities into everyday life balance.

Rest and Sleep
- Assist client to identify role of sleep in daily life activity and modify to best fit individual need (Wood et al., 2015).

Social Participation
- Encourage client to identify socially valued occupations and participate in those occupations with friends.

Sensorimotor
- Assist client to identify and develop plans for engaging in physical activity to promote health and fitness as goals, but not to point of endangering body functions.

Cognitive/Perceptual
- Assist client to set realistic goal and steps to achieve that goal.
- Assist client to establish a daily schedule.
- Set clear, firm limits and boundaries to prevent regression and self-destructive behavior.

Psychosocial
- Provide a structured, reality-oriented program to channel aggression and relieve pain.
- Prepare for impulsivity and unpredictable behavior with a calm voice and prepare redirection plan.
- Assist client to identify positive and negative behaviors and their role in everyday life.
- Provide opportunity to practice positive behaviors in a safe setting.

Context/Environment
- Remove or limit access to physically harmful tools and supplies.
- Address with client the consequences of self-destructive behavior on the family.
- Facilitate coordination of services such as service providers, employment counselor, employment agency, disability manager, insurance provider.

Precautions/Safety Considerations

Person should be monitored at all times using suicide precautions, including para-suicide attempts, which may be a cry for help but may become deadly (Cara, 2013).

Prognosis and Outcome

Recovery is possible but condition is usually chronic. Person continues to have difficulty setting boundaries (too little or too much) and maintaining a balance (variety) of actions and occupations in a regular schedule.

REFERENCES

American Psychiatric Association. (2013). *Diagnostic and statistical manual of mental disorders* (5th ed.). https://doi.org/10.1176/appi.books.9780890425596

Cara, E. (2013). Personality disorders. In E. Cara & A. MacRae (Eds.). *Psychosocial occupational therapy: An evolving practice* (3rd ed., pp. 258–307). Delmar Cengage Learning.

Dahl, K., Larivière, N., & Corbiére, M. (2017). Work participation of individuals with borderline personality disorder: A multiple case study. *Journal of Vocational Rehabilitation, 46*(3), 377–388. https://doi.org/10.3233/JVR-170874

Desrosiers, L., Saint-Jean, M., & Breton, J. J. (2015). Treatment planning: A key milestone to prevent treatment dropout in adolescents with borderline personality disorder. *Psychology and Psychotherapy: Theory, Research and Practice, 88*(2), 178–196. https://doi.org/10.1111/papt.12033

Falklöf, I., & Haglund, L. (2010). Daily occupations and adaptation to daily life described by women suffering from borderline personality disorder. *Occupational Therapy in Mental Health, 26*(4), 354–374. https://doi.org/10.1080/0164212X.2010.518306

Larivière, N., Couture, É., Blackburn, C., Carbonneau, M., Lacombe, C., Schinck, S. A., Pierre, D., & St-Cyr-Tribble, D. (2015). Recovery, as experienced by women with borderline personality disorder. *Psychiatric Quarterly, 86*(4), 555–568. https://doi.org/10.1007/s11126-015-9350-x

Larivière, N., Desrosiers, J., Tousignant, M., & Boyer, R. (2010). Who benefits the most from psychiatric day hospitals? A comparison of three clinical groups. *Journal of Psychiatric Practice, 16*(2), 93–102. https://doi.org/10.1097/01.pra.0000369970.87779.ca

Lee, S., & Harris, M. (2010). The development of an effective occupational therapy assessment and treatment pathway for women with a diagnosis of borderline personality disorder in an inpatient setting: Implementing the model of human occupation. *British Journal of Occupational Therapy, 73*(11), 559–563. https://doi.org/10.4276/030802210X12892992239396

Porter, R. S. (Ed.). (2018). *The Merck manual of diagnosis and therapy* (20th ed.). Merck Sharp & Dohme.

Potvin, O., Vallée, C., & Larivière, N. (2019). Experience of occupations among people living with a personality disorder. *Occupational Therapy International, 2019*, Article 9030897. https://doi.org/10.1155/2019/9030897

Wood, A., Brooks, R., & Beynon-Pindar, C. (2015). The experience of sleep for women with borderline personality disorder: An occupational perspective. *British Journal of Occupational Therapy, 78*(12), 750–756. https://doi.org/10.1177/0308022615587864

BIBLIOGRAPHY

Doughty, K., & Brown, C. (2019). Personality disorders. In C. Brown, V. C. Stoffel, & J. P. Muñoz (Eds.), *Occupational therapy in mental health: A vision for participation* (2nd ed., pp. 169–181). F.A. Davis.

Larivière, N., Denis, C., Payeur, A., Ferron, A., Levesque, S., & Rivard, G. (2016). Comparison of objective and subjective life balance between women with and without a personality disorder. *Psychiatric Quarterly, 87*, 663–673. https://doi.org/10.1007/s11126-016-9417-3

Larivière, N., Desrosiers, J., Tousignant, M., & Boyer, R. (2010). Exploring social participation of people with cluster B personality disorders. *Occupational Therapy in Mental Health*, 26(4), 375–386. https://doi.org/10.1080/0164212X.2010.518307

Conversion Disorder

Also called functional neurological symptom disorder, psychogenic disorder, nonorganic disorder, dissociative disorder, functional movement disorder, somatization.

Description

A conversion disorder is an unconscious defense mechanism that consists of neurologic symptoms or deficits that develop unconsciously and nonvolitionally, usually involving motor or sensory functions. The manifestations are incompatible with known pathophysiologic mechanisms or anatomic structures. Symptoms may include loss of sensation, paralysis, pain, or other dysfunctions of the nervous system (O'Toole, 2017; Porter, 2018).

Cause

Conversion symptoms are commonly attributed to mental factors or emotional conflicts, such as stress or anxiety, which are repressed and transformed into symbolic physical symptoms (O'Toole, 2017; Porter, 2018). Biological, psychological, and social factors including predisposing vulnerabilities, precipitating mechanisms, and perpetuating factors may be involved (Nicholson et al., 2020). Formal criteria for a diagnosis of conversion disorder are listed in the *Diagnostic and Statistical Manual of Mental Disorders* (5th. ed., American Psychiatric Association, 2013).

Typical Motor/Neurological Signs (Gardiner et al., 2018)
- Typical "dragging" gait of functional leg weakness, with the forefoot in contact with the ground and hip externally rotated.
- Fixed dystonic posture seen in function dystonia, typically foot in an inverted and plantar flexed.
- Hoover's sign for functional limb weakness. Weakness of hip extension that returns to normal with contralateral hip flexion against resistance.
- Tremor entrainment test for function tremor, where the tremor disappears transiently or change in rhythm when copying movements made by examiner.

Dissociate (Nonepileptic) Seizures (Gardiner et al., 2018)
- Long duration of attacks more than 3 minutes
- Prolonged sudden motionless unresponsiveness greater that 2 minutes
- Closed eyes
- Crying during/immediately after an attack
- Memory of being in a seizure

Evaluation/Assessment

Areas

In conversion disorders, a wide variety of occupations may be involved or only one or two, depending on the individual client. Not all areas below would be appropriate for all clients. Case analysis is important.

- Activities of Daily Living/Instrumental ADL: self-care skills, functional mobility, functional communication, driving
- Education/Work: school and school activities, homemaking, work skills and job responsibilities
- Play/Leisure: leisure interests and hobbies
- Rest/Sleep: sleep patterns, sleep disruptions

- Social Participation: social roles, community participation
- Sensorimotor: endurance, dexterity, functional range of motion, gross and fine motor coordination, muscle strength and tone, pain and pain tolerance, postural control, sensory processing, sensibility (touch, proprioception, stereognosis, skin temperature)
- Cognitive/Perceptual: attending behavior, learning, memory, executive function (decision making, judgment, mental flexibility, problem solving, time management)
- Psychosocial: self-image, self-esteem, anxiety, frustration tolerance
- Context/Environment: ergonomics at school, home, or work; adaptive equipment and devices; home modification; school schedule adaptation; animal assistants
- Development (Infant, Child, Adolescent only): developmental milestones

Instruments
(Note: the COPM-5 is the only instrument listed in the References by name. Use of other instruments depends on needs of clients.)

Instruments Developed by Occupational Therapy Personnel
- Adolescent/Adult Sensory Profile (AASP; Brown & Dunn, 2002)
- Assessment of Motor and Process Skills (8th ed.; AMPS-8; Fisher & Bray Jones, 2016)
- Canadian Occupational Performance Measure (5th ed.; COPM-5; Law et al., 2014)
- Model of Human Occupational Screening Tool (MHOST. 2.0; Parkinson et al., 2006)
- Occupational Circumstances Assessment Interview and Rating Scale (Version 4.0, OCAIRS; Forsyth et al., 2005)
- Occupational Self-Assessment (Version 2.2; OSA 2.2; Baron et al., 2006)
- Worker Role Interview (Version 10.0; WRI 10.0; Braveman et al., 2005)

Instruments Developed by Other Professionals and Used by Occupational Therapy Personnel
- None identified

Problems/Issues

Activities of Daily Living/Instrumental ADL
- Person may have difficulty performing self-care activities, such as dressing.
- Person may have difficulty with mobility, such as walking.
- Person may have difficulty performing transfers, such as getting in and out of tub.
- Person may have difficulty performing IADL tasks such as meal preparation and cleanup, basic housekeeping, shopping, driving.

Education/Work
- Person may have difficulty performing school or work tasks and routines.
- Person may have difficulty with transportation requirements associated with school or work activities.

Play/Leisure
- Person may have stopped engaging in favorite play or leisure activities.
- Person may have difficulty performing certain tasks associated with play or leisure activities.

Rest/Sleep
- Person may have disrupted sleep patterns.
- Person may have difficulty maintaining a sleep routine.

Social Participation
- Person may have restricted or stopped participation in social activities.
- Person may experience anxiety or stress reactions during participation in certain social activities.

Sensorimotor
- Person may have low or poor endurance in relation to that needed to perform daily tasks.
- Person may lack dexterity needed to perform daily tasks.

- Person may lack functional range of motion needed to perform daily tasks.
- Person may lack gross and fine motor coordination needed to perform daily tasks.
- Person may have decreased muscle strength and tone needed to perform daily tasks.
- Person may experience pain when moving the body to perform certain tasks.
- Person may experience low pain tolerance, which interferes with performing daily tasks.
- Person may have poor postural control.
- Person may experience hyper- or hypo-responses to sensory inputs typically experienced in the individual's environment.
- Person may experience loss of or decreased sensibility (touch, proprioception, stereognosis, skin temperature registration), which may increase risk of injury.

Cognitive/Perceptual
- Person may have difficulty attending to complete tasks.
- Person may experience difficulty learning new or novel information.
- Person may experience difficulty with memory or experience loss of memory.
- Person may experience difficulty with executive functions (decision making, judgment, mental flexibility, problem solving, time management) such as making poor choices in task performance or failing to use effective problem-solving techniques.

Psychosocial
- Person may experience emotional stress or have stressors in daily life.
- Person may experience anxiety generally or in specific situations.
- Person may have reduced self-confidence.

Context/Environment
- Person may have experienced loss of sense of control over built or natural environment situations.

Intervention/Treatment

Models and programs developed by occupational therapy personnel include case studies (Gardiner et al., 2018), discussion summary (Royal College of Occupational Therapists, 2018), and sensory processing (Ranford et al., 2018). Models and programs developed by other professionals but used by occupational therapy personnel include behavioral shaping therapy (Dahlhauser et al., 2017), biopsychosocial etiological framework (Nicholson et al., 2020), and case study (Yam et al., 2016). Team members include physicians, psychiatrists, neurologists, psychologists, nursing personnel, physical therapy personnel, and occupational therapy personnel. The goal is to focus on successful and effective occupational performance without using abnormal movements or techniques or focusing directly on the symptoms and to overcome the effects of disability through practical support to improve performance and satisfaction in activities of daily living (Nicholson et al., 2020).

Activities of Daily Living/Instrumental ADL
- Provide opportunity to perform ADL and IADL tasks under supervision.
- Stop performance of any task if abnormal movements are seen.
- Suggest alternate methods (ergonomic, compensatory, adapted) to perform task.

Education/Work
- Provide opportunity to perform school or work tasks under supervision.
- Stop performance of any task if abnormal movements are seen.
- Suggest alternate methods (ergonomic, compensatory, adapted, occupational rebalancing) to facilitate better task performance.

Play/Leisure
- Provide opportunity to perform play or leisure tasks under supervision.

- Stop performance of any task if abnormal movements are seen.
- Suggest alternate methods (ergonomic, compensatory, adapted, occupational rebalancing) to perform task.

Rest/Sleep
- Review with client sleep routine and patterns.
- Education client about good sleep habits.
- Suggest modifications such as setting a regular sleep schedule, darkening the room, wearing earplugs, changing to cotton nightwear.

Social Participation
- Review with client social situation that may be causing anxiety or stress; using a recording device such as a smartphone may be useful to observe situations.
- Educate client on alternate approaches to situations that cause anxiety or stress.

Sensorimotor
- Focus on occupational (activity, task) performance as opposed to focusing on symptoms; as performance improves, sensorimotor symptoms should abate.
- Educate client about sensory processing responses if hyper- or hypo-responses are identified.
- Functional tremor
  ▸ Superimpose alternative voluntary rhythm (tapping, opening/closing, music/song) over existing tremor and gradually slow all movement to a complete rest.
  ▸ For unilateral tremor, use unaffected limb to dictate a new rhythm (tapping, opening and closing hand, use of music).
  ▸ Assist client to relax muscles in limb to prevent co-contraction.
  ▸ Try to control a tremor with client at rest, before moving on to activity.
  ▸ Use gross rather than fine movement (e.g., handwriting—use a large marker and large piece of paper or whiteboard with big lettering rather than regular size pen/pencil and paper).
  ▸ Discourage co-contraction or tensing of muscles (usually not a helpful long-range strategy).
- Functional jerks
  ▸ Address prejerk cognitions and movements such as anxiety, frustration, or breath-holding.
  ▸ Use general relaxation techniques such as diaphragmatic breathing or progressive muscular relaxation.
  ▸ Use sensory grounding strategy focused on noticing details in environment (sounds, sights, and smells).
  ▸ Encourage learning "slow" movement activities such as yoga or tai chi.
- Dystonia
  ▸ Encourage optimal postural alignment at rest and withing function 24 hours per day.
  ▸ Encourage even distribution of weight in sitting, transfers, standing, and walking to normalize movement patterns and muscle activity.
  ▸ Grade activity to increase time that affected limb is used within functional activities.
  ▸ Avoid postures that promote prolonged position of joints at end of range (full hip, knee, or ankle flexion while sitting).
  ▸ Discourage "nursing" affected limb, but demonstrate and promote therapeutic resting postures and limb use.
  ▸ Use strategies that reduce muscle overactivity, pain, and fatigue (e.g., muscle relaxation strategies, support affected limb at rest, using pillows or furniture to take weight off a limb when sitting or lying down).
  ▸ Address associated problems with pain and hypersensitivity.
- Functional limb weakness
  ▸ Engage client in tasks that promote normal movement, good alignment, and even weight bearing.
  ▸ Joint sessions with physical therapy colleagues may be useful.

- Hypersensitivity
  - ▶ Address symptoms of hypersensitivity to touch, light, sound, or movement.
  - ▶ See Sensory Over-Responsivity in Section 2: Sensory Disorders.

Cognitive/Perceptual

- Focus on cognitive skills needed to perform occupational (activity, task) performance; as performance improves, cognitive performance should improve.
- Educate client about cognitive impairments, if present, that may interfere with effective occupational performance.

Psychosocial

- Educate and when possible, provide opportunity to practice stress management techniques, such as diaphragmatic breathing, progressive muscle relaxation, biofeedback, or other methods of relaxation client may enjoy to increase mind–body awareness.
- Address with client symptoms of anxiety (racing heart rate, tight chest).
- Encourage engagement in occupations client states are enjoyable.

Context/Environment

- Consider if adapted equipment or techniques may facilitate occupational performance if person is unable to engage in treatment; generally, aids and assistive equipment are avoided if client is actively engaged in rehabilitation to avoid compensatory movement patterns (Gardiner et al., 2018).
- Consider whether animal assistance (pet ownership, pet rental) may reduce stress or anxiety.
- Consider whether home modifications or arrangement of furniture and furnishings may reduce stress or anxiety.
- Consider whether changing transportation arrangements in the community (drive less, bus more, bicycle to work) may reduce stress or anxiety.
- Consider whether changing community integration patterns or participation may reduce stress or anxiety.
- Educate family or caregivers about conversion/functional neurological disorder.

Precautions/Safety Considerations

Stop client from using abnormal or unsafe movements. Educate client about safety considerations.

Prognosis and Outcome

Prognosis and outcome have been successful when occupational performance is resolved to the client's satisfaction. Failure to gain client's satisfaction may result in actual tissue damage due to continued lack of activity or use of abnormal movements. Failure to gain client's satisfaction may result in increased symptoms including depression.

Cost Effectiveness

Cost effectiveness of intervention is unknown due to lack of studies. Cost of failure to address client's actual need for emotional support (correct diagnosis) is considered to be high, but actual numbers are estimates.

REFERENCES

American Psychiatric Association. (2013). *Diagnostic and statistical manual of mental disorders* (5th ed.). https://doi.org/10.1176/appi.books.9780890425596

Dahlhauser, S. E., Theuer, A., & Hollman, J. (2017). Satisfaction and occupational performance in patients with functional movement disorder. *Open Journal of Occupational Therapy, 5*(2), Article 5. https://doi.org/10.15453/2168-6408.1287

Gardiner, P., MacGregor, L., Carson, A., & Stone, J. (2018). Occupational therapy for functional neurologic disorders: A scoping review and agenda for research. *CNS Spectrums, 23*(3), 205–212. https://doi.org/10.1017/S1092852917000797

Nicholson, C., Edwards, M. J., Carson, A. J., Gardiner, P., Golder, D., Hayward, K., Humblestone, S., Jinadu, H., Lumsden, C., MacLean, J., Main, L., Macgregor, L., Nielsen, G., Oakley, L., Price, J., Ranford, J., Ranu, J., Sum, E., & Stone, J. (2020). Occupational therapy consensus recommendations for functional neurological disorder. *Journal of Neurology, Neurosurgery and Psychiatry, 91*(10), 1037–1045. https://doi.org/10.1136/jnnp-2019-322281

O'Toole, M. T. (Ed.). (2017). *Mosby's dictionary of medicine, nursing & health professions* (10th ed.). Elsevier.

Porter, R. S. (Ed.). (2018). *The Merck manual of diagnosis and therapy* (20th ed.). Merck Sharp & Dohme.

Ranford, J., Perez, D. L., & MacLean, J. (2018). Additional occupational therapy considerations for functional neurological disorders: A potential role for sensory processing. *CNS Spectrums, 23*(3), 194–195. https://doi.org/10.1017/S1092852918000950

Royal College of Occupational Therapists. (2018). *Discussion summary: Functional neurological disorders/symptoms.*

Yam, A., Rickards, T., Pawlowski, C. A., Harris, O., Karandikar, N., & Yutsis, M. V. (2016). Interdisciplinary rehabilitation approach for functional neurological symptom (conversion) disorder: A case study. *Rehabilitation Psychology, 61*(1), 102–111. https://doi.org/10.1037/rep0000063

Depression and Depressive Disorders

See also Anxiety and General Anxiety Disorder, Bipolar Disorders, Brain Injuries, Cognitive Impairment, Stroke: Chronic, Stroke: Hemiplegia, Substance-Related and Addictive Disorders, Suicide and Suicidal Behavior.

Description

Depressive disorders are characterized by sadness severe enough or persistent enough to interfere with function and decreased interest or pleasure in activities (R. S. Porter, 2018). Depression may be a temporary or chronic mental disorder. Depression may be characterized by feelings of sadness, loneliness, despair, low self-esteem, and self-reproach. Behaviors may include psychomotor retardation, agitation, withdrawal from social contact, and vegetative states such as loss of appetite and insomnia (*Stedman's*, 2011). Depression may result in occupational deprivation as the person restricts and reduces participation and engagement in everyday activities. Depressive symptoms may impede independence in activities of daily living, hinder quality of life, and affect physical functioning (Chippendale & Bear-Lehman, 2012).

Major depressive disorder is considered if five or more of the following are present for 2 weeks or longer, occur almost every day, and represent a change from previous functioning:

- Depressed mood (subjective reports may include feeling sad, empty, or hopeless; child or adolescent may be irritable)
- Marked decreased interest or pleasure
- Significant weight loss when not dieting or weight gain of more than 5% of body weight in a month or decrease or increase in appetite
- Insomnia or hypersomnia
- Psychomotor agitation or retardation
- Fatigue or loss of energy
- Feelings of worthlessness or excessive or inappropriate guilt

- Diminished ability to think or concentrate or indecisiveness
- Recurrent thoughts of death, recurrent suicidal ideation, or suicide attempt (American Psychiatric Association, 2013)

Cause

The exact cause is unknown but probably involves heredity, changes in neurotransmitter levels, alternated neuroendocrine function, and psychosocial factors (R. S. Porter, 2018).

Evaluation/Assessment

Areas

- Activities of Daily Living/Instrumental ADL: basic ADLs (eating, dressing, grooming, shaving, brushing teeth, toileting, transfers, functional communication, functional mobility); independent living (meal preparation, housekeeping, home maintenance, driving, shopping); health maintenance (medication management, physical activity)
- Education/Work: academic performance/failure, work performance (quality, quantity), work attendance
- Play/Leisure: interests, values, frequency, location
- Rest/Sleep: sleep disturbance, sleep routine
- Social Participation: types, frequency, location, with whom
- Sensorimotor: movement speed, accuracy, fatigue, sensory processing
- Cognitive/Perceptual: attention, memory, executive functions
- Psychosocial: mood, affect, anxiety, role performance, sense of competence, quality of life
- Context/Environment: support system, family and caregiver education
- Development (Infant, Child, Adolescent only): increased irritability
- Comorbidities: anxiety, bipolar disorder, brain injury, concussion, diabetes, older adult, physical disabilities, stroke, substance abuse, suicide

Instruments

Instruments Developed by Occupational Therapy Personnel

- Adolescent/Adult Sensory Profile (AASP; Brown & Dunn, 2002)
- Canadian Occupational Performance Measure (5th ed.; COPM-5; Law et al., 2014)
- Occupational Balance Questionnaire (OBQ; Wagman & Håkansson, 2014)
- Occupational Self-Assessment (Version 2.2; OSA 2.2; Baron et al., 2006)
- Satisfaction with Daily Occupations (SDO; Eklund, 2004)

Instruments Developed by Other Professionals and Used by Occupational Therapy Personnel

- Barratt Impulsivity Scale (BIS; Patton et al., 1995)
- Beck Depression Inventory (2nd ed.; BDI-II; Beck et al., 1996)
- Behavioral Activation for Depression Scale (BADS; Kanter et al., 2007)
- Brief Assessment Schedule Depression Cards (BASDEC; Adshead et al., 1992)
- Center for Epidemiology Studies Depression Scale (CES-D; Radloff, 1977)
- Children's Depression Inventory-2 (CDI-2; Kovacs, 2010; see also de la Vega et al., 2016, in References)
- Client Satisfaction Questionnaire (CSQ; Larsen et al., 1979)
- Clinical Outcomes in Routine Evaluation–Outcome Measure (CORE-OM; Evans et al., 2002)
- Depression Intensity Scale Circles (DISCs; Turner-Stokes et al., 2005)
- Empowerment Scale (ES; Rogers et al., 1997)
- Functional Capacity Evaluation (FCE; Ramano & Buys, 2018, in References)
- Hamilton Rating Scale for Depression (HRSD; Hamilton, 1960)
- Helping Alliance Questionnaire II (HAq-II; Luborsky et al., 1996)
- Hospital Anxiety and Depression Scale (HADS; Zigmond & Snaith, 1983)
- Manchester Short Assessment of Quality of Life (MANSA; Priebe et al., 1999)

- Montgomery-Åsberg Depression Self-Rating Scale (MADSR; Montgomery & Åsberg, 1979)
- Multidimensional Assessment of Fatigue (MAF; Belza, 1995)
- Patient Health Questionnaire-9 (PHQ-9; Löwe et al., 2004)
- Pearlin Self-Mastery Scale (PSMS; Pearlin & Schooler, 1978)
- Sense of Coherence Scale (SOC; Antonovsky, 1987)
- Social Support Questionnaire–Short Form (SSQ-SF; Sarason et al., 1987)
- Stroke Aphasic Depression Questionnaire (SADQ; Lincoln et al., 2000, hospital version)
- Symptom Checklist-90-Revised (SC-90-R; Derogatis, 1994)
- Temperament Evaluation of Memphis, Pisa, Paris and San Diego (TEMPS; Akiskal & Akiskal, 2005)
- Toronto Alexithymia Scale (TAS-20; Bagby et al., 1994)
- Work Ability Index (WAI; Ilmarinen, 2007)
- World Health Organization Quality of Life–BREF (WHOQOL-BREF; The WHOQOL Group, 1998)

Problems/Issues
Activities of Daily Living/Instrumental ADL
- Person may report loss of appetite.
- Person may skip meals.
- Person may be neglecting personal hygiene and grooming.
- Person may be dressing inappropriately or failing to change clothing on a regular basis.
- Person may neglect housekeeping tasks (meal preparation, cleaning, doing laundry).
- Person may neglect home maintenance tasks.
- Person may not be shopping for groceries or other household or personal needs.
- Person may not be caring for children or pets.
- Person may not be taking medications as prescribed.

Education/Work
- Person's job performance may diminish or have been cited as unsatisfactory.
- Person's grades may have decreased or person may have received one or more failing grades.
- Person may be failing to attend class or go to work.

Play/Leisure
- Person may have reduced or stopped engagement in favorite leisure occupations.

Rest/Sleep
- Person may report increased difficulty falling asleep, insomnia.
- Person may report waking up in the middle of night and being unable to go back to sleep.
- Person may be sleeping more than usual or necessary, more than 6–8 hours.

Social Participation
- Person may withdrawal from social contact and occupations.

Sensorimotor
- Person may show signs of psychomotor retardation.

Cognitive/Perceptual
- Person may have difficulty paying attention.
- Person may have difficulty remembering facts or events previously well learned.
- Person may have difficulty with executive functions such as problem solving, decision making.

Psychosocial
- Person often appears to be disinterested and lack motivation to engage in doing activities, tasks, or occupations.
- Person often appears withdrawn and disengaged from surroundings.

- Person may express emotions such as feelings of sadness, loneliness, despair, low self-esteem, self-reproach, dejection, hopelessness.
- Person may report anhedonia (inability to feel pleasure).
- Person may report dysphoria (generalized dissatisfaction with life).
- Person may have a condition called alexithymia (an inability to describe one's emotions).
- Person may have difficulty interacting with others and become isolated.
- Person may not be fulfilling roles such as parent, spouse, provider, or other roles.

Context/Environment

- Person may avoid contact with social support system.
- Person, family, or caregivers may lack information about depression, depressive symptoms, and management.
- Person, family, or caregivers may lack information about available resources in the community or on the internet.
- Person, family, or caregivers may lack access to resources (limited transportation, no internet connection).

Intervention/Treatment

Programs developed by occupational therapists include behavioral activation (Drysdale & Boyle, 2019), case study (Cara, 2013), cognitive work hardening program (Wisenthal & Krupa, 2014), occupational therapy and psychosocial interventions program (Çakmak et al., 2016), occupational therapy group (Edel et al., 2017), Share Your Life Story writing workshop (Chippendale & Bear-Lehman, 2012), and Tree Theme Method (Gunnarsson et al., 2018). Programs developed by other professionals but used by occupational therapists include augmented cognitive behavioral therapy (Kootker et al., 2015), cognitive-behavioral therapy (Kootker et al., 2019), individual enabling and support (IES; S. Porter & Bejerholm, 2018), integrative group therapy model (Söchting et al., 2013), quality of life model (Pan et al., 2012), return to work (Hees et al., 2013; Ramano et al., 2016), telerehabilitation (Linder et al., 2015), and work hardening (Wisenthal & Krupa, 2013, 2014; Wisenthal et al., 2018). The focus of intervention through occupational therapy is to support and encourage activation of graded behavioral change through engaging or reengaging the person in meaningful values, interests, and occupation. Different areas of the brain may be activated by using occupations that focus on cognitively demanding tasks versus those focused on emotional responses (Palmer et al., 2015).

Activities of Daily Living/Instrumental ADL

- Practice self-care and instrumental activities through functional performance in natural environment and usual time of day (do not rely on verbal report).

Education/Work

- Cognitive work hardening program (Wisenthal & Krupa, 2014).
  - ▶ Work with client to identify return-to-work barriers and develop an intervention plan agreeable to the client.
  - ▶ Assist client to develop the work tolerance (mental stamina) needed to meet minimally required work hours (may be graded from part-time to full-time).
  - ▶ Assist client to develop the cognitive skills needed to meet the job demands.
  - ▶ Assist client to develop fatigue management strategies such as pacing work and rest cycles or changing tasks on a specific time schedule.
  - ▶ Assist client to develop coping skills and strategies to deal with workplace interpersonal, organizational, and task demands.
  - ▶ Assist client to learn relevant ergonomic principles to facilitate job performance.
  - ▶ Assist client to gain or regain the confidence in ability to return to work.
  - ▶ Work with employer to develop a gradual return-to-work program designed and agreed upon by all stakeholders.

▶ Ensure that workplace accommodations are provided.

▶ Facilitate matching of client's strengths and limitations to the job requirements.

• Individual enabling and support (S. Porter & Bejerholm, 2018).

▶ Phase 1: Enabling—Clients attend hour-long weekly session to facilitate motivational, cognitive, and lifestyle strategies.

▶ Phase 2: Assessment—Hour-long appointments to complete a vocational profile and plan.

▶ Phase 3: Job seeking.

▶ Phase 4: Supported employment—Client undergoes a 1-hour session once every 3rd week to receive further support to help client maintain employment based on individual needs.

▶ Weekly log books are required of the client and questionnaires are completed at 6 and 12 months.

Play/Leisure

• Occupational therapy and psychosocial interventions program used handcrafts, drawing, sports activities, and morning group meetings (Note: largest group of clients were diagnosed as depressed, but other diagnoses were included in the study).

Rest/Sleep

• See Sleep–Wake Disorders in Section 13: Lifestyle Conditions.

Social Participation

• Encourage person (and family or caregivers as available) to participate in social activities with family, friends, and colleagues.

• Consider adjustments to social occupations such as passive versus active, time limited, close to home or in home, fewer people, familiar activities.

Sensorimotor

• See Sensory-Based Problems in Adults in Section 2: Sensory Disorders.

Cognitive/Perceptual

• Help client learn what depression is as a disorder and how the disorder feeds on itself creating a loop.

• Help client learn to consider the link between doing versus not doing, and how each makes the person feel.

• Help client to begin to challenge the behaviors and actions that reinforce depression.

• Help client learn how to approach and solve situations/problems that appear difficult rather than avoiding the issue(s).

• Support client in making small changes to habits, rituals, or routines.

• Support client to identify and explore individual values.

• Support client to identify new or renewed interests.

• Support client to learn self-management skills that are effective for the individual.

• Help client set graded goals to produce small behavior change toward achieving larger goals.

Psychosocial

• Behavioral activation program (Drysdale & Boyle, 2019).

▶ Week 1: Client identifies behavioral patterns and starts to change them.

▶ Week 2: Client focuses on getting out of TRAPS (trigger, response, avoidance pattern) and back on TRAC (trigger response, alternative coping).

▶ Week 3: Client takes action: a problem-solving approach.

▶ Week 4: Client focuses on values: the guide to who he or she is.

▶ Week 5: Client develops responses to thinking, worry, and rumination.

▶ Week 6: Focus on making changes one step at a time.

▶ Week 7: Focus on freeing the self from mood dependence.

▶ Week 8: Building the relationships the client wants and tying everything together.

- Tree Theme Method (Gunnarsson et al., 2018).
  - ▶ Session 1: Session begins with progressive relaxation. Client paints tree representing current life situation followed by life storytelling.
  - ▶ Session 2: Progressive relaxation. Client paints a tree representing childhood followed by continued life storytelling.
  - ▶ Session 3: Progressive relaxation. Client paints a tree representing adolescence followed by continued life storytelling.
  - ▶ Session 4: Progressive relaxation. Client paints a tree representing adulthood followed by continued life storytelling.
  - ▶ Session 5: Progressive relaxation. Client paints a tree representing the future followed by a dialogue in which the client makes plans for the future by identifying the need for change and how to incorporate the changes into everyday life.

Context/Environment
- Provide information about depression to family, employers, and others.
- Assist in making modifications to the work environment such as ergonomic changes.
- Increase accessibility to resources.

Precautions/Safety Considerations
Clients with depressive symptoms should be monitored for suicidal ideation or behavior.

Prognosis and Outcome
Variable depending on the type of depression. Medication is successful for some clients but others do not respond well to medication and the depression may become chronic (persistent depressive disorder or dysthymia; R. S. Porter, 2018).

REFERENCES
American Psychiatric Association. (2013). *Diagnostic and statistical manual of mental disorders* (5th ed.). https://doi.org/10.1176/appi.books.9780890425596

Çakmak, S., Süt, H., Öztürk, S., Tamam, L., & Bal, U. (2016). The effects of occupational therapy and psychosocial interventions on interpersonal functioning and personal and social performance levels of corresponding patients. *Archives of Neuropsychiatry, 53*(3), 234–240. https://doi.org/10.5152/npa.2015.10130

Cara, E. (2013). Mood disorders. In E. Cara, & A. MacRae (Eds.), *Psychosocial occupational therapy: An evolving practice* (3rd ed., pp. 221–257). Delmar Cengage Learning.

Chippendale, T., & Bear-Lehman, J. (2012). Effect of life review writing on depressive symptoms in older adults: A randomized controlled trial. *American Journal of Occupational Therapy, 66*(4), 438–446. https://doi.org/10.5014/ajot.2012.004291

de la Vega, R., Racine, M., Sánchez-Rodríguez, E., Solé, E., Castarlenas, E., Jensen, M. P., Engel, J., & Miró, J. (2016). Psychometric properties of the short form of the Children's Depression Inventory (CDI-S) in young people with physical disabilities. *Journal of Psychosomatic Research, 90,* 57–61. https://doi.org/10.1016/j.jpsychores.2016.09.007

Drysdale, L., & Boyle, C. (2019). Delivering behavioural activation to beat depression. *OT News, 27*(1), 18–19.

Edel, M. A., Blackwell, B., Schaub, M., Emons, B., Fox, T., Tornau, F., Vieten, B., Roser, P., Haussleiter, I. S., & Juckel, G. (2017). Antidepressive response of inpatients with major depression to adjuvant occupational therapy: A case-control study. *Annals of General Psychiatry, 16,* Article 1. https://doi.org/10.1186/s12991-016-0124-0

Gunnarsson, A. B., Wagman, P., Hedin, K., & Håkansson, C. (2018). Treatment of depression and/or anxiety–Outcomes of a randomised controlled rail of the Tree Theme Method versus regular occupational therapy. *BMC Psychology, 6,* Article 25. https://doi.org/10.1186/s40359-018-0237-0

Hees, H. L., de Vries, G., Koeter, M. W., & Schene, A. H. (2013). Adjuvant occupational therapy improves long-term depression recovery and return-to-work in good health in sick-listed employees with major depression: Results of a randomised controlled trial. *Occupational and Environmental Medicine, 70*(4), 252–260. https://doi.org/10.1136/oemed-2012-100789

Kootker, J. A., Rasquin, S. M. C., Smits, P., Geurts, A. C., van Heugten, C. M., & Fasotti, L. (2015). An augmented cognitive behavioural therapy for treating post-stroke depression: Description of a treatment protocol. *Clinical Rehabilitation, 29*(9), 833–843. https://doi.org/10.1177/02 69215514559987

Kootker, J. A., van Heugten, C. M., Kral, B., Rasquin, S. M. C., Geurts, A. C., & Fasotti, L. (2019). Caregivers effects of augmented cognitive-behavioural therapy for post-stroke depressive symptoms in patients: Secondary analyses to a randomized controlled trial. *Clinical Rehabilitation, 33*(6), 1056–1065. https://doi.org/10.1177/0269215519833013

Linder, S. M., Rosenfeldt, A. B., Bay, R. C., Sahu, K., Wolf, S. L., & Alberts, J. L. (2015). Improving quality of life and depression after stroke through telerehabilitation. *American Journal of Occupational Therapy, 69*(2), Article 6902290020. https://doi.org/10.5014/ajot.2015.014498

Palmer, S. M., Crewther, S. G., Carey, L. M., & the START Project Team. (2015). A meta-analysis of changes in brain activity in clinical depression. *Frontiers in Human Neuroscience, 8*, Article 1045. https://doi.org/10.3389/fnhum.2014.01045

Pan, A.-W., Chen, Y.-L., Chung, L.-I., Wang, J.-D., Chen, T.-J., & Hsiung, P.-C. (2012). A longitudinal study of the predictors of quality of life in patients with major depressive disorder utilizing a linear mixed effect model. *Psychiatry Research, 198*(3), 412–419. https://doi.org/10.1016/j.psychres.2012.02.001

Porter, R. S. (Ed.). (2018). *The Merck manual of diagnosis and therapy* (20th ed.). Merck Sharp & Dohme.

Porter, S., & Bejerholm, U. (2018). The effect of individual enabling and support on empowerment and depression severity in persons with affective disorders: Outcome of a randomized control trial. *Nordic Journal of Psychiatry, 72*(4), 259–267. https://doi.org/10.1080/080394 88.2018.1432685

Ramano, E., & Buys, T. (2018). Occupational therapists' views and perceptions of function capacity evaluation of employees suffering from major depressive disorders. *South African Journal of Occupational Therapy, 48*(1), 9–15. https://doi.org/10.17159/2310-3833/2017/vol48n1a3

Ramano, E., Buys, T., & de Beer, M. (2016). Formulating a return-to-work decision for employees with major depressive disorders: Occupational therapists' experiences. *African Journal of Primary Health Care & Family Medicine, 8*(2), Article a954. https://doi.org/10.4102/phcfm.v8i2.954

Söchting, I., O'Neal, E., Third, B., Rogers, J., & Ogrodniczuk, J. (2013). An integrative group therapy model for depression and anxiety in later life. *International Journal of Group Psychotherapy, 63*(4), 502–523. https://doi.org/10.1521/ijgp.2013.63.4.502

Stedman's medical dictionary for the health professions and nursing (7th ed.). (2011). Wolters Kluwer.

Wisenthal, A., & Krupa, T. (2013). Cognitive work hardening: A return-to-work intervention for people with depression. *Work, 45*(4), 423–430. https://doi.org/10.3233/WOR-131635

Wisenthal, A., & Krupa, T. (2014). Using intervention mapping to deconstruct cognitive work hardening: A return-to-work intervention for people with depression. *BMC Health Services Research, 14*, Article 530. https://doi.org/10.1186/s12913-014-0530-4

Wisenthal, A., Krupa, T. Kirsh, B. H., & Lysaght, R. (2018). Cognitive work hardening for return to work following depression: An intervention study. *Canadian Journal of Occupational Therapy, 85*(1), 21–32. https://doi.org/10.1177/0008417417733275

BIBLIOGRAPHY

Albert, S. M., Bear-Lehman, J., & Burkhardt, A. (2012). Mild depressive symptoms, self-reported disability, and slowing across multiple functional domains. *International Psychogeriatrics, 24*(2), 253–260. https://doi.org/10.1017/S1041610211001499

American Occupational Therapy Association. (2012). *School mental health toolkit: Depression.* https://www.aota.org/-/media/Corporate/Files/Practice/Children/SchoolMHToolkit/Depression.pdf

Bingham, K. S., Kumar, S., Dawson, D. R., Mulsant, B. H., & Flint, A. J. (2018). A systematic review of the measurement of function in late-life depression. *American Journal of Geriatric Psychiatry, 26*(1), 54–72. https://doi.org/10.1016/j.jagp.2017.08.011

Duncan, M., & Prowse, C. (2014). Occupational therapy with mood disorders. In R. Crouch & L. Wegner (Eds.), *Occupational therapy in psychiatry and mental health* (5th ed., pp. 389–407). Wiley.

Engel-Yeger, B., Muzio, C., Rinosi, G., Solano, P., Geoffroy, P. A., Pompili, M., Amore, M., & Serafini, G. (2016). Extreme sensory processing patterns and their relation with clinical conditions among individuals with major affective disorders. *Psychiatry Research, 236,* 112–118. https://doi.org/10.1016/j.psychres.2015.12.022

Ghaffari, A., Akbarfahimi, M., & Forough, B. (2017). A comparison of the relation of depression, and cognitive, motor and functional deficits in chronic stroke patients: A pilot study. *Advances in Bioscience & Clinical Medicine, 5*(4). http://dx.doi.org/10.7575/aiac.abcmed.17.05.04.01

Hoshino, A., Amano, S., Suzuki, K., & Suwa, M. (2016). Relationships between depression and stress factors in housework and paid work among Japanese women. *Hong Kong Journal of Occupational Therapy, 27*(1), 35–41. https://doi.org/10.1016/j.hkjot.2016.03.001

Kim, D. (2017). Relationships between caregiving stress, depression, and self-esteem in family caregivers of adults with a disability. *Occupational Therapy International, 2017,* Article 1686143. https://doi.org/10.1155/2017/1686143

Kneebone, I., Baker, J., & O'Malley, H. (2010). Screening for depression after stroke: Developing protocols for the occupational therapist. *British Journal of Occupational Therapy, 73*(2), 71–76. https://doi.org/10.4276/030802210X12658062793843

Kneebone, I., Stone, N., Robertson, S., & Walker-Samuel, N. (2013). Screening for depression after stroke: Occupational therapists' performance to protocols. *Occupational Therapy in Mental Health, 29*(2), 106–113. https://doi.org/10.1080/0164212X.2013.788971

Lin, F.-H., Yih, D. N., Shih, F.-M., & Chu, C.-M. (2019). Effect of social support and health education on depression scale scores of chronic stroke patients. *Medicine, 98*(44), Article e17667. https://doi.org/10.1097/MD.0000000000017667

Mulholland, F., & Jackson, J. (2018). The experience of older adults with anxiety and depression living in the community: Aging, occupation and mental wellbeing. *British Journal of Occupational Therapy, 81*(11), 657–666. https://doi.org/10.1177/0308022618777200

Pan, A. W., Chung, L., Chen, T. J., Hsiung, P. C., & Rao, D. (2011). Occupational competence, environmental support and quality of life for people with depression: A path analysis. *American Journal of Psychiatric Rehabilitation, 14*(1), 40–54. https://doi.org/10.1080/15487768.2011.546282

Paniccia, M., Paniccia, D., Thomas, S., Taha, T., & Reed, N. (2017). Clinical and non-clinical depression and anxiety in young people: A scoping review on heart rate variability. *Autonomic Neuroscience, 208,* 1–14. https://doi.org/10.1016/j.autneu.2017.08.008

Pascoe, M. C., Crewther, S. G., Carey, L. M., & Crewther, D. P. (2011). Inflammation and depression: Why poststroke depression may be the norm and not the exception. *International Journal of Stroke, 6*(2), 128–135. https://doi.org/10.1111/j.1747-4949.2010.00565.x

Roush, S., Monica, C., Carpenter-Song, E., & Drake, R. E. (2015). First-person perspectives on dual diagnosis anonymous (DDA): A qualitative study. *Journal of Dual Diagnosis, 11*(2), 136–141. https://doi.org/10.1080/15504263.2015.1025215

Serafini, G., Gonda, X., Canepa, G., Pompili, M., Rihmer, Z., Amore, M., & Engel-Yeger, B. (2017). Extreme sensory processing patterns show a complex association with depression, and impulsivity, alexithymia, and hopelessness. *Journal of Affective Disorders, 210,* 249–257. https://doi.org/10.1016/j.jad.2016.12.019

Serafini, G., Engel-Yeger, B., Vazquez, G. H., Pompili, M., & Amore, M. (2017). Sensory processing disorders are associated with duration of current episode and severity of side effects. *Psychiatry Investigation, 14*(1), 51–57. https://doi.org/10.4306/pi.2017.14.1.51

Stahl, S. T., Rodakowski, J., Saghafi, E. M., Park, M., Reynolds, C. F., & Dew, M. A. (2016). Systematic review of dyadic and family-oriented interventions for late-life depression. *International Journal of Geriatric Psychiatry, 31*(9), 963–973. https://doi.org/10.1002/gps.4434

Stazyk, K. DeMatteo, C., Moll, S., & Missiuna, C. (2017). Depression in youth recovering from concussion: Correlates and predictors. *Brain Injury, 31*(5), 631–638. https://doi.org/10.1080/02699052.2017.1283533

Tse, S., & Spangler, N. W. (2019). Mood disorders. In C. Brown, V. C. Stoffel, & J. P. Muñoz (Eds.), *Occupational therapy in mental health: A vision for participation* (2nd ed., pp. 182–196). F.A. Davis.

Wu, C. Y., Terhorst, L., Karp, J. F., Skidmore, E. R., & Rodakowski, J. (2018). Trajectory of disability in older adults with newly diagnosed diabetes: Role of elevated depressive symptoms. *Diabetes Care, 41*(10), 2072–2078. https://doi.org/10.2337/dc18-0007

Early or First Psychosis

Description

Early psychosis refers to identification of the psychosis and the start of intervention when symptoms of psychosis were recognized by professionals (physicians, psychologists, psychiatrists). First psychosis is treatment of no more than 12 months following the first episode illness (Hui et al., 2014). The terms *early* and *first* refer to the initial diagnosis and the start of intervention, not necessarily to the beginning of symptoms. As Brown (2011) reported, some symptoms may have existed since early childhood but were not recognized and identified until later when the symptoms became more severe (disabling) or a traumatic event occurred that triggered the display of symptoms to others.

Cause

The specific cause is unknown. Heredity and early childhood trauma may contribute.

Evaluation/Assessment

Areas

- Activities of Daily Living/Instrumental ADL: financial management, home management independent living skills
- Education/Work: work schedule
- Play/Leisure: interests, values, frequency of engagement, location
- Rest/Sleep: habits, disturbances
- Social Participation: interests, frequency, location, with whom
- Sensorimotor: akathisia (motor restlessness)
- Cognitive/Perceptual: attention span, concentration
- Psychosocial: avolition, anhedonia, apathy, hallucinations, delusions, interpersonal relationship, anxiety, depression, self-esteem
- Context/Environment: social support
- Development (Infant, Child, Adolescent only): developmental profile
- Comorbidity: substance abuse

Instruments

Instruments Developed by Occupational Therapy Personnel

- Adolescent/Adult Sensory Profile (AASP; Brown & Dunn, 2002)
- Allen Cognitive Level Screen (5th ed.; ACLS-5; Allen et al., 2007)
- Contextual Memory Test (CMT; Toglia, 1993)
- Life Functioning Assessment Inventory (L-FAI; Hui et al., 2013, in References)
- Occupational Self-Assessment (Version 2.2; OSA 2.2; Baron et al., 2006)

Instruments Developed by Other Professionals and Used by Occupational Therapy Personnel
- Abnormal Involuntary Movement Scale (AIMS; Guy, 1976)
- Assessment of Premorbid Schizoid-Schizotypal Traits (APSST; Foerster et al., 1991)
- Azima Battery (AB; Azima & Azima, 1959; Note: developed for occupational therapy, but not by occupational therapy personnel.)
- Barnes Akathisia Rating Scale (BARS; Barnes, 1989)
- Beck Cognitive Insight Scale (BCIS; Beck et al., 2004)
- Calgary Depression Scale for Schizophrenia (CDSS; Addington et al., 1992)
- Green Paranoid Thought Scales (GPTS; Green et al., 2008)
- Interview of the Retrospective Assessment of the Onset of Schizophrenia (IRAOS; Häfner et al., 1992)
- Positive and Negative Syndrome Scale (PANSS; Kay et al., 1987)
- Premorbid Adjustment Scale (PAS; Cannon-Spoor et al., 1982)
- Psychosis Recovery Inventory (PRI; Chen et al., 2005)
- Role Functioning Scale (RFS; Goodman et al., 1993)
- Scale for Assessment of Negative Symptoms (SANS; Andreasen, 1983)
- Scale for Assessment of Positive Symptoms (SAPS; Andreasen, 1984)
- Simpson Angus Scale (SAS; Simpson & Angus, 1970)
- Social and Occupational Functioning Assessment Scale (SOFAS; Morosini et al., 2000)

Problems/Issues

Activities of Daily Living/Instrumental ADL
- Person may have acquired substantial debt or loss of financial support, such as loss of a student loan or scholarship due to leaving school.
- Person may have difficulty managing medication schedule leading to skipping dosages.
- Person may experience weight gain related to certain medications.

Education/Work
- Person may have uncharacteristically poor or failing grades.
- Person may have been dismissed from school (flunked out) or quit suddenly.
- Person may have been disciplined at work for absenteeism, failure to perform job duties, or interpersonal conflicts/disagreements.
- Person may have been dismissed (fired) from work.
- Person may have started and quit a number of jobs in a short period of time.

Play/Leisure
- Person may have discontinued engaging in favorite leisure activities.

Rest/Sleep
- Person may report sleep disturbances.
- Person may spend many more hours in bed than necessary for adequate sleep.

Social Participation
- Person may restrict participation or disengage in social activities.

Sensorimotor
- Person may display akathisia (restlessness, agitation due to side effects of some medications).

Cognitive/Perceptual
- Person may report the voices are directing/controlling behavior.
- Person may have difficulty correctly assessing current level of ability with selected occupation, often overestimating capacity.

Psychosocial
- Person may report that activities/occupations no longer have any meaning or purpose.

- Person may report feelings of apathy and anhedonia (loss of sense of pleasure).
- Person may have hallucinations.
- Person may have delusions.
- Person may experience difficulty maintaining interpersonal relationships related to perceived "strange behaviors" by others.

Context/Environment
- Person may have a community or interpersonal restraining order because of past behavior.

Intervention/Treatment

Models and programs developed by occupational therapy personnel include the Canadian Model of Occupational Performance (CMOP; Brown, 2011), Case Study—The Lived Experience (Roush & Read, 2019), Early Assessment Service for Young People with Psychosis (EASY; Poon et al., 2010), and Jockey Club Early Psychosis (JCEP; Hui et al., 2014). Models and programs developed by other professionals but used by occupational therapy personnel include the constructivist, grounded theory (Krupa et al., 2010; Lal et al., 2013), developmental framework (Brown, 2011), Job in Jeopardy (Williams & Lloyd, 2016), early assessment and support alliance (Waite, 2014; Wen & Roush, 2017), metacognitive training (Pos et al., 2018), PhotoVoice (Roush & Read, 2019), projective techniques (Zafran et al., 2017; Zafran et al., 2012; Zafran et al., 2018), and sculpting (Roush & Read, 2019). Team members include physicians, psychiatrists, social workers, psychologists, and occupational therapy personnel. The goal is on assisting the client to "learn by doing" and to understand how to maintain autonomy (Brown, 2011).

Activities of Daily Living/Instrumental ADL
- Assist client to develop and maintain a medication schedule.
- Assist client to develop and maintain independent living skills: meal planning and preparation, housekeeping, laundry, shopping, transportation.

Education/Work
- Provide opportunity to develop career plans through activities such as volunteering.
- Suggest modification of work schedule for those employed such as working half time, working a flex schedule, or working at home.

Play/Leisure
- Assist client to reengage and reconnect with previously known leisure activities and interests.
- Assist client to explore and develop new leisure activities, especially if previous activities or interests are not feasible.

Rest/Sleep
- Assist client to develop and maintain consistent sleep habits and routines.

Social Participation
- Assist client to reestablish participation in positive social and cultural activities but not negative (related to substance abuse, violence, criminal behavior).
- Assist client to explore and develop new social and cultural activities.

Sensorimotor
- Assist client to develop and maintain a physical fitness program (exercises, walking, running, engaging in sports activities).

Cognitive/Perceptual
- Assist client to develop an awareness of disability and its implications for daily life such as carefully matching current level of ability and capacity with selected occupation or activity.
- Assist client in maintaining control over occupational choices.
- Assist client to make new plans, especially if previous goals and activities are not feasible.

- Assist client to develop and implement self-advocacy skills to maintain rights to services and community resources.
- Assist client to talk about negative interactions with others and how to address the issue.
- Assist client to develop a crisis management program to manage symptoms.

Psychosocial

- Assist client to focus on productive roles.
- Use of photographs, videos, and participation in familiar activities may assist in reconnecting person with previously valued activities.

Context/Environment

- Consider referral to Alcoholics Anonymous or Narcotics Anonymous for substance abuse, if present.
- Educate family, peers, educators, employers about mental illness.
- Assist client and social support group to take advantage of community and internet resources.
- Advocate for improved services for persons with mental illness.

Precautions/Safety Considerations

Relapse is possible. Learning to managing symptoms is critical.

Prognosis and Outcome

Mental illness is often a chronic disorder but can be managed when client learns to identify triggers and take action to reduce the stressors. Paid and nonpaid work attained by post-illness is an important role performance in determining the extent of maintaining well-being, recovery, and social inclusion (Turner et al., 2015).

REFERENCES

Brown, J. A. (2011). Talking about life after early psychosis: The impact on occupational performance. *Canadian Journal of Occupational Therapy, 78*(3), 156–163. https://doi.org/10.2182/cjot.2011.78.3.3

Hui, C. L. M., Chang, W. C., Chan, S. K. W., Lee, E. H. M., Tam, W. W. Y., Lai, D. C., Wong, G. H. Y., Tang, J. Y. M., Li, F. W. S., Leung, K. F., McGhee, S. M., Sham, P. C., & Chen, E. Y. H. (2014). Early intervention and evaluation for adult-onset psychosis: The JCEP study rationale and design. *Early Intervention in Psychiatry, 8*(3), 261–268. https://doi.org/10.1111/eip.12034

Hui, C. L.-M., Li, Y.-K., Leung, K.-F., Tang, J. Y.-M., Wong, G. H.-Y., Chang, W.-C., Chan, S. K.-W., Lee, E. H.-M., & Chen, E. Y.-H. (2013). Reliability and validity of the Life Functioning Assessment Inventory (L-FAI) for patients with psychosis. *Social Psychiatry and Psychiatric Epidemiology, 48*, 1687–1695. https://doi.org/10.1007/s00127-013-0679-x

Krupa, T., Woodside, H., & Pocock, K. (2010). Activity and social participation in the period following a first episode of psychosis and implications for occupational therapy. *British Journal of Occupational Therapy, 73*(1), 13–20. https://doi.org/10.4276/030802210X12629548272628

Lal, S., Ungar, M., Leggo, C., Malla, A., Frankish, J., & Suto, M. J. (2013). Well-being and engagement in valued activities: Experiences of young people with psychosis. *OTJR: Occupation, Participation and Health, 33*(4), 190–197. https://doi.org/10.3928/15394492-20130912-02

Poon, M. Y. C., Siu, A. M. H., & Ming, S. Y. (2010). Outcome analysis of occupational therapy programme for persons with early psychosis. *Work, 37*(1), 65–70. https://doi.org/10.3233/WOR-2010-1057

Pos, K., Meijer, C. J., Verkerk, O., Ackema, O., Krabbendam, L., & de Haan, L. (2018). Metacognitive training in patients recovering from a first psychosis: An experience sampling study testing treatment effects. *European Archives of Psychiatry and Clinical Neuroscience, 268*, 57–64. https://doi.org/10.1007/s00406-017-0833-7

Roush, S., & Read, H. (2019). Early psychosis programs for adolescents and young adults. In C. Brown, V. C. Stoffel, & J. P. Muñoz (Eds.), *Occupational therapy in mental health: A vision for participation* (2nd ed., pp. 585–600). F.A. Davis.

Turner, N., O'Mahony, P., Hill, M., Fanning, F., Larkin, C., Waddington, J., O'Callaghan, E., & Clarke, M. (2015). Work life after psychosis: A detailed examination. *Work, 51*(1), 143–152. https://doi.org/10.3233/WOR-141865

Waite, A. (2014). On the brink: Occupational therapy program helps address early psychosis. *OT Practice, 19*(11), 9–12.

Wen, V., & Roush, S. (2017). Occupational therapy in early psychosis intervention: A manual for an emerging practice. *OT Practice, 22*(15), 14–18.

Williams, P. L., & Lloyd, C. (2016). A review of job tenure under the Job in Jeopardy programme in first episode psychosis. *The British Journal of Occupational Therapy, 79*(5), 284–289. https://doi.org/10.1177/0308022615625649

Zafran, H., Mazer, B., Tallant, B., Chilingaryan, G., & Gelinas, I. (2017). Detecting incipient schizophrenia: A validation of the Azima battery in first episode psychosis. *Psychiatric Quarterly, 88*(3), 585–602. https://doi.org/10.1007/s11126-016-9482-7

Zafran, H., Tallant, B., & Gelinas, I. (2012). A first-person exploration of the experience of academic reintegration after first episode psychosis. *International Journal of Psychosocial Rehabilitation, 16*(1), 27–43.

Zafran, H., Tallant, B., Gelinas, I., & Jordan, S. (2018). The phenomenology of early psychosis elicited in an occupational therapy expressive evaluation. *Occupational Therapy in Mental Health, 34*(1), 3–31. https://doi.org/10.1080/0164212X.2017.1338982

Eating Disorders

Includes anorexia nervosa, bulimia nervosa, binge eating.

Description

Eating disorders are a group of behaviors related to unresolved emotional conflicts that involve a persistent disturbance of eating that alters consumption or absorption of food or significantly impairs physical health and/or psychosocial functioning (O'Toole, 2017; Porter, 2018). Eating disorders arise from "entrenched maladaptive cognitions that lead to negative coping mechanisms and irrational body perceptions that become habitual" (Biddiscombe et al., 2018, p. 99).

Anorexia nervosa "is characterized by a relentless pursuit of thinness, a morbid fear of obesity, a distorted body image, and restriction of intake relative to requirements, leading to a significantly low body weight" (Porter, 2018, p. 1754). Nutritional deficiency disorders are common. Patients are preoccupied with food, including studying diets and calories; hoarding, concealing, and wasting food; collecting recipes; and preparing elaborate meals for other people. "Many patients with anorexia nervosa also exercise excessively to control weight" (Porter, 2018, pp. 1754–1755). Anorexia nervosa is a disorder characterized by a prolonged refusal to eat, resulting in emaciation, amenorrhea, emotional disturbance concerning body image, and fear of becoming obese (O'Toole, 2017).

Bulimia nervosa "is characterized by recurrent episodes of binge eating followed by some form of inappropriate compensatory behavior," such as purging, fasting, or driven exercise (Porter, 2018, p. 1756). The individual tends to be consistently overconcerned about body shape and weight. Unlike individuals with anorexia nervosa, those with bulimia nervosa are usually of normal or above-normal weight and tend to consume sweet, high-fat foods. The amount of food consumed sometimes involves thousands of calories. Physical signs may include swollen parotid glands, scars on the knuckles (from induced vomiting), and dental erosion (Porter, 2018). Formal criteria for a diagnosis of anorexia nervosa and bulimia nervosa are listed in the *Diagnostic and Statistical Manual of Mental Disorders* (5th ed.; *DSM-5*; American Psychiatric Association, 2013).

Cause

Etiology of anorexia nervosa (AN) is unknown other than being female. Bulimia nervosa (BN) is often triggered by psychosocial stress. Certain biological traits may be involved (Brand-Gothelf et al., 2016).

Evaluation/Assessment

Areas

- Activities of Daily Living/Instrumental ADL: eating habits, meal preparation, dressing and clothing, shopping, budgeting
- Education/Work: school or work activities, volunteering
- Play/Leisure: leisure activities and interests
- Rest/Sleep: not discussed
- Social Participation: social and community activities
- Sensorimotor: sensory modulation to taste/gustatory, vestibular/kinesthetic, somatosensory/tactile, proprioception input
- Cognitive/Perceptual: executive functions including beliefs, values, and knowledge about food portions, calories, calorie counting, diets and dieting, effects of exercise, being fat or thin, normal weight, rituals regarding meal preparation; problem solving, decision making, perceptions regarding hunger and fatigue
- Psychosocial: body image and awareness, self-image, level of self-confidence, anxiety, depression, role choice and performance, quality of life
- Context/Environment: family expectations, cultural and religious rituals, media coverage
- Comorbidities: diagnosis of anxiety, depression, obsessive compulsive disorder, borderline personality disorder

Instruments

Instruments Developed by Occupational Therapy Personnel

- Canadian Occupational Performance Measure (5th ed; COPM-5; Law et al., 2014)
- Eating and Meal Preparation Skills Questionnaire (EMPSQ; Lock et al., 2012; in References)
- Role Checklist (RC; Oakley et al., 1986)
- Sensory Responsiveness Questionnaire (SRQ; Bar-Shalita et al., 2009)

Instruments Developed by Other Professionals and Used by Occupational Therapy Personnel

- Eating Attitudes Test (EAT-26; Garner et al., 1982)
- Eating Disorder Inventory-3 (EDI-3; Garner, 2004)

Problems/Issues

Activities of Daily Living/Instrumental ADL

- Person may restrict food input.
- Person may binge eat and then purge food.
- Person may have a list of "good" (acceptable to eat) foods and "bad" or "feared" foods (avoid, do not eat).
- Person may have rituals about eating (cutting food into X number of pieces, eating X number of pieces per time unit, using only certain utensils to serve or pans for cooking).
- Person may choose to eat alone to hide eating rituals.
- Person may skip meals by planning daily schedule so that time to eat is not available.
- Person may only wear certain clothes that "make a person look thin" or cover body with baggy or loose-fitting garments.
- Person may take a long time getting dressed because the "just right" garments must be located for the "just right look."

- Person may take a long time to shop for groceries because labels must be read carefully.
- Person may tend to hoard or restrict finances (AN) or be impulsive and overspend (BN).
- Person may have lost functional mobility (AN).
- Person may have dental decay and gum disease due to purging.

Education/Work
- Person tends to be a perfectionist and avoids tasks where he or she may not excel.
- Person's choice of work may coincide with eating disorder (dancers tend to be thin).
- Person may avoid volunteering in situations where food is served or alternately be a food server without eating any of the food.

Play/Leisure
- Person may restrict leisure activities to physical activities and exercise.
- Person may prefer individual or solo activities such as running.

Social Participation
- Person may avoid engaging in social activities that involve food, such as eating at a party or restaurant, because of concerns related to controlling calorie input or choice of foods.
- Person may attend only those social activities where food is not served or can be avoided by stating lack of hunger or planning to eat later.

Sensorimotor
- Person may have a reduced ability to modulate sensory, physiological, and affective responses (Brand-Gothelf et al., 2016).
- Person may have a sensory modulation disorder such as overresponsiveness (AN) or under-responsiveness (BN).
- Person may have difficulty identifying various food tastes including sweets.
- Person may have dental problems related to purging behavior.

Cognitive/Perceptual
- Person usually has inaccurate information and beliefs about the number of calories needed to attain and maintain normal weight and healthy diet, portion sizes, proper preparation of certain foods, when foods should be discarded, how long a meal should take to consume, size of food bites, number of food bites in an average meal, diets and dieting, etc.
- Person may have distorted sense of hunger or fatigue (Note: distortion may be a somatosensory deficit, a long-held belief and habit, or both).
- Person may experience difficulty with attention, concentration, and memory, which are side effects of starvation.
- Person may focus solely on food and food-related activities to the exclusion of almost all other activities.

Psychosocial
- Person may express guilt about overeating.
- Person may express concern about becoming fat.
- Person may express anxiety and fear about eating certain foods.
- Person may have low or poor self-esteem.
- Person may have a distorted body image in which the person "sees" him- or herself as fat.
- Person may lack self-confidence.
- Person may express feelings of being out of control except around food.
- Person may have few or no friends because of the restricted acceptable list of activities the person will accept.
- Person may have role deficit performance as a child, sibling, friend, peer, student, coworker because of time and energy devoted to eating and food-related tasks.
- Person with anorexia nervosa diagnosis may have role performance deficits in worker, friend, and amateur/hobbyist (Quiles-Cestari & Ribeiro, 2012).

- Personality traits for anorexia nervosa: compulsivity, perfectionism, desire to conform, lack of initiative and spontaneity, introversion and limited expression of emotions, tendency to avoid risk or danger, high need for validation from others, excessive self-control, impaired ability to permit self-gratification (Lock & Pépin, 2019).
- Personality traits for bulimia nervosa: impulsivity, seeking sensory stimulation and/or heightened mood states, extroversion, inadequate self-control, impaired ability to cope with delayed or denied self-gratification (Lock & Pépin, 2019).
- Personality traits for binge eating: low self-esteem, harm avoidance, socially prescribed perfectionism and depressive personality (Lock & Pépin, 2019).

Context/Environment
- Person may have family expectations that he or she feels cannot be met.
- Person may be listening or looking at media coverage (magazine, TV, social) stating that a certain look is desirable.
- Person may be subject to certain cultural beliefs, rituals, and traditions about what should or should not be done relating to the body and food.

Intervention/Treatment

Models and programs developed by occupational therapy personnel include Ayres Sensory Integration (ASI; Gardiner & Brown, 2010), Canadian Model of Occupational Performance (CMOP; Gardiner & Brown, 2010; Mack, 2019), case studies (Wagenfeld & Olsen, 2017), ecology of human performance (EHP; Mack, 2019), model of human occupation (MOHO; Gardiner & Brown, 2010; Lock et al., 2012; Mack, 2019), person-environmental-occupational-performance (PEOP; Mack, 2019), and sensory activity group (Wheatley, 2019). Models and programs developed by other professionals but used by occupational therapy personnel include cognitive behavior therapy (CBT; Lock et al., 2012; Mack, 2019; Seymour, 2015, 2016), figured world (Elliot, 2012), and the recovery model (Clark & Nayar, 2012). The recovery model focused on improving motivation and ability to participate in meaningful activities, increased caloric intake and weight restoration, and a reduction in maladaptive body perceptions and eating disorder behaviors (Biddiscombe et al., 2018). Working with a dietician or nutritionist is important in building a team approach along with a physician and nurse. A physical therapist may help with a safe exercise group. Goals are to assist client to find meaning and purpose in life through engaging in social and community activity to bolster self-esteem and increase socialization (Wagenfeld & Olson, 2017).

Activities of Daily Living/Instrumental ADL
- Use functional activities (meal preparation, grocery shopping, shopping for clothes, budgeting) to address issues and concerns.
- Have client plan "safe" meals (foods the person will eat) and gradually encourage client to add "feared, challenged, or unsafe" foods to the menu.
- Have client add dessert (sweets) to planned menu of expected calorie count.
- Have client practice planning three meals a day for 7 days = 21 meals.
- Encourage client to finish eating within a given time period (AN).
- Develop a life skills group focusing on independent living skills such as shopping, budgeting, finances, housekeeping, doing laundry, and other skills person may have missed.

Education/Work
- Explore with client job opportunities including observing job tasks being performed.
- Explore volunteer opportunities in the community that may become a focus.

Play/Leisure
- Explore client's interests and abilities.
- Provide opportunity to practice previously learned activities and to learn new ones.

- Explore with client if physical activity and exercise could be expanded into a new area of interest such as competitive running (bicycling, swimming, etc.).

Social Participation
- Encourage client to participate in social activities with family and friends.
- Encourage client to eat with others and in public.

Sensorimotor
- Explore sensory responsivity (over- or under-responsivity) and recommend compensatory techniques as useful (see Sensory Processing Disorders: Child and Ayres Sensory Integration Approach in Section 2: Sensory Disorders).

Cognitive/Perceptual
- Provide factual information about eating and food including calories, portions, weight, diets, healthy foods, healthy balance of different types of food, proper preparation of foods, proper storage and discarding of foods, etc.
- Provide opportunity to discuss values and beliefs, including distortions and inaccuracies, about food, eating, meal preparation, grocery shopping, and discarding of food.
- Assist client to develop a daily schedule of activities that includes time for eating.
- Develop or participate in a self-reflection or contemplation group designed to examine an eating disorder as a friend and an enemy through writing letters or advertisements as a means of examining what an eating disorder does to the person's life.
- An example of the cognitive task:
  - Have client(s) identify target beliefs (number of calories, size of portions, weight gain, types of diets, amount and type of exercise, etc.).
  - Have client(s) predict the outcome of the food challenge.
  - Challenge the prediction through exposure (provide factual information).
  - Have client(s) observe whether the beliefs are valid.
  - Have client(s) reflect on experience.

Psychosocial
- Small groups may provide opportunities to learn to work with others and learn from other's experiences.
- Help client to identify the emotional situations that trigger the eating disorder behaviors.
- Help client to develop coping strategies to avoid the eating disorder behaviors.
- Encourage resumption of role performances previously held by client.
- Support corrective role performance related to food and meal preparation, including eating with others.

Context/Environment
- Explore with client possible conflicts with family over expectations.
- Work with client to provide information about eating disorders to family, caregivers, and friends and how they can help.
- Explore with client what community services might be useful to improve the client's quality of life.

Precautions/Safety Considerations

Health conditions should be monitored including cardiovascular, body mass index, dental issues, and bone mass (Waugh et al., 2011). Person with anorexia nervosa is at risk for cardiovascular disorders due to malnutrition. Person with bulimia nervosa diagnosis is at risk for substance use, self-harm, and risky sexual relationships (Lock & Pépin, 2019).

Prognosis and Outcome

Recovery is possible, averaging 57 to 79 months (Mack, 2019), but for many clients the condition becomes chronic, and signs of relapse must be monitored closely.

REFERENCES

American Psychiatric Association. (2013). *Diagnostic and statistical manual of mental disorders* (5th ed.). https://doi.org/10.1176/appi.books.9780890425596

Biddiscombe, R. J., Scanlan, J. N., Ross, J., Horsfield, S., Aradas, J., & Hart, S. (2018). Exploring the perceived usefulness of practical food groups in day treatment for individuals with eating disorders. *Australian Occupational Therapy Journal, 65*(2), 98–106. https://doi.org/10.1111/1440-1630.12442

Brand-Gothelf, A., Parush, S., Eitan, Y., Admoni, S., Gur, E., & Stein, D. (2016). Sensory modulation disorder symptoms in anorexia nervosa and bulimia nervosa: A pilot study. *International Journal of Eating Disorders, 49*(1), 59–68. https://doi.org/10.1002/eat.22460

Clark, M., & Nayar, S. (2012). Recovery from eating disorders: A role for occupational therapy. *New Zealand Journal of Occupational Therapy, 59*(1), 13–17.

Elliot, M. L. (2012). Figured world of eating disorders: Occupations of illness. *Canadian Journal of Occupational Therapy, 79*(1), 15–22. https://doi.org/10.2182/cjot.2012.79.1.3

Gardiner, C., & Brown, N. (2010). Is there a role for occupational therapy within a specialist child and adolescent mental health eating disorder service? *British Journal of Occupational Therapy, 73*(1), 38–43. https://doi.org/10.4276/030802210X12629548272745

Lock, L., & Pépin, G. (2019). Eating disorders. In C. Brown, V. C. Stoffel, & J. P. Muñoz (Eds.), *Occupational therapy in mental health: A vision for participation* (2nd ed., pp. 154–168). F.A. Davis.

Lock, L., Williams, H., Bamford, B., & Lacey, J. H. (2012). The St George's eating disorders service meal preparation group for inpatients and day patients pursuing full recovery: A pilot study. *European Eating Disorders Review, 20*(3), 218–224. https://doi.org/10.1002/erv.1134

Mack, R. (2019). Treating eating disorders: An inside look at occupation-based interventions. *OT Practice, 24*(5), 16–21.

O'Toole, M.T. (Ed.). (2017). *Mosby's dictionary of medicine, nursing & health professions* (10th ed.). Elsevier.

Porter, R. S. (Ed.). (2018). *The Merck manual of diagnosis and therapy* (20th ed.). Merck Sharp & Dohme.

Quiles-Cestari, L. M., & Ribeiro, R. P. P. (2012). The occupational roles of women with anorexia nervosa. *Revista Latino-Americana de Enfermagem, 20*(2), 235–242. https://doi.org/10.1590/S0104-11692012000200004

Seymour, A. (2015). Integrated eating disorder services in Wales. *OT News, 23*(12), 38–39.

Seymour, A. (2016). Occupational engagement and participation. *OT News, 24*(12), 22–24.

Wagenfeld, A., & Olson, L. M. (2017). Feeding and eating disorders. In B. J. Atchison& D. P. Dirette (Eds.), *Conditions in occupational therapy* (5th ed., pp. 241–256). Wolters Kluwer.

Waugh, E. J., Woodside, D. B., Beaton, D. E., Coté, P., & Hawker, G. A. (2011). Effects of exercise on bone mass in young women with anorexia nervosa. *Medicine and Science in Sports and Exercise, 43*(5), 755–763. https://doi.org/10.1249/MSS.0b013e3181ff3961

Wheatley, R. (2019). Supporting adolescents on an inpatient eating disorder ward. *OT News, 27*(9), 34–36.

BIBLIOGRAPHY

Crouch, R., & Alers, V. (2014). The treatment of eating disorders in occupational therapy. In R. Crouch & V. Alers (Eds.), *Occupational therapy in psychiatry and mental health* (5th ed., pp. 408–418). Wiley.

Devery, H., Scanlan, J. N., & Ross, J. (2018). Factors associated with professional identity, job satisfaction and burnout for occupational therapists working in eating disorders: A mixed methods study. *Australian Occupational Therapy Journal, 65*(6), 523–532. https://doi.org/10.1111/1440-1630.12503

Emotionally Disturbed Children and Adolescents

Also called emotional disturbance in children, youth, and adolescence; mental illness in children, youth, and adolescence; behavioral disorders in children, youth, and adolescence.

See also Eating Disorders, Anxiety and General Anxiety Disorder, Attention-Deficit/Hyperactivity Disorder, Bipolar Disorders, Depression, Schizophrenia, Substance-Related and Addictive Disorders.

Description

The Individuals with Disabilities Education Improvement Act (IDEA) defines *emotionally disturbed* (ED) as a condition exhibiting one or more of the following characteristics over a long period of time and to a marked degree that adversely affects a child's education performance:

- an inability to learn that cannot be explained by intellectual, sensory, or health factors;
- an inability to build or maintain satisfactory interpersonal relationships with peers and teachers;
- inappropriate types of behavior or feelings under normal circumstances;
- a general pervasive mood of unhappiness or depression; and
- a tendency to develop physical symptoms or fears associated with personal or school problems (IDEA, 2004, § 300.8[c][4][i-ii]).

The term includes schizophrenia but does not apply to children who are socially maladjusted, unless it is determined that they also qualify as having an emotional disturbance. Examples of disorders include anxiety disorders, bipolar disorder, conduct disorder, eating disorders, obsessive-compulsive disorder, and psychotic disorders in children, youth, or adolescence. Examples of behaviors include hyperactivity, impulsiveness, verbal outbursts, short attention span, aggression, self-injurious behavior, acting out, fighting, negative peer relationships, inability to interpret social situations, social anxiety, withdrawal, excessive fear or anxiety, immaturity, inappropriate crying, temper tantrums, or poor coping skills that are continued over long periods of time. The behavior signals that the child or adolescent is not coping with his or her environment or with peers. Children with the most serious emotional disturbances may exhibit distorted thinking, excessive anxiety, bizarre motor acts, and abnormal mood swings. The term *emotional disturbed* does not appear in the American Psychiatric Association (2013) classification of mental disorders.

Cause

Exact cause is unknown but several factors contribute: heredity, brain disorder, diet, stress, family functioning, and environmental factors (Porter, 2018). Examples of person factors include genetic influences, low intelligence, learning difficulties, specific developmental delay, community difficulties, certain mental and emotional traits, chronic physical illness, poor academic performance, and low self-esteem (Evans & Banovic, 2014). Examples of environmental factors include parental conflict, family breakdown, inconsistent disciplines, hostile and rejecting relationships, physical and emotional abuse, parental psychiatric illness, parental criminality, parental substance abuse, death and loss, socioeconomic disadvantage, homelessness, disaster, discrimination, and other significant life events (Evans & Banovic, 2014).

Evaluation/Assessment

Areas
- Activities of Daily Living/Instrumental ADL: basic ADLs, independent living skills
- Education/Work: academic performance, classroom or school behavior, vocational interests

- Play/Leisure: interests, play skills, engagement in leisure occupations, frequency, location
- Rest/Sleep: sleep disturbances
- Social Participation: type, frequency, location, with whom
- Sensorimotor: gross and fine motor skills
- Cognitive/Perceptual: attention, memory (working memory, prospective memory), learning, executive functions (problem solving, decision making, planning, judgment of safety, time management)
- Psychosocial: anxiety, depression, self-esteem, self-efficacy, role performance, interpersonal relations, social skills, quality of life
- Context/Environment: social support, community resources, cultural values and beliefs
- Development (Preschooler, Child, Adolescent only): developmental profile is uneven, development regression has occurred
- Comorbidities: anxiety, attention-deficit/hyperactivity disorder, autistic spectrum disorder, bipolar disorder, conduct disorder, depression, schizophrenia, sensory processing dysfunction, substance abuse

Instruments
Instruments Developed by Occupational Therapy Personnel
- Adolescent/Adult Sensory Profile (AASP; Brown & Dunn, 2002)
- Assessment of Communication and Interaction Skills (ACIS; Forsyth et al., 1998)
- Assessment of Motor and Process Skills (8th ed.; AMPS-8; Fisher & Bray Jones, 2016)
- Canadian Occupational Performance Measure (5th ed.; COPM-5; Law et al., 2014)
- Child Occupational Self-Assessment (COSA; Kramer et al., 2014)
- Children's Assessment of Participation and Enjoyment and Preferences for Activities of Children (CAPE/PAC; King et al., 2004)
- Functional Behavior Assessment Data Collection Tool (Scheibel, 2019, in References)
- Scatterplot (Scheibel, 2019, in References)
- Sensory Integration and Praxis Tests (SIPT; Ayres, 1989)
- Short Child Occupational Profile (Version 2.2; SCOPE; Bowyer et al., 2008)

Instruments Developed by Other Professionals and Used by Occupational Therapy Personnel
- Avoidance and Fusion Questionnaire for Youth (AFQ-Y; Greco et al., 2005; Greco et al., 2008)
- Child Behavior Checklist (CBCL; Achenbach, 2001)

Problems/Issues
Activities of Daily Living/Instrumental ADL
- Preschooler has lost previously mastered basic ADL skills (eating with a spoon, dressing and undressing, bladder and bowel control, washing face and hands independently).
- Preschooler, child, or adolescent may restrict diet and eat only certain foods (consider eating disorder).
- Preschooler, child, or adolescent may have a poor appetite and refuse to eat foods previously eaten (consider eating disorder).
- Child or adolescent may refuse to take medication.
- Child or adolescent may express little interest or actual performance of self-care activities although capable of performing the tasks.
- Child or adolescent may not follow any general routine.
- Adolescent may act out sexually.

Education/Work
- Child or adolescent may have marked change in academic performance from receiving good grades and behavioral conduct scores to poor or failing grades and conduct scores.
- Child or adolescent may be behind in academic performance due to difficulty with subject matter, failure to complete assignments, behavioral self-regulation, or absenteeism.

- Child or adolescent may be dismissed from school because of aggressive, argumentative, disruptive, or destructive behavior in the classroom or school building.
- Child or adolescent may refuse to go to school and become truant.
- Adolescent may not have explored potential vocational interest.

Play/Leisure

- Preschooler may lose previously mastered play skills.
- Preschooler or child may have poorly developed, impoverished, or missing play skills.
- Child or adolescent may have limited or no engagement in leisure occupations.
- Child or adolescent may refuse to engage in play or leisure occupations that are age appropriate.

Rest/Sleep

- Preschooler or child may have frequent and persistent nightmares or bad dreams.
- Preschooler or child may refuse to sleep in certain rooms or bedding.
- Child or adolescent may have sleep disturbances (difficulty falling asleep or staying asleep).
- Adolescent may have marked changes in sleep habits (stay up all night, sleep during the day, sleep most of the day).
- Note: Medications can affect sleep patterns.

Social Participation

- Child or adolescent may have limited or no participation in social activities.

Sensorimotor

- Child or adolescent may demonstrate poor development of gross motor skills such as skipping, jumping, hopping, throwing, catching, balancing on one foot, coordination of two sides of the body.
- Child or adolescent may demonstrate poor development of fine motor skills such as dexterity, coordination of two hands, in-hand manipulation. (Note: Medication may reduce fine motor skills performance. Changes in medication may improve performance.)
- Child or adolescent may demonstrate low energy level and endurance.
- Child or adolescent may complain of pain such as headaches or stomachaches.
- Child or adolescent may demonstrate sensory processing dysfunction: sensory seeking, sensory avoiding, low registration, sensory sensitivity. Children at clinical high risk tend to demonstrate active sensory avoidance, heightened sensory sensitivity, reduced sensory seeking, and reduced low registration (Parham et al., 2019).
- Child or adolescent may experience visual or auditory hallucinations.

Cognitive/Perceptual

- Child or adolescent may have difficulty with attending behavior: concentration, dividing attention.
- Child or adolescent may have difficulty maintaining reality orientation to time, place, and person.
- Child or adolescent may have difficulty with memory, especially working memory and prospective memory.
- Child or adolescent may have difficulty with executive functions such as problem solving, planning ahead, mental flexibility, judgment of safety, time management.
- Child or adolescent may express paranoid ideation.
- Child or adolescent may demonstrate difficulty with visual-perceptual tasks or visual motor perception.

Psychosocial

- Preschooler may become fidgety or in constant motion beyond regular play activities.
- Preschooler or child may have frequent and unexpected temper tantrums (meltdowns).
- Preschooler, child, or adolescent may become withdrawn and prefer being alone.
- Preschooler, child, or adolescent may express feelings of anxiety or fearfulness.

- Preschooler, child, or adolescent may be depressed.
- Preschooler may display self-destructive behavior, such as head banging, or have frequent bodily injuries.
- Child or adolescent may have difficulty coping with everyday (normal) problems and activities such as getting dressed for school, organizing backpack for day's schedule, answering a friend's request for help with an assignment, etc.
- Child or adolescent may be persistently disobedient or show aggression.
- Child or adolescent may demonstrate provocative opposition to authority figures.
- Child or adolescent may threaten to run away or have made actual attempts to run away.
- Child or adolescent may deliberately self-harm or attempt suicide.
- Child or adolescent may be experiencing violence (at home or school, on the playground, on the bus, through social media).
- Child or adolescent may have difficulty performing roles as expected.
- Child or adolescent may have delays or missing social skills.
- Child or adolescent may have poor quality of life and life satisfaction.
- Adolescent may engage in substance abuse (alcohol or drugs).
- Adolescent may engage in criminal behavior (thefts, vandalism).
- Adolescent may express strange thoughts, beliefs, feelings, or unusual behaviors.

Context/Environment
- Child or adolescent may have limited or no social support from family, peers, or friends.
- Parents or caregivers may lack information on managing a child or adolescent with emotionally disturbed behavior.
- Community resources (services, agencies, programs) may be limited or nonexistent.
- Cultural values, beliefs, and traditions may interfere with or limit participation in potential treatment including stigmatization, marginalization, and occupational deprivation.
- Governmental laws, regulations, and policies may hinder access to services.
- Lack of insurance coverage and reimbursement may hinder access to services.

Intervention/Treatment

Models and programs developed by occupational therapy personnel include Doing, Being, Becoming and Belonging (Rouse & Hitch, 2014); groups in community practice (Champagne, 2012); PhotoVoice (Greco et al., 2017); safety tools (MacLachlan & Stromberg, 2018); school to work transition program (Nochajski & Schweitzer, 2014); sensory-based intervention (Yunus et al., 2015); social and emotional learning (American Occupational Therapy Association, 2013b); and strengths-based program (American Occupational Therapy Association, 2012). Models and programs developed by other personnel but used by occupational therapy personnel include Acceptance and Commitment Therapy (ACT; Makki et al., 2018), alternative educational environments (Barnes et al., 2011), bulling prevention (American Occupational Therapy Association, 2013a), interdisciplinary mental health services (Bream, 2010), nurturing interventions (Champagne & Caldwell, 2018), and participation program (Tokolahi et al., 2018). Team members include psychiatrists, nursing personnel, psychologists, educators, vocational counselors, social workers, and occupational therapy personnel. Goal is to address mental health issues that have an impact on the meaningful engagement and purposeful participation in the occupations of children and youth at home, school, and community (Petryk, 2014). The focus is on social and life skills (Arbesman et al., 2013).

Activities of Daily Living/Instrumental ADL
- Encourage client and family to develop a schedule and routine with clear expectations for each member of the family so everyone knows their role and what occupations are to be performed.
- Encourage client to develop and follow a plan for taking medications. Explore with physician and client if adjustments in medications may reduce objectionable side effects.

- Facilitate learning and implementing independent living skills including meal preparation, housekeeping, doing laundry, maintaining clothing in good condition, shopping, learning to drive or use public transportation, looking for and securing an apartment or other housing arrangement.

Education/Work

- Assist client to continue and complete academic program if client has not graduated from high school.
- Assist client to determine if college or vocational training is best course of action.
- Assist client to explore and apply for paid and/or volunteer work.

Play/Leisure

- Assist client to develop and implement play skills, especially symbolic, cooperative, and interactive play skills.
- Encourage client to renew interest and engagement in previously enjoyed leisure occupations.
- Assist client to explore and develop new leisure occupations.

Rest/Sleep

- Assist client to develop and implement sleep habits and routine.
- Explore with physician and client if adjustments in medications may reduce sleep disturbances or if sleeping medications need to be added.

Social Participation

- Encourage client to reestablish contacts with family and friends to participate in social and cultural activities; discourage contacts with negative influences (substance abuse, criminal activities).
- Assist client to explore and develop new social and culture activities.

Sensorimotor

- Assist client to develop and implement a physical fitness program consist with client's interests and abilities.
- Assist client to develop a "safe place" where he or she can retreat when overstimulated by environmental demands or arranging seating so client can escape when overwhelmed by learning task or teacher expectations.
- Select occupations that provide a sensory diet addressing client's needs such as heavy muscle work. Example: sweeping, drumming, kneading clay, making bread as calming occupations.
- Use sensory-based approaches such as sensory process and sensory integration with equipment such as balls as seating devices, rocking chairs, scooter boards, mats.
- Provide a structured schedule of daily occupation with input from the client.

Cognitive/Perceptual

- Provide opportunity to practice problem solving starting with simple problems with two or three steps and working toward more difficult or complex problems.
- Provide opportunity to practice decision making starting with yes/no items and increasing to multiple choice.
- Client may find keeping a diary or photo journal of thoughts and reactions to events useful to record feelings that he or she finds difficult to express to other people.
- Use pictures and simple words to outline the daily schedule.

Psychosocial

- Have client complete the "What helps you feel better?" and "What makes you feel upset?" worksheets in "Safety Tools" (MacLachlan & Stromberg, 2018).
- Increase client's coping skills through deep breathing, relaxation exercises, mindfulness, yoga, tai chi.

- Provide opportunity to improve self-esteem and self-confidence by using client's interests to encourage engagement and participation.
- Use behavior management techniques to analyze existing skills to be modified and new skills to be learned based on understanding antecedent events (set up prior to initiating action), behavior to be modified (may require several steps to be learned), and consequences (rewards, benefits, outcomes).
- Understand and use concept of simultaneous (conflicting) behaviors: If child is performing desired behavior, he or she is not performing undesired behavior. Example: If child is in his seat, he is not out of his seat. Reward in-seat behavior. Set up environment to encourage and facilitate desired behavior.
- Assist client to identify "triggers" that make the client uncomfortable, retreat, or act out and plan a list of options to reduce the impact of the triggers.
- Assist client to practice role performance of roles identified as important to the client starting with those most important and expanding as client is able to manage role expectations successfully (student, worker, family member, hobbyist, organizational member, etc.).
- Assist client to increase and improve social skills in environments client typically encounters or would encounter, if a new role sought, through role playing or narrative stories.

Context/Environment

- Encourage and support parental involvement in service program. Family can plan activities to do together and to do apart.
- With client, plan sessions to help teachers and other adults to understand child's needs and how to address those needs to facilitate occupational behavior.
- Advocate for accessible services and early intervention.
- Advocate for reducing the stigma and discrimination associated with negative cultural values, beliefs, and traditions associated with mental, emotional, and behavioral health disorders.
- Advocate and participate in prevention programs to promote good mental health.
- Assist in training other professionals including teachers and caregivers about mental, behavioral, and emotional health.

Precautions/Safety Considerations

Self-harming, suicidal behavior, or suicide attempts are always possible and should be monitored, especially if one or more of behaviors has been previously noted.

Prognosis and Outcome

Variable. Successful outcomes are possible if the person is able to learn and maintain the habits, routines, and occupations that work best for him or her. However, mental illness is often a chronic disorder that must be monitored regularly including maintaining a strict medication schedule.

REFERENCES

American Occupational Therapy Association. (2012). *School mental health toolkit: Promoting strengths in children and youth.* https://www.aota.org/-/media/Corporate/Files/Practice/Children/School MHToolkit/Promoting%20Strengths%20REVISED.pdf

American Occupational Therapy Association. (2013a). *School mental health toolkit: Bullying prevention and friendship promotion.* https://www.aota.org/-/media/Corporate/Files/Practice/Children/SchoolMHToolkit/BullyingPreventionInfoSheet.pdf

American Occupational Therapy Association. (2013b). *School mental health toolkit: The cafeteria: Creating a positive mealtime experience.* https://www.aota.org/-/media/Corporate/Files/Practice/Children/Cafeteria-Mealtime-Info-Sheet.pdf

American Psychiatric Association. (2013). *Diagnostic and statistical manual of mental disorders* (5th ed.). https://doi.org/10.1176/appi.books.9780890425596

Arbesman, M., Bazyk, S., & Nochajski, S. M. (2013). Systematic review of occupational therapy and mental health promotion, prevention, and intervention for children and youth. *American Journal of Occupational Therapy, 67*(6), e120–e130. https://doi.org/10.5014/ajot.2013.008359

Barnes, K., Vogel, K., & Beck, A. (2011). Occupational therapy for children with severe emotional disturbance in alternative educational settings. In S. Bazyk (Ed.), *Mental health promotion, prevention, and intervention with children and youth: A guiding framework for occupational therapy* (pp. 207–229). AOTA Press.

Bream, S. (2010). Meeting the mental health needs of adolescents. *OT Practice, 15*(11), 15–18.

Champagne, T. (2012). Creating occupational therapy groups for children and youth in community-based mental health practice. *OT Practice, 17*(14), 13–18.

Champagne, T., & Caldwell, B. (2018). Nurturing interventions. In. J. Mikula (Commissioner), *Creating positive cultures of care resource guide* (4th ed.). Massachusetts Department of Mental Health. https://www.mass.gov/doc/section-one-nurturing-interventions/download

Evans, S., & Banovic, J. (2014). Emotional health and wellbeing of children and young people. In W. Bryant, J. Fieldhouse, & K. Bannigan (Eds.), *Creek's occupational therapy and mental health* (5th ed., pp. 389–404). Churchill Livingstone/Elsevier.

Greco, V., Lambert, H. C., & Park, M. (2017). Being visible: PhotoVoice as assessment for children in a school-based psychiatric setting. *Scandinavian Journal of Occupational Therapy, 24*(3), 222–232. https://doi.org/10.1080/11038128.2016.1234642

Individuals with Disabilities Education Improvement Act of 2004, 20 U.S.C. § 1400 *et seq.* (2004).

MacLachlan, J., & Stromberg, N. (2018). Safety tools. In J. Mikula (Commissioner), *Creating positive cultures of care resource guide* (4th ed.). Massachusetts Department of Mental Health. https://www.mass.gov/doc/section-two-safety-tools/download

Makki, M., Hill, J. F., Bounds, D. T., McCammon, S., McFall-Johnsen, M., & Delaney, K. R. (2018). Implementation of an ACT curriculum on an adolescent inpatient psychiatric unit: A quality improvement project. *Journal of Child and Family Studies, 27*, 2918–2924. https://doi.org/10.1007/s10826-018-1132-2

Nochajski, S. M., & Schweitzer, J. A. (2014). Promoting school to work transition for students with emotional/behavioral disorders. *Work, 48*(3), 413–422. https://doi.org/10.3233/WOR-131790

Parham, L. D., Roush, S., Downing, D. T., Michael, P. G., & McFarlane, W. R. (2019). Sensory characteristics of youth at clinical high risk for psychosis. *Early Intervention in Psychiatry, 13*(2), 942–946. https://doi.org/10.1111/eip.12475

Petryk, A. L. (2014). An occupational perspective on child and youth mental health: Reflections from a school-based occupational therapist. *Occupational Therapy Now, 16*(3), 16–18.

Porter, R. S. (Ed.). (2018). *The Merck manual of diagnosis and therapy* (20th ed.). Merck Sharp & Dohme.

Rouse, J., & Hitch, D. (2014). Occupational therapy led activity based group interventions for young people with mental illness: A literature review. *New Zealand Journal of Occupational Therapy, 61*(2), 58–63.

Scheibel, G. (2019). Best practices in supporting students with emotional disturbance. In G. Frolek Clark, J. E. Rioux, & B. E. Chandler (Eds.), *Best practices for occupational therapy in schools* (2nd ed., pp. 253–262). AOTA Press.

Tokolahi, E., Vandal, A. C., Kersten, P., Pearson, J., & Hocking, C. (2018). Cluster-randomised controlled trial of an occupational therapy intervention for children aged 11-13 years, designed to increase participation to prevent symptoms of mental illness. *Child and Adolescent Mental Health, 23*(4), 313–327. https://doi.org/10.1111/camh.12270

Yunus, F. W., Liu, K. P., Bissett, M., & Penkala, S. (2015). Sensory-based intervention for children with behavioral problems: A systematic review. *Journal of Autism and Developmental Disorders, 45*, 3556–3579. https://doi.org/10.1007/s10803-015-2503-9

BIBLIOGRAPHY

American Occupational Therapy Association. (2010). Specialized knowledge and skills in mental health promotion, prevention, and intervention in occupational therapy practice. *American Journal of Occupational Therapy, 64*(6, Suppl.), S30–S43. https://doi.org/10.5014/ajot.2010.64S30

American Occupational Therapy Association. (2011). *Fact sheet: Mental health in children and youth: The benefit and role of occupational therapy.*

American Occupational Therapy Association. (2012). *School mental health toolkit: Social and emotional learning.* https://www.aota.org/-/media/Corporate/Files/Practice/Children/SchoolMH Toolkit/Social-and-Emotional-Learning-Info-Sheet.pdf

American Occupational Therapy Association. (2017). Mental health promotion, prevention and intervention in occupational therapy practice. *American Journal of Occupational Therapy, 71*(Suppl. 2), Article 7112410035. https://doi.org/10.5014/ajot.2017.716S03

Bazyk, S. (Ed.). (2011). *Mental health promotion, prevention, and intervention with children and youth: A guiding framework for occupational therapy.* AOTA Press.

Bazyk, S., & Arbesman, M. (2013). *Occupational therapy practice guidelines for mental health promotion, prevention, and intervention for children and youth.* AOTA Press.

Bream, S. (2013). The history of occupational therapy in adolescent mental health practice. *OT Practice, 18*(5), CE-1–CE-8.

Cronin, A. (2012). Emotional and behavioral disorders. In S. J. Lane & A. C. Bundy (Eds.), *Kids can be kids: A childhood occupations approach* (pp. 507–524). F.A. Davis.

Honey, A., Alchin, S., & Hancock, N. (2014). Promoting mental health and wellbeing for a young person with a mental illness: Parent occupations. *Australian Occupational Therapy Journal, 61*(3), 194–203. https://doi.org/10.1111/1440-1630.12111

Moeeni, Z. S., Arshadi, F. K., & Behrouzmanesh, P. (2015). Study of relationship between behavioral and emotional aspects of working memory and symptoms of sensory processing disorder, behavioral disorders, and social skills. *Journal of Applied Environmental and Biological Sciences, 4*(12S), 134–141.

Nielsen, S. K., & Hektner, J. M. (2014). Understanding the psychosocial knowledge and attitudes of school-based occupational therapists. *Journal of Occupational Therapy, Schools & Early Intervention, 7*(2), 136–150. https://doi.org/10.1080/19411243.2014.930615

Read, H., Roush, S., & Downing, D. (2018). Early intervention in mental health for adolescents and young adults: A systematic review. *American Journal of Occupational Therapy, 72*(5), Article 7205190040. https://doi.org/10.5014/ajot.2018.033118

Sattari, M., Ali Hosseini, S., Rassafiani, M., Gharaei, M. J. M., Biglarian, A., & Esfahani, N. T. (2017). Prevalence of comorbidity behavioral disorders in children with attention deficit hyperactivity. *Journal of Rehabilitation, 18*(1), 25–32. https://doi.org/10.21859/jrehab-180125

Tseng, M. H., Fu, C. P., Cermak, S. A., Lu, L., & Shieh, J. Y. (2011). Emotional and behavioral problems in preschool children with autism: Relationship with sensory processing dysfunction. *Research in Autism Spectrum Disorders, 5*(4), 1441–1450. https://doi.org/10.1016/j.rasd.2011 .02.004

Forensic Mental Health

See also Bipolar Disorders, Early or First Psychosis, Personality Disorders, Schizophrenia, Serious Mental Illness.

Description

Forensic mental health occupational therapy services work with adults (18 years and above) in secure hospitals and facilities.

Cause

Individuals have committed crimes or offenses for which the criminal justice system has incarcerated them, but they also have been judged insane and in need of mental health services while being incarcerated in secure or locked settings such as prisons, jails, correctional facilities, detention centers, or special units for the "criminally insane" in community, state, or federal hospitals. Some patients may be diverted to community services such as halfway houses, transition houses, or community reentry programs (Muñoz, 2019).

Evaluation/Assessment

Areas

- Activities of Daily Living/Instrumental ADL: home management, shopping, transportation
- Education/Work: education level, literacy (reading level), numeracy (math skills), work history, work skills, career interests and choices
- Play/Leisure: interests, abilities, values, frequency, location, level of satisfaction
- Rest/Sleep: sleep disturbance
- Social Participation: types, frequency, location, with whom
- Sensorimotor: coordination and dexterity, mobility, movement, gross motor skills
- Cognitive/Perceptual: working memory, executive functions, time management
- Psychosocial: life satisfaction, roles and role performance, motivation, interaction and social skills, confidence, self-esteem, values and beliefs, emotional regulation
- Context/Environment: occupational deprivation, family separation
- Comorbidities: dementia, diabetes, homelessness, human immunodeficiency virus (HIV), hypertension, intellectual disability, obesity, poverty, sensory processing disorder, substance abuse

Instruments

Instruments Developed by Occupational Therapy Personnel

- Adolescent/Adult Sensory Profile (AASP; Brown & Dunn, 2002)
- Allen Cognitive Level Screen (5th ed.; ACLS-5; Allen et al., 2007)
- Assessment of Awareness of Ability (A3; Kottorp et al., 2013, in References)
- Assessment of Communication and Interaction Skills (ACIS; Forsyth et al., 1998)
- Assessment of Motor and Process Skills (8th ed.; AMPS-8; Fisher & Bray Jones, 2016)
- Canadian Occupational Performance Measure (5th ed.; COPM-5; Law et al., 2014)
- Capacity to Perform Daily Occupations (CPDO; Schult et al., 2000)
- Comprehensive Occupational Therapy Evaluation Scale (COTES; Brayman et al., 1976)
- Double OT (DOT; Haworth & Cyrs, 2017)
- Engagement in Meaningful Activity Survey (EMAS; Eakman et al., 2010)
- Engagement in OTTP Activities Questionnaire (EOAQ; Shea & Siu, 2016, in References)
- Evaluation of Social Interaction (ESI; Fisher & Griswold, 2015; see also Williams & Chard, 2016, in References)
- Executive Function Performance Test (EFPT; Baum & Wolf, 2013)
- Importance scale (IMP; Lindstedt et al., 2004)
- Interest Checklist (ICL; Matsutsuyu, 1969)
- Interview Schedule for Social Interaction (ISSI; Eklund et al., 2007)
- Kawa Model Interview Process (KMIP; Iwama, 2006)
- Kohlman Evaluation of Living Skills (4th ed.; KELS-4; Kohlman-Thompson & Robnett, 2016)
- Model of Human Occupation Screening Tool (Version 2.0; MOHOST 2.0; Parkinson et al., 2006)
- Occupational Circumstances Assessment Interview and Rating Scale (Version 4.0; OCAIRS; Forsyth et al., 2005)
- Occupational Performance History Interview II (OPHI-II; Kielhofner et al., 2004)

- Occupational Questionnaire (OQ; Smith et al., 1986)
- Occupational Self-Assessment (Version 2.2; OSA 2.2; Baron et al., 2006)
- Occupational Therapy Task Observation Scale (OTTOS; Margolis et al., 1996)
- Role Checklist (RC9; Oakley et al., 1986)
- Volitional Questionnaire (Version 4.1; VO 4.1; de las Heras et al., 2007)

Instruments Developed by Other Professionals and Used by Occupational Therapy Personnel
- Essen Climate Evaluation Schema (EssenCES; Schalast et al., 2008)
- Illness Management and Recovery (IMR) Scales (Mueser et al., 2005)
- Independent Living Scales (ILS; Loeb, 1996)
- Level of Service Inventory–Revised (LSI-R; Lowenkamp et al., 2009)
- Manchester Short Assessment of Quality of Life (MANSA; Priebe et al., 1999)
- Montreal Cognitive Assessment (MoCA; Nasreddine et al., 2005)
- Offender Reintegration Scale (ORS; Liptak, 2008)
- Self-Efficacy Scale (SES; Altmaier et al., 1993)
- Social and Occupational Functioning Assessment Scale (SOFAS; Morosini et al., 2000)
- Texas Functional Living Scale (TFLS: Cullum et al., 2009)
- World Health Organization Quality of Life–BREF (WHOQOL-BREF; The WHOQOL Group, 1998)

Problems/Issues

Activities of Daily Living/Instrumental ADL
- Person may demonstrate limited motor and process skills to perform ADLs, especially community-based skills (Kottorp et al., 2013).
- Person may lack home management skills such as meal preparation, doing laundry, shopping for groceries and supplies.
- Person may lack community living skills such as finding living quarters, shopping, using public transportation, driving a car.
- Person may be overweight due to poor nutritional habits or side effects of medications.

Education/Work
- Person may lack basic educational and work-related skills.
- Person may be unemployed.

Play/Leisure
- Person may have few interests or leisure skills.

Rest/Sleep
- Person may experience sleep disturbance due to conditions in secure facility such as lights on at night, noise from other inmates or staff, or noise from air conditioner or heating system in the building.

Social Participation
- Person may lack skills necessary to participate in social activities.

Sensorimotor
- Person may not engage in regular exercise.
- Person may have sensory processing disorders including over- or under-responsiveness.

Cognitive/Perceptual
- Person may have difficulty concentrating (paying attention).
- Person may have difficulty organizing time effectively (time management; O'Connell et al., 2010).
- Person may have difficulty with problem solving and planning ahead.

Psychosocial

- Person may have difficulty performing and maintaining roles and role performance.
- Person may have poor self-esteem.
- Person may experience idleness and boredom (occupational deprivation) due to lack of motivation, lack of responsibilities, or lack of occupation in the secure environment (Bowser et al., 2018).
- Person may experience a sense of hopelessness in terms of prospects of leaving the secure environment.
- Person may lack motivation and present apathy toward participation in occupation.
- Person may exhibit resistive and acting out behaviors such as violence or aggression.
- Person may try to harm self (suicide behaviors).
- Person may lack self-awareness of and insight into mental illness and degree of disability related to the mental illness.
- Person may overestimate and have high confidence in ability and level of skill in performing occupations but demonstrate low performance in actual situation.
- Person may feel disempowered and feel a lack of autonomy.
- Person may experience a poor quality of life (O'Flynn et al., 2018).
- Person may feel that "treatment" and "therapy" are punishment for having a mental illness.

Context/Environment

- Person usually loses contact with the community from which the person came and from the outside world including possessions, friends, and events.
- Person may not have a social support system or may lose contact while in a secure environment.
- Person may not have access to community resources.
- Person may become "institutionally dependent" due to the highly structured management style that occurs in secure environment.
- Person may have difficulty evaluating environmental conditions that constitute a safe environment.

Intervention/Treatment

Models and programs developed by occupational therapy personnel include the Canadian Model of Occupational Performance (Chui et al., 2016), case study (Moore, 2014), family work (Fitzgerald et al., 2012), Kawa model (Muñoz, 2019), Model of Human Occupation (MOHO; Connell, 2015, 2016; Gibson & Allen, 2019; Jamieson, 2016; McNeill & Bannigan, 2014; Moore, 2014; Ozkan et al., 2018; Royal College of Occupational Therapists, 2017; Williams & Chard, 2016), occupational behavior (Moore, 2014), occupation-focused practice (Perkes et al., 2015), occupational engagement (Morris et al., 2016; Morris & Ward, 2018), occupational therapy informal education program (Crabtree et al., 2016), occupational performance process model (Cronin-Davis, 2017), occupational therapy service program (Axford, 2014; Bate et al., 2019; Camus, 2016), occupational therapy training program (Shea & Siu, 2016), sensory processing (Brooker, 2017; Wiglesworth & Farnworth, 2016), and the Vona du Toit Model of Creative Ability (Moore, 2014). Models and programs developed by other professionals but used by occupational therapy personnel include the Good Lives Model (GLM; Ozkan et al., 2018), Serious Game format (Fitzgerald & Kirk, 2013; Fitzgerald et al., 2011), peer support (Brooker & Bowditch, 2019), social inclusion program (Fitzgerald, 2011), work program (Carpenter, 2019; Smith et al., 2010), and Wii Fit program (Bacon et al., 2012). Team members include prison or guard personnel, physicians, psychiatrists, psychologists, nursing personnel, social workers, educators, and occupational therapy personal. The goal is on developing services that (a) address recovery from having committed a criminal offence, (b) mitigate the effects of incarceration on occupational performance by generating opportunities for occupational engagement, and (c) assist the client return to community life including dealing with stigma and discrimination related to having a criminal record (Muñoz et al., 2016). The goal is enable the client to reintegrate or resettle in the community through building performance skills and enabling engagement in the activities of daily life (Muñoz et al., 2016). A related goal is to reduce recidivism both to forensic facilities and mental health services (Note: forensic facilities use the term "service user" rather than inmate, prisoner, criminal, offender, or similar term).

Activities of Daily Living/Instrumental ADL
- Assist in development of medication management program for service users in minimum security or release programs.
- Facilitate management of basic self-care skills.
- Life Skills Program (Moore, 2014)
  - ▶ Communication skills
  - ▶ Conflict management and criticism handling skills
  - ▶ Problem-solving skills
  - ▶ Money management
  - ▶ Work skills (job seeking, completing application, writing a curriculum vitae or resume, participating in a work interview through role playing)

Education/Work
- Assist in providing prevocational training.
- Assist in implementing an individual placement and support (IPS) program (Talbot et al., 2018).
- Assist in providing supported employment such as working in a café (Carpenter, 2019) or shopping mall (Devereaux & Butterworth, 2011).

Play/Leisure
- Serious Game format (adapted from Snakes and Ladders game; Fitzgerald & Kirk, 2013).
  - ▶ Service programs
    - ○ Engagement and Assessment Unit: game focuses on need for service users to engage in the initial assessment process and to start developing a healthy routine (Fitzgerald & Kirk, 2013).
    - ○ Recovery Unit: game focuses on behaviors needed to promote recovery process.
    - ○ Social Inclusion Unit: game focuses on behaviors needed to engage in the community and person's responsibility for participating in the rehabilitation program leading to discharge.
  - ▶ Game adaptations
    - ○ 100 Squares: described activities and events that could have a positive or negative effect on a service user's progress through the pathways.
    - ○ Squares With Ladders: items asked questions or described events that can facilitate movement through the pathway and cause the player to advance in the game (e.g., You attend occupational therapy sessions).
    - ○ Squares With Snakes: items described activities and events that could have a negative effect on progress, causing the play to move backwards in the game (e.g., You did not attend the morning meeting and stayed in bed).
    - ○ Prizes: music vouchers, toiletries, candy.
- Encourage service user to engage in leisure activities.

Rest/Sleep
- See Sleep–Wake Disorders in Section 13: Lifestyle Conditions.

Social Participation
- Focus social participation activities to promote positive interests and engagement to decrease opportunities for violence and aggression.
- Social inclusion program's (Fitzgerald, 2011) five different groups:

- ▶ Leisure group: access to sports, swimming, movies, fishing, gym, tournaments, women's groups, conservation activities.
- ▶ Literacy group: develop literacy skills and entry-level qualifications for job or college; computer use; and accessing public libraries.
- ▶ Stepping stone education group: progress from prevocational training to supported education and employment, and to unsupported services.
- ▶ Precollege: foundation courses in creative writing, cooking, music, drama, information technology, or skills for life and remedial courses in reading and math to pass high-school equivalency exam.
- ▶ Work (paid or voluntary): maintain and develop roles, habits, and identity that support work activities in the community.

Sensorimotor
- Assist in developing a healthy living program stressing exercise as activity to benefit health and well-being (Bacon et al., 2012).

Cognitive/Perceptual
- Promote executive functioning skills including problem solving and goal setting.
- Provide opportunity for control over decision making and choosing.
- Provide time management training.
- Assist person in planning for future engagement in occupations.

Psychosocial
- Assist service user to develop and implement coping skills including self-control (emotional regulation), anger management.
- Provide stress management training such as deep-breathing exercises and relaxation training.
- Support development of self-esteem and self-worth through positive experiences in engagement of occupations.
- Support development of a sense of purpose through doing and participating in meaningful activities.
- Assist development of self-awareness (strengths and weaknesses).
- Support role functions and performance including parenting.
- Provide opportunity to discuss issues such as socializing with known criminals, making amends to victims, or reuniting with family and friends.

Context/Environment
- Assist service user to navigate legal system.
- Promote participation in social support system including family and friends.

Precautions/Safety Considerations (see Muñoz, 2019)

Watch for items that can be used as weapons. Establish a procedure to monitor and count tools and small equipment at end of each activity session. Monitor for signs of suicide behavior. Follow policies and procedures for safety of people and possessions (Moore, 2014).

Prognosis and Outcome

Variable. Factors depend on the length of the sentence imposed by the court, the type of mental illness, and the response to intervention. Some service users may return to the community and independent living. Others may require a degree of supervised living for many years, especially if comorbidity conditions exist such as dementia (du Toit & McGrath, 2018).

REFERENCES
Axford, K. (2014). Setting up a new occupational therapy service in prison. *Occupational Therapy News, 22*(11), 22–23.

Bacon, N., Farnworth, L., & Boyd, R. (2012). The use of the Wii Fit in forensic mental health: Exercise for people at risk of obesity. *British Journal of Occupational Therapy*, 75(2), 61–68. https://doi.org/10.4276/030802212X13286281650992

Bate, S., Marriott, T., & Vanstone, A. (2019). The transition to an occupation therapy-led service. *OT News*, 27(4), 24–26.

Bowser, A., Link, W., Dickson, M., Collier, L., & Donovan-Hall, M. K. (2018). A qualitative study exploring the causes of boredom for men with a psychosis in a forensic setting. *Occupational Therapy in Mental Health*, 34(1), 32–48. https://doi.org/10.1080/0164212X.2017.1331151

Brooker, J. (2017). Sensory approaches within a young offenders prison. *OT News*, 25(10), 36–38.

Brooker, R., & Bowditch, L. (2019). Peer support and how we do it. *OT News*, 27(3), 38–39.

Camus, E. (2016). Occupational therapy on a forensic ward. *Lancet Psychiatry*, 3(1), 22–23. https://doi.org/10.1016/S2215-0366(15)00572-6

Carpenter, C. (2019). A real work environment to build skills and confidence. *OT News*, 27(4), 27–29.

Chui, A. L., Wong, C. I., Maraj, S. A., Fry, D., Jecker, J., & Jung, B. (2016). Forensic occupational therapy in Canada: The current state of practice. *Occupational Therapy International*, 23(3), 229–240. https://doi.org/10.1002/oti.1426

Connell, C. (2015). Case report: An integrated case formulation approach to forensic practice: The contribution of occupational therapy to risk assessment and formulation. *Journal of Forensic Psychiatry & Psychology*, 26(1), 94–106. https://doi.org/10.1080/14789949.2014.981566

Connell, C. (2016). Forensic occupational therapy to reduce risk of reoffending: A survey of practice in the United Kingdom. *Journal of Forensic Psychiatry & Psychology*, 27(6), 907–928. https://doi.org/10.1080/14789949.2016.1237535

Crabtree, J. L., Ohm, D., Wall, J. M., & Ray, J. (2016). Evaluation of a prison occupational therapy informal education program: A pilot study. *Occupational Therapy International*, 23(4), 401–411. https://doi.org/10.1002/oti.1442

Cronin-Davis, J. (2017). Forensic mental health: Creating occupational opportunities. In C. Long, J. Cronin-Davis, & D. Cotterill (Eds.), *Occupational therapy evidence in practice for mental health* (2nd ed., pp. 139–163). Wiley-Blackwell. https://doi.org/10.1002/9781119378785.ch7

Devereaux, S., & Butterworth. (2011). Answering women's vocational needs in a forensic setting. *Mental Health Occupational Therapy*, 16(1), 30.

du Toit, S. H., & McGrath, M. (2018). Dementia in prisons—Enabling better care practices for those ageing in correctional facilities. *British Journal of Occupational Therapy*, 81(8), 460–462. https://doi.org/10.1177/0308022617744509

Fitzgerald, M. (2011). An evaluation of the impact of a social inclusion programme on occupational functioning for forensic service users. *British Journal of Occupational Therapy*, 74(10), 465–472. https://doi.org/10.4276/030802211X13182481841903

Fitzgerald, M., & Kirk, G. (2013). Serious games: An intervention in low-secure settings. *Mental Health Practice*, 17(3), 14–19. https://doi.org/10.7748/mhp2013.11.17.3.14.e813

Fitzgerald, M., Ratcliffe, G., & Blythe, C. (2012). Family work in occupational therapy: A case study from a forensic service. *British Journal of Occupational Therapy*, 75(3), 152–155. https://doi.org/10.4276/030802212X13311219571864

Fitzgerald, M. M., Kirk, G. D., & Bristow, C. A. (2011). Description and evaluation of a serious game intervention to engage low secure service users with serious mental illness in the design and refurbishment of their environment. *Journal of Psychiatric and Mental Health Nursing*, 18(4), 316–322. https://doi.org/10.1111/j.1365-2850.2010.01668.x

Gibson, A., & Allen, H. (2019). Recovery through activity in an adult forensic service. *OT News*, 27(5), 42–43.

Jamieson, L. (2016). Building occupational skills in the prison population. *OT News*, 24(6), 14–16.

Kottorp, A., Heuchemer, B., Lie, I. P., & Gumpert, C. H. (2013). Evaluation of activities of daily living ability and awareness among clients in a forensic psychiatry evaluation unit in Sweden. *British Journal of Occupational Therapy, 76*(1), 23–30. https://doi.org/10.4276/030802 213X13576469254658

McNeill, S., & Bannigan, K. (2014). Forensic and prison services. In W. Bryant, J. Fieldhouse, & K. Bannigan (Eds.), *Creek's occupational therapy and mental health* (5th ed., pp. 424–438). Churchill-Livingston/Elsevier.

Moore, M. (2014). Forensic psychiatry and occupational therapy. In R. Crouch & V. Alers (Eds.), *Occupational therapy in psychiatry and mental health* (5th ed., pp. 106–114). Wiley & Sons. https://doi.org/10.1002/9781118913536.ch7

Morris, K., Cox, D., & Ward, K. (2016). Exploring stories of occupational engagement in a regional secure unit. *Journal of Forensic Psychiatry & Psychology, 27*(5), 684–697. https://doi.org/10.1080/14789949.2016.1187759

Morris, K., & Ward, K. (2018). The implementation of a new conceptual framework for occupational engagement in forensic settings: Feasibility and application to occupational therapy practice. *Mental Health Review Journal, 23*(4), 308–319. https://doi.org/10.1108/MHRJ-03-20 18-0007

Muñoz, J. P. (2019). Mental health practice in criminal justice systems. In C. Brown, V. C. Stoffel, & J. P. Muñoz (Eds.), *Occupational therapy in mental health: A vision for participation* (2nd ed., pp. 615–641). F.A. Davis.

Muñoz, J., Farnworth, L., & Dieleman, C. (2016). Harnessing the power of occupation to meeting the needs of people in criminal justice settings. *Occupational Therapy International, 23,* 221–228. https://doi.org/10.1002/oti.1439

O'Connell, M., Farnworth, L., & Hanson, E. (2010). Time use in forensic psychiatry: A naturalistic inquiry into two forensic patients in Australia. *International Journal of Forensic Mental Health, 9*(2), 101–109. https://doi.org/10.1080/14999013.2010.499558

O'Flynn, P., O'Regan, R., O'Reilly, K., & Kennedy, H. G. (2018). Predictors of quality of life among inpatients in forensic mental health: Implications for occupational therapists. *BMC Psychiatry, 18,* Article 16. https://doi.org/10.1186/s12888-018-1605-2

Ozkan, E., Belhan, S., Yaran, M., & Zarif, M. (2018). Occupational therapy in forensic settings. In M. Huri (Ed.), *Therapeutic and creative use of activity* (pp. 51–70). IntechOpen. https://doi .org/10.5772/intechopen.79366

Perkes, D., Whiteford, G., Charlesworth, G., Weekes, G., Jones, K., Brindle, S., Hoare, L., Todd, E., & Ray, M. (2015). Occupation-focused practice in justice health and forensic mental health: Using a practice-based enquiry approach. *World Federation of Occupational Therapists Bulletin, 71*(2), 101–107. https://doi.org/10.1080/14473828.2015.1103464

Royal College of Occupational Therapists. (2017). *Occupational therapists' use of occupation-focused practice in secure hospitals* (2nd ed.).

Shea, C. K., & Siu, A. M. (2016). Engagement in play activities as a means for youth in detention to acquire life skills. *Occupational Therapy International, 23*(3), 276–286. https://doi.org/10.1002/ oti.1432

Smith, A., Petty, M., Oughton, I., & Alexander, R. T. (2010). Establishing a work-based learning programme: Vocational rehabilitation in a forensic learning disability setting. *British Journal of Occupational Therapy, 73*(9), 431–436. https://doi.org/10.4276/030802210X12839367526174

Talbot, E., Bird, Y., Russell, J., Sahota, K., Schneider, J., & Khalifa, N. (2018). Implementation of individual placement and support (IPS) into community forensic mental health settings: Lessons learned. *British Journal of Occupational Therapy, 81*(6), 338–347. https://doi.org/10 .1177/0308022618756593

Wiglesworth, S., & Farnworth, L. (2016). An exploration of the use of a sensory room in a forensic mental health setting: Staff and patient perspectives. *Occupational Therapy International, 23*(3), 255–264. https://doi.org/10.1002/oti.1428

Williams, B., & Chard, G. (2016). Using the Evaluation of Social Interaction (ESI) with men in a low secure forensic unit. *British Journal of Occupational Therapy, 79*(4), 206–211. https://doi .org/10.1177/0308022615615890

BIBLIOGRAPHY

Craik, C., Bryant, W., Ryan, A., Barclay, S., Brooke, N., Mason, A., & Russell, P. (2010). A qualitative study of service user experiences of occupation in forensic mental health. *Australian Occupational Therapy Journal, 57*(5), 339–344. https://doi.org/10.1111/j.1440-1630.2010.00857.x

Cronin-Davis, J., & Spybey, M. (2011). Forensic occupational therapy: A survey. *Mental Health Occupational Therapy, 16*(1), 20–26.

Donovan, J., & Mason, K. (2010). The impact of dedicated occupational therapy on a forensic intensive care unit: Service user and staff views. *Mental Health Occupational Therapy, 15*(2), 47–49.

Dumont, M., Dumais, A., Briand, C., Côté, G., Lesage, A., & Dubreucq, J. L. (2012). Clinical characteristics of patients deemed to require long-term hospitalization in a civil or forensic psychiatric setting. *International Journal of Forensic Mental Health, 11*(2), 110–118. https://doi.org/10.1080/14999013.2012.690019

Dumont, M., Thériault, J., Briand, C., Dumais, A., & Potvin, S. (2018). Psychosocial approaches for individuals with schizophrenia in correctional and forensic psychiatric settings: A rapid review. *Journal of Forensic Practice, 20*(3), 152–166. https://doi.org/10.1108/JFP-11-2017-0049

Heard, C. P., Scott, J., Tetzlaff, A., & Lumley, H. (2019). Transitional housing in forensic mental health: Considering consumer lived experience. *Health & Justice, 7*(1), Article 8. https://doi.org/10.1186/s40352-019-0091-z

Hitch, D., Hii, Q., & Davey, I. (2016). Occupational therapy in forensic psychiatry: Recent developments in our understandings (2007–2013). *British Journal of Occupational Therapy, 79*(4), 197–205. https://doi.org/10.1177/0308022615591018

Kamanga, E., & Schurgers, J. (2010). Forensic occupational therapy in Africa for women and children. In V. Alers & R. Crouch (Eds.), *Occupational therapy: An African perspective* (pp. 170–189). Sarah Shorten.

Lindstedt, H., Grann, M., & Söderlund, A. (2011). Mentally disordered offenders' daily occupations after one year of forensic care. *Scandinavian Journal of Occupational Therapy, 18*(4), 302–311. https://doi.org/10.3109/11038128.2010.525720

Muñoz, J. P., Farnworth, L., Hamilton, T., Rogers, S., White, J., & Prioletti, G. (2011). Crossing borders in correctional institutions. In F. Kronenberg, N. Pollard, & D. Sakellarous (Eds.), *Occupational therapy without borders: Towards an ecology of occupation-based practices* (2nd ed., pp. 235–246). Elsevier.

Muñoz, J. P., Moreton, E. M., & Sitterly, A. M. (2016). The scope of practice of occupational therapy in U.S. criminal justice settings. *Occupational Therapy International, 23*(3), 241–254. https://doi.org/10.1002/oti.1427

Tan, B. L., Kumar, V. R., & Devaraj, P. (2015). Development of a new occupational therapy service in Singapore prison. *British Journal of Occupational Therapy, 78*(8), 525–529. https://doi.org/10.1177/0308022615571083

White, J., Dieleman, C., Hamilton, T., & Rogers, S. (2013). Occupational therapy in criminal justice. In E. Cara & A. MacRae (Eds.), *Psychosocial occupational therapy: An evolving practice* (3rd ed., pp. 715–773). Delmar.

Withers, P., Boulton, N., Morrison, J., & Jones, A. (2012). Occupational therapy in a medium secure intellectual disability and personality disorder service. *Journal of Learning Disabilities and Offending Behaviour, 3*(4), 206–218. https://doi.org/10.1108/20420921211327356

Hoarding Disorder

See also Autism Spectrum Disorders, Obsessive Compulsive Disorder, Personality Disorders.

Description

Hoarding disorder is characterized by persistent difficulty discarding or parting with possessions, regardless of their actual value or potential threat to health and safety. The result is an accumulation of possessions that congest and clutter living areas to the point that the intended use of the areas is substantially compromised or lost. The disorder is typically chronic, with little or no waxing and waning of symptoms or spontaneous remission. The person experiences extreme distress if the suggestion is made to throw anything away (Grapczynski, 2019; Porter, 2018). The description in Porter (2018) follows the description in the *Diagnostic and Statistical Manual of Mental Disorders* (5th ed.; *DSM-5*; American Psychiatric Association, 2013). However, hoarding can also be described from an occupational therapy perspective as an activity that encompasses a series of tasks that relate to the collection and saving of meaningful and valued items. Hoarding can include habits and routines that structure the tasks and become a person's daily occupation that occupies the person's waking hours and time with roles that have purpose to the individual (Clarke, 2019). Although the accumulation of items may appear disorganized and compromise the usual intended use of living space, to the individual, items are organized in a manner satisfactory to the person (Grapczynski, 2019). A subset of the hoarding disorder is animal hoarding, in which individuals accumulate a large number of animals to the point that the animals do not have adequate nutrition, sanitation, or veterinary care (Doughty & Brown, 2019). Characteristics are listed in the *DSM-5* (American Psychiatric Association, 2013).

Cause

The exact cause is unknown. Several ideas have been suggested. One possible cause is a distorted cognitive belief including fear that harm will come to the individual if the objects are not retained. Another possible cause is that the person believes memories will be lost or emotional and physical discomfort will be experienced if objects are discarded. A third possible cause is that hoarding is the result of poor cognitive skills, especially executive dysfunction, that reduces attention and the ability to problem solve, make decisions, and complete spatial tasks. These deficits reduce the person's ability to focus, organize, sort, and categorize objects resulting in the accumulation of objects and inability to manage them (Clarke, 2019; Dissanayake et al., 2017). Grapczynski (2019) stated that the cause appears to be genetic without specific genes identified but may still have a familial component.

Evaluation/Assessment

Areas

- Activities of Daily Living/Instrumental ADL: self-care, transportation, functional mobility, functional communication
- Education/Work: work attendance, work performance
- Play/Leisure: types of leisure activities, frequency, location
- Rest/Sleep: sleep habits and disturbances
- Social Participation: social activities, frequency of engagement, location, with whom
- Sensorimotor: no specific issues; check general physical fitness
- Cognitive/Perceptual: attention, memory, executive function skills, problem solving, information processing, insight, judgment, categorization
- Psychosocial: self-image, self-identity, depression, anxiety, emotional states (such as shame, embarrassment, and rejection), marginalization, stigma, role performance
- Context/Environment: home safety, unsanitary conditions, legal issues related to public health, justice, economic costs
- Comorbidities: generalized anxiety, social anxiety, depression

Instruments

Instruments Developed by Occupational Therapy Personnel

- Model of Human Occupation Screening Tool (Version. 2.0; MOHOST 2.0; Parkinson et al., 2006)
- Occupational Performance History Inventory (Version 2.1; OPHI-II; Kielhofner et al., 2004)

Instruments Development by Other Professionals and Used by Occupational Therapy Personnel
- Activities of Daily Living in Hoarding Scale (ADL-H; Frost et al., 2013)
- Hoarding Rating Scale-Interview (HRSI; Tolin et al., 2010)

Problems/Issues

Activities of Daily Living/Instrumental ADL
- Person may not be performing routine ADLs because hoarding tasks are taking up all the time.
- Person may be unable to perform some ADL tasks such as bathing because the bathroom is full of hoarded items.
- Person may be unable to maintain a home living environment that is clean and safe because the accumulated items are piled everywhere and only narrow pathways are available to move about the living space.

Education/Work
- Person may be absent from work to complete hoarding tasks.
- Person may be neglecting work tasks to complete hoarding tasks.
- Person may be unable to work and qualify for disability insurance.

Play/Leisure
- Person may not engage in previously enjoyed leisure activities because completing hoarding tasks have become a full-time occupation.
- Person may be unable to locate items associated with leisure activities among the accumulated items or may not have space available to pursue the occupation.

Rest/Sleep
- See Sleep–Wake Disorders in Section 13: Lifestyle Conditions.

Social Participation
- Person may not be participating in social or community activities.

Sensorimotor
- No identified problems directly related to hoarding, but problems may be present due to other coexisting conditions, such as diabetes.

Cognitive/Perceptual
- Person may have difficulty with executive functioning skills including problem solving and decision making.
- Person may have difficulty organizing and sorting.

Psychosocial
- Person usually has limited or no social relationships.
- Person usually has decreased quality of life.
- Person may have a fear of wasting materials.
- Person may have a fear of losing valued information.
- Person may feel ashamed or embarrassed by inability to manage accumulated objects.
- Person may feel rejected by family and friends who do not seem to understand why the objects are important and meaningful.
- Person may be depressed.
- Person may be anxious that something bad will happen if objects are removed.
- Person may have lost life roles because the person is too busy with hoarding tasks.
- Person may have poor insight into the real or potential problem(s) posed by the hoarding.
- Person does not see any need for help from others (family, friends, colleagues, health-care professions, lawyers, or police).

Context/Environment
- Person may have objects in the home stacked to the ceiling such as newspapers, pizza boxes, books, mail, or other objects.

- Person may have objects piled on beds, chairs, tables, or other objects so that intended use is impossible.
- Person may encounter difficulty with housing rules about having too much stuff/clutter in the housing unit.
- Person may encounter difficulty with public health rules and regulations about unsafe and unsanitary living conditions.
- Person may encounter medical personnel who removed objects from the home to declutter the living areas and spaces without consideration of the meaning or value to the person.
- Person and others may be unable to use areas of the home as intended because the area is full of collected objects making access or use impossible.
- Person may be restricted in the type of activities that can be performed in the home because the collected objects take up the space used for such activities.
- Person may be at increased risk of injury or falls in the home because objects must be moved or rearranged just to get from one place to another.

Intervention/Treatment

Models and programs developed by occupational therapy personnel include model of doing, being, belonging, and becoming (Wilcock & Hocking, 2015); model of human occupation (Kielhofner, 2008); person, environment, and occupation model (Law et al., 1996); and case study (Grapczynski, 2019). Models and programs developed by other professionals but used by occupational therapy personnel include cognitive behavioral therapy (Grapczynski, 2019) and "friendly visitor approach" (Spear, 2014). Team members include psychiatrists, nursing personnel, psychologists, social workers, and occupational therapy personnel. The goal is to help the person better manage the hoarding behavior and to engage in roles, habits, and routines not associated with hoarding.

Activities of Daily Living/Instrumental ADL
- Assist person to engage in and complete ADL tasks.
- Assist person to sort and organize hoarded items so that there is access to important areas of the home such as the bathroom and kitchen.

Education/Work
- Assist person to engage in and complete work tasks.
- Assist person to perform homework or other educational activity.

Play/Leisure
- Assist person to identify and reengage in previously enjoyed leisure activities.
- Assist person to identify and engage in new leisure activities.

Rest/Sleep
- See Sleep–Wake Disorders in Section 13: Lifestyle Conditions.

Social Participation
- Encourage person to participate in community activities.

Sensorimotor
- No specific interventions.

Cognitive/Perceptual
- Help person organize, sort, and store objects (Spear, 2014).

Psychosocial
- Encourage person to renew engagement in life roles such as parent, sibling, friend.
- Assist client to clarify values and beliefs regarding saved objects such as what is safe (contamination), what is orderly (sequencing), what is repugnant (unacceptable behavior, harmful), or what is moral (sexual and religious beliefs; Grapczynski, 2019).
- Assist person to develop a sense of power over hoarding behavior.

Context/Environment
- Stress safety and sanitation concerns (Khoo, 2017).

Precautions/Safety Considerations
Person is at risk for falling due to clutter and lack of clear pathways. Unsanitary conditions may exist, with food and food containers not disposed of properly. Unsafe conditions may exist with the piles high enough to bury a person, making escape difficult.

Prognosis and Outcome
Condition tends to be chronic, but intervention can increase the person's ability to manage life roles.

REFERENCES

American Psychiatric Association. (2013). *Diagnostic and statistical manual of mental disorders* (5th ed.). https://doi.org/10.1176/appi.books.9780890425596

Clarke, C. (2019). Can occupational therapy address the occupational implications of hoarding? *Occupational Therapy International, 2019,* Article 5347403. https://doi.org/10.1155/2019/5347403

Dissanayake, S., Barnard, E., & Willis, S. (2017). The emerging role of occupational therapists in the assessment and treatment of compulsive hoarding: An exploratory study. *New Zealand Journal of Occupational Therapy, 64*(2), 22–30.

Doughty, K., & Brown, C. (2019). Personality disorders. In C. Brown, V. C. Stoffel, & J. P. Muñoz (Eds.), *Occupational therapy in mental health: A vision for participation* (2nd ed., pp. 169–181). F.A. Davis.

Grapczynski, C. A. (2019). Obsessive-compulsive and related disorders. In B. J. Atchison & D. P. Dirette (Eds.), *Conditions in occupational therapy* (5th ed., pp. 209–227). Wolters Kluwer.

Khoo, X. Y. (2017). Older adults with hoarding disorder: A harm-reduction approach. *Occupational Therapy Now, 19*(6), 19–20.

Kielhofner, G. (2008). *Model of human occupation* (4th ed.). Wolters Kluwer.

Law, M., Cooper, B., Strong, S., Stewart, D., Rigby, P., & Letts, L. (1996). The person-environment-occupation model: A transactive approach to occupational performance. *Canadian Journal of Occupational Therapy, 63*(1), 9–23. https://doi.org/10.1177/000841749606300103

Porter, R. S. (Ed.). (2018). *The Merck manual of diagnosis and therapy* (20th ed.). Merck Sharp & Dohme.

Spear, S. (2014). "Friendly visitor": An occupational therapist's experiences of supporting a person with compulsive hoarding behavior. *OT Practice, 19*(4), 16–19.

Wilcock, A. A., & Hocking, C. (2015). *An occupational perspective of health* (3rd ed.). Slack.

BIBLIOGRAPHY

Dissanayake, S. (2012). Clearing the clutter. *OT News, 20*(2), 24–25.

Obsessive-Compulsive Disorder
See also Anxiety and General Anxiety Disorder, Depression and Depressive Disorders, Sensory Over-Responsivity.

Description

Obsessive-compulsive disorder (OCD) is characterized by recurrent, persistent, unwanted, and intrusive thoughts, urges, or images (obsessions) and/or by repetitive, ritualistic behaviors or mental acts that the client feels driven to do (compulsions) to try to lessen or prevent the anxiety that obsessions cause. The obsessions and/or compulsions are clinically significant when one or both is time-consuming, causes significant distress, or impairs functioning in daily life (Porter, 2018). Disorders included under OCD include body dysmorphic disorder, hoarding, trichotillomania (hair-pulling disorder), excoriation (skin-picking disorder), substance/medication induced obsessive-compulsive and related disorder, or other medical condition (American Psychiatric Association, 2013).

OCD is not the same as obsessive-compulsive personality disorder (OCPD). The essential feature of OCPD is the preoccupation with order, perfection, and mental and interpersonal control. Characteristics include attempts to maintain control of situations through detailed attention and adherence to rules, trivial details, procedures, lists, and schedules to the extent that the purpose of the occupation or activity may be lost. People with OCPD view their thinking as normal and find pleasure in carrying out orderly and perfectionistic behavior (Doughty & Brown, 2019). The focus of this chapter is on OCD, although the overlap with aspects of OCPD is unavoidable.

Cause

The cause is anxiety based, but the exact cause in an individual client may not always be clearly identifiable (O'Toole, 2017).

Terminology (O'Toole, 2017; Porter, 2018)

- *Compulsion:* An irresistible, repetitive irrational impulse to perform an act that is usually contrary to one's ordinary judgment or standards, yet results in overt anxiety if it is not completed. The compulsion acts to decrease anxiety. The impulse is usually the result of an obsession. Examples include:
  - ▸ checking (stove is turned off, doors are locked),
  - ▸ counting (repeating a behavior a certain number of times),
  - ▸ ordering/organizing (arranging tableware or workspace items in a specific pattern), and
  - ▸ washing (handwashing, bathing, showering).
- *Compulsive ritual:* A series of acts a person feels must be carried out even though the person recognizes that the behavior is useless and inappropriate. Failure to complete the acts causes extreme tension or anxiety. Most rituals are observable, but some mental rituals such as silent repetitive counting may not be directly observed.
- *Obsession:* A persistent and recurrent thought or idea with which the mind is continually and involuntarily preoccupied and that cannot be expunged by logic or reasoning. The dominant theme may be harm avoidance, safety concerns, risk to self or others, danger, contamination, doubt, discomfort, loss, or aggression.
- *Sensory over-responsivity symptoms:* Refers to negative intensive and rapid responses toward daily sensory stimuli (Ben-Sasson et al., 2017).

Evaluation/Assessment

Areas

- Activities of Daily Living/Instrumental ADL
  - ▸ Total amount of time spent on a specific activity per day beyond typical or average (e.g., showering for 5–10 minutes per day may be typical; showering for 55 minutes a day is not)
  - ▸ Number of times per day an activity is repeated beyond typical or average (e.g., showering once or twice a day may be typical; showering 10 times every day is not)
- Education/Work
  - ▸ Total amount of time spent on a specific activity per study period or work shift beyond typical or average
  - ▸ Number of times per study period or work shift activity is repeated beyond typical or average
- Play/Leisure: interests, values, frequency, location, level of satisfaction

- Rest/Sleep: rituals regarding sleep habits or routines
- Social Participation: type, frequency, location, with whom
- Sensorimotor: sensory over-responsivity, modality specific overresponsivity (auditory, gustatory, olfactory, proprioceptive, tactile, vestibular, visual)
- Cognitive/Perceptual: "not just right experiences" (Ben-Sasson et al., 2017)
- Psychosocial: depression, distress, insight, self-stigmatization, fears, role performance
- Context/Environment: family or community stigma, community resources
- Comorbidities: anxiety, autism spectrum disorder, bipolar disorder, cardiac disorders, depression, eating disorders, sensory over-responsivity, substance abuse

Instruments
Instruments Developed by Occupational Therapy Personnel
- None identified.

Instruments Developed by Other Professionals and Used by Occupational Therapy Personnel
- Not Just Right Experiences (NJRE; Summers et al., 2014, in vivo assessment)
- Obsessive-Compulsive Inventory (OCI; Foa et al., 1998)
- Sensory Perception Quotient (SPQ; Tavassoli et al., 2014)
- Visual Analogue Scale for Anxiety (VAS-A; Hornblow & Kidson, 1976)

Problems/Issues
Activities of Daily Living/Instrumental ADL
- Person may bathe or shower several times a day resulting in dry skin.
- Person may wash hands and face several times a day resulting in dry, scaly, and bleeding skin on hands, face, or both.
- Person may only eat food cleaned and prepared by self to avoid contamination.
- Person may have difficulty maintaining normal weight due to limitations in types of food consumed.

Education/Work
- Person may be unable to attend classes or complete education due to obsessive thoughts or demands of compulsive behaviors.
- Person may be unable to find or continue employment due to obsessive thoughts or demands of compulsive behavior.

Play/Leisure
- Person may have stopped engaging in leisure occupations to avoid equipment or situations which cause distress, anxiety, or demand compulsive behavior.
- Person may feel unable to meet some standard of performance expected in engaging in the leisure occupation.
- Person may not engage in leisure occupations because all time and effort is expended in work and productivity occupations.

Rest/Sleep
- Person may report difficulty sleeping due to recurrent thoughts or need to perform compulsive actions.

Social Participation
- Person may stop or decrease participation in social situations due to demands of compulsive behavior and stigmatization.

Sensorimotor
- Person may be overly responsive to certain sensory stimuli (auditory, tactile, visual).

Cognitive/Perceptual
- Person usually has some insight into the disorder but may not be aware of how much the obsessive thoughts or compulsive behaviors have changed life habits and interpersonal behavior.
- Person may have significant difficulty in making decisions.

Psychosocial
- Person may become anxious, distressed, or fearful in situations related to the obsessions.
- Person may be depressed.
- Person may self-stigmatized.
- Person may be self-critical.
- Person may be unable to perform roles consistent with age and sex due to obsessive thoughts or compulsive behaviors.

Context/Environment
- Person may lose contact with family and family support due to obsessive thoughts or compulsive behaviors.
- Person may lose friends and community support due to obsessive thoughts or compulsive behaviors.
- Person may be viewed by others as rigid, controlling, and stubborn.

Intervention/Treatment

Models and programs developed by occupational therapy personnel include the stigmatization program (Akyurek et al., 2019). Models and programs developed by other professionals but used by occupational therapy personnel include cognitive behavioral therapy (Akyurek et al., 2019) and behavioral group treatment (Söchting & Third, 2011). Team members include psychiatrists, psychologists, and occupational therapy personnel. Goals are to refocus or redirect attention away from obsessive thoughts and compulsive actions toward participation in activities of daily living, education, work, leisure, social occupations, and other important areas of functioning.

Activities of Daily Living/Instrumental ADL
- May be used to refocus, redirect, or substitute for compulsive actions.

Education/Work
- May be used to refocus, redirect, or substitute for compulsive actions.

Play/Leisure
- May be used to refocus, redirect, or substitute for compulsive actions.

Rest/Sleep
- Not discussed (see Sleep–Wake Disorders in Section 13: Lifestyle Conditions).

Social Participation
- May be used to refocus, redirect, or substitute for compulsive actions.

Sensorimotor
- Education in energy conservation may be useful to provide information on interaction with environment.
- Assist client to determine if overresponsivity to stimuli is a factor and provide techniques to manage responses.

Cognitive/Perceptual
- Promote self-awareness about wrong beliefs or thoughts about self.
- Assist person to learn that self-control and self-regulation is possible.
- Instruct in time-processing awareness and time management.
- Support completion of project over perfectionism.

Psychosocial
- Promote awareness of how beliefs and thoughts are contributing to difficulty in performing roles and participating in daily activities.
- Provide instruction in relaxation therapy and mindfulness.
- Promote the emotions of enjoyment, fun, and the positive impact these feelings have on mood, thought, and action (Nott, 2014).

Context/Environment
- Provide correct information to family, friends, employers, and others about the disorder.

Precautions/Safety Considerations

Person is at risk of suicide ideation or suicide behavior, especially during depressive episodes.

Prognosis and Outcome

OCD is often chronic with symptoms that wax and wane. OCD has a significant impact on social and occupational functioning. The disorder may be misdiagnosed resulting in inadequate intervention. The most effective intervention is a combination of cognitive behavioral therapy, exposure response prevention therapy, and pharmacotherapy (Grapczynski, 2017). Degree of client's insight as to whether thoughts and beliefs are true or not may be relevant to successful intervention.

REFERENCES

Akyurek, G., Sezer, K. S., Kaya, L., & Temucin, K. (2019). Stigma in obsessive compulsive disorder. In N. Kocabasoglu & J. B. Caglayan (Eds.), *Anxiety disorders* (pp. 87–112). IntechOpen.

American Psychiatric Association. (2013). *Diagnostic and statistical manual of mental disorders* (5th ed.). https://doi.org/10.1176/appi.books.9780890425596

Ben-Sasson, A., Dickstein, N., Lazarovich, L., & Ayalon, N. (2017). Not just right experiences: Association with obsessive compulsive symptoms and sensory over-responsivity. *Occupational Therapy in Mental Health, 33*(3), 217–234. https://doi.org/10.1080/0164212X.2017.1303418 (Note: Study subjects did not have a clinical diagnosis of OCD. OCD symptoms were based on assessments used in the study.)

Doughty, K., & Brown, C. (2019). Personality disorders. In C. Brown, V. C. Stoffel, & J. P. Muñoz (Eds.), *Occupational therapy in mental health: A vision for participation* (2nd ed., pp. 169–181). F.A. Davis.

Grapczynski, C. A. (2017). Obsessive-compulsive and related disorders. In B. J. Atchison & D. P. Dirette (Eds.), *Conditions in occupational therapy* (5th ed., pp. 209–227). Wolters Kluwer.

O'Toole, M. T. (Ed.). (2017). *Mosby's dictionary of medicine, nursing & health professions* (10th ed.). Elsevier.

Nott, A. (2014). Understanding persons with personality disorders: Intervention in occupational therapy. In R. Crouch & V. Alers (Eds.), *Occupational therapy in psychiatry and mental health* (5th ed., pp. 419–434). Wiley. https://doi.org/10.1002/9781118913536.ch26

Porter, R. S. (Ed.). (2018). *The Merck manual of diagnosis and therapy* (20th ed.). Merck Sharp & Dohme.

Söchting, I., & Third, B. (2011). Behavioral group treatment for obsessive-compulsive disorder in adolescence: A pilot study. *International Journal of Group Psychotherapy, 61*(1), 84–97. Https://doi.org/10.1521/ijgp.2011.61.1.84

BIBLIOGRAPHY

Ben-Sasson, A., & Podoly, T. Y. (2017). Sensory over responsivity and obsessive compulsive symptoms: A cluster analysis. *Comprehensive Psychiatry, 73*, 151–159. https://doi.org/10.1016/j.comp

psych.2016.10.013 (Note: Study subjects did not have a clinical diagnosis of OCD. OCD symptoms were based on assessments used in the study.)

Davis, J., & Noyes, S. (2019). Anxiety, obsessive-compulsive, and related disorders. In C. Brown, V. C. Stoffel, & J. P. Muñoz (Eds.), *Occupational therapy in mental health: A vision for participation* (2nd ed., pp. 197–210). F.A. Davis.

Personality Disorders
See also Borderline Personality Disorder and Type B Personality Disorders, Substance-Related and Addictive Disorders.

Description

Personality disorders in general are pervasive, enduring patterns of perceiving, reacting, and relating that cause significant distress or functional impairment (Porter, 2018). Personality disorders exist when personality traits (patterns of thinking, perceiving, reacting, and relating) become so pronounced, rigid, and maladaptive that they impair work and/or interpersonal functioning (Porter, 2018). The social maladaptive behaviors can cause significant distress to the individual and to those who live and work around the individual. The primary problems are self-identity and interpersonal relationships.

Cause

The cause is believed to be a combination of genetic and environmental factors (Porter, 2018). Men are more likely to have diagnoses of antisocial and obsessive-compulsive disorders. Women are more likely to have diagnoses of avoidant and borderline personality disorders (Nott, 2014). Twelve models have been described, although some concepts or constructions may overlap (Cara, 2013; Nott, 2014):

- Behavioral model: Emphasized environment influences and leaning from social environment.
- Biological model: Personality is ascribed to genetic or biological predispositions.
- Biophysical model: Chemical deficiencies or other physiological defects in the central nervous system account for symptoms.
- Biopsychosocial/evolutionary model: Behavior is the result of interaction of biology and environment, which determines whether traits become disorder.
- Cognitive model: Individuals react to the world depending on their perception of it and personal construction of the world determines behavior.
- Dynamic model: Personality is based on internal organizing psychological factors resulting from conflict experienced early in life with emphasis on developmental behaviors.
- Interpersonal model: Personality is understood in relation to interpersonal tendencies that are the social product of interactions with significant others.
- Neurobiological/temperaments model: Biological constitutional dispositions are central to understanding personality disorders.
- Neuropsychiatric model: Neuroanatomical (functional) and neurochemical (operational) cause or amplifying symptoms.
- Psychodynamic model: Emphasizing impact of early experiences and past events. Symptoms depend on whether id, ego, or superego is most predominant—id predominated for erotic behavior, ego for narcissistic behavior, and superego for compulsive behavior.
- Sociological model: Personality is considered to be shaped by social circumstance and pathology is based on deviance from social norms and harm to society.
- Trait model: Personality is shaped by a variety of personality types with interpersonal behavior as the core feature.

Cluster types (Nott, 2014; Porter, 2018):

- Cluster A: Characterized by appearing odd or eccentric.
  - Paranoid: Mistrust and suspicion.
  - Schizoid: Disinterest in others.
  - Schizotypal: Eccentric ideas and behavior.
- Cluster B: Characterized by appearing dramatic, emotional or erratic, extrovert.
  - Antisocial: Social irresponsibility, disregard for others, deceitfulness, manipulative of others for personal gain, does not care about the law or the rights of others.
  - Borderline: Intolerance of being alone and emotional dysregulation, lack of stability in relationships, identity and behavioral patterns.
  - Histrionic: Attention seeking.
  - Narcissistic: Underlying dysregulated, fragile self-esteem and over grandiosity, need for attention and lack of empathy for others.
- Cluster C: Characterized by appearing anxious or fearful, introvert.
  - Avoidant: Avoids interpersonal contact due to rejection sensitivity, low self-esteem and extremely sensitive to criticism.
  - Dependent: Submissiveness and need to be take care of.
  - Obsessive-compulsive: Perfectionism, rigidity and obstinacy, shows strict conformity to rules, moral codes, and order.

Other classifications (Cara, 2013):

- Pleasure deficient/detached: Schizoid, avoidant.
- Interpersonality imbalanced: Dependent, narcissistic, antisocial, histrionic.
- Structurally defective: Schizotypical, borderline paranoid.
- Intrapsychically conflicted: Obsessive-compulsive.

Evaluation/Assessment

Areas
- Activities of Daily Living/Instrumental ADL: basic ADLs, independent living
- Education/Work: academic performance, work history
- Play/Leisure: interests, values, frequency, location
- Rest/Sleep: sleep disturbance
- Social Participation: type, frequency, location, with whom
- Sensorimotor: consider if dysfunction may be present due to comorbidities
- Cognitive/Perceptual: attention, memory, executive functions
- Psychosocial: self-identity, self-esteem, self-concept, self-worth, interpersonal relationships, role performance, quality of life
- Context/Environment: social relations
- Comorbidities: anxiety, depression

Instruments
Instruments Developed by Occupational Therapy Personnel
- None identified.

Instruments Developed by Other Professionals and Used by Occupational Therapy Personnel
- Functional Independence Measure (FIM; Uniform Data System for Medical Rehabilitation, 1997)

Problems/Issues

Activities of Daily Living/Instrumental ADL
- Person may have restricted or limited dietary habits.
- Person may lack skills in independent living tasks.

Education/Work
- Person may be absent from class or work frequently.
- Person may have been dismissed from work and have an inconsistent work history.

Play/Leisure
- Person may have a limited list of leisure occupations and infrequent engagement.

Rest/Sleep
- Person may have sleep disturbance.

Social Participation
- Person may limit or rarely participate in social occupations.
- Person may engage in socially disapproved or unsanctioned occupations as coping mechanisms (Potvin et al., 2019).

Sensorimotor
- Consider if physical fitness should be addressed.

Cognitive/Perceptual
- Person's thinking tends to be rigid, extreme, and distorted.
- Person may lack executive functioning skills including problem solving and decision making.

Psychosocial
- Person usually has reduced social skills.
- Person may lack assertiveness skills.
- Person may have feelings of inadequacy.
- Person may have impulse control problems (behaviors).
- Personal may struggle to cope with stressful situations.
- Person may be lonely and feel isolated.
- Person may have fluctuating labile moods.
- Person's behavior may be inappropriate or maladaptive to the situation.
- Person may have a poor self-concept with low self-esteem.
- Person may be unable to cope with responsibilities.
- Person may struggle to form mature relationships.
- Person may use certain defense mechanisms (Nott, 2014).
  - ▶ Splitting: Person divides people into "good" and "bad" and then plays one off against the other. Common in narcissistic personality. Caution: If regarded as "good," occupational therapy personnel can be emotionally seduced and start colluding with the client to the detriment of progress and therapeutic intervention. Conversely, occupational therapy personnel may withdraw or avoid client in therapy because the interchange is negative, thus denying client skills development.
  - ▶ Denial: Person denies that problems exist and avoids taking responsibility for any disruption caused in occupational or social setting. Common in Cluster C disorders.
  - ▶ Projection: Person may try to merge and manipulate personal boundaries with the therapy personnel and point out faults, rather than face confronting individual problems. Common in Cluster B subtypes. Caution: Awareness of the manipulative mechanism intended toward domination allows occupational therapy personnel to avoid involvement with overintrusive client and avoid pathological dynamics.
  - ▶ Introversion: Person participates in self-damaging acts including self-mutilation, which result in an internal struggle against depression, anger, and frustration. Common in borderline personality. Caution: Allow externalization of aggression in a constructive method to relieve internal struggles and pain.

Context/Environment
- Family may lack knowledge of available community or internet resources.

Intervention/Treatment

Models and programs developed by occupational therapy personnel include individual occupational therapy (Nott, 2014), occupational group therapy (Nott, 2014), and skill approaches (leisure, work, social participation, self-care; Cara, 2013). Models and programs developed by other professionals but used by occupational therapy personnel include cognitive behavioral therapy (Nott, 2014) and therapeutic community model (Nott, 2014). Team members include psychiatrists, physicians, nursing personnel, psychologists, social workers, and occupational therapy personnel. Goals are to reduce subjective distress, enable person to understand that the problems are internal to the self, to decrease maladaptive and socially undesirable behaviors, and to modify problematic personality traits (Porter, 2018). Nott (2014) stated the goals are to stabilize fluctuating mood, improve self-concept and self-esteem, improve insight and judgment, assist in forming mature interpersonal relationships, teach constructive ways of coping with stress and anxiety, allow for appropriate expression and ventilation of feelings, bring about conflict resolution, develop social and assertiveness skills, and promote behavioral change.

Activities of Daily Living/Instrumental ADL
- Consider consequences of behavior in independent living tasks that require interpersonal skills such as shopping, caring for children or pets, sexual relations, or driving.
- Medication management may be a challenge. First, persons with personality disorder may continue to experience symptoms even with medications. Second, keeping a medication schedule may be difficult to maintain outside an institutional setting.

Education/Work
- Cluster A: Clients are generally hard working but are most suited to jobs that require minimal interaction and interpersonal focus. Consider permissive environment with few boundaries.
- Cluster B: Most difficult to maintain work situations due to manipulative behavior and inability to related to peers constructively. Persons need a specific work situation requiring specific skills training along with adapted behaviors such as "pause techniques" to calm down or "halt" overreactions.
- Cluster C: Generally, clients function well at work but may be susceptible to stress reactions due to long hours or being manipulated by others in the workplace. Focus on client's work rights and creating a fairer working environment (to manage anxiety, burnout), assertiveness training, and focusing on job tasks without distractions.

Play/Leisure
- Sports activities (volleyball, board games, tennis, swimming, baseball).
- Outings: movies, picnics, hikes, and cultural outings.
- Clinic or ward barbecues, cookouts, or baking.
- Parties and dances.
- Concerts with talent shows.
- Creative activities.

Rest/Sleep
- See Sleep–Wake Disorders in Section 13: Lifestyle Conditions.

Social Participation Using Groups
- Self-awareness group: Topics such as "draw a river of my life," narrative life stories, shoebox/cakebox with "inside of self" depicted inside box and "outside of self" depicted on exterior of box.
- Dialectical behavior therapy (five problem areas).
  - Dysregulation and lability of emotions by teaching regulation skills.
  - Interpersonal dysregulation in relationship by teaching effective interpersonal skills.
  - Behavioral dysregulation focused on maladaptive behaviors and effective problem solving.

- ▶ Dysregulation of self focused on dealing effectively with feelings of emptiness, poor self-esteem, poor self-confidence.
- ▶ Depersonalization by teaching "mindfulness skills."
- Social skills groups.
  - ▶ Dyads: Decisions are made in pairs with therapist as guide and facilitator.
  - ▶ Role playing: Learning to deal with stressful social situations using assertive behavioral techniques.
  - ▶ Challenging situations: Coping with difficult to manage tasks such as introducing people in a group situation, initiating and maintaining a conversation, returning defective article, dealing with a person who tries to get ahead in line.
  - ▶ Personal situations such as expressing affection, asking for help, coping with destructive criticism, and negotiating or compromising.
- Value clarification groups.
  - ▶ Focus on reassess values, resolve conflict, and promote insight.
  - ▶ Exercises: "My values"—Influence of others on my values, alternative values, and consequence of accepting or rejecting alternatives.
- Stress management and relaxation therapy.
  - ▶ Identify stressors including stress-inducting events.
  - ▶ Develop a stress tolerance profile for stressors.
  - ▶ Identify and practice stress management techniques.

Sensorimotor
- Not addressed.

Cognitive/Perceptual
- Intervention for Cluster A.
  - ▶ Early intervention: Consider one-on-one treatment to manage the personality constructs and problems.
  - ▶ Later group intervention may be considered but be aware of difficulty with social and interpersonal relations. Group probably should be small.
  - ▶ Focus should be on developing strengths using a nonthreatening, structured task-centered approach.
  - ▶ Introduce social skills gradually starting with individual based or assigned tasks and gradually providing more individual choice.
  - ▶ Be prepared to provide support to decrease potential withdrawal or defensive actions if too much demand is made.
  - ▶ Model unconditional acceptance of client's limitations, including strange beliefs, to ensure acceptance by other group members.
- Intervention for Cluster B.
  - ▶ Encourage positive coping and stress management mechanisms.
  - ▶ Clarify with client and help client verbalize real feelings.
  - ▶ Establish a firm, empathic but resolved rapport that encourages empathy, awareness of feelings, and others' point of view.
  - ▶ For borderline personality, a structured, reality-oriented approach is more useful and interpretations of behavior. See chapter on Borderline Personality Disorder.
- Intervention for Cluster C.
  - ▶ Avoidant personality.
    - ○ Develop trust by conveying an accepting attitude.
    - ○ Assist client to make decisions and take responsibility for own actions.
    - ○ Support exploration of appropriate social behavior and assertiveness.
    - ○ Provide information about the negative consequence of avoidance.
  - ▶ Obsessive-compulsive personality disorder (OCPD).
    - ○ Create a relaxed atmosphere.

    ○ Use perfectionism constructively in choice of task and activities but stress completion.
    ○ Encourage client to develop awareness that focus on perfectionism may alienate others.
    ○ Promote enjoyment, fun, and positive feelings and discuss the impact on mood, thoughts, and action.
- Principles of intervention (adapted from Nott, 2014).
  - Focus on observed description and consequences of behavior, not on explaining rationale for behavior.
  - Establish with client a collaborative sharing of and working on problem(s) together.
  - Confront defense mechanisms by description but do not interpret the mechanism.
  - Set limits on behavior and provide structure and organization.
  - Allow and encourage participation in group settings and help everyone to participate.
  - Assist clients to understand and process the consequence of intended actions.
- Principles to avoid (adapted from Nott, 2014).
  - Do not listen to repetitious complaints, change the subject or engage in action (occupation, tasks, activity).
  - Do not insist on a contract that client may not be able to achieve.
  - Do not attempt to save face if fooled and resort to blame and punitive actions to clients. Face up to situation and move on.
  - Do not try to rescue or encourage dependency of clients. Encourage independent thinking and actions.
  - Do not lie or present conflicting nonverbal messages.
  - Do not present self as an emotionless screen that can tolerate all manner of behavior. Set limits.
  - Do not ridicule cults or strange beliefs. Change subject or move to action.

Psychosocial
- Assist client to stabilize fluctuating mood and emotions.
- Assist client to improve self-concept and self-esteem through skill development.
- Assist client to form mature interpersonal relationships.
- Teach client constructive ways of coping with stress and anxiety (mindfulness, deep breathing, yoga, tai chi).
- Allow and encourage expression and ventilation of feelings in appropriate and constructive methods.
- Assist in bringing about conflict resolution.
- Assist client to develop social skills and appropriate assertiveness skills.
- Promote behavioral change toward social and culturally accepted standards.

Context/Environment
- Assist client to identify support groups in the community or online.
- Assist family to identify and learn to support constructive behavior and avoid manipulative behavior.

Precautions/Safety Considerations

Persons with antisocial personality may engage in illegal activities and be incarcerated. Persons with borderline personality disorder are at risk for suicide attempts and behaviors.

Prognosis and Outcome

Persons with personality disorders are often reluctant to seek and remain in treatment (Doughty & Brown, 2019). Although previous literature has suggested that personality disorders were lifelong patterns that were resistant to change, newer literature suggests that change can occur (Doughty & Brown, 2019).

REFERENCES

Cara, E. (2013). Personality disorders. In E. Cara & A. MacRae (Eds.), *Psychosocial occupational therapy: An evolving practice* (3rd ed., pp. 308–339). Delmar Cengage Learning.

Doughty, K., & Brown, C. (2019). Personality disorders. In C. Brown, V. C. Stoffel, & J. P. Muñoz (Eds.), *Occupational therapy in mental health: A vision for participation* (2nd ed., pp. 169–181). F.A. Davis.

Nott, A. (2014). Understanding persons with personality disorders: Intervention in occupational therapy. In R. Crouch & V. Alers (Eds.), *Occupational therapy in psychiatry and mental health* (5th ed., pp. 419–434). Wiley. https://doi.org/10.1002/9781118913536.ch26

Porter, R. S. (Ed.). (2018). *The Merck manual of diagnosis and therapy* (20th ed.). Merck Sharp & Dohme.

Potvin, O., Vallée, C., & Larivière, N. (2019). Experience of occupations among people living with a personality disorder. *Occupational Therapy International, 2019*, Article 9830897. https://doi.org/10.1155/2019/9030897

BIBLIOGRAPHY

Birken, M., & Harper, S. (2017). Experiences of people with a personality disorder or mood disorder regarding carrying out daily activities following discharge from hospital. *British Journal of Occupational Therapy, 80*(7), 409–416. https://doi.org/10.1177/0308022617697995

Larivière, N., Denis, C., Payeur, A., Ferron, A., Levesque, S., & Rivard, G. (2016). Comparison of objective and subjective life balance between women with and without a personality disorder. *Psychiatric Quarterly, 87*, 663–673. https://doi.org/10.1007/s11126-016-9417-3

Larivière, N., Desrosiers, J., Tousignant, M., & Boyer, R. (2010a). Exploring social participation of people with cluster B personality disorders. *Occupational Therapy in Mental Health, 26*(4), 375–386. https://doi.org/10.1080/0164212X.2010.518307

Larivière, N., Desrosiers, J., Tousignant, M., & Boyer, R. (2010b). Who benefits the most from psychiatric day hospitals? A comparison of three clinical groups. *Journal of Psychiatric Practice, 16*(2), 93–102.

O'Toole, M. T. (Ed.). (2017). *Mosby's dictionary of medicine, nursing & health professions* (10th ed.). Elsevier.

Posttraumatic Stress Disorder (PTSD)

Also called posttraumatic stress disorder.
See also Childhood Trauma and Maltreatment.

Description

Posttraumatic stress disorder (PTSD) is recurring, intrusive recollections of an overwhelming traumatic event, with recollection lasting more than 1 month and beginning within 6 months of the event. Symptoms include avoidance of stimuli associated with the traumatic event, nightmares, and flashbacks (Porter, 2018). Persons diagnosed with PTSD also have high rates of comorbidity conditions associated with cardiovascular, gastrointestinal, hepatic (liver), and respiratory systems (Edgelow et al., 2019). Formal criteria for a diagnosis of PTSD are listed in the *Diagnostic and Statistical Manual of Mental Disorders* (5th. ed.; *DSM-5*; American Psychiatric Association, 2013).

Cause

The pathophysiology of the disorder is incompletely understood. Generally, events likely to evoke PTSD are those that invoke feelings of fear, helplessness, or horror. Combat, sexual assault, and natural or man-made disasters are common causes of PTSD (Porter, 2018).

Evaluation/Assessment

Areas

- Activities of Daily Living/Instrumental ADL: self-care, home management, driving
- Education/Work: work history, work performance
- Play/Leisure: interests, values, frequency, location
- Rest/Sleep: sleep disturbance, sleep disorder
- Social Participation: type, frequency, location, with whom
- Sensorimotor: sensory processing
- Cognitive/Perceptual: executive function (problem solving, decision making)
- Psychosocial: emotions (anger, guilt, rage), self-image, self-worth, self-efficacy
- Context/Environment: social support, resources, military service
- Comorbidities: anxiety, brain injury, depression, polytrauma, sensory processing dysfunction

Instruments

Instruments Developed by Occupational Therapy Personnel

- Adolescent/Adult Sensory Profile (AASP; Brown & Dunn, 2002)
- SPOTting PTSD Checklist (see Ash et al., 2015, pp. 20–21, in References)

Instruments Developed by Other Professionals and Used by Occupational Therapy Personnel

- Posttraumatic Stress Disorder Checklist (PSDC; Ventureyra et al., 2002)
- Post-Traumatic Stress Disorder Symptom Scale (PSS; Foa et al., 1993)

Problems/Issues

Activities of Daily Living/Instrumental ADL

- Person may experience loss of appetite.
- Person may experience loss of or changes in libido or fear of intimacy (Engel-Yeger et al., 2015).

Education/Work

- Person may experience disruption of activity.

Play/Leisure

- Person may avoid or change interest in leisure activities.

Rest/Sleep

- Person may have difficulty falling or staying asleep.

Social Participation

- Person may avoid social situations.

Sensorimotor

- Person may experience hypersensitivity to certain stimuli (sounds, sights).
- Person may exhibit low registration to sensory input.
- Person may exhibit avoidance behavior to certain sensory input.

Cognitive/Perceptual

- Person may experience difficulty concentrating.
- Person may lose contact with time and space.

Psychosocial

- Person may use avoidance as a strategy to not encounter situations (e.g., a person who experiences PTSD as a result of a car crash may avoid driving or riding in a car).
- Person may experience intrusive images, thoughts, or memories.
- Person may experience anxiety that is constant causing person to feel hyper-aroused, on edge, overvigilant, easily startled, and irritable.
- Person may experience fear, anger, guilt, grief, numbing, loss of trust, and loss of self-esteem.
- Person may experience loss of or changes in valued life roles.
- Person may feel loss and/or isolation from everyday activities.

- Person may experience flooding.
- Person may experience dissociation.
- Person may experience flashbacks.

Context/Environment
- Person may experience negative attitudes from others that blame the victim.
- Person may lack a social support system from family, friends, or community.
- Person may experience policies/laws within social service agencies that act as deterrents to seeking help.
- Person may live in an area where access to services is limited due to physical barriers or lack of transportation.

Intervention/Treatment

Models and programs developed by occupational therapy personnel include the Canadian Model of Occupational Performance and Enablement and the Person-Environment-Occupation models (Ash et al., 2015), case study (Champagne, 2011; Freedman et al., 2010; Mattila et al., 2011; Precin, 2011b), model of human occupation (Gindi et al., 2016), Redesigning Daily Occupations (ReDo; Eklund & Erlandsson, 2011), occupational therapy life skills program (Beck et al., 2012), return to work (Precin, 2011a, 2011c, 2011d), and the Wilbarger Therapessure Program (Kimball et al., 2018). Models and programs developed by other professionals but used by occupational therapy personnel include aquatic therapy (Herold et al., 2016), collaborative design (Wagenfeld et al., 2013), cranial electrotherapy stimulation (Bracciano et al., 2012), driving intervention (Classen et al., 2014; Classen et al., 2017), driving simulation (Classen et al., 2011), horticultural therapy (Detweiler et al., 2015), interdisciplinary residential treatment (Speicher et al., 2014), ocean therapy (Rogers et al., 2014), service dogs (Crowe, Nguyen, et al., 2018; Crowe, Sánchez, et al., 2018; Yount et al., 2013), therapeutic riding (Lanning et al., 2017), trauma-focused treatment (Torchalla et al., 2019), V-Mart (virtual reality grocery store; Levy et al., 2019), and yoga (Stoller et al., 2012). Team members include physicians, psychologists, social workers, therapeutic recreational specialists, and occupational therapy personnel. Goal is to work with the individual in all phases of recovery, by helping the individual and caregivers to identify recovery-based needs strategies within the context of real-life demands and to participate in significant occupations (Beauchesne & Jacques, 2015; Champagne, 2015).

Activities of Daily Living/Instrumental ADL
- Suggest adaptive or modified self-care and home care to reduce trigger hypersensitivity patterns, dissociation, flooding, or flashbacks.
- Assist veterans to increase awareness of the impact of wartime driving experiences and responses to civilian driving situations.

Education/Work
- Suggest adaptive or modified approaches to work or school-based strategies to reduce triggers, dissociation, flooding, or flashbacks.

Play/Leisure
- Assist client to identify leisure occupations that have been enjoyable in the past.
- Assist client to explore and develop new leisure occupations.

Rest/Sleep
- See Sleep–Wake Disorders in Section 13: Lifestyle Conditions.

Social Participation
- Assist client to participate in social activities starting with those that are familiar from past experience unless those activities involved negative behaviors (substance use, intoxication, high speed car racing).
- Consider if new social activities should be explored and developed.

Sensorimotor
- Provide sensory processing–related techniques.
- Use of a sensory diet may be useful.

Cognitive/Perceptual
- Provide individual and/or group sessions addressing trauma triggers and warning signs.
- Facilitate development of and use of a daily schedule (time management).
- Suggest activity pacing with cycles of rest and activity.
- Assist client to develop a self-management program.
- Assist client to clarify personal values and priorities.
- Assist client to identify and implement satisfying and healthy routines (time management).

Psychosocial
- Provide opportunities to learn new coping strategies for health and wellness.
- Provide programs for stress management and relaxation.
- Encourage person to identify and engage in valued and meaningful roles.
- Provide opportunities to use exposure techniques under supervision and with supportive personnel.

Context/Environment
- Work with clients and families to determine if in-home modifications may reduce situations that trigger PTSD symptoms.
- Provide education and training to family, caregivers, and other professionals on adaptive or modified techniques to address symptoms of PTSD.
- Support transition process (home to community, military to civilian life).

Precautions/Safety Considerations

Person is at increased risk for self-injurious behaviors including substance abuse, self-mutilation, and suicide attempts.

Prognosis and Outcome

Variable. If untreated, chronic PTSD often decreases in severity without disappearing completely, but some people remain severely impaired. With treatment, symptoms usually lessen and person experiences less discomfort (Porter, 2018).

REFERENCES

American Psychiatric Association. (2013). *Diagnostic and statistical manual of mental disorders* (5th ed.). https://doi.org/10.1176/appi.books.9780890425596

Ash, N. P., Bartczak, M., Monteferrante, J., Nurse, A., & Persad, S. (2015). *SPOTting PTSD: A PTSD toolkit for first responders*. McGill University.

Beauchesne, J., & Jacques, C. (2015). From combat to compassion: Enabling change in veterans. *Occupational Therapy Now, 17*(5), 26.

Beck, C. E., Gonzales, F., Jr., Sells, C. H., Jones, C., Reer, T., & Zhu, Y. Y. (2012). The effects of animal-assisted therapy on wounded warriors in an occupational therapy life skills program. *US Army Medical Department Journal*, April–June, 38–45.

Bracciano, A. G., Chang, W. P., Kokesh, S., Martinez, A., Meier, M., & Moore, K. (2012). Cranial electrotherapy stimulation in the treatment of posttraumatic stress disorder: A pilot study of two military veterans. *Journal of Neurotherapy, 16*(1), 60–69. https://doi.org/10.1080/10874208.2012.650100

Champagne, T. (2011). The influence of posttraumatic stress disorder, depression, and sensory processing patterns on occupational engagement: A case study. *Work, 38*(1), 67–75. https://doi.org/10.3233/WOR-2011-1105

Champagne, T. (2015). *Fact sheet: Occupational therapy's role with posttraumatic stress disorder.* American Occupational Therapy Association.

Classen, S., Cormack, N. L., Winter, S. M., Monahan, M., Yarney, A., Lutz, A. L., & Platek, K. (2014). Efficacy of an occupational therapy driving intervention for returning combat veterans. *OTJR: Occupation, Participation and Health, 34*(4), 177–182. https://doi.org/10.3928/15394492-20141006-01

Classen, S., Levy, C., Meyer, D. L., Bewernitz, M., Lanford, D. N., & Mann, W. C. (2011). Simulated driving performance of combat veterans with mild traumatic brain injury and posttraumatic stress disorder: A pilot study. *American Journal of Occupational Therapy, 65*(4), 419–427. https://doi.org/10.5014/ajot.2011.000893

Classen, S., Winter, S., Monahan, M., Yarney, A., Lutz, A. L., Platek, K., & Levy, C. (2017). Driving intervention for returning combat veterans: Interim analysis of a randomized controlled trial. *OTJR: Occupation, Participation and Health, 37*(2), 62–71. https://doi.org/10.1177/1539449216675582

Crowe, T. K., Nguyen, M., Tryon, B., Barger, S., & Sánchez, V. (2018). How service dogs enhance veterans' occupational performance in the home: A qualitative perspective. *Open Journal of Occupational Therapy, 6*(3), Article 12. https://doi.org/10.15453/2168-6408.1468

Crowe, T. K., Sánchez, V., Howard, A., Western, B., & Barger, S. (2018). Veterans transitioning from isolation to integration: A look at veteran/service dog partnerships. *Disability and Rehabilitation, 40*(24), 2953–2961. https://doi.org/10.1080/09638288.2017.1363301

Detweiler, M. B., Self, J. A., Lane, S., Spencer, L., Lutgens, B., Kim, D. Y., Halling, M. H., Rudder, T. C., & Lehmann, L. P. (2015). Horticultural therapy: A pilot study on modulating cortisol levels and indices of substance craving, posttraumatic stress disorder, depression, and quality of life in veterans. *Alternative Therapies in Health and Medicine, 21*(4), 36–41.

Edgelow, M. M., MacPherson, M. M., Arnaly, F., Tam-Seto, L., & Cramm, H. A. (2019). Occupational therapy and posttraumatic stress disorder: A scoping review. *Canadian Journal of Occupational Therapy, 86*(2), 148–157. https://doi.org/10.1177/0008417419831438

Eklund, M., & Erlandsson, L. K. (2011). Return to work outcomes of the Redesigning Daily Occupations (ReDO) program for women with stress-related disorders—A comparative study. *Women & Health, 51*(7), 676–692. https://doi.org/10.1080/03630242.2011.618215

Engel-Yeger, B., Palgy-Levin, D., & Lev-Wiesel, R. (2015). Predicting fears of intimacy among individuals with post-traumatic stress symptoms by their sensory profile. *British Journal of Occupational Therapy, 78*(1), 51–57. https://doi.org/10.1177/0308022614557628

Freedman, S. A., Hoffman, H. G., Garcia-Palacios, A., Weiss, P. L., Avitzour, S., & Josman, N. (2010). Prolonged exposure and virtual reality-enhanced imaginal exposure for PTSD following a terrorist bulldozer attack: A case study. *Cyberpsychology, Behavior, and Social Networking, 13*(1), 95–101. https://doi.org/10.1089/cyber.2009.0271

Gindi, S., Galili, G., Volovic-Shushan, S., & Adir-Pavis, S. (2016). Integrating occupational therapy in treating combat stress reaction within a military unit: An intervention model. *Work, 55*(4), 737–745. https://doi.org/10.3233/WOR-162453

Herold, B., Stanley, A., Oltrogge, K., Alberto, T., Shackelford, P., Hunter, E., & Hughes, J. (2016). Post-traumatic stress disorder, sensory integration, and aquatic therapy: A scoping review. *Occupational Therapy in Mental Health, 32*(4), 392–399. https://doi.org/10.1080/0164212X.2016.1166355

Kimball, J. G., Cao, L., & Draleau, K. S. (2018). Efficacy of the Wilbarger Therapressure Program to modulate arousal in women with post-traumatic stress disorder: A pilot study using salivary cortisol and behavioral measures. *Occupational Therapy in Mental Health, 34*(1), 86–101. https://doi.org/10.1080/0164212X.2017.1376243

Lanning, B. A., Wilson, A. L., Krenek, N., & Beaujean, A. A. (2017). Using therapeutic riding as an intervention for combat veterans: An International Classification of Functioning, Disability, and Health (ICF) approach. *Occupational Therapy in Mental Health, 33*(3), 259–278. https://doi.org/10.1080/0164212X.2017.1283282

Levy, C. E., Miller, D. M., Akande, C. A. Lok, B., Marsiske, M., & Halan, S. (2019). V-Mart, a virtual reality grocery store: A focus group study of a promising intervention for mild traumatic brain injury and posttraumatic stress disorder. *American Journal of Physical Medicine & Rehabilitation, 98*(3), 191–198. https://doi.org/10.1097/PHM.0000000000001041

Mattila, A. M., Crandall, B. D., & Goldman, S. B. (2011). U.S. Army combat operational stress control throughout the deployment cycle: A case study. *Work, 38*(1), 13–18. https://doi.org/10.3233/WOR-2011-1100

Porter, R. S. (Ed.). (2018). *The Merck manual of diagnosis and therapy* (20th ed.). Merck Sharp & Dohme.

Precin, P. (2011a). Expert witness evaluation of posttraumatic stress disorder (PTSD) and return to work. *Work, 38*(1), 83–88. https://doi.org/10.3233/WOR-2011-1107

Precin, P. (2011b). Occupation as therapy for trauma recovery: A case study. *Work, 38*(1), 77–81. https://doi.org/10.3233/WOR-2011-1106

Precin, P. (2011c). Return to work after 9/11. *Work, 38*(1), 3–11. https://doi.org/10.3233/WOR-2011-1099

Precin, P. (2011d). Return to work: A case of PTSD, dissociative identity disorder, and satanic ritual abuse. *Work, 38*(1), 57–66. https://doi.org/10.3233/WOR-2011-1104

Rogers, C. M., Mallinson, T., & Peppers, D. (2014). High-intensity sports for posttraumatic stress disorder and depression: Feasibility study of ocean therapy with veterans of Operation Enduring Freedom and Operation Iraqi Freedom. *American Journal of Occupational Therapy, 68*(4), 395–404. https://doi.org/10.5014/ajot.2014.011221

Speicher, S. M., Walter, K. H., & Chard, K. M. (2014). Interdisciplinary residential treatment of posttraumatic stress disorder and traumatic brain injury: Effects on symptom severity and occupational performance and satisfaction. *American Journal of Occupational Therapy, 68*(4), 412–421. https://doi.org/10.5014/ajot.2014.011304

Stoller, C. C., Greuel, J. H., Cimini, L. S., Fowler, M. S., & Koomar, J. A. (2012). Effects of sensory-enhanced yoga on symptoms of combat stress in deployed military personnel. *American Journal of Occupational Therapy, 66*(1), 59–68. https://doi.org/10.5014/ajot.2012.001230

Torchalla, I., Killoran, J., Fisher, D., & Bahen, M. (2019). Trauma-focused treatment for individuals with posttraumatic stress disorder: The role of occupational therapy. *Occupational Therapy in Mental Health, 35*(4), 386–406. https://doi.org/10.1080/0164212X.2018.1510800

Wagenfeld, A., Roy-Fisher, C., & Mitchell, G. (2013). Collaborative design: Outdoor environments for veterans with PTSD. *Facilities, 31*(9/10), 391–406. https://doi.org/10.1108/02632771311324954

Yount, R., Ritchie, E. C., St. Laurent, M., Chumley, P., & Olmert, M. D. (2013). The role of service dog training in the treatment of combat-related PTSD. *Psychiatric Annals, 43*(6), 292–295. https://doi.org/10.3928/00485713-20130605-11

BIBLIOGRAPHY

American Occupational Therapy Association. (2010). *Fact sheet: Occupational therapy's role with posttraumatic stress disorder*.

Champagne, T. (2019). Trauma and stressor-related disorders. In C. Brown, V. C. Stoffel, & J. P. Muñoz (Eds.), *Occupational therapy in mental health: A vision for participation* (2nd ed., pp. 211–224). F.A. Davis.

Engel-Yeger, B., Palgy-Levin, D., & Lev-Wiesel, R. (2013). The sensory profile of people with post-traumatic stress symptoms. *Occupational Therapy in Mental Health, 29*(3), 266–278. https://doi.org/10.1080/0164212X.2013.819466

Fox, J., Erlandsson, L.-K., & Shiel, A. (2019). A systematic review and narrative synthesis of occupational therapy-led interventions for individuals with anxiety and stress-related disorders. *Occupational Therapy in Mental Health, 35*(2), 179–204. https://doi.org/10.1080/0164212X.2018.1516172

Hossain, M. I., Nahar, N., Nayan, M. J., Ema, A. J., & Alve, M. Y. A. (2013). Experience of Bangladeshi occupational therapists with "Rana Plaza Tragedy" survivors: Recovery and rehabilitation phases of disaster management. *World Federation of Occupational Therapy Bulletin, 68*(1), 14–19. https://doi.org/10.1179/otb.2013.68.1.006

Lopez, A. (2011). Posttraumatic stress disorder and occupational performance: Building resilience and fostering occupational adaptation. *Work, 38*(1), 33–38. https://doi.org/10.3233/WOR-2011-1102

Maxwell, M. (2011). A study in contrasts: Inscriptions of posttraumatic stress disorder (PTSD) in two works of fiction. *Work, 38*(1), 19–32. https://doi.org/10.3233/WOR-2011-1101

Plach, H. L., & Sells, C. H. (2013). Occupational performance needs of young veterans. *American Journal of Occupational Therapy, 67*(1), 73–81. https://doi.org/10.5014/ajot.2013.003871

Precin, P. (2011). Pretraumatic stress prevention (PTSP) versus posttraumatic stress disorder (PTSD). *Work, 38*(1), 89–90. https://doi.org/10.3233/WOR-2011-1108

Rivers, E., & Saunders, S. (2016). Occupational therapy for people with military-related posttraumatic stress disorder: A call for action in Canada. *Occupational Therapy Now, 18*(2), 13–15.

Snedden, D. (2012). Trauma-informed practice: An emerging role of occupational therapy. *Occupational Therapy Now, 14*(6), 26–28.

Sripada, R. K., Henry, J., Yosef, M., Levine, D. S., Bohnert, K. M., Miller, E., & Zivin, K. (2018). Occupational functioning and employment services use among VA primary care patients with posttraumatic stress disorder. *Psychological Trauma, 10*(2), 140–143. https://doi.org/10.1037/tra0000241

Tuchner, M., Meiner, Z., Parush, S., & Hartman-Maeir, A. (2010). Relationships between sequelae of injury, participation, and quality of life in survivors of terrorist attacks. *OTJR: Occupation, Participation and Health, 30*(1), 29–38. https://doi.org/10.3928/15394492-20091214-05

Waldman-Levi, A., Finzi-Dottan, R., & Weintraub, N. (2015). Attachment security and parental perception of competency among abused women in the shadow of PTSD and childhood exposure to domestic violence. *Journal of Child and Family Studies, 24*(1), 57–65. https://doi.org/10.1007/s10826-013-9813-3

Wortman, R. A., Vallone, T., Karnes, M., Walawander, C., Daly, D., & Fox-Garrity, B. (2018). Pinnipeds and PTSD: An analysis of a human-animal interaction case study program for a veteran. *Occupational Therapy International, 2018*, Article 2686728. https://doi.org/10.1155/2018/2686728

Psychosis, Unspecified

See also Schizophrenia, Serious Mental Illness, Bipolar Disorders, Depression.

Description

Psychosis is a mental and behavioral disorder that causes gross distortion or disorganization of a person's mental capacity, affective response, and capacity to recognize reality. Symptoms may include hallucinations and delusions, as well as bizarre motor functioning such as psychomotor agitation (overactivity) or psychomotor inhibition (underactivity). In addition, the person may have difficulty communicating and relating to others to the degree of interfering with the capacity to cope with the ordinary demands of everyday life. Psychosis is a generic term for any of the major mental disorders including schizophrenia, bipolar disorder, and major depression (*Stedman's*, 2011; Strauss et al., 2016).

Cause

Unclear. Contributing factors include heredity, environmental factors, drug interactions, and some neurological disorders (Porter, 2018).

Evaluation/Assessment

Areas
- Activities of Daily Living/Instrumental ADL: basic ADLs—dressing appropriately, wearing makeup, eating regularly, healthy diet
- Education/Work: educational level, work history, work skills
- Play/Leisure: interests, frequency, location
- Rest/Sleep: sleep disturbance
- Social Participation: type, frequency, location, with whom
- Sensorimotor: physical fitness, sensory processing
- Cognitive/Perceptual: executive functions
- Psychosocial: self-efficacy, emotional regulation, role performance, life history, social skills, social isolation
- Context/Environment: community and internet resources, social support
- Comorbidity: substance abuse

Instruments

Instruments Developed by Occupational Therapy Personnel
- Adolescent/Adult Sensory Profile (AASP; Brown & Dunn, 2002)
- Focus Group Questions (FGQ; Makdisi et al., 2013, in References)
- Role Checklist Version 2 Quality Performance (RCV2:QP; Scott et al., 2014)

Instruments Developed by Other Professionals and Used by Occupational Therapy Personnel
- Interpersonal Functionality Scale (IFS), adapted from original Social Functioning Scale (SFS; Birchwood et al., 1990)
- Life Functioning Assessment Inventory (L-FAI; Hui et al., 2013, in References)
- Personal and Social Performance scale (PSP), adapted from original Social and Occupational Functioning Assessment Scale (SOFAS; Morosini et al., 2000)
- Social and Occupational Functioning Assessment Scale (SOFAS, in *Diagnostic and Statistical Manual of Mental Disorders*; 4th ed.; *DSM-IV*; American Psychiatric Association, 1994, p. 760)

Problems/Issues

Activities of Daily Living/Instrumental ADL
- Person may not consistently eat meals or eat nutritious meals.
- Person may not dress consistently or appropriately.
- Person may not bathe or shower on a regular and consistent schedule.
- Person may not groom self (shave, apply makeup, brush and comb hair) regularly.
- Person may have difficulty taking medications on a regular and consistent schedule.
- Person may not attempt to prepare meals, depending on others for food.
- Person may not keep living quarters clean and repaired whether living in a single room, apartment, or home.
- Person may not have private transportation or use public transportation when needed.
- Person may not have a budget or means to manage finances.

Education/Work
- Person may lack basic academic skills.
- Person may have discontinued academic studies (dropped out of school or dismissed due to failing grades, unacceptable behavior on school campus, excessive absenteeism).
- Person may have problems maintaining a paying job due to frequent absences.
- Person may have frequent disagreements or "run ins" with supervisors or fellow workers.
- Person may lack basic work skills.
- Person may be inconsistent in carrying out assigned duties.
- Person may express concern about being let go or fired.

Play/Leisure
- Person may have stopped or limited engagement in most or all leisure occupations.

Rest/Sleep
- Person may experience sleep disturbance.
- Person may not have regular sleep habits and routines.

Social Participation
- Person may have stopped going to or limited participation in most or all social and cultural activities.
- Person may have lost contact with the friends with whom he or she participated in social or cultural activities.

Sensorimotor
- Person may not have a regular physical fitness program.
- Person may have sensory processing dysfunction in all four quadrants of the AASP, including low registration, sensory seeking, sensory sensitivity, and sensory avoiding.

Cognitive/Perceptual
- Person may have difficulty learning new information.
- Person may have difficulty retaining previously learned information and need reminders.
- Person may have difficulty making decisions and planning ahead.
- Person may miss doctors' appointments due to difficulty maintaining and following a schedule.
- Person may have difficulty with following instructions.
- Person may have difficulty with time management (creating a schedule and adhering to the time lines.
- Person may have perceptual dysfunction including visuospatial relations.

Psychosocial
- Person may experience social anxiety and have physically and socially isolated the self from others.
- Person may lack social interaction, social relations, and social management skills.
- Person may feel that other dislike him or her and may want to do harm or violence.
- Person may have difficulty performing expected role functions (student, worker, volunteer, friend, family member, hobbyist, sports player, home maintainer, religious participant, participant in organizations, or other).
- Person may feel isolated from others and feel stuck or lonely.
- Person may have low self-esteem and sense of self-worth.
- Person may have poor sense of self-image, self-efficacy, or self-confidence.
- Person may experience poor quality of life.

Context/Environment
- Person may experience barriers in the home and community to performing occupations (Makdisi et al., 2013).
- Person may experience cultural values and beliefs about mental illness that are negative and discourage social engagement and participation.
- Person may experience social stigma, including feelings of being excluded or devalued.
- Person may lack knowledge about psychosis and its management.
- Person may lack social support from friends, family, or employers.

Intervention/Treatment

Models and programs developed by occupational therapy personnel include the model of human occupation (Aslaksen et al., 2014; Birken et al., 2018), football (soccer exercise) program (Moloney & Rohde 2017), Graduating Living Skills Outside the Ward (GLOW; Birken et al., 2018), and music tempo (Strauss et al., 2016). Models and programs developed by other professionals but used by occupational therapy personnel include Constructivist Grounded Theory (CGT) and Self-Management And Recovery Technology (SMART; Williams et al., 2018). Team members include physicians, psychiatrists, nursing personnel, social workers, psychologists, and occupational therapy personnel. The goal is to increase occupational performance of self-care, productive, and leisure roles (Birken et al., 2018).

Activities of Daily Living/Instrumental ADL
- Assist client in completing basic ADL tasks on a consistent schedule.
- Assist client to develop and maintain a medication schedule.
- Assist client to learn to use public transportation.

Education/Work
- Assist client to address issues that may be reducing ability to work and stay employed; referral to vocational rehabilitation counsel may be useful.
- Assist client to select volunteer opportunities that support increasing sense of making a valued contribution to society while building self-confidence and sense of self-efficacy.

Play/Leisure
- Assist client to reestablish engagement in known or favorite leisure occupations.
- Assist client to explore new or novel leisure occupations.

Rest/Sleep
- See Sleep–Wake Disorders in Section 13: Lifestyle Conditions.

Social Participation
- Assist client to reestablish contact with family and friends to participate in social or cultural activities (avoid reestablishment with those involved in negative occupations such as substance abuse, violence, or criminal behavior).
- Assist client to develop new friendships and participate in new or novel social and cultural activities.

Sensorimotor
- Assist client to develop a consistent physical fitness program (exercises, walking, running, swimming, playing sports).
- Consider if developing a sensory diet program may address sensory processing disorders.
- Consider using music tempo (slow versus fast) as an activity to promote physical motor exercise.

Cognitive/Perceptual
- Grade task and person: balancing ability of the person with the task.
- Assist client to develop a time-management schedule.
- Assist client to plan goals and steps to attain the goals.
- Assist client to assess strengths and weaknesses, purposeful and meaningful occupations.

Psychosocial
- Assist client to develop a positive attitude toward self as a contributing participant to society and increase self-efficacy and self-worth.
- Assist client to make sense of personal experiences and events through participation in occupations and roles that are meaningful to the individual.
- Assist client to engage in self-regulation of negative reactions and emotions through stress reduction (deep breathing, relaxation, imagery, mindfulness, yoga, tai chi).
- Assist client to increase sense of mastery and self-confidence through engagement in purposeful and meaningful activities.
- Assist client to experience sense of belonging through engagement in social activities with acquaintances, family members, peers, friends, and other individuals in the community.

- Assist client to improve social interaction and relations through selected group activities, starting with one-on-one, two or three persons, small (8–10 person), and larger groups, with a specific goal and focus.

Context/Environment

- Assist client to identify barriers and facilitators to occupational performance in the home and community using facilitators to reduce the impact of barriers.
- Use video programs on the internet to help client address social and interpersonal issues (see Williams et al., 2018).

Precautions/Safety Considerations

Person is at risk for suicidal behavior. Person may lack judgment to avoid situations where physical harm may occur.

Prognosis and Outcome

The factors that contribute to mental illness tend to be chronic. Recognition of triggers requires a program to assist the client to recognize the triggering behaviors and to institute a management program to address the behaviors before hospitalization is required.

REFERENCES

American Psychiatric Association. (1994). *Diagnostic and statistical manual of mental disorders* (4th ed.).

Aslaksen, A. M., Scott, P. J., Haglund, L., Ellingham, B., & Bonsaksen, T. (2014). Occupational therapy process in a psychiatric hospital: Using the role checklist version 2: Quality of performance. *Ergoterapeuten*, 4, 38–45.

Birken, M., Henderson, C., & Slade, M. (2018). The development of an occupational therapy intervention for adults with a diagnosed psychotic disorder following discharge from hospital. *Pilot and Feasibility Studies*, 4, Article 81. https://doi.org/10.1186/s40814-018-0267-7

Hui, C. L.-M., Li, Y.-K., Leung, K.-F., Tang, J. Y.-M., Wong, G. H.-Y., Chang, W.-C., Chan, S. K.-W., Lee, E. H.-M., & Chen, E. Y.-H. (2013). Reliability and validity of the life functioning assessment inventory (L-FAI) for patients with psychosis. *Social Psychiatry and Psychiatric Epidemiology*, 48, 1687–1695. https://doi.org/10.1007/s00127-013-0679-x

Makdisi, L., Blank, A., Bryant, W., Andrews, C., Franco, L., & Parsonage, J. (2013). Facilitators and barriers to living with psychosis: An exploratory collaborative study of the perspectives of mental health service users. *British Journal of Occupational Therapy*, 76(9), 418–426. https://doi.org/10.4276/030802213X13782044946346

Moloney, L., & Rohde, D. (2017). Experience of men with psychosis participating in a community-based football programme. *Irish Journal of Occupational Therapy*, 45(2), 100–111. https://doi.org/10.1108/IJOT-06-2017-0015

Porter, R. S. (Ed.). (2018). *The Merck manual of diagnosis and therapy* (20th ed.). Merck Sharp & Dohme.

Strauss, M., van Heerden, S. M., & Joubert, G. (2016). Occupational therapy and the use of music tempo in the treatment of the mental health care user with psychosis. *South African Journal of Occupational Therapy*, 46(1), 21–26. http://dx.doi.org/10.17159/2310-3833/2016/v46n1a6

Stedman's medical dictionary for the health professions and nursing (7th ed., 2011). Wolters Kluwer.

Williams, A., Fossey, E., Farhall, J., Foley, F., & Thomas, N. (2018). Recovery after psychosis: Qualitative study of service user experiences of lived experience videos on a recovery-oriented website. *JMIR Mental Health*, 5(2), Article e37. https://doi.org/10.2196/mental.9934

BIBLIOGRAPHY

Çakmak, S., Süt, H., Öztürk, S., Tamam, L., & Bal, U. (2016). The effects of occupational therapy and psychosocial interventions on interpersonal functioning and personal and social performance levels of corresponding patients. *Archives of Neuropsychiatry, 53*, 234–240. https://doi.org/10.5152/npa.2015.10130

Lal, S., Ungar, M., Leggo, C., Malla, A., Frankish, J., & Suto, M. J. (2013). Well-being and engagement in valued activities: Experiences of young people with psychosis. *OTJR: Occupation, Participation and Health, 33*(4), 190–197. https://doi.org/10.3928/15394492-20130912-02

Parham, L. D., Roush, S., Downing, D. T., Michael, P. G., & McFarlane, W. R. (2019). Sensory characteristics of youth at clinical high risk for psychosis. *Early Intervention in Psychiatry, 13*(2), 264–271. https://doi.org/10.1111/eip.12475

Schizophrenia

Description

Schizophrenia is characterized by a psychosis that results in a loss of contact with reality, hallucinations (false perceptions), delusion (false beliefs), disorganized speech and behavior, flattened flat affect (restricted range of emotions), cognitive deficits (impaired reasoning and problem solving), and occupational and social dysfunction. Symptoms usually begin in adolescence or early adulthood. One or more episodes of symptoms must last at least 6 months or longer before the diagnosis is made (Porter, 2018).

Criteria for diagnosis are listed in the American Psychiatric Association's (2018) *Diagnostic and Statistical Manual of Mental Disorders* (5th ed.).

Cause

The cause is unknown, but evidence for a genetic component is strong.

Evaluation/Assessment

Areas

- Activities of Daily Living/Instrumental ADL: meal planning and preparation, caregiving burden
- Education/Work: work (paid and unpaid) history, work skills
- Play/Leisure: interests, values, frequency of engagement, location
- Rest/Sleep: sleep habits, sleep disorders
- Social Participation: type, location, frequency, with whom
- Sensorimotor: psychomotor retardation, sensory responsiveness
- Cognitive/Perceptual: attention, orientation, memory, executive functions (volition, planning, purposive action, effective performance), conceptual disorganization, difficulty with abstract thinking, stereotyped thinking, judgment, insight
- Psychosocial: coping and stress management, social inclusion, positive symptoms (hallucinations, delusions, bizarre behavior, and thought disorder), negative symptoms (blunting affect, alogia, apathy, anhedonia [decreased ability to experience pleasure from positive stimuli]), delusions, mania, grandiosity, suspiciousness, hostility, anxiety, emotional withdrawal, depression, emotional regulation, and impulse control
- Context/Environment: social support, community resources
- Comorbidities: obesity, pneumonia (associated with clozapine), diabetes

Instruments

Instruments Developed by Occupational Therapy Personnel

- Activities of Daily Living Rating Scale III (ADLRS-III; Chu & Hsieh, 2004, in Chinese; see also Chiu, Lee, Lai, et al., 2015, in References)
- Activity Card Sort (2nd ed.; ACS-2; Baum & Edwards, 2008)
- Adolescent/Adult Sensory Profile (AASP; Brown & Dunn, 2002)
- Adults Subjective Assessment of Participation (ASAP; Jarus et al., 2005)

- Allen Cognitive Level Screen (5th ed.; ACLS-5; Allen et al., 2007)
- Assessment of Motor and Process Skills (8th ed.; AMPS-8; Fisher & Bray Jones, 2016; see also Ayres & John, 2015, in References)
- Assessment of Time Management Skills (ATMS; Janeslätt et al., 2018, in References)
- Canadian Occupational Performance Measure (5th ed.; COPM-5; Law et al., 2014)
- Comprehensive Occupational Therapy Evaluation Scale (COTES; Brayman et al., 1976)
- Computerized Digit Vigilance Test (C-DVT; Lin et al., 2018, in References)
- Dynamic Loewenstein Occupational Therapy Cognitive Assessment (DLOTCA; Katz et al., 2012)
- Executive Functions Performance Test (EFPT; Baum & Wolf, 2013)
- Israeli Adults Assessment of Participation (IAAP; Jarus et al., 2005)
- Kitchen Task Assessment (KTA; Baum & Edwards, 1993)
- Life Functioning Assessment Inventory (L-FAI; Hui et al., 2013, in References)
- Perceive, Recall, Plan, Perform system (PRPP; Chapparo & Ranka, 2014)
- Performance-Based Measure of Executive Functions (PEF; Chiu, Lee, Kuo, et al., 2015, in References)
- Profiles of Occupational Engagement in people with Schizophrenia (POES; Bejerholm et al., 2006)
- Quality of Life Scale for Mental Disorders (QOLMD; Chiu & Lee, 2018, in References)
- Reintegration to Normal Living Index (RNLI; Wood-Dauphinee et al., 1988)
- Routine Task Inventory–Expanded (RTI-E; Katz, 2006)
- Sensory Responsiveness Questionnaire (SRQ; Bar-Shalita et al., 2009)
- Test of Grocery Shopping Skills (TOGSS; Brown et al., 2009)
- Virtual Action Planning–Supermarket (VAP-S; Aubin et al., 2018, in References)
- Weekly Calendar Planning Activity (WCPA; Toglia, 2015)

Instruments Developed by Other Professionals and Used by Occupational Therapy Personnel

- Activity Profile Scale for Patients With Psychiatric Disorders (APS; Kawaguchi et al., 2015)
- Azima Battery (AB; Azima & Azima, 1959)
- Beck Depression Inventory (2nd ed.; BDI-II; Beck et al., 1996)
- Behavioural Assessment of the Dysexecutive Syndrome (BADS; Wilson et al., 1996)
- Brief Assessment of Cognition in Schizophrenia (BACS; Keefe et al., 2004)
- Brief Psychiatric Rating Scale (BPRS; Overall & Gorham, 1962)
- Brief Rating Inventory of Executive Function–Adult Version (BRIEF-A; Roth et al., 2005)
- Brief Scale of Self-Rated Health Condition with Acute Schizophrenia (BsHAS; Ohata et al., 2014)
- Calgary Depression Scale for Schizophrenia (CDSS; Addington et al., 1992)
- Cambridge Neuropsychological Test Automated Battery (CANTAB; Levaux et al., 2007; subtests included Motor Screening, Paired Associate Learning Task, Stockings Cambridge, and Spatial Working Memory)
- Cambridge Prospective Memory Test (Wilson et al., 2005; see also Au et al., 2014; Au et al., 2017, in References)
- Client Satisfaction Questionnaire-8 (CSQ-8; Attkisson & Greenfield, 1994)
- Clinical Global Impression–Severity scale (CGI-S; Busner & Targum, 2007)
- Cognitive Biases Questionnaire for Psychosis (CBQp; Peters et al., 2014; see also Ishikawa et al., 2017, in References)
- Continuous Performance Test (CPT; Rosvold et al., 1956)
- D2 Test of Attention (D2; Bates & Lemay, 2004; see also P. Lee et al., 2018, in References)
- Extrapyramidal Symptom Rating Scale (ESRS; Chouinard & Margolese, 2005)
- Faux Pas Task (FPT; Baron-Cohen et al., 1999)
- Functional Independence Measure (FIM; Uniform Data System for Medical Rehabilitation, 1997)

- Global Assessment of Functioning (GAF) scale (Hall, 1995)
- Instrumental Activities of Daily Living Scale (IADL; Lawton & Brody, 1969; see also Huang et al., 2018, in References)
- Intrinsic Motivation Inventory (IMI; Ryan et al., 1990)
- Lancashire Quality of Life Profile (LQOLP; Oliver et al., 1996)
- Mini-Mental State Examination (MMSE; Folstein et al.,1975)
- Modified Mini-Mental State Examination (3Ms; Teng & Chui, 1987)
- Morisky Medication Adherence Scale-8 (MMAS-8; Morisky et al., 1986)
- Neurobehavioral Cognitive Status Examination (Cognistat; Kiernan et al., 1987)
- Observed Tasks of Daily Living–Revised (OTDL-R; Diehl et al., 2005)
- Personal and Social Performance scale (PSP; Morosini et al., 2000; see also Chiu et al., 2018; S.-C. Lee et al., 2016, in References)
- Positive and Negative Syndromes Scale (PANSS; Kay et al., 1987)
- Quantified Neurological Scale (QNS; Convit et al., 1994)
- Reading the Mind in the Eyes Task (RMET; Baron-Cohen et al., 1997)
- Rey Complex Figure Test (RCFT; Meyers & Meyers, 1995)
- Role Functioning Scale (RFS; Goodman et al., 1993)
- Scale for Assessment of Negative Symptoms (SANS; Andreasen, 1983)
- Scale for Assessment of Positive Symptoms (SAPS; Andreasen, 1984)
- Schizophrenia Cognition Rating Scale (SCoRS; Keefe et al., 2006)
- Schizophrenia Quality of Life Scale Revision 4 (SQLS-R4; Bobes et al., 2005)
- Social Functioning Scale (SFS; Birchwood et al., 1990)
- Social and Occupational Functioning Assessment Scale (SOFAS; Morosini et al., 2000)
- Socially Valued Role Classification Scale (SRCS; Waghorn et al., 2007)
- State Trait Anxiety Inventory (STAI; Spielberger, 2010)
- Strange Stories (SS; Happé, 1994)
- Stroop Color and Word Test (SCWT; Golden & Freshwater, 2002)
- Symbol Digit Modalities Test (SDMT; Smith, 1973)
- Trail Making Test A & B (TMT-A, TMT-B; Reitan & Wolfson, 1995)
- Weintraub Cancellation Test (WCTP; Dawes, 2000)
- Wisconsin Card Sorting Test (WCST; Heaton et al., 1993)
- World Health Organization Disability Assessment Schedule 2.0 (WHODAS-2.0; WHO, 1985; see also R. Chen et al., 2018, in References)

Problems/Issues

Activities of Daily Living/Instrumental ADL

- Person may fail to perform or complete self-maintenance activities including eating, dressing, and bathing. Problem is not due to motor skills but to apathy and lack of motivation.
- Person may be unable to live independently due to failure to have learned and to perform life skills such as handling medications, preparing food, shopping, handling finances, doing laundry, doing housekeeping, using the telephone, and using public transportation.

Education/Work

- Person may have dropped out of school or been dismissed for failing grades.
- Person may have an irregular work history including a history of being fired for not showing up for work assignments or failure to complete assigned work tasks.
- Person may be unable to hold a job due to symptoms associated with schizophrenia.

Play/Leisure

- Person may rarely engage in leisure occupations.
- Person may have few or no identified leisure occupations.
- Person may only engage in passive leisure occupations, such as watching television or listening to music.

Rest/Sleep
- Person may have an irregular sleep schedule.

Social Participation
- Person may avoid or rarely participate in social activities.

Sensorimotor
- Person may experience psychomotor retardation, including changes in movement time, peak velocity, percentage of time to peak velocity, and movement units to infer movement including speed, forcefulness, spatial efficiency (directness), control strategies, and smoothness of movement.
- Person may have impaired visuomotor coordination.

Cognitive/Perceptual
- Person may have impaired ability to shift attention from one task to another.
- Person may demonstrate hemi-inattention on cancellation tests.
- Person may have delayed verbal recall.
- Person may have impaired prospective memory.
- Person may have delayed visual recall.
- Person may have impaired visual-spatial memory and spatial working memory.
- Person may have impaired executive function including ability to plan ahead, use metacognition, time use and management, reasoning, and problem solving.
- Person may experience hallucinations and delusions.
- Person may experience disorganized thinking.

Psychosocial
- Person may have diminished emotional expression.
- Person may lack motivation or volition.
- Person may experience disorganized or catatonic behavior.
- Person may lack self-awareness of illness or need for intervention.

Context/Environment
- Person may lack social support.

Intervention/Treatment

Models and programs developed by occupational therapy personnel include the dynamic interactional model (Kaizerman-Dinerman et al., 2018), Feeling & Doing Group (Revheim et al., 2016), individualized occupational therapy (Shimada et al., 2016a, 2016b; Shimada et al., 2018; Shimada et al., 2017), occupational goal intervention program (Katz & Keren, 2011), social and occupational functioning (Singh et al., 2017), and subject-chosen activities program (Hoshii et al., 2013). Models and programs developed by other professionals but used by occupational therapy personnel include aerobic dance program (M. D. Chen et al., 2016), changes in functional ability (Kawaguchi et al., 2018), frontal/executive program (Miyajima et al., 2018), functional independence (Tanaka et al., 2014), integrated supported employment (Zhang et al., 2017), and trilogy behavioral healthcare program. Team members include psychiatrists, nursing personnel, psychologists, social workers, and occupational therapy personnel. Goals include facilitating occupational performance and promoting quality of life.

Activities of Daily Living/Instrumental ADL
- Home visits to address ADL and IADL issues.
- Practice shopping for groceries in store or online, household management.
- Provide practice in communication skills including eye contact, loudness and pitch of voice, approaching people, initiating conversation.

Education/Work
- Use of background music may facilitate attending behavior in the work setting (Shih et al., 2015).

Play/Leisure
- Explore and expand interests in leisure activities.

Rest/Sleep
- See Sleep–Wake Disorders in Section 13: Lifestyle Conditions.

Social Participation
- Group activities can be used to increase social interactions and participation in social activities.

Sensorimotor
- Provide movement training, including grading and adapting reaching activities by changing object size and distance to enhance movement performance.

Cognitive/Perceptual
- Use a program designed to reteach executive functioning, such as the Occupational Goals Intervention program (stop and think, define the main task, list and partition goal into subgoals, learn steps and monitor).
- Individualized intervention focused on cognitive deficits (attention, memory, and executive functions) in addition to group intervention may provide better results than group intervention alone because individual problems can be the point of focus.
- Executive functions should include activity scheduling, time processing, and time management.

Psychosocial
- Provide program of social skills to facilitate constructive engagement in social activities.
- Use direct engagement in activities to promote self-efficacy.
- Assist clients to participate in pleasurable activities, such as pleasant scents and tastes, using pleasure visual imagery and relaxation, preparing for holidays with simple cooking tasks, playing social games, doing container gardening, learning dance steps, or watching nature programs.
- Encourage clients to transfer learning from pleasurable activities to life situations: "How could you use what we did today to feel better in everyday life?"
- Encourage development of intrinsic motivation by promoting occupational engagement in the activities used in the group activities such as finding and using pleasant smells, cooking tasty meals.
- Self-management instruction to prevent relapse and develop a crisis plan.

Context/Environment
- Consider offering programs for family and caregivers on managing clients with schizophrenia.

Precautions/Safety Considerations
Monitor for suicidal behavior.

Prognosis and Outcome
A study by Minnu and Nalini (2014) did not find occupational therapy intervention effective in reducing negative symptoms of schizophrenia, but Revheim et al. (2016) and Tatsumi et al. (2012) reported positive results. Persons with poor social participation were most likely to be readmitted to the hospital (Smith et al., 2014). Schizophrenia is a chronic disorder but can be managed with medical, family, and community support.

REFERENCES

American Psychiatric Association. (2013). *Diagnostic and statistical manual of mental disorders* (5th ed.). https://doi.org/10.1176/appi.books.9780890425596

Au, R. W. C., Man, D., Shum, D., Lee, E., Xiang, Y. T., Ungvari, G. S., & Tang, W.-K. (2014). Assessment of prospective memory in schizophrenia using the Chinese version of the Cambridge Prospective Memory Test: A controlled study. *Asia-Pacific Psychiatry, 6*(1), 54–61.

Au, R. W. C., Xiang, Y. T., Ungvari, G. S., Lee, E., Shum, D. H. K., Man, D., & Tang, W. K. (2017). Prospective memory performance in persons with schizophrenia and bipolar disorder and healthy persons. *Perspectives in Psychiatric Care, 53*(4), 266–274. https://doi.org/10.1111/ppc.12172

Aubin, G., Béliveau, M. F., & Klinger, E. (2018). An exploration of the ecological validity of the Virtual Action Planning-Supermarket (VAP-S) with people with schizophrenia. *Neuropsychological Rehabilitation, 28*(5), 689–708. https://doi.org/10.1080/09602011.2015.1074083

Ayres, H., & John, A. P. (2015). The Assessment of Motor and Process Skills as a measure of ADL ability in schizophrenia. *Scandinavian Journal of Occupational Therapy, 22*(6), 470–477. https://doi.org/10.3109/11038128.2015.1061050

Chen, M.-D., Kuo, Y.-H., Chang, Y.-C., Hsu, S.-T., Kuo, C.-C., & Chang, J.-J. (2016). Influences of aerobic dance on cognitive performance in adults with schizophrenia. *Occupational Therapy International, 23*, 346–356. https://doi.org/10.1002/oti.1436

Chen, R., Liou, T. H., Chang, K. H., Yen, C. F., Liao, H. F., Chi, W. C., & Chou, K. R. (2018). Assessment of functioning and disability in patients with schizophrenia using the WHO Disability Assessment Schedule 2.0 in a large-scale database. *European Archives of Psychiatry and Clinical Neuroscience, 268*, 65–75. https://doi.org/10.1007/s00406-017-0834-6

Chiu, E. C., Hung, T. M., Huang, C. M., Lee, S. C., & Hsieh, C. L. (2018). Responsiveness of the Personal and Social Performance scale in patients with schizophrenia. *Psychiatry Research, 260*, 338–342. https://doi.org/10.1016/j.psychres.2017.11.053

Chiu, E.-C., & Lee, S.-C. (2018). Factor structure of the Quality of Life Scale for Mental Disorders in patients with schizophrenia. *Journal of Nursing Research, 26*(3), 185–190. https://doi.org/10.1097/jnr.0000000000000236

Chiu, E.-C., Lee, S.-C., Kuo, C.-J., Lung, F.-W., Hsueh, I.-P., & Hsieh, C.-L. (2015). Development of a performance-based measure of executive functions in patients with schizophrenia. *PLOS ONE, 10*(11), Article e0142790. https://doi.org/10.1371/journal.pone.0142790

Chiu, E. C., Lee, Y., Lai, K. Y., Kuo, C. J., Lee, S. C., & Hsieh, C. L. (2015). Construct validity of the Chinese version of the Activities of Daily Living Rating Scale III in patients with schizophrenia. *PLOS ONE, 10*(6), Article e0130702. https://doi.org/10.1371/journal.pone.0130702.

Hoshii, J., Yotsumoto, K., Tatsumi, E., Tanaka, C., Mori, T., & Hashimoto, T. (2013). Subject-chosen activities in occupational therapy for the improvement of psychiatric symptoms of inpatients with chronic schizophrenia: A controlled trial. *Clinical Rehabilitation, 27*(7), 638–645. https://doi.org/10.1177/0269215512473136

Huang, S.-L., Lu, W.-S., Lee, C. C., Wang, H.-W., Lee, S.-C., & Hsieh, C.-L. (2018). Minimal detectable change on the Lawton Instrumental Activities of Daily Living Scale in community-swelling patients with schizophrenia. *American Journal of Occupational Therapy, 72*(5), Article 7205195020. https://doi.org/10.5014/ajot.2018.026898

Hui, C. L.-M., Li, Y.-K., Leung, K.-F., Tang, J. Y.-M., Wong, G. H.-Y., Chang, W.-C., Chan, S. K.-W., Lee, E. H.-M., & Chen, E. Y.-H. (2013). Reliability and validity of the Life Functioning Assessment Inventory (L-FAI) for patients with psychosis. *Social Psychiatry and Psychiatric Epidemiology, 48*, 1687–1695. https://doi.org/10.1007/s00127-013-0679-x

Ishikawa, R., Ishigaki, T., Kikuchi, A., Matsumoto, K., Kobayashi, S., Morishige, S., Hosono, M., Nakamura, Y., Kase, A., Morimoto, T., & Haga, D. (2017). Cross-cultural validation of the Cognitive Biases Questionnaire for psychosis in Japan and examination of the relationships between cognitive biases and schizophrenia symptoms. *Cognitive Therapy and Research, 41*, 313–323. https://doi.org/10.1007/s10608-016-9807-8

Janeslätt, G. K., Holmqvist, K. L., White, S., & Holmefur, M. (2018). Assessment of time management skills: Psychometric properties of the Swedish version. *Scandinavian Journal of Occupational Therapy, 25*(3), 153–161. https://doi.org/10.1080/11038128.2017.1375009

Kaizerman-Dinerman, A., Roe, D., & Josman, N. (2018). An efficacy study of a metacognitive group intervention for people with schizophrenia. *Psychiatry Research, 270,* 1150–1156. https://doi.org/10.1016/j.psychres.2018.10.037

Katz, N., & Keren, N. (2011). Effectiveness of occupational goal intervention for clients with schizophrenia. *American Journal of Occupational Therapy, 65*(3), 287–296. https://doi.org/10.5014/ajot.2011.001347

Kawaguchi, T., Matsunaga, A., Watanabe, A., Suzuki, M., Asano, E., Shirakihara, Y., Shimizu, S., Sawayama, T., Fukuda, M., & Miyaoka, H. (2018). Prediction of changes in functional ability of inpatients with schizophrenia using logarithmic and linear regression modelling. *Hong Kong Journal of Occupational Therapy 31*(2), 76–85. https://doi.org/10.1177/1569186118808431

Lee, P., Lu, W. S., Liu, C. H., Lin, H. Y., & Hsieh, C. L. (2018). Test-retest reliability and minimal detectable change of the D2 test of attention in patients with schizophrenia. *Archives of Clinical Neuropsychology, 33*(8), 1060–1068. https://doi.org/10.1093/arclin/acx123

Lee, S.-C., Tang, S.-F., Lu, W.-S., Huang, S.-L. Deng, N.-Y., Lue, W.-C., & Hsieh, C.-L. (2016). Minimal detectable change of the Personal and Social Performance scale in individuals with schizophrenia. *Psychiatry Research, 246,* 725–729. https://doi.org/10.1016/j.psychres.2016.10.058

Lin, G.-H., Wu, C.-T., Huang, Y.-J., Lin, P., Chou, C.-Y., Lee, S.-C., & Hsieh, C.-L. (2018). A reliable and valid assessment of sustained attention for patients with schizophrenia: The Computerized Digit Vigilance Test. *Archives of Clinical Neuropsychology, 33*(2), 227–237. https://doi.org/10.1093/arclin/acx064

Miyajima, M., Omiya, H., Yamashita, K., Yambe, K., Matsui, M., & Denda, K. (2018). Therapeutic responses to a frontal/executive programme in autism spectrum disorder: Comparison with schizophrenia. *Hong Kong Journal of Occupational Therapy, 31*(2), 69–75. https://doi.org/10.1177/1569186118808217

Minnu, P., & Nalini, M. (2014). Effectiveness of occupational therapy on symptoms of schizophrenia. *International Journal of Nursing, 6*(1), 189–194.

Porter, R. S. (Ed.). (2018). *The Merck manual of diagnosis and therapy* (20th ed.). Merck Sharp & Dohme.

Revheim, N., Han, S., Plattotham, M., Buschbacher, K., & Trémeau, F. (2016). Feelings & doings group: An innovative approach for negative symptoms. *OT Practice Supplement: SIS Quarterly Practice Connections 1*(1), 12–14.

Shih, Y.-N., Chen, C.-S., Chiang, H.-Y., & Liu, C.-H. (2015). Influence of background music on work attention in clients with chronic schizophrenia. *Work, 51*(1), 153–158. https://doi.org/10.3233/WOR-141846

Shimada, T., Nishi, A., Yoshida, T., Tanaka, S., & Kobayashi, M. (2016a). Development of an individualized occupational therapy programme and its effects on the neurocognition, symptoms and social functioning of patients with schizophrenia. *Occupational Therapy International, 23,* 425–435. https://doi.org/10.1002/oti.1445

Shimada, T., Nishi, A., Yoshida, T., Tanaka, S., & Kobayashi, M. (2016b). Factors influencing rehospitalisation of patients with schizophrenia in Japan: A 1-year longitudinal study. *Hong Kong Journal of Occupational Therapy, 28*(1), 7–14. https://doi.org/10.1016/j.hkjot.2016.10.002

Shimada, T., Ohori, M., Inagaki, Y., Shimooka, Y., Sugimura, N., Ishihara, I., Yoshida, T., & Kobayashi, M. (2018). A multicenter, randomized controlled trial of individualized occupational therapy for patients with schizophrenia in Japan, *PLOS ONE, 13*(4), Article e0193869. https://doi.org/10.1371/journal.pone.0193869

Shimada, T., Takamaru, A., Komatsu, S., Sato, Y., Yoshida, T., & Kobayashi, M. (2017). Relationship between recovery and cognitive insight, neurocognition, social functioning, and symptoms in patients with schizophrenia: A cross-sectional study. *Asian Journal of Occupational Therapy, 13*(1), 71–78. https://doi.org/10.11596/asiajot.13.71

Singh, U., Sweta, & Kiran, M. (2017). Efficacy of occupational therapy with supportive techniques on social and occupational functioning among person with schizophrenia. *International Journal of Psychosocial Rehabilitation, 21*(1), 67–74.

Smith, R., De Witt, P., Franzsen, D., Pillay, M., Wolfe, N., & Davies, C. (2014). Occupational performance factors perceived to influence the readmission of mental health care users diagnosed with schizophrenia. *South African Journal of Occupational Therapy, 44*(1), 51–54.

Tanaka, C., Yotsumoto, K., Tatsumi, E., Sasada, T., Taira, M., Tanaka, K., Maeda, K., & Hashimoto, T. (2014). Improvement of functional independence of patients with acute schizophrenia through early occupational therapy: A pilot quasi-experimental controlled study. *Clinical Rehabilitation, 28*(8), 740–747. https://doi.org/10.1177/0269215514521440

Tatsumi, E., Yotsumoto, K., Nakamae, T., & Hashimoto, T. (2012). Effects of occupational therapy on hospitalized chronic schizophrenia patients with severe negative symptoms. *Kobe Journal of Medical Sciences, 57*(4), E145–E154.

Zhang, G. F., Tsui, C. M., Lu, A. J. B., Yu, L. B., Tsang, H. W. H., & Li, D. (2017). Integrated supported employment for people with schizophrenia in mainland China: A randomized controlled trial. *American Journal of Occupational Therapy, 71*(6), Article 7106165020. https://doi .org/10.5014/ajot.2017.024802

BIBLIOGRAPHY

Aubin, G., Lamoureux, J., Gélinas, I., Chapparo, C., Stip, E., & Rainville, C. (2014). Daily task performance and information processing among people with schizophrenia and healthy controls: A comparative study. *British Journal of Occupational Therapy, 77*(9), 466–474. https:// doi.org/10.4276/030802214X14098207541117

Bagul, C., Hadkarni, K., Yadav, J., Abraham, A. K., & Pednekar, S. (2012). Effect of coping strategies on chronic drug resistant auditory hallucination in schizophrenia: A cross over study. *Indian Journal of Occupational Therapy, 44*(1), 20–29.

Bejerholm, U. (2010a). Occupational balance in people with schizophrenia. *Occupational Therapy in Mental Health, 26*(1), 1–17. https://doi.org/10.1080/01642120802642197

Bejerholm, U. (2010b). Relationships between occupational engagement and status of and satisfaction with sociodemographic factors in a group of people with schizophrenia. *Scandinavian Journal of Occupational Therapy, 17*(3), 244–254. https://doi.org/10.3109/11038120 903254323

Chen, K. W., Lee, S. C., Chiang, H. Y., Syu, Y. C., Yu, X. X., & Hsieh, C. L. (2017). Psychometric properties of three measures assessing advanced theory of mind: Evidence from people with schizophrenia. *Psychiatry Research, 257,* 490–496. https://doi.org/10.1016/j.psychres.2017.08.026

Desai, K. (2010). Relationship between cognitive and neurological deficits with psychotic symptoms among schizophrenic patients. *Indian Journal of Occupational Therapy, 42*(3), 23–27.

Foruzandeh, N., & Parvin, N. (2013). Occupational therapy for inpatients with chronic schizophrenia: A pilot randomized controlled trial. *Japan Journal of Nursing Science, 10*(1), 136–141. https://doi.org/10.1111/j.1742-7924.2012.00211.x

Hanzawa, S., Bae, J. K., Tanaka, H., Bae, Y. J, Tanaka, G., Inadomi, H., Nakane, Y., & Ohta, Y. (2010). Caregiver burden and coping strategies for patients with schizophrenia: Comparison between Japan and Korea. *Psychiatry and Clinical Neurosciences, 64*(4), 377–386. https://doi .org/10.1111/j.1440-1819.2010.02104.x

Hellinger, N., Lipskaya-Velikovsky, L., Weizman, A., & Ratzon, N. Z. (2019). Comparing executive functioning and clinical and sociodemographic characteristics of people with schizophrenia who hold a driver's license to those who do not. *Canadian Journal of Occupational Therapy, 86*(1), 70–80. https://doi.org/10.1177/0008417419831399

Kuo, C. J., Yang, S. Y., Liao, Y. T., Chen, W. J., Lee, W. C., Shau, W. Y., Chang, Y. T., Tsai, S. Y., & Chen, C. C. (2013). Second-generation antipsychotic medications and risk of pneumonia in schizophrenia. *Schizophrenia Bulletin, 39*(3), 648–657. https://doi.org/10.1093/schbul/sbr202

Lexén, A., & Bejerholm, U. (2018). Occupational engagement and cognitive functioning among persons with schizophrenia: An explorative study. *Scandinavian Journal of Occupational Therapy*, *25*(3), 172–179. https://doi.org/10.1080/11038128.2017.1290135

Lexén, A., Hofgren, C., Stenmark, R., & Bejerholm, U. (2016). Cognitive functioning and employment among people with schizophrenia in vocational rehabilitation. *Work*, *54*(3), 735–744. https://doi.org/10.3233/WOR-162318

Li, N., Ying, C., & Deng, H. (2012). Cross-sectional assessment of the factors associated with occupational functioning in patients with schizophrenia. *Shanghai Archives of Psychiatry*, *24*(4), 222–230.

Lipskaya, L., Jarus, T., & Kotler, M. (2011). Influence of cognition and symptoms of schizophrenia on IADL performance. *Scandinavian Journal of Occupational Therapy*, *18*(3), 180–187. https://doi.org/10.3109/11038128.2010.490879

Lipskaya-Velikovsky, L., Bar-Shalita, T., & Bart, O. (2015). Sensory modulation and daily-life participation in people with schizophrenia. *Comprehensive Psychiatry*, *58*, 130–137. https://doi.org/10.1016/j.comppsych.2014.12.009

Lipskaya-Velikovsky, L., Jarus, T., Easterbrook, A., & Kotler, M. (2016). Participation in daily life of people with schizophrenia in comparison to the general population. *Canadian Journal of Occupational Therapy*, *83*(5), 297–305. https://doi.org/10.1177/0008417416647158

Lipskaya-Velikovsky, L., Kotler, M., & Jarus, T. (2016). Factors discriminating employment status following in-patient evaluation among persons with schizophrenia. *Work*, *53*(3), 469–478. https://doi.org/10.3233/WOR-152178

Lipskaya-Velikovsky, L., Kotler, M., Weiss, P., Kaspi, M., Gamzo-Sabag, S., & Ratzon, N. (2013). Car driving in schizophrenia: Can visual memory and organization make a difference? *Disability and Rehabilitation*, *35*(20), 1734–1739. https://doi.org/10.3109/09638288.2012.753116

Liu, Y.-C., Chen, K.-C., Yang, Y. K., Chen, Y.-L., & Lin, K.-C. (2011). Relationship between hemi-spatial inattention and performance of activities of daily living in patients with schizophrenia. *Perceptual and Motor Skills*, *112*(3), 703–710. https://doi.org/10.2466/02.09.13.PMS.112.3.703-710

Macedo, M., Marques, A., Queirós, C., & Mariotti, M. C. (2018). Schizophrenia, instrumental activities of daily living and executive functions: A qualitative multidimensional approach. *Cadernos Brasileiros Terapia Ocupacional da UFSCar*, *26*(2), 287–298. https://doi.org/10.4322/2526-8910.ctoAO1153

Masoumi, T., Shafaroodi, N., & Razvan, Z. (2018). Participation of people with schizophrenia in everyday life: Family's perspective. *Iranian Rehabilitation Journal*, *16*(3), 297–306. https://doi.org/10.32598/irj.16.3.297

Moore, K., Merritt, B., & Doble, S. E. (2010). ADL skill profiles across three psychiatric diagnoses. *Scandinavian Journal of Occupational Therapy*, *17*(1), 77–85. https://doi.org/10.3109/11038120903165115

Morimoto, K., Yotsumoto, K., & Hashimoto, T. (2010). Association between psychiatric symptoms and difficulty with computer operation in schizophrenia: Analysis using a questionnaire and a computer operation skills test. *Asian Journal of Occupational Therapy*, *8*(1), 31–38. https://doi.org/10.11596/asiajot.8.31

Nakagawa, Y., & Hoshiyama, M. (2015). Influence of observing another person's action on self-generated performance in schizophrenia. *Cognitive Neuropsychiatry*, *20*(4), 349–360. https://doi.org/10.1080/13546805.2015.1044081

Novak, T., Scanlan, J., McCaul, D., MacDonald, N., & Clarke, T. (2012). Pilot study of a sensory room in an acute inpatient psychiatric unit. *Australasian Psychiatry*, *20*(5), 401–406. https://doi.org/10.1177/1039856212459585

Odes, H., Katz, N., Noter, E., Shamir, Y., Weizman, A., & Valevski, A. (2011). Level of function at discharge as a predictor of readmission among inpatients with schizophrenia. *American Journal of Occupational Therapy*, *65*(3), 314–319. https://doi.org/10.5014/ajot.2011.001362

Ohata, H., Yotsumoto, K., Taira, M., Kochi, Y., & Hashimoto, T. (2014). Reliability and validity of a brief self-rated scale of health condition with acute schizophrenia. *Psychiatry and Clinical Neurosciences, 68*, 70–77. https://doi.org/10.1111/pcn.12105

Perilli, V., Stasolla, F., Maselli, S., & Morelli, I. (2018). Occupational therapy and social skills training for enhancing constructive engagement of patients with schizophrenia: A review. *Clinical Research in Psychology, 1*(1), 1–7. https://doi.org/10.33309/2639-9113.010108

Pongsaksri, M. (2018). Time use for occupation and the expectations of people with schizophrenia and their relatives from the perspective of themselves and their relatives. *Asian Journal of Occupational Therapy, 14*(1), 1–7. https://doi.org/10.11596/asiajot.14.1

Potvin, S., Aubin, G., & Stip, E. (2015). Antipsychotic-induced parkinsonism is associated with working memory deficits in schizophrenia-spectrum disorders. *European Archives of Psychiatry and Clinical Neuroscience, 265*(2), 147–154. https://doi.org/ 10.1007/s00406-014-0511-y

Rempfer, M. V., McDowd, J. M., & Brown, C. E. (2017). Measuring learning potential in people with schizophrenia: A comparison of two tasks. *Psychiatry Research, 258*, 316–321. https://doi .org/10.1016/j.psychres.2017.08.057

Samuel, R., Thomas, E., & Jacob, K. S. (2018). Instrumental activities of daily living dysfunction among people with schizophrenia. *Indian Journal of Psychological Medicine, 40*(2), 134–138. https://doi.org/10.4103/IJPSYM.IJPSYM_308_17

Shahgholi, A., Noori, A. K., Hosseini, S. A., & Sourtigi, H. (2012). The effect of sensory room intervention on perceptual-cognitive performance and the psychiatric status of schizophrenics. *Iranian Rehabilitation Journal, 10*(16), 5–15.

Su, C. Y., Tsai, P. C., Su, W. L., Tang, T. C., & Tsai, A. Y. J. (2011). Cognitive profile difference between Allen Cognitive Levels 4 and 5 in schizophrenia. *American Journal of Occupational Therapy 65*(4), 453–461. https://doi.org/10.5014/ajot.2011.000711

Su, C. T., Yang, A. L., & Lin, C. Y. (2017a). Comparing two schizophrenia-specific quality of life instruments in institutionalized people with schizophrenia. *Psychiatry Research, 258*, 274–282. https://doi.org/10.1016/j.psychres.2017.08.053

Su, C. T., Yang, A. L., & Lin, C. Y. (2017b). The construct of the Schizophrenia Quality of Life Scale Revision 4 for the population of Taiwan. *Occupational Therapy International*, Article 5328101. https://doi.org/10.1155/2017/5328101

Tang, S. F., Chen, I. H., Chiang, H. Y., Wu, C. T., Hsueh, I. P., Yu, W. H., & Hsieh, C. L. (2018). A comparison between the original and Tablet-based Symbol Digit Modalities Test in patients with schizophrenia: Test–retest agreement, random measurement error, practice effect, and ecological validity. *Psychiatry Research, 260*, 199–206. https://doi.org/10.1016/j.psychres.2 017.11.066

Wang, S. M., Kuo, L. C., Ouyang, W. C., Hsu, H. M., & Ma, H. I. (2018). Effects of object size and distance on reaching kinematics in patients with schizophrenia. *Hong Kong Journal of Occupational Therapy, 31*(1), 22–29. https://doi.org/10.1177/1569186118759610

Westcott, C., Waghorn, G., McLean, D., Statham, D., & Mowry, B. (2015). Role functioning among adults with schizophrenia. *British Journal of Occupational Therapy, 78*(3), 158–165. https://doi.org/10.1177/0308022615573372

Zafran, H., Mazer, B., Tallant, B., Chilingaryan, G., & Gelinas, I. (2017). Detecting incipient schizophrenia: A validation of the Azima battery in first episode psychosis. *Psychiatric Quarterly, 88*, 585–602. https://doi.org/10.1007/s11126-016-9482-7

Zayat, E., Rempfer, M., Gajewski, B., & Brown, C. E. (2011). Patterns of association between performance in a natural environment and measures of executive function in people with schizophrenia. *Psychiatry Research 187*(1-2), 1–5. https://doi.org/10.1016/j.psychres.2010.11.011

Zhornitsky, S., Aubin, G., Desfossés, J., Rizkallah, É., Pampoulova, T., Lipp, O., Chiasson, J.-P., Stip, E., & Potvin, S. (2013). Predictors of community functioning in schizophrenia and substance use disorder patients. *Community Mental Health Journal, 49*, 317–322. https://doi .org/10.1007/s10597-012-9525-y

Zhornitsky, S., Potvin, S., Aubin, G., & Stip, E. (2011). Relationship between insight into cognition, extrapyramidal symptoms and mental illness in schizophrenia (Correspondence). *Australian and New Zealand Journal of Psychiatry, 45*(7), 596–597.

Serious Mental Illness

Also called severe mental illness, major mental illness, enduring mental illness, profound mental illness, persistent mental illness, and chronic mental illness.

Description

Serious mental illness is defined by the U.S. Substance Abuse and Mental Health Services Administration (SAMHSA, n.d.) as "someone over 18 having (within the past year) a diagnosable mental, behavior, or emotional disorder that causes serious functional impairment that substantially interferes with or limits one or more major life activities" (para. 1). Alternate names include severe, major, profound, persistent, enduring, long-term, and chronic mental illness. Serious mental illness usually includes disorders such as schizophrenia spectrum disorders, severe bipolar disorder (manic depression), and major depression (unipolar depression). Other countries may list additional disorders. Serious functional impairment may be defined as impairment equivalent to a Global Assessment of Functioning (GAF) score of less than 60.

Cause

Multiple causes are possible, including genetic factors, substance abuse, early life environment, trauma and stress, and other biological factors, including some medical conditions or hormonal changes.

Evaluation/Assessment

Areas

- Activities of Daily Living/Instrumental ADL: weight control, home management, meal planning and preparation, shopping, driving
- Education/Work: academic performance, job skills, work history, occupational identity
- Play/Leisure: interests, frequency, location, level of satisfaction
- Rest/Sleep: sleep habits, sleep patterns
- Social Participation: type, frequency, location, with whom
- Sensorimotor: physical fitness
- Cognitive/Perceptual: arousal, alertness, attention, concentration, memory, executive functions (problem solving, decision making, time management)
- Psychosocial: depression, mania, mood, quality of life, self-efficacy, self-management, self-image, sense of belonging
- Context/Environment: social support, community resources
- Comorbidities: alcohol abuse, coronary heart disease, drug abuse, diabetes, hypertension, obesity or overweight, nicotine dependence, sensory processing dysfunction

Instruments

Instruments Developed by Occupational Therapy Personnel

- Allen Cognitive Level Screen (5th ed.; ACLS-5; Allen et al., 2007)
- Canadian Occupational Performance Measure (5th ed.; COPM-5; Law et al., 2014)
- Comprehensive Occupational Therapy Evaluation Scale (COTES; Brayman et al., 1976)
- Dynamic Loewenstein Occupational Therapy Cognitive Assessment (DLOTCA; Katz et al., 2012)

- Executive Functions Performance Test (EFPT; Baum & Wolf, 2013)
- General Occupational Engagement in people with Severe mental illness (GOES; Eklund & Bejerholm, 2017, in References)
- Observed Tasks of Daily Living–Revised (OTDL-R; Goverover & Josman, 2004)
- Occupational Circumstances Assessment Interview and Rating Scale (Version 4.0; OCAIRS; Forsyth et al., 2005)
- Occupational Performance History Interview (Version 2.1; OPHI-II; Kielhofner et al., 2004)
- Occupational Therapy Task Observation Scale (OTTOS; Margolis et al., 1996)
- Profiles of Occupational Engagement in people with Schizophrenia (POES; Bejerholm et al., 2006; see also Bejerholm & Lundgren-Nilsson, 2015, in References)
- Profiles of Occupational Engagement in People with Severe Mental Illness (POES-P; Tjörn-strand et al., 2013, in References)
- Quality of Life Measure for Persons With Schizophrenia (QOLM-S; Laliberte-Rudman et al., 2004)
- Routine Task Inventory–Expanded (RRI-E; Katz, 2006)
- SÉCuRE (home safety tool; Désormeaux-Moreau et al., 2018b, in References)
- Test of Grocery Shopping Skills (TGSS; Brown et al., 2009)
- Vellore Occupational Therapy Evaluation Scale (VOTES; Samuel et al., 2016, in References)
- Work Environment Impact Scale (WEIS; Moore-Corner et al., 1998)
- Worker Role Interview (Version 10.0; WRI 10.0; Braveman et al., 2005)

Instruments Developed by Other Professionals and Used by Occupational Therapy Personnel
- Adult Hope Scale (AHS; Snyder et al., 1991)
- Behavioral Regulation in Work Questionnaire (BRWQ; Fitzgerald et al., 2015, in References)
- Brief Psychiatric Rating Scale, (BPRS; Overall & Gorham, 1962)
- Empowerment Scale (ES; Rogers et al., 1997)
- Herth Hope Index (HHI; Herth, 1992)
- Lancashire Quality of Life Profile (LQOLP; Oliver et al., 1996)
- Life Stressors and Social Resources Inventory–Adult Form (LISRES-A; Moos & Moos, 1994)
- Manchester Short Assessment of Quality of Life (MANSA; Priebe et al., 1999)
- Multidimensional Scale of Perceived Social Support (MSPSS; Zimet et al., 1988)
- Recovery Assessment Scale (RAS; Corrigan et al., 2004; Hancock et al., 2015; see also Chiba et al., 2010, in References)
- Rejection Experience Scale (RES; Björkman et al., 2007)
- Resilience Scale (RS; Wagnild & Young, 1993)
- Satisfaction with Life Scale (SWLS; Diener et al., 1985)
- Short-Form 36 Health Survey (SF-36; Ware et al., 1993)
- Wide Range Achievement Test (5th ed.; WRAT-5; Wilkinson & Robertson, 2017)
- Wisconsin Card Sorting Test (WCST; Heaton et al., 1993)
- Work Accommodation and Natural Support Scale (WANSS; Corbière et al., 2014)

Problems/Issues
Activities of Daily Living/Instrumental ADL
- Person may fail to complete basic ADL tasks such as eating regularly, dressing, bathing/showering, grooming (Note: failure to complete the tasks is usually not the inability to perform but instead related to motivation).
- Person may experience weight gain related to side effect of some medications.
- Person may have a pattern of unhealthy eating, including eating junk foods, fried foods, and few fruits and vegetables.
- Person may have limited understanding of how unhealthy eating affects health.

- Person may experience difficulty performing IADL tasks, such home management, preparing healthy meals, managing finances, shopping for groceries and household items, driving or using public transportation.
- Person may lack parenting and childcare skills.

Education/Work
- Person may have difficulty completing academic assignments or attending required classes.
- Person may have difficulty locating and maintaining employment.

Play/Leisure
- Person may lack identified leisure activities in which the person engages regularly.
- Person may have identified passive activities (watching TV), but no active engagement activities.

Rest/Sleep
- Person may have sleep disturbances.
- Person may not maintain a regular sleep schedule.

Social Participation
- Person may lack opportunities to participate in social activities.

Sensorimotor
- Person may have low energy level (lethargy, fatigue).
- Person may fail to exercise regularly or maintain physical fitness.
- Person may have low sensory registration or sensory sensitivity.

Cognitive/Perceptual
- Person may have difficulty maintaining attention and concentration.
- Person may have difficulty with memory.
- Person may have difficulty with executive functions such as planning ahead, problem solving, decision making, judgment of safety, organization, time management.

Psychosocial
- Person may lack motivation (low incentive) to change behavior.
- Person may experience anhedonia (lack of pleasure or interest).
- Person may experience stigma related to illness.
- Person may have few coping skills.
- Person may lack social skills including finding mates and friends.
- Women's symptoms of depression tend to be more severe than men's (Bonsaksen & Lerdal, 2012).

Context/Environment
- Person may experience lack of social support from family or friends.
- Person may have a police or criminal record.
- Person may live in a "food desert" with limited access to fresh fruits and vegetables.
- Person may live in a household that does not consider healthy eating a priority.

Intervention/Treatment

Models and programs developed by occupational therapy personnel include action over inertia (Edgelow & Krupa, 2011), Documentation of Occupational Therapy Session during Intervention (D.O.T.S.I.; Bart et al., 2011; Lipskaya-Velikovsky et al., 2014), home-based occupational therapy intervention (Lindström et al., 2012), in-house vocational training program (Lee et al., 2018), modelizing home safety (Désormeaux-Moreau et al., 2018a), Nutrition and Exercise for Wellness and Recovery (NEW-R; Brown et al., 2011; Brown et al., 2015), person-environment-occupation model (Prasad & Acharya, 2014), person-environment-occupation-performance model (PEOP; Tyminski, 2019), prevocational training program (Chuang et al., 2015), and tai chi health promotion program (Chapleau & Dirette, 2013). Models and programs developed by other professionals but used by occupational therapy personnel include Baduanjin exercise program (M. D. Chen et al., 2016), dynamic interactional model (Josman & Regev, 2018), Health Optimisation Program for Employment (HOPE), thinking skills for work (TSW; Contreras et al., 2016; Contreras et al., 2012), individual placement and support (Areberg & Bejerholm, 2013; Bejerholm et al., 2015; Bejerholm & Björkman, 2011; Bejerholm et al., 2011; Lexén & Bejerholm, 2016; Lexén et al., 2013; van Veggel et al., 2015; Williams et al., 2015), Keshet family education program (Weiss et al., 2018), recovery education program (S. P. Chen et al., 2014; S. P. Chen et al., 2013), Transtheoretical Model (TTM; Tyminski, 2019), walking program (Swarbrick et al., 2018), and wellness for life program (Gill et al., 2016). Team members may include physicians (psychiatrist, neurologist), nursing personnel, psychologists, social workers, vocational rehabilitation counselors, and occupational therapy personnel. The goal is focus on time use, activity patterns and occupational engagement to link health and well-being with behavioral activation, time management, and activity promotion (Höhl et al., 2017). Clients found meaning in being socially engaged, feeling competent and accepted, creating routines, being productive, being creative, seeking knowledge, and taking care of body and mind (Argentzell et al., 2012).

Activities of Daily Living/Instrumental ADL
- Assist client in basic ADLs such as dressing on a budget, appropriate dress in the workplace, hair care, bathing and washing, dental care.
- Assist client to participate in a program to manage weight gain and obesity including eating healthy foods, preparing healthy meals, shopping for healthy foods, and sticking to a diet plan (see NEW-R program; Brown et al., 2011).
- Assist client to participate in a homemaking program.
- Assist client to participate in a parenting program if children are involved.
- Encourage health promotion and management including healthy eating, life balance, setting boundaries and crisis management, smoking cessation, sexual education, managing other health issues (diabetes, hypertension).
- Provide assistance in financial management including weekly and monthly budgeting, playing bills, filing taxes, opening a saving/checking account, creating a food budget, understanding a paycheck stub, identifying housing options based on income, understanding Social Security Disability Insurance.
- Assist client in obtaining a driver's license, using public transportation, safety awareness in the community.

Education/Work
- Assist client in obtaining education such as a GED, registering for night classes, improving basic academic skills, improving computer skills, applying for college, referral for tutoring and community academic support services.
- Provide opportunity for prevocational training.
- Explore and pursue realistic employment opportunities including resume writing, interviewing (mock, role playing) and feedback, computer skills training, effective work site communication, volunteering, employee rights and benefits, and general literacy.
- Assist client to participate in a supported employment program using individual placement and support.
- Explore need for work space and environmental adaptations (seating, lighting, desk organization).

Play/Leisure
- Provide opportunity for leisure exploration and engagement such as developing healthy leisure activities, restoring interest in hobbies, developing new interests.

Rest/Sleep

- Assist client to develop and implement a sleep routine and sleep environment to support adequate sleep and rest based on client's health status and lifestyle.

Social Participation

- Provide opportunities and encourage reconnecting with friends and family, planning healthy social activities, developing new friendships, handling stress in busy environments or during the holidays.

Sensorimotor

- Encourage client to participate in an exercise program (more exercise increases quality of life; Bonsaksen & Lerdal, 2012).

Cognitive/Perceptual

- Client may benefit from self-learning programs (see recovery education program applying the appreciate inquiry approach [S. P. Chen et al., 2013; S. P. Chen et al., 2014]).
- Client may need assistance to increase attention skills or in use of visual/verbal cueing aids to assist memory.
- Client may need assistance in using executive functions such as problem solving, decision making, goal setting, planning ahead, judgment of safety, time management.

Psychosocial

- Assist client to change behaviors through the six-step process of precontemplation, contemplation, preparation, action, maintenance, and termination (engagement); therapists can be especially helpful in preparation and action steps.
- Provide opportunity to increase sense of self-competency.
- Provide education in and opportunity to practice coping and stress management techniques (deep breathing, yoga, imagery, visualization).
- Provide opportunity to learn strategies to manage specific symptoms and emotions to reduce incidence of relapse such as dealing with hallucinations (auditory, visual, tactile), anger, depression, grief, and anxiety.

Context/Environment

- Assist client in identifying and using community resources.
- Provide information to family and others regarding serious mental illness and its impact on everyday life.
- Assist client to locate, establish, and maintain a safe living environment to reduce incidence of accidents and injuries.

Precautions/Safety Considerations

Person may be at risk for complications of diabetes including undiagnosed diabetes. Person may be at risk for complications related to obesity and being overweight including cardiac and heart conditions. Person may be at risk of complications from polypharmacy in addition to overdose. Person may be at risk for suicide or suicidal behavior.

Prognosis and Outcome

Serious mental illness is a chronic condition requiring ongoing management throughout the person's life. Specific health problems and life challenges may change over the years, requiring different management approaches.

REFERENCES

Areberg, C., & Bejerholm, U. (2013). The effect of IPS on participants' engagement, quality of life, empowerment, and motivation: A randomized controlled trial. *Scandinavian Journal of Occupational Therapy, 20*(6), 420–428. https://doi.org/10.3109/11038128.2013.765911

Argentzell, E., Håkansson, C., & Eklund, M. (2012). Experience of meaning in everyday occupations among unemployed people with severe mental illness. *Scandinavian Journal of Occupational Therapy, 19*(1), 49–58. https://doi.org/10.3109/11038128.2010.540038

Bart, O., Bar, M. A., Rosenberg, L., Hamudot, V., & Jarus, T. (2011). Development and validation of the Documentation of Occupational Therapy Session during intervention (D.O.T.S.I.). *Research in Developmental Disabilities, 32*(2), 719–726. https://doi.org/10.1016/j.ridd.2010.11.008

Bejerholm, U., Areberg, C., Hofgren, C., Sandlund, M., & Rinaldi, M. (2015). Individual placement and support in Sweden—A randomized controlled trial. *Nordic Journal of Psychiatry, 69*(1), 57–66. https://doi.org/10.3109/08039488.2014.929739

Bejerholm, U., & Björkman, T. (2011). Empowerment in supported employment research and practice: Is it relevant? *International Journal of Social Psychiatry, 57*(6), 588–595. https://doi.org/10.1177/0020764010376606

Bejerholm, U., Larsson, L., & Hofgren, C. (2011). Individual placement and support illustrated in the Swedish welfare system: A case study. *Journal of Vocational Rehabilitation, 35*(1), 59–72. https://doi.org/10.3233/JVR-2011-0554

Bejerholm, U., & Lundgren-Nilsson, Å. (2015). Rasch analysis of the Profiles of Occupational Engagement in people with Severe mental illness (POES) instrument. *Health and Quality of Life Outcomes, 13*, Article 130. https://doi.org/10.1186/s12955-015-0327-0

Bonsaksen, T., & Lerdal, A. (2012). Relationships between physical activity, symptoms and quality of life among inpatients with severe mental illness. *British Journal of Occupational Therapy, 75*(2), 69–75. https://doi.org/10.4276/030802212X13286281651036

Brown, C., Goetz, J., & Hamera, E. (2011). Weight loss intervention for people with serious mental illness: A randomized controlled trial of the RENEW program. *Psychiatric Services, 62*(7), 800–802. https://doi.org/10.1176/ps.62.7.pss6207_0800

Brown, C., Read, H., Stanton, M., Zeeb, M., Jonikas, J. A., & Cook, J. A. (2015). A pilot study of the Nutrition and Exercise for Wellness and Recovery (NEW-R): A weight loss program for individuals with serious mental illnesses. *Psychiatric Rehabilitation Journal, 38*(4), 371–373. https://doi.org/10.1037/prj0000115

Chapleau, A. M., & Dirette, D. P. (2013). An evaluation of the potential effectiveness of a Tai Chi program for health promotion among people with severe mental illness. *Open Journal of Occupational Therapy, 1*(2), Article 4. https://doi.org/10.15453/2168-6408.1036

Chen, M.-D., Yeh, Y.-C., Tsai, Y.-J., Chang, Y.-C., Yu, J.-W., & Hsu, C.-H. (2016). Efficacy of Baduanjin exercise and feasibility of mobile text reminders on follow-up participation in people with severe mental illness: An exploratory study. *Journal of Psychiatric Practice, 22*(3), 241–249. https://doi.org/10.1097/PRA.0000000000000158

Chen, S.-P., Krupa, T., Lysaght, R., McCay, E., & Piat, M. (2013). The development of recovery competencies for in-patient mental health providers working with people with serious mental illness. *Administration and Policy in Mental Health, 40*, 96–116. https://doi.org/10.1007/s10488-011-0380-x

Chen, S.-P., Krupa, T., Lysaght, R., McCay, E., & Piat, M. (2014). Development of a recovery education program for inpatient mental health providers. *Psychiatric Rehabilitation Journal, 37*(4), 329–332. https://doi.org/10.1037/prj0000082

Chiba, R., Miyamoto, Y., & Kawakami, N. (2010). Reliability and validity of the Japanese version of the Recovery Assessment Scale (RAS) for people with chronic mental illness: Scale development. *International Journal of Nursing Studies, 47*(3), 314–322. https://doi.org/10.1016/j.ijnurstu.2009.07.006

Chuang, W.-F., Hwang, E., Lee, H.-L., & Wu, S.-L. (2015). An in-house prevocational training program for newly discharged psychiatric inpatients: Exploring its employment outcomes and the predictive factors. *Occupational Therapy International, 22*(2), 94–103. https://doi.org/10.1002/oti.1388

Contreras, N. A., Fossey, E., Castle, D. J., Harvey, C., Crosse, C., Morgain, D., & Rossell, S. L. (2016). What is the personal experience of jobseekers with severe mental illness undertaking a cognitive remediation program? *Psychosocial Intervention, 25*(3), 195–201. https://doi.org/10.1016/j.psi.2016.02.003

Contreras, N. A., Rossell, S. L., Castle, D. J., Fossey, E., Morgan, D., Crosse, C., & Harvey, C. (2012). Enhancing work-focused supports for people with severe mental illnesses in Australia. *Rehabilitation Research and Practice, 2012*, Article 863203. https://doi.org/10.1155/2012/863203

Désormeaux-Moreau, M., Larivière, N., & Aubin, G. (2018a). Modelizing home safety as experienced by people with mental illness. *Scandinavian Journal of Occupational Therapy, 25*(3), 190–202. https://doi.org/10.1080/11038128.2017.1335343

Désormeaux-Moreau, M., Aubin, G., & Larivière, N. (2018b). SÉCuRE: A clinical tool for comprehensively assessing home safety of people with mental illness. *British Journal of Occupational Therapy, 81*(9), 503–513. https://doi.org/10.1177/0308022618762085 (Note: Assessment in French only)

Edgelow, M., & Krupa, T. (2011). Randomized controlled pilot study of an occupational time-use intervention for people with serious mental illness. *American Journal of Occupational Therapy, 65*(3), 267–276. https://doi.org/10.5014/ajot.2011.001313

Eklund, M., & Bejerholm, U. (2017). Staff ratings of occupational engagement among people with severe mental illness—Psychometric properties of a screening tool in the day center context. *BMC Health Services Research 17*, Article 338. https://doi.org/10.1186/s12913-017-2283-3

Fitzgerald, S., Chan, F., Deiches, J., Umucu, E., Hsu, S.-T., Lee, H.-L., Bezyak, J., & Iwanaga, K. (2015). Assessing self-determined work motivation in people with severe mental illness: A factor-analytic approach. *Australian Journal of Rehabilitation Counselling. 21*(2), 123–136. https://doi.org/10.1017/jrc.2015.12

Gill, K. J., Zechner, M., Zambo Anderson, E., Swarbrick, M., & Murphy, A. (2016). Wellness for life: A pilot of an interprofessional intervention to address metabolic syndrome in adults with serious mental illnesses. *Psychiatric Rehabilitation Journal, 39*(2), 147–153. https://doi.org/10.1037/prj0000172

Höhl, W., Moll, S., & Pfeiffer, A. (2017). Occupational therapy interventions in the treatment of people with severe mental illness. *Current Opinion in Psychiatry, 30*(4), 300–305. https://doi.org/10.1097/YCO.0000000000000339

Josman, N., & Regev, S. (2018). Dynamic interactional model in severe mental illness: Metacognitive and strategy-based intervention. In N. Katz & J. Toglia (Eds.), *Cognition, occupation, and participation across the lifespan* (4th ed., pp. 387–402). AOTA Press.

Lee, H.-L., Hwang, E. J., Wu, S.-L., Tu, W.-M., Wang, M. H., & Chan, F. (2018). Employment outcomes after vocational training for people with chronic psychiatric disorders: A multicenter study. *American Journal of Occupational Therapy, 72*(5), Article 72051950. https://doi.org/10.5014/ajot.2018.028621

Lexén, A., & Bejerholm, U. (2016). Exploring communication and interaction skills at work among participants in individual placement and support. *Scandinavian Journal of Occupational Therapy 23*(4), 314–319. https://doi.org/10.3109/11038128.2015.1105294

Lexén, A., Hofgren, C., & Bejerholm, U. (2013). Reclaiming the worker role: Perceptions of people with mental illness participating in IPS. *Scandinavian Journal of Occupational Therapy, 20*(1), 54–63. https://doi.org/10.3109/11038128.2012.693946

Lindström, M., Hariz, G.-M., & Bernspång, B. (2012). Dealing with real-life challenges: Outcome of a home-based occupational therapy intervention for people with severe psychiatric disability. *OTJR: Occupation, Participation and Health, 32*(2), 5–14. https://doi.org/10.3928/15394492-20110819-01

Lipskaya-Velikovsky, L., Bar, M. A., & Bart, O. (2014). Context and psychosocial intervention in mental health. *Scandinavian Journal of Occupational Therapy, 21*(2), 136–144. https://doi.org/10.3109/11038128.2013.871334

Prasad, H., & Acharya, V. (2014). A cross sectional study of employment pattern in patients with severe mental Illness. *Indian Journal of Occupational Therapy, 46*(2), 35–40.

Samuel, R., Russell, P. S., Paraseth, T. K., Ernest, S., & Jacob, K. S. (2016). Development and validation of the Vellore Occupational Therapy Evaluation Scale to assess functioning in people with mental illness. *International Journal of Social Psychiatry, 62*(7), 616–626. https://doi.org/10.1177/0020764016664754

Substance Abuse and Mental Health Services Administration. (n.d.). *Mental health and substance use disorders.* Retrieved May 20, 2022 from https://www.samhsa.gov/find-help/disorders

Swarbrick, M., Nemec, P. B., Brandow, C. L., & Spagnolo, A. (2018). Strategies to promote walking among community-dwelling individuals with major mental disorders. *Journal of Psychosocial Nursing and Mental Health Services, 56*(3), 25–32. https://doi.org/10.3928/02793695-20171205-01

Tjörnstrand, C., Bejerholm, U., & Eklund, M. (2013). Psychometric testing of a self-report measure of engagement in productive occupations. *Canadian Journal of Occupational Therapy, 80*(2), 101–110. https://doi.org/10.1177/0008417413481956

Tyminski, Q. (2019). Supporting behavior change for persons with serious mental illness: An application of two models. *SIS Quarterly Practice Connections, 4*(3), 19–21.

van Veggel, R., Waghorn, G., & Dias, S. (2015). Implementing evidence-based supported employment in Sussex for people with severe mental illness. *British Journal of Occupational Therapy, 78*(5), 286–294. https://doi.org/10.1177/0308022614567667

Weiss, P., Hadas-Lidor, N., Weizman, A., & Sachs, D. (2018). The effectiveness of a knowledge translation cognitive-educational intervention for family members of persons coping with severe mental illness. *Community Mental Health Journal, 54*(4), 485–495. https://doi.org/10.1007/s10597-017-0169-9

Williams, P. L., Lloyd, C., Waghorn, G., & Machingura, T. (2015). Implementing evidence-based practices in supported employment on the Gold Coast for people with severe mental illness. *Australian Occupational Therapy Journal, 62*(5), 316–325. https://doi.org/10.1111/1440-1630.12202

BIBLIOGRAPHY

Alexandratos, K., Barnett, F., & Thomas, Y. (2012). The impact of exercise on the mental health and quality of life of people with severe mental illness: A critical review. *The British Journal of Occupational Therapy, 75*(2), 48–60. https://doi.org/10.4276/030802212X13286281650956

Arbesman, M., & Logsdon, D. W. (2011). Occupational therapy interventions for employment and education for adults with serious mental illness: A systematic review. *American Journal of Occupational Therapy, 65*(3), 238–246. https://doi.org/10.5014/ajot.2011.001289

Bejerholm, U., & Areberg, C. (2014). Factors related to the return to work potential in persons with severe mental illness. *Scandinavian Journal of Occupational Therapy, 21*(4), 277–286. https://doi.org/10.3109/11038128.2014.889745

Blank, A. A., Harries, P., & Reynolds, F. (2015). "Without occupation you don't exist": Occupational engagement and mental illness. *Journal of Occupational Science, 22*(2), 197–209. https://doi.org/10.1080/14427591.2014.882250

Bonsaksen, T. (2012). Exploring gender differences in quality of life. *Mental Health Review Journal, 17*(1), 39–49. https://doi.org/10.1108/13619321211231815

Briand, C., & Menear, M. (2014). Implementing a continuum of evidence-based psychosocial interventions for people with severe mental illness: Part 2—Review of critical implementation issues. *Canadian Journal of Psychiatry, 59*(4), 187–195.

Brown, C. (2012). *Occupational therapy practice guidelines for adults with serious mental illness.* AOTA Press.

Brown, C., Geiszler, L. C., Lewis, K. J., & Arbesman, M. (2018). Effectiveness of interventions for weight loss for people with serious mental illness: A systematic review and meta-analysis. *American Journal of Occupational Therapy, 72*(5), Article 7205190030. https://doi.org/10.5014/ajot.2018.033415

Carson, N. E., Blake, C. E., & Saunders, R. (2015). Perceptions and dietary intake of self-described healthy and unhealthy eaters with severe mental illness. *Community Mental Health Journal, 51*, 281–288. https://doi.org/10.1007/s10597-014-9806-8

Conn, A., Bourke, N., James, C., & Haracz, K. (2019). Occupational therapy intervention addressing weight gain and obesity in people with severe mental illness: A scoping review. *Australian Occupational Therapy Journal, 66*(4), 446–457. https://doi.org/10.1111/1440-1630.12575

Cook, J. A., Razzano, L., Jonikas, J. A., Swarbrick, M. A., Steigman, P. J., Hamilton, M. M., Carter, T. M., & Santos, A. B. (2016). Correlates of co-occurring diabetes and obesity among community mental health program members with serious mental illnesses. *Psychiatric Services, 67*(11), 1269–1271. https://doi.org/10.1176/appi.ps.201500219

Cook, J. A., Razzano, L. A., Swarbrick, M. A., Jonikas, J. A., Yost, C., Burke, L., Steigman, P. J., & Santos, A. (2015). Health risks and changes in self-efficacy following community health screening of adults with serious mental illnesses. *PLOS ONE, 10*(4), Article e0123552. https://doi.org/10.1371/journal.pone.0123552

D'Amico, M. L., Jaffe, L. E., & Gardner, J. A. (2018). Evidence for interventions to improve and maintain occupational performance and participation for people with serious mental illness: A systematic review. *American Journal of Occupational Therapy, 72*(5), Article 7205190020. https://doi.org/10.5014/ajot.2018.033332

DeAngelis, T., Mollo, K., Giordano, C., Scotten, M., & Fecondo, B. (2019). Occupational therapy programming facilitates goal attainment in a community work rehabilitation setting. *Journal of Psychosocial Rehabilitation and Mental Health, 6*, 107–115. https://doi.org/10.1007/s40737-018-00133-5

Désormeaux-Moreau, M., Aubin, G., & Larivière, N. (2017). Home safety issues experienced by people with mental health conditions: Theoretical reflection on related ethical issues. *Journal of Ethics in Mental Health, 10*, 1–14.

Doroud, N., Fossey, E., & Fortune, T. (2015). Recovery as an occupational journey: A scoping review exploring the links between occupational engagement and recovery for people with enduring mental health issues. *Australian Occupational Therapy Journal, 62*(6), 378–392. https://doi.org/10.1111/1440-1630.12238

Gibson, R. W., D'Amico, M., Jaffe, L., & Arbesman, M. (2011). Occupational therapy interventions for recovery in the areas of community integration and normative life roles for adults with serious mental illness: A systematic review. *American Journal of Occupational Therapy, 65*(3), 247–256. https://doi.org/10.5014/ajot.2011.001297

Gruhl, K. L. R. (2010). The employment rights of people with serious mental illness in Ontario: Considering the influence of dominant ideology on marginalizing practices. *World Federation of Occupational Therapists Bulletin, 62*(1), 33–39. https://doi.org/10.1179/otb.2010.62.1.007

Hasson, H., Andersson, M., & Bejerholm, U. (2011). Barriers in implementation of evidence-based practice: Supported employment in Swedish context. *Journal of Health Organization and Management 25*(3), 332–345. https://doi.org/10.1108/14777261111143563

Jackman, M. M. (2016). Occupational therapy services. In N. N. Sing, J. W. Barber, & S. Van Sant (Eds.), *Handbook of recovery in inpatient psychiatry* (pp. 279–308). Springer Nature.

Kidd, S. A., Virdee, G., Krupa, T., Burnham, D., Hemingway, D., Margolin, I., Patterson, M., & Zabkiewicz, D. (2013). The role of gender in housing for individuals with severe mental illness: A qualitative study of the Canadian service context. *BMJ Open, 3*(6), Article 3002914. https://doi.org/10.1136/bmjopen-2013-002914

McGuire, A. B., Lysaker, P. H., & Wasmuth, S. (2015). Altered self-experience and goal setting in severe mental illness. *American Journal of Psychiatric Rehabilitation, 18*(4), 333–362. https://doi.org/10.1080/15487768.2015.1089800

McKay, E. A. (2010). "Rip that book up, I've changed": Unveiling the experiences of women living with and surviving enduring mental illness. *British Journal of Occupational Therapy, 73*(3), 96–105. https://doi.org/10.4276/030802210X12682330090370

Menear, M., & Briand, C. (2014). Implementing a continuum of evidence-based psychosocial interventions for people with severe mental illness: Part 1—Review of major initiatives and implementation strategies. *Canadian Journal of Psychiatry, 59*(4), 178–186.

Milbourn, B., McNamara, B., & Buchanan, A. (2015). The lived experience of everyday activity for individuals with severe mental illness. *Health Sociology Review, 24*(3), 270–282. https://doi.org/10.1080/14461242.2015.1034747

Milbourn, B., McNamara, B., & Buchanan, A. (2017). A qualitative study of occupational well-being for people with severe mental illness. *Scandinavian Journal of Occupational Therapy, 24*(4), 269–280. https://doi.org/10.1080/11038128.2016.1241824

Noyes, S. (2015). Living in the community with serious mental illness: Occupational therapy's role in a community residential setting. *OT Practice, 20*(21), 23–26.

Noyes, S., Sokolow, H., & Arbesman, M. (2018). Evidence for occupational therapy intervention with employment and education for adults with serious mental illness: A systematic review. *American Journal of Occupational Therapy, 72*(5), Article 7205190010. https://doi.org/10.5014/ajot.2018.033068

Northey, A., & Barnett, F. (2012). Physical health parameters: Comparison of people with severe mental illness with the general population. *British Journal of Occupational Therapy, 75*(2), 100–105. https://doi.org/10.4276/030802212X13286281651199

Pelletier, J. F., Corbière, M., Lecomte, T., Briand, C., Corrigan, P., Davidson, L., & Rowe, M. (2015). Citizenship and recovery: Two intertwined concepts for civic-recovery. *BMC Psychiatry, 15*, Article 37. https://doi.org/10.1186/s12888-015-0420-2

Pfeiffer, B., Brusilovskiy, E., Bauer, J., & Salzer, M. S. (2014). Sensory processing, participation, and recovery in adults with serious mental illnesses. *Psychiatric Rehabilitation Journal, 37*(4), 289–296. https://doi.org/10.1037/prj0000099

Redlich, D., Hadas-Lidor, N., Weiss, P., & Amirav, I. (2010). Mediated learning experience intervention increases hope of family members coping with a relative with severe mental illness. *Community Mental Health Journal, 46*, 409–415. https://doi.org/10.1007/s10597-009-9234-3

Rempfer, M., Brown, C., & Hamera, E. (2011). Learning potential as a predictor of skill acquisition in people with serious mental illness. *Psychiatry Research, 185*(1-2), 293–295. https://doi.org/10.1016/j.psychres.2009.12.009

Rigby, L., & Wilson, I. (2017). Occupational therapy interventions for someone experiencing severe and enduring mental illness. In C. Long, J. Cronin-Davis, & D. Cotterill (Eds.), *Occupational therapy evidence in practice for mental health* (2nd ed., pp. 109–137). Wiley.

Sells, C. H., & Stoffel, V. D. (2011). Strategies to enable meaningful everyday living for people with psychiatric disabilities and other mental health needs. In C. H. Christiansen & K. M. Matuska (Eds.), *Ways of living: Intervention strategies to enable participations* (4th ed., pp. 405–429). AOTA Press.

Sutton, D., Bejerholm, U., & Eklund, M. (2019). Empowerment, self and engagement in day center occupations: A longitudinal study among people with long-term mental illness. *Scandinavian Journal of Occupational Therapy, 26*(1), 69–78. https://doi.org/10.1080/11038128.2017.1397742

Swarbrick, M. (2019). Providing occupational therapy services for persons with major mental disorders: Promoting recovery and wellness. In B. A. B. Schell & G. Gillen (Eds.), *Willard and Spackman's occupational therapy* (13th ed., pp. 1036–1046). Wolters Kluwer.

Tjörnstrand, C., Bejerholm, U., & Eklund, M. (2011). Participation in day centres for people with psychiatric disabilities: Characteristics of occupations. *Scandinavian Journal of Occupational Therapy, 18*(4), 243–253. https://doi.org/10.3109/11038128.2011.583938

Villotti, P., Corbière, M., Fossey, E., Fraccaroli, F., Lecomte, T., & Harvey, C. (2017). Work accommodations and natural supports for employees with severe mental illness in social businesses: An International comparison. *Community Mental Health Journal, 53*, 864–870. https://doi.org/10.1007/s10597-016-0068-5

Waghorn, G., Stephenson, A., & Browne, D. (2011). The importance of service integration in developing effective employment services for people with severe mental health conditions. *British Journal of Occupational Therapy, 74*(7), 339–347. https://doi.org/10.4276/0308022 11X13099513661153

Williams, A. E., Fossey, E., Corbière M., Paluch, T., & Harvey, C. (2016). Work participation for people with severe mental illnesses: An integrative review of factors impacting job tenure. *Australian Occupational Therapy Journal, 63*(2), 65–85. https://doi.org/10.1111/1440-1630.12237

Williams, L., Magin, P., Sultana, J., & Haracz, K. (2016). The role of occupational therapists in the provision of dietary interventions for people with severe mental illness: Results from a national survey. *British Journal of Occupational Therapy, 79*(7), 442–449. https://doi.org/10 .1177/0308022615620680

Substance-Related and Addictive Disorders

Also called addiction, substance abuse, substance addiction, substance dependence, substance use disorder, substance misuse, drug addiction, alcoholism.

See also Fetal Alcohol Spectrum Disorder.

Description

Substance-related disorders involve drugs that directly activate the brain's reward system. The activation of the reward system typically results in feelings of pleasure: The specific pleasurable feelings evoked vary widely depending on the drug (Porter, 2018). Substance-related disorders encompass 10 separate classes of drugs: alcohol; caffeine; cannabis; hallucinogens; inhalants; opioids; sedatives, hypnotics, and anxiolytics; stimulants; tobacco; and other or unknown substances (e.g., gambling; American Psychiatric Association, 2013).

Substance-related disorders are divided into two groups: substance use disorders and substance-induced disorders. *Substance use disorders* involve a pathological pattern of behaviors in which patients continue to use a substance despite experiencing significant problems related to its use. There may also be physiologic manifestations, including changes in brain circuitry. *Substance-induced disorders* include intoxication, withdrawal, and substance or medication-induced mental disorders (psychotic, bipolar, depressive, anxiety, obsessive-compulsive, sleep, sexual dysfunctions, delirium, and neurocognitive disorders). *Substance-induced disorders* involve the direct effects of a drug on the body (American Psychiatric Association, 2013; Porter, 2018).

The classification under substance-related disorders is not based on whether a drug is legal (e.g., alcohol, caffeine), illegal or illicit (e.g., hallucinogens), available by prescription (e.g., morphine, lorazepam), or considered to be a narcotic (e.g., opium, opium derivatives).

Substance use disorders involve negative patterns of behavior, including the following:

- impaired control (e.g., using more than intended or unable to cut down when wanting to do so);
- social impairment (e.g., unable to meet established roles such as worker or parent);
- risky use (e.g., continuing to use despite negative outcomes); and
- pharmacological criteria (tolerance and withdrawal; American Psychiatric Association, 2013).

Cause

Ingestion or inhalation of the substance. Substance is used for various reasons, such as altering or enhance mood, part of religious ceremonies, obtaining spiritual enlightenment, or enhancing performance (Porter, 2018). Lancaster and Chacksfield (2014) suggested seven reasons related to the occupational perspective. The first six reasons are socially sanctioned uses, while the last two are not presently socially sanctioned.

- Enabling occupation: by reducing tension, removing inhibition, stimulating mental alertness, and through imitating others' drug use.
- Coping mechanism: to counter anxiety, to relieve pain, mask distress, increase confidence and peer acceptance, or as self-medication for mental health problems.
- Altering perception: to develop a wider understanding of life, for desired spiritual attainment, as part of a religious ritual, to assist creativity, to enjoy drug-induced perception.
- Adding meaning: through the ritual and habits of drug-taking behavior, the routine of obtaining drugs or drug dealing, the excitement of illegal activities, or through interacting and sharing a culture with associates in a drug-using network.
- Enhancing occupations: by celebrating positive events, enhancing good feelings, or removing negative emotional states.
- Managing occupational risk factors: to cope with occupational deprivation, occupational deficiency, idleness and/or boredom ("killing time"), or coping with occupational imbalance such as the pressure of too many demands on one's time.
- Avoiding occupation: through intoxication, stimulus seeking, denial of responsibility, or through escape into drug culture and addiction status (adapted from Lancaster & Chacksfield, 2014).
- Imposed occupation: culture of drinking and smoking related to payment in wine and tobacco for services in lieu of money (Cloete & Ramugondo, 2015).

Terminology

- *Addiction* is defined as a "disease of brain reward, motivation, memory, and related circuitry. Dysfunction in these circuits leads to characteristic biological, psychological, social and spiritual manifestations. This (dysfunction) is reflected in an individual pathologically pursuing reward and/or relief by substance use and other behaviors" (American Society of Addiction Medicine, 2011, p. 1).
- *Craving:* Desires for the drug that preclude or block thinking about anything else and are associated with specific reward pathways in the brain that are more likely in an environmental context of previous use. Cravings are viewed as a signal of an impending relapse (American Psychiatric Association, 2013).
- *Impaired control:* Taking larger amounts of a substance than intended over time, many unsuccessful attempts to reduce use, persistent desire to decrease or discontinue use, person's daily activities revolve around obtaining the substance and recovering from its use (American Psychiatric Association, 2013).
- *Intoxication disorder:* Short-term symptoms associated with current use of a substance including the problematic behaviors and psychological changes (American Psychiatric Association, 2013).
- *Risky use:* Person consumes substances in spite of being physically hazardous and despite knowing the substance use is causing persistent physical, legal, and/or psychological problems (American Psychiatric Association, 2013).
- *Social impairment:* Persistent substance use associated with inability to carry out major or key occupational roles, serious social and interpersonal problems, and withdrawal from leisure occupations and family activities (American Psychiatric Association, 2013).
- *Tolerance:* Person requires increased amounts of a substance to get the desired effect or experiences a significantly reduced effect when usual dosage is consumed (American Psychiatric Association, 2013).
- *Withdrawal:* Occurs when blood or tissue concentrations decline in a person who has used heavily, which makes the person more likely to consume again to relieve symptoms (American Psychiatric Association, 2013).
- *Withdrawal disorder:* Symptoms that occur immediately and for a longer period after a client who has been heavily using a substance stops ingesting, including problematic behaviors (American Psychiatric Association, 2013).

Evaluation/Assessment

Areas

- Activities of Daily Living/Instrumental ADL: self-care and self-maintenance skills, independent living skills including homemaking, meal preparation, budget and financial management, functional mobility, medication management, shopping, driving and transportation, health literacy
- Education/Work: academic performance, employment status
- Play/Leisure: interests, values, frequency, location, level of satisfaction
- Rest/Sleep: sleep disturbance
- Social Participation: frequency, type, location, with whom
- Sensorimotor: fine motor coordination
- Cognitive/Perceptual: attention, memory, learning, executive functions, metacognition, altered perceptions
- Psychosocial: emotional regulation, social skills and relationships, quality of life
- Context/Environment: social support system, information needs of stakeholders, environmental modification or change
- Comorbidities: mental illness (schizophrenia, bipolar disorders, depression, personality disorder), stress disorder such as posttraumatic stress disorder (PTSD), or other medical conditions such as diabetes, high blood pressure, cardiac disease, pulmonary disorders, gastrointestinal disorders that existed prior to the substance abuse disorder but may be aggravated by the addiction, homelessness, pain and chronic pain

Instruments

Types may include screening assessments, structured questionnaires, interviews, risk assessments, observations, performance-function-based assessments, or physiological assessment (urine, blood analysis, electrocardiogram [ECG]).

Instruments Developed by Occupational Therapy Personnel

- Adolescent/Adult Sensory Profile (AASP; Brown & Dunn, 2002)
- Allen Cognitive Level Screen (5th ed.; ACLS-5; Allen et al., 2007; see also Rojo-Mota et al., 2017, in References)
- Assessment of Motor and Process Skills (8th ed.; AMPS-8; Fisher & Bray Jones, 2016; see also Rojo-Mota et al., 2017, in References)
- Canadian Occupational Performance Measure (5th ed.; COPM-5; Law et al., 2014)
- Dynamic Loewenstein Occupational Therapy Cognitive Assessment (DLOTCA; Katz et al., 2012; see also Rojo-Mota et al., 2017, in References)
- Interest Checklist (ICL; Matsutsuyu, 1969; see also Modified Interest Checklist forms; Kielhofner & Neville, 1983)
- Lifestyle History Questionnaire (LHQ; Martin et al., 2015, in References)
- Model of Human Occupational Screening Tool (Version 2.0; MOHOST 2.0; Parkinson et al., 2006)
- Occupational Circumstances Assessment Interview and Rating Scale (Version 4.0; OCAIRS; Forsyth et al., 2005)
- Occupational Performance History Interview (Version 2.1; OPHI-II; Kielhofner et al., 2004)
- Occupational Self-Assessment (Version 2.2; OSA 2.2; Baron et al., 2006)
- Role Checklist (RC; Oakley et al., 1986; see also Role Checklist Version 3: Participation and Satisfaction [RCv3], Scott, 2019)
- Self-Development Group Survey (SDGS; Peloquin, 2010, in References)
- Test of Grocery Shopping Skills (TOGSS; Brown et al., 2009)
- Volitional Questionnaire (Version 4.1; VQ 4.1; de las Heras et al., 2007)
- Work Environment Impact Scale (WEIS; Moore-Corner et al., 1998)

Instruments Developed by Other Professionals and Used by Occupational Therapy Personnel

- Addiction Severity Index (5th ed.; ASI-5; McLellan et al., 1992)

- Alcohol Problems Questionnaire (APQ; Williams & Drummond, 1994)
- Alcohol Use Disorders Identification Test–Consumption (AUDIT-C; Bush et al., 1998)
- Beck Depression Inventory (2nd ed.; BDI-II; Beck et al., 1996)
- CAGE Alcohol Questionnaire (CAGE; Ewing, 1984)
- Career Exploration Inventory (5th ed.; CEI-5; Liptak, 2015)
- Client Satisfaction Questionnaire-8 (CSQ-8; Attkisson & Greenfield, 1994)
- Coping Responses Inventory (CRI; Adult Form; Moos, 1993)
- Drug Abuse Screening Test (DAST; Gavin et al., 1989)
- Fagerström Test for Nicotine Dependence (FTND; Heatherton et al., 1991)
- Internal/External Locus of Control Scale (I/ELOC; Rotter, 1966)
- Metacognition Assessment Scale–Abbreviated (MAS; Semerari et al., 2003)
- Montreal Cognitive Assessment (MoCA; Nasreddine et al., 2005; see also Sawant et al., 2017, in References)
- Personal Growth Initiative Scale-II (PGIS-II; Robitschek et al., 2012
- Readiness to Return to Work Scale (RRWS; Franche et al., 2007)
- Rosenberg Self-Esteem Scale (RSES; Rosenberg, 1965)
- Severity of Alcohol Dependence Questionnaire (SADQ; Stockwell et al., 1983)
- Short Michigan Alcoholism Screening Instrument Geriatric Version (SMAST-G; Regents, University of Michigan, 1991)
- Short Opiate Withdrawal Scale (SOWS; Gossop, 1990)
- Social Skills Inventory (SSI; Del Prette & Del Prette, 2013)
- Spiritual Well-Being Scale (SWBS; Ellison, 1983)
- Treatment Outcomes Profile (TOP; Marsden et al., 2008)

Problems/Issues

Activities of Daily Living/Instrumental ADL
- Person may neglect to perform basic ADLs, such as changing clothes regularly, bathing or washing, grooming and hygiene, eating regularly.
- Person may have difficulty with finances (money management and budgeting), driving safely and soberly, shopping, securing and maintaining housing.

Education/Work
- Person's attendance may be irregular leading to termination.
- Person's academic or work performance may become substandard (grades decrease, performance evaluation unsatisfactory).
- Person may be engaged in illegal or nonsanctioned work such as prostitution, pimping, selling and distributing drugs, manufacturing or growing illegal crops.
- Person may have difficulty identifying legal, positive, or sanctioned work and productive activities to aid recovery.

Play/Leisure
- Person may discontinue or withdraw from engaging in favorite leisure activities.
- Person may have few or no leisure activities.

Rest/Sleep
- Person may experience sleep disturbances.
- Person may have no established sleep routine.

Social Participation
- Person may discontinue participation in social activities with previous group of friends.
- Person may only participate with persons who share the addiction culture.

Sensorimotor
- Person may have experienced chronic pain and use substances to control the pain.

- Person may have hypersensitivity or hyposensitivity to certain stimuli.
- Person may have a sensory processing disorder (Engel-Yeger, 2014).

Cognitive/Perceptual

- Person may have difficulty paying attention and concentrating.
- Person may experience memory lapses due to blackouts.
- Person may have no set routine, schedule, or time-management system.

Psychosocial

- Person may experience boredom due to lack of participation in meaningful occupations other than securing drugs or alcohol.
- Person may experience stressors that lead to the addicting behaviors and stressors that are a result of the substance abuse, such as loss of employment, divorce, death of loved one, loss of friends, lack of funds to pay rent.
- Person may experience loss of role identity and poor role performance.
- Person may lack motivation to change behavior or experience fluctuating motivation.
- Person may lack awareness of illness or disabilities.
- Person may have lost hope that change is possible and experience a sense of hopelessness and helplessness about life situation.
- Person may have low self-esteem and a sense of worthlessness.
- Person may be ambivalent about participating in an intervention program because change involves giving up the "good" aspects of the addicting behavior as well as "bad."

Context/Environment

- Person may lack social support from family, friends, coworkers, or employer.
- Person may lack knowledge of services available or how to access them.
- Person may challenge the distinction between legal, socially sanctioned drug use as opposed to the position of some drug use viewed as illicit and distribution as being socially unacceptable (Kiepek, 2016).

Intervention/Treatment

Models and programs developed by occupational therapy personnel include case studies (Costa, 2017; Hoppes et al., 2013; Raphael-Greenfield, 2019), cognitive disabilities model (Rojo-Mota et al., 2017), GESTTO (Hermeto et al., 2012), intensive residential program (e.g., ADA House; Hoppes et al., 2013; Peloquin, 2010; Peloquin & Ciro, 2013), life skills group classes (Abaoğlu et al., 2017; Hoppes et al., 2013), medication management (American Occupational Therapy Association, 2017), model of sensory processing (Stols et al., 2013), self-development group (Hoppes et al., 2013), Tree Theme Method (Cardinale et al., 2014), and theory of human need for occupation (Jennings & Cronin-Davis, 2016). Models and programs developed by other professionals but used by occupational therapy personnel include addictions program and career exploration (Darko-Mensah, 2011), Dual Diagnosis Anonymous (Roush et al., 2015), multidisciplinary approach (Crouch & Wegner, 2014), opioid guidelines (Rowe & Breeden, 2018), Solution-Focused Brief Therapy (SFBT; Hoppes et al., 2013), and Stages of Change (Prochaska & DiClemente, 1986, cited in Lancaster & Chacksfield, 2014). Team members include physicians, nursing personnel, psychologists, social workers, peer counselors, and occupational therapy personnel. The goal of intervention is to help individuals to develop life skills and coping strategies, and a more satisfying balanced lifestyle (Lancaster & Chacksfield, 2014). Specific goals including developing coping skills to address frustration, learning to handle stresses and challenges, promoting healthy and meaningful substance-free activities, enhancing occupational performance and life skills, cultivating problem-solving strategies to support life satisfaction, and enhancing communication and self-expression skills (Peloquin, 2010).

Activities of Daily Living/Instrumental ADL

- Provide program or module on regaining activities of daily living habits (e.g., see Precin, 2014).
- Assist client in developing skills to care for others such as parenting classes, caregiving responsibilities, and care of pets.
- Assist client to develop living skills (household management, budgeting, meal preparation, effective communication (letter writing and phone use).

Education/Work

- Assist client to develop work readiness skills such as filling out application forms, mastering local bus schedule, and identifying suitable jobs from the classified ads or online job available databases.
- Assist client to explore and develop productive occupations that are legal and sanctioned, can provide a source of income, and contribute to creating a routine in time management.

Play/Leisure

- Assist client to explore, develop, or redevelop leisure interests and skills.
- Assist client to integrate leisure occupations into daily life schedule.
- Assist client to enhance self-expression through leisure occupations.

Rest/Sleep

- Assist client to identify safe sleep locations.
- Assist client to develop a regular sleep routine and associated habits.
- Discuss with client other ways of dealing with problems than sleeping the day away.

Social Participation

- Assist client to identify and participate in sanctioned social activities related to leisure interests and skills.

Sensorimotor

- Provide an exercise program that is integrated into the client's daily schedule.
- Assist client in participating in a pain management program (see Pain and Chronic Pain in Section 2: Sensory Disorders).
- Assist client to address sensory sensitivities to achieve better control and response to situations in which the stimuli may occur, such as too much light, too much noise, too cold, or too warm.

Cognitive/Perceptual

- Provide program or module on time management (establishing a routine, following a schedule; e.g., see Precin, 2014).
- Provide program or module on executive functions and metacognition including problem solving, planning, setting goals and priorities, and discussion of results.
- Assist client to identify, appreciate, and engage in meaningful and healthy substance-free lifestyle.

Psychosocial

- Provide program or module on stress management that includes identifying stressors, triggers, and management approaches (e.g., see Precin, 2014).
- Provide program or module on building social skills in sobriety (e.g., see Precin, 2014). Role playing is a useful technique to discuss anger management.
- Provide program or module on self-development to target self-discovery, self-expression, and self-management.
- Provide program or module on relaxation training including stretching, visual imagery, progressive muscle relaxation, self-massage, deep breathing, meditative exercises, or yoga.

- Assist client to reestablish a sense of hopefulness through successful completion of occupations, following a schedule, participating in a leisure activity, or successfully solving a personal problem (setting a goal and achieving it).
- Assist client to identify and clarify values.
- Assist client to increase sense of self as capable of insight, change, master, and self-direction.

Context/Environment

- Determine whether an evaluation of the workplace might be helpful to address ergonomic issues contributing to pain and whether modifications might reduce pain.

Precautions/Safety Considerations

Person is at risk for overdose of drugs. Person may lose consciousness due to excessive drinking. Person may be at risk for seizures due to brain response to drugs. Person is at risk for injury to self or others if intoxicated while driving. Person is at risk for suicide or accidental death from overdose.

Prognosis and Outcome

Mixed results. Relapse occurs especially in clients with poor coping and assertion skills (da Silva et al., 2018). Suicide and accidental death have occurred. The consequences of intervention of substance use disorders vary greatly depending on the substance (Porter, 2018).

Cost Effectiveness

Intensive package of care (8 a.m.–5 p.m., 5 days per week, full complement of staff, including occupational therapy) was 18 times more expensive than the nonintensive package of care (one professional visit per week and one weekly group session) in Brazil (Becker & Razzouk, 2018).

REFERENCES

Abaoğlu, H., Cesim, Ö. B., Kars, S., & Çelik, Z. (2017). Life skills in occupational therapy. In M. Huri (Ed.), *Occupational therapy—Occupation focused holistic practice in rehabilitation*. Intech. https://doi.org/10.5772/intechopen.68462

American Occupational Therapy Association. (2017). Occupational therapy's role in medication management. *American Journal of Occupational Therapy, 71*(Suppl. 2), Article 7112410025. https://doi.org/10.5014/ajot.2017.716S02

American Psychiatric Association. (2013). *Diagnostic and statistical manual of mental disorders* (5th ed.). https://doi.org/10.1176/appi.books.9780890425596

American Society of Addiction Medicine. (2011, April 12). *Public policy statement: Definition of addiction.* https://www.asam.org/docs/default-source/public-policy-statements/1definition_of_addiction_long_4-11.pdf?sfvrsn=a8f64512_4

Becker, P., & Razzouk, D. (2018). Cost of a community mental health service: A retrospective study on a psychosocial care center for alcohol and drug users in São Paulo. *Sao Paulo Medical Journal, 136*(5), 433–441. https://doi.org/10.1590/1516-3180.2018.0164310818

Cardinale, J., Malacari, L., Broggi, S., Savignano, J., & Fisher, G. (2014). Model of occupational empowerment and Gunnarsson's Tree Theme: Intervention for mothers in recovery. *Occupational Therapy in Mental Health, 30*(1), 43–68. https://doi.org/10.1080/0164212X.2014.878237

Cloete, L. G., & Ramugondo, E. L. (2015). "I drink": Mothers' alcohol consumption as both individualized and imposed occupation. *South African Journal of Occupational Therapy, 45*(1), 34–40. https://doi.org/10.17159/2310-3833/2015/v45no1a6

Costa, D. (2017). Occupational therapy's role in countering opioid addiction. *OT Practice, 22*(1), 13–16.

Crouch, R., & Wegner, L. (2014). Substance use and abuse: Intervention by a multidisciplinary approach which includes occupational therapy. In R. Crouch & L. Wegner (Eds.), *Occupa-*

tional therapy in psychiatry and mental health (5th ed., pp. 446–464). Wiley. https://doi.org/ 10.1002/9781118913536.ch28

da Silva, M. L., Hatanaka, Y. F., de Cássia Rondina, R., & da Silva, N. R. (2018). Evaluation of the repertory of social skills of users of psychoactive substances under treatment. *Cadernos Brasileiros de Terapia Ocupacional da UFSCar, 26*(4), 849–858. https://doi.org/10.4322/2526-89 10.ctoAO1633

Darko-Mensah, S. (2011). Working addictions: The development, implementation and evaluation of the pilot group Career Exploration 101. *Occupational Therapy Now, 13*(6), 5–6.

Engel-Yeger, B. (2014). Sensory processing disorders among substance dependents. *Cadernos Brasileiros de Terapia Ocupacional da UFSCar, 22*(Suppl.), 111–118. https://doi.org/10.4322/ cto.2014.035

Hermeto, E. M. C., de Araújo Fernandes, L., da Silva, N. M., & de Holanda, I. C. L. C. (2012). Theater as a therapeutic resource for the prevention of substance abuse: Teenagers' perception. *Revista Brasileira em Promoção da saúde, 26*(3), 329–335.

Hoppes, S., Bryce, H. R., & Peloquin, S. M. (2013). Substance abuse and occupational therapy. In E. Cara & A. MacRae (Eds.), *Psychosocial occupational therapy: An evolving practice* (3rd ed., pp. 840–875). Delmar Cengage Learning.

Jennings, H., & Cronin-Davis, J. (2016). Investigating binge drinking using interpretative phenomenological analysis: Occupation for health or harm? *Journal of Occupational Science, 23*(2), 245–254. https://doi.org/10.1080/14427591.2015.1101387

Kiepek, N. (2016). *Licit, illicit, prescribe: Substance use and occupational therapy.* Canadian Association of Occupational Therapists.

Lancaster, J., & Chacksfield, J. (2014). Substance misuse. In W. Bryant, J. Fieldhouse, & K. Bannigan (Eds.), *Creek's occupational therapy and mental health* (5th ed., pp. 439–455). Churchill Livingstone Elsevier.

Martin, L. M., Triscari, R., Boisvert, R. Hipp, K., Gersten, J., West, R. C., Kisling, E., Donham, A., Kollar, N., & Escobar, P. (2015). Development and evaluation of the Lifestyle History Questionnaire (LHQ) for people entering treatment for substance addictions. *American Journal of Occupational Therapy, 69*(3), Article 6903250010. https://doi.org/10.5014/ajot.2015.014050

Peloquin, S. M. (2010). Occupational therapy among women in recovery from addition. *OT Practice, 15*(9), 12–15, 22.

Peloquin, S. M., & Ciro, C. A. (2013). Self-development groups among women in recovery: Client perceptions of satisfaction and engagement. *American Journal of Occupational Therapy, 67*(1), 82–90. https://doi.org/10.5014/ajot.2013.004796

Porter, R. S. (Ed.). (2018). *The Merck manual of diagnosis and therapy* (20th ed.). Merck Sharp & Dohme.

Precin, P. (2014). *Living skills recovery workbook* (2nd ed.). Echo Point Books.

Raphael-Greenfield, E. (2019). Substance-related and addictive disorders. In B. J. Atchison & D. P. Dirette (Eds.), *Conditions in occupational therapy* (5th ed., pp. 257–288). Wolters Kluwer.

Rojo-Mota, G., Pedrero-Pérez, E. J., de León, J. M. R. S., León-Frade, I., Aldea-Poyo, P., Alonso-Rodríguez, M., Pedrero-Aguilar, J., & Morales-Alonso, S. (2017). Loewenstein Occupational Therapy Cognitive Assessment to evaluate people with addictions. *Occupational Therapy International, 2017*, Article 2750328. https://doi.org/10.1155/2017/2750328

Roush, S., Monica, C., Carpenter-Song, E., & Drake, R. E. (2015). First-Person perspectives on dual diagnosis anonymous (DDA): A qualitative study. *Journal of Dual Diagnosis, 11*(2), 136–141. https://doi.org/10.1080/15504263.2015.1025215

Rowe, N. C., & Breeden, K. L. (2018). Opioid guidelines and their implications for occupational therapy. *OT Practice, 23*(15), CE-1–CE-8.

Sawant, P., Gokhale, P., & Ferzandi, A. (2017). Screening of chronic alcoholics for cognitive impairment using Montreal Cognitive Assessment—Occupational therapy perspective. *Journal of Health Management, 19*(4), 634–648. https://doi.org/10.1177/0972063417727620

Stols, D., van Heerden, R., Van Jaarsvel, A., & Nel, R. (2013). Substance abusers' anger behavior and sensory processing patterns: An occupational therapy investigation. *South African Journal of Occupational Therapy*, *43*(1), 25–34.

BIBLIOGRAPHY

Amorelli, C. R. (2016). Psychosocial occupational therapy interventions for substance-use disorders: A narrative review. *Occupational Therapy in Mental Health*, *32*(2), 167–184. https://doi.org/10.1080/0164212X.2015.1134293

Andersson, C., Eklund, M., Sundh, V., Thundal, K. L., & Spak, F. (2012). Women's patterns of everyday occupations and alcohol consumption. *Scandinavian Journal of Occupational Therapy*, *19*(3), 225–238. https://doi.org/ 10.3109/11038128.2010.527013

Bell, T., Wegner, L., Blake, L., Jupp, L., Nyabenda, F., & Turner, T. (2015). Clients' perception of an occupational therapy intervention at a substance use rehabilitation centre in the Western Cape. *South African Journal of Occupational Therapy*, *45*(2), 10–14. https://doi.org/10.17159/2310-3833/2015/v45n2a3

Davies, R., & Cameron, J. (2010). Self-identified occupational competencies, limitations and priorities for change in the occupational lives of people with drug misuse problems. *British Journal of Occupational Therapy*, *73*(6), 251–260. https://doi.org/10.4276/030802210X12759925468907

Gomes, R. R., Ribeiro, M. C., Matlas, E. C., Brěda, M. Z., & Mângla, E. F. (2015). Motivation and expectations in treatment search for abusive use and addiction of crack, alcohol and other drugs. *Revista de Terapia Ocupacional da Universidad of São Paulo*, *26*(3), 326–335. https://doi.org/10.11606/issn.2238-6149.v26i3p326-335

Hoxmark, E., Wynn, T. N., & Wynn, R. (2012). Loss of activities and its effect on the well-being of substance abusers. *Scandinavian Journal of Occupational Therapy*, *19*(1), 78–83. https://doi.org/10.3109/11038128.2011.552120

Kiepek, N. (2016). Exploring legitimacy and authority in the construction of truth regarding personal experiences of drug use. *Journal of Addiction Research & Therapy*, *7*(2), Article 1000273. https://doi.org/10.4172/2155-6105.1000273

Kiepek, N., & Baron, J. L. (2019). Use of substances among professionals and students of professional programs: A review of the literature. *Drugs: Education, Prevention and Policy*, *26*(1), 6–31. https://doi.org/10.1080/09687637.2017.1375080

Kiepek, N., & Beagan, B. (2018). Substance use and professional identity. *Contemporary Drug Problems*, *45*(1), 47–66. https://doi.org/10.1177/0091450917748982

Kiepek, N., Beagan, B., & Harris, J. (2018). A pilot study to explore the effects of substances on cognition, mood, performance, and experience of daily activities. *Performance Enhancement & Health*, *6*(1), 3–11. https://doi.org/10.1016/j.peh.2018.02.003

Kiepek, N., & Magalhães, L. (2011). Addictions and impulse-control disorders as occupation: A selected literature review and synthesis. *Journal of Occupational Science*, *18*(3), 254–276. https://doi.org/10.1080/14427591.2011.581628

Knis-Matthews, L. (2010). The destructive path of addiction: Experiences of six patents who are substance dependent. *Occupational Therapy in Mental Health*, *26*(3), 201–340. https://doi.org/10.1080/0164212X.2010.498728

Leppard, A., Ramsay, M., Duncan, A., Malachowski, C., & Davis, J. A. (2018). Interventions for women with substance abuse issues: A scoping review. *American Journal of Occupational Therapy*, *72*(2), Article 7202205030. https://doi.org/10.5014/ajot.2018.022863

Louie, F. (2012). Occupational therapy and substance abuse: Case study of a teen. *World Federation of Occupational Therapists Bulletin*, *66*(1), 38–39. https://doi.org/10.1179/otb.2012.66.1.014

Luck, K., & Beagan, B. (2015). Occupational transition of smoking cessation in women: "You're restructuring your whole life." *Journal of Occupational Science*, *22*(2), 183–196. https://doi.org/10.1080/14427591.2014.887418

Martin, L. M., Smith, M., Rogers, J., Wallen, T., & Boisvert, R. (2011). Mothers in recovery: An occupational perspective. *Occupational Therapy International, 18*(3), 152–161. https://doi.org/10.1002/oti.318

McCombie, R. P. (2018). Prevalence of alcohol use and reasons for drinking among occupational therapists: An exploratory investigation. *Occupational Therapy in Mental Health, 34*(4), 389–404. https://doi.org/10.1080/0164212X.2018.1440365

McCombie, R. P., & Stirling, J. L. (2018). Opioid substance abuse among occupational therapy clients. *Occupational Therapy in Mental Health, 34*(1), 49–60. https://doi.org/10.1080/0164212x.2017.1360827

Mirza, M., Harrison, E. A., Chang, H. C., Salo, C., & Birman, D. (2018). Community perspectives on substance use among Bhutanese and Iraqi refugees resettled in the United States. *Journal of Prevention & Intervention in the Community, 46*(1), 43–60. https://doi.org/10.1080/10852352.2018.1385956

Morris, D. N., Johnson, A., Losier, A., Pierce, M., & Sridhar, V. (2013). Spirituality and substance abuse recovery. *Occupational Therapy in Mental Health, 29*(1), 78–84. https://doi.org/10.1080/0164212x.2013.761112

Moyers, P., & Stoffel, V. C. (2010). Preventing substance abuse in adolescents and adults. In M. E. Scoffa, S. M. Reitz, & M. A. Pizzi (Eds.), *Occupational therapy in the promotion of health and wellness* (pp. 280–306). F.A. Davis.

Narain, N., Liu, W., Mahmood, Z., & Duncan, A. (2018). Women's perspectives related to occupational performance following participation in substance use recovery programs. *Occupational Therapy in Mental Health, 34*(1), 61–74. https://doi.org/10.1080/0164212X.2017.1395309

Plach, H., & Stoffel, V. C. (2019). Substance abuse and co-occurring disorders. In C. Brown, V. C. Stoffel, & J. P. Muñoz (Eds.), *Occupational therapy in mental health: A vision for participation* (2nd ed., pp. 238–249). F.A. Davis.

Rojo-Mota, G., Pedrero-Pérez, E. J., de León, J. M. R. S., & Page, J. C. M. (2014). Assessment of motor and process skills in daily life activities of treated substance addicts. *Scandinavian Journal of Occupational Therapy, 21*(6), 458–464. https://doi.org/10.3109/11038128.2014.922610

Rojo-Mota, G., Pedrero-Pérez, E. J., & Huertas-Hoyas, E. (2017). Systematic review of occupational therapy in the treatment of addiction: Models, practice, and qualitative and quantitative research. *American Journal of Occupational Therapy, 71*(5), Article 7105100030. https://doi.org/10.5014/ajot.2017.022061

Rojo-Mota, G., Pedrero-Pérez, E. J., Huertas-Hoyas, E., Merritt, B., & MacKenzie, D. (2017). Allen Cognitive Level Screen for the classification of subjects treated for addiction. *Scandinavian Journal of Occupational Therapy, 24*(4), 290–298. https://doi.org/10.3109/11038128.2016.1161071

Scaffa, M. E., Riels, L. A., Moyers, P., & Stoffel, V. C. (2014). Community-based approaches for substance abuse disorders. In E. M. Scaffa & S. M. Reitz (Eds.), *Occupational therapy in community-based practice settings* (2nd ed., pp. 318–344). F.A. Davis.

Silver, M. (2015). Alcohol use in older adults: How occupational therapy can help. *OT Practice, 20*(9), 17–20.

Suarez, M., Horton-Bierema, W., & Bodine, C. (2018). Challenges and resources available for mothers in opiate recovery: A qualitative study. *Open Journal of Occupational Therapy, 6*(2), Article 2. https://doi.org/10.15453/2168-6408.1483

Swarbrick, M. A., Cook, J. A., Razzano, L. A., Jonikas, J. A., Gao, N., Williams, J., & Yudof, J. (2017). Correlates of current smoking among adults served by the public mental health system. *Journal of Dual Diagnosis, 13*(2), 82–90. https://doi.org/10.1080/15504263.2017.1296603

Sy, M. P., Ohshima, N., & Roraldo, P. N. R. (2018). The role of Filipino occupational therapists in substance addiction and rehabilitation: A Q-methodology. *Occupational Therapy in Mental Health, 34*(4), 367–388. https://doi.org/10.1080/0164212X.2018.1446206

Sznitman, S., & Engel-Yeger, B. (2017). Sensation seeking and adolescent alcohol use: Exploring the mediating role of unstructured socializing with peers. *Alcohol and Alcoholism, 52*(3), 396–401. https://doi.org/10.1093/alcalc/agx008

Wasmuth, S., Crabtree, J. L., & Scott, P. J. (2014). Exploring addiction-as-occupation. *British Journal of Occupational Therapy, 77*(12), 605–613. https://doi.org/10.4276/030802214X14176260335264

Wasmuth, S., Pritchard, K., & Kaneshiro, K. (2016). Occupation-based intervention for addictive disorders: A systematic review. *Journal of Substance Abuse Treatment, 62*, 1–9. https://doi.org/10.1016/j.jsat.2015.11.011

Wasmuth, S., Outcalt, J., Buck, K., Leonhardt, B. L., Vohs, J., & Lysaker, P. H. (2015). Metacognition in persons with substance abuse: Findings and implications for occupational therapists. *Canadian Journal of Occupational Therapy, 82*(3), 150–159. https://doi.org/10.1177/0008417414564865

Wegner, L., Arend, T., Bassadein, R., Bismath, A., & Cros, L. (2014). Experience of mothering drug-dependent youth: Influences on occupational performance patterns. *South African Journal of Occupational Therapy, 44*(2), 6–11.

Williams, R. M., & Privott, C. R. (2018). Experiences of postpartum women in one residential treatment facility for substance use disorders: A qualitative case study. *International Journal of Interdisciplinary Social & Community Studies, 13*(1), 1–12. https://doi.org/10.18848/2324-7576/CGP/v13i01/1-12

Suicide and Suicidal Behavior

Description

Suicidal behavior includes completed suicide and attempted suicide. Thoughts and plans about suicide are referred to as suicide ideation. Completed suicide or death by suicide is a suicidal act, voluntarily and intentionally, that results in death. Attempted suicide is a nonfatal, self-directed, potentially injurious act intended to result in death. A suicide attempt may or may not result in injury (Porter, 2018). A suicide survivor or suicide bereaved refers to a person who has lost someone to suicide (Novalis, 2017). The term *committed suicide* is considered to be a judgmental term and thus is generally avoided in the literature.

Cause

Suicidal behaviors usually result from the interaction of several factors. The primary remediable risk factor in suicide is depression. Other risk factors include the following:

- Serious mental disorders
- Use of alcohol, abuse of drugs, and prescription pain drugs
- Previous suicide attempts
- Serious physical disorders, especially in the elderly and in persons with chronic pain
- Personality disorders such as borderline personality disorder
- Unemployment and economic downturns
- Traumatic childhood experiences including maltreatment and bullying
- Family history of suicide and/or mental disorders
- Suicidal ideations (thoughts)
- Talking about wanting to die or to kill oneself
- Looking up different ways to kill oneself
- Talking about feeling hopeless or having no reason/purpose to live
- Talking about feeling trapped, or in unbearable pain
- Talking about being a burden to others
- Increased use of drugs or alcohol

- Being anxious or agitated; behaving recklessly
- Sleeping too little or too much
- Withdrawing, feeling isolated
- Showing rage; talking about seeking revenge
- Displaying extreme mood swings
- Giving away prize possessions and/or making a will
- Reconnecting with old friends and extended family as if to say good-bye
- Culture or religious beliefs that suicide is a noble resolution to a dilemma
- Unwillingness to seek help for a physical and/or mental health problem (Ash et al., 2015; Lambert & Carley, 2013; Novalis, 2017; Porter, 2018)

Evaluation/Assessment
Areas
- Activities of Daily Living/Instrumental ADL: changes in habits and routines
- Education/Work: employment history, especially unwanted termination
- Play/Leisure: interests, types, location, frequency; especially changes
- Rest/Sleep: sleep patterns (too much, too little)
- Social Participation: type, frequency, location, with whom; especially changes
- Sensorimotor: chronic pain, chronic motor or sensory deficit
- Cognitive/Perceptual: attention, memory, executive functions (planning ahead)
- Psychosocial: depression, suicide behavior (looking for a means to kill self, talking about killing or harming self, about death and dying), sense of hopelessness (such as feeling trapped), anger or rage, anxious or agitated behavior, mood changes, lack of purpose or goal, withdrawal
- Context/Environment: social support system, knowledge of resources
- Comorbidities or Risk Factors: anxiety, borderline personality disorder, depression, posttraumatic stress disorder, serious mental illness, substance abuse, terminal diagnosis or illness

Instruments
Instruments Developed by Occupational Therapy Personnel
- Allen Cognitive Level Screen (5th ed.; ACLS-5; Allen et al., 2007)
- Assessment of Communication and Interaction Skills (Version 4.0; ACIS; Forsyth et al., 1998)
- Assessment of Motor and Process Skills (8th ed.; AMPS-8; Fisher & Bray Jones, 2016)
- Canadian Occupational Performance Measure (5th ed.; COPM-5; Law et al., 2014)
- Model of Human Occupation Screening Tool (Version 2.0; MOHOST 2.0; Parkinson et al., 2006)
- Occupational Circumstances Assessment Interview and Rating Scale (Version 4.0; OCAIRS; Forsyth et al., 2005)
- Occupational Performance History Interview (Version 2.1; OPHI-II; Kielhofner et al., 2004)
- Occupational Self-Assessment (Version 2.2; OSA 2.2; Baron et al., 2006)
- Volitional Questionnaire (Version 4.1; VQ 4.1; de las Heras et al., 2007)
- Work Environment Impact Scale (Version 2.0; WEIS; Moore-Corner et al., 1998)

Instruments Developed by Other Professionals and Used by Occupational Therapy Personnel
- Questions That Leaders Can Use to Help Evaluate Suicide Risk (see Mummert et al., 2014, in References)

Problems/Issues
Activities of Daily Living/Instrumental ADL
- Person may be unable or unwilling to drive or take advantage of public transportation leading to isolation (associated with PTSD).
- Person may need assistance in developing healthy life habits, including eating, which decreases overall health status.

- Person may have limited financial resources.
- Person may be homeless or living in temporary housing.

Education/Work
- Person may discontinue academic education.
- Person may have inadequate work habits or skills.

Play/Leisure
- Person may have few or no leisure activities.
- Person may have disengaged in favorite leisure activities.

Rest/Sleep
- Person may have sleep disturbances, including poor sleep habits.

Social Participation
- Person may discontinue participation in social situations.
- Person may withdraw (disengage) from family and friends.

Sensorimotor
- Person may have changes in sleep patterns.

Cognitive/Perceptual
- Person may experience changes in cognitive and perceptual functions, especially if substance abuse, psychiatric illness, or trauma causing brain injury is present.

Psychosocial
- Person may talk about or threaten to kill or harm self.
- Person may talk or write about death, suicide, or harming self.
- Person may express feelings of hopelessness and helplessness.
- Person may express feelings of being trapped or stuck.
- Person may express feeling anxious and agitated.
- Person may increase use of alcohol and/or drug use.
- Person may experience dramatic mood changes.
- Person may express a lack of purpose in life (nothing is worth doing or has meaning).
- Person may lack or have poor coping skills.
- Person may be socially isolated and not feel he or she belongs with any group of persons or place.
- Person may experience changes in roles and role performance (some may be unwanted).
- Person may feel he or she is a burden to others requiring more care due to loss of functional abilities related to aging or chronic disease.
- Person may have problems with interpersonal relationships (divorce, breakup, dispute with supervisor/employer/family members).

Context/Environment
- Person may lack knowledge and information about available resources.
- Person may lack a social support system.
- Person may live in an area with limited access to resources.

Intervention/Treatment

Models and programs developed by occupational therapy personnel include case study (Lee & West, 2014), "Orange Cone Project" (Mummert et al., 2014), and person-environment-occupation (Kashiwa et al., 2017). Models and programs developed by other professionals but used by occupational therapy personnel include Operation Your Life Counts (Mummert et al., 2014). Team members include physicians, nursing personnel, psychologists and counselors, social workers, and occupational therapy personnel. The goal is to promote adaptive coping strategies including meaningful relationships with family and friends, and to reduce feelings of social isolation and lack of belonging and participation in meaningful occupations (Kashiwa et al., 2017; Lambert & Carley, 2013).

Activities of Daily Living/Instrumental ADL
- Provide opportunity to practice specific ADL or IADL skills that client identifies as needing development or redevelopment, such as planning and preparing well-balanced meals, practicing driving, or getting an apartment.

Education/Work
- Explore with client academic and work skills that may need development or improvement.

Play/Leisure
- Assist client to explore new leisure activities or redevelop previously known activities.
- Use of creative arts (writing, poetry) may assist person to express feelings.
- Facilitate occupational engagement in meaningful leisure activities.

Rest/Sleep
- See Sleep–Wake Disorders in Section 13: Lifestyle Conditions.

Social Participation
- Facilitate occupational engagement in social activities.
- Facilitate social inclusion in social situations.
- Provide opportunities to practice social interaction skills.

Sensorimotor
- Develop or recommend access to pain management program if person has chronic pain.
- Assist client to develop an exercise plan as part of a wellness and health living program.

Cognitive/Perceptual
- Provide opportunity to practice problem solving.

Psychosocial
- Increase adaptive coping skills and resiliency to improve sense of self-efficacy and social inclusion using group or individual intervention.
- Provide opportunity to role play situations that cause distress or anger to try different approaches to responding to situations.
- Provide stress and anger management techniques such as relaxation training, deep-breathing exercises, or yoga.

Context/Environment
- Provide information and access to community resources.
- Participate in or assist in developing a suicide prevention program.

Precautions/Safety Considerations

Be aware of items in the environment that may be used to injure or harm the client. Be aware of the importance of reporting concerns to other team members of client behaviors that may suggest suicide is being considered by the client. Know how to summon emergency support if suicide attempt to made during an occupational therapy session or in any situation where an occupational therapy practitioner may be present.

Prognosis and Outcome

Variable. Maintaining a suicide prevention program is useful.

REFERENCES
Ash, N. P., Bartczak, M., Monteferrante, J., Nurse, A., & Persad, S. (2015). *SPOTting PTSD: A PTSD toolkit for first responders*. McGill University.

Kashiwa, A., Sweetman, M. M., & Helgeson, L. (2017). Occupational therapy and veteran suicide: A call to action. *American Journal of Occupational Therapy, 71*(5), Article 710510001. https://doi.org/10.5014/ajot.2017.023358

Lambert, W. L., & Carley, E. (2013). Mental health of adolescents. In E. Cara & A. MacRae (Eds.), *Psychosocial occupational therapy: An evolving practice* (3rd ed., pp. 427–472). Delmar Cengage Learning.

Lee, S., & West, R. (2014). Cognitive approaches to intervention. In W. Bryant, J. Fieldhouse, & K. Bannigan (Eds.), *Creek's occupational therapy and mental health* (5th ed., pp. 224–239). Churchill Livingstone.

Mummert, C., Wilson, A., & Yancosek, K. (2014). Helping prevent military suicides—Operation your life counts. *OT Practice, 19*(22), 13–15.

Novalis, S. D. (2017). Suicide awareness and occupational therapy for suicide survivors. *OT Practice, 22*(21), CE-1–CE-8.

Porter, R. S. (Ed.). (2018). *The Merck manual of diagnosis and therapy* (20th ed.). Merck Sharp & Dohme.

BIBLIOGRAPHY

Bergson, K. (2016). Should occupational therapists be trained to talk about suicide? *OT News, 24*(9), 25.

Haertl, K. (2019). Coping and resilience. In C. Brown, V. C. Stoffel, & J. P. Muñoz (Eds.), *Occupational therapy in mental health: A vision for participation* (2nd ed., pp. 342–365). F.A. Davis.

Hewitt, K., & Boniface, G. (2014). CAOT Professional Issue forum: Suicide prevention and the role of occupational therapy. *Occupational Therapy Now, 16*(4), 13–15.

Reel, K., Hewitt, K., & Drolet, M. J. (2018). CAOT Professional issue forum: Medical assistance in dying (MAiD) and suicide prevention: Navigating potential professional and ethical tension. *Occupational Therapy Now, 20*(5), 11–12.

Lifestyle Conditions

Asylum Seekers, Human Displacement, Immigrants, Migrants, and Refugees

Also called displaced persons.

Description

Individual is unable to remain or chooses not to remain in their country or locale of origin.

Cause

Economic loss, natural disasters, famine, social change, political change, climate change, religious beliefs, declared or undeclared war, armed conflict, gang conflict, territorial disputes, human rights violations, physical or psychological torture, marginalization, or persecution (perceived or real threats to personal or family safety) are all potential reasons for a person to leave one country or locale and move to another (World Federation of Occupational Therapists, 2019).

Terminology

- *Asylum seeker:* A person who has fled the country of origin in order to seek refuge in another country, but has yet to receive a residence permit to live as a citizen in the new country (Morville & Erlandsson, 2017). A person seeking sanctuary (World Federation of Occupational Therapists, 2019).
- *Human displacement:* Refers to the forced movement of people from their homes, locality, environment, and occupational activities due to situations such as war, persecution, and disaster (World Federation of Occupational Therapists, 2014, 2019).
- *Immigrant:* A person who comes from another country to take up residence.
- *Occupational alienation:* The imposition of activities that do not have a positive meaning or do not promote health (World Federation of Occupational Therapists, 2019).
- *Occupational deprivation:* A state of preclusion from engagement in occupations due to factors that are not within the immediate control of the individual (Morville & Erlandsson, 2017). Factors may be environmental, political, environmental, economic, geographic, or interpersonal (World Federation of Occupational Therapists, 2019).
- *Occupational disruption:* Act of delaying or interrupting continuity of everyday life; result is disorder (Morville & Erlandsson, 2017).
- *Occupational imbalance:* A disproportionate amount of time is spent on one occupation at the expense of another, affecting both the quality and quantity of time spent on other occupations (World Federation of Occupational Therapists, 2019).
- *Occupational justice:* Right of every individual to be able to meet basic needs and to have equal opportunities and life changes to reach toward her or his potential, but specific to the individual's engagement in diverse and meaningful occupation (World Federation of Occupational Therapists, 2019).
- *Occupational rights:* A person has the right to participate in a range of occupations that enable the individual to flourish, fulfill potential, and experience satisfaction in a way consistent with the person's culture and beliefs (World Federation of Occupational Therapists, 2019).
- *Refugee:* A person fleeing conflict or persecution (World Federation of Occupational Therapists, 2019).
- *Relocation:* Adaption of individuals from a particular cultural context to another (Bennett et al., 2012).

Evaluation/Assessment

Areas

- Activities of Daily Living/Instrumental ADL: communication skills (ability to speak and understand English or access to translator), dressing and clothing choice (e.g., following clothing rules for attending school), food and meal preparation habits and preferences, locating

housing and housekeeping skills, money management, getting a driver's license, transportation skills to take public transit, access to health-care services
- Education/Work: academic achievement, literacy in reading English, work permit (green card), work skills, qualifications to pass testing requirements for state license
- Play/Leisure: interests, types, frequency, location (in country of origin, in present location)
- Rest/Sleep: sleep cycles including afternoon rest breaks
- Social Participation: types, frequency, location, with whom (in country of origin, in present location)
- Sensorimotor: physical fitness (Note: traumatic injuries or chronic illnesses may be present that require additional assessment of sensorimotor functions)
- Cognitive/Perceptual: problem solving, mental flexibility, planning, time management (routines, schedules)
- Psychosocial: anxiety, stress management, coping skills, self-image, self-confidence, self-identity, social isolation, role status loss (family and friends, work related, leisure related, community based), sense of meaning and purpose, role performance, quality of life
- Context/Environment: customs, values, beliefs, barriers (legal, institutional, geographic, social, cultural), health literacy, resources (support groups, training programs, community programs)
- Development (Infant, Child, Adolescent only): development milestones, developmental regression or delay (check attention, concentration, gross and fine-motor coordination)
- Comorbidity: depression

Instruments
(Note: Most studies used an interview format developed by the authors.)

Instruments Developed by Occupational Therapy Personnel
- Canadian Occupational Performance Measure (5th ed.; COPM-5; Law et al., 2014)

Instruments Developed by Other Professionals and Used by Occupational Therapy Personnel
- European Health Literacy Survey Questionnaire (EHLSQ; Sørensen et al., 2013)

Problems/Issues
Activities of Daily Living/Instrumental ADL
- Person may experience language barrier to expressing and receiving accurate communication.
- Person may lack knowledge on how to prepare foods available in the United States.
- Person may lack knowledge of how to shop for groceries, clothing, and other necessities.
- Person may lack skills on money management and banking system in the United States.
- Person may lack information on how to get a driver's license or the requirements to apply.
- Person may lack information on how to use public transportation.

Education/Work
- Child may not be able to speak and understand language well enough to participate in school activities.
- Person may not have the academic credentials needed for a job or occupation in the United States.
- Person may not know how to apply to take a required test to qualify for a license.

Play/Leisure
- Child may have little opportunity to play with peers or with toys that are age appropriate.
- Person may find that previous leisure occupations are not common in the United States (playing cricket, carving tusks, playing games with elephants).

Rest/Sleep
- Child may experience nightmares or other sleep disturbance.
- Person may be used to much longer afternoon breaks than the 30- to 60-minute break provided by most work settings in the United States.

Social Participation
- Child may have limited opportunity to play with peers or participate in age-appropriate occupations.
- Person may be unfamiliar with United States social activities such as attending or watching American football games, including tailgating.
- Person may be unfamiliar with "bar hopping" especially if the person comes from a country or society that does not condone liquor.

Sensorimotor
- Person may become deconditioned and lack physical fitness due to lack of a regular routine or physical exercise program.

Cognitive/Perceptual
- Person may lack cognitive and perceptual skills expected of a child or adult in the United States.
- Person may have difficulty setting long-term goals due to uncertainty about status as an immigrant.
- Person may have difficulty with time management due to lack of structure and routine.

Psychosocial
- Person may express anxiety about the future.
- Person may experience stress due to issues of acculturation.
- Person may experience role loss due to separation from family, friends, and community in country of origin.
- Person may experience decreased sense of self-identity and self-efficacy.
- Person may experience loss of self-confidence and self-worth.
- Person may experience decreased motivation as challenges continue to arise.
- Person may experience decreased quality of life.

Context/Environment
- Person may experience "cultural shock" regarding the differences in cultural and social beliefs in the United States and differences in values and beliefs from those observed and followed in the country of origin.
- Person may be unfamiliar with how to access the health care system or social services.
- Person may lack social support.
- Person may experience stigma, racism, or other types of discrimination.
- Facilities for programs may be lacking, unavailable, or inaccessible such as school for refugee or migrant children, health services, sanitation, or other basic services.

Intervention/Treatment

Models and programs developed by occupational therapy personnel include case study–bipolar (Maroney et al., 2014), case study–depression (Maroney et al., 2014; Pooremamali, Östman, et al., 2011), case study–asylum seeker (Pollard, 2015), case study–weaving (Stephenson et al., 2013), community-based occupational therapy (Black, 2011), cultural brokerage care (Lindsay et al., 2014), life skills program (Crandall & Smith, 2015; Suleman & Whiteford, 2013), music making and singing (Adrian, 2013; Raanaas et al., 2019), occupational justice model (Smith, 2017; Trimboli, 2017), occupational performance process model (OPPM; De Koker et al., 2019), occupational therapy program for high school refugees (Copley et al., 2011), participatory occupational justice framework (Suleman & Whiteford, 2013), and person-environment-occupation model (Trimboli, 2017). Models and programs developed by other professionals but used by occupational therapy personnel include grounded theory (Pooremamali, Persson, & Eklund, 2011), health literacy (Wångdahl et al., 2015; Wångdahl et al., 2019), holistic model (Stickley & Stickley, 2010), social inclusion (Morville & Jessen-Winge, 2019), and therapeutic horticulture (Bishop & Purcell, 2013). Team members include immigration personnel, physicians, nursing personnel, psychologists, social workers, vocational counselors, and occupational therapy personnel. Goals include rebuilding the individual's capacity roles, routines, and self-efficacy to address occupational imbalance, deprivation, and adaptation requirements, and develop social networks through community-based programs that are strength-based, client-centered, and context specific (World Federation of Occupational Therapists, 2014, 2019).

Activities of Daily Living/Instrumental ADL

- Assist client to communicate. Language is important but art (drawing and painting), music (singing and playing instruments), photography, pantomime, and drama may also facilitate effective communication.
- Assist client to locate foods familiar to the person or substitutes to eat and prepare for meals.
- Assist client to locate clothing familiar to the person but also meet any special rules required of a local school district.
- Assist client to locate housing within access to potential educational or work settings.
- Assist client to learn to use public transportation and/or get a driver's license.
- Assist client to learn core skills such as money management, home management, shopping, parenting within new culture.

Education/Work

- Assist in determining child's academic level and learning skills.
- Assist person to get academic transcript evaluated for potential enrollment in an educational institution or application for employment.
- With assistance of a vocational counselor assist person to develop a resume for employment, evaluate work skills, improve work skills if need be, practice applying for employment.
- Assist client to identify possible volunteer opportunities.

Play/Leisure

- Assist client to determine which leisure occupations can be applied in the new community.
- Assist person to explore and develop new leisure occupations common in both country of origin and new community (e.g., gardening, needle arts, rug making, woodwork).

Rest/Sleep

- Assist client to adjust rest and sleep cycles to new community.

Social Participation

- Assist client to participate in social activities within the community.

Sensorimotor

- Assist child to develop gross and fine motor skills to age-appropriate level.
- Assist client to develop and maintain a physical fitness program.

Cognitive/Perceptual

- Assist child to develop attention, concentration, and executive skills to age-appropriate level.
- Assist client to develop and maintain a schedule of daily activity, develop routines, and manage time.

Psychosocial

- Assist client to find meaning and purpose in occupations.
- Assist client to develop sense of self-efficacy and self-worth.
- Assist client to develop role performance expected in society and culture of new country.

Context/Environment

- Assist client to identify and use available resources.
- Assist client to identify and understand legislation and policies regarding immigration status, whether temporary or permanent, including rights and responsibilities.
- Advocate for additional resources to facilitate integration into the community.

Precautions/Safety Considerations

Personal safety should be monitored.

Prognosis and Outcome

Variable. Some asylum seekers, immigrants, and refugees make good adjustment to their new country but others struggle for many years.

REFERENCES

Adrian, A. (2013). An exploration of Lutheran music-making among US immigrants and refugee populations. *Journal of Occupational Science, 20*(2), 160–172. https://doi.org/10.1080/14427591.2013.775690

Bennett, K. M., Scornaiencki, J. M., Brzozowski, J., Denis, S., & Magalhaes, L. (2012). Immigration and its impact on daily occupations: A scoping review. *Occupational Therapy International, 19*, 185–203. https://doi.org/10.1002/oti.1336

Bishop, R., & Purcell, E. (2013). The value of an allotment group for refugees. *British Journal of Occupational Therapy, 76*(6), 264–269. https://doi.org/10.4276/030802213X13706169932824

Black, M. (2011). From kites to kitchens: Collaborative community-based occupational therapy for refugee survivors of torture. In F. Kronenberg, N. Pollard, & D. Sakellariou (Eds.), *Occupational therapies without borders* (Vol. 2, pp. 217–225). Churchill Livingstone/Elsevier.

Copley, J., Turpin, M., Gordon, S., & McLaren, C. (2011). Development and evaluation of an occupational therapy program for refugee high school students. *Australian Occupational Therapy Journal, 58*(4), 310–316. https://doi.org/10.1111/j.1440-1630.2011.00933.x

Crandall, J., & Smith, Y. J. (2015). Life skills program: Occupational therapy among resettled refugees in an urban context. *OT Practice, 20*(22), 18–20.

De Koker, R., Lambers, S., & Vercruysse, L. (2019). Occupational therapy at "Klein Kasteeltje" in Brussels for children of asylum seekers who cannot participate in the Belgian schooling system. *World Federation of Occupational Therapists Bulletin, 75*(1), 34–42. https://doi.org/10.1080/14473828.2019.1570703

Lindsay, S., Tétrault, S., Desmaris, C., King, G. A., & Piérart, G. (2014). The cultural brokerage work of occupational therapists in providing culturally sensitive care. *Canadian Journal of Occupational Therapy, 81*(2), 114–123. https://doi.org/10.1177/0008417413520441

Maroney, P., Potter, M., & Thacore, V. R. (2014). Experiences in occupational therapy with Afghan clients in Australia. *Australian Occupational Therapy Journal, 61*(1), 13–19. https://doi.org/10.1111/1440-1630.12094

Morville, A., & Erlandsson, L. K. (2017). Occupational deprivation for asylum seekers. In D. Sakellariou & N. Pollard (Eds.), *Occupational therapies without borders* (2nd ed., pp. 381–389). Elsevier.

Morville, A. L., & Jessen-Winge, C. (2019). Creating a bridge: An asylum seeker's ideas for social inclusion. *Journal of Occupational Science, 26*(1), 53–64. https://doi.org/10.1080/14427591.2018.1500933

Pollard, N. (2015). Seeking asylum in the UK. In N. Rushford & K. Thomas (Eds.), *Disaster and development: An occupational perspective* (pp. 95–102). Churchill Livingstone.

Pooremamali, P., Östman, M., Persson, D., & Eklund, M. (2011). An occupational therapy approach to the support of a young immigrant female's mental health: A story of bicultural personal growth. *International Journal of Qualitative Studies on Health and Well-Being, 6*(3), Article 7084. https://doi.org/10.3402/qhw.v6i3.7084

Pooremamali, P., Persson, D., & Eklund, M. (2011). Occupational therapists' experience of working with immigrant clients in mental health care. *Scandinavian Journal of Occupational Therapy, 18*(2), 109–121. https://doi.org/10.3109/11038121003649789

Raanaas, R. K., Aase, S. Ø., & Huot, S. (2019). Finding meaningful occupation in refugees' re-settlement: A study of amateur choir singing in Norway. *Journal of Occupational Science. 26*(1), 65–76. https://doi.org/10.1080/14427591.2018.1537884

Smith, Y. J. (2017). Occupational justice and advocacy: Working with former refugees and asylum seekers at personal and community levels. In D. Sakellariou & N. Pollard (Eds.), *Occupational therapies without borders* (2nd ed., pp. 433–440). Elsevier.

Stephenson, S. M., Smith, Y. J., Gibson, M., & Watson, V. (2013). Traditional weaving as an oc-cupation of Karen refugee women. *Journal of Occupational Science, 20*(3), 224–235. https://doi.org/10.1080/14427591.2013.789150

Stickley, A., & Stickley, T. (2010). A holistic model for the rehabilitation and recovery of inter-nally displaced people in war-torn Uganda. *British Journal of Occupational Therapy, 73*(7), 335–338. https://doi.org/10.4276/030802210X12759925544461

Suleman, A., & Whiteford, G. E. (2013). Understanding occupational transitions in forced mi-gration: The importance of life skills in early refugee resettlement. *Journal of Occupational Science, 20*(2), 201–210. https://doi.org/10.1080/14427591.2012.755908

Trimboli, C. (2017). Occupational justice for asylum seeker and refugee children: Issues, effects and action. In D. Sakellariou & N. Pollard (Eds.), *Occupational therapies without borders* (2nd ed., pp. 460–467). Elsevier.

Wångdahl, J., Lytsy, P., Mårtensson, L., & Westerling, R. (2015). Health literacy and refugees' experiences of the health examination for asylum seekers—A Swedish cross-sectional study. *BMC Public Health, 15*, Article 1162. https://doi.org/10.1186/s12889-015-2513-8

Wångdahl, J., Westerling, R., Lytsy, P., & Mårtensson, L. (2019). Perspectives on health examina-tion for asylum seekers in relation to health literacy—Focus group discussions with Arabic and Somali speaking participants. *BMC Health Services Research, 19*, Article 676. https://doi.org/10.1186/s12913-019-4484-4

World Federation of Occupational Therapists. (2014). *Position statement: Human displacement.* https://wfot.org/resources/human-displacement

World Federation of Occupational Therapists. (2019). *Resource manual: Occupational therapy for dis-placed persons.* https://www.wfot.org/resources/wfot-resource-manual-occupational-therapy-for-displaced-persons

BIBLIOGRAPHY

Arola, L. A., Dellenborg, L., & Häggblom-Kronlöf, G. (2018). Occupational perspective of health among persons ageing into the context of migration. *Journal of Occupational Science, 25*(1), 65–75. https://doi.org/10.1080/14427591.2017.1368411

Berr, K., Marotzki, U., & Schiller, S. (2019). Broadening the understanding of employment and identity of Syrian women living in Germany: A biographical study. *Journal of Occupational Science, 26*(2), 294–307. https://doi.org/10.1080/14427591.2018.1540356

Blankvoort, N., Arslan, M., Tonoyan, A., Damour, A., & Mpabanzi, L. (2018). A new you: A collaborative exploration of occupational therapy's role with refugees. *World Federation of Occupational Therapists Bulletin, 74*(2), 92–98. https://doi.org/10.1080/14473828.2018.1526560

Burchett, N., & Matheson, R. (2010). The need for belonging: The impact of restricts on working on the well-being of an asylum seeker. *Journal of Occupational Science, 17*(2), 85–91. https://doi.org/10.1080/14427591.2010.9686679

Campbell, E. J., & Turpin, M. J. (2010). Refugee settlement workers' perspectives on home safety issues for people from refugee backgrounds. *Australian Occupational Therapy Journal, 57*(6), 425–430. https://doi.org/10.1111/j.1440-1630.2010.00882.x

Crawford, E., Turpin, M., Nayar, S., Steel, E., & Durand, J.-L. (2016). The structural-personal in-teraction: Occupational deprivation and asylum seekers in Australia. *Journal of Occupational Science, 23*(3), 321–338. https://doi.org/10.1080/14427591.2016.1153510

Darawsheh, W. B. (2019). Exploration of occupational deprivation among Syrian refugees displaced in Jordan. *American Journal of Occupational Therapy, 73*(4), Article 7304205030. https://doi.org/10.5014/ajot.2019.030460

Driver, C., & Beltran, P. O. (1998). Impact of refugee trauma on children's occupational role as school students. *Australian Occupational Therapy Journal, 45*(1), 23–38.

Eckemoff, E., Sudha, S., & Wang, D. (2018). End of life care for older Russian immigrants–Perspectives of Russian immigrants and hospice staff. *Journal of Cross-Cultural Gerontology, 33*(3), 229–245. https://doi.org/10.1007/s10823-018-9353-9

Gupta, J. (2012). Human displacement, occupational disruptions, and reintegration: A case study. *World Federation of Occupational Therapists Bulletin, 66*(1), 27–26. https://doi.org/10.1179/otb.2012.66.1.010

Gupta, J., & Sullivan, C. (2013). The central role of occupation in the doing, being and belonging of immigrant women. *Journal of Occupational Science, 20*(1), 23–35. https://doi.org/10.1080/14427591.2012.717499

Hocking, C., Townsend, E., Gerlach, A., Huot, S., Laiberte Rudman, D., & van Bruggen, H. (2015). "Doing" human rights in diverse occupational therapy practice. *Occupational Therapy Now, 17*(4), 18–20.

Huot, S. (2016). The production of precariousness through policy: Occupational injustice faced by forced migrants in Canada. *Occupational Therapy Now, 18*(1), 23–24.

Huot, S., Kelly, E., & Park, S. J. (2016) Occupational experiences of forced migrants: A scoping review. *Australian Occupational Therapy Journal, 63*(3), 186–205. https://doi.org/10.1111/1440-1630.12261

Huot, S., & Veronis, L. (2018). Examining the role of minority community spaces for enabling migrants' performance of intersectional identities through occupation. *Journal of Occupational Science, 25*(1), 37–50. https://doi.org/10.1080/14427591.2017.1379427

Ingvarsson, L., Egilson, S. T., & Skaptadottir, U. D. (2016). "I want a normal life like everyone else": Daily life of asylum seekers in Iceland. *Scandinavian Journal of Occupational Therapy, 23*(6), 416–424. https://doi.org/10.3109/11038128.2016.1144787

Kielsgaard, K., Kristensen, H. K., & Nielsen, D. S. (2018). Everyday life and occupational deprivation in single migrant mothers living in Denmark. *Journal of Occupational Science, 25*(1), 19–36. https://doi.org/10.1080/14427591.2018.1445659

Lintner, C., & Elsen, S. (2018). Getting out of the seclusion trap: Work as meaningful occupation for the subjective well-being of asylum seekers in South Tyrol, Italy. *Journal of Occupational Science, 25*(1), 76–86. https://doi.org/10.1080/14427591.2017.1373256

Mayne, J., Lowrie, D., & Wilson, J. (2016). Occupational experiences of refugees and asylum seekers resettling in Australia: A narrative review. *OTJR: Occupation, Participation and Health, 36*(4), 204-215. https://doi.org/10.1177/1539449216668648

Mirza, M. (2012). Occupational upheaval during resettlement and migration: Findings of global ethnography with refugees with disabilities. *OTJR: Occupation, Participation and Health, 32*(Suppl. 1), S6–S14. https://doi.org/10.3928/15394492-20110906-04

Mirza, M. Q., Harrison, E. A., Chang, H. C., Salo, C. D., & Birman, D. (2018). Community perspectives on substance use among Bhutanese and Iraqi refugees resettled in the United States. *Journal of Prevention & Intervention in the Community, 46*(1), 43–60. https://doi.org/10.1080/10852352.2018.1385956

Mirza, M., Luna, R., Mathews, B., Hasnain, R., Hebert, E., Niebauer, A., & Mishra, U. D. (2014). Barriers to healthcare access among refugees with disabilities and chronic health conditions resettled in the US Midwest. *Journal of Immigrant and Minority Health, 16*(4), 733–742. https://doi.org/10.1007/s10903-013-9906-5

Morville, A., Amris, K., Eklund, M., Danneskiold-Samsøe, B., & Erlandsson, L. (2015). A longitudinal study of changes in asylum seekers ability regarding activities of daily living during their stay in the asylum center. *Journal of Immigrant and Minority Health, 17*(3), 852–859. https://doi.org/10.1007/s10903-014-0004-0

Morville, A., & Erlandsson, L. (2013). The experience of occupational deprivation in an asylum centre: The narratives of three men. *Journal of Occupational Science, 20*(3), 212–223. https://doi.org/10.1080/14427591.2013.808976

Morville, A. L., Erlandsson, L. K., Danneskiold-Samsøe, B., Amris, K., & Eklund, M. (2015). Satisfaction with daily occupations amongst asylum seekers in Denmark. *Scandinavian Journal of Occupational Therapy, 22*(3), 207–215. https://doi.org/10.3109/11038128.2014.982702

Morville, A., Erlandsson, L. Eklund, M., Danneskiold-Samsøe, B., Christensen, R., & Amris, K. (2014). Activity of daily living performance amongst Danish asylum seekers: A cross-sectional study. *Torture: Quarterly Journal on Rehabilitation of Torture Victims and Prevention of Torture, 24*(1), 49–64.

Mpofu, C., & Hocking, C. (2013). "Not made here": Occupational deprivation of non-English speaking background immigrant health professionals in New Zealand. *Journal of Occupational Science, 20*(2), 131–145. https://doi.org/10.1080/14427591.2012.729500

Nayar, S., & Wright-St Clair, V. A. (2018). Strengthening community: Older Asian immigrants' contributions to New Zealand society. *Journal of Cross-Cultural Gerontology, 33*(4), 355–368. https://doi.org/10.1007/s10823-018-9357-5

Peralta-Catipon, T. (2012). Collective occupations among Filipina migrant workers: Bridging disrupted identities. *OTJR: Occupation, Participation and Health, 32*(2), 14–21. https://doi.org/10.3928/15394492-20110805-01

Rivas-Quarneti, N., Movilla-Fernández, J.-J., & Magalhães, L. (2018). Immigrant women's occupational struggles during the socioeconomic crisis in Spain: Broadening occupational justice cocenptualization. *Journal of Occupational Science, 25*(1), 6–18. https://doi.org/10.1080/14427591.2017.1366355

Roos, K., Wenger, I., Sowe, R., & Indermühle, Y. (2018). Addressing barriers to work for asylum seekers: Report from Switzerland. *World Federation of Occupational Therapists Bulletin, 74*(2), 123–127. https://doi.org/10.1080/14473828.2018.1540100

Smith, H. C. (2015). An exploration of the meaning of occupation to people who seek asylum in the United Kingdom. *British Journal of Occupational Therapy, 78*(10), 614–621. https://doi.org/10.1177/0308022615591174

Smith, H. C. (2018). Finding purpose through altruism: The potential of "doing for others" during asylum. *Journal of Occupational Science, 25*(1), 87–99. https://doi.org/10.1080/14427591.2017.1371633

Smith, Y. (2017). Occupational justice and advocacy: Working with former refugees and asylum seekers at personal and community levels. In D. Sakellariou & N. Pollard (Eds.), *Occupational therapies without borders* (2nd ed., pp. 433–440). Elsevier.

Smith, Y. J. (2013). We all Bantu—We have each other: Preservation of social capital strengths during forced migration. *Journal of Occupational Science, 20*(2), 173–184. https://doi.org/10.1080/14427591.2013.786647

Smith, Y. J., Cornella, E., & Williams, N. (2014). Working with populations from a refugee background: An opportunity to enhance the occupational therapy educational experience. *Australian Occupational Therapy Journal, 61*(1), 20–27. https://doi.org/10.1111/1440-1630.12037

Smith, Y. J., Stephenson, S., & Gibson-Satterthwaite, M. (2013). The meaning and value of traditional occupational practice: A Karen woman's story of weaving in the United States. *Work, 45*(1), 25–30. https://doi.org/10.3233/WOR-131600

Sterling, K., & Nayar, S. (2013). Changes to occupation for Indian immigrant men: Questions for practice. *New Zealand Journal of Occupational Therapy, 60*(2), 21–26.

Thornton, M., & Spalding, N. (2018). An exploration of asylum seeker and refugee experiences of activity: A literature review. *World Federation of Occupational Therapists Bulletin, 74*(2), 114–122. https://doi.org/10.1080/14473828.2018.1539282

Trimboli, C., & Halliwell, V. (2018). A survey to explore the interventions used by occupational therapists and occupational therapy students with refugees and asylum seekers. *World Fed-*

eration of Occupational Therapists Bulletin, 74(2), 106–113. https://doi.org/10.1080/144738 28.2018.1535562

Trimboli, C., Rivas-Quarneti, N., Blankvoort, N., Roosen, I., Algado, S. S., & Whiteford, G. (2019). The current and future contribution of occupational therapy and occupational science to transforming the situation of forced migrants: Critical perspectives from a think tank. *Journal of Occupational Science, 26*(2), 323–328. https://doi.org/10.1080/14427591.2019.1604408

Trimboli, C., & Taylor, J. (2016). Addressing the occupational needs of refugees and asylum seekers. *Australian Occupational Therapy Journal, 63*(6), 434–437. https://doi.org/10.1111/1440-16 30.12349

Werge-Olsen, I., & Vik, K. (2012). Activity as a tool in language training for immigrants and refugees. *Scandinavian Journal of Occupational Therapy, 19*(6), 530–541. https://doi.org/10.3 109/11038128.2012.661455

Winlaw, K. (2017). Making the connection: Why refugees and asylum seekers need occupational therapy services. *Occupational Therapy Now, 19*(4), 18–19.

Wright-St Clair, V. A., Nayar, S., Kim, H., Wang, S. M., Sodhi, S. K., Chung, A., Suchdev, J., & Hu, C. (2018). Late-life Asian immigrants managing wellness through contributing to socially embedded networks. *Journal of Occupational Science, 25*(1), 51–64. https://doi.org/10.1080/1 4427591.2017.1370607

Yamamoto, S., & Matsuo, H. (2017). Current situation and challenges regarding the social participation of Syrian refugees with disabilities in urban areas of Jordan. *Asian Journal of Occupational Therapy, 13*(1), 87–93.

Yazdani, F., Rassafiani, M., Tune, K., Pollard, N., Sakellariou, D., Fani, M., Nobakht, L., & Firuzi, S. (2018). Immigration, participation in health services and social occupations: A literature review. *International Journal of Travel Medicine and Global Health, 6*(2), 36–47. https://doi.org/10 .15171/IJTMGH.2018.09

Disaster Management

See also Asylum Seekers, Human Displacement, Immigrants, Migrants, and Refugees; Anxiety and General Anxiety Disorder; Posttraumatic Stress Disorder (PTSD).

Description

A disaster is a sudden and universal phenomenon that seriously disrupts the quality of life of individuals, families, and communities in both the short and long terms (Jeong et al., 2016). The American Occupational Therapy Association has prepared two documents concerned with disaster (American Occupational Therapy Association, 2011, 2017). The 2011 document was rescinded in 2017 (American Occupational Therapy Association, 2018).

Cause

Two causes are recognized: natural and technological. Natural disasters occur when community abilities cannot cope with devastating geographical, meteorological, or biological events (floods, fires, hurricanes, earthquakes, droughts, epidemics, pandemics). Technological disasters are triggered by human activities (ferryboat sinking, school bus crash, building or bridge collapsing) or terrorist attacks (9/11 in New York City; Jeong et al., 2016).

Stages of Disaster Management (Jeong et al., 2016)

- Prevention: evaluating the possibility of a disaster and its potential impacts.
- Preparedness: preparing a plan to address the effects of a disaster.
- Response: providing resources for humanitarian aid to victims.
- Recovery: supporting communities and assisting with reconstruction of physical and mental well-being of its citizens.

Evaluation/Assessment
Areas
- Activities of Daily Living/Instrumental ADL: shelter (private home, apartment, hotel, motel, community center), finances (cash, credit card, electronic banking), clothing, minor health problems, household furnishings, laundry services, communication (telephone, cell phone, email, social media), transportation (car, truck, bus, train, airplane)
- Education/Work: academic performance, work history, job loss
- Play/Leisure: interests, frequency, location
- Rest/Sleep: sleep disturbance
- Social Participation: type, frequency, location, with whom
- Sensorimotor: (if physical injury is present) muscle strength, joint range of motion, endurance, sensory loss, pain
- Cognitive/Perceptual: attention, concentration, memory, executive functions
- Psychosocial: anxiety, stress reactions, self-identity, role performance, quality of life
- Context/Environment: housing availability, community resources, state and national resources
- Development (Infant, Child, Adolescent only): development delay, developmental regression

Instruments
Instruments Developed by Occupational Therapy Personnel
- Interview Questions (Sima et al. 2017, in References)
- Signs of Critical Incident Stress (checklist; World Federation of Occupational Therapists, 2019, in References)
- Signs of Danger Versus Safety (Red Flag–Green Flag; World Federation of Occupational Therapists, 2019, in References)

Instruments Developed by Other Professionals and Used by Occupational Therapy Personnel
- None identified in references to this chapter

Problems/Issues
Activities of Daily Living/Instrumental ADL
- Person may be displaced after losing shelter and living arrangements.
- Person may lose clothing and other possessions through displacement or damage from fire or mold.
- Person may experience financial loss.
- Person may experience short-term health problems such as nausea, upset stomach, sweating, chills, diarrhea, dizziness, light headedness, rapid pulse, heart pounding, rapid breathing or panting, headaches, increased blood pressure, dry mouth, flushed face, feeling warm or hot.
- Person may not have access to basic health care and medications.
- Person may lose access to child care and pet care services.
- Person may lose access to transportation (loss of personal vehicle, disruption in mass transportation system).

Education/Work
- Child may not be able to attend school (lack of transportation, damage to school building, no direction from teacher regarding assignments or learning tasks to be completed).
- Person may not be able to work at regular job (lack of transportation, damage to work site, no direction from employer or supervisor regarding tasks to be completed.

Play/Leisure
- Child may not be able to engage in favorite play activities with favorite play objects or favorite playmates (play objects lost or destroyed, playmates separated by distance or injured).

- Person may not be able to engage in favorite leisure occupations (supplies and equipment lost or damaged, loss of access to location, other priorities leave little time, space, or energy).

Rest/Sleep
- Person may experience sleep disturbance.
- Person may report distressing dreams.

Social Participation
- Child or person may not be able to participate in familiar social activities (injury, loss of life, no access to location, loss of supplies and equipment, other priorities limit time, space, or energy).

Sensorimotor
- Person may experience muscle tremors as a reaction to stress.
- Person may experience loss of muscle coordination as a reaction to stress.
- Person may experience muscle aches and pains as a reaction to stress.
- Person may experience numbness or tingling as a reaction to stress.
- Person may experience actual physical injury (fractures, dislocations, cuts, bruises, abrasions).
- Person may experience sensory limitation (loss of glasses or hearing aids), injury, or loss.

Cognitive/Perceptual
- Person may have difficulty paying attention and concentrating on a specific task or conversation (low or short attention span).
- Person may think more slowly than normal for individual.
- Person may demonstrate confusion and difficulty with naming objects.
- Person may make simple errors in calculation.
- Person may demonstrate impaired decision making.
- Person may demonstrate difficulty with problem solving.
- Person may have difficulty structuring time and actions as a consequence of the disaster disrupting normal habits and routines.

Psychosocial
- Person may experience anxiety, worry, and fearfulness.
- Person may express feelings of sadness and depression.
- Person may feel lost and isolated.
- Person may experience feelings of guilt for not be being able to do more to mitigate the extent of damage.
- Person may express feelings of anger or have angry outbursts and emotional tirades.
- Person may be grieving for loss of or injury to family members, friends, colleagues.
- Person may be emotionally numb or shocked.
- Person may be on edge, be irritable, or express feelings of nervousness or panic.
- Person may express feelings of loss of control.
- Person may become withdrawn, defensive, or attempt to hide self and feelings.
- Person may become hyperactive or hypoactive.
- Person may be easily startled.

Context/Environment
- Person may lack information or knowledge about what type of disaster has occurred and what actions can or should occur.
- Person may lack knowledge of available resources or how to access those resources.

Intervention/Treatment
Models and programs developed by occupational therapy personnel include case study–COVID-19 (Whitney & Walsh, 2020), case study–earthquake (Lee, 2014), case study–flooding (Duque et al.,

2012), case study–tsunami (Rushford & Thomas, 2011), case studies–other (Rushford & Thomas, 2015a), Disaster and Development Occupational Perspective (DDOP; Rushford & Thomas, 2015a, 2015b; Thomas & Rushford, 2015), disaster preparedness program (Duque et al., 2014), guide for occupational therapy first responders to disasters and trauma (World Federation of Occupational Therapists, 2019), and occupational stewardship (Rushford, 2015; Rushford & Thomas, 2015b). Models and programs developed by other professionals but used by occupational therapy personnel include disaster preparedness, response, and recovery (DPRR; Nair & Tyagi, 2014; Rushford & Thomas, 2011); multidisciplinary team (Hossain et al., 2013); and recovery model (Pizzi, 2015). Team members include physicians, psychiatrics, psychologists, nursing personnel, life style coaches, and occupational therapy personnel. Goal is to facilitate the engagement in meaningful routines and occupations that may be disrupted by disaster (World Federation of Occupational Therapists, 2014).

Activities of Daily Living/Instrumental ADL

- Identify which basic ADL tasks are causing the most stress at the moment such as eating and food preparation, dressing and clothing, toileting and available facilities and toilet supplies, bathing/showering and access to facilities and supplies, getting and managing medications, shelter and sleeping quarters.
- Identify which IADL tasks are causing the most stress: acquiring groceries or finding places to eat, washing and drying clothes, access to transportation, child and pet care, electricity and gas services, communication systems (postal, electronic, social).

Education/Work

- Assist client to develop and implement a study program (what subjects, how much time, who will assist and evaluate results?) to continue academic studies.
- Assist client to identify work skills acquired throughout including those that have not been used recently.
- Assist in updating resume or curriculum vitae.
- Assist in exploring what work opportunities are available in present circumstances or may be available in a given time period or location.
- Facilitate the reestablishment of livelihoods.

Play/Leisure

- Assist client to identify favorite leisure occupations, especially those than can be engaged in given the present circumstances and conditions of disaster recovery.
- Assist client to identify new or novel leisure occupations that meet the current circumstances and conditions of disaster recovery.
- Consider if group leisure performance is possible (can some group members teach others?).
- Consider what materials (toys, games, sports equipment, etc.) may be available on-site that can be used for leisure occupations including adaptations and modifications.

Rest/Sleep

- See Sleep–Wake Disorders in Section 13: Lifestyle Conditions.

Social Participation

- Assist client to identify social activities that the individual has previously enjoyed participating in. Can those social activities be reconstructed or adapted in the current conditions?
- Assist client to identify new or novel social activities. Consider who is available to form a social group and what supplies and equipment can be used or adapted.

Sensorimotor

- Neurological conditions: splint fabrication, edema control, wound and scar management.
- Deconditioning: muscle force exercises to increase strength, manual manipulation and joint mobilization to increase range of motion.

Cognitive/Perceptual

- Assist client to set goals and develop action plans (e.g., Action Plan in World Federation of Occupational Therapists, 2019, p. 12; Note: family member, friend, colleague or other professional could be substituted for first responder).

Psychosocial

- Assist client to identify stress reactions and those that cause the most intense feelings (e.g., use checklist "Signs of Critical Incidence Stress" in World Federation of Occupational Therapists, 2019, p. 9).
- Assist client to identify reactions to feelings of danger or safety (e.g., use checklist "Red Flag–Green Flag Strategy" in World Federation of Occupational Therapists, 2019, p. 10).
- Assist client to increase sense of resilience (e.g., worksheet in reliving a disturbing memory in World Federation of Occupational Therapists, 2019, p. 11).
- Assist client to reduce stress and increase coping strategies: meditation methods (World Federation of Occupational Therapists, 2019, p. 13); diaphragmatic breathing (World Federation of Occupational Therapists, 2019, p. 14); describe, interpret, evaluate (DIE) model (World Federation of Occupational Therapists, 2019, p. 14); Automatic Negative Thoughts (ANTS) method (World Federation of Occupational Therapists, 2019, p. 15); tapping points method (World Federation of Occupational Therapists, 2019, pp. 16–18); grounding (World Federation of Occupational Therapists, 2019, p. 19); and quotations from the field (World Federation of Occupational Therapists, 2019, pp. 20–23).

Context/Environment

- Assist client to identify and use community, state, and federal resources.
- Ensuring accessible environment such as assisting in rebuilding homes and community facilities.
- Increase self-preparedness (Jeong et al., 2016).
  - ▶ Design specific plans to address different issues (home, workplace, shelter).
  - ▶ Survey risks and resources in the community.
  - ▶ Educate community personnel about evacuation of people with disabilities.
  - ▶ Know function of key agencies and organizations involved in responding to and recovering from disasters.
  - ▶ Inform stakeholders and public about role of occupational therapy in disasters.
  - ▶ Partner with key stakeholders and organizations to respond to disasters.
- Provide information, education, and services to community members and other professionals.

Precautions/Safety Considerations

- Injury due to unsafe environments: unstable buildings, exposed or leaking electrical wires or gas pipes, unsanitary conditions (sewage, waste materials, unclean or contaminated water).
- Lack of institutional services: police, fire, hospitals, transportation.

Prognosis and Outcome

Variable. Response depends in part on the resources of the individual and in part on the social and governmental services available to respond and address the needs for recovery, rehabilitation, and reconstruction.

REFERENCES

American Occupational Therapy Association. (2011). The role of occupational therapy in disaster preparedness, response, and recovery. *American Journal of Occupational Therapy, 65*(Suppl. 1), S11–S25. https://doi.org/10.5014/ajot.2011.65S11

American Occupational Therapy Association. (2017). AOTA's societal statement on disaster response and risk reduction. *American Journal of Occupational Therapy, 71*(Suppl. 2), Article 7112410060. https://doi.org/10.5014/ajot.2017.716S11

American Occupational Therapy Association. (2018). *Reference manual of the official documents of the American Occupational Therapy Association, Inc.*

Duque, R. L., Ching, P. E., & Amihan-Bayas, C. (2012). Occupational therapy within layers of disasters, poverty and conflict: A case study. *World Federation of Occupational Therapists Bulletin, 66*(1), 24–26. https://doi.org/10.1179/otb.2012.66.1.009

Duque, R. L., Grecia, A., & Ching, P. E. (2013). Development of a national occupational therapy disaster preparedness and response plan: The Philippine experience. *World Federation of Occupational Therapists Bulletin, 68*(1), 26–30. https://doi.org/10.1179/otb.2013.68.1.008

Hossain, M. I., Nahar, N., Nayan, M. J., Ema, A. J., & Alve, M. Y. A. (2013). Experience of Bangladeshi occupational therapists with "Rana Plaza Tragedy" survivors: Recovery and rehabilitation phases of disaster management. *World Federation of Occupational Therapy Bulletin, 68*(1), 14–19. https://doi.org/10.1179/otb.2013.68.1.006

Jeong, Y., Law, M., DeMatteo, C., Stratford, P., & Kim, H. (2016). The role of occupational therapists in the contexts of a natural disaster: A scoping review. *Disability and Rehabilitation, 38*(16), 1620–1631. https://doi.org/10.3109/09638288.2015.1106597

Lee, H. C. (2014). The role of occupational therapy in the recovery stage of disaster relief: A report from earthquake stricken areas in China. *Australian Occupational Therapy Journal, 61*(1), 28–31. https://doi.org/10.1111/1440-1630.12106

Nair, P., & Tyagi, N. (2014). Occupational therapy: Metamorphosis with vision in public health for disaster preparedness, response and recovery. *Indian Journal of Occupational Therapy, 46*(3), 71–76.

Pizzi, M. A. (2015). Hurricane Sandy, disaster preparedness, and the recovery model. *American Journal of Occupational Therapy, 69*(4), Article 6904250020. https://doi.org/10.5014/ajot.2015.015990

Rushford, N. (2015). Occupational stewardship and collaborative engagement: A practice model. In N. Rushford & K. Thomas (Eds.), *Disaster and development: An occupational perspective* (pp. 243–248). Edinburgh: Churchill Livingstone.

Rushford, N. A., & Thomas, K. A. (2011). Natural disasters: Challenging occupational therapists. In F. Kronenberg, N. Pollard, & D. Sakellariou (Eds.), *Occupational therapies without borders* (Vol. 2, pp. 185–193). Churchill Livingstone/Elsevier.

Rushford, N., & Thomas, K. (2015a). Disaster and development: A call to action. In N. Rushford & K. Thomas (Eds.), *Disaster and development: An occupational perspective* (pp. 3–19). Churchill Livingstone.

Rushford, N., & Thomas, K. (2015b). An occupational perspective on disaster and development and a conceptual framework. In N. Rushford & K. Thomas (Eds.). *Disaster and development: An occupational perspective* (pp. 235–241). Churchill Livingstone.

Sima, L., Thomas, Y., & Lowrie, D. (2017). Occupational disruption and natural disaster: Finding a "new normal" in a changed context. *Journal of Occupational Science, 24*(2), 128–139. https://doi.org/10.1080/14427591.2017.1306790

Thomas, K., & Rushford, N. (2015). Disaster and development: Practical considerations in promoting an occupational perspective. In N. Rushford & K. Thomas (Eds.), *Disaster and development: An occupational perspective* (pp. 239–262). Churchill Livingstone.

Whitney, R. V., & Walsh, W. E. (2020). *Occupational therapy's role in time of disaster: Addressing periods of occupational disruption.* American Occupational Therapy Association.

World Federation of Occupational Therapists. (2014). *Position statement: Occupational therapy in disaster preparedness and response (DP&R).* https://www.wfot.org/resources/occupational-therapy-in-disaster-preparedness-and-response-dp-r

World Federation of Occupational Therapists. (2019). *Guide for occupational therapy first responders to disasters and trauma.* https://www.wfot.org/resources/wfot-guide-for-occupational-therapy -first-responders-to-disasters-and-trauma

BIBLIOGRAPHY

Bulan, P. M. P., & Eturma, C. M. (2018). Practising occupational therapists' attitudes towards disaster management. *World Federation of Occupational Therapists Bulletin, 74*(2), 99–105. https://doi.org/10.1080/14473828.2018.1533154

Habib, M. M., Uddin, M. J., Sahrman, S. U., Jahan, N., & Akter, S. (2013). Occupational therapy role in disaster management in Bangladesh. *World Federation of Occupational Therapy Bulletin, 68*(1), 33–37. https://doi.org/10.1179/otb.2013.68.1.010

Moore, M. (2017). Regaining control after an uncontrollable event. *OT News, 25*(9), 16–18.

Parente, M., Tofani, M., De Santis, R., Esposito, G., Santilli, V., & Galeoto, G. (2017). The role of the occupational therapist in disaster areas: Systematic review. *Occupational Therapy International 2017,* Article 6475761. https://doi.org/10.1155/2017/6474761

Rushford, N. (2015). Lost in the mix: A case for inclusive and participatory approaches to disaster and development. In N. Rushford & K. Thomas (Eds.), *Disaster and development: An occupational perspective* (pp. 41–49). Churchill Livingstone.

Rushford, N., & Thomas, K. (2015). Disaster, development and occupational therapy: Historical perspectives and possibilities. In N. Rushford & K. Thomas (Eds.), *Disaster and development: An occupational perspective* (pp. 11–19). Churchill Livingstone.

Rushford, N., & Thomas, K. (2015). Disaster risk, vulnerability and resilience: An emergent socio-ecological perspective. In N. Rushford & K. Thomas (Eds.), *Disaster and development: An occupational perspective* (pp. 21–32). Churchill Livingstone.

Sakellariou, D., & Ullberg, S. B. (2015). Disaster, daily life and meaning. In N. Rushford & K. Thomas (Eds.), *Disaster and development: An occupational perspective* (pp. 33–40). Churchill Livingstone.

Santosa, T. B. (2013). Occupational therapy fieldwork experience in disaster response and recovery. *World Federation of Occupational Therapists Bulletin, 68*(1), 31–43. https://doi.org/10.1179/otb.2013.68.1.009

Shiino, Y., & Hasegawa, K. (2017). Disaster support activities after the great east Japan earthquake in Fukushima. In D. Sakellariou & N. Pollard (Eds.), *Occupational therapies without borders* (2nd ed., pp. 506–512). Elsevier.

Sinclair, K., & Thomas, K. (2010). Occupational therapy in disaster response. *World Federation of Occupational Therapists Bulletin, 61*(1), 64–68. https://doi.org/10.1179/otb.2010.61.1.016

Smith, T. M., Drefus, A., & Hersch, G. (2011). Habits, routines and roles of graduate students: Effects of Hurricane Ike. *Occupational Therapy in Health Care, 25*(4), 283–297. https://doi.org/10.3109/07380577.2011.600426

Smith, T. M., & Picone, N. M. (2019). Providing occupational therapy for disaster survivors. In B. A. Boyt Schell & G. Gillen (Eds.), *Willard and Spackman's occupational therapy* (13th ed., pp. 1065–1075). Wolters Kluwer.

Smith, T. M., & Scaffa, M. (2014). Providing occupational therapy for disaster survivors. In B. Schell, G. Gillen, & M. Scaffa (Eds.), *Willard & Spackman's occupational therapy* (12th ed., pp. 962–971). Wolters Kluwer.

Stark, S. (2013). Stories from the field: Reflections on occupational therapy experiences in Haiti following the earthquake. *World Federation of Occupational Therapists Bulletin, 68*(1), 20–25. https://doi.org/10.1179/otb.2013.68.1.007

Taylor, E., Jacobs, R., & Marsh, E. D. (2011). First year post-Katrina: Changes in occupational performance and emotional response. *Occupational Therapy in Mental Health, 27*(1), 3–25.

Driving Cessation and Driving Retirement

See also Driving Fitness.

Also called cessation of driving, driving disruption, loss of driver's license, nondriving, retiring from driving, retirement from driving, stop driving, stopping driving, unfit driver.

Description

Driving cessation is the process by which a person stops driving. Driving cessation can be voluntary when a person decides on his or her own to stop driving or involuntary when a driver's license is revoked by the vehicle licensing board (e.g., Department of Transportation, Department of Motor Vehicles). Driving retirement occurs before driving cessation and is described as the transition from operating a vehicle to becoming a passenger or using alternative types of transportation (Bridge et al., 2017). Additional terminology includes the term *driver restrictions*, usually items stated on a driver's license listing conditions which must be followed under penalty of law, such as wearing glasses or driving in daylight hours only; *driving interruption*, a term used to describe a period of time in which the person is not driving, such as during an acute period of illness or confinement to a facility such as a hospital or prison without access to a vehicle; and *unlicensed driving*, a term used to describe driving behavior that occurs when the person does not have a valid driver's license due to the license being revoked or expired (lapsed, not renewed by expiration date). Driving cessation involves balancing the benefits of safety to the person, pedestrians, and other drivers against the cost to the individual of social isolation, decreasing functional status, impaired quality of life, clinical depression and possible loss of independence (Porter, 2018).

Cause

Reason for voluntarily giving up driving may include the costs associated with driving a vehicle, anxiety about driving, loss of enjoyment of driving, concerns about safety, and availability of other forms of transportation. Reasons for involuntary driving cessation may include poor vision, chronic health limitations, poor memory, poor hearing, history of at-fault accidents and citations, and unsafe driving practices (Brzuz, 2018).

Warning Signs of Unsafe Driving (Alzheimer's Association, n.d.)
- Becoming angry or confused while driving
- Confusing the gas and brake pedals
- Driving at an inappropriate speed
- Forgetting how to locate familiar destinations
- Forgetting the destination during a drive
- Hitting curbs
- Making errors at intersections
- Making slow or poor decisions while driving
- Not keeping within lanes
- Not obeying traffic signs
- Returning late from a routine drive

Evaluation/Assessment

Areas
- Activities of Daily Living/Instrumental ADL: medication management, shopping, transfers, mobility, transportation
- Education/Work: transportation needs
- Play/Leisure: interests, values, type, frequency, location
- Rest/Sleep: sleep disturbance, sleep disorder, sleep habits
- Social Participation: type, location, frequency, with whom

- Sensorimotor: reaction time, muscle weakness, range of motion, endurance, pain, visual impairment
- Cognitive/Perceptual: dementia, attention and concentration, memory, executive functions, such as mental flexibility, problem solving and planning ahead, visual perception
- Psychosocial: social isolation, depression, coping, quality of life, self-confidence, sense of dependency, locus of control, loss of life roles
- Context/Environment: social support, alternative transportation systems, community resources for the disabled, alternate driver availability, housebound
- Comorbidities: amputation, arthritis, attention-deficit/hyperactivity disorder, autism spectrum disorder, carpal tunnel syndrome, cerebral palsy, cognitive impairment, dementia, diabetes, epilepsy, multiple sclerosis, Parkinson's disease, polytrauma, serious mental illness, pulmonary disorders, scleroderma, spina bifida, spinal cord injury, stroke, substance abuse, traumatic brain injury, visual impairment (age-related macular degeneration, cataracts, decreased contrast sensitivity, decreased acuity, diabetic retinopathy, glaucoma, loss of visual field, presbyopia)

Instruments
Instruments Developed by Occupational Therapy Personnel
- Canadian Occupational Performance Measure (5th ed.; COPM-5; Law et al., 2014)
- Driver Identity Survey (DIS; Pachana et al., 2017, in References)
- Occupational Therapy–Driver Off-Road Assessment Battery (OT-DORA Battery; Unsworth et al., 2012, in References)
- Preroad DriveABLE Competence Screen (PDCS; Korner-Bitensky et al., 2011, in References)

Instruments Developed by Other Professionals and Used by Occupational Therapy Personnel
- Digit Vigilance Test (DVT; Lewis, 1995)
- Geriatric Depression Scale (GDS; Yesavage et al.,1982–1983)
- Judgment of Line Orientation (JOLO; Benton et al., 1983)
- Montreal Cognitive Assessment (MoCA; Nasreddine et al., 2005)
- Road Sign Recognition Test (RSRT; Lincoln & Fanthrone, 1994)
- Short-Form 36 Health Survey (SF-36; Ware et al., 1993)
- SIMARD Screening Tool (Dobbs & Schopflocher, 2010; see also Bédard et al., 2011)
- Trail Making Test Part B (TMT-B; Reitan & Wolfson, 1995)

Problems/Issues
Activities of Daily Living/Instrumental ADL
- Person may experience a change in health status.
- Person may have difficulty with transfers, especially getting in/on and out/off of a vehicle.

Education/Work
- Person may have difficulty getting to paid or volunteer work setting.

Play/Leisure
- Person may have to give up engagement in favorite leisure occupations.

Rest/Sleep
- Person may have a sleep disorder.

Social Participation
- Person may be unable to participate in preferred social activities.

Sensorimotor
- Person may have visual changes due to ocular diseases such as age-related macular degeneration, uncorrected cataracts, untreated glaucoma, diabetic retinopathy.
- Person may have loss of visual acuity and peripheral vision.
- Person may have decreased ability to adapt to changes in light and heightened sensitivity to glare.

Cognitive/Perceptual

- Person may have difficulty planning ahead to organize and perform occupations using alternative transportation systems.
- Person may have presbyopia (decreased ability to accommodate, which impairs depth perception).

Psychosocial

- Person may display little or no insight into the risk posed to self or others due to decreased motor, sensory, cognitive, perceptual, or behavior skills.
- Person may be unable to self-regulate to restrict driving to safe levels.
- Person may resist or reject recommendation or requirement to stop driving.
- Person may experience social isolation after ceasing driving.
- Person may become depressed after ceasing driving.
- Person may experience decreased quality of life.
- Person may experience decreased sense of independence.
- Person may report feeling "stuck" or "housebound" when unable to drive independently.
- Person may report feeling older than actual age because driving cessation is viewed as a sign of "getting old" in the person's mind.
- Person may be unable to perform some life roles.
- Person may experience loss of self-identity as the "family driver" and "owner in charge of the family vehicle."

Context/Environment

- Person may lose access to the community.
- Family members may lack information as to how the person's diagnosis can affect safe driving ability.
- Person and family may lack knowledge to access a professional who can evaluate person's driving ability and make recommendations.
- Health-care professionals may fail to refer a person for a driving assessment even when signs or symptoms are apparent.
- Person, family, and caregivers may lack information about availability and accessibility of alternative transportation systems.
- Alternative transportation systems may be unavailable where person lives, unreliable, expensive, and require booking in advance.
- Person may need adapted equipment to access alternative transportation systems such as a swivel seat or grab bar over window.

Intervention/Treatment

Models and programs developed by occupational therapy personnel include case study (Haltiwanger & Underwood, 2011), driver retirement program (Chan et al., 2015), and model of human occupation (Haltiwanger & Underwood, 2011). Models and programs developed by other professionals but used by occupational therapy personnel include driving cessation system (Kristalovich, 2010), group intervention (Liddle, Haynes, Pachana, et al., 2014), Knowledge Enhances Your Safety (KEYS) program (Coxon & Keay, 2015), traveling a new road (Fry et al., 2013), and University of Queensland Driver Retirement Initiative (UQDRIVE; Gustafsson et al., 2012; Gustafsson et al., 2011; Liddle, Haynes, Gustafsson, et al., 2014; Liddle et al., 2015). Team members include general physicians, neurologists, ophthalmologists, psychologists, physical therapists, driving rehabilitation specialists, licensing organizations and boards, family and friends, and occupational therapy personnel. Goal is to increase consumer knowledge about safe driving and driving cessation/retirement and determine if the person should stop driving a vehicle. The goal is to reduce the negative outcome of driving retirement by assisting with planning for and adjustment to driving retirement, as well as by promoting community engagement and personal control (Bridge et al., 2017).

Activities of Daily Living/Instrumental ADL

- Assist client to determine how shopping for groceries and other essentials can be accomplished, such as using alternative transportation systems or using delivery systems.
- Assist client to shop online if person has not previously mastered online shopping skills. (Note: May require applying for a credit card.)
- Assist client to determine what physical, motor, sensory, and cognitive skills might be needed to use alternate transportation.

Education/Work

- Assist client to determine what alternative transportation systems might be available to permit person to continue paid or volunteer work.
- Assist client to explore work (paid or volunteer) that could be done at home or within short walking distance.

Play/Leisure

- Assist client to determine what alternative transportation systems are available to permit person to continue engaging in favorite leisure occupation.
- Assist client to explore new leisure occupations that can be done at home, within walking distance, or using available transportation systems.

Rest/Sleep

- Assist in adapting or modifying sleeping habits to provide rest before driving.

Social Participation

- Assist client to determine what alternative transportation systems are available to permit person to continue participation in social activities.
- Assist client to explore new social activities that can be done at home, within walking distance, or using available transportation systems.

Sensorimotor

- Provide exercise program to maintain physical fitness (in clinic, in home, using online programs).

Cognitive/Perceptual

- Provide or refer client to a cognitive rehabilitation program if cognition is a factor.
- Provide or refer client to a visual rehabilitation program if vision is a factor.

Psychosocial

- Encourage client to talk about feelings depression.
- Discuss with client and family members changes in life roles such as spouse or children having to do more of the driving and being more dependent on others for transportation.
- Discuss with client changes that may affect quality of life and lifestyle.

Context/Environment

- Discuss with client and family members state licensing requirements and reporting regulations applicable to state of residence.
- Explore community resources, including alternative transportation systems available, with client, family, and caregivers (Oakes & Gandiaga, 2018).
  - ▶ Public transportation (fixed route buses and trains with fixed schedules; some buses or trains may have wheelchair lifts or ground level entrance platforms).
  - ▶ Taxi service (national or local companies; fees are usually based on miles traveled, but some fixed rates may be applied by local governments).

- ▶ Paratransit (services via vans or taxis available for people with disabilities who cannot use fixed route transportation; some vehicles have adaptations for wheelchair users; service may require booking in advance).
- ▶ Independent Transportation Network (ITN; a not-for-profit service for older adults where pay is based on miles driven; may require booking in advance).
- ▶ Uber or Lyft (drivers are called via a smartphone, and no cash is exchanged).
- ▶ Go-Go Grandparent (ride sharing service designed for people without smartphones who have a landline; may require booking in advance).
- ▶ Private drivers (driver is hired by the individual client; usually, arrangements must be made in advance).
- ▶ Community vans (some senior retirement communities have free van service available to residents to local shopping centers and some scheduled social events, and fee-for-service to other destinations, such as doctor or dentist appointments).
- ▶ Veterans Administration Medical Centers (available transportation for those veterans who have appointments at a veterans medical facility).
- • Explore with client, family, and caregivers if adapted devices might facilitate transfers (getting in and out of a vehicle).

Precautions/Safety Considerations

Dizziness has been reported by some clients when being tested in a simulator. A vehicle used for on-road testing must be equipment with dual brakes at a minimum.

Prognosis and Outcome

Variable. Planning ahead is helpful but clients' adaptation to non-driving status depends on individual characteristics and environmental alternatives.

REFERENCES

Alzheimer's Association. (n.d.). *Dementia and driving.* Retrieved April 27, 2022, from https://www .alz.org/help-support/caregiving/safety/dementia-driving#.~:text=Signs_of_unsafe_driving

Bédard, M., Weaver, B., Man-Son-Hing, M., Classen, S., Porter, M., & Candrive Investigators. (2011). The SIMARD screening Tool to identify unfit drivers: Are we there now? *Journal of Primary Care & Community Health, 2*(2), 133–135. https://doi.org/10.1177/2150131910397704

Bridge, K., Lapointe, J., & Craik, J. (2017). Occupational therapists' role in driving retirement: Supporting engagement in times of transition. *Occupational Therapy Now, 19*(3), 8–10.

Brzuz, A. (2018). Older drivers' perceptions of driving cessation. *OT Practice, 23*(13), 8–11.

Chan, M. L., Gustafsson, L., & Liddle, J. (2015). An intervention to support professional driver retirement transition: Results of a pilot study for older taxi drivers in Singapore. *British Journal of Occupational Therapy, 78*(6), 391–400. https://doi.org/10.1177/0308022614562400

Coxon, K., & Keay, L. (2015). Behind the wheel: Community consultation informs adaptation of safe-transport program for older drivers. *BMC Research Notes, 8,* Article 764. https://doi.org/ 10.1186/s13104-015-1745-0

Fry, D., Fox, B., & Donnelly, C. (2013). Traveling a new road: A driving cessation group in primary care. *Occupational Therapy Now, 15*(6), 25–26.

Gustafsson, L., Liddle, J., Liang, P., Pachana, N., Hoyle, M., Mitchell, G., & McKenna, K. (2012). A driving cessation program to identify and improve transport and lifestyle issues of older retired and retiring drivers. *International Psychogeriatrics, 24*(5), 794–802. https://doi.org/10.10 17/S1041610211002560

Gustafsson, L., Liddle, J., Lua, S., Hoyle, M., Pachana, N. A., Mitchell, G. K., & McKenna, K. T. (2011). Participant feedback and satisfaction with the UQDRIVE groups for driving cessation. *Canadian Journal of Occupational Therapy, 78*(2), 110–117. https://doi.org/10.2182/cjot .2011.2.6

Haltiwanger, E. P., & Underwood, N. S. (2011). Life after driving: A community-dwelling senior's experience. *Physical & Occupational Therapy in Geriatrics, 29*(2), 156–167. https://doi.org/10.3109/02703181.2011.563416

Korner-Bitensky, N., Audet, T., Man-Son-Hing, M., Benoit, D., Kaizer, F., & Gélinas, I. (2011). Test–retest reliability of the Preroad DriveABLE Competence Screen. *Physical & Occupational Therapy in Geriatrics, 29*(3), 202–212. https://doi.org/10.3109/02703181.2011.573619

Kristalovich, L. (2010). Dementia and driving: From diagnosis to driving cessation and beyond. *Occupational Therapy Now, 12*(5), 20–22.

Liddle, J., Hayes, R., Gustafsson, L., & Fleming, J. (2014). Managing driving issues after an acquired brain injury: Strategies used by health professionals. *Australian Occupational Therapy Journal, 61*(4), 215–223. https://doi.org/10.1111/1440-1630.12119

Liddle, J., Haynes, M., Pachana, N. A., Mitchell, G., McKenna, K., & Gustafsson, L. (2014). Effect of a group intervention to promote older adults' adjustment to driving cessation on community mobility: A randomized controlled trial. *The Gerontologist, 54*(3), 409–422. https://doi.org/10.1093/geront/gnt019

Liddle, J., Liu, X., Aplin, T., & Gustafsson, L. (2015). The experiences of peer leaders in a driving cessation programme. *British Journal of Occupational Therapy, 78*(6), 383–390. https://doi.org/10.1177/0308022614562403

Oakes, C. E., & Gandiaga, E. (2018). Role of occupational therapy in driving cessations: Helping older adults navigate the options. *OT Practice: SIS Quarterly Practice Connections, 3*(2), 21–25.

Pachana, N. A., Jetten, J., Gustafsson, L., & Liddle, J. (2017). To be or not to be (an older driver): Social identify theory and driving cessation in later life. *Aging & Society, 37*(8), 1597–1608. https://doi.org/10.1017/S0144686X16000507

Porter, R. S. (Ed.). (2018). *The Merck manual of diagnosis and therapy* (20th ed.). Merck Sharp & Dohme.

Unsworth, C., Baker, A., Taitz, C., Chan, S.-P., Pallant, J., Russell, K., & Odell, M. (2012). Development of a standardised Occupational Therapy–Driver Off-Road Assessment Battery to assess older and/or functionally impaired drivers. *Australian Occupational Therapy Journal, 59*(1), 23–36. https://doi.org/10.1111/j.1440-1630.2011.00979.x

BIBLIOGRAPHY

Al-Hassani, S. B., & Alotaibi, N. M. (2014). The impact of driving cessation on older Kuwaiti adults: Implications to occupational therapy. *Occupational Therapy in Health Care, 28,* 264–276. https://doi.org/10.3109/07380577.2014.917779

Blane, A., Lee, H. C., Lee, M., Parsons, R., & Falkmer, T. (2016). The cognitive and sociodemographic influences on driving performance and driving cessation in post-stroke drivers. *Advances in Transportation Studies, 38,* 75–90.

Chacko, E. E., Wright, W. M., Worrall, R. C., Adamson, C., & Cheung, G. (2015). Reactions to driving cessation: A qualitative study of people with dementia and their families. *Australasian Psychiatry 23*(5), 496–499. https://doi.org/10.1177/1039856215591326

Dickerson, A. E., Molnar, L. J., Bédard, M., Eby, D. W., Berg-Weger, M., Choi, M., Grigg, J., Horowitz, A., Meuser, T., Myers, A., O'Connor, M., & Silverstein, N. M. (2019). Transportation and aging: An updated research agenda to advance safe mobility among older adults transitioning from driving to non-driving. *The Gerontologist, 59*(2), 215–221. https://doi.org/10.1093/geront/gnx120

Fleming, J., Liddle, J., Nalder, E., Weir, N., & Cornwell, P. (2014). Return to driving in the first 6 months of community integration after acquired brain injury. *NeuroRehabilitation, 34*(1), 157–166. https://doi.org/10.3233/NRE-131012

Holmes, J. D., Alvarez, L., Johnson, A. M., Robinson, A. E., Gilhuly, K., Horst, E., Kowalchuk, A., Rathwell, K., Reklitis, Y., & Wheildon, N. (2019). Driving with Parkinson's disease: Exploring lived experience. *Parkinson's Disease, 2019,* Article 3169679. https://doi.org/10.1155/2019/3169679

Liang, P., Fleming, J., Gustafsson, L., Griffin, J., & Liddle, J. (2017). Family members' experiences of driving disruption after acquired brain injury. *Brain Injury, 31*(4), 517–525. https://doi.org/10.1080/02699052.2017.1283058

Liang, P., Gustafsson, L., Liddle, J., & Fleming, J. (2015). Family members' needs and experiences of driving disruption due to health conditions or ageing. *Disability and Rehabilitation, 37,* 2114–2129.

Liang, P., Gustafsson, L., Liddle, J., & Fleming, J. (2017). Family members' needs and experiences of driving disruption over time following an acquired brain injury: An evolving issue. *Disability and Rehabilitation, 39*(14), 1398–1407. https://doi.org/10.1080/09638288.2016.1196397

Liang, P., Liddle, J., Fleming J., & Gustafsson, L. (2016). Family members' narratives of lifespace: Mapping changes before and after a brain injury causing driving disruption. *Australian Occupational Therapy Journal, 63*(3), 164–174. https://doi.org/10.1111/1440-1630.12258

Liddle, J., Bennett, S., Allen, S., Lie, D. C., Standen, B., & Pachana, N. A. (2013). The stages of driving cessation for people with dementia: Needs and challenges. *International Psychogeriatrics, 25*(12), 2033–2046. https://doi.org/10.1017/S1041610213001464

Liddle, J., Fleming, J., McKenna, K., Turpin, M., Whitelaw, P., & Allen, S. (2011). Driving and driving cessation after traumatic brain injury: Processes and key times of need. *Disability and Rehabilitation, 33*(25-26), 2574–2586. https://doi.org/10.3109/09638288.2011.582922

Liddle, J., Fleming, J., McKenna, K., Turpin, M., Whitelaw, P., & Allen, S. (2012). Adjustment to loss of the driving role following traumatic brain injury: A qualitative exploration with key stakeholders. *Australian Occupational Therapy Journal, 59*(1), 79–88. https://doi.org/10.1111/j.1440-1630.2011.00978.x

Liddle, J., Gustafsson, L., Bartlett, H., & McKenna, K. (2012). Time use, role participation and life satisfaction of older people: Impact of driving status. *Australian Occupational Therapy Journal, 59*(5), 384–392. https://doi.org/10.1111/j.1440-1630.2011.00956.x

Liddle, J., Gustafsson, L., Mitchell, G., & Pachana, N. A. (2017). A difficult journey: Reflections on driving and driving cessation from a team of clinical researchers. *The Gerontologist, 57*(1), 82–88. https://doi.org/10.1093/geront/gnw079

Liddle, J., Reaston, T., Pachana, N., Mitchell, G., & Gustafsson, L. (2014). Is planning for driving cessation critical for the well-being and lifestyle of older drivers? *International Psychogeriatrics, 26*(7), 1111–1120. https://doi.org/10.1017/S104161021400060X

Liddle, J., Tan, A., Liang, P., Bennett, S., Allen, S., Lie, D. C., & Pachana, N. A. (2016). "The biggest problem we've ever had to face": How families manage driving cessation with people with dementia. *International Psychogeriatrics, 28*(1), 109–122. https://doi.org/10.1017/s1041610215001441

Mullen, N. W., Parker, B., Wiersma, E., Stinchcombe, A., & Bédard, M. (2017). Looking forward and looking back: Older adults' views of the impacts of stopping driving. *Occupational Therapy in Health Care, 31*(3), 188–204. https://doi.org/10.1080/07380577.2017.1337282

Niewoehner, P. M., & Thomas, F. P. (2011). Motor vehicle operation in the setting of multiple sclerosis with myelopathy: Assessment, adaptive equipment, counseling, and cessation of driving. *Continuum, 17*(4), 877–881. https://doi.org/10.1212/01.CON.0000403800.95364.3a

Scott, T., Liddle, J., Pachana, N., Beattie, E., & Mitchell, G. (2020). Managing the transition to non-driving in patients with dementia in primary care settings: Facilitators and barriers reported by primary care physicians. *International Psychogeriatrics, 32*(12), 1419–1428. https://doi.org/10.1017/S1041610218002326

Sinnott, C., Foley, T., Horgan, L., McLoughlin, K., Sheehan, C., & Bradley, C. (2019). Shifting gears versus sudden stops: Qualitative study of consultations about driving in patients with cognitive impairment. *BMJ Open, 9*(8), Article e024452. https://doi.org/10.1136/bmjopen-2018-024452

Sullivan, C., & Buckley, S. (2013). A survey examining the impact of driving cessation on people with epilepsy in Ireland. *British Journal of Occupational Therapy, 76*(9), 399–408. https://doi.org/10.4276/030802213X13782044946265

Turner, L. M., Liddle, J., & Pachana, N. A. (2017). Parkinson's disease and driving cessation: A journey influenced by anxiety. *Clinical Gerontologist, 40*(3), 220–229. https://doi.org/10.10 80/07317115.2016.1215365

Wheatley, C. J., Carr, D. B., & Marottoli, R. A. (2014). Consensus statements on driving for persons with dementia. *Occupational Therapy in Health Care, 28*(2), 132–139. https://doi.org/10 .3109/07380577.2014.903583

Driving Fitness

See also Driver Cessation and Driving Retirement.

Description

Driving fitness is a multidimensional occupation that requires the integration of motor, sensory, cognitive, perceptual, and behavioral processes and competencies that permits a person to control, operate, and maneuver a vehicle safely toward a preselected destination while observing and following applicable laws. Driving is classified as an instrumental activity of daily living. The role of practitioners is to do functional assessments to help determine overall driving safety and communicate recommendations effectively to drivers and their family members or caregivers (Porter, 2018). Porter (2018) recommended that older persons with a history of falls, cardiac disorders, neurological disorders, diabetes mellitus, sleep disorders, and drugs be considered candidates for driver evaluation.

Cause

The cause of unsafe or impaired driving involves multiple factors such as the person's functional status of motor, sensory, cognitive, and emotional regulation abilities; disease-related changes; drug abuse; failure to observe and follow applicable laws; or failure to maintain the vehicle in good working order (Porter, 2018).

Evaluation/Assessment

Areas

- Activities of Daily Living/Instrumental ADL: transfer skills (especially getting in and out of a vehicle), mobility devices (especially storing and retrieving from a vehicle), use of private versus public transportation
- Education/Work: driving requirements (if any), parking location, getting to and from workstation
- Play/Leisure: interests, values, type, frequency, location, level of satisfaction
- Rest/Sleep: sleep habits
- Social Participation: type, location, frequency, with whom
- Sensorimotor: muscle strength (grip strength), range of motion, endurance (stamina), coordination of two sides of body, reaction time, reflexes, body flexibility and mobility (trunk and neck rotation, moving foot from gas to break quickly), stiffness (especially in the fingers), fatigue, headaches, dizziness, visual impairments (both focal/focused and peripheral vision), pain
- Cognitive/Perceptual: attention, concentration, memory, executive functions: decision making, planning, anticipation, information processing speed, spatial awareness and orientation, visual searching/scanning
- Psychosocial: anxiety, anger management, self-efficacy, quality of life, sense of independence
- Context/Environment: knowledge of traffic laws, availability of transportation systems
- Comorbidities: amputation, arthritis, attention-deficit/hyperactivity disorder, autism spectrum disorder, bipolar disorders, cardiac diseases, carpal tunnel syndrome, cerebral palsy, cognitive

impairment, dementia, diabetes, epilepsy, Huntington's disease, multiple sclerosis, Parkinson's disease, polytrauma, pulmonary disorders, schizophrenia, scleroderma, serious/severe mental illness, sleep disorders, spina bifida, spinal cord injuries, stroke, substance abuse, traumatic brain injury, visual impairment

Instruments

(Note: Includes both off-road and on-road instruments.)

Instruments Developed by Occupational Therapy Personnel

- Cognitive Performance Test, Revised (CPT-R; Burns, 2018; see also Burns et al., 2018, in References)
- DriveAware/DriveSafe (Kay et al., 2009; see also Allan et al., 2016, in References)
- Driving Observation Schedule (DOS; Vlahodimitrakou et al., 2013, in References)
- (Electronic) Driving Observation Schedule (eDOS; Koppel et al., 2013, in References)
- Fitness to Drive Screen Measure (FDSM; Classen et al., 2015, in References)
- Occupational Therapy–Driver Off-Road Assessment Battery (OT-DORA; Unsworth et al., 2012, in References)
- Occupational Therapy Driving Assessment (OTDA; Alberta Health Services [AHS] Provincial Occupational Therapy Driving Working Group, 2017, in References)
- Occupational Therapy Driving Evaluation Report (OTDER; Alberta Health Services [AHS] Provincial Occupational Therapy Driving Working Group, 2017, in References)
- Occupational Therapy Risk Propensity Test (OT-RiPT; Bruce et al., 2015, in References)
- Preroad DriveABLE Competence Screen (PDCS; Korner-Bitensky et al., 2011, in References)
- Road Law and Road Craft Test (RLRCT; Unsworth et al., 2010, in References)
- Record of Driving Errors (RODE; Barco, Baum, et al., 2015; and Barco, Carr, et al., 2015, in References)
- Safe Driving Behavior Measure (SDBM; Classen, Wang, Winter, et al., 2013; Classen et al., 2012a, 2012b; Classen et al., 2010; and Crizzle, Classen, Winter, et al., 2012, in References)
- Saskatchewan Psychiatric Occupational Therapy Driving Screen (SPOTDS; Carey et al., 2018, in References)
- Western University On-Road Assessment (WUORA; Classen, Krasniuk, et al., 2017; Classen et al., 2016, in References)

Instruments Developed by Other Professionals and Used by Occupational Therapy Personnel

- Adelaide Driving Self-Efficacy Scale (ADSES; George et al., 2007)
- Assessment of Driving-Related Skills (ADReS; Wang et al., 2003; see also Woolnough et al., 2013, in References)
- Beck Anxiety Inventory (BAI; Beck & Steer, 1993)
- Beck Depression Inventory (2nd ed.; BDI–II; Beck et al., 1996)
- Benton Visual Retention Task (BVRT; Eslinger et al., 1985)
- Clinical Dementia Rating Scale (CDR; Morris, 1997)
- Cognitive Behavioral Driver's Inventory (CBDI; Engum et al., 1988; see also Duquette et al., 2010, in References)
- Decisional Balance Scale (DBS; Nigg et al., 1998; see also Sukhawathanakul et al., 2015, in References)
- DriveABLE (Dobbs, 1997; Dobbs et al., 1998)
- Driver Behaviour Questionnaire (DBQ; Reason et al., 1990; see also Koppel et al., 2018, in References)
- Driving Comfort Scales (Daytime [DCS-D], Nighttime [DCS-N]; Myers et al., 2008)
- Driving Habits and Intensions Questionnaire (DHIQ; Kowalski et al., 2012; see also Song et al., 2015; and Song et al., 2016, in References)
- Driving Habits Questionnaire (DHQ; Owsley et al., 1999)
- Fatigue Severity Scale (FSS; Krupp et al., 1989)

- Hopkins Verbal Learning Test–Revised (HVLT-R; Benedict et al., 1998)
- Mini-Mental State Examination (MMSE; Folstein et al., 1975; see also Crizzle, Classen, Bédard, et al., 2012, in References)
- Minimal Assessment of Cognitive Function in Multiple Sclerosis (MACFIMS; Benedict et al., 2006)
- Montreal Cognitive Assessment (MoCA; Nasreddine et al., 2005; see also Kwok et al., 2015; Rapoport et al., 2013, in References)
- Motor-Free Visual Perception Test (4th ed.; MVPT-4; Colarusso & Hamill, 2015)
- Neuropsychological Assessment Battery (NAB; Stern & White, 2003)
- OSCAR (Levasseur et al., 2015, in References; assessment in French)
- Pelli-Robson Contrast Sensitivity Test (PRCST; Mäntyjärvi & Laitnen, 2001)
- Perceived Driving Abilities scale (PDAS; Blanchard & Myers, 2010; MacDonald et al., 2008)
- Posttraumatic Stress Disorder Checklist (PSDC; Ventureyra et al., 2001)
- Post-Concussion Symptom Scale (PSS; Lovell et al. 2006)
- Rapid Pace Walk (Person is instructed to walk as quickly as possible along a 10-foot tape measure, turn around, and walk back [20 feet]. Time over 7.5 seconds is significant for safe driving.)
- Rey Auditory Verbal Learning Test (RAVLT; Schmidt, 1996)
- Rey-Osterrieth Complex Figure Test (ROCF; Meyers & Meyers, 1995)
- Sequential Finger-Thumb Opposition (SF-TO; Person is instructed to move thumb toward each finger sequentially and back; Water & Burns, 1995)
- SIMARD Screening Tool (Dobbs & Schopflocher, 2010; see also Bédard et al., 2013; Bédard et al., 2011, in References)
- Situational Driving Avoidance (SDA; Blanchard & Myers, 2010; MacDonald et al., 2008)
- Situational Driving Frequency (SDF; Blanchard & Myers, 2010; MacDonald et al., 2008)
- Symbol Digit Modalities Test (SDMT; Smith, 1973)
- Trail Making Test Parts A & B (Trails A, Trails B; Reitan & Wolfson, 1995; see also Papandonatos et al., 2015, in References)
- Useful Field of View (UFOV; Edwards et al., 2006; see also Classen, Wang, Crizzle, et al., 2013, in References)

Problems/Issues

Activities of Daily Living/Instrumental ADL
- Person may not have the financial resources to pay for modifications needed to make vehicle safe given person's current health status.
- Person may not find a vehicle that fits needs especially if person has disabilities.

Education/Work
- Person may be unable to get to or experience difficulty getting to paid or volunteer work without driving.

Play/Leisure
- Person may experience activity limitations and limitations on ability to engage in favorite leisure occupations without being able to drive.

Rest/Sleep
- Person may experience drowsiness or fall asleep while driving resulting in unsafe driving.

Social Participation
- Person may experience participation restrictions if he or she is unable to drive.

Sensorimotor
- Person may have reduced reflexes and response times.
- Person may have restricted range of motion of upper or lower extremities or neck.

- Person may have muscle weakness or paralysis and be unable to depress accelerator and brake pedals, turn steering wheel, or operate turn signals.
- Person may lack trunk rotation necessary to reach for the seat belt.
- Person may experience discomfort while wearing seat belt.
- Person may have stiffness in fingers that makes undoing (unlocking, unlatching) the seat belt difficult.
- Person may experience fatigue while driving.

Cognitive/Perceptual

- Person may become confused as to what is expected of a driver.
- Person may fail to obey traffic signs.
- Person may be slow to make decision or make poor decisions while driving.
- Person may drive at an inappropriate speed for the conditions (road, weather, traffic).
- Person may not stay within the driving lanes.
- Person may hit the curb.
- Person may make errors at intersections such as turning left when there is a posted no left turn signal.
- Person may confuse the gas and brake pedals.
- Person may forget the destination during a drive.

Psychosocial

- Person may get angry or irritable quickly and make aggressive actions toward other drivers.
- Person may be impulsive (not waiting turn, making unsafe lane changes or turns).
- Person may become anxious or fearful (in high traffic situations, poor weather conditions).
- Person may be fearful that he or she cannot get out of vehicle quickly in an emergency (difficulty rotating trunk, difficulty standing up, difficulty unlocking seat belt).

Context/Environment

- Person may become lost in local familiar surroundings.
- Person may be unfamiliar with the road conditions such as road closures.
- Person may fail to consider weather conditions before driving.
- Person be unaware of alternative transportation availability.

Intervention/Treatment

Models and programs developed by occupational therapy personnel include the driving readiness program (Lafrance et al., 2017) and driving simulation program (Classen et al., 2011; Mazer et al., 2015; Naveh et al., 2015). Models and programs developed by other professionals but used by occupational therapy personnel include CarFit (Belagamage et al., 2014; Craik et al., 2015; Stav, 2010), Stay SHARP (Korner-Bitensky & Kua, 2010), Drive Safe initiatives/practices (Dun, Baker, et al., 2015; Dun, Bull, et al., 2015), OSCAR program (Levasseur et al., 2015), Veterans Driving Intervention program (Classen, Cormack, et al., 2014; Classen, Monahan, et al., 2014; Classen, Winter, et al., 2017), and vehicle modification (Di Stefano, Stuckey, & Kinsman, 2019; Di Stefano, Stucky, Kinsman, & Lavender, 2019). Team members include general physicians, neurologists, ophthalmologists, psychologists, physical therapists, driving rehabilitation specialists, and occupational therapy personnel. Goal is to improve person-to-vehicle fit, increase consumer knowledge about safe driving, and determine if the person can drive safely and obey applicable laws.

Activities of Daily Living/Instrumental ADL

- Assist client in determining needs for driving.

Education/Work

- Assist client to determine best routes for driving to paid or volunteer work.

Play/Leisure

- Assist client to plan driving needs for leisure occupations. Consider alternative transportation.

Rest/Sleep

- Review with client sleeping habits to avoid sleepiness while driving.
- Suggest client take a nap or rest period before driving.

Social Participation

- Assist client to plan driving needs to participate in social occupations. Consider alternative transportation.

Sensorimotor

- Recommend client avoid driving when fatigued.
- Recommend client avoid driving when client has a headache.
- Recommend client consider reducing driving distance or arrange to change drivers.
- Recommend client reduce amount of time of continuous driving or take breaks while driving.
- Recommend client reduce or abstain from driving at night, especially in unfamiliar places.
- Recommend learning to use Global Positioning System (GPS) and provide instruction and practice as needed.
- Recommend client avoid talking with others while driving.
- Recommend client reduce speed while driving.
- Recommend client minimize lane changes.
- Recommend client reduce number of turns required, especially left-hand turns without signal lights.
- Recommend client allow more distance between vehicles.
- Recommend tying a ribbon to the seat belt, which may ease retrieval for persons with reduced trunk rotation.

Cognitive/Perceptual

- Assist client to avoid taking risks. Reduce number of left turns, reduce driving in poor weather, reduce nighttime driving, avoid rush hour driving.
- Assist client to review driving laws.
- Assist client to plan driving trips when traffic is lighter such as midmorning or early on weekends.

Psychosocial

- Discuss with client situations that are frustrating or result in anger and how to avoid or manage such situations.
- Facilitate client's learning to self-identify, self-regulate, and compensate for decreased driving abilities.

Context/Environment

- Assist client to create and follow a regular vehicle maintenance program including any state or local required vehicle inspections.
- Assist client to review safety conditions before driving such as correct height of seat, rearview mirror adjustment, clean windows front and back, tire pressure.
- Assist client to learn to use GPS.
- Assist client to use local traffic system alerts regarding road closures or unsafe weather conditions.
- Assist client to determine if adaptations to vehicle will be necessary before driving can be accomplished safely and provide resources for securing the adaptations.
  - ▶ Steering additions: knobs (spinner, stationery), palm grip, tri-pin grip.
  - ▶ Accelerator and brake controls: left foot pedal, gas pedal block, hand controls.
  - ▶ Mirrors: additional mirrors or extended mirrors.

- Seating and positioning: cushions, swivel base seat.
- Hand bars: removable grab bar which hooks onto door latch.
- Leg lift strap: helps lift legs into vehicle.
- Navigation: wireless or GPS technology.
- Backup camera.

Precautions/Safety Considerations

Dizziness has been reported when using simulators. On-road testing requires a vehicle modified with dual controls, especially dual brake pedals.

Prognosis and Outcome

Variable. Many factors must be considered during driver evaluation and any recommendation for return to unrestricted driving, driving with new or existing restrictions, or driver cessation.

REFERENCES

Alberta Health Services (AHS) Provincial Occupational Therapy Driving Working Group. (2017). *Occupational therapy practice guide for enabling participation in driving* (2nd ed.).

Allan, C., Coxon, K., Bundy, A., Peattie, L., & Keay, L. (2016). DriveSafe and DriveAware assessment tools are a measure of driving-related function and predicts self-reported restriction for older drivers. *Journal of Applied Gerontology, 35*(6), 583–600. https://doi.org/10.1177/0733464815570666

Barco, P. P., Baum, C. M., Ott, B. R., Ice, S., Johnson, A., Wallendorf, M., & Carr, D. B. (2015). Driving errors in persons with dementia. *Journal of the American Geriatrics Society, 63*(7), 1373–1380. https://doi.org/10.1111/jgs.13508

Barco, P. P., Carr, D. B., Rutkoski, K., Xiong, C., & Roe, C. M. (2015). Interrater reliability of the Record of Driving Errors (RODE). *American Journal of Occupational Therapy, 69*(2), Article 6902350020. https://doi.org/10.5014/ajot.2015.013128

Bédard, M., Marshall, S., Man-Son-Hing, M., Weaver, B., Gélinas, I., Korner-Bitensky, N., Mazer, B., Naglie, G., Porter, M. M., Rapoport, M. J., Tuokko, H., & Vrkljan, B. (2013). It is premature to test older drivers with the SIMARD-MD. *Accident Analysis & Prevention, 61*, 317–321. https://doi.org/10.1016/j.aap.2013.04.001

Bédard, M., Weaver, B., Man-Son-Hing, M., Classen, S., Porter, M., & Candrive Investigators. (2011). The SIMARD screening tool to identify unfit drivers: Are we there now? *Journal of Primary Care & Community Health, 2*(2), 133–135. https://doi.org/10.1177/2150131910397704

Belagamage, L., Lapointe, J., & McCarthy, N. (2014) CarFit: Helping mature drivers find their safest fit. *Occupational Therapy Now, 16*(4), 7–8.

Bruce, C., Unsworth, C. A., Tay, R., & Dillon, M. P. (2015). Development and validation of the Occupational Therapy Risk Propensity Test (OT-RiPT) for drivers with disability. *Scandinavian Journal of Occupational Therapy, 22*(2), 147–152. https://doi.org/10.3109/11038128.2014.992952

Burns, T., Lawler, K., Lawler, D., McCarten, J. R., & Kuskowski, M. (2018). Predictive value of the Cognitive Performance Test (CPT) for staging function and fitness to drive in people with neurocognitive disorders. *American Occupational Therapy Association, 72*(4), Article 7204205040. https://doi.org/10.5014/ajot.2018.027052

Carey, A., Burton, C., Grochulski, A., Pinay, P., & Remillard, A. J. (2018). Development of the Saskatchewan psychiatric occupational therapy driving screen. *British Journal of Occupational Therapy, 81*(4), 187–195. https://doi.org/10.1177/0308022617752065

Classen, S., Cormack, N. L. Winter, S. M., Monahan, M., Yarney, A., Lutz, A. L., & Platek, K. (2014). Efficacy of an occupational therapy driving intervention for returning combat veterans. *OTJR: Occupation, Participation and Health, 34*(4), 177–182. https://doi.org/10.3928/15394492-20141006-01

Classen, S., Krasniuk, S., Alvarez, L., Monahan, M., Morrow, S. A., & Danter, T. (2017). Development and validity of Western University's on-road assessment. *OTJR: Occupation, Participation and Health, 37*(1), 14–29. https://doi.org/10.1177/1539449216672859

Classen, S., Krasniuk, S., Knott, M., Alvarez, L., Monahan, M., Morrow, S., & Danter, T. (2016). Interrater reliability of Western University's on-road assessment. *Canadian Journal of Occupational Therapy, 83*(5), 317–325. https://doi.org/10.1177/0008417416663228

Classen, S., Levy, C., Meyer, D. L., Bewernitz, M., Lanford, D. N., & Mann, W. C. (2011). Simulated driving performance of combat veterans with mild traumatic brain injury and posttraumatic stress disorder: A pilot study. *American Journal of Occupational Therapy, 65*(4), 419–427. https://doi.org/10.5014/ajot.2011.000893

Classen, S., Monahan, M., Canonizado, M., & Winter, S. (2014). Utility of an occupational therapy driving intervention for a combat veteran. *American Journal of Occupational Therapy, 68*(4), 405–411. https://doi.org/10.5014/ajot.2014.010041

Classen, S., Velozo, C. A., Winter, S. M., Bédard, M., & Wang, Y. (2015). Psychometrics of the Fitness-to-Drive Screening Measure. *OTJR: Occupation, Participation and Health, 35*(1), 42–52. https://doi.org/10.1177/1539449214561761

Classen, S., Wang, Y., Crizzle, A. M., Winter, S. M., & Lanford, D. N. (2013). Predicting older driver on-road performance by means of the Useful Field of View and Trail Making Test Part B. *American Journal of Occupational Therapy, 67*(5), 574–582. https://doi.org/10.5014/ajot.2013.008136

Classen, S., Wang, Y., Winter, S. M., Velozo, C. A., Lanford, D. N., & Bédard, M. (2013). Concurrent criterion validity of the Safe Driving Behavior Measure: A predictor of on-road driving outcomes. *American Journal of Occupational Therapy, 67*(1), 108–116. https://doi.org/10.5014/ajot.2013.005116

Classen, S., Wen, P. S., Velozo, C. A., Bédard, M., Winter, S. M., Brumback, B., & Lanford, D. N. (2012a). Psychometrics of the self-report Safe Driving Behavior Measure for older adults. *American Journal of Occupational Therapy, 66*(2), 233–241. https://doi.org/10.5014/ajot.2012.001834

Classen, S., Wen, P. S., Velozo, C. A., Bédard, M., Winter, S. M., Brumback, B. A., & Lanford, D. N. (2012b). Rater reliability and rater effects of the Safe Driving Behavior Measure. *American Journal of Occupational Therapy, 66*(1), 69–77. https://doi.org/10.5014/ajot.2012.002261

Classen, S., Winter, S., Monahan, M., Yarney, A. Link Lutz, A., Platek, K., & Levy, C. (2017). Driving intervention for returning combat veterans. *OTJR: Occupation, Participation and Health, 37*(2), 62–71. https://doi.org/10.1177/1539449216675582

Classen, S., Winter, S. M., Velozo, C. A., Bédard, M., Lanford, D. N., Brumback, B., & Lutz, B. J. (2010). Item development and validity testing for a self- and proxy report: The Safe Driving Behavior Measure. *American Journal of Occupational Therapy, 64*(2), 296–305. https://doi.org/10.5014/ajot.64.2.296

Craik, J., Stern, E., Lapointe, J., McCarthy N., & Schold Davis, E. (2015). CarFit Canada: Lessons learned from an international collaboration. *World Federation of Occupational Therapists Bulletin, 71*(1), 22–25. https://doi.org/10.1179/1447382815Z.0000000006

Crizzle, A. M., Classen, S., Bédard, M., Lanford, D., & Winter, S. (2012). MMSE as a predictor of on-road driving performance in community dwelling older drivers. *Accident Analysis and Prevention, 49*, 287–292. https://doi.org/10.1016/j.aap.2012.02.003

Crizzle, A. M., Classen, S., Winter, S. M., Silver, W., LaFranca, C., & Eisenschenk, S. (2012). Associations between clinical tests and simulated driving performance in persons with epilepsy. *Epilepsy & Behavior, 23*(3), 241–246. https://doi.org/10.1016/j.yebeh.2011.12.019

Di Stefano, M., Stuckey, R., & Kinsman, N. (2019). Understanding characteristics and experiences of drivers using vehicle modifications. *American Journal of Occupational Therapy, 73*(1), Article 7302205150. https://doi.org/10.5014/ajot.2019.023721

Di Stefano, M., Stuckey, R., Kinsman, N., & Lavender, K. (2019). Vehicle modification prescription: Australian Occupational Therapy consensus-based guidelines. *American Journal of Occupational Therapy, 73*(2), Article 7302205140. https://doi.org/10.5014/ajot.2019.024331

Dun, C., Baker, K., Swan, J., Vlachou, V., & Fossey, E. (2015). "Drive Safe" initiatives: An analysis of improvements in mental health practices (2005-2013) to support safe driving. *British Journal of Occupational Therapy, 78*(6), 364–368. https://doi.org/10.1177/0308022614562785

Dun, C., Bull, B., Hitch, D., Lhuede, K., Vlachou, V., & Swan, J. (2015). Supporting safe driving practices among consumers of mental health services: Guidelines for assessment. *Psychiatric Services, 66*(5), 536–538. https://doi.org/10.1176/appi.ps.201400224

Duquette, J., McKinley, P., Mazer, B., Gélinas, I., Vanier, M., Benoit, D., & Gresset, J. (2010). Impact of partial administration of the Cognitive Behavioral Driver's Inventory on concurrent validity for people with brain injury. *American Journal of Occupational Therapy, 64*(2), 279–287. https://doi.org/10.5014/ajot.64.2.279

Koppel, S., Charlton, J., Langford, J., Vlahodimitrakou, Z., Di Stefano, M., Macdonald, W., Mazer, B., Gelinas, I., Vrkljan, B., & Marshall, S. (2013). The relationship between older drivers' performance on the driving observation schedule (eDOS) and cognitive performance. *Annals of Advances in Automotive Medicine, 57*, 67–76.

Koppel, S., Stephens, A. N., Charlton, J. L., Di Stefano, M., Darzins, P., Odell, M., & Marshall, S. (2018). The Driver Behaviour Questionnaire for older drivers: Do errors, violations and lapses change over time? *Accident Analysis & Prevention, 113*, 171–178. https://doi.org/10.1016/j.aap.2018.01.036

Korner-Bitensky, N., Audet, T., Man-Son-Hing, M., Benoit, D., Kaizer, F., & Gélinas, I. (2011). Test-Retest reliability of the Preroad DriveABLE Competence Screen. *Physical & Occupational Therapy in Geriatrics, 29*(3), 202–212. https://doi.org/10.3109/02703181.2011.573619

Korner-Bitensky, N., & Kua, A. (2010). The occupational therapist's role in keeping older drivers safe: Refreshing driving skills—The stay SHARP program. *Occupational Therapy Now, 12*(5), 7–8.

Kwok, J. C. W., Gélinas, I., Benoit, D., & Chilingaryan, G. (2015). Predictive validity of the Montreal Cognitive Assessment (MoCA) as a screening tool for on-road driving performance. *British Journal of Occupational Therapy, 78*(2), 100–108. https://doi.org/10.1177/0308022614562399

Lafrance, M. E., Benoit, D., Dahan-Oliel, N., & Gélinas, I. (2017). Development of a driving readiness program for adolescents and young adults with cerebral palsy and spina bifida. *British Journal of Occupational Therapy, 80*(3), 173–182. https://doi.org/10.1177/0308022616672480

Levasseur, M., Audet, T., Gélinas, I., Bédard, M., Langlais, M. E., Therrien, F. H., Renaud, J., Coallier, J. C., & D'Amours, M. (2015). Awareness tool for safe and responsible driving (OSCAR): A potential educational intervention for increasing interest, openness and knowledge about the abilities required and compensatory strategies among older drivers. *Traffic Injury Prevention, 16*(6), 578–586. https://doi.org/10.1080/15389588.2014.994742

Mazer, B., Gélinas, I., Duquette, J., Vanier, M., Rainville, C., & Chilingaryan, G. (2015). A randomized clinical trial to determine effectiveness of driving simulator retraining on the driving performance of clients with neurological impairment. *British Journal of Occupational Therapy, 78*(6), 369–376. https://doi.org/10.1177/0308022614562401

Naveh, Y., Shapira, A., & Ratzon, N. Z. (2015). Using a driving simulator during vehicle adaptation. *British Journal of Occupational Therapy, 78*(6), 377–382. https://doi.org/10.1177/0308022614562404

Papandonatos, G. D., Ott, B. R., Davis, J. D., Barco, P. P., & Carr, D. B. (2015). Clinical utility of the Trail-Making Test as a predictor of driving performance in older adults. *Journal of the American Geriatrics Society, 63*(11), 2358–2364. https://doi.org/10.1111/jgs.13776

Porter, R. S. (Ed.). (2018). *The Merck manual of diagnosis and therapy* (20th ed.). Merck Sharp & Dohme.

Rapoport, M. J., Naglie, G., Weegar, K., Myers, A., Cameron, D, Crizzle, A., Korner-Bitensky, N., Tuokko, H., Vrkljan, B., Bédard, M., Porter, M. M., Mazer, B., Gélinas, I., Man-Son-Hing, M., &

Marshall, S. (2013). The relationship between cognitive performance, perceptions of driving comfort and abilities, and self-reported driving restrictions among healthy older drivers. *Accident Analysis & Prevention, 61*, 288–295.

Song, C. S., Chun, B. Y., & Chung, H. S. (2015). Test-retest reliability of the Driving Habits Questionnaire in older self-driving adults. *Journal of Physical Therapy Science, 27*(11), 3597–3599.

Song, C. S., Lee, J. H., & Han, S. W. (2016). Test-retest reliability of the safe driving behavior measure for community-dwelling elderly drivers. *Journal of Physical Therapy Science, 28*(6), 1716–1719.

Stav, W. (2010). CarFit: An evaluation of behavior change and impact. *British Journal of Occupational Therapy, 73*(12), 589–597. https://doi.org/10.4276/030802210X12918167234208

Sukhawathanakul, P., Tuokko, H., Rhodes, R. E., Marshall, S. C., Charlton, J., Koppel, A., S., Gélinas, I., Naglie, G., Mazer, B., Vrkljan, B., Myers, A., Man-Son-Hing, M., Bédard, M., Rapoport, M., Korner-Bitensky, N., & Porter, M. M. (2015). Measuring driving-related attitudes among older adults: Psychometric evidence for the decisional balance scale across time and gender. *The Gerontologist, 55*(6), 1068–1078. https://doi.org/10.1093/geront/gnv077

Unsworth, C. A., Baker, A., Taitz, C., Chan, S. P., Pallant, J. F., Russell, K. J., & Odell, M. (2012). Development of a standardised Occupational Therapy–Driver Off-Road Assessment Battery to assess older and/or functionally impaired drivers. *Australian Occupational Therapy Journal, 59*(1), 23–36. https://doi.org/10.1111/j.1440-1630.2011.00979.x

Unsworth, C. A., Pallant, J. F., Russell, K. J., Germano, C., & Odell, M. (2010). Validation of a test of road law and road craft knowledge with older or functionally impaired drivers. *American Journal of Occupational Therapy, 64*(2), 306–315. https://doi.org/10.5014/ajot.64.2.306

Vlahodimitrakou, Z., Charlton, J. L., Langford, J., Koppel, S., Di Stefano, M., Macdonald, W., Mazer, B., Gelinas, I., Vrkljan, B., Porter, M. M., Smith, G. A., Cull, A. W., & Marshall, S. (2013). Development and evaluation of a Driving Observation Schedule (DOS) to study everyday driving performance of older drivers. *Accident Analysis & Prevention, 61*, 253–260. https://doi.org/10.1016/j.aap.2013.03.027

Woolnough, A., Salim, D., Marshall, S. C., Weegar, K., Porter, M. M., Rapoport, M. J., Man-Son-Hing, M., Bédard, M., Gélinas, I., Korner-Bitensky, N., Mazer, B., Naglie, G., Tuokko, H., & Vrkljan, B. (2013). Determining the validity of the AMA guide: A historical cohort analysis of the assessment of driving related skills and crash rate among older drivers. *Accident Analysis & Prevention, 61*, 311–316. https://doi.org/10.1016/j.aap.2013.03.020

BIBLIOGRAPHY

Alosco, M. L., Penn, M. S., Spitznagel, M. B., Cleveland, M. J., Ott, B. R., & Gunstad, J. (2015). Reduced physical fitness in patients with heart failure as a possible risk factor for impaired driving performance. *American Journal of Occupational Therapy, 69*(2), Article 6902260010. https://doi.org/10.5014/ajot.2015.013573

Alvarez, L., & Classen, S. (2018). Driving with Parkinson's disease: Cut points for clinical predictors of on-road outcomes. *Canadian Journal of Occupational Therapy, 85*(3), 232–241. https://doi.org/10.1177/0008417418755458

American Occupational Therapy Association. (2012). *Fact sheet: Driving and transportation options for older adults.*

American Occupational Therapy Association. (2016). Driving and community mobility. *American Journal of Occupational Therapy, 70*(Suppl. 2), Article 7012410050. https://doi.org/10.5014/ajot.2016.706S04

Asimakopulos, J., Boychuck, Z., Sondergaard, D., Poulin, V., Ménard, I., & Korner-Bitensky, N. (2012). Assessing executive function in relation to fitness to drive: A review of tools and their ability to predict safe driving. *Australian Occupational Therapy Journal, 59*(6), 402–427. https://doi.org/10.1111/j.1440-1630.2011.00963.x

Bédard, M., & Dickerson, A. E. (2014). Consensus statements for screening and assessment tools. *Occupational Therapy in Health Care, 28*(2), 127–131. https://doi.org/10.3109/07380577.201 4.903017

Bédard, M., Parkkari, M., Weaver, B., Riendeau, J., & Dahlquist, M. (2010). Assessment of driving performance using a simulator protocol: Validity and reproducibility. *American Journal of Occupational Therapy, 64*(2), 336–340. https://doi.org/10.5014/ajot.64.2.336

Bottari, C., Lamothe, M. P., Gosselin, N., Gélinas, I., & Ptito, A. (2012). Driving difficulties and adaptive strategies: The perception of individuals having sustained a mild traumatic brain injury. *Rehabilitation Research and Practice, 2012,* Article 837301. https://doi.org/10.1155/2012/ 837301

Cameron, D. H., Zucchero Sarracini, C., Rozmovits, L., Naglie, G., Herrmann, N., Molnar, F., Jordan, J., Byszewski, A., Tang-Wai, D., Dow, J., Frank, C., Henry, B., Pimlott, N., Seitz, D., Vrkljan, B., Taylor, R., Masellis, M., & Rapoport, M. J. (2017). Development of a decision-making tool for reporting drivers with mild dementia and mild cognitive impairment to transportation administrators. *International Psychogeriatrics, 29*(9), 1551–1563. https://doi.org/10.1017/S1 041610217000242

Cammarata, M., Mueller, A. S., Harris, J., & Vrkljan, B. (2017). The role of the occupational therapist in driver rehabilitation after stroke. *Physical & Occupational Therapy in Geriatrics, 35*(1), 20–33. https://doi.org/10.1080/02703181.2016.1277443

Campos, J., Bédard, M., Classen, S., Delparte, J. J., Hebert, D. A., Hyde, N., Law, G., Naglie, G., & Yung, S. (2017). Guiding framework for driver assessment using driving simulators. *Frontiers in Psychology, 8,* Article 1428. https://doi.org/10.3389/fpsyg.2017.01428

Chee, D. Y., Lee, H. C., Patomella, A.-H., & Falkmer, T. (2017). Driving behaviour profile of drivers with autism spectrum disorder (ASD). *Journal of Autism and Developmental Disorders, 47,* 2658–2670. https://doi.org/10.1007/s10803-017-3178-1

Chee, J. N., Hawley, C., Charlton, J. L., Marshall, S., Gillespie, I., Koppel, S., Vrkljan, B., Ayotte, D., & Rapoport, M. J. (2019). Risk of motor vehicle collision or driving impairment after traumatic brain injury: A collaborative international systematic review and meta-analysis. *Journal of Head Trauma Rehabilitation, 34*(1), E27–E38. https://doi.org/10.1097/HTR.0000000000000400

Chiu, C. W. C., Law, C. K. M., & Cheng, A. S. K. (2019). Driver assessment service for people with mental illness. *Hong Kong Journal of Occupational Therapy, 32*(2), 77–83. https://doi.org/ 10.1177/1569186119886773

Choi, S. Y., Yoo, D. H., & Lee, J. S. (2015). Usefulness of the DriveABLE cognitive assessment in predicting the driving risk factor of stroke patients. *Journal of Physical Therapy Science, 27*(10), 3133–3135.

Classen, S. (2014). Summary of an evidence based review on interventions for medically at risk older drivers. *Occupational Therapy in Health Care, 28*(2), 223–228. https://doi.org/10.3109 /07380577.2014.896490

Classen, S., Brumback, B., Monahan, M., Malaty, I. I., Rodriguez, R. L., Okun, M. S., & McFarland, N. R. (2014). Driving errors in Parkinson's disease: Moving closer to predicting on-road outcomes. *American Journal of Occupational Therapy, 68*(1), 77–85. https://doi.org/105014/ ajot.2014.008698

Classen, S., Crizzle, A. M., Winter, S. M., Silver, W., & Eisenschenk, S. (2012). Evidence-based review on epilepsy and driving. *Epilepsy & Behavior, 23*(2), 103–112. https://doi.org/org/10 .1016/j.yebeh.2011.11.015

Classen, S., Jeghers, M., Morgan-Daniel, J., Winter, S., King, L., & Struckmeyer, L. (2019). Smart in-vehicle technologies and older drivers: A scoping review. *OTJR: Occupation, Participation and Health, 39*(2), 97–107. https://doi.org/10.1177/1539449219830376

Classen, S., Krasniuk, S., Morrow, S. A., Alvarez, L., Monahan, M., Danter, T., & Rosehart, H. (2018). Visual correlates of fitness to drive in adults with multiple sclerosis. *OTJR: Occupation, Participation and Health, 38*(1), 15–27. https://doi.org/10.1177/1539449217718841

Classen, S., & Monahan, M. (2013). Evidence-based review on interventions and determinants of driving performance in teens with attention deficit hyperactivity disorder or autism spectrum disorder. *Traffic Injury Prevention, 14*(2), 188–193. https://doi.org/10.1080/1538958 8.2012.700747

Classen, S., Monahan, M., Auten, B., & Yarney, A. (2014). Evidence-based review of interventions for medically at-risk older drivers. *American Journal of Occupational Therapy, 68*(4), e107–e114. https://doi.org/10.5014/ajot.2014.010975

Classen, S., Monahan, M., Brown, K. E., & Hernandez, S. (2013). Driving indicators in teens with attention deficit hyperactivity and/or autism spectrum disorder. *Canadian Journal of Occupational Therapy, 80*(5), 274–283. https://doi.org/10.1177/0008417413501072

Classen, S., Monahan, M., & Wang, Y. (2013). Driving characteristics of teens with attention deficit hyperactivity and autism spectrum disorder. *American Journal of Occupational Therapy, 67*(6), 664–673. https://doi.org/10.5014/ajot.2013.008821

Classen, S., Shechtman, O., Awadzi, K. D., Joo, Y., & Lanford, D. N. (2010). Traffic violations versus driving errors of older adults: Informing clinical practice. *American Journal of Occupational Therapy, 64*(2), 233–241. https://doi.org/10.5014/ajot.64.2.233

Classen, S., Wang, Y., Crizzle, A. M., Winter, S. M., & Lanford, D. N. (2013). Gender differences among older drivers in a comprehensive driving evaluation. *Accident Analysis & Prevention, 61*, 146–152. https://doi.org/10.1016/j.aap.2012.10.010

Classen, S., Winter, S., Brown, C., Morgan-Daniel, J., Medhizadah, S., & Agarwal, N. (2019). An integrative review on teen distracted driving for model program development. *Frontiers in Public Health, 7*, Article 111. https://doi.org/10.3389/fpubh.2019.00111

Classen, S., Witter, D. P., Lanford, D. N., Okun, M. S., Rodriguez R. L., Romrell, J., Malaty, I., & Fernandez, H. H., (2011) Usefulness of screening tools for predicting driving performance in people with Parkinson's disease. *American Journal of Occupational Therapy, 65*(5), 579–588. https://doi.org/10.5014/ajot.2011.001073

Cochran, L. M., & Dickerson, A. E. (2019). Driving while navigating: On-road driving performance using GPS or printed instructions. *Canadian Journal of Occupational Therapy, 86*(1), 61–69. https://doi.org/10.1177/0008417419831390

Crizzle, A. M., Classen, S., LaFranca, C., Winter, S. M., Roper, S. N., & Eisenschenk, S. (2013). Assessing the driving performance of a person with epilepsy presurgery and postsurgery. *American Journal of Occupational Therapy, 67*(3), e24–e29. https://doi.org/10.5014/ajot.2013 .006569

Crizzle, A. M., Classen, S., & Uc, E. Y. (2012). Parkinson disease and driving: An evidence-based review. *Neurology, 79*(20), 2067–2074. https://doi.org/10.1212/WNL.0b013e3182749e95

Crizzle, A. M., Classen, S., Lanford, D., Malaty, I. A., Okun, M. S., Wang, Y., Wagle Shukla, A., Rodriguez, R. L., & McFarland, N. R. (2013). Postural/gait and cognitive function as predictors of driving performance in Parkinson's disease. *Journal of Parkinson's Disease, 3*(2) 153–160. https://doi.org/10.3233/JPD-120152

Crizzle, A. M., Classen, S., Lanford, D., Malaty, I. A., Okun, M. S., Wagle Shukla, A., & McFarland, N. R. (2013). Driving performance and behaviors: A comparison of gender differences in Parkinson's disease. *Traffic Injury Prevention, 14*(4), 340–345. https://doi.org/10.1080/15389 588.2012.717730

Dalchow, J. L., Niewoehner, P. M., Henderson, R. R., & Carr, D. B. (2010). Test acceptability and confidence levels in older adults referred for fitness-to-drive evaluations. *American Journal of Occupational Therapy, 64*(2), 252–258. https://doi.org/10.5014/ajot.64.2.252

Davis, E. S. (2012). Transportation holds key to successful aging in place. *Rehab Management, 25*(3), 22–25.

Di Stefano, M., & Macdonald, W. (2010). Australian occupational therapy driver assessors' opinions on improving on-road driver assessment procedures. *American Journal of Occupational Therapy, 64*(2), 325–335. https://doi.org/10.5014/ajot.64.2.325

Di Stefano, M., & Macdonald, W. (2012). Design of occupational therapy on-road test routes and related validity issues. *Australian Occupational Therapy Journal, 59*(1), 37–46. https://doi.org/10.1111/j.1440-1630.2011.00990.x

Dickerson, A. E. (2014). Screening and assessment tools for determining fitness to drive: A review of the literature for the pathways project. *Occupational Therapy in Health Care, 28*(2), 82–121. https://doi.org/10.3109/07380577.2014.904535

Dickerson, A. E., & Bédard, M. (2014). Decision tool for clients with medical issues: A framework for identifying driving risk and potential to return to driving. *Occupational Therapy in Health Care, 28*(2), 194–202. https://doi.org/10.3109/07380577.2014.903357

Dickerson, A. E., Meuel, D. B., Ridenour, C. D., & Cooper, K. (2014). Assessment tools predicting fitness to drive in older adults: A systematic review. *American Journal of Occupational Therapy, 68*(6), 670–680. https://doi.org/10.5014/ajot.2014.011833

Dickerson, A. E., Reistetter, T., Davis, E. S., & Monahan, M. (2011). Evaluating driving as a valued instrumental activity of daily living. *American Journal of Occupational Therapy, 65*(1), 64–75. https://doi.org/10.5014/ajot.2011.09052

Elgin, J., McGwin, G., Wood, J. M., Vaphiades, M. S., Braswell, R. A., DeCarlo, D. K., Kline, L. B., & Owsley C. (2010). Evaluation of on-road driving in people with hemianopia and quadrantanopia. *American Journal of Occupational Therapy, 64*(2), 268–278. https://doi.org/10.5014/ajot.64.2.268

Fields, S. M., & Unsworth, C. A. (2017). Revision of the competency standards for occupational therapy driver assessors: An overview of the evidence for the inclusion of cognitive and perceptual assessments within fitness-to-drive evaluations. *Australian Occupational Therapy Journal, 64*(4), 328–339. https://doi.org/10.1111/1440-1630.12379

Frith, J., Hubbard, I. J., James, C. L., & Warren-Forward, H. (2015). Returning to driving after stroke: A systematic review of adherence to guidelines and legislation. *British Journal of Occupational Therapy, 78*(6), 349–355. https://doi.org/10.1177/0308022614562795

Gagnon, S., Marshall, S., Kadulina, Y., Stinchcombe, A., Bédard, M., Gélinas, I., Man-Son-Hing, M., Mazer, B., Naglie, G., Porter, M. M., Rapoport, M., Tuokko, H., Vrkljan, B., & Candrive Research Team. (2016). CIHR Candrive cohort comparison with Canadian household population holding valid driver's licenses. *Canadian Journal on Aging, 35*(Suppl. 1), 99–109. https://doi.org/10.1017/S0714980816000052

Gagnon, S., Stinchcombe, A., Curtis, M., Kateb, M., Polgar, J., Porter, M. M., & Bédard, M. (2019). Driving safety improves after individualized training: An RCT involving older drivers in an urban area. *Traffic Injury Prevention, 20*(6), 595–600. https://doi.org/10.1080/15389588.2019.1630826

George, S., Crotty, M., Gelinas, I., & Devos, H. (2014). Rehabilitation for improving automobile driving after stroke. *Cochrane Database of Systematic Reviews, 2*, Article CD008357.

Gish, J. A., & Vrkljan, B. (2016). Aging embodiment and the somatic work of getting into and out of a car. *Journal of Aging Studies, 36*, 33–46. https://doi.org/10.1016/j.jaging.2015.12.004

Golisz, K. (2014a). Occupational therapy and driving and community mobility for older adults. *American Journal of Occupational Therapy, 68*(6), 654–656. https://doi.org/10.5014/ajot.2014.013144

Golisz, K. (2014b). Occupational therapy interventions to improve driving performance in older adults: A systematic review. *American Journal of Occupational Therapy, 68*(6), 662–669. https://doi.org/10.5014/ajot.2014.011247

Hannold, E. M., Classen, S., Winter, S., Lanford, D. N., & Levy, C. E. (2013). Exploratory pilot study of driving perceptions among OIF/OEF veterans with mTBI and PTSD. *Journal of Rehabilitation Research and Development, 50*(10), 1315–1330. https://doi.org/10.1682/JRRD.2013.04.0084

Hawley, C. (2015). Knowledge and attitudes of occupational therapists to giving advice on fitness to drive. *British Journal of Occupational Therapy, 78*(6), 339–348. https://doi.org/10.1177/0308022614562402

Hellinger, N., Lipskaya-Velikovsky, L., Weizman, A., & Ratzon, N. Z. (2019). Comparing executive functioning and clinical and sociodemographic characteristics of people with schizophrenia who hold a driver's license to those who do not. *Canadian Journal of Occupational Therapy, 86*(1), 70–80. https://doi.org/10.1177/0008417419831399

Hickey, A. J., Weegar, K., Kadulina, Y., Gagnon, S., Marshall, Myers A., Tuokko, H., Bédard, M., Gélinas, I., Man-Son-Hing, M., Mazer, B., Naglie, G., Porter, M., Rapoport, M., Vrkljan, B., & Candrive Research Team. (2013). The impact of subclinical sleep problems on self-reported driving patterns and perceived driving abilities in a cohort of active older drivers. *Accident Analysis & Prevention, 61*, 296–303. https://doi.org/10.1016/j.aap.2013.02.032

Hunt, L. (2010). Driving rehabilitation: Frequently asked questions and answers. *Occupational Therapy Now, 12*(5), 19.

Hunt, L., Brown, A. E., & Gilman, I. P. (2010). Drivers with dementia and outcomes of becoming lost while driving. *American Journal of Occupational Therapy, 64*(2), 225–232. https://doi.org/10.5014/ajot.64.2.225

Jouk, A., Sukhawathanakul, P., Tuokko, H., Myers, A., Naglie, G., Vrkljan, B., Porter, M. M., Rapoport, M., Marshall, S., Mazer, B., Man-Son-Hing, M., Korner-Bitensky, N., Gélinas, I., & Bedard, M. (2016). Psychosocial constructs as possible moderators of self-reported driving restrictions. *Canadian Journal on Aging, 35*(Suppl. 1), 32–43. https://doi.org/10.1017/S0714980816000027

Kajaks, T., Vrkljan, B., MacDermid, J., & Godwin, A. (2016). Using simulation to better understand the effects of aging on driver visibility. *Canadian Journal on Aging, 35*(Suppl. 1), 110–116. https://doi.org/10.1017/S0714980816000106

Kay, L. G., Bundy, A. G., Clemson, L., Cheal, B., & Glendenning, T. (2012). Contribution of off-road tests to predicting on-road performance: A critical review of tests. *Australian Occupational Therapy Journal, 59*(1), 89–97. https://doi.org/10.1111/j.1440-1630.2011.00989.x

Koppel, S., Charlton, J. L., Hua, P., Liu, P. Y., Pham, H., Stephan, K., Logan, D., St Louis, R. M., Gao, G., Griffiths, D., Williams, G., Witharanage, T., Di Stefano, M., Darzins, P., Odell, M., Porter, M. M., Mazer, B., Gelinas, I., Vrkljan, B., & Marshall, S. (2018). Are older drivers' driving patterns during an on-road driving task representative of their real-world driving patterns? *Traffic Injury Prevention, 19*(Suppl. 2), S173–S175. https://doi.org/10.1080/15389588.2018.1532219

Koppel, S., Charlton, J., Langford, J., Di Stefano, M., MacDonald, W., Vlahodimitrakou, Z., Mazer, B. L., Gelinas, I., Vrkljan, B., Eliasz, K., Myers, A., Tuokko, H. A., & Marshall, S. C. (2016). Driving task: How older drivers' on-road driving performance relates to abilities, perceptions, and restrictions. *Canadian Journal on Aging, 35*(Suppl. 1), 15–31. https://doi.org/10.1017/S0714980816000015

Koppel S., Charlton, J. L., Richter, N., Di Stefano, M., Macdonald, W., Darzins, P., Newstead, S. V., D'Elia, A., Mazer, B., Gelinas, I., Vrkljan, B., Eliasz, K., Myers, A., & Marshall, S. (2017). Are older drivers' on-road driving error rates related to functional performance and/or self-reported driving experiences? *Accident Analysis & Prevention, 103*, 1–9. https://doi.org/10.1016/j.aap.2017.03.006

Koppel, S., Stephens, A. N., Bédard, M., Charlton, J. L., Darzins, P., Stefano, M. D., Gagnon., S., Gélinas, I., Hua, P., MacLeay, L., Man-Son-Hing, M., Mazer, B., Myers, A., Naglie, G., Odell, M., Porter, M. M., Rapoport, M. J., Stinchcombe, A., Tuokko, H., ... Marshall, S. (2019). Self-reported violations, errors and lapses for older drivers: Measuring the change in frequency of aberrant driving behaviours across five time-points. *Accident Analysis & Prevention, 123*, 132–139. https://doi.org/10.1016/j.aap.2018.11.009

Korner-Bitensky, N., Menon, A., von Zweck, C., & Van Benthem, K. (2010). Occupational therapists' capacity-building needs related to older driver screening assessment, and intervention: A Canadawide survey. *American Journal of Occupational Therapy, 64*(2), 316–324. https://doi.org/10.5014/ajot.64.2.316

Korner-Bitensky, N., Toal-Sullivan, D., & vonZweck, C. (2011). Driving and older adults: Towards a national occupational therapy strategy for screening. *Occupational Therapy Now, 9*(4), 3–5.

Krasniuk, S., Classen, S., Morrow, S. A., Monahan, M., Danter, T., Rosehart, H., & He, W. (2017). Driving errors that predict on-road outcomes in adults with multiple sclerosis. *OTJR: Occupation, Participation and Health, 37*(3), 115–124. https://doi.org/10.1177/15394492177 08554

Kristalovich, L., & Ben Mortenson, W. (2019). Visual field impairment and driver fitness: A 1-year review of crashes and traffic violations. *American Journal of Occupational Therapy, 73*(5), Article 7305345010. https://doi.org/10.5014/ajot.2019.030973

Langford J., Charlton J. L., Koppel, S., Myers, A., Tuokko, H., Marshall, S., Man-Son-Hing, M., Darzins, P., Di Stefano, M., & Macdonald, W. (2013). Findings from the Candrive/Ozcandrive study: Low mileage older drivers, crash risk and reduced fitness to drive. *Accident Analysis & Prevention, 61*, 304–310. https://doi.org/10.1016/j.aap.2013.02.006

Lee, H. C., Yanting Chee, D., Selander, H., & Falkmer, T. (2012). Is it reliable to assess visual attention of drivers affected by Parkinson's disease from the backseat?–a simulator study. *Emerging Health Threats Journal, 5*(1), Article 15343. https://doi.org/10.3402/ehtj.v5i0.15343

Mazer, B., Laliberté, M., Hunt, M., Lemoignan, J., Gélinas, I., Vrkljan, B., Naglie, G., & Marshall, S. (2016). Ethics of clinical decision-making for older drivers: Reporting health-related driving risk. *Canadian Journal on Aging, 35*(Suppl. 1), 69–80. https://doi.org/10.1017/S0714980 816000088

McGuire, M. J., & Schold Davis, E. (2012). *Driving and community mobility: Occupational therapy across the lifespan.* AOTA Press.

McNamara, A., George, S., Ratcliffe, J., & Walker, R. (2015). Older people's attitudes towards resuming driving in the first four months post-stroke. *Australasian Journal on Ageing, 34*(1), E13–E18. https://doi.org/10.1111/ajag.12135

McNamara, A., Ratcliffe, J., & George, S. (2014). Brief report: Evaluation of driving confidence in post-stroke older drivers in South Australia. *Australasian Journal on Ageing, 33*(3), 205–207. https://doi.org/10.1111/ajag.12117

McNamara, A., Walker, R., Ratcliffe, J., & George, S. (2015). Perceived confidence relates to driving habits post-stroke. *Disability and Rehabilitation, 37*(14), 1228–1233. https://doi.org/10.3109/ 09638288.2014.958619

McNamara, C., & Buckley, S. E. (2015). The road to recovery: Experiences of driving with bipolar disorder. *British Journal of Occupational Therapy, 78*(6), 356–363. https://doi.org/10.1177/ 0308022614562581

Ménard, I., Benoit, M., Boule-Laghzali, N., Hébert, M.-C., Parent-Taillon, J., Pérusse, J., Rouleau, S., & Korner-Bitensky, N. (2012). Occupational therapists' perceptions of their role in the screening and assessment of the driving capacity of people with mental illnesses. *Occupational Therapy in Mental Health, 28*(1), 36–50. https://doi.org/10.1080/0164212X.2011.650962

Metwa, L., Classen, S., & van Niekerk, L. (2016). The lived experience of drivers with a spinal cord injury: A qualitative inquiry. *South African Journal of Occupational Therapy, 46*(3), 55–62.

Monahan, M., Classen, S., & Helsel, P. V. (2013). Pre-driving evaluation of a teen with attention deficit hyperactivity disorder and autism spectrum disorder. *Canadian Journal of Occupational Therapy, 80*(1), 35–41. https://doi.org/10.1177/0008417412474221

Morrow, S. A., Classen, S., Monahan, M., Danter, T., Taylor, R., Krasniuk, S., Rosehart, H., & He, W. (2018). On-road assessment of fitness-to-drive in persons with MS with cognitive impairment: A prospective study. *Multiple Sclerosis Journal, 24*(11), 1499–1506. https://doi .org/10.1177/1352458517723991

Motta, K., Lee, H., & Falkmer, T. (2014). Post-stroke driving: Examining the effect of executive dysfunction. *Journal of Safety Research, 49*, 33–38. https://doi.org/10.1016/j.jsr.2014.02.005

Mullen, N. W., Weaver, B., Riendeau, J. A., Morrison, L. E., & Bédard, M. (2010). Driving performance and susceptibility to simulator sickness: Are they related? *American Journal of Occupational Therapy, 64*(2), 288–295. https://doi.org/10.5014/ajot.64.2.288

Ng, K. C., & Lovell, R. (2012). Survey on Victorian driver assessors' experience of critical incidents. *Australian Occupational Therapy Journal, 59*(1), 47–55. https://doi.org/10.1111/j.1440-1630.2010.00895.x

Niewoehner, P. M., Henderson, R. R., Dalchow, J., Beardsley, T. L., Stern, R. A., & Carr, D. B. (2012). Predicting road test performance in adults with cognitive or visual impairment referred to a Veterans Affairs Medical Center driving clinic. *Journal of the American Geriatrics Society, 60*(11), 2070–2074. https://doi.org/10.1111/j.1532-5415.2012.04201.x

Patterson, L., Mullen, N., Stinchcombe, A., Weaver, B., & Bédard, M. (2019). Measuring the impact of driving status: The Centre for Research on Safe Driving-Impact of Driving Status on Quality of Life (CRSD-IDSQoL) tool. *Canadian Journal of Occupational Therapy, 86*(1), 30–39. https://doi.org/10.1177/0008417418824980

Pearce, A. M., Smead, J. M., & Cameron, I. D. (2012). Retrospective cohort study of accident outcomes for individuals who have successfully undergone driver assessment following stroke. *Australian Occupational Therapy Journal, 59*(1), 56–62. https://doi.org/10.1111/j.1440-1630.2011.00981.x

Porter, M. M., Smith, G. A., Cull, A. W., Myers, A. M., Bédard, M., Gélinas, I., Mazer, B. L., Marshall, S. C., Naglie, G., Rapoport, M. J., Tuokko, H. A., & Vrkljan, B. H. (2015). Older driver estimates of driving exposure compared to in-vehicle data in the Candrive II study. *Traffic Injury Prevention, 16*(1), 24–27. https://doi.org/10.1080/15389588.2014.894995

Rapoport, M. J., Naglie, G., Herrmann, N., Zucchero Sarracini, C., Mulsant, B. H., Frank, C., Kiss, A., Seitz, D., Vrkljan, B., Masellis, M., Tang-Wai, D., Pimlott, N., & Molnar, F. (2014). Developing physician consensus on the reporting of patients with mild cognitive impairment and mild dementia to transportation authorities in a region with mandatory reporting legislation. *American Journal of Geriatric Psychiatry, 22*(12), 1530–1543. https://doi.org/10.1016/j.jagp.2013.12.002

Rapoport, M. J., Plonka, S. C., Finestone, H., Bayley, M., Chee, J. N. Vrkljan, B., Koppel, S., Linkewich, E., Charlton, J. L., Marshall, S., delCampo, M., Boulos, M. I., Swartz, R. H., Bhangu, J., Saposnik, G., Comay, J., Dow, J., Ayotte, D., & O'Neill, D. (2019). A systematic review of the risk of motor vehicle collision after stroke or transient ischemic attack. *Topics in Stroke Rehabilitation, 26*(3), 226–235. https://doi.org/10.1080/10749357.2018.1558634

Rapoport, M. J., Sukhawathanakul, P., Naglie, G., Tuokko, H., Myers, A., Crizzle, A., Korner-Bitensky, N., Vrkljan, B., Bédard, M., Porter, M. M., Mazer, B., Gélinas, I., Man-Son-Hing, M., & Marshall, S. (2016). Cognitive performance, driving behavior, and attitudes over time in older adults. *Canadian Journal on Aging, 35*(Suppl. 1), 81–91. https://doi.org/10.1017/S07149808081600009X

Rapoport, M. J., Weegar, K., Kadulina, Y., Bédard, M., Carr, D., Charlton, J. L., Dow, J., Gillespie, I. A., Hawley, C. A., Koppel, S., McCullagh, S., Molnar, F., Murie-Fernández, M., Naglie, G., O'Neill, D., Shortt, S., Simpson, C., Tuokko, H. A., Vrkljan, B. H., & Marshall, S. (2015). An international study of the quality of national-level guidelines on driving with medical illness. *QJM: An International Journal of Medicine, 108*(11), 859–869. https://doi.org/10.1093/qjmed/hcv038

Ratzon, N. Z., Lunievsky, E. K., Ashkenasi, A., Laks, J., & Cohen, H. A. (2017). Simulated driving skills evaluation of teenagers with attention deficit hyperactivity disorder before driving lessons. *American Journal of Occupational Therapy, 71*(3), Article 7103220010. https://doi.org/10.5014/ajot.2017.020164

Riendeau, J. A., Maxwell, H., Patterson, L., Weaver, B., & Bédard, M. (2016). Self-rated confidence and on-road driving performance among older adults. *Canadian Journal of Occupational Therapy, 83*(3), 177–183. https://doi.org/10.1177/0008417416645912

Ross, P., Ponsford, J. L., Di Stefano, M., Charlton, J., & Spitz, G. (2016). On the road again after traumatic brain injury: Driver safety and behaviour following on-road assessment and rehabilitation. *Disability and Rehabilitation, 38*(10), 994–1005. https://doi.org/10.3109/09638288.2015.1074293

Ross, P. E., Di Stefano, M., Charlton, J., Spitz, G., & Ponsford, J. L. (2018). Interventions for resuming driving after traumatic brain injury. *Disability and Rehabilitation, 40*(7), 757–764. https://doi.org/10.1080/09638288.2016.1274341

Ross, P. E., Ponsford, J. L., Di Stefano, M., & Spitz, G. (2015). Predictors of on-road driver performance following traumatic brain injury. *Archives of Physical Medicine and Rehabilitation, 96*(3), 440–446. https://doi.org/10.1016/j.apmr.2014.09.027

Rouleau, S., Mazer, B., Ménard, I., & Gautier, M. (2010). A survey on driving in clients with mental health disorders. *Occupational Therapy in Mental Health, 26*(1), 85–95. https://doi.org/10.1080/01642120903515318

Samuelsson, K., Modig-Arding, I., & Wressle, E. (2018). Driving after an injury or disease affecting the brain: An analysis of clinical data. *British Journal of Occupational Therapy, 81*(7), 376–383. https://doi.org/10.1177/0308022618755999

Sawada, T., Fujita, Y., Shiratori, M., & Shibuya, M. (2016). Driving risk in a stroke patient with mild cognitive deficits could not be predicted by neuropsychological testing: A case report. *Asian Journal of Occupational Therapy, 12*(1), 61–66.

Sawula, E., Polgar, J., Porter, M. M., Gagnon, S., Weaver, B., Nakagawa, S., Stinchcombe, A., & Bédard, M. (2018). The combined effects of on-road and simulator training with feedback on older drivers' on-road performance: Evidence from a randomized controlled trial. *Traffic Injury Prevention, 19*(3), 241–249. https://doi.org/10.1080/15389588.2016.1236194

Shaw, L., Polgar, J., Vrkljan, B., & Jacobson, J. (2010). Seniors' perceptions of vehicle safety risks and needs. *American Journal of Occupational Therapy, 64*(2), 215–224. https://doi.org/10.5014/ajot.64.2.215

Shechtman, O., Awadzi, K. D., Classen, S., Lanford, D. N., & Joo, Y. (2010). Validity and critical driving errors of on-road assessment for older drivers. *American Journal of Occupational Therapy, 64*(2), 242–251. https://doi.org/10.5014/ajot.64.2.242

Silvestdri, K. E. (2013). Safe and steady in the driver's seat. *Rehab Management, 26*(3), 22–25.

Sinnott, C., Foley, T., Forsyth, J., McLoughlin, K., Horgan, L., & Bradley, C. P. (2018). Consultations on driving in people with cognitive impairment in primary care: A scoping review of the evidence. *PLOS ONE, 13*(10), Article e0205580. https://doi.org/10.1371/journal.pone.0205580

Smith, A., Marshall, S., Porter, M., Ha, L., Bédard, M., Gélinas, I., Man-Son-Hing, M., Mazer, B., Rapoport, M., Tuokko, H., & Vrkljan, B. (2013). Stability of physical assessment of older drivers over 1 year. *Accident Analysis & Prevention, 61*, 261–266. https://doi.org/10.1016/j.aap.2013.02.007

Stack, A. H., Duggan, O., & Stapleton, T. (2018). Assessing fitness to drive after stroke. *Irish Journal of Occupational Therapy, 46*(2), 106–129. https://doi.org/10.1108/IJOT-03-2018-0006

Stapleton, T., & Connelly, D. (2010). Occupational therapy practice in predriving assessment post stroke in the Irish context: Findings from a nominal group technique meeting. *Topics in Stroke Rehabilitation, 17*(1), 58–68. https://doi.org/10.1310/tsr1701-58

Stapleton, T., Connolly, D., & O'Neill, D. (2012). Exploring the relationship between self-awareness of driving efficacy and that of a proxy when determining fitness to drive after stroke. *Australian Occupational Therapy Journal, 59*(1), 63–70. https://doi.org/10.1111/j.1440-1630.2011.00980.x

Stinchcombe, A., Gagnon, S., Kateb, M., Curtis, M., Porter, M. M., Polgar, J., & Bédard, M. (2017). Letting in-vehicle navigation lead the way: Older drivers' perceptions of and ability to follow a GPS navigation system. *Accident Analysis and Prevention, 106*, 515–520. https://doi.org/10.1016/j.aap.2016.10.022

Tuokko, H., Jouk, A., Myers, A., Marshall, S., Man-Son-Hing, M., Porter, M. M., Bédard, M., Gélinas, I., Korner-Bitensky, N., Mazer, B., Naglie, G., Rapoport, M., & Vrkljan, B. (2014). A re-examination of driving-related attitudes and readiness to change driving behavior in older adults. *Physical & Occupational Therapy in Geriatrics, 32*(3), 210–227. https://doi.org/10.3109/02703181.2014.931503

Tuokko, H., Sukhawathanakul, P., Walzak, L., Jouk, A., Myers, A., Marshall, S., Naglie, G., Rapoport, M., Vrkljan, B., Porter, M., Man-Son-Hing, M., Mazer, B., Korner-Bitensky, N., Gélinas, I., & Bédard, M. (2016). Attitudes: Mediators of the relation between health and driving in older adults. *Canadian Journal on Aging, 35*(Suppl. 1), 44–58. https://doi.org/10.1017/S0714 980816000076

Unsworth, C. A. (2010). Issues surrounding driving and driver assessment for people with mental health problems. *Mental Health Occupational Therapy, 15*(2), 41–44.

Unsworth, C. A. (2011). Gaining insights to the clinical reasoning that supports an on-road driver assessment. *Canadian Journal of Occupational Therapy, 78*(2), 97–102. https://doi.org/10.2182/cjot.2011.78.2.4

Unsworth, C. A., & Baker, A. (2014). Driver rehabilitation: A systematic review of the types and effectiveness of interventions used by occupational therapists to improve on-road fitness-to-drive. *Accident Analysis and Prevention, 71*, 106–114. https://doi.org/10.1016/j.aap.2014 .04.017

Unsworth, C. A., Baker, A. M., So, M. H., Harries, P., & O'Neill, D. (2017). A systematic review of evidence for fitness-to-drive among people with the mental health conditions of schizophrenia, stress/anxiety disorder, depression, personality disorder and obsessive compulsive disorder. *BMC Psychiatry, 17*, Article 318. https://doi.org/1186/s12888-017-1481-1

Unsworth, C., & Chan, S. P. (2016). Determining fitness to drive among drivers with Alzheimer's disease or cognitive decline. *British Journal of Occupational Therapy, 79*(2), 102–111. https://doi.org/10.1177/0308022615604645

Unsworth, C., Harries, P., & Davies, M. (2015). Using social judgment theory method to examine how experienced occupational therapy driver assessors use information to make fitness-to-drive recommendations. *British Journal of Occupational Therapy, 78*(2), 109–120. https://doi .org/10.1177/0308022614562396

Vernon, S. (2010). Driving and mental illness. *Mental Health Occupational Therapy, 14*(1), 18–19.

Vrkljan, B. H., Cranney, A., Worswick, J., O'Donnell, S., Li, L. C., Gélinas, I., Byszewski, A., Man-Son-Hing, M., & Marshall, S. (2010). Supporting safe driving with arthritis: Developing a driving toolkit for clinical practice and consumer use. *American Journal of Occupational Therapy, 64*(2), 259–267. https://doi.org/10.5014/ajot.64.2.259

Vrkljan, B. H., McGrath, C. E., & Letts, L. J. (2011). Assessment tools for evaluating fitness to drive: A critical appraisal of evidence. *Canadian Journal of Occupational Therapy, 78*(2), 80–96. https://doi.org/10.2182/cjot.2011.78.2.3

Vrkljan, B. H., Myers, A. M., Blanchard, R. A., Crizzle, A. M., & Marshall, S. (2015). Practices used by occupational therapists and others in driving assessment centers for determining fitness-to drive: A case-based approach. *Physical & Occupational Therapy in Geriatrics, 33*(2), 163–174. https://doi.org/10.3109/02703181.2015.1016647

Vrkljan, B. H., Myers, A. M., Crizzle, A. M., Blanchard, R. A., & Marshall, S. C. (2013). Evaluating medically at-risk drivers: A survey of assessment practices in Canada. *Canadian Journal of Occupational Therapy, 80*(5), 295–303. https://doi.org/10.1177/0008417413511788

Winter, S. M., Classen, S., Bédard, M., Lutz, B. J., Velozo, C. A., Lanford, D. N., & Brumback, B. A. (2011). Focus group findings for the self-report safe driving behaviour measure. *Canadian Journal of Occupational Therapy, 78*(2), 72–79. https://doi.org/10.2182/cjot.2011.7 8.2.2

Yi, J., Lee, H. C.-Y., Parsons, R., & Falkmer, T. (2015). The effect of the global positioning system on the driving performance of people with mild Alzheimer's disease. *Gerontology, 61*(1), 79–88. https://doi.org/10.1159/000365922

Yuval-Greenberg, S., Keren, A., Hilo, R., Paz, A., & Ratzon, N. (2019). Gaze control during simulator driving in adolescents with and without attention deficit hyperactivity disorder. *American Journal of Occupational Therapy, 73*(3), Article 7303345030. https://doi.org/10.5014/ajot.2019.031500

Emergency Occupational Therapy Services
Also called occupational therapy primary care services.

Description

Occupational therapists are part of an interprofessional health-care team that provides assessments, rehabilitation services, and quality of care to assist in making complex decisions on admissions and discharges, and eliminate unnecessary admissions to the hospital. Occupational therapists ensure "the safety of clients by assessing the client's capacity for activities of daily living, recommending appropriate equipment and services and educating the client and family on their use to ensure safety" (Canadian Association of Occupational Therapists, 2015, p. 1). However, occupational therapists need clarity in their role in the emergency department (Chown et al., 2016).

Cause

People coming to emergency departments for services related to illness and injuries, some of which may be life-threatening while others may result in less serious health risks.

Examples of High-Risk Factors Identifiable in the Emergency Service Assessments

- Person (or caregiver) reports need for regular assistance to perform activities of daily living tasks (eating, bathing, dressing, toileting, taking medications).
- Person (or caregiver) reports need for additional assistance recently because of a "new" illness, infection, or injury such as a fracture, cardiac arrest, or stroke.
- Person (or caregiver) reports a sudden change in functional ability (ADL/IADL performance), functional mobility, or functional cognition, especially due to the progression of the disease (neurodegenerative, neurocognitive).
- Person has been hospitalized within the past 3–6 months for 1 or more nights.
- Person has recently experienced a decrease in vision (new glasses, new diagnosis of visual impairment).
- Person (or caregiver) reports increased difficulty remembering recent information (losing or misplacing things, or forgetting appointments) or confusion.
- Person has a history of cognitive impairment (poor recall) or not oriented to person, place, or time (day, month, season) as reported by the person, caregiver, or recorded in the medical record.
- Person is taking five or more medications as reported by the person, caregiver, or recorded in the medical record.
- Person has difficulty walking (poor balance) or transferring from bed to chair as demonstrated on-site.
- Person has a recent history of falls (within last 6 months) as reported by the person, caregiver, or recorded in the medical record.
- Person has previously been in the emergency service department within the last 30 days as reported by the person, caregiver, or recorded in the medical record.
- Person lives alone and has no available caregiver that could stay with the person temporarily.

Source: Based on statements in assessments used in the emergency service department.

Evaluation/Assessment

Areas

- Activities of Daily Living/Instrumental ADL: self-maintenance (eating and drinking, bathing including washing and drying, toileting including bowel and bladder, medications, functional mobility, functional communication, transfers); IADLs including shopping, meal preparation, housekeeping, driving or use of transportation systems
- Education/Work: return to school or work

- Play/Leisure: interests, hobbies, values, frequency, location
- Rest/Sleep: sleep disturbances, sleep disorder
- Social Participation: location, frequency, type, with whom
- Sensorimotor: balance and coordination, muscle strength, range of motion, endurance, history of falls, positioning
- Cognitive/Perceptual: attention, memory, learning, executive functions
- Psychosocial: emotional regulation, reality orientation, substance abuse, social isolation, violence, interpersonal and social skills
- Context/Environment: home layout (rooms, stairs), safety equipment, adapted devices, social support, social services available
- Comorbidities: chronic medical conditions (diabetes, high blood pressure), chronic mental health conditions (schizophrenia, bipolar), fractures, homeless, older adult, substance abuse and disorders, traumatic brain injury, and issues related to instrumental activities of daily living

Instruments

Instruments Developed by Occupational Therapy Personnel

- ADL Taxonomy (Törnquist & Sonn, 2014)
- Elder-Friendly Emergency Department Tool (EFEDT; McCusker, Vu, et al., 2018, in References)
- Functional Status Assessment of Seniors in Emergency Departments (FSAS-ED; Veillette et al., 2009)
- Scales Measuring Problematic Emergency Department Experiences (SMPESE; McCusker, Cetin-Sahin, et al., 2018, in References)

Instruments Developed by Other Professionals and Used by Occupational Therapy Personnel

- Barthel Index (BI; Mahoney & Barthel, 1965)
- Canadian Study of Health and Aging–Clinical Frailty Scale (CSHA-CFS; Rockwood et al., 2005)
- Clinical Frailty Scale (CFS; see Canadian Study of Health and Aging–Clinical Frailty Scale)
- Rockwood Frailty Scale (RFS; see Clinical Frailty Scale)
- Frenchay Activities Index (FAI; Holbrook & Skilbeck,1983)
- Geriatric Depression Scale (GDS; Yesavage et al., 1982–1983)
- Get Up and Go Test (GUGT; Mathias et al., 1986)
- Identification of Seniors at Risk (ISAR; Asomaning & Loftus, 2014)
- Mini-Mental Status Exam (MMSE; Folstein et al., 1975)
- Triage Risk Stratification Tool (TRST; Meldon et al., 2003)

Problems/Issues

Activities of Daily Living/Instrumental ADL

- Person may not be able to perform basic ADLs safely, such as transfers.
- Person may not be able to drive safely following traffic rules and using judgment to avoid injury or accident.

Education/Work

- Not discussed.

Play/Leisure

- Person may have stopped engaging in all leisure occupations including those considered favorites according to family or caregiver report.

Rest/Sleep

- Person may not be sleeping.
- Person may be sleepwalking, wandering, or leaving the residence at night.

Social Participation

- Person may refuse to participate in any social activities although was previously socially active according to family or caregiver report.

Sensorimotor
- Person may demonstrate lack of balance or ability to walk without risk of falling.
- Person may demonstrate lack of muscle strength and/or functional range of motion.

Cognitive/Perceptual
- Person may demonstrate difficulty maintaining a state of arousal or alertness.
- Person may demonstrate cognitive impairment in the areas of attention, memory, or executive functions.
- Person may demonstrate moderate or severe signs of dementia.

Psychosocial
- Person may demonstrate lack of emotional regulation (emotional instability).
- Person may demonstrate difficulty maintaining contact with reality (illusions, delusions, hallucinations).
- Person may demonstrate signs of severe depression.
- Person may have become isolated from others.

Context/Environment
- Person may need referral for services such as homelessness, mental health, substance abuse disorders (Lloyd et al., 2017).
- Person may need to have home check for safety and modification.
- Family or other caregivers may need instructions in caring for the person.
- Family or other caregivers may need information on other services available in the community to assist with caring for the person being seen in the emergency service.

Intervention/Treatment

Models and programs developed by occupational therapy personnel include case study (James, 2016), emergency department visit program (James, 2016), fall prevention program (Harper et al., 2017), and fall reduction home visit program (Chu et al., 2017). Models and programs developed by others but used by occupational therapy personnel include frailty team (Bennett & Fuller, 2019) and general review of interventions (Gagnon-Roy et al, 2018). Team members may include physicians, nursing personnel, social workers, physical therapy personnel, dietitians or nutritionists, and occupational therapy personnel. Goals include determining a client's capacity to perform activities of daily living safely and effectively (fall prevention), making recommendations for appropriate equipment and services, educating client and family on client's functional status, and making recommendations to staff regarding need for further assessment or admission.

Activities of Daily Living/Instrumental ADL
- Recommend person have a caregiver or caregivers assigned (family members, agency personnel).
- Provide specific training and education in assisting with self-maintenance activities.
- Recommend review of medications and modify schedule, organizers, and reminders.
- Review nutritional status and recommend referral to dietitian or nutritionist.
- Recommend review of driving status to restrict or stop driving.
- Assist client to schedule regular medical checkups for chronic conditions.

Education/Work
- No specific recommendations.

Play/Leisure
- No specific recommendations.

Rest/Sleep
- Review sleep hygiene.
- Recommend modifications in sleep habits and environmental status.

Social Participation
- No specific recommendations.

Sensorimotor
- Recommend or provide specific mobility device and equipment (walker, cane, scooter, wheelchair).
- Recommend balance and strength exercises.

Cognitive/Perceptual
- Recommend use of memory aids (calendars, smartphones, organizers, labels).
- Review vision and visuospatial perception as factors in mobility and driving.

Psychosocial
- Provide information to client on ways to reduce fear of falling by taking proactive steps to modify environment or use mobility aids.
- Provide information to client and caregivers to avoid self-harm related to over- or undermedication, side effects of polymedications including use of over-the-counter drugs, injury due to falls, potential burns from scalding water or flames from hot stove, frostbite or heat exhaustion while wandering, unreported medical condition, failure to follow instructions on use of equipment.

Context/Environment
- Recommend installation of safety equipment such as grab bars, railings or bannisters, ramps, "rocker" light switches, lever handles on doors.
- Recommend person receive additional evaluation by other professional (dietitian or nutritionist, physical therapist, speech pathologist, psychiatrist, psychologist, home health nurse).
- Person may need referral to other community resources such as shops for inexpensive clothing, free or low-cost food pantries, free or low-cost medical services, free or low-cost rooms and showers.
- Consider recommending a home safety check evaluation to reduce risk of falling and other injuries.
- Educate client and caregivers regarding medications value, risks, and prevention.
- Educate client and caregivers on cognitive disorders such as dementia, including ways to prevent wandering.
- Educate client and caregivers on prevention of falls.
- Educate client and caregivers on mobility devices, antislip shoes and socks, removal of throw rugs, increased lighting, removing clutter to improve mobility safety.

Precautions/Safety Considerations

Older individuals presenting at an emergency service should be evaluated for risk of falling. Chronic medical and mental health conditions should be considered in discharge plan such as mental health disorder, substance abuse disorder, terminal illness (Rosenwax et al., 2011).

Prognosis and Outcome

Comprehensive discharge planning and follow-up can reduce repeat visits to the emergency service, including correct referral to other agencies.

Cost Effectiveness

A falls prevention intervention program for older individuals is cost effective (Harper et al., 2019). A falls prevention intervention program reduced hospital admissions (Harper et al, 2017). Occupational therapy can reduce the number of admissions (College of Occupational Therapists, 2013; Edwards, 2015; Lucking & Shields, 2015; Robinson et al., 2014).

REFERENCES

Bennett, S., & Fuller, J. (2019). The ever growing frailty team. *OT News, 27*(4), 36–37.

Canadian Association of Occupational Therapists. (2015). *Fact sheet: Occupational therapy in the emergency department.* https://www.caot.ca/document/4053/Emergency%20Department%20-%20Fact%20Sheet.pdf

Chown, G., Soley, T., Moczydlowski, S., Chimento, C., & Smoyer, A. (2016). A phenomenological study on the perception of occupational therapists practicing in the emergency department. *Open Journal of Occupational Therapy, 4*(1), Article 3. https://doi.org/10.15453/2168-6408.1126

Chu, M. M.-L., Fong, K. N.-K., Lit, A. C.-H., Rainer, T. H., Cheng, S. W.-C., Au, F. L.-Y., Fung, H. K.-K., Wong, C.-M., & Tong, H.-K. (2017). An occupational therapy fall reduction home visit program for community-dwelling older adults in Hong Kong after an emergency department visit for a fall. *Journal of the American Geriatrics Society, 65*(2), 364–372. https://doi.org/10.1111/jgs.14527

College of Occupational Therapists. (2013). *Fact sheet: Occupational therapists working in A&E teams help reduce admissions and re-admissions to hospital.*

Edwards, T. (2015). A collaborative approach to reducing A&E admissions. *OT News, 23*(7), 36–37.

Gagnon-Roy, M., Hami, B., Généreux, M., Veillette, N., Sirois, M. J., Egan, M., & Provencher, V. (2018). Preventing emergency department (ED) visits and hospitalisations of older adults with cognitive impairment compared with the general senior population: What do we know about avoidable incidents? Results from a scoping review. *BMJ Open, 8*(4), Article e019908. https://doi.org/10.1136/bmjopen-2017-019908

Harper, K. J., Arendts, G., Geelhoed, E. A., Barton, A. D., & Celenza, A. (2019). Cost analysis of a brief intervention for the prevention of falls after discharge from an emergency department. *Journal of Evaluation in Clinical Practice, 25*(2), 244–250. https://doi.org/10.1111/jep.13041

Harper, K. J., Barton, A. D., Arendts, G., Edwards, D. G., Petta, A. C., & Celenza, A. (2017). Controlled clinical trial exploring the impact of a brief intervention for prevention of falls in an emergency department. *Emergency Medicine Australasia, 29*(5), 524–530. https://doi.org/10.1111/1742-6723.12804

James, K. (2016). Occupational therapists in emergency departments. *Emergency Medicine Journal, 33*(6), 442–443. https://doi.org/10.1136/emermed-2015-205536

Lloyd, C., Hilder, J., & Williams, P. L. (2017). Emergency department presentations of people who are homeless: The role of occupational therapy. *British Journal of Occupational Therapy, 80*(9), 533–538. https://doi.org/10.1177/0308022617706679

Lucking, A., & Shields, S. (2015). OT in emergency and acute medicine. *OT News, 23*(10), 33.

McCusker, J., Cetin-Sahin, D., Cossette, S., Ducharme, F., Vadeboncoeur, A., Vu, T. T. M., Veillette, N., Ciampi, A., Belzile, E., Berthelot, S., Lachance, P.-A., & Mah, R. (2018). How older adults experience an emergency department visit: Development and validation of measures. *Annals of Emergency Medicine, 71*(6), 755–766. https://doi.org/10.1016/j.annemergmed.2018.01.009

McCusker, J., Vu, T. T. M., Veillette, N., Cossette, S., Vadeboncoeur, A., Ciampi, A., Cetin-Sahin, D., & Belzile, E. (2018). Elder-friendly emergency department: Development and validation of a quality assessment tool. *Journal of the American Geriatrics Society, 66*(2), 394–400. https://doi.org/10.1111/jgs.15137

Robinson, A., Lord-Vince, H., & Williams, R. (2014). The need for a 7-day therapy service on an emergency assessment unit. *British Journal of Occupational Therapy, 77*(1), 19–23. https://doi.org/10.4276/030802214X13887685335508

Rosenwax, L. K., McNamara, B. A., Murray, K., McCabe, R. J., Aoun, S. M., & Currow, D. C. (2011). Hospital and emergency department use in the last year of life: A baseline for future modifications to end-of-life care, *Medical Journal of Australia, 194*(11), 570–573. https://doi.org/10.5694/j.1326-5377.2011.tb03106.x

BIBLIOGRAPHY

Baker, A., Unsworth, C. A., & Lannin, N. A. (2015). What information is provided in Australian emergency departments about fitness-to-drive after mild traumatic brain injury: A national survey. *Australian Occupational Therapy Journal, 62*(1), 50–55. https://doi.org/10.1111/1440 -1630.12172

Bissett, M., Cusick, A., & Lannin, N. A. (2013). Functional assessments utilised in emergency departments: A systematic review. *Age and Ageing, 42*(2), 163–172. https://doi.org/10.1093/ ageing/afs187

College of Occupational Therapists. (2015). *Urgent care: the value of occupational therapy.* https:// www.rcot.co.uk/sites/default/files/Urgent%20care%20-%20The%20value%20of%20Occu pational%20Therapy.pdf

Cusick, A., Johnson, L., & Bissett, M. (2010). Continuing professional development for occupational therapy emergency department services. *Australian Occupational Therapy Journal, 57*(6), 380–385. https://doi.org/10.1111/j.1440-1630.2010.00874.x

Edwards, A. (2010). Demonstrating quality and efficiency in A&E. *OT News, 18*(5), 24.

Harper, K. J., Gibson, N. P., Barton, A. D., Petta, A. C., Pearson, S. K., & Celenza, A. (2013). Effects of emergency department care coordination team referrals in older people presenting with a fall. *Emergency Medicine Australasia, 25*(4), 324–333. https://doi.org/10.1111/1742-6723.12098

Howard, M. (2010). OTs in accident and emergency: A slightly different perspective. *OT News, 18*(5), 27 28.

James, K., Jones, D., Kempenaar, L., Preston, J., & Kerr, S. (2016). Occupational therapy and emergency departments: A critical review of the literature. *British Journal of Occupational Therapy, 79*(8), 459–466. https://doi.org/10.1177/0308022616629168

Rutter, S., & Blakey, V. (2010). The emergency care therapy team. *OT News, 18*(5), 35.

Sirois, M. J., Griffith, L., Perry, J., Daoust, R., Veillette, N., Lee, J., Pellerier, M., Wilding, L., & Émond, M. (2017). Measuring frailty can help emergency departments identify independent seniors at risk of function decline after minor injuries. *Journals of Gerontology: Series A, 72*(1), 68–74. https://doi.org/10.1093/gerona/glv152

Spang, L., & Holmqvist, K. (2015). Occupational therapy practice in emergency care: Occupational therapists' perspectives. *Scandinavian Journal of Occupational Therapy, 22*(5), 345–354. https://doi.org/10.3109/11038128.2015.1033455

Falls

Description

Falls are defined as unintentionally coming to rest on the ground, floor, or other lower level (Chase et al., 2012). Some of the major consequences of falls are hip fractures, brain injuries, decline in functional abilities, and reductions in social and physical activities (Barbour et al, 2014). People at risk for falls include those with diseases or disorders such as arthritis or stroke. Falls threaten the independence of older individuals and may cause a cascade of individual and socioeconomic consequences (Porter, 2018). Falls are not random accidents but are the result of numerous risk factors and compromised medical conditions (Lampiasi & Jacobs, 2010).

Cause

Falls are caused by physical factors such as poor neuromuscular function, sensory factors such as poor vision, and environmental factors such as slippery surfaces or unexpected changes in the height or type of surface. Age is a factor beginning in middle age. Postsurgery is also a risk factor. Causes of falls can be grouped as intrinsic (individual factors), extrinsic (environmental hazards), or situational (related to an activity being done; Porter, 2018).

Evaluation/Assessment
Areas
- Activities of Daily Living/Instrumental ADL: hazards associated with performance of self-maintenance skills
- Education/Work: hazards at work setting (paid or unpaid)
- Play/Leisure: hazards associated with engaging in favorite leisure occupations (occupation itself such as equipment used or setting in which occupation occurs)
- Rest/Sleep: sleep habits and routines, sleepiness, sleep disorders
- Social Participation: hazards associated with participation in favorite social activities
- Sensorimotor: history of previous falls, muscle strength, grip strength, postural stability, unsteady gait, poor coordination, balance, sarcopenia, visual acuity, contrast sensitivity, dark adaptation
- Cognitive/Perceptual: attention, memory, executive functions, mental flexibility, dementia, depth perception
- Psychosocial: fear of falling, anxiety about losing independence, self-efficacy, quality of life
- Context/Environment: environmental hazards (unfamiliar environment, uneven or slippery surface, wet floor, inadequate lighting, loose rugs, unsecured cords, lack of hand rails, broken or missing steps, high overhead shelves, unstable or broken chairs), adapted devices and equipment (mobility, safety, easier to use)
- Comorbidities: blood pressure regulation, cognitive impairment, neuromotor disorders, osteoporosis, diabetes, peripheral neuropathy, joint disorders/diseases, vestibular disorders, visual impairment, blind, human immunodeficiency virus (HIV) infection, drug or alcohol addition, individuals 65 and older, medications that affect the central nervous system

Instruments
Instruments Developed by Occupational Therapy Personnel
- Canadian Occupational Performance Measure (5th ed.; COPM-5; Law et al., 2014)
- Falls Behavioral Scale (FaB; Clemson et al., 2003)
- Guidetomeasure-OT (3D measurement system; Hamm et al., 2019a, 2019b, in References)
- Home Falls and Accidents Screening Tool (HOMEFAST; Mackenzie et al., 2000; see also Mackenzie, 2017, and Romli et al., 2017, in References)
- Home Falls and Accidents Screening Tool for Health Professionals (HOME FAST-HP; Mackenzie & Byles, 2018, and Vu & Mackenzie, 2012, in References)
- Home Safety Self-Assessment Tool (HSSAT; Horowitz et al., 2013, and Tomita et al., 2014, in References)
- In-Home Occupational Performance Evaluation (I-HOPE; Stark et al., 2010)
- Obstacle: A Tool to Assess the Home Environment (Lemmens et al., 2017, in References)
- Safe at Home (SAH; Robnett et al., 2003)
- Safety Assessment of Function and the Environment for Rehabilitation–Health Outcome Measurement and Evaluation (3th ed.; SAFER-HOME 3; Chiu & Oliver, 2006)
- Westmead Home Safety Assessment (WeHSA; Clemson et al., 1992)

Instruments Developed by Other Professionals and Used by Occupational Therapy Personnel
- Control, Autonomy, Self-realization, Pleasure-19 (CASP-19; Hyde et al., 2003)
- Fall Harm Risk Screen (FHRS; Breisinger et al., 2014)
- Functional Independence Measure (FIM; Uniform Data System for Medical Rehabilitation, 1997)
- Home Assessment Checklist (Porter, 2018, pp. 2864–2865)
- Home Environment Assessment for the Visual Impaired (HEAVI; Swenor et al., 2016, in References)
- Mini-Mental State Examination (MMSE; Folstein et al., 1975)
- Modified Falls-Efficacy Scale (M-FES; Edwards & Lockett, 2008)

- Outdoor Falls Questionnaire (OFQ; Chippendale, 2015)
- Performance-Oriented Assessment of Mobility (POAOM; Tinetti, 1986)
- Social Provision Scale (SPS; Cutrona & Russell, 1987)
- Stroke Assessment of Fall Risk (SAFR; Breisinger & Campbell, 2011; see also Breisinger et al., 2014, in References)
- Timed Up and Go test (TUG; Podsiadlo & Richardson, 1991; see Harper et al., 2020, in References)

Problems/Issues

Activities of Daily Living/Instrumental ADL

- Person may be at risk for falls while performing self-maintenance occupations due to intrinsic (personal factors such limited mobility or dizziness when standing up), extrinsic (environment such as poor lighting or cords that can trip), or situational (hurrying to answer the phone or carrying too heavy a load down stairs).

Education/Work

- Person may be at risk for falls while working at a paid or unpaid position.

Play/Leisure

- Person may be at risk for falls while engaging in favorite leisure occupation.

Rest/Sleep

- Person may be at risk for falls due to inadequate sleep resulting in drowsiness.
- Person may be at risk for falls due to getting up in the middle of night without turning on the lights or slipping on the floor while hurrying to the bathroom.

Social Participation

- Person may be at risk for falls while participating in social activities.

Sensorimotor

- Person is at increased risk of falling if there is a history of previous falls.
- Person may be at risk for falls due to lack of muscle strength, incoordination, poor balance, dizziness.
- Person may be at risk for falls due to visual impairments including lack of acuity, poor contrast sensitivity, or eye disorders such as glaucoma, retinopathy.

Cognitive/Perceptual

- Person may be at risk for falls due cognitive impairment that restricts person's ability to evaluate danger of situation.
- Person may be at risk for falls due to perceptual disorder such difficulty with depth perception leading to misjudging distance to, height of, or drop off of curb or stair.

Psychosocial

- Person may have a fear of falling and avoid locations or situations, such as going outdoors where fear is greatest.
- Person may have a decreased quality of life.

Context/Environment

- Person may be unaware of dangers that exist in home.
- Person may be aware of dangers in the home such as stairs and limit activity to lower level.
- Person may need to use adapted devices.

Intervention/Treatment

Models and programs created by occupational therapy personnel include environmental assessment and modification (Pighills et al., 2011), exercise education program (Chang et al.,

2011), home environmental audit (Currin et al., 2012), occupational therapy fall reduction home visit program (Chu et al., 2017), Stroll Safe outdoor program (Chippendale, 2019), and Westmead Home Visit Program (Clemson et al., 2014). Models and programs created by other professionals but used by occupational therapy personnel include cognitive therapy (Segev-Jacubovski et al., 2011), day hospital falls prevention program (Irvine et al., 2010), fall prevention intervention protocol (Mackenzie & Clemson, 2014; Mackenzie et al., 2020; Mackenzie et al., 2013), Falls Sensei (Money et al., 2019), LIFE Pilot Study (Clemson et al., 2012; Clemson et al., 2010), Nintendo Wii (Bell et al., 2011), multidisciplinary fall-prevention program (Bleijlevens et al., 2010), mulifactorial falls-prevention program (Johansson et al., 2018), self-management (Espiritu, 2013), Stepping On (Xu et al., 2019), and tailored prevention program (Wesson et al., 2013). Team members include physicians, psychologists, computer specialists, architects, physical therapists, and occupational therapy personnel. The goal is to prevent falls and increase safety by adding safer equipment or devices where appropriate, subtracting/getting rid of unsafe conditions or objects, transforming/changing use of environment and objects to safer use, or changing behavior to promote a safer living environment.

Activities of Daily Living/Instrumental ADL
- Review medications with client to determine if each is being taken correctly. Medications may need to reviewed by a physician or pharmacist to determine if dosage is correct and side effects that may cause dizziness or loss of motor control can be controlled.
- Assist client to assess everyday activities for potential risk factors that may cause falls such as footwear (high heels).

Education/Work
- Review with client any paid or volunteer work setting for hazards or unsafe conditions and recommend changes to promote safer work conditions.
- Consider if consulting with employer or supervisor could improve safer working conditions for all employees.

Play/Leisure
- Review with client favorite leisure occupations to determine if any hazards or unsafe conditions are present.
- Recommend exploring new leisure occupations with client that are less hazardous.

Rest/Sleep
- Review bedroom and bathroom safety to determine if pathway from bed to bathroom is clear and can be well lit at night.
- Consider if changing sleep quarters to main floor could reduce use of stairs.

Social Participation
- Review with client if locations of social activities present any hazards or unsafe conditions.
- Consider making recommendations to improve social participation in the home and community.

Sensorimotor
- Client should engage in regular exercise program to maintain or increase strength, balance, and postural stability, which are integrated into daily and meaningful occupations.
- Review with client if visual system should be evaluated for visual impairment and corrections as needed to acuity, alignment, and contrast sensitivity.
- Tips for getting up from a fall.
  - Locate a secure chair or other piece of furniture.
  - Roll onto side. Most people start by turning the head, then the shoulder, arms, hips, and legs.
  - Push up onto hands and knees (all fours position).
  - Crawl to the sturdy chair or furniture and place hands on the chair or furniture.
  - Using chair or furniture for balance, come to a half-kneeling position.

▸ Slowing rise from half-kneeling position by pushing with hips and arms.

▸ Stand up and turn to sit down on chair or furniture (adapted from Bearden, 2017).

Cognitive/Perceptual

- Programs to improve functional cognition may be useful.
- Encourage clients to think of ways to minimize risk of falling when performing occupations in everyday life.
- Assist client to develop a regular schedule of meaningful occupations in which to engage and participate.
- Client may benefit from practicing visual-perceptual skills.

Psychosocial

- Discussion with client about reducing the fear of falling and how to better ensure safety while engaging in all occupational areas.
- Encourage client, family, and caregivers to adopt a positive attitude about reducing risk of falling.
- Assist client to feel in control of the falls intervention program.
- Recommendations for changes should account for the client's beliefs regarding ability and personal motivation, which may influence the client's participation in falls intervention.

Context/Environment

- Discuss with client, family, or caregivers making home or living environment safer.
- If a client has a history of falls, offer to conduct a home hazard assessment, including recommendations.
- Offer to make a home hazard assessment and make recommendations to any client at risk of falls for home modification such as adding grab bars, railings or lighting, reducing clutter, clearing and straightening pathways, securing cords.
- Consider if a recommendation for a home hazard assessment should be routine at discharge for any client with reduced functional ability at discharge.
- Make available information, advice, and instruction to all clients and anyone living in the community on how to reduce risk of falls. Recommendations should be tailored to individual fall risk factors, lifestyles, and preferences.
- Make information, advice, and instruction available in multiple formats and language (web based, written, presentation).
- Assist policy makers, program managers, educators, and other health professionals to adopt strategies to make routine fall prevention screening a regular part of the health care delivery system.

Precautions/Safety Considerations

Perioperative falls may be underreported (Kronzer et al., 2016). See also Context/Environments under Evaluation/Assessment.

Prognosis and Outcome

Fall prevention continues to be a work in progress. A variety of approaches are needed to meet the different needs of people with different lifestyles, living environments, and living situations.

Cost Effectiveness

A day hospital falls prevention program was cost effective (Irvine et al., 2010).

REFERENCES

Barbour, K. E., Stevens, J. A., Helmick, C. G., Luo, Y. H., Murphy, L. B., Hootman, J. M., Theis, K., Anderson, L. A., Baker, N. A, Sugerman, D. E., & the Centers for Disease Control and Prevention

(CDC). (2014). Falls and fall injuries among adults with arthritis—United States, 2012. *MMWR: Morbidity and Mortality Weekly Report, 63*(17), 379–383.

Bearden, A. D. (2017). National patient safety goals and fall prevention techniques. In H. Smith-Gabai & S. E. Holm (Eds.), *Occupational therapy in acute care* (2nd ed., pp. 107–111). AOTA Press.

Bell, C. S., Fain, E., Daub, J., Warren, S. H., Howell, S. H., Southard, K. S., Sellers, C., & Shadoin, H. (2011). Effects of Nintendo Wii on quality of life, social relationships, and confidence to prevent falls. *Physical & Occupational Therapy in Geriatrics, 29*(3), 213–221. https://doi.org/10.31 09/02703181.2011.559307

Bleijlevens, M. H. C., Hendriks, M. R. C., Van Haastregt, J. C. M. N., Crebolder, H. F. J. M., & van Eijk, J. T. M. (2010). Lessons learned from a multidisciplinary fall-prevention programme: The occupational-therapy element. *Scandinavian Journal of Occupational Therapy, 17*(4), 319–325. https://doi.org/10.3109/11038120903419038

Breisinger, T. P., Skidmore, E. R., Niyonkuru, C., Terhorst, L., & Campbell, G. B. (2014). The Stroke Assessment of Fall Risk (SAFR): Predictive validity in inpatient stroke rehabilitation. *Clinical Rehabilitation, 28*(12), 1218–1224. https://doi.org/10.1177/0269215514534276

Chang, M., Huang, Y. H., & Jung, H. (2011). The effectiveness of the exercise education programme on fall prevention of the community-dwelling elderly: A preliminary study. *Hong Kong Journal of Occupational Therapy, 21*(2), 56–63. https://doi.org/10.1016/j.hkjot.2011 .10.002

Chase, C. A., Mann, K., Wasek, S., & Arbesman, M. (2012). Systematic review of the effect of home modification and fall prevention programs on falls and the performance of community-dwelling older adults. *American Journal of Occupational Therapy, 66*(3), 284–291. https:// doi.org/10.5014/ajot.2012.005017

Chippendale, T. (2019). Feasibility of the Stroll Safe outdoor fall prevention program. *American Journal of Occupational Therapy, 73*(4), Article 7304205060. https://doi.org/10.5014/ajot.2019 .031294

Chu, M. M., Fong, K. N., Lit, A. C., Rainer, T. H., Cheng, S. W., Au, F. L., Fung, H. K. K., Wong, C. M., & Tong, H. K. (2017). An occupational therapy fall reduction home visit program for community-dwelling older adults in Hong Kong after an emergency department visit for a fall. *Journal of the American Geriatrics Society, 65*(2), 364–372. https://doi.org/ 10.1111/jgs.14527

Clemson, L., Donaldson, A., Hill, K., & Day, L. (2014). Implementing person-environment approaches to prevent falls: A qualitative inquiry in applying the Westmead approach to occupational therapy home visits. *Australian Occupational Therapy Journal, 61*(5), 325–334. https://doi.org/10.1111/1440-1630.12132

Clemson, L., Fiatarone Singh, M. A., Bundy, A., Cumming R. G., Manollaras, K., O'Loughlin, P., & Black, D. (2012). Integration of balance and strength training into daily life activity to reduce rate of falls in older people (the LiFE study): Randomised parallel trial. *BMJ, 345,* Article e7879. https://doi.org/10.1136/bmj.e4547

Clemson, L., Fiatarone Singh, M., Bundy, A., Cumming, R. G., Weissel, E., Munro, J., Manollaras, K., & Black, D. (2010). LiFE pilot study: A randomised trial of balance and strength training embedded in daily life activity to reduce falls in older adults. *Australian Occupational Therapy Journal, 57*(1), 42–50. https://doi.org/10.1111/j.1440-1630.2009.00848.x

Currin, M. L., Comans, T. A., Heathcote, K., & Haines, T. P. (2012). Staying safe at home. Home environmental audit recommendations and uptake in an older population at high risk of falling. *Australasian Journal on Ageing, 31*(2), 90–95. https://doi.org/10.1111/j.1741-6612.20 11.00545.x

Espiritu, E. W. (2013). Standing tall: A self-management approach to fall prevention intervention. *OT Practice, 18*(16), 14–18.

Hamm, J., Money, A., & Atwal, A. (2019a). Enabling older adults to carry out paperless falls-risk self-assessments using guidetomeasure-3D: A mixed methods study. *Journal of Biomedical Informatics, 92,* Article 103135. https://doi.org/10.1016/j.jbi.2019.103135

Hamm, J., Money, A. G., & Atwal, A. (2019b). Guidetomeasure-OT: A mobile 3D application to improve the accuracy, consistency, and efficiency of clinician-led home-based falls-risk assessments. *International Journal of Medical Informatics, 129*, 349–365. https://doi.org/10.1016/j.ij medinf.2019.07.004

Harper, K. J., Riley, V., Petta, A., Jacques, A. Spendier, N., & Ingram, K. (2020). Occupational therapist use of the "Timed Up and Go" test in a memory clinic to compare performance between cognitive diagnoses and screen for falls risk. *Australian Occupational Therapy Journal, 67*(1), 13–21. https://doi.org/10.1111/1440-1630.12617

Horowitz, B. P., Nochajski, S. M., & Schweitzer, J. A. (2013). Occupational therapy community practice and home assessments: Use of the Home Safety Self-Assessment Tool (HSSAT) to support aging in place. *Occupational Therapy in Health Care, 27*(3), 216–227.

Irvine, L., Conroy, S. P., Sach, T., Gladman, J. R. F., Harwood, R. H., Kendrick, D., Coupland, C., Drummond, A., Barton, G., & Masud, T. (2010). Cost-effectiveness of a day hospital falls prevention programme for screened community-dwelling older people at high risk of falls. *Age and Ageing, 39*(6), 710–716. https://doi.org/10.1093/ageing/afq108

Johansson, E., Jonsson, H., Dahlberg, R., & Patomella, A. H. (2018). The efficacy of a multi-factorial falls-prevention programme, implemented in primary health care. *British Journal of Occupational Therapy, 81*(8), 474–481. https://doi.org/10.1177/0308022618756303

Kronzer, V. L., Wildes, T. M., Stark, S. L., & Avidan, M. S. (2016). Review of perioperative falls. *British Journal of Anaesthesia, 117*(6), 720–732. https://doi.org/10.1093/bja/aew377

Lampiasi, N., & Jacobs, M., (2010). The role of physical and occupational therapies in fall prevention and management in the home setting. *Care Management Journals, 11*(2), 122–127. https://doi.org/10.1891/1521-0987.11.2.122

Lemmens, R., Gielen, C., & Spooren, A. (2017). Obstacle: A tool to assess the home environment designed for all. *Studies in Health Technology and Informatics, 242*, 168–174. https://doi .org/10.3233/978-1-61499-798-6-168

Mackenzie, L. (2017). Evaluation of the clinical utility of the Home Falls and Accidents Screening Tool (HOME FAST). *Disability and Rehabilitation, 39*(15), 1489–1501. https://doi.org/10 .1080/09638288.2016.1204015

Mackenzie, L., & Byles, J. (2018). Scoring the Home Falls and Accidents Screening Tool for health professionals (HOME FAST-HP): Evidence from one epidemiological study. *Australian Occupational Therapy Journal, 65*(5), 346–353. https://doi.org/10.1111/1440-1630.12467

Mackenzie, L., & Clemson, L. (2014). Can chronic disease management plans including occupational therapy and physiotherapy services contribute to reducing falls risk in older people? *Australian Family Physician, 43*(4), 211–215.

Mackenzie, L., Clemson, L., & Irving, D. (2020). Fall prevention in primary care using chronic disease management plans: A process evaluation of provider and consumer perspectives. *Australian Occupational Therapy Journal, 67*(1), 22–30. https://doi.org/10.1111/1440-1630.12618

Mackenzie, L., Clemson, L., & Roberts, C. (2013). Occupational therapists partnering with general practitioners to prevent falls: Seizing opportunities in primary health care. *Australian Occupational Therapy Journal, 60*(1), 66–70. https://doi.org/10.1111/1440-1630.12030

Money, A. G., Atwal, A., Boyce, E., Gaber, S., Windeatt, S., & Alexandrou, K. (2019). Falls Sensei: A serious 3D exploration game to enable the detection of extrinsic home fall hazards for older adults. *BMC Medical Informatics and Decision Making, 19*, Article 85. https://doi.org/10.1186/ s12911-019-0808-x

Pighills, A. C., Torgerson, D. J., Sheldon, T. A., Drummond, A. E., & Bland, J. M. (2011). Environmental assessment and modification to prevent falls in older people. *Journal of the American Geriatrics Society, 59*(1), 26–33. https://doi.org/10.1111/j.1532-5415.2010.03221.x

Porter, R. S. (Ed.). (2018). *The Merck manual of diagnosis and therapy* (20th ed.). Merck Sharp & Dohme.

Romli, M. H., Mackenzie, L., Lovarini, M., Tan, M. P., & Clemson, L. (2017). The interrater and test-retest reliability of the Home Falls and Accidents Screening Tool (HOME FAST) in Malaysia: Using raters with a range of professional backgrounds. *Journal of Evaluation in Clinical Practice, 23*(3), 662–669. https://doi.org/10.1111/jep.12697

Segev-Jacubovski, O., Herman, T., Yogev-Seligmann, G., Mirelman, A., Giladi, N., & Hausdorff, J. M. (2011). The interplay between gait, falls and cognition: Can cognitive therapy reduce fall risk? *Expert Review of Neurotherapeutics, 11*(7), 1057–1075. https://doi.org/10.1586/ern.11.69

Swenor, B. K., Yonge, A. V., Goldhammer, V., Miller, R., Gitlin, L. N., & Ramulu, P. (2016). Evaluation of the Home Environment Assessment for the Visually Impaired (HEAVI): An instrument designed to quantify fall-related hazards in the visually impaired. *BMC Geriatrics, 16*, Article 214. https://doi.org/10.1186/s12877-016-0391-2

Tomita, M. R., Saharan, S., Rajendran, S., Nochajski, S. M., & Schweitzer, J. A. (2014). Psychometrics of the Home Safety Self-Assessment Tool (HSSAT) to prevent falls in community-dwelling older adults. *American Journal of Occupational Therapy, 68*(6), 711–718. https://doi.org/10.5014/ajot.2014.010801

Vu, T. V., & Mackenzie, L. (2012). The inter-rater and test-retest reliability of the Home Falls and Accidents Screening Tool. *Australian Occupational Therapy Journal, 59*(3), 235–242. https://doi.org/10.1111/j.1440-1630.2012.01012.x

Wesson, J., Clemson, L., Brodaty, H., Lord, S., Taylor, M., Gitlin, L., & Close, J. (2013). A feasibility study and pilot randomized trial of a tailored prevention program to reduce falls in older people with mild dementia. *BMC Geriatrics, 13*, Article 89. https://doi.org/10.1186/1471-2318-13-89

Xu, T., O'loughlin, K., Clemson, L., Lannin, N. A., Koh, G., & Dean, C. (2019). Therapists' perspectives on adapting the Stepping On falls prevention programme for community-dwelling stroke survivors in Singapore. *Disability and Rehabilitation, 41*(21), 2528–2537. https://doi.org/10.1080/09638288.2018.1471168

BIBLIOGRAPHY

Ballinger, C., & Brooks, C. (2013). *An overview of best practice for falls prevention from an occupational therapy perspective.* Health Foundation.

Blaylock, S. E., & Vogtle, L. K. (2017). Falls prevention interventions for older adults with low vision: A scoping review. *Canadian Journal of Occupational Therapy, 84*(3), 139–147. https://doi.org/10.1177/0008417417711460

Chase, C. A., Mann, K., Wasek, S., & Arbesman, M. (2012). Systematic review of the effect of home modification and fall prevention programs on falls and the performance of community-dwelling older adults. *American Journal of Occupational Therapy, 66*(3), 284–291. https://doi.org/10.5014/ajot.2012.005017

Chippendale, T., Gentile, P. A., & James, M. K. (2017). Characteristics and consequences of falls among older adult trauma patients: Considerations for injury prevention programs. *Australian Occupational Therapy Journal, 64*(5), 350–357. https://doi.org/10.1111/1440-1630.12380

College of Occupational Therapists. (2015). *Occupational therapy in the prevention and management of falls in adults: Practice guideline.*

de Groot, G. C., & Fagerström, L. (2011). Older adults' motivating factors and barriers to exercise to prevent falls. *Scandinavian Journal of Occupational Therapy, 18*(2), 153–160. https://doi.org/10.3109/11038128.2010.487113

Elliott, S., & Leland, N. E. (2018). Occupational therapy fall prevention interventions for community-dwelling older adults: A systematic review. *American Journal of Occupational Therapy, 72*(4), Article 7204190040. https://doi.org/10.5014/ajot.2018.030494

Elliott, S. J., Ivanescu, A., Leland, N. E., Fogo, J., Painter, J. A., & Trujillo, L. G. (2012). Feasibility of interdisciplinary community-based fall risk screening. *American Journal of Occupational Therapy, 66*(2), 161–168. https://doi.org/10.5014/ajot.2012.002444

Erlandson, K. M., Plankey, M. W., Springer, G., Cohen, H. S., Cox, C., Hoffman, H. J., Yin, M. T., & Brown, T. T. (2016). Fall frequency and associated factors among men and women with or at risk for HIV infection. *HIV Medicine, 17*(10), 740–748. https://doi.org/10.1111/hiv.12378

Gotzmeister, D., Zecevic, A. A., Klinger, L., & Salmoni, A. (2015). "People are getting lost a little bit": Systemic factors that contribute to falls in community-dwelling octogenarians. *Canadian Journal on Aging, 34*(3), 397–410. https://doi.org/10.1017/S071498081500015X

Grant, A., Mackenzie, L., & Clemson, L. (2015). How do general practitioners engage with allied health practitioners to prevent falls in older people? An exploratory qualitative study. *Australasian Journal on Ageing, 34*(3), 149–154. https://doi.org/10.1111/ajag.12157

Gutman, S. A., Amarantos, K., Berg, J., Aponte, M., Gordillo, D., Rice, C., Smith, J., Perry, A., Wills, T., Chen, E., Peters, R., & Schluger, Z. (2018). Home safety fall and accident risk among prematurely aging, formerly homeless adults. *American Journal of Occupational Therapy, 72*(4), 72419503. https://doi.org/10.5014/ajot.2018.028050

Hägvide, M. L., Larsson, T. J., & Borell, L. (2013). Fall scenarios in causing older women's hip fractures. *Scandinavian Journal of Occupational Therapy, 20*(1), 21–28. https://doi.org/10.3109/11038128.2012.661456

Haltiwanger, E. P. (2013). Preventing falls. *Diabetes Self-Management, 30*(2), 10–12, 14.

Hamm, J., Money, A., Atwal, A., & Ghinea, G. (2019). Mobile three-dimensional visualisation technologies for clinician-led fall prevention assessments. *Health Informatics Journal, 25*(3), 788–810. https://doi.org/10.1177/1460458217723170

Hamm, J., Money, A., Atwal, A., & Paraskevopoulos, I. (2016). Fall prevention intervention technologies: A conceptual framework and survey of the state of the art. *Journal of Biomedical Informatics, 59*, 319–345. https://doi.org/10.1016/j.jbi.2015.12.013

Jensen, L. E., & Padilla, R. (2011). Effectiveness of interventions to prevent falls in people with Alzheimer's disease and related dementias. *American Journal of Occupational Therapy, 65*(5), 532–540. https://doi.org/10.5014/ajot.2011.002626

Jensen, L., & Padilla, R. (2017). Effectiveness of environment-based interventions that address behavior, perception, and falls in people with Alzheimer's disease and related major neurocognitive disorders: A systematic review. *American Journal of Occupational Therapy, 71*(5), Article 7105180030. https://doi.org/10.5014/ajot.2017.027409

Johansson, E., Borell, L., & Jonsson, H. (2014). Letting go of an old habit: Group leaders' experiences of a client-centred multidisciplinary falls-prevention programme. *Scandinavian Journal of Occupational Therapy, 21*(2), 98–106. https://doi.org/10.3109/11038128.2013.868515

Johnston, K., Barras, S., & Grimmer-Somers, K. (2010). Relationship between pre-discharge occupational therapy home assessment and prevalence of post-discharge falls. *Journal of Evaluation in Clinical Practice, 16*(6), 1333–1339. https://doi.org/10.1111/j.1365-2753.2009.01339.x

Lee, I., & Leland, N. (2013). Fall prevention for community-living older adults: A tale of two systematic reviews. *OT Practice, 18*(16), 19–22.

Leland, N. E., Elliott, S. J., O'Malley, L., & Murphy, S. L. (2012). Occupational therapy in fall prevention: Current evidence and future directions. *American Journal of Occupational Therapy, 66*(2), 149–160. https://doi.org/10.5014/ajot.2012.002733

Leland, N. E., Gozalo, P., Teno, J., & Mor, V. (2012). Falls in newly admitted nursing home residents: A national study. *Journal of the American Geriatrics Society, 60*(5), 939–945. https://doi.org/10.1111/j.1532-5415.2012.03931.x

Leland, N. E., Kaldenberg, J., & Lee, I. (2012). Watching their steps: Integrating vision intervention into daily practice to limit fall risk at skilled nursing facilities. *OT Practice, 17*(11), 7–16.

Liddle, J., Lovarini, M., Clemson, L., Mackenzie, L., Tan, A., Pit, S. W., Poulos, R., Tiedemann, A., Sherrington, C., Roberts, C., & Willis, K. (2018). Making fall prevention routine in primary care practice: perspectives of allied health professionals. *BMC Health Services Research, 18*, Article 598. https://doi.org/10.1186/s12913-018-3414-1

Maggi, P., de Almeida Mello, J., Delye, S., Cès, S., Macq, J., Gosset, C., & Declercq, A. (2018). Fall determinants and home modifications by occupational therapists to prevent falls. *Canadian Journal of Occupational Therapy, 85*(1), 79–87. https://doi.org/10.1177/0008417417714284

Middlebrook, S., & Mackenzie, L. (2012). The Enhanced Primary Care program and falls prevention: Perceptions of private occupational therapists and physiotherapists, *Australasian Journal on Ageing, 31*(2), 72–77. https://doi.org/10.1111/j.1741-6612.2011.00527.x

Painter, J. A., Allison, L., Dhingra, P., Daughtery, J., Cogdill, K., & Trujillo, L. G. (2012). Fear of falling and its relationship with anxiety, depression and activity engagement among community-dwelling older adults. *American Journal of Occupational Therapy, 66*(2), 169–176. https://doi.org/10.5014/ajot.2012.002535

Peterson, E. W. (2011). Reducing fall risk: A guide to community-based programs. *OT Practice, 16*(16), 15–20.

Peterson, E. W., Finlayson, M., Elliott, S. J., Painter, J. A., & Clemson L. (2012). Unprecedented opportunities in fall prevention for occupational therapy practitioners. *American Journal of Occupational Therapy, 66*(2), 127–130. https://doi.org/10.5014/ajot.2012.003814

Sampaio, R. A. C., Sampaio, P. Y. S., Castaño, L. A. A., Barbieri, J. F., Júnior, H. J. C., Arai, H., Uchida, M. C., & Guiterrez, G. L. (2017). Cutoff values for appendicular skeletal muscle mass and strength in relation to fear of falling among Brazilian older adults: Cross-sectional study. *Sao Paulo Medical Journal, 135*(5), 434–443. https://doi.org/10.1590/1516-3180.2017.0049030517

Schepens, S., Sen, A., Painter, J. A., & Murphy S. L. (2012). Relationship between fall-related efficacy and activity engagement in community-dwelling older adults: A meta-analytic review. *American Journal of Occupational Therapy, 66*(2), 137–148. https://doi.org/10.5014/ajot.2012.001156

Schepens, S. L., Panzer, V., & Goldberg, A. (2011). Randomized controlled trial comparing tailoring methods of multimedia-based fall prevention education for community-dwelling older adults. *American Journal of Occupational Therapy, 65*(6), 702–709. https://doi.org/10.5014/ajot.2011.001180

Schmid, A. A., Arnold, S. E., Jones, V. A., Ritter, M. J., Sapp, S. A., & Van Puymbroeck, M. (2015). Fear of falling in people with chronic stroke. *American Journal of Occupational Therapy, 69*(3), Article 6903350020. https://doi.org/10.5014/ajot.2015.016253

Schmid, A. A., Van Puymbroeck, M., Knies, K., Spangler-Morris, C., Watts, K., Damush, T., & Williams, L. S. (2011). Fear of falling among people who have sustained a stroke: A 6-month longitudinal pilot study. *American Journal of Occupational Therapy, 65*(2), 125–132. https://doi.org/10.5014/ajot.2011.000737

Stark, S. L., Roe, C. M., Grant, E. A., Hollingsworth, H., Benzinger, T. L., Fagan, A. M., Buckles, V. D., & Morris, J. C. (2013). Preclinical Alzheimer disease and risk of falls. *Neurology, 81*(5), 437–443. https://doi.org/10.1212/WNL.0b013e31829d8599

Stark, S. L., Silianoff, T. J., Kim, H. L., Conte, J. W., & Morris, J. C. (2015). Tailored calendar journals to ascertain falls among older adults. *OTJR: Occupation, Participation and Health, 35*(1), 53–59. https://doi.org/10.1177/1539449214561764

Steinman B. A., Nguyen, A. Q. D., Pynoos, J., & Leland, N. E. (2011). Falls-prevention interventions for persons who are blind or visually impaired. *Insight, 4*(2), 83–91.

Swink, L. A., Schmid, A. A., Atler, K., Klinedinst, T., Marchant, T. P., Marchant, D. R., & Malcolm, M. P. (2020). Fall risk factors for individuals under the age of 65 years with type 2 diabetes mellitus. *British Journal of Occupational Therapy, 83*(3), 191–196. https://doi.org/10.1177/0308022619876552

Taylor, S. F., Coogle, C. L., Cotter, J. J., Welleford, E. A., & Copolillo, A. (2019). Community-dwelling older adults' adherence to environmental fall prevention recommendations. *Journal of Applied Gerontology, 38*(6), 755–774. https://doi.org/10.1177/0733464817723087

Thomas, A., Saroyan, A., & Lajoie, S. P. (2012). Creation of an evidence-based practice reference model in falls prevention: Findings from occupational therapy. *Disability and Rehabilitation, 34*(4), 311–328. https://doi.org/10.3109/09638288.2011.607210

Toto, P. (2012). *Fact sheet: Occupational therapy and the prevention of falls.* American Occupational Therapy Association.

Tzingounakis, A. (2012). Falls prevention: Investigating best practice for community occupational therapists. *Occupational Therapy Now, 14*(3), 9–12.

Waqar, A., & Begum, R. (2019). To find out the prevalence and various risk factors for falls in older adults (60–75 years) community NCR Delhi. *Indian Journal of Physiotherapy and Occupational Therapy, 13*(1) 1–5. https://doi.org/10.5958/0973-5674.2019.00001.7

Wheeler, E., Coogle, C. L., Fix, R. C., Owens, M. G., & Waters, L. H. (2018). Physical and occupational therapy practice improvement following interprofessional evidence-based falls prevention training. *Journal of Allied Health, 47*(1), 9–18.

Williams, G. R., Deal, A. M., Nyrop, K. A., Pergolotti, M., Guerard, E. J., Jolly T. A., & Muss, H. B. (2015). Geriatric assessment as an aide to understanding falls in older adults with cancer. *Supportive Care in Cancer, 23*(8), 2273–2280. https://doi.org/10.1007/s00520-014-2598-0

Frailty and Frail Conditions
Also called frail elder, frail elderly.
See also Falls, Incontinence, Low Vision, Older Adults, Visual Impairment.

Description

Frailty has been described as a "clinically recognizable state of increased vulnerability resulting from a decline in reserve and function across multiple physiologic systems such that the ability to cope with everyday or acute stressors is compromised" (Wyrko, 2015, p. 377). Although age, especially 80 years or older, is a high risk factor, age is not the defining criterion, nor is overall physical condition. Frailty is more adequately explained as a "dynamic pre-disability state that includes losses in physical, psychological and/or social domains" (Coelho et al., 2015, p. 1).

Cause

Specific problems known to lead to frailty are muscle weakness, slowness, exhaustion/fatigue, low physical activity, and weight loss (Provencher et al., 2017). Components that can result in frailty include five interrelated domains:

- Physical environment: appearance of home, bathroom and toilet facilities, fall hazards, heights of windows, kitchen surfaces, stairs, type of housing.
- Physical health: activities of daily living, appearance, comorbidities, mobility, polypharmacy.
- Economic factors: cost of adaptations, cost of access to services, home management costs, living expenses.
- Social environment: carer burden, loneliness, overprotective or overly supportive loved ones, social isolation.
- Mental health and psychological factors: cognitive impairment, emotional state, perception of individual's health and well-being, personality traits such as independent or dependent, positive outlook or negative, and proactive or passive (Coker et al., 2019).

Evaluation/Assessment
Areas
- Activities of Daily Living/Instrumental ADL: basic ADLs (bathing, toileting); independent living skills (medication, finances, housekeeping, home management, shopping, driving)
- Education/Work: usually not a factor because person is retired or not employed
- Play/Leisure: interests, values, frequency, location
- Rest/Sleep: sleep disturbance, sleep disorders

- Social Participation: type, frequency, location, with whom
- Sensorimotor: physical fitness, muscle and grip strength, endurance, sensory functions
- Cognitive/Perceptual: attention, memory and learning, executive functions
- Psychosocial: motivation, mood (anxiety, depression, apathy), quality of life, role performance
- Context/Environment: social support, accessibility, resources, cultural perspectives
- Comorbidities: existing or preexisting chronic diseases and/or disorders, acute or recent traumatic events

Instruments

Note: Authors have suggested that assessment in the home environment may provide a more accurate evaluation of function than in a clinical environment, especially for tasks such as cooking or meal preparation (Provencher, Demers, Gagnon, & Gélinas, 2012; Provencher, Demers, & Gélinas, 2012; Provencher et al., 2013).

Instruments Developed by Occupational Therapy Personnel

- Assessment of Motor and Process Skills (8th ed.; AMPS-8; Fisher & Bray Jones, 2016)
- Community Dependency Index (CDI; Eakin & Baird, 1995)
- Performance Assessment of Self-Care Skills (Version 4.1; PASS 4.1; Rogers et al., 2016)

Instruments Developed by Other Professionals and Used by Occupational Therapy Personnel

- Barthel Index (BI; Mahoney & Barthel, 1965)
- Berg Balance Scale (BBS; Berg et al., 1989)
- Canadian Study of Health and Aging–Clinical Frailty Scale (CSHA-CFS; Rockwood et al., 2005)
- Cardiovascular Health Study frailty index (CHSfi; Fried et al., 2001)
- Edmonton Frail Scale (EFS; Rolfson et al., 2006; see also Wyrko, 2015, in References)
- European Quality of Life 5-Dimension Scale (EuroQol5; EuroQol Group, 1990)
- Free and Cued Selective Reminding Test (FCSRT; Grober et al., 2009)
- Functional Independence Measure (FIM; Uniform Data System for Medical Rehabilitation, 1997)
- Geriatric Depression Scale (GDS; Yesavage et al., 1982–1983)
- Göteborg Quality of Life Instrument (GQoL; Tibblin et al., 1990)
- Grip strength (Wang et al., 2018)
- Groningen Frailty Indicator (GFI; Steverink et al., 2001)
- Index of Activities of Daily Living (K-ADL; Katz et al., 1970)
- Instrumental Activities of Daily Living (IADL; Lawton & Brody, 1969)
- interRAI Home Care (HC; Landi et al., 2000)
- Katz Index of Activities of Daily Living (Katz ADL Index; see Index of Activities of Daily Living)
- KM Visual Acuity Chart (KM Chart; Moutakis et al., 2004)
- Mini-Mental State Examination (MMSE; Folstein et al., 1975)
- Mobility-Tiredness Scale (Mob-T; Fieo et al., 2013)
- Montreal Cognitive Assessment (MoCA; Nasreddine et al., 2005)
- Pearlin Self-Mastery Scale (PSMS; Pearlin & Schooler, 1978)
- PRISMA-7 (Raiche et al., 2008)
- Short Form 36 Health Survey (SF-36; Ware et al., 1993)
- State-Trait Anxiety Inventory (STAI; Spielberger, 1983)
- Stroop Color and Word Test (SCWT; Golden & Freshwater, 2002)
- Tilburg Frailty Indicator (TFI; Gobbens et al., 2010)
- Tinetti Performance Oriented Mobility Assessment (POMA; Tinetti, 1986)
- Tower of London (ToL; Shallice, 1982)
- Trail Making Test A and B (TMT-A, TMT-B; Reitan & Wolfson, 1995)
- Wechsler Memory Scale (4th ed.; WMS-IV; Wechsler, 2009)

Problems/Issues

Activities of Daily Living/Instrumental ADL

- Person may have difficulty performing basic ADL tasks such a bathing, toileting, eating, dressing.
- Person may have lost weight over past 3 months.
- Person may have difficulty performing independent living tasks such as taking medications, managing finances, housekeeping, shopping, driving safely.

Education/Work

- Not discussed.

Play/Leisure

- Person may be unable to continue or have lost interest in continuing engagement in previously enjoyed leisure occupations.

Rest/Sleep

- Person may experience sleep disturbances.

Social Participation

- Person may limit or stop participation in favorite social occupations.

Sensorimotor

- Person usually has decreased grip strength.
- Person usually has poor balance, is at risk for falls.
- Person usually has slow gait (walking) speed.
- Person may express fatigue and/or lack of endurance.
- Person may have identified or unidentified visual impairment (acuity, loss of visual field).

Cognitive/Perceptual

- Person may have cognitive impairment.
- Person may have visual perceptual deficit such as poor spatial relations.

Psychosocial

- Person may lack motivation or have apathy.
- Person may be anxious or depressed.
- Person may have decreased role performance.
- Person may have decreased quality of life and life satisfaction.
- Person may report feelings of decreased self-worth or self-efficacy.

Context/Environment

- Home or living arrangements may have issues with accessibly and safety.
- Caregivers may be unaware of the extent to which they are compensating for person's deficits and that person would experience significant disability if caregiver suddenly was unavailable.
- Person and caregivers may lack information about assistive devices or technology.
- Person and caregivers may lack information about available community or internet resources.

Intervention/Treatment

Models and programs developed by occupational therapy personnel include the life goal-setting technique (Yuri et al., 2016). Models and programs developed by other professionals but used by occupational therapy personnel include client-centered and activity-oriented program (De Vriendt et al., 2016), elderly persons in the risk zone (Gustafsson et al., 2013; Gustafsson et al., 2012), prevention of care (Metzelthin et al., 2013), Preventive Home Visit (PHV; Behm et al., 2016; Dahlin-Ivanoff et al., 2010), and multiprofessional senior group meetings (Behm et al., 2016; Dahlin-Ivanoff et al., 2010). Team members include physicians, geriatric specialists, nursing personnel, psychologists, recreational personnel, social workers, dietitians or nutritionists, pharmacists, physical therapy personnel, and occupational therapy personnel. Goals are to improve the functioning (occupational performance) of clients that will enable engagement in meaningful occupations of everyday living (De Coninck et al., 2017).

Activities of Daily Living/Instrumental ADL

- Person may need assistance in medication management including a review of medications with physician or pharmacist to determine which are necessary and what side effects could be reduced, such as "brain fog" or psychomotor signs.
- Person may need assistance with incontinence.
- Person may need assistance with nutrition including meal preparation and grocery shopping.
- Person may need assistance with home maintenance and home management.
- Person may need a review of driving including best fit of car to driver and driver fitness and safety.
- Provide information and advice, and practice use, if needed, on available public transportation including transport for disabled/handicapped.

Education/Work

- Provide information on available continuing education in the community (gardening, art history, budget and finance).

Play/Leisure

- Provide opportunity to reengage in previously enjoyed occupations, perhaps with modifications or adaptations such as added light, use of magnification, adapted equipment or supplies.
- Provide opportunity to "try out" new leisure occupations.

Rest/Sleep

- Provide information and advice on improving sleep habits and sleeping arrangements.
- Provide information on sleep disorders and refer client to sleep specialist, if needed.

Social Participation

- Provide opportunity to participate in previous social occupations by modifying or adapting aspects such as in-home versus in community, fewer participants, shorter time period, reduced active participation.
- Provide opportunity to "try out" new social occupations.

Sensorimotor

- Provide information and advice about and, when appropriate, instructions in a basic home exercise program including balance exercises.
- Provide training to reduce incidence of falls and fall recovery strategies.

Cognitive/Perceptual

- Person may need assistance with use of memory aids.
- Provide practice in use of executive functions such as problem solving, decision making, setting priorities.

Psychosocial

- Provide advice and training in stress management and coping strategies (mindfulness, relaxation, deep breathing, yoga).

Context/Environment

- Provide information and assistance in home modification to improve safety (fall risk, fire danger, smoke alarms) and accessibility.
- Provide information and advice, and training, if needed, in use of assistive devices and technology.

- Provide training to family members or other caregivers to promote function and safety.
- Provide information and advice on how to prevent identified fall risks.
- Provide information about available community and internet resources.

Precautions/Safety Considerations

Person is at risk for falls. Person is at risk for negative or harmful side effects of medication. Person and caregivers may be unaware of potential hazards and unsafe conditions in the home or approaches to minimize or eliminate the hazards.

Prognosis and Outcome

Frailty can progress to functional disability and dependency. Preventive measures can stop or slow the progress toward disablement and dependent status (Metzelthin et al., 2013).

REFERENCES

Behm, L., Eklund, K., Wilhelmson, K., Ziden, L., Gustafsson, S., Falk, K., & Dahlin-Ivanoff, S. (2016). Health promotion can postpone frailty: Results from the RCT—Elderly Persons in the Risk Zone. *Public Health Nursing, 33*(4), 303–315. https://doi.org/10.1111/phn.12240

Coelho, T., Paúl, C., Gobbens, R. J. J., & Fernandes, L. (2015). Determinants of frailty: The added value of assessing medication. *Frontiers in Aging Neuroscience, 7*, Article 56. https://doi .org/10.3389/fnagi.2015.00056

Coker, J. F., Martin, M. E., Simpson, R. M., & Lafortune, L. (2019). Frailty: An in-depth qualitative study exploring the views of community care staff. *BMC Geriatrics, 19*, Article 47. https://doi.org/10.1186/s12877-019-1069-3

Dahlin-Ivanoff, S., Gosman-Hedström, G., Edberg, A.-K., Wilhelmson, K., Eklund, K., Duner A., Ziden, L., Welmer, A.-K., & Landahl, S. (2010). Elderly persons in the risk zone. Design of a multidimensional, health-promoting, randomised three-armed controlled trial for "prefrail" people of 80+ years living at home. *BMC Geriatrics, 10*, Article 27. https://doi.org/10.1186/ 1471-2318-10-27

De Coninck, L., Bekkering, G. E., Bouckaert, L., Declercq, A., Graff, M. J. L., & Aertgeerts, B. (2017). Home- and community-based occupational therapy improves functioning in frail older people: A systematic review. *Journal of the American Geriatrics Society, 65*(8), 1863–1869. https://doi.org/10.1111/jgs.14889

De Vriendt, P., Peersman, W., Florus, A., Verbeke, M., & Van de Velde, D. (2016). Improving health related quality of life and independence in community dwelling frail older adults through a client- centred and activity-oriented program. A pragmatic randomized controlled trial. *Journal of Nutrition, Health & Aging, 20*(1), 35–40. https://doi.org/10.1007/s12603-016-0673-6

Gustafsson, S., Eklund, K., Wilhelmson, K., Edberg, A.-K., Johansson, B., Kronlöf, G. H., Gosman-Hedström, G., & Dahlin-Ivanoff, S. (2013). Long-term outcome for ADL following the health-promoting RCT—Elderly Persons in the Risk Zone. *The Gerontologist, 53*(4), 654–663. https:// doi.org/10.1093/geront/gns121

Gustafsson, S., Wilhelmson, K., Eklund, K., Gosman-Hedström, G., Zidén, L., Kronlöf, G. H., Højgaard, B., Slinde, F., Rothenberg, E., Landahl, S., & Dahlin-Ivanoff, S. (2012). Health-promoting interventions for persons aged 80 and older are successful in the short term— Results from the randomized and three-armed Elderly Persons in the Risk Zone study. *Journal of the American Geriatrics Society, 60*(3), 447–454. https://doi.org/10.1111/j.1532-54 15.2011.03861.x

Metzelthin, S., van Rossum, E., de Witte, L. P., Ambergen, A. W., Hobma, S. O., Sipers, W., & Kempen, G. I. J. M. (2013). Effectiveness of interdisciplinary primary care approach to reduce disability in community dwelling frail older people: Cluster randomised controlled trial. *BMJ, 347*, Article f5264. https://doi.org/10.1136/bmj.f5264

Provencher, V., Béland, F., Demers, L., Desrosiers, J., Bier, N., Avila-Funes, J. A., Galand, C., Julien, D., Fletcher, J. D., Trottier, L., & Hami, B. (2017). Are frailty components associated with disability in specific activities of daily living in community-dwelling older adults? A multicenter Canadian study. *Archives of Gerontology and Geriatrics, 73*, 187–194. https://doi.org/10.1016/j.archger.2017.07.027

Provencher, V., Demers, L., Gagnon, L., & Gélinas, I. (2012). Impact of familiar and unfamiliar settings on cooking task assessments in frail older adults with poor and preserved executive functions. *International Psychogeriatrics, 24*(5), 775–783. https://doi.org/10.1017/S104161021100216X

Provencher, V., Demers, L., & Gélinas, I. (2012). Factors that may explain differences between home and clinic meal preparation task assessments in frail older adults. *International Journal of Rehabilitation Research, 35*(3), 248–255. https://doi.org/10.1097/MRR.0b013e3283544cb8

Provencher, V., Demers, L., Gélinas, I., & Giroux, F. (2013). Cooking task assessment in frail older adults: Who performed better at home and in the clinic? *Scandinavian Journal of Occupational Therapy, 20*(5), 374–383. https://doi.org/10.3109/11038128.2012.743586

Wyrko, Z. (2015). Frailty at the front door. *Clinical Medicine, 15*(4), 377–381.

Yuri, Y., Takabatake, S., Nishikawa, T., Oka, M., & Fujiwara, T. (2016). The effects of a life goal-setting technique in a preventive care program for frail community-dwelling older people: A cluster nonrandomized controlled trial. *BMC Geriatrics, 16*, Article 101. https://doi.org/10.1186/s12877-016-0277-3

BIBLIOGRAPHY

Bennett, S., & Fuller, J. (2019). The ever growing frailty team. *OT News, 27*(4), 36–37.

de Almeida Mello, J., Declercq, A., Cès, S., Van Durme, T., Van Audenhove, C., & Macq, J. (2016). Exploring home care interventions for frail older people in Belgium: A comparative effectiveness study. *Journal of the American Geriatrics Society, 64*(11), 2251–2256. https://doi.org/10.1111/jgs.14410

Fritz, H., Seidarabi, S., Barbour, R., & Vonbehren, A. (2019). Occupational therapy intervention to improve outcomes among frail older adults: A scoping review. *American Journal of Occupational Therapy, 73*(3), Article 7303205130. https://doi.org/10.5014/ajot.2019.030585

Roland, K., Theou, O., Jakobi, J., Swan, L., & Jones, G. R. (2011). Exploring frailty: Community physical and occupational therapists' perspectives. *Physical & Occupational Therapy in Geriatrics, 29*(4), 270–286. https://doi.org/10.3109/02703181.2011.616986

Roland, K., Theou, O., Jakobi, J., Swan, L., & Jones, G. R. (2014). How do community physical and occupational therapists classify frailty? A pilot study. *Journal of Frailty & Aging, 3*(4), 247–250. https://doi.org/10.14283/jfa.2014.32

Shears, M., Takaoka, A., Rochwerg, B., Bagshaw, S. M., Johnstone, J., Holding, A., Tharmalingam, S., Millen, T., Clarke, F., Rockwood, K., Li, G., Thabane, L., Muscedere, J., Stelfox, H. T., Cook, D. J., & Canadian Critical Care Trials Group. (2018). Assessing frailty in the intensive care unit: A reliability and validity study. *Journal of Critical Care, 45*, 197–203. https://doi.org/10.1016/j.jcrc.2018.02.004

Homeless Person

Also called homelessness, persons who are homeless.

Description

A homeless person (or family) is an individual (or group of individuals) who lacks a fixed, regular, and adequate nighttime residence, and a person who has a nighttime residence that is (a) supervised publicly or privately in an operated shelter designed to provide temporary living accommodations, (b) an institution that provides a temporary residence for individuals intended to be institutionalized, or (c) a public or private place not designed for, nor ordinarily used as, a regular sleeping accommodation for human beings (McKinney-Vento Homeless Assistance Act, 1987). Australian authors have suggested a slightly different categorization, as follows: (a) primary homelessness are persons without conventional accommodation, including improvised dwellings, who are called "rough sleepers"; (b) secondary homelessness includes couch or sofa surfers with friends or relatives, and people who move frequently from one form of temporary shelter to the next; and (c) tertiary homelessness are persons with medium- to long-term boarding arrangements (Slatter et al., 2012).

Cause

Two types of causes are recognized, although often aspects of both coexist at the same time: socio-environmental (structural) and personal. Socio-environmental factors include poverty, lack of housing including lack of affordable housing, lack of job opportunities especially unskilled positions, limited salaries and benefits, and welfare regulations that may restrict eligibility or amount of benefits received. Personal factors include drug and alcohol misuse, poor mental and physical health, lack of social support, and relationship breakdown (Boland & Cunningham, 2019). Other personal factors may be inadequate job skills, especially in the area of interpersonal skills, an intermittent job history resume, loss of employment, failure to pass drug screening tests, an arrest and conviction history, and extended total amount of time spent in institutions (hospitals, clinics, jails, prisons, detention centers, etc.).

Evaluation/Assessment

Areas

- Activities of Daily Living/Instrumental ADL: nutritional status, clothing, finances, housekeeping, transportation
- Education/Work: academic achievement, work skills, work resume
- Play/Leisure: interests, values, frequency, location
- Rest/Sleep: sleep hygiene, sleep location
- Social Participation: type, frequency, location, with whom
- Sensorimotor: gross and fine motor skills
- Cognitive/Perceptual: attention, memory, learning, executive functions
- Psychosocial: emotional regulation, social skills, quality of life
- Context/Environment: community resources, social support
- Comorbidities: physical and mental health conditions, substance abuse, poverty, legal status

Instruments

Instruments Developed by Occupational Therapy Personnel

- Allen Cognitive Level Screen (5th ed.; ACLS-5; Allen et al., 2007)
- Assessment of Motor and Process Skills (8th ed.; AMPS-8; Fisher & Bray Jones, 2016)
- Canadian Occupational Performance Measure (5th ed.; COPM-5; Law et al., 2014)
- Executive Function Performance Test (EFPT; Baum & Wolf, 2013)
- Kohlman Evaluation of Living Skills (4th ed.; KELS-4; Kohman Thompson & Robnett, 2016)
- Large Allen Cognitive Level Screen (5th ed.; LACLS-5; Allen et al., 2007)
- Manage Med Screening (MMS; Robnett et al., 2007)
- Occupational Circumstances Assessment Interview and Rating Scale (Version 4.0; OCAIRS 4.0; Forsyth et al., 2005)
- Performance Assessment of Self-Care Skills (Version 4.1; PASS 4.1; Chisholm et al., 2016)
- Practical Skills Test (PST; Helfrich & Fogg, 2007; see also Chang et al., 2013, in References)

Instruments Developed by Other Professionals and Used by Occupational Therapy Personnel

- Impact of Event Scale-Revised (IES-R; Weiss, 2004)
- Manchester Short Assessment of Quality of Life (MANSA; Priebe et al., 1999)

- Perceived Stress Scale (PSS; Cohen et al., 1983)
- University of Rhode Island Change Assessment (URICA; McConnaughy et al., 1983)
- World Health Organization Quality of Life Scale–Abbreviated Version (WHOQOL-BREF; WHOQOL Group, 1998)

Problems/Issues

Activities of Daily Living/Instrumental ADL

- Person may have poor dietary habits leading to poor nutritional status and possible health related conditions.
- Person may need a weight management program to monitor weight gain (obesity) or loss (not eating enough) or control of diabetes.
- Person may not know how or have the resources to maintain clothing in good (wearable) and clean condition.
- Person may have limited financial resources and/or limited skills in managing/budgeting those resources.
- Person may lack skills in home care and management.
- Person may have child care responsibilities or responsibilities for caring for other persons.
- Person may have responsibilities for caring for a pet or companion animal.
- Person may lack access to or knowledge of transportation systems.

Education/Work

- Person may have poor literacy skills.
- Person may not have employable work skills.
- Person may lack access to equipment needed to apply for a position such as phone, computer, scanner, or printer.
- Person may be unable to get to job sites to interview for positions because no vehicle or public transportation is available.
- Person may have a poor work history with frequent terminations.

Play/Leisure

- Person may lack opportunity (occupational deprivation) to engage in leisure activities.
- Person may lack leisure interests or skills.

Rest/Sleep

- Person may have poor sleep habits and hygiene.
- Person may lack a consistent and safe place to sleep.
- Person may sleep during the day, and stay up at night to achieve sense of safety.

Social Participation

- Person may have limited opportunity for social activities.

Sensorimotor

- Person may have deficits in gross or fine motor skills.
- Person may have sensory deficits, especially in vision or hearing.

Cognitive/Perceptual

- Person may have cognitive impairments.
- Person may have time management issues including insufficient occupation during parts of the day leading to boredom.
- Person may experience occupational imbalance in which there is excessive engagement in one occupation or group of occupations to the exclusion of other occupations.
- Person may have perceptual deficits especially in visual perception.

Psychosocial

- Person may have difficulty in emotional regulation including aggression, anger, irritability, or flat affect.

- Person may lack skills in self-management including coping skills and stress management.
- Person may have decreased sense of self-concept, self-worth, and self-confidence.
- Person may experience sense of loss of control over everyday life.
- Person may have deficits in social skills and interpersonal relations.
- Person may have a limited or poor quality of life.
- Person may have a mental health diagnosis or symptoms congruent with mental health disorder including posttraumatic stress disorder, schizophrenia, bipolar disorder, personality disorder, depression, anxiety, paranoia, or phobia.

Context/Environment
- Person may lack knowledge of how to maintain a safe environment in the home.
- Person may lack knowledge of community resources.
- Person may have limited or no social support system.
- Person may have experienced domestic or street violence.
- Person may experience barriers (policies, regulations, "red tape") to accessing social or government services.
- Person may experience occupational apartheid behavior in which restrictions from occupational pursuits are imposed by others because of perceived personal characteristics.
- Person may experience occupational alienation in which the he or she is not able to engage in meaningful occupations and instead must engage in tasks that do not reflect the person's full capacities.
- Person may experience occupational deprivation in which an illness or disability prohibits engagement in meaningful occupations.
- Person may experience occupational marginalization in which everyday options or choices are not available to the individual due to certain restrictions imposed by society based on attributes such as gender or age.
- Services person needs may be underfunded or unavailable or both.

Intervention/Treatment

Models and programs developed by occupational therapy personnel include the Apartment Living Program (Gutman, Raphael-Greenfield, Berg et al., 2018), case study, environment safety modification program (Gutman, Douglas, et al., 2018), Housing Transition Program (Gutman et al., 2016), intervention service (Fieldhouse et al., 2011), life skills acquisition exercise (Helfrich & Synovec, 2019), model of human occupation (Bradley et al., 2011), occupational justice (Schultz-Krohn & Tyminski, 2018), person-environment-occupation model (Faulkner, 2016), stress management program (Gutman et al., 2019), and Supporting Many to Achieve Residential Transition (SMART; Gutman & Raphael-Greenfield, 2017). Models and programs developed by other professions but used by occupational therapy personnel include the Assertive Community Treatment (ACT) model (Lloyd & Bassett, 2010, 2012; Lloyd et al., 2010), Geographic Information Systems (GIS; Chan, Gopal, & Helfrich, 2014; Chan, Helfrich, et al., 2014), goal attainment scaling (Gutman & Raphael-Greenfield, 2017), harm reduction program (Helfrich & Synovec, 2019), mobile outreach street health (Marval & Townsend, 2013), situated learning theory (Helfrich & Synovec, 2019), transtheoretical model (TTM; Helfrich et al., 2012), and trauma-informed care (Helfrich & Synovec, 2019). Team members may include staff members in homeless shelters or adult daycare centers, community charity social service workers, psychologists or counselors, dietitians or nutritionists, nursing personnel, on-call physicians, and occupational therapy personnel. The goal of occupational therapy is to establish or reestablish participation in a balance of the occupations of everyday living including self-maintenance (especially shelter and housing), productivity, and leisure.

Activities of Daily Living/Instrumental ADL
- Provide program or module on food, diet, and nutrition (see Gutman et al., 2019; Helfrich, 2014—note that all programs and modules are facilitated by the addition of opportunities to

practice, use of homework assignments for outpatients, role playing situations and events, and group discussion).

- Provide program or module on maintaining an apartment or apartment living skills (see Gutman & Raphael-Greenfield, 2017; Helfrich, 2014).
- Provide program or module on money management and finances (see Gutman & Raphael-Greenfield, 2017; Helfrich, 2014).
- Provide program or module on securing shelter or getting an apartment (see Gutman & Raphael-Greenfield, 2017).
- Provide program or module on maintaining general health and wellness (see Gutman & Raphael-Greenfield, 2017).

Education/Work
- Assist person to get additional education.
- Provide opportunity to increase literacy skills.
- Provide opportunity to practice work skills in sheltered employment or supportive employment.
- Provide opportunity to practice job interview skills, creating a resume, and identifying possible employment sites.

Play/Leisure
- Provide program or module on leisure and recreation.

Rest/Sleep
- Provide program or module on sleep hygiene (see Gutman et al., 2019).

Social Participation
- Provide program or module on community participation.

Sensorimotor
- Provide program or module on exercises and physical fitness.

Cognitive/Perceptual
- Provide program or module on Wellness Recovery Action Plan construction (WRAP).
- Provide program or module on planning ahead, setting and achieving goals.

Psychosocial
- Provide program or module on anger management and conflict resolution (see Gutman et al., 2019).
- Provide program or module on relaxation techniques such as meditation, deep-breathing exercises, yoga.

Context/Environment
- Provide program or module on community living (see Gutman & Raphael-Greenfield, 2017).
- Provide program or module on being a good tenant and neighbor (see Gutman & Raphael-Greenfield, 2017).

Precautions/Safety Considerations

Person may be at risk for suicide behavior. Person may need medical management to adjust or change medications.

Prognosis and Outcome

There is no standard for prognosis or outcome because individual situations vary widely. Ideally, person should be placed in permanent housing but such arrangements are not always possible due to individual choice or available housing limitations.

REFERENCES

Boland, L., & Cunningham, M. (2019). Homelessness: Critical reflections and observations from an occupational perspective. *Journal of Occupational Science, 26*(2), 308–315. https://doi.org/10.1080/14427591.2018.1512006

Bradley, D. M., Hersch, G., Reistetter, T., & Reed, K. (2011). Occupational participation of homeless people. *Occupational Therapy in Mental Health, 27*(1), 26–35. https://doi.org/10.1080/0164212X.2010.518311

Chan, D. V., Gopal, S., & Helfrich, C. A. (2014). Accessibility patterns and community integration among previously homeless adults: A Geographic Information Systems (GIS) approach. *Social Science & Medicine, 120*, 142–152. https://doi.org/10.1016/j.socscimed.2014.09.005

Chan, D. V., Helfrich, C. A., Hursh, N. C., Rogers, E. S., & Gopal, S. (2014). Measuring community integration using Geographic Information Systems (GIS) and participatory mapping for people who were once homeless. *Health & Place, 27*, 92–101. https://doi.org/10.1016/j.healthplace.2013.12.011

Chang, F. H., Helfrich, C. A., & Coster, W. J. (2013). Psychometric properties of the Practical Skills Test (PST). *American Journal of Occupational Therapy, 67*(2), 246–253. https://doi.org/10.5014/ajot.2013.006627

Fieldhouse, J., Parmenter, V., Peregrine, D., & Barham, R. (2011). *Evaluation of an occupational therapy intervention service within homeless services in Bristol.* University of the West of England.

Faulkner, T. (2016). From street life to lodging: Reflections on time's occupational journey. *Occupational Therapy Now, 18*(3), 25–26.

Gutman, S. A., Barnett, S., Fischman, L., Halpern, J., Hester, G., Kerrisk, C., McLaughlin, T., Ozel, E., & Wang, H. (2019). Pilot effectiveness of a stress management program for sheltered homeless adults with mental illness: A two-group controlled study. *Occupational Therapy in Mental Health, 73*(4, Suppl. 1), Article 7311520431. https://doi.org/10.5014/ajot.2019.73S1-PO5034

Gutman, S. A., Douglas, D., Carmiencke, A., Freudman, L., Huerta, M., McCaa, M., Miller, S., Sherpa, A., Viant, M., & Schreibman, D. (2018). Assessing environmental safety modifications in the chronically ill sheltered homeless population: A pilot study. *Annals of International Occupational Therapy, 1*(2), 95–102. https://doi.org/10.3928/24761222-20180620-04

Gutman, S. A., & Raphael-Greenfield, E. I. (2017). Effectiveness of a supportive housing program for homeless adults with mental illness and substance use: A two-group controlled trial. *British Journal of Occupational Therapy, 80*(5), 286–293. https://doi.org/10.1177/0308022616680368

Gutman, S. A., Raphael-Greenfield, E. I., Berg, J., Agnese, A., Gross, S., Ashmi, S., Ogunye, O., Shin, C., & Weiss, D. (2018). Feasibility and satisfaction of an apartment living program for homeless adults with mental illness and substance use disorder. *Psychiatry, 81*(3), 228–239. https://doi.org/10.1080/00332747.2018.1502555

Gutman, S. A., Raphael-Greenfield, E. I., & Simon, P. M. (2016). Feasibility and acceptability of a pilot housing transition program for homeless adults with mental illness and substance use. *Occupational Therapy in Health Care, 30*(2), 124–138. https://doi.org/10.3109/07380577.2015.1060660

Helfrich, C. (2014). *Life skills manual: Strategies for maintaining residential stability.* National Rehabilitation Information Center. https://naric.com/?q=en/content/order-life-skills-manual

Helfrich, C. A., Chan, D. V., Simpson, E. K., & Sabol, P. (2012). Readiness-to-change cluster profiles among adults with mental illness who were homeless participating in a life skills intervention. *Community Mental Health Journal, 48*(6), 673–681. https://doi.org/10.1007/s10597-011-9383-z

Helfrich, C. A., & Synovec. (2019). Homeless and women's shelters. In C. Brown, V. C. Stoffel, & J. P. Muñoz (Eds.), *Occupational therapy in mental health* (2nd ed., pp. 672–690). Davis.

Lloyd, C., & Bassett, H. (2010). The role of an Australian Homeless Health Outreach Team: Background, Part 1. *International Journal of Therapy and Rehabilitation, 17*(7), 376–384.

Lloyd, C., & Bassett, H. (2012). The role of occupational therapy in working with the homeless population: An assertive outreach approach. *New Zealand Journal of Occupational Therapy, 59*(1), 18–23.

Lloyd, C., Bassett, H., & King, R. (2010). The Queensland Homeless Health Outreach teams: Do they use the Assertive Community Treatment model? *Advances in Mental Health, 9*(2), 130–137. https://doi.org/10.5172/jamh.9.2.130

Marval, R., & Townsend, E. (2013). Homelessness: Enabling solutions in primary health-care occupational therapy. *Occupational Therapy Now, 15*(5), 17–19.

McKinney-Vento Homeless Assistance Act of 1987, 42 U.S.C. ch. 119 § 11301 et seq.

Schultz-Krohn, W., & Tyminski, Q. (2018). *Community-built occupational therapy services or those who are homeless.* American Occupational Therapy Association.

Slatter, J., Lloyd, C., & King, R. (2012). Homelessness and companion animals: More than just a pet? *British Journal of Occupational Therapy, 75*(8), 377–383. https://doi.org/10.4276/030 802212X13433105374350

BIBLIOGRAPHY

Andersen, J., Kot, N., Ennis, N., Colantonio, A., Ouchterlony, D., Cusimano, M. D., & Topolovec-Vranic, J. (2014). Traumatic brain injury and cognitive impairment in men who are homeless. *Disability and Rehabilitation, 36*(26), 2210–2215. https://doi.org/10.3109/09638288.20 14.895870

Chang, F. H., Helfrich, C. A., Coster, W. J., & Rogers, E. S. (2015). Factors associated with community participation among individuals who have experienced homelessness. *International Journal of Environmental Research and Public Health, 12*(9), 11364–11378. https://doi.org/ 10.3390/ijerph120911364

Cunningham, M. J., & Slade, A. (2019). Exploring the lived experience of homelessness from an occupational perspective. *Scandinavian Journal of Occupational Therapy, 26*(1), 19–32. https:// doi.org/10.1080/11038128.2017.1304572.

Gutman, S. A., Amarantos, K., Berg, J., Aponte, M., Gordillo, D., Rice, C., Smith, J., Perry, A., Wills, T., Chen, E., Peters, R., & Schluger, Z. (2018). Home safety fall and accident risk among prematurely aging, formerly homeless adults. *American Journal of Occupational Therapy, 72*(4), Article 7204195030. https://doi.org/10.5014/ajot.2018.028050

Helfrich, C. A., & Chan, D. V. (2013). Changes in self-identified priorities, competencies, and values of recently homeless adults with psychiatric disabilities. *American Journal of Psychiatric Rehabilitation, 16*(1), 22–49. https://doi.org/10.1080/15487768.2013.762298

Helfrich, C. A., Chan, D. V., & Sabol, P. (2011). Cognitive predictors of life skill intervention outcomes for adults with mental illness at risk for homelessness. *American Journal of Occupational Therapy, 65*(3), 277–286. https://doi.org/10.5014/ajot.2011.001321

Helfrich, C. A., Peters, C. Y., & Chan, D. V. (2011). Trauma symptoms of individuals with mental illness at risk for homelessness participating in a life skills intervention. *Occupational Therapy International, 18*(3), 115–123. https://doi.org/10.1002/oti.308

Helfrich, C. A., Simpson, E. K., & Chan, D. V. (2014). Change patterns of homeless individuals with mental illness: A multiple case study. *Community Mental Health Journal, 50*(5), 531–537. https://doi.org/10.1007/s10597-013-9647-x

Illman, S. C., Spence, S., O'Campo, P. J., & Kirsh, B. H. (2013). Exploring the occupations of homeless adults living with mental illnesses in Toronto. *Canadian Journal of Occupational Therapy, 80*(4), 215–223. https://doi.org/10.1177/0008417413506555

Lloyd, C., Hilder, J., & Williams, P. L. (2017). Emergency department presentations of people who are homeless: The role of occupational therapy. *British Journal of Occupational Therapy, 80*(9), 533–538. https://doi.org/10.1177/0308022617706679

Lloyd, C., King, R. Hilder, J., & Bassett, H. (2012). A profile of homeless people seen in the Gold Coast Hospital Emergency Department. *Australasian Psychiatry, 20*(3), 255–256. https://doi .org/10.1177/1039856212447664

Marshall, C. A., Davidson, L., Li, A., Gewurtz, R., Roy, L., Barbic, S., Kirsh, B., & Lysaght, R. (2019). Boredom and meaningful activity in adults experiencing homelessness: A mixed-methods study. *Canadian Journal of Occupational Therapy, 86*(5), 357–370. https://doi.org/10.1177/0008417419833402

Marshall, C. A., Lysaght, R., & Krupa, T. (2017). The experience of occupational engagement of chronically homeless persons in a mid-sized urban context. *Journal of Occupational Science, 24*(2), 165–180. https://doi.org/10.1080/14427591.2016.1277548

Marshall, C. A., Lysaght, R., & Krupa, T. (2018). Occupational transition in the process of becoming housed following chronic homelessness. *Canadian Journal of Occupational Therapy, 85*(1), 33–45. https://doi.org/10.1177/0008417417723351

Marshall, C. A., & Rosenberg, M. W. (2014). Occupation and the process of transition from homelessness. *Canadian Journal of Occupational Therapy, 81*(5), 330–338. https://doi.org/10.1177/0008417414548573

Murtagh, L., Lloyd, C., & Bassett, H. (2010). The role of an Australian Homeless Health Outreach Team: Part 2: A case study. *International Journal of Therapy and Rehabilitation, 17*(8), 436–443.

Parmenter, V., Fieldhouse, J., & Barham, R. (2013). An occupational therapy intervention service to hostels for homeless people: An overview. *British Journal of Occupational Therapy, 76*(5), 242–245. https://doi.org/10.4276/030802213X13679275042807

Raphael-Greenfield, E. (2012). Assessing executive and community functioning among homeless persons with substance use disorders using the Executive Function Performance Test. *Occupational Therapy International, 19*(3), 135–143. https://doi.org/10.1002/oti.1328

Raphael-Greenfield, E. J., & Gutman, S. A. (2015). Understanding the lived experience of formerly homeless adults as they transition to supportive housing. *Occupational Therapy in Mental Health, 31*(1), 35–49. https://doi.org/10.1080/0164212X.2014.1001011

Roy, L., Vallée, C., Kirsh, B. H., Marshall, C. A., Marval, R., & Low, A. (2017). Occupation-based practices and homelessness: A scoping review. *Canadian Journal of Occupational Therapy, 84*(2), 98–110. https://doi.org/10.1080/0164212X.2017.1344901

Rybski, D., & Israel, H. (2017). Impact of social determinants on parent sense of competency in mothers who are homeless or poor housed. *Occupational Therapy in Mental Health, 33*(4), 342–359. https://doi.org/10.1080/0164212X2017.1344901

Rybski, D., & Israel, H. (2019). Social skills and sensory processing in preschool children who are homeless or poor housed. *Journal of Occupational Therapy, Schools & Early Intervention, 12*(2), 170–181. https://doi.org/10.1080/19411243.2018.1523768

Salsi, S., Awadallah, Y., Leclair, A. B., Breault, M.-L., Duong, D.-T., & Roy, L. (2017). Occupational needs and priorities of women experiencing homelessness. *Canadian Journal of Occupational Therapy, 84*(4-5), 229–241. https://doi.org/10.1177/0008417417719725

Silva, C. R., Silvestrini, M. S., Von Poellnitz, J. C., Prado, A. C. D. S. A., & Junior, J. D. L. (2018). Creative strategies and homeless people: Occupational therapy, art, culture and sensitive displacement. *Cadernos Brasileiros Terapia Ocupacional São Carlos, 26*(2), 489–500. https://doi.org/10.4322/2526-8910.cto1128

Simpson, E. K., Conniff, B. G., Faber, B., & Semmelhack, E. F. (2018). Daily occupations routines, and social participation of homeless young people. *Occupational Therapy in Mental Health, 34*(3), 203–227. https://doi.org/10.1080/0164212X.2017.1421491

Thomas, Y., Gray, M., & McGinty, S. (2010). Homelessness and the right to occupation and inclusion: An Australian perspective. *WFOT Bulletin, 62*(1), 19–25. https://doi.org/10.1179/otb.2010.62.1.005

Thomas, Y., Gray, M., & McGinty, S. (2011). A systematic review of occupational therapy interventions with homeless people. *Occupational Therapy in Health Care, 25*(1), 38–53. https://doi.org/10.3109/07380577.2010.528554

Thomas, Y., Gray, M., & McGinty, S. (2012). An exploration of subjective wellbeing among people experiencing homelessness: A strengths-based approach. *Social Work in Health Care, 51*(9), 780–797. https://doi.org/10.1080/00981389.2012.686475

Thomas, Y., Gray, M., & McGinty, S. (2017). The occupational well-being of people experiencing homelessness. *Journal of Occupational Science, 24*(2), 181–192. https://doi.org/10.1080/14427591.2017.13018288

Thomas, Y., Gray, M., McGinty, S., & Ebringer, S. (2011). Homeless adults engagement in art: First steps towards identity, recovery and social inclusion. *Australian Occupational Therapy Journal, 58*(6), 429–436. https://doi.org/10.1111/j.1440-1630.2011.00977.x

Topolovec-Vranic, J., Ennis, N. Colantonio, A., Cusimano, M. D., Hwang, S. W., Kontos, P., Ouchterlony, D., & Stergiopoulos, V. (2012). Traumatic brain injury among people who are homeless: A systematic review. *BMC Public Health, 12*, Article 1059. https://doi.org/10.1186/1471-2458-12-1059

Topolovec-Vranic, J., Ennis, N., Howatt, M., Ouchterlony, D., Michalak, A., Masanic, C., Colantonio, A., Hwang, S. W., Kontos, P., Stergiopoulos, V., & Cusimano, M. D. (2014). Traumatic brain injury among men in an urban homeless shelter: Observational study of rates and mechanisms of injury. *CMAJ Open, 2*(2), e69–e76. https://doi.org/10.9778/cmajo.20130046

Tsang, A., Davis, J. A., & Polatajko, H. J. (2013). On the edge of the possible: Considering homelessness. *Canadian Journal of Occupational Therapy, 80*(4), 200–204. https://doi.org/10.1177/0008417413505422

Van Oss, T., Condoluci, S., & Annino, R. (2018). Homelessness and the role of occupational therapy. *SIS Quarterly Practice Connections, 3*(2), 11–13.

LGBTQ Population

Description

Lesbian, Gay, Bisexual, Transgender and Queer population. Gender dysphoria is included in this chapter.

Cause

Biologic factors such as genetic complement or prenatal hormonal milieu largely determine gender identity. However, gender identity and gender role are also influenced by social factors, such as the character of the parents' emotional bond, and the relationship each parent has with the child (Porter, 2018).

Terminology

- *Bisexual:* Sexual attraction to or sexual behavior with both men and women (VandenBos, 2015).
- *Cissexism:* Ideology based on the belief that biological characteristics related to sex correspond to psychosocial characteristics related to gender (Silva et al., 2015).
- *"Coming out":* Revealing that one is LGBTQ to family, friends, coworkers, employers, or others (VandenBos, 2015).
- *"Doing gender":* The creation and re-creation of one's own gender by acing as an individual, guided by social norms and expectations (Schneider et al., 2019).
- *FTM:* Female-to-male transsexualism (Porter, 2018).
- *Gay:* Denoting individuals, especially males, who are sexually attracted to and aroused by members of their own sex (VandenBos, 2015).
- *Gender dysphoria:* Characterized by strong, persistent cross-gender identification; person feels imprisoned in a body incompatible with the subjective gender identity (Porter 2018).
- *Gender expression:* A person's appearance and behavior according to social expectation of a given gender depending on the culture in which the person lives (Silva et al., 2015).
- *Gender identity:* Subjective sense of knowing to which gender one belongs; in other words, whether the person regards him- or herself as male, female, bisexual, transgender or other term (Porter, 2018). The gender with which the person identifies, which may or may not correspond to the gender assigned at birth (Silva et al., 2015).

- *Gender role:* The objective, public expression of gender identity and includes everything a person says and does to indicate to the individual and to others the degree to which the person is the gender to which the individual identifies (Porter, 2018).
- *Homophobia:* Fear, prejudice, anger, and hatred of gay men and lesbians (VandenBos, 2015).
- *Homosexual, Homosexuality:* Sexual attraction or activity between members of the same sex. Most often applied to men. The term *lesbian* is more applied to women (VandenBos, 2015).
- *Lesbian:* Female–female sexual orientation or behavior (VandenBos, 2015).
- *MTF:* Male-to-female transsexualism (Porter, 2018).
- *Queer:* Refers to gays and lesbians or related to same-sex sexual orientation (VandenBos, 2015). Queer theory considers that masculine and feminine are present in both men and women, so that each person has characteristics that can qualify as masculine or feminine apart from biological sex (Silva et al., 2015).
- *Sexual identity:* The sex to which a person is sexually attracted (Porter, 2018); the sense of one-self as man or woman (Silva et al., 2015).
- *Sexual orientation:* The affective-sexual attraction for someone, an internal state regarding sexuality (heterosexual, homosexual, or bisexual; Silva et al., 2015).
- *Transition:* Process of transforming from one gender to another typically including cross-dressing, a change of legal identification, psychological and medical counseling, and surgical and medical intervention to change physical sex characteristics (Avrech Bar et al., 2016).
- *Transgender:* Relating to gender identified that differs from culturally determined gender roles and biological sex (VandenBos, 2015). An individual whose gender identity is not congruent with the sex assigned to the person at birth (Schneider et al., 2019).
- *Transphobia:* Negative attitudes or feelings toward people who are transsexual or transgender.
- *Transsexuality or Transsexualism:* A gender identity disorder consisting of a persistent sense of discomfort relating to one's anatomical sex with a persistent wish to be rid of one's genitals and to live as a member of the other sex (VandenBos, 2015).

Evaluation/Assessment

Areas

- Activities of Daily Living/Instrumental ADL: dressing (as male, female, neutral), grooming (skin care, makeup), meal preparation, doing laundry, shopping for clothing, sexual practices
- Education/Work: gendered related job skills (masculine, feminine), gender disclosure at school or work (coming out, stay in the closet)
- Play/Leisure: interests, types, frequency, location
- Rest/Sleep: no information identified
- Social Participation: type, frequency, location, with whom
- Sensorimotor: no information identified
- Cognitive/Perceptual: no information identified
- Psychosocial: anxiety, self-identity, self-acceptance, suicide behavior, social isolation, role performance, family relations, peer relations, quality of life
- Context/Environment: cultural norms and expectations, social attitudes, social discrimination, social prejudice, social sigma, physical safety, community and internet resources
- Development (Infant, Child, Adolescent only): play skills, social development
- Comorbidities: substance use disorders, depression

Instruments

Instruments Developed by Occupational Therapy Personnel

- Occupational Performance History Interview (Version 2.1; OPHI-II; Kielhofner et al., 2004)

Instruments Developed by Other Professionals and Used by Occupational Therapy Personnel

- Satisfaction with Life Scale (SWLS; Diener et al., 1985)
- Short Form 36 Health Survey (SF-36; Ware et al., 1993)

Problems/Issues

Activities of Daily Living/Instrumental ADL
- Adolescent may have left home (run away) or have been kicked out of the family home and be homeless (living on the street).
- Person may lack finances for basic living: food, clothing, shelter, transportation.
- Person may have experienced discrimination in housing if landlord knows or learns that the person is or may be LGBTQ. Although such discrimination is not legal, the person may not have the resources to challenge the action.

Education/Work
- Child may be harassed, bullied, teased, threatened, insulted, rejected, humiliated, or experience other negative behavior at school if LGBTQ status is known or suspected.
- Child may have difficulty making or keeping friends if LGBTQ status is known or suspected.
- Child may encounter rules at school that discriminate, such as being required to use the bathroom and wear clothing based on the assigned sex on the birth certificate.
- Adolescent may have dropped out of school before graduating to avoid real or perceived discrimination and other negative behaviors.
- Person may lack job training and job skills due to lack of education and/or work opportunities.
- Person may be denied employment or be let go if status as LGBTQ is known to employer.
- Person may be limited to low paying jobs or prostitution because of LGBTQ status.

Play/Leisure
- Child may prefer to play with toys considered more appropriate for a child of the other sex such as a boy who prefers dress up dolls or a girl who prefers racing toy cars and trucks.
- Child may prefer to assume role in games more appropriate for child of the other sex such as boy preferring to assume the role of mother or female in pretend games.
- Child may prefer to play with peers who are of the preferred sex as oppose to playing with those of birth assigned sex.

Rest/Sleep
- Not discussed.

Social Participation
- Child/adolescent/person may be excluded from social activities or events because of sexual orientation.

Sensorimotor
- No specific issues related to LGBTQ status but problems may exist in any given individual.

Cognitive/Perceptual
- Person with comorbid substance disorder may experience cognitive impairment related to the drug or drugs used.

Psychosocial
- Child may insist that "he" is actually a girl or the "she" is actually a boy.
- Child may complain about anatomy and genitals that are of the "wrong" sex according to the child's preference and a desire for the "right" anatomy and genitals.
- Child often has experienced rejection and exclusion from parents and other family members when the child started to change appearance or refused to play with toys or games considered sex appropriate and expressed a desire to change sex.
- Person may have lost contact with family and friends because family cannot accept LGBTQ status.
- Person may be anxious about immediate and future needs.
- Person may lack a positive sense of self-identity.
- Person may lack self-confidence and self-efficacy.
- Person may experience poor quality of life.

Context/Environment

- Person may not feel safe in the community due to potential physical abuse, aggression, violence, and stigmatization.
- Person may not know about or have access to community social support services.
- Person may need an advocate to obtain access to services.

Intervention/Treatment

Models and programs developed by occupational therapy personnel: None. Models and programs developed by other professionals but used by occupational therapy personnel: None. The literature is primarily interviews and suggestions for programs but not programs actually implemented. Team members include physicians, psychiatrists, nursing personnel, social workers, psychologists, vocational rehabilitation counselors, physical therapists, and occupational therapy personnel. Goals: Clients who describe themselves as lesbian, gay, bisexual, or queer are not usually referred to occupational therapy for their sexual orientation but for a coexisting condition such as substance abuse. The LGBTQ status should be considered in the selection of the intervention program. Clients who identify themselves as transgender may receive direct services to facilitate the transformation from MTF or FTM to promote occupational identity and competence (Avrech Bar et al., 2016).

Activities of Daily Living/Instrumental ADL

- FTM: Assist client to learn basic ADLs performed by men: shaving or trimming a beard, haircut or style, selecting and buying men's clothing and shoes (size and fit, worn on which occasions), selecting a wallet and men's hat, washing and caring for men's clothing.
- MTF: Assist client to learn basic ADLs performed by women: selecting and putting on makeup, hair styling and washing, use of deodorant and perfume, selecting and buying women's clothing and shoes (size and fit, worn on which occasions), selecting accessories (purse, jewelry, women's hat), washing and caring for women's clothing.

Education/Work

- MTF or FTM: Assist client to improve or increase level of education and training.
- MTF: Assist client to evaluate whether the same job may be possible to continue or if a different job will be required or preferred. Example: Client was an accountant before MTF so can continue in same profession. Client was construction worker typically considered men's work. Client may need to change jobs such as working in a construction office rather than on construction sites directly.
- FTM: Assist client to evaluate whether the same job may be possible to continue or if a different job will be required or preferred. Example: Client was a hairdresser before FTM so can continue in same profession. Client was a clerk in a woman's clothing store. Client may need to change jobs such as learning to sell men's clothing.
- Consider if referral to a vocational rehabilitation counselor or work hardening program may be useful to the client.

Play/Leisure

- Assist MTF or FTM to determine if current leisure occupations are acceptable to new lifestyle.
- Assist MTF or FTM to explore and develop new leisure occupations that may be more compatible with new sexual orientation.

Rest/Sleep

- Not discussed.

Social Participation

- Assist MTF or FTM to determine if current social activities are acceptable to new lifestyle and whether current friends and colleagues are accepting of change of sexual orientation.
- Assist MTF or FTM to explore and develop new social activities that are compatible with change of sexual orientation.

Sensorimotor

- Assist MTF or FTM to determine if current physical fitness program is acceptable to new lifestyle. Example: Jogging or running in the community park can continue without modification. Workout at the local fitness center will require shifting from the men's changing room to the women's or vice versa and may require changing which equipment is used such as weight lifting equipment.

Cognitive/Perceptual

- Assist MTF or FTM with problem-solving strategies to explore options.
- Assist MTF or FTM with planning ahead to anticipate changes that may be required in housing, employment, physical safety, and lifestyle.

Psychosocial

- Assist MTF or FTM to develop stress and coping strategies: deep breathing, relaxation, yoga, mindfulness, tai chi.
- Assist MTF or FTM to identify occupations that can increase sense of self-identity and self-efficacy.
- Assist MTF or FTM to engage or participate in occupations that improve self-confidence and sense of self-worth.

Context/Environment

- Assist client to identify and participate in a local transgender support group.
- Assist client to identify and use community and internet resources.
- Advocate for improved health care and social services for all LGBTQ individuals.

Precautions/Safety Considerations

All LGBTQ individuals are at risk for violence (physical and verbal; domestic or in the community).

Prognosis and Outcome

According to Porter (2018), FTM reassignment surgeries are generally more successful than MTF. Socially, MTF transgender individuals are more at risk for violence.

REFERENCES

Avrech Bar, M., Jarus, T., Wada, M., Rechtman, L., & Noy, E. (2016). Male-to-female transition: Implications for occupational performance, health, and life satisfaction. *Canadian Journal of Occupational Therapy, 83*(2), 72–82. https://doi.org/10.1177/0008417416635346

Porter, R. S. (Ed.). (2018). *The Merck manual of diagnosis and therapy* (20th ed.). Merck Sharp & Dohme.

Schneider, J., Page, J., & van Nes, F. (2019). "Now I feel much better than in my previous life": Narratives of occupational transitions in young transgender adults. *Journal of Occupational Science, 26*(2), 219–232. https://doi.org/10.1080/14427591.2018.1550726

Silva, R. G. L. B., Bezerra, W. C., & Queiroz, S. B. (2015). The impacts of transgender identities in sociability of travesties and transsexual women. *Revista de Terapia Ocupacional da Universidade de São Paulo, 26*(3), 364–372. https://doi.org/10.11606/issn.2238-6149.v26i3p364-372

VandenBos, G. (Ed.). (2015). *APA dictionary of psychology* (2nd ed.). American Psychological Association.

BIBLIOGRAPHY

Baker, K., & Beagan, B. (2014). Making assumptions, making space: An anthropological critique of cultural competency and its relevance to queer patients. *Medical Anthropology Quarterly, 28*(4), 578–598. https://doi.org/10.1111/maq.12129

Beagan, B., Chiasson, A., Fiske, C. A., Forseth, S. D., Hosein, A. C., Myers, M. R., & Stang, J. E. (2013). Working with transgender clients: Learning from physicians and nurses to improve occupational therapy practice. *Canadian Journal of Occupational Therapy, 80*(2), 82–91. https://doi.org/10.1177/0008417413484450

Beagan, B. L., De Souza, L., Godbout, C., Hamilton, L., MacLeod, J., Paynter, E., & Tobin, A. (2012). "This is the biggest thing you'll ever do in your life": Exploring the occupations of transgendered people. *Journal of Occupational Science, 19*(3), 226–240. https://doi.org/10.1080/14427591.2012.659169

Beagan, B., Fredericks, E., & Bryson, M. (2015). Family physician perceptions of working with LGBTQ patients: Physician training needs. *Canadian Medical Education Journal, 6*(1), e14–e22. https://doi.org/10.36834/cmej.36647

Beagan, B. L., Fredericks, E., & Goldberg, L. (2012). Nurses' work with LGBTQ patients: "They're just like everybody else, so what's the difference"? *Canadian Journal of Nursing Research, 44*(3), 44–63.

Falzarano, M., & Pizzi, M. (2015). Experiences of lesbian and gay occupational therapists in the healthcare system. *Journal of Allied Health, 44*(2), 65–72.

Harbin, A., Beagan, B., & Goldberg, L. (2012). Discomfort, judgment, and health care for queers. *Journal of Bioethical Inquiry, 9*(2), 149–160. https://doi.org/10.1007/s11673-012-9367-x

Hattie, B., & Beagan, B. (2013). Reconfiguring spirituality and sexual/gender identify: "It's a feeling of connection to something bigger, It's part of a wholeness." *Journal of Religion & Spirituality in Social Work, 32*(3), 244–268. https://doi.org/10.1080/15426432.2013.801733

Jenkins, C. L., Edmundson, A., Averett, P., & Yoon, I. (2014). Older lesbians and bereavement: Experiencing the loss of a partner. *Journal of Gerontological Social Work, 57*(2-4), 273–287. https://doi.org/10.1080/01634372.2013.850583

Kottorp, A., Johansson, K., Aase, P., & Rosenberg, L. (2016). Housing for ageing LGBTQ people in Sweden: A descriptive study of needs, preferences, and concerns. *Scandinavian Journal of Occupational Therapy, 23*(5), 337–346. https://doi.org/10.3109/11038128.2015.1115547

Kwong, J., Bockting, W., Gabler, S., Abbruzzese, L. D., Simon, P., Fialko, J., III., Bonaparte, S., Malark, A., Towe, M., Weber, T., & Hall, P. (2017). Development of an interprofessional collaborative practice model for older LGBT adults (Letter to the Editor). *LGBT Health, 4*(6), 442–444. https://doi.org/10.1089/lgbt.2016.0160

Leite, J. D., Jr., & Lopes, R. E. (2017). Transvestility, transsexuality and demands for occupational therapists training. *Cadernos Brasileiros Terapia Ocupacional São Carlos, 25*(3), 481–495. http://dx.doi.org/10.4322/2526-8910.ctoAO1060

McCave, E. L., Aptaker, D., Hartmann, K. D., & Zucconi, R. (2019). Promoting affirmative transgender health care practice within hospitals: An IPE standardized patient simulation for graduate health care learners. *MedEdPORTAL, 15*, Article 10861. https://doi.org/10.15766/mep_2374-8265.10861

Meach, L. (2017). The occupational experiences of lesbian, gay, bisexual and transgender (LGBT) individuals during the coming out process: An analysis of self-acceptance, disclosure, and occupational change. *OCCUPATION, 2*(1), Article 2.

O'Toole, M. T. (Ed.). (2017). *Mosby's dictionary of medicine, nursing & health professions* (10th ed.). Elsevier.

Phoenix, N., & Ghul, R. (2016). Gender transition in the workplace: An occupational therapy perspective. *Work, 55*(1), 197–205. https://doi.org/10.3233/WOR-162386

Rosenberg, L., Kottorp, A., & Johansson, K. (2018). LGBQ-specific elderly housing as a "sparkling sanctuary": Boundary work on LGBQ identity and community in relationship to potential LGBQ-specific elderly housing in Sweden. *Journal of Homosexuality, 65*(11), 1484–1506. https://doi.org/10.1080/00918369.2017.1377487

Simpson, E. K., & Helfrich, C. A. (2014). Oppression and barriers to service for black, lesbian survivors of intimate partner violence. *Journal of Gay & Lesbian Social Services, 26*(4), 441–465. https://doi.org/10.1080/10538720.2014.951816

Twinley, R. (2014). Sexual orientation and occupation: Some issues to consider when working with older gay people to meet their occupational needs. *British Journal of Occupational Therapy*, 77(12), 623–625. https://doi.org/10.4276/030802214X14176260335381

Twinley, R., & Price, L. (2017). Appreciating the lived experience of some older gay people: Considerations for contemporary occupational therapy practice. In D. Sakellariou & N. Pollard (Eds.), *Occupational therapies without borders* (2nd ed., pp. 109–117). Elsevier.

Obesity and Overweight Conditions

Description

Obesity and overweight are determined by body mass index—that is, by measuring overall weight and height. Obesity is defined as having a body mass index (BMI) of 30 kg/m2 or greater (O'Toole, 2017). Obesity is subdivided into types as follows: Class I (BMI 30–34.9), Class II (BMI 35–39.9), and Class III (BMI 40 or more). Overweight is determined by a BMI of 25 to 29.9 kg/m2 (O'Toole, 2017). Obesity in children, aged between 5–19 years, is defined as a BMI-for-age greater than 2 standard deviations above the WHO Growth Reference median. Overweight is defined as a BMI-for-age greater than 1 standard deviation above the WHO growth reference median (World Health Organization, 2021).

Cause

Causes of obesity are probably multifactorial and include genetic predisposition. Ultimately, obesity results from a long-standing imbalance between energy intake and energy expenditure, including energy utilization for basic metabolic processes and energy expenditure from physical activity. However, many other factors appear to increase a person's predisposition to obesity, including endocrine disruptors, sleep and wake cycles disturbances, and environmental factors (Porter, 2018).

Evaluation/Assessment

Areas

- Activities of Daily Living/Instrumental ADL: basic ADLs such as bathing, dressing and toileting, mobility, transfers, meal planning and preparation, shopping (buying clothes), driving, transportation, child care (parents and grandparents),
- Education/Work: job absenteeism, work history, workplace bias
- Play/Leisure: interests, values, types, location, frequency
- Rest/Sleep: sleep disturbances, sleep apnea
- Social Participation: type, location, frequency, with whom
- Sensorimotor: endurance and activity tolerance, reaching range of motion, movement flexibility, posture and postural control, skin integrity
- Cognitive/Perceptual: executive functions
- Psychosocial: stigmatization, discrimination, depression, quality of life, mood disorder
- Context/Environment: social support, adapted devices, equipment modification, occupational deprivation, accessibility (narrow chairs)
- Development (Infant, Child, Adolescent only): developmental milestones
- Comorbidities: cancer, cardiovascular disease, diabetes, eating disorders, hyperlipidemia, hypertension, musculoskeletal disorders, osteoarthritis, serious mental illness, side effects of medications, spinal cord injury, stroke, substance addition and abuse, psychosocial and societal problems including restricted access to health care

Instruments
Instruments Developed by Occupational Therapy Personnel
- Canadian Occupational Performance Measure (5th ed.; COPM-5; Law et al., 2014)
- Occupational Questionnaire (OQ; Smith et al., 1986)
- Pizzi Healthy Weight Management Assessment (PHWMA; Kuo et al., 2016, in References)

Instruments Developed by Other Professionals and Used by Occupational Therapy Personnel
- Attitudes Toward Obese Persons Scale (ATOP; Allison et al., 1991)
- Beck Anxiety Inventory (BAI; Beck & Steer, 1993)
- Beck Depression Inventory (2nd ed.; BDI-II; Beck et al., 1996)
- Eating Disorder Evaluation Questionnaire (EDE-Q; Fairburn & Beglin, 1994)
- Rosenberg Self-Esteem Scale (RSES; Rosenberg, 1965)

Problems/Issues
Activities of Daily Living/Instrumental ADL
- Person may have difficulty performing basic ADL tasks related to bathing, dressing, and toileting because of insufficient reach and flexibility to wash and dry buttocks, back, and feet.
- Person may have difficulty transferring safely in and out of a vehicle, or use public transportation due to insufficient space, lack of seat belt extenders, or weight restrictions on scooters and wheelchairs.
- Person may have difficulty planning and preparing nutritious and healthy meals including portion control.

Education/Work
- Person may have difficulty performing certain tasks at work.
- Person may have lost a job due to absenteeism.
- Person may have experienced discrimination in hiring due to being overweight.

Play/Leisure
- Person may have restricted ability or be unable to engage in favorite leisure occupations.

Rest/Sleep
- Person may experience sleep apnea.
- Person may experience sleep disturbance due to pain.
- Person may experience sleep disturbance due to decreased bed mobility.

Social Participation
- Person may restrict or avoid social participation due to stigma or feelings of discrimination.

Sensorimotor
- Person may have decreased endurance and activity tolerance.
- Person may be in danger of skin breakdown due to comorbid conditions.

Cognitive/Perceptual
- Person may have difficulty with memory functions and learning skills.
- Person may have difficulty with executive functions including planning ahead, making decisions, problem solving.

Psychosocial
- Person may experience stigmatization.
- Person may have reduced sense of self-efficacy.
- Person may be depressed.
- Person may experience decreased quality of life.

Context/Environment

- Person may have multiple cultural and environments factors which support obesity (eating fatty foods, peer pressure, cultural rituals).
- Person may need adapted devices and equipment.
- Person may need environmental access.
- Person may need equipment modification to ensure safety while seated or being transported.

Intervention/Treatment

Models and programs developed by occupational therapy personnel include bariatrics (Hamby, 2011); Canadian Model of Occupational Performance (Barclay & Forwell, 2018); case studies (Ardanowski & Pasch, 2010; Blanchard, 2017; Dahl-Popolizio et al., 2017); ecology of human performance (Kuczmarski et al., 2010); lifestyle change or modification (American Occupational Therapy Association, 2013, Dieterle, 2018); person, environment, occupation, and performance model (Forhan & Gill, 2013); and Wii Fit (Bacon et al., 2012). Models and programs developed by other professionals but used by occupational therapy personnel include community-based approach (Cantal, 2019), Godoy method (RAGodoy device; de Godoy et al., 2017), home-health intervention (Cantal, 2019; Pizzi & Orloff, 2015), independent living service (Gregory, 2014), interdisciplinary team-based approach (Cantal, 2019), multitiered approach (Bazyk & Winne, 2013), Nutrition and Exercise for Wellness and Recovery (NEW-R; Brown et al., 2015; Brown et al., 2014), pediatric weight management program (Kuo et al., 2013), prevention programs (Cantal, 2019; Lau et al., 2013), and primary care (Cantal, 2019). Team members include bariatric physicians, nursing personnel, dieticians, social workers, case managers, pharmacists, physical therapy personnel, and occupational therapy personnel. Goals include helping clients change lifestyles, engage in meaningful activities, and learn to manage body weight by focusing on health promotion, disease prevention, advocacy, remediation, adaptation, and maintenance approaches (Allen, 2015; Brewster et al., 2014). All approaches to occupational therapy are used: health promotion to prevent obesity or to promote weight loss, remediation and restoration of function despite obesity and related comorbidities, compensation and adaption to increase function and participation despite obesity and disability prevention (Dieterle, 2018).

Activities of Daily Living/Instrumental ADL

- Assist client and dietician to plan, secure, and prepare healthy, nutritious meals with portion control in mind.
- Assist client in developing a food tracking and eating routine diary (when, where, what, why, how much, with whom).
- Assist person to improve mobility and access to transportation.

Education/Work

- Provide job-site analysis and make recommendations for workplace modification that reduces range of motion needed to acquire needed items or eliminates certain motions and movements.
- Assist client to explore if other vocational interests and abilities may be useful in identifying new work site potentials such as working from home, using voice activation computer programs.

Play/Leisure

- Assist client to make modifications or adaptations that may permit client to continue to engage in favorite leisure occupations.
- Assist client to identify and explore new leisure interests and occupations that are within client's ability to function.

Rest/Sleep

- Review with client sleep patterns and positions included in bed mobility.

- Assist client to review bedding and bed clothes to determine if silk or satin sheets and pajamas might increase bed mobility.
- Review with client if environmental factors are reducing quality and quantity of sleep such as lighting, noise, or temperature regulation.

Social Participation
- Encourage client to participate in social activities including identifying and exploring new options for social participation.

Sensorimotor
- Assist client to develop and implement an exercise program to improve strength and functional movement for walking and stair climbing.
- Assist client to develop and use a pain management program (see Pain and Chronic Pain in Section 2: Sensory Disorders).

Cognitive/Perceptual
- Modify program based on cognitive level and abilities.
- Facilitate development and achievement of client-centered goals.
- Allow, but guide as needed, client to make informed decisions.

Psychosocial
- Facilitate development or redevelopment of self-esteem through success in meeting goals or completing projects.

Context/Environment
- Provide education about obesity and its management.
- Provide instruction and practice in lifestyle modification.
- Consider cultural differences regarding diet and weight (Ristovski-Slijepcevic et al., 2010).

Precautions/Safety Considerations

Environmental conditions (furniture, beds, transport equipment, and any modifications must be constructed or reinforced to account for weight of client).

Prognosis and Outcome

Obesity can become a chronic disease which requires ongoing intervention and management including lifestyle modification, pharmacotherapy, and sometimes surgery (Brewster et al., 2014; Canadian Association of Occupational Therapists, 2015).

REFERENCES
Adult
Allen, M. (2015). *Fact sheet: Occupational therapy's role in bariatric care.* American Occupational Therapy Association.

American Occupational Therapy Association. (2013). Obesity and occupational therapy. *American Journal of Occupational Therapy, 67*(6, Suppl.), S39–S46.

Ardanowski, C., & Pasch, P. (2011). Spinal cord injury and the bariatric patient: Overcoming treatment barriers through innovative solutions. *Rehab Management, 24*(6), 18–21.

Bacon, N., Farnworth, L., & Boyd, R. (2012). Use of the Wii Fit in forensic mental health: Exercise for people at risk of obesity. *British Journal of Occupational Therapy, 75*(2), 61–68. https://doi .org/10.4276/030802212X13286281650992

Barclay, K. S., & Forwell, S. J. (2018). Occupational performance issues of adults seeking bariatric surgery for obesity. *American Journal of Occupational Therapy, 72*(5), Article 7205195030. https://doi.org/10.5014/ajot.2018.025924

Blanchard, S. (2017). Obesity. In B. J. Atchison & D. P. Dirette (Eds.), *Conditions in occupational therapy* (5th ed., pp. 541–558). Wolters Kluwer.

Brewster, K. Z., Nowrouzi, B., & Davis, L. C. (2014). The role of occupational therapy in obesity management. *University of Toronto Medical Journal, 91*(1), 33–35.

Brown, C., Goetz, J., Hamera, E., & Gajewski, B. (2014). Treatment response to the RENEW weight loss intervention in schizophrenia: Impact of intervention setting. *Schizophrenia Research, 159*(2-3), 421–425. https://doi.org/10.1016/j.schres.2014.09.018

Brown, C., Read, H., Stanton, M., Zeeb, M., Jonikas, J. A., & Cook, J. A. (2015). A pilot study of the Nutrition and Exercise for Wellness and Recovery (NEW-R): A weight loss program for individuals with serious mental illnesses. *Psychiatric Rehabilitation Journal, 38*(4), 371–373. https://doi.org/10.1037/prj0000115

Canadian Association of Occupational Therapists. (2015). *CAOT Position statement: Obesity and healthy occupation.*

Dahl-Popolizio, S., Rogers, O., Muir, S., Carroll, J. K., & Manson, L. (2017). Interprofessional primary care: The value of occupational therapy. *Open Journal of Occupational Therapy, 5*(3), Article 11. https://doi.org/10.15453/2168-6408.1363

de Godoy, J. M. P., de Godoy, A. C. P., & de Fatima Guerreiro Godoy, M. (2017). Considering the hypothesis of the pathophysiology of cellulite in its treatment. *Dermatology Reports, 9*(2), Article 7352. https://doi.org/10.4081/dr.2017.7352

Dieterle, C. (2018). Managing obesity in adults: A role for occupational therapy. *OT Practice,* Article CEA1118, CE1–CE8.

Forhan, M., & Gill, S. (2013). Cross-border contributions to obesity research and interventions: A review of Canadian and American occupational therapy contributions. *Occupational Therapy in Health Care, 27*(2), 129–141. https://doi.org/10.3109/07380577.2013.785642

Gregory, S. (2014). Obesity: A permanent and substantial disability? *OT News, 22*(8), 27.

Hamby, J. R. (2011). Appendix G. Bariatrics: Implication for acute care practice. In H. Smith-Gabai & S. E. Holm (Eds.), *Occupational therapy in acute care* (pp. 625–638). AOTA Press.

O'Toole, M. T. (Ed.). (2017). *Mosby's dictionary of medicine, nursing & health professions* (10th ed.). Elsevier.

Porter, R. S. (Ed.). (2018). *The Merck manual of diagnosis and therapy* (20th ed.). Merck Sharp & Dohme.

Ristovski-Slijepcevic, S., Bell, K., Chapman, G. E., & Beagan, B. (2010). Being "thick" indicates you are eating, you are healthy and you have an attractive body shape: Perspectives on fatness and food choice amongst Black and White men and women in Canada. *Health Sociology Review, 19*(3), 317–329.

Child/Adolescent

Bazyk, S., & Winne, R. (2013). A multi-tiered approach to addressing the mental health issues surrounding obesity in children and youth. *Occupational Therapy in Health Care, 27*(2), 84–98. https://doi.org/ 10.3109/07380577.2013.785643

Cantal, A. (2019). Managing obesity in pediatrics: A role for occupational therapy. *OT Practice, 24*(1), CE1–CE7.

Kuczmarski, M., Reitz, S. M., & Pizzi, M. A. (2010). Weight management and obesity reduction. In M. E. Scaffa, S. M. Reitz, & M. A. Pizzi (Eds.), *Occupational therapy in the promotion of health and wellness* (pp. 253–279). F.A. Davis.

Kuo, F., Goebel, L. A., Satkamp, N., Beauchamp, R., Kurrasch, J. M. Smith, A. R., & Maguire, J. M. (2013). Service learning in a pediatric weight management program to address childhood obesity. *Occupational Therapy in Health Care, 27*(2), 142–162. https://doi.org/10.3109/073 80577.2013.780318

Kuo, F., Pizzi, M. A., Chang, W. P., Koning, S. J., & Fredrick, A. S. (2016). Exploratory study of the clinical utility of the Pizzi Healthy Weight Management Assessment (PHWMA) among Burmese high school students. *American Journal of Occupational Therapy, 70*(5), Article 7005180040. https://doi.org/10.5014/ajot.2016.021659

Lau, C., Stevens, D., & Jia, J. (2013). Effects of an occupation-based obesity prevention program for children at risk. *Occupational Therapy in Health Care, 27*(2), 163–175. https://doi.org/10.3109/07380577.2013.783725

Pizzi, M., & Orloff, S. (2015). Childhood obesity as an emerging area of practice for occupational therapists: A case report. *New Zealand Journal of Occupational Therapy, 62*(1), 29–38.

World Health Organization. (2021). *Obesity and overweight.* https://www.who.int/news-room/fact-sheets/detail/obesity-and-overweight

BIBLIOGRAPHY

Adult

American Occupational Therapy Association. (2013). Obesity and occupational therapy. *American Journal of Occupational Therapy, 67*, S39–S46. https://doi.org/10.5014/ajot.2013.67S39

Blanchard, S., & Mosley, L. J. (2010). Geriatric obesity. *Gerontology Special Interest Section Quarterly, 3*(2), 1–4.

Bonsaksen, T., Fagermoen, M. S., & Lerdal, A. (2015). Factors associated with self-esteem in persons with morbid obesity and in persons with chronic obstructive pulmonary disease: A cross-sectional study. *Psychology, Health & Medicine, 20*(4), 431–442. https://doi.org/10.1080/13548506.2014.959529

Brown, C., Geiszler, L. C., Lewis, K. J., & Arbesman, M. (2018). Effectiveness of interventions for weight loss for people with serious mental illness: A systematic review and meta-analysis. *American Journal of Occupational Therapy, 72*(5), Article 7205190030. https://doi.org/10.5014/ajot.2018.033415

Conn, A., Bourke, N., James, C., & Haracz, K. (2019). Occupational therapy intervention addressing weight gain and obesity in people with severe mental illness: A scoping review. *Australian Occupational Therapy Journal, 66*(4), 446–457. https://doi.org/10.1111/1440-1630.12575

Cook, J. A., Razzano, L., Jonikas, J. A., Swarbrick, M. A., Steigman, P. J., Hamilton, M. M., Carter, T. M., & Santos, A. B. (2016). Correlates of co-occurring diabetes and obesity among community mental health program members with serious mental illnesses. *Psychiatric Services, 67*(11), 1269–1271. https://doi.org/10.1176/appi.ps.201500219

Forhan, M. (2014). Weight loss interventions for rehabilitation patients with obesity. *Current Obesity Reports 3*(3), 330–335. https://doi.org/10.1007/s13679-014-0113-z

Forhan, M., Bhambhani, Y., Dyer, D., Ramos-Salas, X., Ferguson-Pell, M., & Sharma, A. (2010). Rehabilitation in bariatrics: Opportunities for practice and research. *Disability and Rehabilitation, 32*(11), 952–959. https://doi.org/10.3109/09638280903483885

Forhan, M., & Gill, S. V. (2013). Obesity, functional mobility and quality of life. *Best Practice & Research. Clinical Endocrinology & Metabolism, 27*(2), 129–137. https://doi.org/10.1016/j.beem.2013.01.003

Forhan, M., Law, M., Taylor, V. H., & Vrkljan, B. H. (2012). Factors associated with the satisfaction of participation in daily activities for adults with Class III obesity. *OTJR: Occupation, Participation and Health, 32*(3), 70–78. https://doi.org/10.3928/15394492-20111028-01

Forhan, M., Law, M., Vrkljan, B. H., & Taylor, V. H. (2010a). The experience of participation in everyday occupations for adults with obesity. *Canadian Journal of Occupational Therapy, 77*(4), 210–218. https://doi.org/10.2182/cjot.2010.77.4.3

Forhan, M., Law, M., Vrkljan, B. H., & Taylor, V. H. (2011). Participation profile of adults with class III obesity. *OTJR: Occupation, Participation and Health, 31*(3), 135–142. https://doi.org/10.3928/15394492-20101025-02

Forhan, M., Risdon, C., & Solomon, P. (2013). Contributors to patient engagement in primary health care: Perceptions of patients with obesity. *Primary Health Care Research and Development, 14*(4), 367–372. https://doi.org/10.1017/S1463423612000643

Forhan, M., & Salas, X. R. (2013). Inequities in healthcare: A review of bias and discrimination in obesity treatment. *Canadian Journal of Diabetes, 37*(3), 205–209. https://doi.org/10.1016/j.jcjd.2013.03.362

Forhan, M., Vrkljan, B., & MacDermid, J. (2010). A systematic review of the quality of psychometric evidence supporting the use of an obesity-specific quality of life measure for use with persons who have class III obesity. *Obesity Reviews, 11*(3) 222–228. https://doi.org/10.1111/j.1467-789X.2009.00612.x

Forhan, M., Zagorski, B. M., Marzonlini, S., Oh, P., & Alter, D. A. (2013). Predicting exercise adherence for patients with obesity and diabetes referred to a cardiac rehabilitation and secondary prevention program. *Canadian Journal of Diabetes, 37*(3), 189–194. https://doi.org/10.1016/j.jcjd.2013.03.370

Haracz, K., Ryan, S., Hazelton, M., & James, C. (2013). Occupational therapy and obesity: An integrative literature review. *Australian Occupational Therapy Journal, 60*(5), 356–365. https://doi.org/10.1111/1440-1630.12063

Lang, J., James, C., Ashby, S., Plotnifkoff, R., Guest, M., Kable, A., Collins, C., & Snodgrass, S. (2013). The provision of weight management advice: An investigation into occupational therapy practice. *Australian Journal of Occupational Therapy Journal, 60*(6), 387–394. https://doi.org/10.1111/1440-1630.12073

Leemhuis, K., & Cozzolino, M. (2010). Obesity, stigma, and occupational therapy. *Physical Disabilities Special Interest Section Quarterly, 33*(4), 1–3.

Lundgren, J. D., Rempfer, M. V., Brown, C. E., Goetz, J., & Hamera, E. (2010). The prevalence of night eating syndrome and binge eating disorder among overweight and obese individuals with serious mental illness. *Psychiatry Research, 175*(3), 233–236. https://doi.org/10.1016/j.psychres.2008.10.027

Mata, H., Mikkola, A., Loveland, J., & Hallowell, P. T. (2015). Occupational therapy and bariatric surgery: Discovering occupation after weight-loss surgery. *OT Practice, 20*(1), 11–15.

Miyake, Y., Eguchi, E., Ito, H., Nakamura, K., Ito, T., Nagaoka, K., Ogino, N., & Ogino, K. (2018). Association between occupational dysfunction and metabolic syndrome in community-dwelling Japanese adults in a cross-sectional study: Ibara study. *International Journal of Environmental Research and Public Health, 15*(11), Article 2572. https://doi.org/10.3390/ijerph15112575

Nielsen, S. S., & Christensen, J. R. (2018). Occupational therapy for adults with overweight and obesity: Mapping interventions involving occupational therapists. *Occupational Therapy International, 2018*, Article 7412686. https://doi.org/10.1155/2018/7412686

Nossum R., Johansen, A. E., & Kjeken, I. (2018). Occupational problems and barriers reported by individuals with obesity. *Scandinavian Journal of Occupational Therapy, 25*(2), 136–144. https://doi.org/10.1080/11038128.2017.1279211

Pizzi, M. A. (2013). Obesity, health and quality of life: A conversation to further the vision in occupational therapy. *Occupational Therapy in Health Care, 27*(2), 78–83. https://doi.org/10.3109/07380577.2013.778442

Puhl, R. M., Latner, J. D., O'Brien, K., Luedicke, J., Danielsdottir, S., & Forhan, M. (2015). A multinational examination of weight bias: Predictors of anti-fat attitudes across four countries. *International Journal of Obesity, 39*(7), 1166–1173. https://doi.org/10.1038/ijo.2015.32

Ramos Salas, X., Alberga, A. S., Cameron, E., Estey, L., Forhan, M., Kirk, S. F. L., Russell-Mayhew, S., & Sharma, A. M. (2017). Addressing weight bias and discrimination: Moving beyond raising awareness to creating change. *Obesity Reviews, 18*(11), 1323–1335. https://doi.org/10.1111/obr.12592

Ramos Salas, X., Forhan, M., Caulfield, T., Sharma, A. M., & Raine, K. D. (2019). Addressing internalized weight bias and changing damaged social identities for people living with obesity. *Frontiers in Psychology, 10*, Article 1409. https://doi.org/10.3389/fpsyg.2019.01409

Ramos Salas, X., Forhan, M., Caulfield, T., Sharma, A. M., & Raine, K. (2017). A critical analysis of obesity prevention policies and strategies. *Canadian Journal of Public Health, 108*(5-6), e598–e608. https://doi.org/10.17269/cjph.108.6044

Ramos Salas, X., Forhan, M., & Sharma, A. M. (2014). Diffusing obesity myths. *Clinical Obesity, 4*(3), 189–196. https://doi.org/10.1111/cob.12059

Seida, J. C., Sharma, A. M., Johnson, J. A., & Forhan, M. (2018). Hospital rehabilitation for patients with obesity: A scoping review. *Disability and Rehabilitation, 40*(2), 125–134. https://doi.org/10.1080/09638288.2016.1243163

Sharma, S., Wharton, S., Forhan, M., & Kuk, J. L. (2011). Influence of weight discrimination on weight loss goals and self-selected weight loss interventions. *Clinical Obesity, 1*(4-6), 153–160. https://doi.org/10.1111/j.1758-8111.2011.00028.x

Taylor, V. H., Forhan, M., Vigod, S. N., McIntyre, R. S., & Morrison, K. M. (2013). The impact of obesity on quality of life. *Best Practice & Research Clinical Endocrinology & Metabolism, 27*(2), 139–146. https://doi.org/10.1016/j.beem.2013.04.004

Tessier, A., Mayo, N. E., & Cieza, A. (2011). Content identification of the IWQOL-Lite with the International Classification of Functioning, Disability and Health. *Quality of Life Research, 20*, 467–477. https://doi.org/10.1007/s11136-010-9787-1

Vroman, K., & Cote, S. (2011). Prejudicial attitudes toward clients who are obese: Measuring implicit attitudes of occupational therapy students. *Occupational Therapy in Health Care, 25*(1), 77–90. https://doi.org/10.3109/07380577.2010.533252

Child/Adolescent

Cairney, J., Hay, J., Veldhuizen, S., Missiuna, C., Mahlberg, N., & Faught, B. E. (2010). Trajectories of relative weight and waist circumference among children with and without developmental coordination disorder. *Canadian Medical Association Journal, 182*(11), 1167–1172. https://doi.org/10.1503/cmaj.091454

Cermak, S. A., Katz, N., Weintraub, N., Steinhart, S., Raz-Silbiger, S., Munoz, M., & Lifshitz, N. (2015). Participation in physical activity, fitness, and risk for obesity in children with developmental coordination disorder: A cross-cultural study. *Occupational Therapy International, 22*, 163–173. https://doi.org/10.1002/oti.1393

Hong, I., Coker-Bolt, P., Anderson, K. R., Lee, D., & Velozo, C. A. (2016). Relationship between physical activity and overweight and obesity in children: Findings from the 2012 National Health and Nutrition Examination Survey National Youth Fitness Survey. *American Journal of Occupational Therapy, 70*(5), Article 7005180060. https://doi.org/10.5014/ajot.2016.021212

Lin, C.-Y., Su, C.-T., & Ma, H.-I. (2012). Physical activity patterns and quality of life of overweight boys: A preliminary study. *Hong Kong Journal of Occupational Therapy, 22*(1), 31–37. https://doi.org/10.1016/j.hkjot.2012.06.001

Orban, K., Edberg, A.-K., Thorngren-Jerneck, K., Önnerfält, J., & Erlandsson, L. K. (2014). Changes in parents' time use and its relationship to child obesity. *Physical & Occupational Therapy in Pediatrics, 34*(1), 44–61. https://doi.org/10.3109/01942638.2013.792311

Pizzi, M. A. (2013). Obesity, health and quality of life: A conversation to further the vision in occupational therapy. *Occupational Therapy in Health Care, 27*(2), 78–83. https://doi.org/10.3109/07380577.2013.778442

Pizzi, M. A. (2016). Promoting health, well-being, and quality of life for children who are overweight or obese and their families. *American Journal of Occupational Therapy, 70*(5), Article 7005170010. https://doi.org/10.5014/ajot.2016.705001

Pizzi, M. A., & Vroman, K. (2013). Childhood obesity: Effects on children's participation, mental health, and psychosocial development. *Occupational Therapy in Health Care, 27*(2), 99–112. https://doi.org/10.3109/07380577.2013.784839

Pizzi, M., Vroman, K. G., Lau, C., Gill, S. V., Bazyk, S., Suarez-Balcazar, Y., & Orloff, S. (2014). Occupational therapy and the childhood obesity epidemic: Research, theory and practice. *Journal of Occupational Therapy, Schools, & Early Intervention, 7*(2), 87–105. https://doi.org/1 0.1080/19411243.2014.930605

Poulsen, A. A., Desha, L., Ziviani, J., Griffiths, L., Heaslop, A., Khan, A., & Leong, G. M. (2011). Fundamental movement skills and self-concept of children who are overweight. *International Journal of Pediatric Obesity, 6*(2-2), e464–e471. https://doi.org/10.3109/17477166.2 011.575143

Puhl, R. M., Latner, J. D., O'Brien, K., Luedicke, J., Forhan, M., & Danielsdottir, S. (2016). Cross-national perspectives about weight-based bullying in youth: Nature, extent and remedies. *Pediatric Obesity, 11*(4), 241–250. https://doi.org/10.1111/ijpo.12051

Suarez-Balcazar, Y., Friesema, J., & Lukyanova, V. (2013). Culturally competent interventions to address obesity among African American and Latino children and youth. *Occupational Therapy in Health Care, 27*(2), 113–128. https://doi.org/10.3109/07380577.2013.785644

Todd, A. S., Street, S. J., Ziviani, J., Byrne, N. M., & Hills, A. P. (2015). Overweight and obese adolescent girls: The importance of promoting sensible eating and activity behaviors from the start of the adolescent period. *International Journal of Environmental Research and Public Health, 12*(2), 2306–2329. https://doi.org/10.3390/ijerph120202306

Older Adults

See also Driving Cessation, Driving Fitness, Frailty and Frail Conditions, and Retirement.

Description

Older adults are usually those 65 years or older. The oldest old are those 85 years or older (O'Toole, 2017). This chapter focuses on preventative strategies and health promotion for older adults living in the community as opposed to being hospitalized and treated for specific disorders.

Cause

Living 65 years or longer (or celebrating lots of birthdays).

Evaluation/Assessment

Areas

- Activities of Daily Living/Instrumental ADL: basic ADLs (eating, dressing, grooming bathing/showering, toileting, cutting toenails, transfers); independent living occupations: food purchasing and meal preparation, light housekeeping and maintenance, doing laundry and storing clothing, shopping for groceries and household supplies, budgeting and maintaining finances, keeping track of medications, using communication systems including telephone or smartphone, using private and public transportation, providing child and pet care
- Education/Work: academic achievement (education level completed), work history, vocational interests including volunteering
- Play/Leisure: interests, skills, values, frequency, location, level of satisfaction
- Rest/Sleep: sleep habits and routines, sleep disorders
- Social Participation: types, frequency, location, with whom
- Sensorimotor: physical fitness, exercise program, muscle strength, joint range of motion, endurance, sensory acuity and discrimination (auditory, gustatory, olfactory, proprioception, tactile, temperature, vision)
- Cognitive/Perceptual: attention, memory, executive functions, visual perception, auditory perception

- Psychosocial: depression, anxiety, self-efficacy, self-identity, self-confidence, self-worth, role performance, isolation, social relations, quality of life
- Context/Environment: home modification, adapted devices, community services and resources, social support
- Comorbidities: obesity, diabetes, chronic pulmonary obstructive disease (COPD), dementia, visual impairment, hearing loss, physical disability, psychological disability

Instruments

Note: Results of assessment in a clinic or unfamiliar environment may be lower than results in a home or familiar environment (Provencher, Demers, Gagnon, & Gélines, 2012; Provencher, Demers, & Gélines, 2012).

Instruments Developed by Occupational Therapy Personnel
- Activities of Daily Living Index (ADL Index; Gitlin et al., 2006)
- Activity Card Sort (2nd ed.; ACS-2; Baum & Edwards, 2008)
- Adolescent/Adult Sensory Profile (AASP; Brown & Dunn, 2002)
- Assessment of Motor and Process Skills (8th ed.; AMPS-8; Fisher & Bray Jones, 2016)
- Canadian Occupational Performance Measure (5th ed.; COPM-5; Law et al., 2014)
- Engagement in Meaningful Activities Survey (EMAS; Goldberg et al., 2002; see also Eakman et al., 2010, in References)
- Everyday Technology Use Questionnaire (ETUQ; Rosenberg et al., 2009)
- Health Enhancement Lifestyle Profile (HELP; J. E. Hwang, 2010a, 2010b, 2012a, in References)
- Health Enhancement Lifestyle Profile–Screener (HELP-Screener; E. J. Hwang & Peralta-Catipon, 2015, and J. E. Hwang, 2012a, 2012b, 2013, in References)
- In-Home Occupational Performance Evaluation (I-HOPE; Stark et al., 2010, in References)
- Instrumental Activities of Daily Living Index (IADL Index; Gitlin et al., 2006)
- Instrumental Activities of Daily Living Profile (IADLP; Bottari et al., 2009; see also Bier et al., 2016, in References)
- Klein-Bell ADL Scale (KB-ADL; Klein & Bell, 1982)
- Life Satisfaction Questionnaire (LISAT-9; Fugl-Meyer et al., 1991)
- Management of Everyday Technology Assessment (META; Malinowsky et al., 2010; Malinowsky et al., 2012; and Malinowsky et al., 2011, in References)
- Modified Interest Checklist (MIC; Kielhofner & Neville, 1983)
- Nottingham Extended Activities of Daily Living (NEADL; Nouri & Lincoln, 1987)
- Performance Assessment of Self-Care Skills (Version 4.1; PASS 4.1; Chisholm et al., 2016)
- Reintegration to Normal Living Index (RNLI; Wood-Dauphinee et al., 1988)
- Safety Assessment of Function and the Environment for Rehabilitation–Health Outcome Measurement and Evaluation (3rd ed.; SAFER-HOME 3; Chiu & Oliver, 2006)
- Self-Report Safe Driving Behavior Measure (SRSDBM; Classen et al., 2012, in References)
- Sunnaas Index of Activities of Daily Living (Sunnaas Index; Vandeberg et al., 1991)
- Westmead Home Safety Assessment (WeHSA; Clemson et al., 1992; see also Hasegawa & Kamimura, 2018, in References)

Instruments Developed by Other Professionals and Used by Occupational Therapy Personnel
- Activities-Specific Balance Confidence (ABC) Scale (Powell & Myers, 1995)
- Adelaide Activities Profile (AAP; Clark & Bond, 1995)
- Assessment of Life Habits (LIFE-H; Fourgeyrollas & Noreau, 2005)
- Barthel Index (BI; Mahoney & Barthel, 1965)
- Caregiver Assessment of Function and Upset (CAFU; Gitlin et al., 2005)
- Disability Rating Scale (DRS; Rappaport et al., 1982)
- Early Treatment in Diabetic Retinopathy Study (ETDRS) chart (Ferris et al., 1982)
- European Quality of Life 5-Dimension Scale (EuroQol 5 Dimension, EQ-5D; EuroQol Group, 1990)

- Frenchay Activities Index (FAI; Holbrook & Skilbeck, 1983)
- Functional Independence Measure (FIM; Uniform Data System for Medical Rehabilitation, 1997)
- Functional Status Questionnaire (FSQ; Jette et al., 1986)
- Groningen Activity Restriction Scale (GARS; Suurmeijer et al., 1994)
- Health Assessment Questionnaire–Disability Index (HAQ-DI; Bruce & Fries, 2005)
- Hospital Anxiety and Depression Scale (HADS; Zigmond & Snaith, 1983)
- Index of Activities of Daily Living (K-ADL; Katz et al., 1963)
- Instrumental Activities of Daily Living (Lawton IADL, Lawton-Brody IADL; Lawton & Brody, 1969)
- Instrumental Activity Measure (IAM; Grimby et al., 1996)
- Interpersonal Support Evaluation List (ISEL; Heitzman & Kaplan, 1988)
- Interview of Deterioration in Daily Activities in Dementia (IDDAD; Voigt-Radloff et al., 2012)
- Inventory of Coping Strategies (ICS; Robichaud & Lamarre, 2002)
- Katz Index of Activities of Daily Living (Katz ADL; see Index of Activities of Daily Living)
- Late Life Function and Disability Index (LLFADI; Jette et al., 2002)
- Lawton-Brody Instrumental Activities of Daily Living (see Instrumental Activities of Daily Living)
- Life-Space Assessment (LSA; Baker et al., 2003)
- Modified Barthel Index (MBI; Collin et al., 1988)
- Montreal Cognitive Assessment (MoCA; Nasreddine et al., 2005)
- Myers-Briggs Type Indicator (MBTI Step III; Myers & Brigs Foundation, 2009)
- Mini-Mental State Examination (MMSE; Folstein et al., 1975; see also Crizzle et al., 2012, in References)
- Northwick Park Index of Independence in Activities of Daily Living (Northwick Park Index of Independence in ADL, Northwick Park ADL Scale; Benjamin, 1976)
- Performance Oriented Mobility Assessment (POMA; see Tinetti Performance Oriented Mobility Assessment)
- Rivermead Activities of Daily Living Assessment (Rivermead ADL; Whiting & Lincoln, 1980)
- Satisfaction with Life Scale (SWLS; Diener et al., 1985)
- Short Falls Efficacy Scale-International (S-FES-I; Kempen et al., 2008)
- Short Form 36 Health Survey (SF-36; Ware et al., 1993)
- Timed Up and Go test (TUG; Podsiadlo & Ricardson, 1991)
- Tinetti Performance Oriented Mobility Assessment (POMA; Tinetti, 1986)
- Trail Making Test (TMT) Part B (Reitan, 1958; see also Classen et al., 2013, in References)
- Useful Field of View (UFOV; Ball & Owsley, 1993; see also Classen et al., 2013, in References)

Problems/Issues

Activities of Daily Living/Instrumental ADL

- Person may have difficulty performing basic ADL tasks due to physical, cognitive, or emotional problems.
- Person may have difficulty performing independent living skills due to physical, cognitive, or emotional problems. Especially important are meal preparation and nutritional status, medication management, financial management, shopping, driving.

Education/Work

- Person may need to plan for retirement.
- Person may need to find supplemental income.
- Person may need to explore voluntary and unpaid options for occupational balance.

Play/Leisure

- Person may have stopped engaging in formally enjoyed leisure occupations.

- Person may need to reengage in known leisure occupations with modifications to accommodate physical, cognitive, or emotional limitations.
- Person may want to develop or expand leisure occupations but need advice and guidance.

Rest/Sleep
- Person may experience sleep disturbance due to physical, cognitive, or emotional problems.
- Person may experience disruption in sleep habits and routine.

Social Participation
- Person may have stopped or limited participation in previously enjoyed social and cultural activities due to real or perceived physical, cognitive, or emotional problems.
- Person may need assistance to overcome limitations to participation (environmental modification, adapted devices).

Sensorimotor
- Person may have decreased muscle strength in core muscle groups including decreased hand grip strength.
- Person may have limitations in joint range of motion due to stiffness and joint deterioration.
- Person may be deconditioned due to lack of participation in a regular physical fitness program.
- Person may have decreased sensory acuity and discrimination in all sensory systems.

Cognitive/Perceptual
- Person may have decreased ability to attend and concentrate.
- Person may have decreased memory and ability to learn new information.
- Person may have decreased skills in executive functioning (problem solving, planning, judgment of safety, time management).
- Person may have decreased auditory and visual perception.

Psychosocial
- Person may be depressed or anxious.
- Person may have decreased sense of self-efficacy and self-worth.
- Person may have decreased sense of self-confidence and self-identity.
- Person usually experiences changes in role function if retired from paid work or when the children are no longer living at home.
- Person may experience decreased quality of life.

Context/Environment
- Person may struggle to use everyday technology (microwave, electric can opener, smartphone, computer).
- Person may have limited knowledge about aging process, maintaining good health, planning for retirement, role performance as a retired person.
- Person may have limited knowledge about available community and internet resources.
- Person may have limited knowledge about environmental modifications to make home more accessible.
- Person may have limited knowledge about adapted devices that may make performing everyday tasks easier and safer.

Intervention/Treatment

Models and programs developed by occupational therapy personnel include the activity-pacing program (Timmer et al., 2019), biofeedback and ball exercise program (Jahagirdar & Kenkre, 2010), computer tablet technology (Benham, 2019; Kaldenberg & Smallfield, 2017), home arrangements (Altuntaş et al., 2017), home visit occupational therapy (Imanishi et al., 2017), intensive client-centered occupational therapy in the home (Nielsen et al., 2019), lifestyle redesign (Clark et al., 2015), lively living (Slaughter et al., 2018), medication adherence (Sanders & Van Oss, 2013), predischarge home visits (Clemson et al., 2016), and upstream living (Fowler,

2019). Models and programs developed by other professionals but used by occupational therapy personnel include Advancing Better Living for Elders (ABLE; Jutkowitz et al., 2012), aging in place (Sheffield et al., 2013), assistive technology intervention (Mortenson et al., 2013), elderly persons in the risk zone (Dahlin-Ivanoff et al., 2016), preventive home visits (Behm et al., 2013), reablement program (Tuntland et al., 2015; Tuntland et al., 2017), technology acceptance model (Money et al., 2015), and vision self-management (Girdler et al., 2010). Team members include physicians, surgeons, ophthalmologists, audiologists, dieticians, nursing personnel, pharmacists, physical therapy personnel, social workers, speech pathologists, vocational counselors, and occupational therapy personnel. Goals are to maintain or improve general health status and promote wellness and well-being in occupational performance of self-care, productivity, and leisure.

Activities of Daily Living/Instrumental ADL

- Assist person to develop and follow healthy habits regarding diet including reading labels for nutritional content, eating fresh fruit and vegetables, avoiding foods high in fat, and so forth. Consultation with a dietician or nutritionist may be helpful.
- Assist person to develop a routine for taking medication focusing on the time to take medication (meal based, wake up, going to bed, specific time during the day, during work hours), location for storing medication (kitchen, bathroom, bedroom, family room), location for administration (in plain sight, easily accessible, where client spends most time, table where meals are eaten), total routine (breakfast, dinner, lunch, work, nap).

Education/Work

- Consider adult education programs (local Y, local museum, local community college, video recording, internet based.
- Consider part-time work: consultation, teaching, home-based business.
- Consider unpaid or volunteer work in community, city, state, national, international.

Play/Leisure

- Continue or renew engagement in previously performed leisure occupations with modifications, if needed.
- Explore and engage in new or novel interests and leisure occupations (arts and crafts, writing, photography, scrapbooking, gardening, computer games, card and board games, outside games and sports).

Rest/Sleep

- Review sleep habits and routines.
- Address sleep disturbances including referral to sleep specialists if major problems are detected.

Social Participation

- Social activities: card games, dinner (breakfast, lunch) club, discussion groups, movie night, gardening.
- Cultural activities: concerts, opera, ballet, theater, museum, religious.

Sensorimotor

- Activity pacing group program (five 45-minute sessions)
  - ▸ Day 1—self-monitory (listening to the body)
  - ▸ Day 2—balancing rest and activity
  - ▸ Day 3—activity-pacing group education
  - ▸ Day 4—prioritizing tasks and alternating high- and low-energy tasks
  - ▸ Day 5—maintaining a level of activity and gradually increasing activity
- Exercises: Swiss ball exercises, TheraBand exercises, walking program, dancing, swimming, fitness training, aerobics, Pilates
- Hearing
  - ▸ Background noise reduction: add rugs and curtains, arrange seating away from windows and doors, close windows and doors that do not need to be open.

- ▶ Volume adjustment: increase volume of television, telephone, smartphone, and appliances; sit closer to television; use headphones if audio output plug is available; use closed captioning on television.
  - ▶ Other technologies: strobe or flashing doorbell and fire alarms, flashing alerts on smartphone, use motion detectors with lights.
- Vision
  - ▶ Adequate light: add task lights under counters or needed work spaces, increase lighting in hallways and stairs, use adjustable lamps with hoods.
  - ▶ Glare reduction: use blinds or shades to decrease glare, have glasses coated with glare reduction coating.
  - ▶ Adequate contrast: use bold line paper, use black on white or white on black for contrasting surface versus task.
  - ▶ Other technologies: use adjustable mirrors for grooming, use voice output microwaves, add tactile textures to items, use lighted keyholes or doorbells, use motion detectors with bright lights.
- Smell (olfactory)
  - ▶ Provide opportunity to practice sense of smell and track results (loss of sense of smell in a warning sign for dementia).

Cognitive/Perceptual

- Memory: provide practice in using memory (memory games, remembering dates and events past and present).
- Executive function: practice problem solving, planning, scheduling, personal and home safety.
- Perception: practice in visual, spatial, and auditory perceptual tasks.

Psychosocial

- Stress reduction strategies: deep breathing, relaxation, imagery, mindfulness, yoga, tai chi.
- Assist client to identify accomplishments to increase sense of self-efficacy, self-identify, and self-worth.
- Assist client to identify actions that would improve quality of life.

Context/Environment

- Provide information and resources on successful aging, and health promotion and maintenance.
- Assist client to improve home safety through environmental modifications (add lighting, add railings, add banisters, less clutter, clean pathways, remove small rugs, replace broken steps, etc.).
- Assist client to increase ability to master everyday technology (electronic gadgets, computer, smartphone).
- Discuss with client fall prevent program (see chapter on Falls in this section).

Precautions/Safety Considerations

- Falls: see Falls in this section.
- Cognitive impairment: see Cognitive Impairment, Memory Impairment, and Executive Dysfunction in Section 11: Cognitive-Perceptual Disorders.
- Personal safety from violence to person and family members.

Prognosis and Outcome

Variable. Some community dwelling residents are open to learning to better manage their health and safety in daily living, others not so much. Availability of resources (financial, community, internet) is another major consideration.

Cost Effectiveness

Preventative programs in occupational therapy are cost effective such as aging in place program (Jutkowitz et al., 2012), fall prevention and dementia (Nagayama et al., 2016), occupation-focused health promotion discussion group (Zingmark et al., 2016) and preventing bathing disability (Zingmark et al., 2017).

REFERENCES

Altuntaş, O., Torpil, B., & Uyanik, M. (2017). Occupational therapy for elderly people. In M. Huri (Ed.), *Occupation focused holistic practice in rehabilitation* (pp. 195–206). IntechOpen.

Behm, L., Dahlin Ivanoff, S., & Zidén, L. (2013). Preventive home visits and health—Experiences among very old people. *BMC Public Health, 13*, Article 378. https://doi.org/10.1186/1471-24 58-13-378

Benham, S. (2019). Using technology to promote occupational performance in older adults. *SIS Quarterly Practice Connections, 4*(2), 28–30.

Bier, N., Belchior, P. C., Paquette, G., Beauchemin, E., Lacasse-Champagne, A., Messier, C., Pellerin, M.-L., Petit, M., Mioshi, E., & Bottari, C. (2016). The Instrumental Activity of Daily Living Profile in Aging: A feasibility study. *Journal of Alzheimer's Disease, 52*(4), 1361–1371. https://doi.org/10.3233/JAD-150957

Clark, F., Blanchard, J., Sleight, A., Cogan, A., Florindez, L., Gleason, S., Heymann, R., Hill, V., Holden, A., Murphy, M., Proffitt, R., Niemiec, S. S., & Vigen, C. (2015). *Lifestyle redesign: The intervention tested in the USC well elderly studies* (2nd ed.). AOTA Press.

Classen, S., Wang, Y., Crizzle, A. M., Winter, S. M., & Lanford, D. N. (2013). Predicting older driver on-road performance by means of the Useful Field of View and Trail Making Test Part B. *American Journal of Occupational Therapy, 67*(5), 574–582. https://doi.org/10.5014/ ajot.2013.008136

Classen, S., Wen, P. S., Velozo, C. A., Bédard, M., Winter, S. M., Brumback, B., & Lanford, D. N. (2012). Psychometrics of the Self-Report Safe Driving Behavior Measure for older adults. *American Journal of Occupational Therapy, 66*(2), 233–241. https://doi.org/10.5014/ajot.20 12.001834

Clemson, L., Lannin, N. A., Wales, K., Salkeld, G., Rubenstein, L., Gitlin, L., Barris, S., Mackenzie, L., & Cameron, I. D. (2016). Occupational therapy predischarge home visits in acute hospital care: A randomized trial. *Journal of the American Geriatrics Society, 64*(10), 2019–2026. https://doi.org/10.1111/jgs.14287

Crizzle, A. M., Classen, S., Bédard, M., Lanford, D., & Winter, S. (2012). MMSE as a predictor of on-road driving performance in community dwelling older drivers. *Accident Analysis & Prevention, 49*, 287–292. https://doi.org/10.1016/j.aap.2012.02.003

Dahlin-Ivanoff, S., Eklund, K., Wilhelmson, K., Behm, L., Häggblom-Kronlöf, G., Zidén, L., Landahl, S., & Gustafsson, S. (2016). For whom is a health-promoting intervention effective? Predictive factors for performing activities of daily living independently. *BMC Geriatrics, 16*, Article 171. https://doi.org/10.1186/s12877-016-0345-8

Eakman, A. M., Carlson, M., & Clark, F. (2010). Factor structure, reliability and convergent validity of the Engagement in Meaningful Activities Survey for older adults. *OTJR: Occupation, Participation and Health, 30*(3), 111–121. https://doi.org/10.3928/15394492-20090518-01

Fowler, N. L. (2019). Upstream living: Occupation-based health promotion for community-dwelling older adults. *SIS Quarterly Practice Connections, 4*(4), 23–25.

Girdler, S. J., Boldy, D. P., Dhaliwal, S. S., Crowley, M., & Packer, T. L. (2010). Vision self-management for older adults: A randomised controlled trial. *British Journal of Ophthalmology, 94*(2), 223–228. https://doi.org/10.1136/bjo.2008.147538

Hasegawa, A., & Kamimura, T. (2018). Development of the Japanese version of the Westmead Home Safety Assessment for the elderly in Japan. *Hong Kong Journal of Occupational Therapy, 31*(1), 14–21. https://doi.org/10.1177/1569186118764065

Hwang, E. J., & Peralta-Catipon, T. (2015). A review and case exemplifications of Health Enhancement Lifestyle Profile (HELP) and its Screener (HELP-Screener) for older adults. *Open Journal of Occupational Therapy, 3*(3) Article 8. https://doi.org/10.15453/2168-6408.1170

Hwang, J. E. (2010a). Promoting healthy lifestyles with aging: Development and validation of the Health Enhancement Lifestyle Profile (HELP) using the Rasch Measurement Model. *American Journal of Occupational Therapy, 64*(5), 786–795. https://doi.org/10.5014/ajot.20 10.09088

Hwang, J. E. (2010b). Reliability and validity of the Health Enhancement Lifestyle Profile (HELP). *OTJR: Occupational, Participation & Health, 30*(4), 158–168. https://doi.org/10.3928/ 15394492-20091225-01

Hwang, J. E. (2012a). Development and validation of a 15-item lifestyle screening for community-dwelling older adults. *American Journal of Occupational Therapy, 66*(6), e98–e106. https://doi .org/10.5014/ajot.2012.005181

Hwang, J. E. (2012b). Validity of the Health Enhancement Lifestyle Profile-screener (HELP-Screener). *OTJR: Occupation, Participation and Health, 32*(4), 135–141. https://doi.org/10.392 8/15394492-20120217-01

Hwang, J. E. (2013). Reliability of the Health Enhancement Lifestyle Profile–Screener (HELP-Screener). *American Journal of Occupational Therapy, 67*(1), e6–e10. https://doi.org/10.5014/ ajot.2013.005934

Imanishi, M., Tomohisa, H., & Higaki, K. (2017). Quantifying the effect of home visit occupational therapy on the quality of life of elderly individuals. *Asian Journal of Occupational Therapy, 13*(1), 1–6. https://doi.org/10.11596/asiajot.13.1

Jahagirdar, S. S., & Kenkre, I. R. (2010). Training elderly for mobility and strength using EMG-biofeedback and Swiss ball/peanut ball exercises. *Indian Journal of Occupational Therapy, 42*(1), 17–25.

Jutkowitz, E., Gitlin, L. N., Pizzi, L. T., Lee, E., & Dennis, M. (2012). Cost effectiveness of a home-based intervention that helps functionally vulnerable older adults age in place at home. *Journal of Aging Research, 2012*, Article 680265. https://doi.org/10.1155/2012/680265

Kaldenberg, J., & Smallfield, S. (2017). Training older adults with low vision to use a computer tablet: A feasibility study. *British Journal of Occupational Therapy, 80*(2), 117–122. https:// doi.org/10.1177/0308022616648172

Malinowsky, C., Almkvist, O., Kottorp, A., & Nygård, L. (2010). Ability to manage everyday technology: A comparison of persons with dementia or mild cognitive impairment and older adults without cognitive impairment. *Disability and Rehabilitation: Assistive Technology, 5*(6), 462–469. https://doi.org/10.3109/17483107.2010.496098

Malinowsky, C., Almkvist, O., Nygård, L., & Kottorp, A. (2012). Individual variability and environmental characteristics influence older adults' abilities to manage everyday technology. *International Psychogeriatrics, 24*(3), 484–495. https://doi.org/10.1017/S1041610211002092

Malinowsky, C., Nygård, L., & Kottorp, A. (2011). Psychometric evaluation of a new assessment of the ability to manage technology in everyday life. *Scandinavian Journal of Occupational Therapy, 18*(1), 26–35. https://doi.org/10.3109/11038120903420606

Money, A. G., Atwal, A., Young, K. L., Day, Y., Wilson, L., & Money, K. G. (2015). Using the Technology Acceptance Model to explore community dwelling older adults' perceptions of a 3D interior design application to facilitate pre-discharge home adaptations. *BMC Medical Informatics and Decision Making, 15*, Article 73. https://doi.org/10.1186/s12911-015-0190-2

Mortenson, W. B., Demers, L., Fuhrer, M. J., Jutai, J. W., Lenker, J., & DeRuyter, F. (2013). Effects of an assistive technology intervention on older adults with disabilities and their informal caregivers: An exploratory randomized control trial. *American Journal of Physical Medicine & Rehabilitation, 92*(4), 297–306. https://doi.org/10.1097/PHM.0b013e31827d65bf

Nagayama, H., Tomori, K., Ohno, K., Takahashi, K., & Yamauchi, K. (2016). Cost-effectiveness of occupational therapy in older people: Systematic review of randomized controlled trials. *Occupational Therapy International, 23*, 103–120. https://doi.org/10.1002/oti.1408

Nielsen, T. L., Andersen, N. T., Petersen, K. S., Polatajko, H., & Nielsen, C. V. (2019). Intensive client-centred occupational therapy in the home improves older adults' occupational performance: Results from a Danish randomized controlled trial. *Scandinavian Journal of Occupational Therapy, 26*(5), 325–342. https://doi.org/10.1080/11038128.2018.1424236

O'Toole, M. T. (Ed.). (2017). *Mosby's dictionary of medicine, nursing & health professions* (10th ed.). Elsevier.

Provencher, V., Demers, L., Gagnon, L., & Gélinas, I. (2012). Impact of familiar and unfamiliar settings on cooking task assessments in frail older adults with poor and preserved executive functions. *International Psychogeriatrics, 24*(5), 775–783. https://doi.org/10.1017/S1041610 21100216X

Provencher, V., Demers, L., & Gélinas, I. (2012). Factors that may explain differences between home and clinic meal preparation task assessments in frail older adults. *International Journal of Rehabilitation Research, 35*(3), 248–255. https://doi.org/10.1097/MRR.0b013e3283544cb8

Sanders, M. J., & Van Oss, T. (2013). Using daily routines to promote medication adherence in older adults. *American Journal of Occupational Therapy, 67*(1), 91–99. https://doi.org/10.50 14/ajot.2013.005033

Sheffield, C., Smith, C. A., & Becker, M. (2013). Evaluation of an agency-based occupational therapy intervention to facilitate aging in place. *The Gerontologist, 53*(6), 907–918. https://doi.org/10.1093/geront/gns145

Slaughter, B., McGowan, K., Metheny, A., Underdown, H., Wingerter, K., & Clarke, L. (2018). Lively living: An occupation-based intervention to enhance participation in community-dwelling older adults. *SIS Quarterly Practice Connections, 3*(3), 23–25.

Stark, S. L., Somerville, E. K., & Morris, J. C. (2010). In-home occupational performance evaluation (I-HOPE). *American Journal of Occupational Therapy, 64*(4), 580–589. https://doi.org/10.5014/ ajot.2010.08065

Timmer, A. J., Unsworth, C. A., & Browne, M. (2019). A randomized controlled trial protocol investigating effectiveness of an activity-pacing program for deconditioned older adults. *Canadian Journal of Occupational Therapy, 86*(2), 136–147. https://doi.org/10.1177/0008417419830374

Tuntland, H., Aaslund, M. K., Espehaug, B., Førland, O., & Kjeken, I. (2015). Reablement in community-dwelling older adults: A randomised controlled trial. *BMC Geriatrics, 15*, Article 145. https://doi.org/10.1186/s12877-015-0142-9

Tuntland, H., Kjeken, I., Langeland, E., Folkestad, B., Espehaug, B., Førland, O., & Aaslund, M. K. (2017). Predictors of outcomes following reablement in community-dwelling older adults. *Clinical Interventions in Aging, 12*, 55–63. https://doi.org/10.2147/CIA.S125762

Zingmark, M., Nilsson, I., Fisher, A. G., & Lindholm, L. (2016). Occupation-focused health promotion for well older people—A cost-effectiveness analysis. *British Journal of Occupational Therapy, 79*(3), 153–162. https://doi.org/10.1177/0308022615609623

Zingmark, M., Nilsson, I., Norström, F., Sahlén, K. G., & Lindholm, L. (2017). Cost effectiveness of an intervention focused on reducing bathing disability. *European Journal of Ageing, 14*, 233–241. https://doi.org/10.1007/s10433-016-0404-1

BIBLIOGRAPHY

Albert, S. M., Bear-Lehman, J., & Anderson, S. J. (2015). Declines in mobility and changes in performance in the instrumental activities of daily living among mildly disabled community-dwelling older adults. *Journals of Gerontology: Series A, 70*(1), 71–77. https://doi.org/10.1093 /gerona/glu088

American Occupational Therapy Association. (2016). *Fact Sheet: Occupational therapy services for persons with visual impairment.*

Anaby, D., Miller, W. C., Jarus, T., Eng, J. J., Noreau, L., & PACC Research Group. (2011). Participation and well-being among older adults living with chronic conditions. *Social Indicators Research, 100*(1), 171–183. https://doi.org/10.1007/s11205-010-9611-x

Arbesman, M., & Mosley, L. J. (2012). Systematic review of occupation- and activity-based health management and maintenance interventions for community-dwelling older adults. *American Journal of Occupational Therapy 66*(3), 277–283. https://doi.org/10.5014/ajot.2012.003327

Auger, C., Demers, L., Gélinas, I., Miller, W. C., Jutai, J. W., & Noreau, L. (2010). Life-space mobility of middle-aged and older adults at various stages of usage of power mobility devices. *Archives of Physical Medicine and Rehabilitation, 91*(5), 765–773. https://doi.org/10.1016/j.apmr.2010.01.018

Bear-Lehman, J., & Albert, S. M. (2018). Occupational performance and subclinical disability in community dwelling older adults. *Annals of International Occupational Therapy, 1*(2), 61–72. https://doi.org/10.3928/24761222-20180409-02

Berger, S., Escher, A., Mengle, E., & Sullivan, N. (2018). Effectiveness of health promotion, management, and maintenance interventions within the scope of occupational therapy for community-dwelling older adults: A systematic review. *American Journal of Occupational Therapy, 72*(4), Article 7204190010. https://doi.org/10.5014/ajot.2018.030346

Bonder, B. R., & Dal Bello-Haas, V. (Eds.). (2018). *Functional performance in older adults* (4th ed.). F.A. Davis.

Brown, C. L., & Finlayson, M. L. (2013). Performance measures rather than self-report measures of functional status predict home care use in community-dwelling older adults. *Canadian Journal of Occupational Therapy, 80*(5), 284–294. https://doi.org/10.1177/0008417413501467

Chippendale, T., & Boltz, M. (2015). Living legends: Effectiveness of a program to enhance sense of purpose and meaning in life among community-dwelling older adults. *American Journal of Occupational Therapy, 69*(4), Article 6904270010. https://doi.org/10.5014/ajot.2015.014894

Clark, F., Blanchard, J., Sleight, A., Cogan, A., Florindez, L., Gleason, S., Heymann, R., Hill, V., Holden, A., Murphy, M., Proffitt, R., Niemiec, S. S., & Vigen, C. (2015). *Lifestyle redesign: The intervention tested in the USC well elderly studies* (2nd ed.). AOTA Press.

Classen, S., Monahan, M., Auten, B., & Yarney, A. (2014). Evidence-based review of interventions for medically at-risk older drivers. *American Journal of Occupational Therapy, 68*(4), e107–e114. https://doi.org/10.5014/ajot.2014.010975

Cohen, H. S., Stitz, J., Sangi-Haghpeykar, H., & Williams, S. P. (2018). Vision screening in adults across the life span. *Southern Medical Journal, 111*(2), 109–112. https://doi.org/10.14423/SMJ.0000000000000762

DeLaney, L. H., Hu, Y. L., Keglovits, M., Somerville, E. K., Baum, C. M., & Stark, S. L. (2016). Predictors of engagement in home activities among community-dwelling older adults. *Physical & Occupational Therapy in Geriatrics, 34*(4), 205–220. https://doi.org/10.1080/02703181.2016.1268237

Demecs, I. P., & Miller, E. (2019). Participatory art in residential aged care: A visual and interpretative phenomenological analysis of older residents' engagement with tapestry weaving. *Journal of Occupational Science, 26*(1), 99–114. https://doi.org/10.1080/14427591.2018.1515649

Engel-Yeger, B., & Rosenblum, S. (2017). The relationship between sensory-processing patterns and occupational engagement among older persons. *Canadian Journal of Occupational Therapy, 84*(1), 10–21. https://doi.org/10.1177/0008417417690415

Gitlow, L. (2014). Technology use by older adults and barriers to using technology. *Physical & Occupational Therapy in Geriatrics, 32*(3), 271–280. https://doi.org/10.3109/02703181.2014.946640

Golding-Day, M., Whitehead, P., Radford, K., & Walker, M. (2017). Interventions to reduce dependency in bathing in community dwelling older adults: A systematic review. *Systematic Reviews, 6*(1), Article 198. https://doi.org/10.1186/s13643-017-0586-4

Hovbrandt, P., Carlsson, G., Nilsson, K., Albin, M. & Håkansson, C. (2019). Occupational balance as described by older workers over the age of 65. *Journal of Occupational Science, 26*(1), 40–52. https://doi.org/10.1080/14427591.2018.1542616

Hunt, L. A., & Wolverson, C. E. (Eds.). (2015). *Work and the older person: Increasing longevity and well-being.* Slack.

Hunter, E. G., & Kearney, P. J. (2018). Occupational therapy interventions to improve performance of instrumental activities of daily living for community-dwelling older adults: A systematic review. *American Journal of Occupational Therapy, 72*(4), Article 7204190050. https://doi.org/10.5014/ajot.2018.031062

Juang, C., Knight, B. G., Carlson, M., Niemiec, S. L. S., Vigen, C., & Clark, F. (2018). Understanding the mechanisms of change in a lifestyle intervention for older adults. *The Gerontologist, 58*(2), 353–361. https://doi.org/10.1093/geront/gnw152

Juckett, L. A., & Robinson, M. L. (2018). Implementing evidence-based interventions with community-dwelling older adults: A scoping review. *American Journal of Occupational Therapy, 72*(4), Article 7204095010. https://doi.org/10.5014/ajot.2018.031583

Korp, K. E., Taylor, J. M., & Nelson, D. L. (2012). Bathing area safety and lower extremity function in community dwelling older adults. *OTJR: Occupation, Participation & Health, 32*(2), 22–29. https://doi.org/10.1177/153944921203200201

Levy, L. (2018). Cognitive aging: Considerations for adults and older adults. In N. Katz & J. Toglia (Eds.), *Cognition, occupation, and participation across the lifespan* (4th ed., pp. 29–50). AOTA Press.

Liu, C. J., Chang, W. P., & Chang, M. C. (2018). Occupational therapy interventions to improve activities of daily living for community-dwelling older adults: A systematic review. *American Journal of Occupational Therapy, 72*(4), Article 7204190060. https://doi.org/10.5014/ajot.2018.031252

Lowman, L. S. (2017). *Clinical review: Home modifications: Occupational therapy.* CINAHL Information Systems.

McPeek, R., Nichols, A. L., Classen, S., & Breiner, J. (2011). Bias in older adults' driving self-assessments: The role of personality. *Transportation Research Part F: Traffic Psychology and Behaviour, 14*(6), 579–590. https://doi.org/10.1016/j.trf.2011.06.001

Nastasi, J. A. (2018). Maximizing independence in older adults with visual impairment and hearing loss. *SIS Quarterly Practice Connections, 3*(3), 20–22.

Nikolova, R., Demers, L., Béland, F., & Giroux, F. (2011). Transitions in the functional status of disabled community-living older adults over a 3-year follow-up period. *Archives of Gerontology and Geriatrics, 52*(1), 12–17. https://doi.org/10.1016/j.archger.2009.11.003

Nygård, L., Pantzar, M., Uppgard, B., & Kottorp, A. (2012). Detection of activity limitations in older adults with MCI or Alzheimer's disease through evaluation of perceived difficulty in use of everyday technology: A replication study. *Aging & Mental Health, 16*(3), 361–371. https://doi.org/10.1080/13607863.2011.605055

Orellano, E., Colón, W. I., & Arbesman, M. (2012). Effect of occupation and activity-based interventions on instrumental activities of daily living performance among community-dwelling older adults: A systematic review. *American Journal of Occupational Therapy, 66*(3), 292–300. https://doi.org/10.5014/ajot.2012.003053

Papageorgiou, N., Marquis, R., Dare, J., & Batten, R. (2016). Occupational therapy and occupational participation in community dwelling older adults: A review of the evidence. *Physical & Occupational Therapy in Geriatrics, 34*(1), 21–42. https://doi.org/10.3109/02703181.2015.1109014

Petty, L. S., Foster, J. E. G., & Rigby, P. (2019). Identifying community-dwelling older adults' vision loss during mobility assessments: A scoping review. *Canadian Journal of Occupational Therapy 86*(2), 95–105. https://doi.org/10.1177/0008417419831800

Provencher, V., Desrosiers, J., Demers, L., & Carmichael, P. H. (2016). Optimizing social participation in community-dwelling older adults through the use of behavioral coping strategies. *Disability and Rehabilitation, 38*(10), 972–978. https://doi.org/10.3109/09638288.2015.1070297

Sanders, M. J., Van Oss, T., Hussey, B., Eich, A., Kapilow, L., & Santoro, D. (2014). Community-based interprofessional experiences in education: Real-life learning about older adults. *Gerontology Special Interest Section Quarterly, 37*(2), 1–4.

Smallfield, S., & Molitor, W. L. (2018). Occupational therapy interventions supporting social participation and leisure engagement for community-dwelling older adults: A systematic review. *American Journal of Occupational Therapy, 72*(4), Article 7204190020. https://doi.org/10.5014/ajot.2018.030627

Wales, K., Clemson, L., Lannin, N., & Cameron, I. (2016). Functional assessments used by occupational therapists with older adults at risk of activity and participation limitations: A systematic Review. *PLOS ONE, 11*(2), Article e0147980. https://doi.org/10.1371/journal.pone.0147980

Wesson, J., Clemson, L., Brodaty, H., & Reppermund, S. (2015). Estimating functional cognition in older adults using observational assessments of task performance in complex everyday activities: A systematic review and evaluation of measurement properties. *Neuroscience & Biobehavioral Reviews, 68,* 335–360. https://doi.org/10.1016/j.neubiorev.2016.05.024

Yu, S. T. S., Yu, M.-L., Brown, T., & Andrews. H. (2018). Association between older adults' functional performance and their scores on the Mini Mental State Examination (MMSE) and Montreal Cognitive Assessment (MoCA). *Irish Journal of Occupational Therapy, 46*(1), 4–23. https://doi.org/10.1108/IJOT-07-2017-0020

Zingmark, M., Fisher, A. G., Rocklöv, J., & Nilsson, I. (2014). Occupation-focused interventions for well older people: An exploratory randomized controlled trial. *Scandinavian Journal of Occupational Therapy, 21*(6), 447–457. https://doi.org/10.3109/11038128.2014.927919

Poverty

Description

Poverty can be viewed from four approaches: monetary, subjective, living conditions, and lack of capacities (Simó Algado et al., 2017). Monetary is the most common and may be described as the condition of not having the means to afford basic human needs such as health care, education, clothing, and shelter as well as lack of material wealth (income, money) needed to maintain existence (Crouch, 2010; O'Toole, 2017). Money can buy health insurance, better nutrition, and housing in safer neighborhoods with play areas, access to good schools, and opportunity to participate in activities to stay physically fit. The subjective approach is based on perceptions of poverty, such as what clothes a person wears or whether the person can provide the children with a good education. Living conditions focus on material deprivation such as food, clothing, housing, employment conditions, health literacy, neighborhood environment, and leisure activities. Lack of capacities involves lack of control over one's life and vulnerability when there is limited access to good paying jobs, adequate housing, quality food, clean water, or other services usually offered by society and communities. Poverty also undermines the ability of a child to develop his or her full capability to achieve essential functioning (Crouch, 2010; Trani et al., 2018).

Cause

Children, older adults, new immigrants, persons with disabilities, and members of ethnic minorities are at greatest risk of poverty (Semega et al., 2017).

Terminology

- *Absolute poverty:* Refers to subsistence below minimum socially acceptable living conditions and requirements for physical well-being (Duncan et al., 2011).
- *Chronic poverty:* People who experience poverty for the duration of their lives or for considerable periods of time (Eidelman et al., 2010).
- *Extreme poverty:* Family cannot fulfill survival needs (Simó Algado et al., 2017).
- *Moderate poverty:* Basic needs are covered but living conditions are precarious (Simó Algado et al., 2017).

- *New poor:* People who have been recently classified as living below the poverty line because of sudden or unexpected circumstances such as serious illness, divorce, or sudden job layoffs (Lysack & Adamo, 2019).
- *Poverty line:* A level of personal or family income below which one is classified as poor according to governmental standards (Semega et al., 2017, reported that 40.6 million Americans were living in poverty).
- *Relative poverty:* People live in rich countries but without access to quality health care, educational services, or leisure and cultural activities (Simó Algado et al., 2017). Relative poverty is described as a level of income or deprivation that falls below a threshold that society deems acceptable (Leadley & Hocking, 2017).
- *Structural poverty:* Person's position in society remains static due to limited access to resources available within the existing social power relations (Eidelman et al., 2010).
- *Working poor:* People who work full time but whose wages do not raise them above the poverty line (Lysack & Adamo, 2019).

Evaluation/Assessment

Areas

- Activities of Daily Living/Instrumental ADL: nutrition, housing, health care
- Education/Work: education level, work history, work skills, employment status
- Play/Leisure: interests, frequency, location
- Rest/Sleep: sleep habits and routines
- Social Participation: type, frequency, location, with whom
- Sensorimotor: physical fitness, sensory stimulation, visual and hearing acuity
- Cognitive/Perceptual: attention, memory, executive functions (problem solving, planning, time management)
- Psychosocial: depression, stress and coping strategies, anxiety, self-identity, self-worth, sense of hopelessness and helplessness, role performance, quality of life
- Context/Environment: political power and politics, societal trends, legal regulations and policies, religious beliefs and traditions, health literacy, neighborhood crime and safety, geographical limitations to accessible resources for food, housing, education, health care, sociocultural and leisure occupations
- Development (Infant, Child, Adolescent only): developmental delay
- Comorbidities: diabetes, obesity, hypertension, cardiovascular disease, substance abuse, asthma, violence, HIV/AIDS, intellectual disability, psychiatric disability, physical disability

Instruments

Instruments Developed by Occupational Therapy Personnel

- Questionnaire of Biopsychosocial Child Characteristics (QBCC; Costa et al., 2018, in References)

Instruments Developed by Other Professionals and Used by Occupational Therapy Personnel

- Denver Developmental Screening Test (2nd ed.; Denver II; Frankenburg et al., 1992)

Problems/Issues

Activities of Daily Living/Instrumental ADL

- Child may be less likely to eat fresh fruit and vegetables on a daily basis.
- Child may have experienced rationing and lack of choice in clothing and footwear.
- Child or person may have experienced lack of a permanent home, shift frequently from one place to another, from one school to another, disrupting schooling and socialization.
- Child or person may have had to delay medical treatment or access to medication because of limited finances.

- Person may have experienced a lack of good nutrition for many years.
- Person may lack access to good housing in safe neighborhood.
- Person may lack access to public transportation.
- Person may report chronic limited finances and high level of debt.
- Person may not have access to regular health care such as a family physician or have health insurance.

Education/Work
- Child may be behind grade level in academic performance.
- Person may not have attained an educational level required for many jobs.
- Person may have limited work skills.
- Person may have a work history of many low paying (minimum wage) jobs.

Play/Leisure
- Child may have limited play skills (imaginative, cooperative).
- Child and person may have limited opportunity to engage in physical activities such as sports and games.
- Person may have limited repertoire of leisure occupations.

Rest/Sleep
- Child and person may have sleep disturbances related to living situation.
- Child may have to share a bed with other siblings or adults.

Social Participation
- Child may have limited opportunity to participate in social activities and may experience social exclusion due to lack of funds or other resources available to children living in middle- or upper-income families.
- Person may have few opportunities due to work schedule to participate in social activities.

Sensorimotor
- Child may demonstrate delay in gross and fine motor skills.
- Child may be less physically active and spend more time in sedentary activities.
- Person may not maintain an exercise or physical fitness program.

Cognitive/Perceptual
- Child may have poor attending behavior.
- Person may have limited problem-solving skills, ability to plan ahead, or ability to create a time schedule.

Psychosocial
- Child or person is likely to have witnessed or have been the victim of maltreatment or violence.
- Person may report high levels of stress including chronic stress related to finances.
- Person may express feelings of anxiety and depression.
- Person may have poor self-concept, self-efficacy, self-identity.
- Person may have poor sense of self-worth or self-confidence.
- Person may have poor quality of life and life satisfaction.

Context/Environment
- Child or person may live in housing that is damp and cold, placing person at higher risk for respiratory illnesses.
- Person may live in high crime area, limiting opportunities for play activities for children and outside activities for adults.
- Person may have limited health literacy about health conditions that person already has or may be at risk for incurring in the future.

- Person may live in a "food desert" where there is limited or no access to fresh fruit, vegetables, or meat within miles of the dwelling or is accessible by public transit.
- Person may have limited access to health care services that are affordable or free.
- Person may have a history of religious or cultural traditions that limit thinking about health and health-care services.
- Person may have limited knowledge of available community resources or access to those resources.
- Person may not have access to internet or other computer-based resources.

Intervention/Treatment

Models and programs developed by occupational therapy personnel include Doing, Being, and Becoming (Duncan et al., 2011) and occupational justice (Simó Algado et al., 2017). Models and programs developed by other professionals but used by occupational therapy personnel include the Moli Mierons Project in Spain (Simó Algado et al., 2017). Team members include physicians, psychiatrists, psychologists, nursing personnel, educators, public health workers, social workers, city planners, politicians, and occupational therapy personnel. Goals are to address the needs for improved access to and performance of self-care, productive, and leisure occupations and to improve quality of life and life satisfaction.

Activities of Daily Living/Instrumental ADL
- Assist adult client or clients to access, plan, and prepare meals that include fresh fruits, vegetables, and meat within a limited budget.
- Assist adult client to manage finances including budgeting and financial planning.
- Tailor intervention options in accordance with the person's financial ability.

Education/Work
- Assist child to perform academic tasks including modifying tasks or using adapted equipment.
- Assist child to participate in school activities.
- Assist adult client to explore and develop work skills and employment opportunities.

Play/Leisure
- Assist child to develop play skills including imaginative and cooperative play.
- Assist adult client to explore and develop leisure occupations.

Rest/Sleep
- Assist child and adult clients to review sleep habits and routines to improve quality of sleep.

Social Participation
- Assist child and adult to participate in social and cultural activities available within available finances such as free concerts or practice sporting events open to the public.

Sensorimotor
- Assist child to develop gross and fine motor skills.
- Assist adult client to develop and maintain a physical fitness program including home exercises.
- Group exercise programs can be used.

Cognitive/Perceptual
- Assist child to develop cognitive skills (attending, memory, learning, executive skills).
- Assist adult client to develop and implement problem-solving strategies.
- Group planning sessions can be used.

Psychosocial
- Assist adult client to explore which of the following extrinsic coping strategies can be useful (Duncan et al., 2011).

- ▶ Bartering/bargaining/begging: Strategy for acquiring marketable good for a business or acquiring material goods for subsistence by offering something in exchange (other than money), such as cleaning a house in exchange for items of clothing.
- ▶ Borrowing and lending: Asking for or extending loans in cash or in-kind from and to people who are related (family or boarders) to the borrower or lender. However, running a lending business is different and usually requires a business license and/or access to an account.
- ▶ Caring: Caring for other people's children (caring for family member's children is most common; however, running a daycare or nursery school program is different. Many states require a facility license and/or specialized training required for the person operating the facility).
- ▶ Laboring: Selling homemade objects such as soap, candy, cookies, cakes, items of clothing or jewelry.
- ▶ Networking: Involves building and maintaining an informal economy of family and friends that supports the exchange of cash and in-kind services. Each member is known to provide a given service, which others can request at a stated price in money or in-kind services.
- ▶ Preserving: Strategy to turn discarded objects into functional ones or finding ways to make produce last longer, such as using tin cans instead of buying flower pots.
- ▶ Pursuing: Following up leads for potential sources of income such as odd jobs as day workers, and often in addition, looking for ways to bypass regulatory structures to avoid paying fees for public services such as bus or train fares.
- ▶ Saving: Strategies to "stretch the money or dollar" such as buying in bulk, looking for advertised or unadvertised specials, joining an informal saving association or co-op, or being judicious in use of goods including reusing items intended for single use such as washing plastic utensils.
- ▶ Trading: Short-term pick-up work in return for needed service such as sweeping for floor of a restaurant for 15 minutes in return for lunch.
- ● Assist adult client to explore the importance of intrinsic coping strategies to life situation (Duncan et al., 2011).
  - ▶ Dignity stance: "Refers to the innate sense of pride and self-worth" that enables a person "to keep the indignity and dehumanizing effects of poverty at bay" (Duncan, 2011, p. 67).
  - ▶ Moral stance: Provides the cultural and spiritual value base from which the person operates, such as commitment to family, honoring parents, or spirit of self-discipline.
  - ▶ Preemptive stance: Planning in advance to ensure "proactive management of anticipated or imminent set backs related to health, social events and household dynamics" (Duncan, 2011, p. 67). Examples: Choosing not to work outside (as a day laborer) when it's raining, having fellow workers remind person to take medications when he became quarrelsome.
  - ▶ Opportunistic stance: Demonstrating cunning in reading, interpreting and anticipating situations or events as potentially income generating such as checking dates of upcoming sporting events and making arrangements for paid parking at a vacant lot nearby, or making special objects to sell to commemorate a certain event.
  - ▶ Trade-off stance: "Doing a favour or helping someone to bank goodwill in anticipation of trading in on it at a later stage" (Duncan, 2011, p. 67). Trade-offs are sometimes viewed as manipulative, exploitative, or immoral, especially if the favor is viewed as taking advantage of someone's condition (disability) or immediate situation (car breaks down; Duncan, 2011).

Context/Environment

- ● Educate clients about available services within personal financial means, especially among older individuals who may have less access to information about available services (Walsh, 2016).
- ● Advocate for "children's right to education, and to engage in leisure, play, artistic and cultural activities" (Leadley & Hocking, 2017).
- ● Act as an advocate for improved services for people living in poverty.

- Advocate for policies to reduce economic disparities to ensure equal access to health-care services.
- Identify stakeholders that can be approached and organized to improve services for people living in poverty.
- Assist client or clients to become advocates in their own right to improve services in their neighborhood.

Precautions/Safety Considerations

Assist clients to improve or increase safety in the neighborhood generally, and for the individual, safety is a consideration. Therapists must be realistic about working with clients who live in poverty with the goal of improving clients' ability to survive within the poverty environment, but not expect that intervention will result in the client getting out of poverty. The exception is a client who has temporarily experienced poverty but who previously had the resources to live above the poverty level.

Prognosis and Outcome

Clients can learn to make better use of existing resources but usually remain within the poverty level.

REFERENCES

Costa, E. F., Chaves Cavalcante, L. I., Said de Lima, S., & de Nazaré Alencar, C. (2018). Family poverty, neuropsychomotor development and children's play in the insular and continental regions of Belém. *Revista de Terapia Ocupacional da Universidade de São Paulo, 29*(2), 179–186. https://doi.org/10.11606/issn.2238-6149.v29i2p179-186

Crouch, R. (2010) The impact of poverty on the service delivery of occupational therapy in Africa. In V. Alers & R. Crouch (Eds.), *Occupational therapy: An African perspective* (pp. 98–111). Sarah Shorten.

Duncan, M., Swartz, L., & Kathard, H. (2011). The burden of psychiatric disability on chronically poor households: Part 2 (coping). *South African Journal of Occupational Therapy, 41*(2), 64–70.

Eidelman, T., Gouws, V., Howe, C., Kulber, T., Küm, J., Schoenfeld, L., & Duncan, M. (2010). Women surviving chronic poverty and psychiatric disability. *South African Journal of Occupational Therapy, 40*(3), 4–8.

Leadley, S., & Hocking, C. (2017). An occupational perspective of childhood poverty. *New Zealand Journal of Occupational Therapy, 64*(1), 23–31.

Lysack, C. L., & Adamo, D. E. (2019). Social, economic, and political factors that influence occupational performance. In B. A. Boyt Schell & G. Gillen (Eds.), *Willard and Spackman's occupational therapy* (13th ed., pp. 240–255). Wolters Kluwer.

O'Toole, M. T. (Ed.). (2017). *Mosby's dictionary of medicine, nursing & health professions* (10th ed.). Elsevier.

Semega, J. L., Fontenot, K. R., & Kollar, M. A. (2017). *Income and poverty in the United States: 2016.* U.S. Census Bureau. https://census.gov/content/dam/Census/library/publications/2017/demo/P60-259.pdf

Simó Algado, S., de San Eugenio, J., & Ginesta, X. (2017). Promoting active citizenship against poverty through a participatory community intervention In D. Sakellariou & N. Pollard (Eds.), *Occupational therapies without borders* (2nd ed., pp. 355–362). Elsevier.

Trani, J. F., Bakhshi, P., Brown, D., Lopez, D., & Gall, F. (2018). Disability as deprivation of capabilities: Estimation using a large-scale survey in Morocco and Tunisia and an instrumental variable approach. *Social Science & Medicine, 211*, 48–60. https://doi.org/10.1016/j.socscimed.2018.05.033

Walsh, H. A. (2016). Examining the impact of poverty on older adults' occupations and health care. *Occupational Therapy Now*, 18(2), 28-30.

BIBLIOGRAPHY

Duncan, M., Swartz, K., & Kathard, H. (2010). The burden of psychiatric disability on chronically poor households: Part 1 (costs). *South African Journal of Occupational Therapy*, 41(3), 55–63.

Retirement

Description

Retirement is the exit from the labor force taken by an individual and taken with the intention of reducing or ceasing the psychological commitment to (full-time paid) work thereafter (Brown, 2018). Retirement is often the first major transition faced by the elderly. Work has been a major occupation in the individual's life for 40 to 50 years. The occupational transition from worker role to retiree affects physical and mental health depending on the person's attitude toward and reason for retiring (Porter, 2018). Habits, routines, and time management are all affected, and the transition to retirement may be a period of significant readjustment (Pettican & Prior, 2011). For some individuals the transitions are welcomed, but for other individuals the process of adapting to full-time retiree is accompanied by the unwelcomed loss of values and meaning in life (Jonsson, 2010). Cutchin et al. (2010) identified the 10 most common occupations for persons after moving to a retirement community: reading, eating out at a restaurant, grocery shopping, watching television, visiting friends or family, exercising outside of the home, attending concerts, shopping (nongrocery), attending parties, and attending movies. Note that some individuals may continue to engage in in work-related activities by participating in part-time paid work or volunteer and unpaid work.

Cause

Some people choose to retire, having looked forward to quitting work (voluntary retirement); others are forced to retire because of health problems or job loss (involuntary retirement; Porter, 2018).

Terminology

- *Bridge employment:* Changing jobs or moving to part-time employment as a means of transitioning to retirement (Braveman et al., 2018).
- *Disability retirement:* Cessation from work that occurs earlier than expected in the person's life course because of a chronic health issue (Brown, 2018).
- *Phased retirement:* Person stays with the same employer while gradually reducing work hours and effort (Braveman et al., 2018).
- *Senior residential care settings:* Facilities that provide continuing care and housing for older individuals such as assisted living and skilled nursing care facilities.
- *Retirement center:* A facility or organized program to provide social services and activities for senior citizens who generally do not require ongoing health care (O'Toole, 2017).

Evaluation/Assessment

Areas

- Activities of Daily Living/Instrumental ADL: health status, financial resources and management, caregiving, habits, and routines
- Education/Work: paid work, unpaid or volunteer work, workplace accommodation
- Play/Leisure: interests, types, frequency, location

- Rest/Sleep: no information identified
- Social Participation: type, frequency, location, with whom
- Sensorimotor: physical strength, grip strength, endurance, balance, reaction time, temperature (thermal) tolerance, visual acuity, hearing acuity
- Cognitive/Perceptual: attention, memory, learning, executive functions (problem solving, planning, time management)
- Psychosocial: self-concept, self-image, self-identity, self-worth, attitudes, stress, role performance, isolation, spirituality, sense of meaningfulness, quality of life
- Context/Environment: cultural values and beliefs, social expectations, environmental modification, community resources
- Comorbidities: multiple sclerosis, other chronic health conditions

Instruments
Instruments Developed by Occupational Therapy Personnel
- Model of Human Occupation Screening Tool (Version 2.0; MOHOST 2.0; Parkinson et al., 2006)
- National Institutes of Health (NIH) Activity Record (ACTRE; Gerber & Furst, 1992)
- Occupational Performance History Interview (Version 2.1; OPHI-II; Kielhofner et al., 2004)
- Work Environment and Impact Scale (WEIS; Moore-Corner et al., 1998)
- Worker Role Interview (Version 10.0; WRI 10.0; Braveman et al., 2005)

Instruments Development by Other Professionals and Used by Occupational Therapy Personnel
- None identified

Problems/Issues
Activities of Daily Living/Instrumental ADL
- Person may have difficulty managing finances.
- Person may have difficulty performing caregiving activities.

Education/Work
- Person may need workplace accommodation.

Play/Leisure
- Person may to adapt or modify engagement in leisure occupations.
- Person may need to explore new leisure occupation.

Rest/Sleep
- No information identified.

Social Participation
- Person may lose social contacts from work setting after retirement.
- Person may be unable to participate in certain social activities due to changes in health status.

Sensorimotor
- Person may need an exercise program to maintain physical fitness.

Cognitive/Perceptual
- Person may have cognitive impairments due to health conditions.
- Person may have difficulty with time management when use of time must be self-managed.
- Person may have difficulty with problem solving.
- Person may have difficulty planning ahead.

Psychosocial
- Person may feel a loss of self-worth and self-identity after retirement (as though a part of the person's being had been amputated; Jonsson, 2010).

- Person may become isolated with few or no social companions that are not connected to former work settings.
- Person may report that everyday life is boring and there is nothing to do without the routine and structure that working provided.
- Person may report a loss of connectedness and "team player" that working with others provided.
- Person may experience a reduced quality of life and life satisfaction.
- Person may have negative attitudes toward retirement resulting in failure to plan and participate in available resources.
- Person may feel stressed and unable to cope with tradition from worker role to retiree role.

Context/Environment

- Person may have negative values and beliefs about retirement.
- Person may lack knowledge about available resources.
- Person may benefit from environmental modification.

Intervention/Treatment

Models and programs developed by occupational therapy personnel include the Model of Human Occupation (MOHO; Brown, 2018; Eagers et al., 2016, 2019; Hewitt et al., 2010; Pepin & Deutscher, 2011), Canadian Model of Performance–Engagement (CMOP-E; Brown, 2018), incorporating technology (Emas et al., 2018), Lifestyle Redesign (Mountain & Craig, 2011), person-environment-occupation model (Walker & McNamara, 2013), and technology training (Emas et al., 2018). Models and programs developed by other professionals but used by occupational therapy personnel include continuity theory (Braveman et al., 2018; Eagers et al., 2016; Hewitt et al., 2010), embodiment (Laliberte Rudman, 2015), Foucauldian theory (Laliberte Rudman, 2015), life-course approach (Braveman et al., 2018), life-span development (Braveman et al., 2018), resource-based dynamic longitudinal perspective (Brown, 2018), and stage theory (Braveman et al., 2018). Team members include physicians, psychologists, recreation specialists, vocational rehabilitation counselors, social workers, case managers, and occupational therapy personal. Goal is to facilitate a successful transition from the role of paid worker to a satisfactory balance of productivity and leisure occupations while maintaining self-care and maintenance occupations (Braveman et al., 2018).

Activities of Daily Living/Instrumental ADL

- Review with client if adaptations or modifications are needed to perform self-care skills. Example: bathrooms (Morales et al., 2012).
- Review with client if adaptations or modifications are needed to perform independent living skills such as housekeeping tasks, grocery shopping, transportation, eating at restaurants, entertaining friends and family, caring for grandchildren or pets.
- Assist client to manage finances including budgeting.
- Assist client to plan for moving from a home or apartment to a retirement community.

Education/Work

- Assist client to explore if adult education programs may be of interest.
- Assist client to decide if part-time work in the same occupation or different occupation may be of interest.
- Review with client possible part-time or temporary options to consider such as job sharing, reduced work schedules, rehiring retirees on a part-time or temporary basis, using retirees as contractors or consultants on an as-needed basis.
- Assist client to identify and try out voluntary, charity, or other unpaid work.
- Assist employers to develop work-to-nonwork transition programs.

Play/Leisure
- Assist client to maintain or expand engagement in existing leisure occupations.
- Consider if existing leisure occupations need to be modified or adapted to better fit client's existing abilities and capacities.
- Assist client to explore and develop new leisure occupations.

Rest/Sleep
- No information identified.

Social Participation
- Assist client to maintain participation in existing social or cultural activities.
- Assist client to explore and develop new social or cultural activities (movies, concerts, social clubs, organizational meetings, museums, religious services).

Sensorimotor
- Assist client to develop and implement an exercise plan and physical fitness program.

Cognitive/Perceptual
- Assist client to plan ahead for retirement (total retirement, working part-time, volunteering a number of hours, identified leisure and social activities, exercise program, budget).
- Assist client with time management skills (scheduling, organizing activities, making lists).

Psychosocial
- Assist client to identify occupations that have meaning and purpose whether paid or unpaid, work or leisure, social or alone, mental or physical or other dimension.

Context/Environment
- Assist client to identify and explore available resources in the community.

Precautions/Safety Considerations
No information identified.

Prognosis and Outcome
Prognosis of clients with persistent deficits is typically poor. Clients with minimally conscious state tend to improve (Porter, 2018). Cole and Macdonald (2011) suggested three roles for retired occupational therapy personnel: promote volunteer exploration and participation for older adults with disabilities, provide group interventions for persons transitioning to retirement, and consult with organizations that depend on volunteers to guide them in revising the way they define and organize volunteer roles.

REFERENCES
Braveman, B., Bowyer, P., & Fogerty, R. E. (2018). Work and retirement. In B. R. Bonder & V. D. Bello-Haas (Eds.), *Functional performance in older adults* (4th ed., pp. 313–325). F.A. Davis.
Brown, C. L. (2018). Expanding the occupational therapy role to support transitions from work to retirement for people with progressive health conditions. *American Journal of Occupational Therapy, 72*(6), Article 7206347010. https://doi.org/10.5014/ajot.2018.028407
Cole, M. B., & Macdonald, K. C. (2011). Retired occupational therapists' experiences in volunteer occupations. *Occupational Therapy International, 18*(1), 18–31. https://doi.org/10.1002/oti.307
Cutchin, M. P., Marshall, V. W., & Aldrich, R. (2010). Moving to a continuing care retirement community: Occupations in the therapeutic landscape process. *Journal of Cross-Cultural Gerontology, 25*, 117–132. https://doi.org/10.1007/s10823-010-9113-y
Eagers, J., Franklin, R. C., Broome, K., & Yau, M. K. (2016). A review of occupational therapy's contribution to and involvement in the work-to-retirement transition process: An Australian

perspective. *Australian Occupational Therapy Journal, 63*(4), 277–292. https://doi.org/10.1111/1440-1630.12300

Eagers, J., Franklin, R. C., Broome, K., & Yau, M. K. (2019). The experiences of work: Retirees' perspectives and the relationship to the role of occupational therapy in the work-to-retirement transition process. *Work, 64*(2), 341–354. https://doi.org/10.3233/WOR-192996

Emas, S., Montoya, L., Chen, A., Tran, C., Tran, P., & Dharni, A. (2018). Empowering older adults: Incorporating technology for retirement adjustment. *Physical & Occupational Therapy in Geriatrics, 36*(2-3), 245–257. https://doi.org/10.1080/02703181.2018.1497747

Hewitt, A., Howie, L., & Feldman, S. (2010). Retirement: What will you do? A narrative inquiry of occupation-based planning for retirement: Implications for practice. *Australian Occupational Therapy Journal, 57*(1), 8–16. https://doi.org/10.1111/j.1440-1630.2009.00820.x

Jonsson, H. (2010). Occupational transitions: Work to retirement. In C. H. Christiansen & E. A. Townsend (Eds.), *Introduction to occupation: The art and science of living* (2nd ed., pp. 211–230). Pearson.

Laliberte Rudman, D. (2015). Embodying positive aging and neoliberal rationality: Talking about the aging body within narratives of retirement. *Journal of Aging Studies, 34*, 10–20. https://doi.org/10.1016/j.jaging.2015.03.005

Morales, E., Rousseau, J., & Passini, R. (2012). Bathrooms in retirement residences: Perceptions and experiences of seniors and caregivers. *Physical & Occupational Therapy in Geriatrics, 30*(1), 1–21. https://doi.org/10.3109/02703181.2011.644656

Mountain, G. A., & Craig, C. L. (2011). The lived experience of redesigning lifestyle post-retirement in the UK. *Occupational Therapy International, 18*, 48–58. https://doi.org/10.1002/oti.309

O'Toole, M. T. (Ed.). (2017). *Mosby's dictionary of medicine, nursing & health professions* (10th ed.). Elsevier.

Pepin, G., & Deutscher, B. (2011). The lived experience of Australian retirees: "I'm retired, what do I do now?" *British Journal of Occupational Therapy, 74*(9), 419–426. https://doi.org/10.4276/030802211X13153015305556

Pettican, A., & Prior, S. (2011). "It's a new way of life": An exploration of the occupational transition of retirement. *British Journal of Occupational Therapy, 74*(1), 12–19. https://doi.org/10.4276/030802211X12947686093521

Porter, R. S. (Ed.). (2018). *The Merck manual of diagnosis and therapy* (20th ed.). Merck Sharp & Dohme.

Walker, E., & McNamara, B. (2013). Relocating to retirement living: An occupational perspective on successful transitions. *Australian Occupational Therapy Journal, 60*(6), 445–453. https://doi.org/10.1111/1440-1630.12038

BIBLIOGRAPHY

Eagers, J., Franklin, R. C., Yau, M. K., & Broome, K. (2018). Pre-retirement job and the work-to-retirement occupational transition process in Australia: A review. *Australian Occupational Therapy Journal, 65*(4), 314–328. https://doi.org/10.1111/1440-1630.12452

Embrey, E., & Zur, B. (2017). Continuing the mind and spirit of occupational therapy in retirement. *Occupational Therapy Now, 19*(3), 22–24.

Goods, N., & Millsteed, J. (2016). Understanding retirement for ageing adults with a disability in supported employment. *British Journal of Occupational Therapy, 79*(11), 713–721. https://doi.org/10.1177/0308022616662051

Jonsson, H. (2011). The first steps into the third age: The retirement process from a Swedish perspective. *Occupational Therapy International, 18*, 32–38. https://doi.org/10.1002/oti.311

Laliberte Rudman, D. (2014). Reflecting on the socially situated and constructed nature of occupation: A research program addressing the contemporary restructure of retirement. In D. Pierce (Ed.), *Occupational science for occupational therapy* (pp. 143–156). Slack.

Laliberte Rudman, D. (2015). Situating occupation in social relations of power: Occupational possibilities, ageism and the retirement "choice." *South African Journal of Occupational Therapy*, 45(1), 27–33. http://dx.doi.org/10.17159/2310-3833/2015/v45no1a5

Oakman, J., & Howie, L. (2013). How can organisations influence their older employees' decision of when to retire? *Work, 45*(3), 389–397. https://doi.org/10.3233/WOR-2012-1403

Sleep–Wake Disorders

Description

Sleep is a physiological state of relative unconsciousness and inaction of the voluntary or skeletal muscles, the need for which recurs periodically (*Stedman's*, 2011). Metabolism is also depressed (O'Toole, 2017). The stages of sleep have been variously defined in terms of depth (light, deep), electroencephalographic characteristics (delta waves, synchronization), physiologic characteristics, and presumed anatomic level (pontine, mesencephalic, rhombencephalic, and rolandic (*Stedman's*, 2011). Porter (2018) described two states of sleep: nonrapid eye movement (NREM) constituting about 75% to 80% of total sleep time in adults with three stages (N1, N2, and N3) in increasing depth of sleep, and rapid eye movement (REM) sleep that follows each cycle of NREM sleep. During N1, the brain waves are of the theta type, followed in N2 by the appearance of distinctive sleep spindles, and N3 in which delta waves appear (O'Toole, 2017). Sleep–wake disorders include insomnia disorder, hypersomnolence disorder, narcolepsy, obstructive sleep apnea hypopnea, central sleep apnea, sleep-related hypoventilation, circadian rhythm disorders, nonrapid eye movement sleep arousal disorders, nightmare disorder, rapid eye movement sleep behavior disorder, restless legs syndrome, and substance/medication-induced sleep disorder (American Psychiatric Association, 2013). Disordered sleep can cause emotional disturbance, memory difficulty, poor motor skills, decreased work efficiency, and increased risk of traffic accidents. It can also contribute to cardiovascular disorders and mortality (Porter, 2018). The most common sleep-related symptoms are insomnia (difficulty falling or staying asleep, early awaking or a sensation of unrefreshing sleep) and excessive daytime sleepiness (EDS), a tendency to fall asleep during normal waking hours (Porter, 2018).

Cause

Multiple causes are known including structural changes to the breathing system, pain, brain injury, physical injury, neurological changes, mental health problems, and development and aging issues. Causes of insomnia include inadequate sleep hygiene, adjustment insomnia, psychophysiologic insomnia, physical or mental sleep disorders, drug-dependent and drug-induced sleep disorders, central sleep apnea syndrome, circadian rhythm sleep disorders, periodic limb movement disorder, and restless legs syndrome. Cause of excessive daytime sleepiness include inadequate sleep hygiene, physical or mental sleep disorders, insufficient sleep syndrome, drug-dependent and drug-induced sleep disorders, obstructive sleep apnea, circadian rhythm sleep disorders, narcolepsy, and periodic limb movement disorder (Porter, 2018).

Terminology (Adapted from Porter, 2018, except where noted)

- *Adjustment insomnia:* Results from acute emotional stressors that disrupt sleep, such as loss of job, hospitalization.
- *Central sleep apnea:* Consists of repeated episodes of breathing cessation or shallow breathing during sleep, lasting at least 10 seconds and caused by diminished respiratory effort and manifested as insomnia or disturbed and unrefreshing sleep.
- *Circadian rhythm disorders:* Result in misalignment between endogenous sleep–wake rhythms and environmental light–darkness cycle, such as may occur with jet lag or shift work.

- *Drug-related sleep disorders:* "Result from chronic use of or withdrawal from various drugs" (Porter, 2018, p. 2014).
- *Hypersomnolence disorder:* Self-reported excessive sleepiness despite a main sleep period lasting at least seven hours occurring on a repeated sequence during a day, week or month (American Psychiatric Association, 2013).
- *Idiopathic hypersomnia:* Excessive daytime sleepiness with or without a long sleep time. Disorder is differentiated by lack of cataplexy, hypnogogic hallucinations, or sleep paralysis.
- *Inadequate sleep hygiene:* Refers to behaviors that are not conducive to sleep, including consumption of caffeine or other stimulant drugs, exercise or excitement, or an irregular sleep–wake schedule.
- *Insufficient sleep syndrome:* "Involves not sleeping enough at night despite adequate opportunity to do so, typically because of various social or employment commitments" (Porter, 2018, p. 2014).
- *Major mental disorders:* Most depression and mood disorders are associated with insomnia or excessive daytime sleepiness.
- *Narcolepsy:* Characterized by chronic excessive daytime sleepiness with cataplexy (sudden loss of muscle tone), sleep paralysis, and hypnagogic or hypnopompic hallucinations ("vivid auditory or visual illusions or hallucinations that occur when just falling asleep [hypnagogic] or immediately after awakening [hypnopompic]"; Porter, 2018, p. 2015).
- *Nightmare disorder:* Characterized by repeated occurrence of extended, extremely dysphoric, and well-remembered dreams that usually involve efforts to avoid threats to survival, security, or physical integrity and generally occur during second half of major sleep episode (American Psychiatric Association, 2013).
- *Nonrapid eye movement sleep arousal disorder:* Characterized by recurrent episodes of incomplete awakening from sleep, usually occurring during the first third of a major sleep episode accompanied by either sleepwalking or sleep terrors (American Psychiatric Association, 2013).
- *Obstructive sleep apnea (OSA):* "Consists of episodes of partial or complete closure of the upper airway during sleep, leading to cessation of breathing" for 10 seconds or longer (Porter, 2018, p. 2014). Person may snore or wake up gasping and report unrefreshing sleep or excessive daytime sleepiness.
- *Periodic limb movement disorder (PLMD):* Characterized by repetitive twitching or kicking of the lower extremities during sleep. Person is typically unaware of the movements and brief arousal that may follow but may complain of interrupted nocturnal sleep or excessive daytime sleepiness.
- *Psychophysiologic insomnia:* Insomnia that "persists well beyond resolution of precipitating factors," such as anticipatory anxiety about another sleepless night (Porter, 2018, p. 2014).
- *Physical disorders:* Those that cause pain or discomfort, such as arthritis, cancer, or herniated disk, particularly those that worsen with movement.
- *Rapid eye movement sleep behavior disorder:* Characterized by repeated episodes or arousal during sleep associated with vocalization and/or complex motor behaviors (American Psychiatric Association, 2013).
- *Restless legs syndrome:* Characterized by an irresistible urge to move the legs that may be accompanied by paresthesia in the limbs when reclining; as a result, person may have difficulty falling asleep, have repeated nocturnal awakenings, or both.
- *Sleep deprivation:* Result of interference with basic physiological urge to sleep that can cause significant reduction in performance and alertness (O'Toole, 2017).
- *Sleep disorder:* "A persistent disturbance of typical sleep patterns (including the amount, quality, and timing of sleep) or the chronic occurrence of abnormal events or behavior during sleep" (VandenBos, 2015, p. 987).
- *Sleep hygiene:* "Techniques for the behavioral treatment of insomnia that involve instructions given to the client to follow certain routines aimed at improving sleep patterns," such using

bed for sleep and sex only, not napping during the day, decreasing caffeine intake, going to bed at a regular set time, and keeping a sleep diary (VandenBos, 2015. p. 988).

- *Sleep-related hypoventilation:* Demonstrated by episodes of decreased respiration associated with elevated CO_2 levels (American Psychiatric Association, 2013).
- *Sleep–wake schedule disorder:* A form of dyssomnia caused by a conflict between a person's circadian rhythm and socioeconomic demands of society, such as work or travel schedules (O'Toole, 2017).
- *Substance/medication-induced sleep disorder:* Characterized by a prominent and severe disturbance in sleep with evidence of history, physical examination, or laboratory findings of substance intoxication or withdrawal from or exposure to a medication capable of producing the symptoms.

Evaluation/Assessment
Areas
- Activities of Daily Living/Instrumental ADL: self-care (effective performance), driving, meal preparation
- Education/Work: work tasks (effective performance), child care
- Play/Leisure: engagement
- Rest/Sleep: symptoms of sleep disturbances and/or disorders
- Social Participation: engagement
- Sensorimotor: auditory, visual, tactile, proprioception, hypersensitivity
- Cognitive/Perceptual: awareness, arousal, memory, time management/scheduling
- Psychosocial: role performance, anxiety, depression
- Context/Environment: light, noise/sound, bedding
- Comorbidities:
  - Acquired/traumatic brain injury (Biajar et al., 2017; Duclos et al., 2015; Fogelberg et al., 2012; Fogelberg et al., 2016; Mollayeva et al., 2013; Mollayeva, Mollayeva, & Colantonio, 2016; Mollayeva, Mollayeva, et al., 2016; Mollayeva, Pratt, et al., 2016; Picard, 2017; Wiseman-Hakes et al., 2013)
  - Affective disorders, including bipolar (Engel-Yeger et al., 2017)
  - Attention-deficit/hyperactivity disorder (Brown et al., 2012)
  - Autistic spectrum disorder (American Occupational Therapy Association, 2017; Brown et al., 2012; Cuomo et al., 2017; Schoen et al., 2017; Weaver, 2015)
  - Borderline personality disorder (Wood et al., 2015)
  - Cerebral palsy (Brown et al., 2012)
  - Chronic obstructive pulmonary disease (Oh et al., 2016)
  - Chronic pain (Barnhouse, 2019)
  - Depression (Hamera et al., 2013)
  - Developmental delay (Brown et al., 2012; Casey et al., 2019)
  - Down syndrome (Brown et al., 2012)
  - Infants (Thomas et al., 2015)
  - Intellectual disability (Casey et al., 2019)
  - Multiple sclerosis (Fogelberg et al., 2016)
  - Older adults (American Occupational Therapy Association, 2017; Leland et al., 2016; Leland et al., 2014; Picard, 2017; Sheth & Thomas, 2019; Smallfield & Molitor, 2018)
  - Parkinson's disease (Johnson & Westlake, 2018)
  - Posttraumatic stress disorder (Mollayeva et al., 2017)
  - Psychiatric or mental health conditions (Barnhouse, 2019; Gardner et al., 2017)
  - Sensory integration dysfunction (Milton & Lovett, 2014)
  - Sensory processing patterns (Engel-Yeger & Shochat, 2012)
  - Sjögren's syndrome (Hackett et al., 2018; Hackett et al., 2017)

▸ Spinal cord injury (Fogelberg et al., 2016; Fogelberg et al., 2017)
▸ Stroke (Park, 2019a, 2019b)

Instruments

Instruments Developed by Occupational Therapy Personnel

- Adolescent/Adult Sensory Profile (AASP; Brown & Dunn, 2002)
- Canadian Occupational Performance Measure (5th ed.; COPM-5; Law et al., 2014)
- Daily Cognitive-Communication and Sleep Profile (DCCASP; Fung et al., 2013, in References)
- Occupational Profile of Sleep (OPOS; Pierce & Summers, 2011, 2019, in References)

Instruments Developed by Other Professionals and Used by Occupational Therapy Personnel

- ActiGraph Accelerometer (measurement instrument)
- Beck Depression Inventory (2nd ed.; BDI-II; Beck et al., 1996)
- Dysfunctional Beliefs and Attitudes about Sleep Scale (DBAS-16; Morin et al., 2007)
- Dysfunctional Beliefs and Attitudes about Sleep Scale (DBAS-28; Morin et al., 1993)
- Epworth Sleepiness Scale (ESS; Johns, 1991)
- Functional range of motion (especially ability to turn/roll body from supine to prone and back again)
- General Sleep Disturbance Scale (GSDS; Lee, 1992)
- Patient-Reported Outcomes Measurement Information System (PROMIS; Hahn et al., 2014)
- Pittsburgh Sleep Quality Index (PSQI, Buysse et al., 1989)
- Polysomnography (measurement instrument)

Problems/Issues

Activities of Daily Living/Instrumental ADL

- Person may fail to perform or perform poorly certain self-care activities due to lack of sleep or drowsiness.
- Person may be eating a full meal just before going to bed or preparing to go to sleep.
- Person may experience urinary frequency that requires getting out of bed frequently during sleep cycle.
- Person may endanger self and others while preparing or serving meals due to lack of sleep or drowsiness.
- Person may endanger self and others when driving a vehicle while drowsy.

Education/Work

- Person may fail to perform or perform poorly certain work tasks due to lack of sleep or drowsiness.
- Person may endanger self and others while operating equipment when drowsy.
- Person may have a night job which forces the person to sleep during the day when most people are awake and moving about.
- Person may fall asleep during time he or she is responsible for watching and caring for young children thus endangering their safety.

Play/Leisure

- Person may not engage in leisure activities due to lack of sleep or drowsiness.

Rest/Sleep

- Person may fall asleep during the daytime hours (not due to narcolepsy).
- Person may use sleep to avoid performing undesirable tasks or situations.
- Person may report that sleep disturbances are interfering with daily activities performance.

Social Participation

- Person may use lack of sleep as an avoidance technique to avoid engaging in social activities.

Sensorimotor

- Person may be sensitive to visual stimuli such as bright lights, blue light from screens, blinking lights from traffic lights or electronic devices.
- Person may be sensitive to sounds or noises such as people talking, traffic noise, animal noises, electronic devices.
- Person may be sensitive to touch, such as bedding that is perceived to be scratchy or itchy.
- Person may be sensitive to perceived hardness or softness of the mattress or other sleeping surface.
- Person may experience pain while trying to sleep, which delays going to sleep or wakes the person up during sleep cycle.
- Person may demonstrate hypersensitivity to certain stimuli (Engel-Yeger et al., 2017).

Cognitive/Perceptual

- Person may have difficulty paying attention to what is being said by other people.
- Person may have difficulty maintaining level of arousal needed to perform tasks.
- Person may experience difficulty with memory tasks.
- Person may experience difficulty with executive functions such as judgment, problem solving, decision making.

Psychosocial

- Person may experience nightmares, night terrors, or flashbacks.
- Person may be aware that performance is not "up to par."
- Person may avoid social situations because of past experience where family or friends complained about poor attending behavior or tasks performance.

Context/Environment

- Person's environment may contain elements that are barriers to good sleep habits and routines.
  - Person may experience the effects of lights or lighting that may be too bright or provide intermittent brightness including electronic devices, outside security lights, advertising signs, traffic lights.
  - Person may experience noises or unwanted sounds that interfere with sleep.
  - Person may experience temperatures that are too hot or cold to promote sleep.
  - Person may have bedding or sleeping conditions that are uncomfortable to body positions.
  - Person may have bedding that is uncomfortable due to tactile stimuli, such as does not stay in place when person changes positions.
- Person, family, caregivers, and others may lack information on the importance of sleep habits and routines and the environmental factors that contribute to promoting restful and refreshing sleep.

Intervention/Treatment

Models and programs developed by occupational therapy personnel include lifestyle redesign (Blanchard et al., 2015; Leland et al., 2016), person-environment-occupation (Biajar et al., 2017), and person-environment-occupation-performance (PEOP; Ho & Siu, 2018). Models and programs developed by other professionals but used by occupational therapy personnel include music (Harris, 2014), oral-pharyngeal motor training (Cheng et al., 2017), positioning (Inncente, 2014; Jarus et al., 2011), Restoring Effective Sleep Tranquility (REST; Eakman et al., 2017), and sleep tool education (Farrehi et al., 2016). Team members include physicians, nursing personnel, psychologists, and occupational therapy personnel. The goal of intervention is to create sleep habits and routines, and a sleeping environment that promotes sleep that is restful and refreshing to the individual and promotes optimal occupational performance, participation, and engagement in daily life (Picard, 2017). Occupational therapy personnel should always refer a client to a physician, psychiatrist, or sleep specialist if a sleep disorder—such as obstructed sleep apnea, narcolepsy, or chronic obstructive pulmonary disease—is suspected.

Activities of Daily Living/Instrumental ADL

- Eating/drinking: Advise person that eating a full or large meal just before bedtime may interfere with going to sleep. Limiting fluid intake before bedtime may reduce number of bathroom visits during the night.
- Food choices: Advise person that drinking stimulants (caffeine, coffee) just before bedtime may interfere with going to sleep.
- Driving: Advise person of dangers of driving when drowsy or sleep deprived.

Education/Work

- Work equipment: Advise person of the dangers of operating equipment when sleep deprived.

Play/Leisure

- Engagement in favorite leisure activity before bedtime may facilitate relaxation.
- Avoid or reduce screen time on electronic devices with strong light.
- Playing soft, rhythmic music may be helpful (Harris, 2014).

Rest/Sleep

- Rest during the day may be useful but napping during the day may interfere with nighttime sleeping.
- If the client has trouble falling asleep, suggest getting up, leaving the bedroom, and doing some boring chore until feeling sleepy. Then, go back to bed. Same suggestion if person goes to sleep but wakes up in the middle of the night (Gentry & Loveland, 2013).

Social Participation

- Support participation in social activities.

Sensorimotor

- Auditory
  - ▸ Wearing earplugs may decrease effects of unwanted sounds.
  - ▸ Installing sound-reducing items such as curtains or carpeting, running a fan to produce a "white noise" effect.
  - ▸ Turning off the heating/cooling system at night or adjusting the cycle.
  - ▸ Help client analyze environment for sources of unwanted sounds and determine if the sounds can be eliminated or muted (e.g., buzzing or humming sounds from electronic devices, traffic noises, turning down or turning off televisions or gaming equipment).
- Visual
  - ▸ Wearing night shades may decrease effects of visual stimuli.
  - ▸ Installing a blackout curtain.
  - ▸ Fully closing the window shades.
  - ▸ Reducing amount of ambient light from electronic devices.
  - ▸ Help client analyze environment for sources of unwanted light.
- Tactile
  - ▸ Explore with client if bedding is considered to cause itchiness or to be scratchy.
  - ▸ Recommend bedding be of smooth materials such as soft cotton or silk.
- Proprioception/positioning
  - ▸ Body should be in a neutral or symmetrical position with the spine straight. An asymmetrical sleeping position may contribute to asymmetrical body positions, especially of the hip joints, during the day (Casey et al., 2019; Inncente, 2014). Note that neutral/symmetrical positioning is also important to consider when engaging in resting.
  - ▸ Explore with client if bedding mattress or other sleep surface is too soft or too hard for comfort.
  - ▸ Determine if client is able to move about the bed without waking up (bed mobility).
- Vibration, rocking
  - ▸ Gentle vibration or rhythm may be helpful.
  - ▸ A pillow with built-in vibration may be tried.

- Exercise
  - ▶ Recommend person get regular exercise during the day.
  - ▶ Recommend person not engage in vigorous exercise within 2 hours of bedtime to avoid overstimulation.
- Pain
  - ▶ Determine if pain is a factor in reducing sleep time and effectiveness.
  - ▶ Recommend client seek advice from a physician to reduce pain.

Cognitive/Perceptual

- Habits/routines/rituals
  - ▶ Assist client to achieve sleep hygiene: defined as the habits and practices necessary for quality nighttime sleep and daytime alertness (Gentry & Loveland, 2013, p. 11).
  - ▶ Explore with client which habits/routines/rituals tend to facilitate sleep and which act as barriers.
  - ▶ Assist client to identify changes that can be made to reduce the barriers.
  - ▶ Help client create a bedtime routine including any helpful ideas such as guided meditation, deep breathing, progressive muscle relaxation, and visualization techniques.
  - ▶ Be sure client, family members, or caregivers understand purpose and placement instructions of any positioning equipment.
- Time management
  - ▶ Explore with client what a typical day and week encompasses using a time chart.
  - ▶ Explore with client if changes in use of time and time management could be made.
  - ▶ Suggest establishing a regular scheduled routine for going to bed and getting up. Setting and keeping a regular sleep schedule can take 2 to 3 weeks. Encourage client to stick with the plan.
- Pacing cycles of rest and activity
  - ▶ Suggest client practice pacing activities to reduce overactivity and overstimulation.
  - ▶ Suggest organizing activities so that those that require the most energy are performed when person feels he or she has the most energy to apply to the task(s) including use of morning, afternoon, or evening time.
  - ▶ Suggest client alternate activity cycles and rest periods (Fung et al., 2014).
- Sleep diary
  - ▶ Recommend client keep a sleep diary: record bedtime, wake times, time actually gotten out of bed, sleep medications, and any problems occurring during sleep.
  - ▶ Review with client effectiveness of any changes made in relation to reports in sleep diary.

Psychosocial

- Assist client to identify recurrent negative/bad dream themes or nightmares.
- Suggest client not do tasks just before bedtime that tend to promote worry or anxiety, such as paying bills.
- A meditation program may be helpful (Gutman et al, 2017).
- Suggest making a list of worries/problems before going to bed and put the list aside to be dealt with in the morning or other specified time.

Context/Environment

- Assistive technology
  - ▶ Low tech: pillows, wedges, rolled up towels, teddy bears, soft toys.
  - ▶ High tech: continuous positive airway pressure (CPAP), adaptive servo ventilator, nasotracheal suction mechanical ventilation, positioning devices, light therapy, acupuncture, temperature control sheets, vacuum bags.
- Lighting: Suggest soft lights for sleep quarters. Avoid florescent lights or yard lights directly outside the bedroom window. Restrict light with blackout curtains or window shades. Check for sources of ambient light.

- Sound/noise: Suggest sound reducing fabrics, check for recurrent sounds.
- Temperature control: Check temperature control at night. Also check if bedding adds too much heat or not enough.
- Bedding: Check for comfortable bedding that supports the client's body but does not restrict movement in bed. Check for sheets and pillowcases that are smooth and soft, not rough or scratchy.
- Bedroom: Use the bedroom for sleep preparation and sleep itself.
- Consider recommending the National Sleep Foundation sleep hygiene program: Avoid food intake, alcohol, caffeine, and screen time before bed.

Precautions/Safety Considerations: (Red Flag Warning)

- Falling asleep while driving or other potentially dangerous situation.
- Repeated sleep attacks (falling asleep without warning).
- Breathing interruptions or awakening with gasping reported by partner or family member.
- Unstable cardiac or pulmonary status.
- History of a recent stroke.
- Continuous cataplexy attacks (status cataplecticus).
- History of violent behavior or injury to self or others while asleep.
- Frequent sleepwalking or other out-of-bed behavior (Porter, 2018).
- Abandonment of positioning equipment.

Prognosis and Outcome

Variable. Both good and poor outcomes have been reported.

REFERENCES

American Occupational Therapy Association. (2017). *Fact sheet: Occupational therapy's role with sleep.*

American Psychiatric Association. (2013). *Diagnostic and statistical manual of mental disorders* (5th ed.). https://doi.org/10.1176/appi.books.9780890425596

Barnhouse, J. (2019). The issue with sleep. *OT News, 27*(3), 28–29.

Biajar, A., Mollayeva, T., Sokoloff, S., & Colantonio, A. (2017). Assistive technology to enable sleep function in patients with acquire brain injury: Issues and opportunities. *British Journal of Occupational Therapy, 80*(4), 225–249. https://doi.org/10.1177/0308022616688017

Blanchard, J., Leland, N. E., Vigen, C., Mallinson, T., Fogelberg, D., Carlson, M., Clark, F., & Sleight, A. (2015). Does sleep change after an occupation-based lifestyle intervention? A pilot study. *American Journal of Occupational Therapy, 69*(Suppl. 1), Article 6911515045. https://doi.org/10.5014/ajot.2015.69S1-RP102B

Brown, C., Swedlove, F., Beery, R., & Turlapati, L. (2012). Occupational therapists' health literacy interventions for children with disordered sleep and/or pain. *New Zealand Journal of Occupational Therapy, 59*(2), 9–17.

Casey, J., Hoffman, L. A., Hutson, J., & Kittelson-Aldred, T. (2019). Supporting the occupation of sleep through night time positioning equipment. *SIS Quarterly Practice Connections, 4*(2), 7–9.

Cheng, S. Y., Kwong, S. H. W., Pang, W. M., & Wan, L. Y. (2017). Effects of an oral-pharyngeal motor training programme on children with obstructive sleep apnea syndrome in Hong Kong: A retrospective pilot study. *Hong Kong Journal of Occupational Therapy, 30*(1), 1–5. https://doi.org/10.1016/j.hkjot.2017.09.001

Cuomo, B. M., Vaz, S., Lee, E. A. L., Thompson, C., Rogerson, J. M., & Falkmer, T. (2017). Effectiveness of sleep-based interventions for children with autism spectrum disorder: A meta-synthesis. *Pharmacotherapy, 37*(5), 555–578. https://doi.org/10.1002/phar.1920

Duclos, C., Beauregard, M. P., Bottari, C., Ouellet, M. C., & Gosselin, N. (2015). The impact of poor sleep on cognition and activities of daily living after traumatic brain injury: A review. *Australian Occupational Therapy Journal, 62*(1), 2–12. https://doi.org/10.1111/1440-1630.12164

Eakman, A., Schmid, A. A., Henry, K. L., Rolle, N. R., Schelly, C. Pott, C. E., & Burns, J. E. (2017). Restoring effective sleep tranquility (REST): A feasibility and pilot study. *British Journal of Occupational Therapy, 80*(6), 350–360. https://doi.org/10.1177/0308022617691538

Engel-Yeger, B., & Shochat, T. (2012). The relationship between sensory processing patterns and sleep quality in healthy adults. *Canadian Journal of Occupational Therapy, 79*(3), 134–141. https://doi.org/10.2182/cjot.2012.79.3.2

Engel-Yeger, B., Gonda, X., Walker, M., Rihmer, Z., Pompili, M., Amore, M., & Serafini, G. (2017). Sensory hypersensitivity predicts reduced sleeping quality in patients with major affective disorders. *Journal of Psychiatric Practice, 23*(1), 11–24. https://doi.org/10.1097/PRA.000000 0000000210

Farrehi, P. M., Clore, K. R., Scott, J. R., Vanini, G., & Clauw, D. J. (2016). Efficacy of sleep tool education during hospitalization: A randomized controlled trial. *American Journal of Medicine, 129*(12), 1329.e9–1329.e17. https://doi.org/10.1016/j.amjmed.2016.08.001

Fogelberg, D. J., Hoffman, J. M., Dikmen, S., Temkin, N. R., & Bell, K. R. (2012). Association of sleep and co-occurring psychological conditions at 1 year after traumatic brain injury. *Archives of Physical Medicine and Rehabilitation, 93*(8), 1313–1318. https://doi.org/10.1016/j.a pmr.2012.04.031

Fogelberg, D. J., Hughes, A. J., Vitiello, M. V., Hoffman, J. M., & Amtmann, D. (2016). Comparison of sleep problems in individuals with spinal cord injury and multiple sclerosis. *Journal of Clinical Sleep Medicine, 12*(5), 695–701. https://doi.org/10.5664/jcsm.5798

Fogelberg, D. J., Leland, N. E., Blanchard, J., Rich, T. J., & Clark, F. A. (2017). Qualitative experience of sleep in individuals with spinal cord injury. *OTJR: Occupation, Participation and Health, 37*(2), 89–97. https://doi.org/10.1177/1539449217691978

Fung, C., Wiseman-Hakes, C., Stergiou-Kita, M., Nguyen, M., & Colantonio, A. (2013). Opinion: Time to wake up: Bridging the gap between theory and practice for sleep in occupational therapy. *British Journal of Occupational Therapy, 76*(8), 384–386. https://doi.org/10.4276/03 0802213X13757040168432

Fung, C. H. L., Nguyen, M., Moineddin, R., Colantonio, A., & Wiseman-Hakes, C. (2014). Reliability and validity of the Daily Cognitive–Communication and Sleep Profile: A new instrument for monitoring sleep, wakefulness and daytime function. *International Journal of Methods in Psychiatric Research, 23*(2), 217–228. https://doi.org/10.1002/mpr.1422

Gardner, J., Swarbrick, M., Ackerman, A., Church, T., Rios, V., Valente, L., & Rutledge, J. (2017). Effects of physical limitations on daily activities among adults with mental health disorders: Opportunities for nursing and occupational therapy interventions. *Journal of Psychosocial Nursing and Mental Health Services, 55*(10), 45–51. https://doi.org/10.3928/02793695-2017 0818-05

Gentry, T., & Loveland, J. (2013). Sleep: Essential to living life to its fullest. *OT Practice, 18*(1), 9–14.

Gutman, S. A., Gregory, K. A., Sadlier-Brown, M. M., Schlissel, M. A., Schubert, A. M., Westover, L. A., & Miller, R. C. (2017). Comparative effectives of three occupational therapy sleep interventions: A randomized controlled study. *OTJR: Occupation, Participation and Health, 37*(1), 5–13. https://doi.org/10.1177/1539449216673045

Hackett, K. L., Deary, V., Deane, K. H. O., Newton, J. L., Ng, W. F., & Rapley, T. (2018). Experience of sleep disruption in primary Sjögren's syndrome: A focus group study. *British Journal of Occupational Therapy, 81*(4), 218–226. https://doi.org/10.1177/0308022617745006

Hackett, K. L., Gotts, Z. M., Ellis, J., Deary, V., Rapley, T., Ng, W. F., Newton, J. L., & Deane, K. H. O. (2017). An investigation into the prevalence of sleep disturbances in primary Sjögren's syndrome: A systematic review of the literature. *Rheumatology, 56*(4), 570–580. https://doi .org/10.1093/rheumatology/kew443

Hamera, E., Brown, C., & Goetz, J. (2013). Objective and subjective sleep disturbances in individuals with psychiatric disabilities. *Issues in Mental Health Nursing, 34*(2), 110–116. https://doi.org/10.3109/01612840.2012.729648

Harris, M. J. (2014). Music as a transition for sleep. *Occupational Therapy Now, 16*(6), 11–13.

Ho, E. C. M., & Siu, A. M. H. (2018). Occupational therapy practice in sleep management: A review of conceptual models and research evidence. *Occupational Therapy International, 2018*, Article 8637498. https://doi.org/10.1155/2018/8637498

Inncente, R. (2014). Night-time positioning equipment: A review of practices. *New Zealand Journal of Occupational Therapy, 61*(1), 13–19.

Jarus, T., Bart, O., Rabinovich, G., Sadeh, A., Bloch, L., Dolfin, T., & Litmanovitz, I. (2011). Effects of prone and supine positions on sleep state and stress responses in preterm infants. *Infant Behavior and Development, 34*(2), 257–263. https://doi.org/10.1016/j.infbeh.2010.12.014

Johnson, B. P., & Westlake, K. P. (2018). Link between Parkinson disease and rapid eye movement sleep behavior disorder with dream enactment: Possible implications for early rehabilitation. *Archives of Physical Medicine and Rehabilitation, 99*(2), 411–415. https://doi.org/10.1016/j.apmr.2017.08.468

Leland, N. E., Fogelberg, D., Sleight, A., Mallinson, T., Vigen, C., Blanchard, J., Carlson, M., & Clark, F. (2016). Napping and nighttime sleep: Findings from an occupation-based intervention. *American Journal of Occupational Therapy, 70*(4), Article 7004270010. https://doi.org/10.5014/ajot.2016.017657

Leland, N. E., Marcione, N., Schepens Niemiec, S. L., Kelkar, K., & Fogelberg, D. (2014). What is occupational therapy's role in addressing sleep problems among older adults? *OTJR: Occupation, Participation and Health, 34*(3), 141–149. https://doi.org/10.3928/15394492-20140513-01

Milton, L. E., & Lovett, B. E. (2014). Sleep, occupation, and dysfunction in sensory integration. In J. M. Hereford (Ed.), *Sleep and rehabilitation: A guide for health professions* (pp. 265–278). Slack.

Mollayeva, T., D'Souza, A., Mollayeva, S., & Colantonio, A. (2017). Post-traumatic sleep–wake disorders. *Current Neurology and Neuroscience Reports, 17*(4), 38. https://doi.org/10.1007/s11910-017-0744-z

Mollayeva, T., Kendzerska, T., & Colantonio, A. (2013). Self-report instruments for assessing sleep dysfunction in an adult traumatic brain injury population: A systematic review. *Sleep Medicine Reviews, 17*(6), 411–423. https://doi.org/10.1016/j.smrv.2013.02.001

Mollayeva, T., Mollayeva, S., & Colantonio, A. (2016). The risk of sleep disorder among persons with mild traumatic brain injury. *Current Neurology and Neuroscience Reports, 16*(6), Article 55. https://doi.org/10.1007/s11910-016-0657-2

Mollayeva, T., Mollayeva, S., Shapiro, C. M., Cassidy, J. D., & Colantonio, A. (2016). Insomnia in workers with delayed recovery from mild traumatic brain injury. *Sleep Medicine, 19*, 153–161. https://doi.org/10.1016/j.sleep.2015.05.014

Mollayeva, T., Pratt, B., Mollayeva, S., Shapiro, C. M., Cassidy, J. D., & Colantonio, A. (2016). The relationship between insomnia and disability in workers with mild traumatic brain injury/concussion: Insomnia and disability in chronic mild traumatic brain injury. *Sleep Medicine, 20*, 157–166. https://doi.org/10.1016/j.sleep.2015.09.008

Oh, H. W., Kim, S. H., & Kim, K. U. (2016). The effects a respiration rehabilitation program on IADL, satisfaction with leisure, and quality of sleep of patients with chronic obstructive pulmonary disease. *Journal of Physical Therapy Science, 28*(12), 3357–3360.

O'Toole, M. T. (Ed.). (2017). *Mosby's dictionary of medicine, nursing & health professions* (10th ed.). Elsevier.

Park, J. (2019a). Effects of the sleep quality of chronic stroke outpatients on patterns of activity performance and quality of life. *Sleep and Hypnosis, 21*(3), 228–232. https://doi.org/10.5350/Sleep.Hypn.2019.21.0190

Park, J. (2019b). A study on the sleep quality, pain, and instrumental activities of daily living of outpatients with chronic stroke. *Journal of Physical Therapy Science, 31*(2), 149–152. https://doi.org/10.1589/jpts.31.149

Picard, M. M. (2017). *Fact sheet: Occupational therapy's role in sleep*. American Occupational Therapy Association.

Pierce, D., & Summers, K. (2011). Rest and sleep. In C. Brown & V. C. Stoffel (Eds.). *Occupational therapy in mental health: A vision for participation* (pp. 736–758). F.A. Davis.

Pierce, D., & Summers, K. (2019). Rest and sleep. In C. Brown & V. C. Stoffel (Eds.), *Occupational therapy in mental health: A vision for participation* (2nd ed., pp. 909–930). F.A. Davis.

Porter, R. S. (Ed.). (2018). *The Merck manual of diagnosis and therapy* (20th ed.). Merck Sharp & Dohme.

Schoen, S. A., Man, S., & Spiro, C. (2017). A sleep intervention for children with autism spectrum disorder: A pilot study. *Open Journal of Occupational Therapy, 5*(2), Article 3. https://doi.org/10.15453/2168-6408.1293

Sheth, M., & Thomas, N. (2019). Managing sleep deprivation in older adults: A role for occupational Therapy. *OT Practice, 24*(3), CE-1–CE-8.

Smallfield, S., & Molitor, W. L. (2018). Occupational therapy interventions addressing sleep for community-dwelling older adults: A systematic review. *American Journal of Occupational Therapy, 72*(4), Article 7204190030. https://doi.org/10.5014/ajot.2018.031211

Stedman's medical dictionary for the health professions and nursing (7th ed.). (2011). Wolters Kluwer.

Thomas, S., Bundy, A. C., Black, D., & Lane, S. J. (2015). Toward early identification of sensory over-responsivity (SOR): A construct for predicting difficulties with sleep and feeding in infants. *OTJR: Occupation, Participation and Health, 35*(3), 178–186. https://doi.org/10.1177/1539449215579855

VandenBos, G. R. (Ed.). (2015). *APA dictionary of psychology* (2nd ed.). American Psychological Association.

Weaver, L. L. (2015). Effectiveness of work, activities of daily living, education, and sleep interventions for people with autism spectrum disorder: A systematic review. *American Journal of Occupational Therapy, 69*(5), Article 6905180020. https://doi.org/10.5014/ajot.2015.017962

Wiseman-Hakes, C., Murray, B., Moineddin, R., Rochon, E., Cullen, N., Gargaro, J., & Colantonio, A. (2013). Evaluating the impact of treatment for sleep/wake disorders on recovery of cognition and communication in adults with chronic TBI. *Brain Injury, 27*(12), 1364–1376. https://doi.org/10.3109/02699052.2013.823663

Wood, A., Brooks, R., & Beynon-Pindar, C. (2015). The experience of sleep for women with borderline personality disorder: An occupational perspective. *British Journal of Occupational Therapy, 78*(12), 750–756. https://doi.org/10.1177/0308022615587864

BIBLIOGRAPHY

Green, A., Brown, C., & Iwana, M. (Eds.). (2015). *An occupational therapist's guide to sleep and sleep problems*. Jessica Kingsley.

Mollayeva, T., Colantonio, A., Mollayeva, S., & Shapiro, C. M. (2013). Screening for sleep dysfunction after traumatic brain injury. *Sleep Medicine, 14*(12), 1235–1246. https://doi.org/10.1016/j.sleep.2013.07.009

Mollayeva, T., Thurairajah, P., Burton, K., Mollayeva, S., Shapiro, C. M., & Colantonio, A. (2016). The Pittsburgh Sleep Quality Index as a screening tool for sleep dysfunction in clinical and non-clinical samples: A systematic review and meta-analysis. *Sleep Medicine Reviews, 25*, 52–73. https://doi.org/10.1016/j.smrv.2015.01.009

O'Donoghue, N., & McKay, E. A. (2012). Exploring the impact of sleep apnoea on daily life and occupational engagement. *British Journal of Occupational Therapy, 75*(11), 509–516. https://doi.org/10.4276/030802212X13522194759932

Solet, J. (2014). Sleep and rest. In B. Schell, G. Gillen, & M. Scaffa (Eds.), *Willard and Spackman's occupational therapy* (12th ed., pp. 714–730). Wolters Kluwer.

Solet, J. (2019). Sleep and rest. In B. Schell & G. Gillen (Eds.), *Willard and Spackman's occupational therapy* (13th ed., pp. 727–846). Wolters Kluwer.

Tester, N. J., & Foss, J. J. (2018). Sleep as an occupational need. *American Journal of Occupational Therapy, 72*(1), Article 7201347010. https://doi.org/10.5014/ajot.2018.020651

Watson, M., Garden, J., Swedlove, F., & Brown, C. A. (2014). Back to the basics: Sleep and occupation. *Occupational Therapy Now, 16*(6), 8–10.

Terminal Illness, End of Life, Palliative Care, and Hospice

Description

Four trajectories constitute terminal illness and end of life:

- Sudden or unexpected death: trauma (accidents, gunshots, stabbing), cardiac arrest (heart attack), or cardiovascular accident (stroke), which is the initial incident; death occurs within hours or days, leaving little or no time for rehabilitation efforts.
- Chronic organ failure: heart failure, chronic pulmonary obstructive disease; function that decreases irregularly, caused by periodic and sometimes unpredictable acute exacerbations of the underlying disorder.
- Dementia/frailty trajectory: multiple organ failure; a prolonged indefinite period of severe dysfunction that may not be steadily progressive such as occurs with a disabling stroke, progressive neurological disorder, severe dementia, or frailty.
- Cancer trajectory: a limited period of steadily progressive functional decline (Chow, 2018; Porter, 2018).

Cause

See conditions listed above. Note: Conditions such as schizophrenia and mental health conditions may be underrepresented in the programs discussed (McNamara et al., 2018).

Terminology

- *End-of-life care:* Program aims to relieve distress that is often associated with death and improve the quality of life for both those diagnosed with an advanced or terminal illness and their loved ones (Canadian Association of Occupational Therapists, 2011).
- *Hospice:* A program of care and support for people who are likely to die within a few months. Hospice care focuses on comfort and meaningfulness, not on a cure. Services may include physical care, counseling, drugs, and medical equipment and supplies (Porter, 2018).
- *Palliative care:* An interdisciplinary team approach to care for people with serious or life-threatening illnesses aimed at improving quality of life by helping relieve bothersome physical symptoms, such as pain and psychosocial and spiritual distress. The goal is to offer pain relief and symptom management, and to offer support systems to clients and their families (American Occupational Therapy Association, 2015; Porter, 2018).

Position Statements

Several occupational therapy associations have prepared position statements on terminal illness, end of life, palliative care, or hospice, including the American Occupational Therapy Association (2016), the Canadian Association of Occupational Therapists (2011), Occupational Therapy Australia (2015), Occupational Therapy New Zealand (2013), and the World Federation of Occupational Therapists (2014).

Evaluation/Assessment

Areas

- Activities of Daily Living/Instrumental ADL: self-maintenance skills (bathing, dressing, feeding, toileting), driving
- Education/Work: work history
- Play/Leisure: interests, types, frequency, occupational deprivation
- Rest/Sleep: sleep disturbance
- Social Participation: with whom, location, frequency
- Sensorimotor: mobility, cachexia (weakness), dyspnea (breathlessness), fatigue, pain
- Cognitive/Perceptual: problem solving
- Psychosocial: anger, denial, depression, grief and loss, role performance, sense of self-competence and self-worth, self-confidence, hopelessness, loss of control, disempowerment, loss of dignity, lack of choice, quality of life
- Context/Environment: home safety, home modification, adaptive devices
- Development (Infant, Child, Adolescent only): no information identified

Instruments

Instruments Developed by Occupational Therapy Personnel

- Canadian Occupational Performance Measure (5th ed.; COPM-5; Law et al., 2014)
- Functional Assessment of Chronic Illness Therapy-Palliative Care (FACIT-Pal; Lyons et al., 2009)
- Occupational Circumstances Assessment Interview and Rating Scale (OCAIRS; Forsyth et al., 2005)

Instruments Development by Other Professionals and Used by Occupational Therapy Personnel

- Center for Epidemiological Studies Depression Scale (CES-D; Radloff, 1977)
- Functional Assessment of Chronic Illness Therapy (FACIT; Webster et al., 2003)
- Inventory of Complicated Grief (ICG; Prigerson et al., 1995)
- Measuring Your Concerns and Wellbeing (MYCaW; Patterson et al., 2003)
- Philadelphia Geriatric Center Moral Scale (PGCMS; Lawton, 1972)

Problems/Issues

Activities of Daily Living/Instrumental ADL

- Person may have increasing difficulty performing self-maintenance skills as functional ability decreases.

Education/Work

- Not discussed.

Play/Leisure

- Person may decrease engaging in favorite leisure activities.

Rest/Sleep

- Person may experience changes in sleep/wake patterns.

Social Participation

- Person may decrease participation in social activities.

Sensorimotor

- Person may experience fatigue and feelings of being tired.
- Person may experience pain.
- Person may experience dyspnea (breathlessness).
- Person may experience loss of muscle strength.
- Person may experience decreased joint range of motion.

Cognitive/Perceptual
- Person may lack problem-solving skills.
- Person may lack basic knowledge and information about available resources.

Psychosocial
- Person may experience the cycle of grief: anger, bargaining, denial, depression, and acceptance.
- Person may feel a sense of hopelessness, helplessness, and loss of control.
- Person may experience decreased motivation to engage in activities feeling that nothing matters or is important anymore.
- Person may experience loss of role performance and self-worth as functional ability decreases.
- Person may experience decreased quality of life.
- Person may experience loss of self-confidence and self-competence as functional ability decreases.
- Person may experience decreased sense of dignity as others must assist in performing self-maintenance activities.

Context/Environment
- Family members and caregivers may require information, education, and training on physical management of the person such as safe transfers.
- Family members and caregivers may require education and training on the use and maintenance of adaptive equipment such as scooters, wheelchairs, hoists, and lifts.

Intervention/Treatment

Models and programs developed by occupational therapy personnel include the Canadian Model of Occupational Performance (Finlay, 2019); doing, being, and becoming (Pickens et al., 2010); living well group (Biggerstaff & O'Donnell, 2014); and rehabilitation program (Kasven-Gonzalez et al., 2010). Models and programs developed by other professionals but used by occupational therapy personnel include ENABLE II (Bakitas et al., 2013; Maloney et al., 2013), ENABLE III (Bakitas et al., 2015; Dionne-Odom et al., 2015; Dionne-Odom et al., 2016), and mindful hand (Finlay, 2019). Team members include physicians, nursing personnel, social workers, chaplains, physical therapists, and occupational therapy personnel. The goal is to alleviate pain and suffering, maintain or improve safety, provide comfort, prevent injuries, and enhance quality of life by encouraging people to participate in meaningful occupations and rewarding experiences (Canadian Association of Occupational Therapists, 2011).

Activities of Daily Living/Instrumental ADL
- Bathing and showering: safety focus (grab bars, shower bench/chair, handheld showerhead), energy conservation.
- Dressing: adaptive devices, modified techniques, work simplification, energy conservation, fatigue management, safety focus (e.g., getting dressed in bed, using elastic or Velcro fasteners, slip on shoes such as loafers or sandals, T-shirts or polo shirts).
- Meal preparation: energy conservation, activity modification, reorganizing storage; plan and eat healthy diet; eat smaller, more frequent meals.
- Home management: use good body mechanics, energy conservation, activity tolerance, adaptive equipment.

Education/Work
- No information identified.

Play/Leisure
- Identify and support engagement in enjoyable and meaningful leisure activities with modifications as needed to adjust in changing functional status.

Rest/Sleep
- Assist client to develop presleep routines to facilitate longer periods of sleep.
- Encourage use of good bed positions and bedding to improve rest and reduce skin breakdown.

Social Participation
- Facilitate social activities with modifications such as amount of time, location, and type of activity.

Sensorimotor
- *Pain management:* Assist clinic to create a pain management program that encourages activities when pain medications are most effective or when occupation is most effective in countering the sensation of pain.
- *Fatigue management:* Assist clinic to develop a fatigue management program that includes pacing activities, alternating action and occupation with rest cycles, and clustering "must do" activities when energy level is highest.
- *Posture and body mechanics:* Assist client to maintain good posture and alignment in static positions and dynamic movement.

Cognitive/Perceptual
- *Anxiety diary:* Encourage client to create and use a diary to write down feelings and worries both emotionally and physically. Use the diary to reflect when person is feeling better to find ways (problem solve) to deal with anxiety cycle in the future.
- *Distraction:* Assist client to identify occupations that distract or shift attention away from feelings of anxiety. The occupations should be ones that are personally enjoyable to the client.
- *Mindfulness:* Have reassuring phrases available to repeat, shift focus to deep breathing, focus on the environment around the client and looking at the view outside the window.
- *Problem solving:* Provide opportunity to solve problems raised by the client.
- *Time management:* Assist in creating a time schedule that integrates highest energy level with the activities of greatest importance to the client.
- *Visualization:* Encourage client to imagine going to a "happy place" or "peaceful place" to help calm the person.

Psychosocial
- *Stress management:* Assist client in learning to manage stress through techniques such as relaxation training, yoga, or similar techniques.
- *Coping skills:* Encourage communication and discussion about feelings, fears, and anxieties.
- *Quality of life:* Assist client in achieving the maximum life satisfaction by supporting goals with modifications as needed to account for changes in functional status.
- *Life roles:* Assist client to identify life roles that are important and meaningful and assist in addressing barriers to performing the activities associated with those roles.

Context/Environment
- Make recommendations for home safety and modification.
- Make recommendations for adaptive devices and equipment to facilitate engagement and participation.
- Provide information, education, coaching, and training to family and caregivers.
- Assist in identifying community resources that may be useful to the client, family, and caregivers.

Precautions/Safety Considerations

Client is at increased risk of injury due to reduced functional ability. Fall prevention should be observed. Client is at increased risk for bedsores (pressure sores, decubitus ulcers) due to increased time resting and possible decreased nutritional status.

Prognosis and Outcome

Outcome is death, but the prognosis may be variable depending on the course of the disease, disorder, or condition. Some clients may be discharged because immediate needs are met but be seen again because further decline has occurred. Other clients may be seen only once before their death.

REFERENCES

American Occupational Therapy Association. (2015). *Fact sheet: The role of occupational therapy in palliative and hospice care.*

American Occupational Therapy Association. (2016). The role of occupational therapy in end-of-life care. *American Journal of Occupational Therapy, 70*(Suppl. 2), Article 7212410075. https://doi.org/10.5014/ajot.2016.706S17

Bakitas, M., Lyons, K. D., Hegel, M. T., & Ahles, T. (2013). Oncologists' perspectives on concurrent palliative care in a National Cancer Institute-designated comprehensive cancer center. *Palliative & Supportive Care, 11*(5), 415–423. https://doi.org/10.1017/S1478951512000673

Bakitas, M. A., Tosteson, T. D., Li, Z., Lyons, K. D., Hull, J. G., Li, Z., Dionne-Odom, J. N., Frost, J., Dragnev, K. H., Hegel, M. T., Azuero, A., & Ahles, T. A. (2015). Early versus delayed initiation of concurrent palliative oncology care: Patient outcomes in the ENABLE III randomized controlled trial. *Journal of Clinical Oncology, 33*(13), 1438–1445. https://doi.org/10.1200/JCO.2014.58.6362

Biggerstaff, B., & O'Donnell, J. (2014). Living well, step by step. *OT News, 22*(6), 32–33.

Canadian Association of Occupational Therapists. (2011). CAOT *Position statement: Occupational therapy and end-of-life care.* https://www.caot.ca/document/3705/O%20-%20OT%20and%20End%20of%20Life%20Care.pdf

Chow, J. K. (2018). Occupational therapy in hospice and palliative care. In H. M. Pendleton & W. Schultz-Krohn (Eds.), *Pedretti's occupational therapy* (8th ed., pp. 1195–1213). Elsevier.

Dionne-Odom, J. N., Azuero, A., Lyons, K. D., Hull, J. G., Tosteson, T., Li, Z., Li, Z., Frost, J., Dragnev, K. H., Akyar, I., Hegel, M. T., & Bakitas, M. A. (2015). Benefits of early versus delayed palliative care to informal family caregivers of patients with advanced cancer: Outcomes from the ENABLE III randomized controlled trial. *Journal of Clinical Oncology, 33*(13), 1446–1452. https://doi.org/10.1200/JCO.2014.58.7824

Dionne-Odom, J. N., Azuero, A., Lyons, K. D., Hull, J. G., Prescott, A. T., Tosteson, T., Frost, J., Dragnev, K. H., & Bakitas, M. A. (2016). Family caregiver depressive symptom and grief outcomes from the ENABLE III randomized controlled trial. *Journal of Pain and Symptom Management, 52*(3), 378–385. https://doi.org/10.1016/j.jpainsymman.2016.03.014

Finlay, A. (2019). Life enhancing work. *OT News, 27*(5), 18–20.

Kasven-Gonzalez, N., Souverain, R., & Miale, S. (2010). Improving quality of life through rehabilitation in palliative care: Case report. *Palliative & Supportive Care, 8*(3), 359–369. https://doi.org/10.1017/S1478951510000167

Maloney, C., Lyons, K. D., Li, Z., Hegel, M., Ahles, T. A., & Bakitas, M. (2013). Patient perspectives on participation in the ENABLE II randomized controlled trial of a concurrent oncology palliative care intervention: Benefits and burdens. *Palliative Medicine, 27*(4), 375–383. https://doi.org/10.1177/0269216312445188

McNamara, B., Same, A., Rosenwax, L., & Kelly, B. (2018). Palliative care for people with schizophrenia: A qualitative study of an under-serviced group in need. *BMC Palliative Care, 17*, Article 53. https://doi.org/10.1186/s12904-018-0309-1

Occupational Therapy Australia. (2015). Position statement: Occupational therapy in palliative care. *Australian Occupational Therapy Journal, 62*(6), 459–461. https://doi.org/10.1111/1440-1630.12264

Occupational Therapy New Zealand. (2013). *End of life/palliative care position statement.* https://www.otnzwna.co.nz/otnz-wna/otnz-wna-documents/otnz-wna-position-statements/

Pickens, N. D., O'Reilly, K. R., & Sharp, K. C. (2010). Holding on to normalcy and overshadowed needs: Family caregiving at end of life. *Canadian Journal of Occupational Therapy,* *77*(4), 234–240. https://doi.org/10.2182/cjot.2010.77.4.5

Porter, R. S. (Ed.). (2018). *The Merck manual of diagnosis and therapy* (20th ed.). Merck Sharp & Dohme.

World Federation of Occupational Therapists. (2014). *Position statement: Occupational therapy in end of life care.* https://wfot.org/assets/resources/Occupational-Therapy-in-End-of-Life-Care.pdf

BIBLIOGRAPHY

Ashworth, E. (2014). Utilizing participation in meaningful occupation as an intervention approach to support the acute model of inpatient palliative care. *Palliative & Supportive Care,* *12*(5), 409–412. https://doi.org/10.1017/S1478951513000734

Badger, S., Macleod, R., & Honey, A. (2016). "It's not about treatment, it's how to improve your life": The lived experience of occupational therapy in palliative care. *Palliative & Supportive Care, 14*(3), 225–231. https://doi.org/10.1017/S1478951515000826

Davis, J., Asuncion, M., Rabello, J., Silangcruz, C., & van Dyk, E. (2013). A qualitative review of occupational therapists' listening behaviors and experiences when caring for patients in palliative or hospice care. *OTJR: Occupation, Participation and Health, 33*(1), 12–20. https://doi.org/10.3928/15394492-20121012-01

Dionne-Odom, J. N., Lyons, K. D., Akyar, I., & Bakitas, M. A. (2016). Coaching family caregivers to become better problem solvers when caring for persons with advanced cancer. *Journal of Social Work in End-of-Life & Palliative Care. 12*(1-2), 63–81. https://doi.org/10.1080/15524 256.2016.1156607

Eva, G., & Morgan, D. (2018). Mapping the scope of occupational therapy practice in palliative care: A European Association for Palliative Care cross-sectional survey. *Palliative Medicine, 32*(5), 960–968. https://doi.org/10.1177/0269216318758928

Falardeau, M., Lambert, E., & Arpin, J. (2013). Reflections on services for people in palliative or end-of-life care. *Occupational Therapy Now, 15*(2), 19–21.

Halkett, G. K. B., Ciccarelli, M., Keesing, S., & Aoun, S. (2010). Occupational therapy in palliative care: Is it under-utilised in Western Australia? *Australian Occupational Therapy Journal, 57*(5), 301–309. https://doi.org/10.1111/j.1440-1630.2009.00843.x

Hammill, K., Bye, R., & Cook, C. (2014). Occupational therapy for people living with a life-limiting illness: A thematic review. *British Journal of Occupational Therapy, 77*(11), 582–589. https://doi.org/10.4276/030802214X14151078348594

Keesing, S., & Rosenwax, L. (2011). Is occupation missing from occupational therapy in palliative care? *Australian Occupational Therapy Journal, 58*(5), 329–336. https://doi.org/10.1111/ j.1440-1630.2011.00958.x

Keesing, S., & Rosenwax, L. (2013). Establishing a role for occupational therapists in end-of-life care in Western Australia. *Australian Occupational Therapy Journal, 60*(5), 370–373 https://doi.org/10.1111/1440-1630.12058

Lala, A. P., & Kinsella, E. A. (2011). A phenomenological inquiry into the embodied nature of occupation at end of life. *Canadian Journal of Occupational Therapy, 78*(4), 246–254. https://doi.org/10.2182/cjot.2011.78.4.6

Lyons, K. D., Padgett, L. S., Marshall, T. F., Greer, J. A., Silver, J. K., Raj, V. S., Zucker, D. S., Fu, J. B., Pergolotti, M., Sleight, A. G., & Alfano, C. M. (2019). Follow the trail: Using insights from the growth of palliative care to propose a roadmap for cancer rehabilitation. *CA: A Cancer Journal for Clinicians, 69*(2), 113–126. https://doi.org/10.3322/caac.21549

Matovu, S. (2010). Occupational therapy in palliative care in an African setting. In V. Alers & R. Crouch (Eds.), *Occupational therapy: An African perspective* (pp. 252–267). Sarah Shorten.

Mills, K., & Payne, A. (2015). Enabling occupation at the end of life: A literature review. *Palliative & Supportive Care, 13*(6), 1755–1769. https://doi.org/10.1017/S1478951515000772

Morgan, D. D., & White, K. M. (2012). Occupational therapy interventions for breathlessness at the end of life. *Current Opinion in Supportive and Palliative Care, 6*(2), 138–143. https://doi.org/10.1097/SPC.0b013e3283537d0e

O'Hara, R. E., Hull, J. G., Lyons, K. D., Bakitas, M., Hegel, M. T., Li, Z., & Ahles, T. A. (2010). Impact on caregiver burden of a patient-focused palliative care intervention for patients with advanced cancer. *Palliative & Supportive Care, 8*(4), 395–404. https://doi.org/10.1017/S1478951510000258

Pizzi, M. (2010a). Promoting health and wellness in end-of-life care. *Gerontology Special Interest Section Quarterly, 33*, 1–4.

Pizzi, M. (2010b). Promoting wellness in end-of-life care. In M. E. Scaffa, S. M. Reitz, & M. A. Pizzi (Eds.), *Occupational therapy in the promotion of health and wellness* (pp. 493–511). F.A. Davis.

Pizzi, M. A. (2014). Promoting health, wellness and quality of life at the end of life: Hospice interdisciplinary perspectives on creating a good death. *Journal of Allied Health, 43*(4), 212–220.

Pizzi, M. A. (2015). Promoting health and well-being at the end of life through client-centered care. *Scandinavian Journal of Occupational Therapy, 22*(6), 442–449. https://doi.org/10.3109/11038128.2015.1025834

Prescott, A. T., Hull, J. G., Dionne-Odom, J. N., Tosteson, T. D., Lyons, K. D., Li, Z., Li, Z., Dragnev, K. H., Hegel, M. T., Steinhauser, K. E., Ahles, T. A., & Bakitas, M. A. (2017). The role of a palliative care intervention in moderating the relationship between depression and survival among individuals with advanced cancer. *Health Psychology, 36*(12), 1140–1146. https://doi.org/10.1037/hea0000544

Razavi, C., & Gaylor, M. (2016). Smarter working for palliative care in the community. *OT News, 24*(8), 40–42.

Şahin, S., Akel, S., & Zarif, M. (2017). Occupational therapy in oncology and palliative care. In M. Huri (Ed.), *Occupation focused holistic practice in rehabilitation.* IntechOpen. https://doi.org/10.5772/intechopen.68463

Sleight, A. G., Lyons, K. D., Vign, C., Macdonald, H., & Clark, F. (2018). The association of health-related quality of life with unmet supportive care needs and sociodemographic factors in low-income Latina breast cancer survivors: A single-centre pilot study. *Disability and Rehabilitation, 41*(26), 3151–3156. https://doi.org/10.1080/09638288.2018.1485179

Svidén, G. A., Tham, K., & Borell, L. (2010). Involvement in everyday life for people with a life-threatening illness. *Palliative & Supportive Care, 8*(3), 345–352. https://doi.org/10.1017/S1478951510000143

Taylor, A., & Ford, R. (2019). Linking hospital to home at end of life. *OT News, 27*(5), 22–24.

Woods, J., & Cowpo, L. (2019). Palliative care—Whose responsibility is it to deliver? *OT News, 27*(4), 20–22.

Violence and Abuse

Includes: Domestic Violence, Workplace Violence, Elder Abuse, Intimate Partner Abuse.

Also called domestic abuse, battered woman or women, elder neglect, intimate partner violence.

See also Childhood Trauma and Maltreatment.

Description

Categories

• *General: Violence* is a broad term which is open to subjective and social interpretation, and often depends on the context to determine what is socially acceptable or not. Meaning and value are determined by personal and societal consequences (Aldrich & White, 2012). Persons who experience violence may experience occupational injustice (unable to participate and engage in desired occupations), occupational deprivation (lack of access to occupations), and occupational imbalance (limited range of occupations) due to the power and control dynamics within the abusive relationship (American Occupational Therapy Association, 2017).

- *Domestic violence:* Physical, psychological, or sexual abuse between people who are living together. The abuse may occur between intimate partners, parents and children, grandparents and children, or siblings (Porter, 2018). Women and girls are most often involved but not exclusively. Domestic violence involves the willful intimidation, physical assault, battery, sexual assault, or other abuse behavior as part of a systematic pattern of power and control perpetrated by one partner against another (American Occupational Therapy Association, 2017).

- *Workplace violence:* Four subtypes are recognized (Brown & Kain, 2019):
  - ▶ Type 1: Criminal intent—Perpetrator has no relationship to workers or business and is usually committing a crime.
  - ▶ Type II: Customer/client—Perpetrator is a customer, client, or visitor of the work setting.
  - ▶ Type III: Worker on worker—Perpetrator is a coworker.
  - ▶ Type IV: Personal relationship—Perpetrator has or had a personal relationship with the victim.

- *Elder abuse:* Physical or psychological mistreatment, neglect, or financial exploitation of the elderly (Porter, 2018). Also defined as "harm to an adult aged 65 or older caused by another individual" including physical violence, nonconsensual sex, psychological or emotional distress, improper use of belongings or finances, or failure to provide needed care (VandenBos, 2015, p. 356). Elder abuse may be "a single, or repeated act, or lack of appropriate action occurring within any relationship where there is an expectation of trust which causes harm or distress" (Canadian Association of Occupational Therapists, 2012, p. 2).

- *Intimate partner abuse*: Focuses on abuse between two intimate partners inclusive of spouses, boyfriends, girlfriends, dating partners, and sexual partners (American Occupational Therapy Association, 2017).

Types of Violence or Abuse

- *Captive bystanders:* Usually children who cannot escape the violence and may hear or witness the violence with no perceived exit or remission from the situation (Gabriel et al., 2018).
- *Denial of entitlements protected by law:* Includes "censoring or interfering with a person's mail; withholding information to which the person is entitled; restricting liberties," such as not letting the person go out and socialize, and "denying privacy, visitors, phone calls or religious worship and spiritual practice" (Canadian Association of Occupational Therapists, 2013, p. 14).
- *Expressive violence:* Frustrations arising from experience (no financial gain; Aldrich & White, 2012).
- *Financial or economic abuse:* "Exploitation of or inattention to a person's possessions or funds" including "swindling, pressuring a person to distribute assets, and managing a person's money irresponsibly" (Porter, 2018, p. 2858).
- *Instrumental violence:* Violence that is incorporated into an act to achieve some desired outcome such as financial (Aldrich & White, 2012).
- *Neglect:* "Failure or refusal to provide food, medicine, personal care, or other necessities" and also abandonment (Porter, 2018, p. 2858; see also Canadian Association of Occupational Therapists, 2013).
- *Physical abuse or violence:* Use of force resulting in physical or psychological injury or discomfort which may include beating, biting, breaking bones, bruising, confining, cutting, deprivation of food or sleep, force feeding, gunshot, hitting, kicking, pinching, poking, pulling hair, punching, pushing, restraining, scratching, shaking, shoving, slapping, spitting, stabbing,

strangling, striking, twisting arms or legs, or unwanted administration of drugs (Canadian Association of Occupational Therapists, 2013; Porter, 2018).

- *Psychological abuse or violence:* Use of words, acts, or other means to cause emotional stress or anguish including any nonphysical behavior that may belittle, degrade, humiliate, intimidate, or undermine the person and acts to increase control of one person over another. Examples include abusive language, financial control, and social isolation from family, friends, or other people including all forms of communication (email, phone, letters, or visits; Canadian Association of Occupational Therapists, 2013; Porter, 2018). May also be called emotional abuse.
- *Perpetrator:* The abuser (Scaffa et al., 2010).
  - ▶ Domineering or bullying type: Person feels entitled to exert power and authority. Person may have insight into nature of maladaptive behavior, but tends to neglect, engage in financial abuse or sexual abuse.
  - ▶ Impaired type: Person has mental or physical problems him- or herself that prevent individual from delivering expected services. Person may be unaware of deficits and control the victim through abuse especially neglect.
  - ▶ Narcissistic type: Person into relationship to meet his or her needs. Person is more likely to steal and neglect.
  - ▶ Overwhelmed type: Person is well intended but when situation exceeds what the person can provide, physical or verbal abuse occurs but person does not look for victims.
  - ▶ Sadistic or psychopathic type: Person takes pleasure in mistreating victims and feels power and importance when he or she abuses others.
- *Sexual abuse or violence:* Includes unwanted touching, grabbing, or kissing and the use of threats or force to coerce sexual activity (Porter, 2018).
- *Survivor:* Individual who is currently in an abusive relationship (recipient) or who has overcome the abuse (American Occupational Therapy Association, 2017).

Cause

Divided into three types of triggers and examples (Brown & Kain, 2019):

- Physical triggers: hunger or lack of food, need to use bathroom, threatening body language or tone of voice, unwanted touch or restraint.
- Emotional triggers: emotional needs not addressed, feeling unsafe, medication side effects, sense of powerlessness, and being yelled at.
- Environmental triggers: clutter, color choice, crowds, noise or sounds, types of lighting.

Evaluation/Assessment

Areas

- Activities of Daily Living/Instrumental ADL: basic ADLs, independent living skills
- Education/Work: work environment, employment history
- Play/Leisure: interests, values, frequency, location
- Rest/Sleep: sleep disturbances
- Social Participation: types, frequency, location, with whom
- Sensorimotor: repeated physical injuries such as bruising or fractures
- Cognitive/Perceptual: attention, memory, executive functions
- Psychosocial: depression, self-efficacy, role performance, quality of life
- Context/Environment: social support, environmental barriers, resources
- Comorbidities: posttraumatic stress disorder, anxiety, depression, dementia, traumatic brain injury

Instruments
Instruments Developed by Occupational Therapy Personnel

- Adolescent/Adult Sensory Profile (AASP; Brown & Dunn, 2002)

- Canadian Occupational Performance Measure (5th ed.; COPM-5; Law et al., 2014)
- Health Enhancement Lifestyle Profile–Screener (HELP-Screener; Hwang, 2012)
- Occupational Profile (OP; American Occupational Therapy Association, 2020)
- Test of Playfulness (Version 4.2; ToP 4.2; Bundy, 2010)

Instruments Developed by Other Professionals and Used by Occupational Therapy Personnel
- Coding Interactive Behavior (CIB; Feldman, 1998)
- Experiences in Close Relationship (ECR; Brennan et al., 1998)
- Parenting Sense of Competence Scale (PSOC; Johnston & Mash, 1989)
- Posttraumatic Diagnostic Scale (PTDS; Foa et al., 1997)

Problems/Issues

Activities of Daily Living/Instrumental ADL
- Person, especially if elderly, may have difficulty managing basic ADLs: eating, toileting, bathing, dressing, grooming, functional communication, functional mobility including transfers.
- Person may lack skills in child rearing and parenting.
- Person may lack knowledge of or access to community mobility services.
- Person may lack knowledge of or access to money management and financial services.
- Person may lack skills in home management (house cleaning, doing laundry, simple clothing repair).
- Person may lack skills in shopping (groceries, clothing, sundries, furniture).
- Person may lack skills in meal planning and preparation.
- Person may lack skills in health management such as healthy diet, home safety.

Education/Work
- Person may lack basic academic skills including speaking English, printing or writing, computer skills, basic mathematic skills.
- Person may lack basic work skills including those needed to explore and obtain employment such as preparing a resume, filling out an application, making and keeping an interview date.
- Person may lack knowledge of opportunities to explore or participate in volunteer services.

Play/Leisure
- Person may lack knowledge of developmental play skills for children under his or her care.
- Person may lack opportunity to engage in known leisure occupations.
- Person may lack opportunity to explore and engage in new leisure occupations.

Rest/Sleep
- Person may lack regular sleep habits and routines.
- Person may have a sleep disorder.

Social Participation
- Person may lack opportunity to participate in familiar social occupations.
- Person may lack opportunity to explore and participate in new social occupations.

Sensorimotor
- Person may have bruises or evidence of repeated physical injury (bruises, lacerations, fractures), which should be identified and reported to appropriate persons (physician, charge nurse, legal guardian, legal authorities).

Cognitive/Perceptual
- Person may have difficulty maintaining attention and concentration.
- Person may lack executive functions skills such as decision making, problem solving, time management.

Psychosocial
- Person may be anxious or depressed.

- Person may lack self-esteem, self-efficacy, self-worth.
- Person may be unable to perform expected role functions: parent, spouse, partner.
- Person may experience role confusion including role reversal, role conflict, and lack of positive role models (Gabriel et al., 2018).
- Person may have poor quality of life.

Context/Environment
- Person may have a history of abuse.
- Person may lack knowledge of available resources: community, internet.
- Person may want to connect or reconnect with spiritual or religious events.

Intervention/Treatment

Models and programs developed by occupational therapy personnel include beauty and massage salon (Eagles, 2019), case examples (American Occupational Therapy Association, 2017), Kawa model (Humbert et al., 2013), and clinical vignette (Bonder & Anetzberger, 2018). Models and programs developed by other professionals but used by occupational therapy personnel include attachment theory (Waldman-Levi et al., 2015). Team members include physicians, nursing personnel, psychologists, social workers, lawyers, legal guardians, and occupational therapy personnel. Goals are to assist survivors to create opportunities to rebuild lives and regain life skills free from abuse (American Occupational Therapy Association, 2017; Javaherian-Dysinger et al., 2016).

Activities of Daily Living/Instrumental ADL
- Review with client, especially with elderly person, if assistance is needed to perform basic ADLs such as eating, dressing, grooming, toileting, bathing/showering, communication, mobility.
- Assist learning and implementation of effective parenting, child care, and child rearing skills for age of children being cared for.
- Provide education and practice in budgeting and financial management.
- Provide opportunity to practice home management skills (cleaning, doing laundry, mending clothes, minor home repair, home safety).
- Provide opportunity to plan meals and engage in meal preparation.
- Provide opportunity to shop for groceries, clothing, home furnishings.
- Explore with client community mobility options including use of public transportation or getting a driver's license.
- Provide education in health management: healthy diet, exercise, safety.

Education/Work
- Assist client to engage in adult learning classes (English as a Second Language, reading, math skills).
- Assist in selection of employment opportunities based on skill assessment.
- Assist in evaluating employment barriers.
- Assist in locating and participating in volunteer or unpaid occupations.

Play/Leisure
- Assist parent to provide age-appropriate play skills.
- Assist client to review and reconnect, if client wishes, with favorite leisure occupations.
- Assist client to explore and engage in new leisure occupations.

Rest/Sleep
- Provide information about establishing and maintaining sleep habits and routines.
- Review with client barriers to sleep such as too much light, noise, or smells; inadequate bedding.

Social Participation
- Assist client to review and reconnect, if client wishes, with familiar social occupations.
- Assist client to explore and participate in new social occupations with family, peers, friends, and community organizations.

Sensorimotor

- Assist client to develop and maintain physical fitness and exercise program.

Cognitive/Perceptual

- Facilitate development of attention and concentration.
- Facilitate use of executive functioning skills including effective decision making, problem solving, time management, organization.

Psychosocial

- Provide practice in stress and anxiety management techniques such as breathing exercises, mindfulness training, yoga.
- Provide practice in assertiveness skill.
- Provide opportunity to discuss and role play healthy interpersonal relationships.
- Provide opportunity to develop positive self-esteem.

Context/Environment

- Provide information about and assistance in using local, regional, national, or internet resources.
- Provide information about and access to legal services for reporting violence and abuse.
- Provide assistance in accessing other legal services as needed: divorce, legal guardianship, immigration.

Precautions/Safety Considerations

Therapists should know the warning signs of elder abuse and actions to take in identified cases (Canadian Association of Occupational Therapists, 2013).

Prognosis and Outcome

Variable. Prognosis and outcome are dependent on identification and intervention. Violence and abuse can become a chronic condition, especially for the perpetrator, and is likely to continue if intervention does not occur. The survivor may be unable to escape without help because the abusive relationship shapes attitudes, values, and beliefs (Twinley & Addidle, 2012).

REFERENCES

General

Aldrich, R. M., & White, N. (2012). Reconsidering violence: A response to Twinley and Addidle (2012) and Morris (2012). *British Journal of Occupational Therapy, 75*(11), 527–529. https://doi.org/10.4276/030802212X13522194760057

Porter, R. S. (Ed.). (2018). *The Merck manual of diagnosis and therapy* (20th ed.). Merck Sharp & Dohme.

Scaffa, M. E., Chromiak, B., Reitz, S. M., Blair-Newton, A. Murphy, L., & Wallis, C. B. (2010). Unintentional injury and violence prevention. In M. E. Scaffa, S. M. Reitz, & M. A. Pizzi (Eds.), *Occupational therapy in the promotion of health and wellness* (pp. 350–375). F.A. Davis.

Twinley, R., & Addidle, G. (2012). Considering violence: The dark side of occupation. *British Journal of Occupational Therapy, 75*(4), 202–204. https://doi.org/10.4276/030802212X13336366278257

VandenBos, G. (Ed.). (2015). *APA dictionary of psychology* (2nd ed.). American Psychological Association.

Domestic

American Occupational Therapy Association. (2017). Occupational therapy services for individuals who have experienced domestic violence. *American Journal of Occupational Therapy, 71*(Suppl. 2), Article 7112410037. https://doi.org/10.5014/ajot.2017.716s10

Eagles, L. (2019). Promoting health and wellbeing with domestic violence survivor. *OT News,* *27*(11), 30–32.

Gabriel, L., Tizro, Z., James, H., Cronin-Davis, J., Beetham, T., Corbally, A., Lopez-Moreno, E., & Hill, S. (2018). "Give me some space": Exploring youth to parent aggression and violence. *Journal of Family Violence, 33,* 161–169. https://doi.org/10.1007/s10896-017-9928-1

Javaherian-Dysinger, H., Krpalek, D., Huecker, E., Hewitt, L., Cabrera, M., Brown, C., Francis, J., Rogers, K., & Server, S. (2016). Occupational needs and goals of survivors of domestic violence. *Occupational Therapy in Health Care, 30*(2), 175–186. https://doi.org/10.3109/07380 577.2015.1109741

Waldman-Levi, A., Finzi-Dottan, R., & Weintraub, N. (2015). Attachment security and parental perception of competency among abused women in the shallow of TRSD and childhood exposure to domestic violence. *Journal of Child and Family Studies, 24,* 57–65. https://doi .org/10.1007/s10826-013-9813-3

Workplace Violence

Brown, B., & Kain, E. (2019). A role for occupational therapy practitioners in mitigating episodes of workplace violence in health care. *SIS Quarterly Practice Connections, 4*(2), 31–33.

Elder Abuse

Bonder, B., & Anetzberger, G. J. (2018). Culture, ethics, and elder abuse. In B. R. Bonder & V. D. Bello-Haas (Eds.), *Functional performance in older adults* (4th ed., pp. 75–90). F.A. Davis.

Canadian Association of Occupational Therapists. (2012). *CAOT position statement: Elder abuse prevention and management and occupational therapy.*

Canadian Association of Occupational Therapists. (2013). *Strategies for interprofessional health care providers to address elder abuse/mistreatment.*

Intimate Partner Violence

Humbert, T. K., Bess, J. L., & Mowery, A. B. (2013). Exploring women's perspectives of overcoming intimate partner violence: A phenomenological study. *Occupational Therapy in Mental Health, 29*(3), 246–265. https://doi.org/10.1080/0164212X.2013.819465

BIBLIOGRAPHY

American Occupational Therapy Association. (2018). AOTA's societal statement on youth violence. *American Journal of Occupational Therapy, 72*(Suppl. 2), Article 7212410090. https:// doi.org/10.5014/ajot.2018.72S209

Gabriel, L., James, H., Cronin-Davis, J., Tizro, Z., Beetham, T., Hullock, A., & Raynar, A. (2017). Reflexive research with mothers and children victims of domestic violence. *Counselling & Psychotherapy Research, 17*(2), 157–165. https://doi.org/10.1002/capr.12117

Mollayeva, T., Mollayeva, S., Lewko, J., & Colantonio, A. (2016). Sex differences in work-related traumatic brain injury due to assault. *Work, 54*(2), 415–423. https://doi.org/10.3233/WOR -162339

Njelesani, J. (2019). "A child who is hidden has no rights": Responses to violence against children with disabilities. *Child Abuse & Neglect, 89,* 58–69. https://doi.org/10.1016/j.chiabu.20 18.12.024

Njelesani, J., Hashemi, G., Cameron, C., Cameron, D., Richard, D., & Parnes, P. (2018). From the day they are born: A qualitative study exploring violence against children with disabilities in West Africa. *BMC Public Health, 18,* Article 153. https://doi.org/10.1186/s12889-018-5057-x

Waldman-Levi, A., Bundy, A., & Katz, N. (2015). Playfulness and interaction: An exploratory study of past and current exposure to domestic violence. *OTJR: Occupation, Participation, & Health, 35*(2), 89–94. https://doi.org/10.1177/1539449214561762

Single- or Two-Article Disorders

Single- or Two-Article Disorders

Acute Flaccid Myelitis

Kornafel, T., Tsao, E. Y., Sabelhaus, E., Surges, L., & Apkon, S. D. (2017). Physical and occupational therapy for a teenager with acute flaccid myelitis: A case report. *Physical & Occupational Therapy in Pediatrics, 37*(5), 485–595. https://doi.org/10.1080/01942638.2016.1255289

Adult Brachial Plexus Injuries

Chinchalkar, S. J., Larocerie-Salgado, J., Cepek, J., & Grenier M. L. (2018). The use of dynamic assist orthosis for muscle reeducation following brachial plexus injury and reconstruction. *Journal of Hand and Microsurgery, 10*(3), 172–177. https://doi.org/10.1055/s-0038-1642068

Wellington, B., & McGeehan, C. (2015). A case study from a nursing and occupational therapy perspective—Providing care for a patient with a traumatic brachial plexus injury. *International Journal of Orthopaedic and Trauma Nursing, 19*(1), 15–23. https://doi.org/10.1016/j.ijotn.2014.01.001

Adhesive Capsulitis

Gupta, D., Desai, O. P., & Rastogi, S. (2019). To compare the effect of home based program and supervised occupational therapy program in adhesive capsulitis patients with diabetes mellitus. *Indian Journal of Physiotherapy and Occupational Therapy 13*(1), 48–53. https://doi.org/10.5958/0973-5674.2019.00010.8

von der Heyde, R. L. (2011). Occupational therapy interventions for shoulder conditions: A systematic review. *American Journal of Occupational Therapy, 65*(1), 16–23. https://doi.org/10.5014/ajot.2011.09184

Age-Related Macular Degeneration

Deemer, A. D., Massof, R. W., Rovner, B. W., Casten, R. J., & Piersol, C. V. (2017). Functional outcomes of the low vision depression prevention trial in age-related macular degeneration. *Investigative Ophthalmology & Visual Science, 58*, 1514–1520. https://doi.org/10.1167/iovs.16-20001

Agenesis of the Corpus Callosum

Demopoulos, C., Arroyo, M. S., Dunn, W., Strominger, Z., Sherr, E. H., & Marco, E. (2015). Individuals with agenesis of the corpus callosum show sensory processing differences as measured by the sensory profile. *NeuroRehabilitation, 29*(5), 751–758. https://doi.org/10.1037/neu0000165

Ankylosing Spondylitis

Kjeken, I., Bø, I., Rønningen, A., Spada, C., Mowinckel, P., Hagen, K. B., & Dagfinrud, H. (2013). A three-week multidisciplinary in-patient rehabilitation programme had positive long-term effects in patients with ankylosing spondylitis: Randomized controlled trial. *Journal of Rehabilitation Medicine, 45*(3), 260–267. https://doi.org/10.2340/16501977-1078

Anterior Cruciate Ligament Reconstruction

Burland, J. P., Toonstra, J., Werner, J. L., Mattacola, C. G., Howell, D. M., & Howard, J. S. (2018). Decision to return to sport after anterior cruciate ligament reconstruction, Part I: A qualitative investigation of psychosocial factors. *Journal of Athletic Training, 53*(5), 452–463. https://doi.org/10.4085/1062-6050-313-16

Asthma

Engel-Yeger, B., Almog, M., & Kessel, A. (2014). The sensory profile of children with asthma. *Acta Paediatrics, 103*(11), e490–e494. https://doi.org/10.1111/apa.12746

Bálint Syndrome

Sunagawa, K., Nakagawa, Y., & Funayama, M. (2015). Effectiveness of use of button-operated electronic devices among persons with Bálint Syndrome. *American Journal of Occupational Therapy, 69*(2), Article 6902290050. https://doi.org/10.5014/ajot.2015.014522

Benign Joint Hypermobility Syndrome

Smith, T. O., Bacon, H., Jerman, E., Easton, V., Armon, K., Poland, F., & Macgregor, A. (2014). Physiotherapy and occupational therapy interventions for people with benign joint hypermobility syndrome: A systematic review of clinical trials. *Disability and Research, 36*(10), 797–803. https://doi.org/10.3109/09638288.2013.819388

Bereavement

Dahdah, D. F., & Joaquim, R. H. V. T. (2018). Occupational therapy in the bereavement process: A meta-synthesis. *South African Journal of Occupational Therapy, 48*(3), 12–18. https://doi.org/10.17159/2310-3833/2017/vol48n3a3

Fluegeman, J. E., Schrauben, A. R., & Cleghorn, S. M. (2013). Bereavement support for children: Effectiveness of Camp Erin from an occupational therapy perspective. *Bereavement Care, 32*(2), 74–81. https://doi.org/10.1080/02682621.2013.812820

Brain Abscess/Empyema

Graddidge, K., Casteleijn, D., & Franzsen, D. (2013). Using the occupational therapy practice framework-II to treat a rare condition—Brain abscess and empyema. *South African Journal of Occupational Therapy, 43*(2), 33–39.

Capitolunate Dissociation

Chinchalkar, S. J., Pipicelli, J. G., & Richards, R. (2010). Controlled active mobilization after dorsal capsulodesis to correct capitolunate dissociation. *Journal of Hand Therapy, 23*(4), 404–411. https://doi.org/10.1016/j.jht.2010.06.002

Caregiver Depression

Dionne-Odom, J. N., Azuero, A., Lyons, K. D., Hull, J. G., Prescott, A. T., Tosteson, T., Frost, J., Dragnev, K. H., & Bakitas, M. A. (2016). Family caregiver depressive symptom and grief outcomes from the ENABLE III randomized controlled trial. *Journal of Pain and Symptom Management, 52*(3), 378–385. https://doi.org/10.1016/j.jpainsymman.2016.03.014

Carpal Instability

Wong, J. M. W., Kwan, M. W. W., Au, F. L. Y., & Ho, P. C. (2010). A dynamic wrist splint for palmer midcarpal instability: An enhanced design. *Hong Kong Journal of Occupational Therapy, 20*(1), 25–29. https://doi.org/10.1016/S1569-1861(10)70055-3

Carpometacarpal (Thumb) Arthroplasty

Crosby, C. A., Reitz, J. L., Mester, E. A., & Grenier, M. L. (2013). Rehabilitation following thumb CMC, radiocarpal, and DRUJ arthroplasty. *Hand Clinics, 29*(1), 123–142. https://doi.org/10.1016/j.hcl.2012.08.025

Poole, J. L., Walenta, M. H., Alonzo, V., Coe, A., & Moneim, M. (2011). A pilot study comparing of two therapy regimens following carpometacarpal joint arthroplasty. *Physical & Occupational Therapy in Geriatrics, 29*(4), 327–336. https://doi.org/10.3109/02703181.2011.613530

Charcot Marie Tooth

Poole, J. L., Huffman, M., Hunter, A., Mares, C., & Siegel, P. (2015). Reliability and validity of the Manual Ability Measure–36 in persons with Charcot-Marie-Tooth disease. *Journal of Hand Therapy, 28*(4), 364–368. https://doi.org/10.1016/j.jht.2015.04.003

Complex Disease: Adult

Pellegrini, M., Formisano, D. Bucciarelli, V., Schiavi, M., Fugazzaro, S., & Costi, S. (2018). Occupational therapy in complex patients: A pilot randomized controlled trial. *Occupational Therapy International, 2018*, Article 3081094. https://doi.org/10.1155/2018/3081094

Complex (Emotional) Trauma: Child
Fraser, K., MacKenzie, D., & Versnel, J. (2019). What is the current state of occupational therapy practice with children and adolescents with complex trauma? *Occupational Therapy in Mental Health, 35*(4), 317–338. https://doi.org/10.1080/0164212X.2019.1652132

Corticobasal Degeneration
Cure PSP. (2016). *What every social worker, physical therapist, occupational therapist, speech-language pathologist should know about progressive supranuclear palsy (PSP), corticobasal degeneration (CBD), multiple system atrophy (MSA): A comprehensive guide to signs, symptoms and management strategies.* https://www.psp.org/wp-content/uploads/2016/08/ALLIED-HEALTH-BROCHURE_web.pdf

Congenital Cytomegalovirus
Muldoon, K. M., Armstrong-Heimsoth, A., & Thomas, J. (2017). Knowledge of congenital cytomegalovirus (cCMV) among physical and occupational therapists in the United States. *PLOS ONE, 12*(10), Article e0185635. https://doi.org/10.1371/journal.pone.0185635

Congenital Diaphragmatic Hernia
Moran, M. M., Gunn-Charlton, J. K., Walsh, J. M., Cheong, J. L. Y., Anderson, P. J., Doyle, L. W., Greaves, S., & Hunt, R. W. (2019). Associations of neonatal noncardiac surgery with brain structure and neurodevelopment: A prospective case-control study. *Journal of Pediatrics, 212,* 93–101. https://doi.org/10.1016/j.jpeds.2019.05.050

Congenital Muscular Torticollis
Chon, S. C., Yoon, S. I., & You, J. H. (2010). Use of the novel myokinetic stretching technique to ameliorate fibrotic mass in congenital muscular torticollis: An experimenter-blinded study with 1-year follow-up. *Journal of Back and Musculoskeletal Rehabilitation, 23*(2), 63–68. https://doi.org/10.3233/bmr-2010-0251

Cri du Chat Syndrome
Kim, M. K. I., & Kim, D. J. (2018). Effects of oral stimulation intervention in newborn babies with Cri du Chat syndrome: Single-subject research design. *Occupational Therapy International, 2018,* Article 6573508. https://doi.org/10.1155/2018/6573508

Cubital Tunnel Syndrome
Szekeres, M., MacDermid, J. C., King, G. J. W., & Grewal, R. (2015). The relationship between the patient-rated ulnar nerve evaluation and the common impairment measures of grip strength, pinch strength, and sensation. *Journal of Hand Therapy, 28,* 39–45. https://doi.org/10.1016/j.jht.2014.10.003

Deafblind
Jaiswal, A., Aldersey, H., Wittich, W., Mirza, M., & Finlayson, M. (2018). Participation experiences of people with deafblindness or dual sensory loss: A scoping review of global deafblind literature. *PLOS ONE, 13*(9), Article e0203772. https://doi.org/10.1371/journal.pone.0203772

de Quervain's
Neiduski, R. (2016). Clinical relevance commentary on: Hand therapy versus corticosteroid injections in the treatment of de Quervain's disease: A systematic review and meta-analysis, *Journal of Hand Therapy, 29*(1), 3–11. https://doi.org/10.1016/j.jht.2015.12.004

Dermatitis
Holness, D. L., Beaton, D., Harniman, E., DeKoven, J., Skotnicki, S., Nixon, R., & Switzer-McIntyre, S. (2013). Hand and upper extremity function in workers with hand dermatitis. *Dermatitis, 24*(3), 131–136. https://doi.org/10.1097/DER.0b013e3182910416

Dissociative Identity Disorder
Precin, P. (2011). Return to work: A case of PTSD, dissociative identity disorder, and satanic ritual abuse. *Work, 38*(1), 57–66. https://doi.org/10.3233/wor-2011-1104

Duchenne Muscular Dystrophy
Bray, P., Bundy A. C., Ryan, M. M., & North, K. N. (2017). Can in-the-moment diary methods measure health-related quality of life in Duchenne muscular dystrophy? *Quality of Life Research 26*, 1145–1152. https://doi.org/10.1007/s11136-016-1442-z

Elbow Dislocation/Fracture
Grenier, M. L., & Shankland, B. (2020). The use of static progressive and serial static orthoses in the management of elbow contractures after complex fracture dislocation injuries: A pediatric case study. *Journal of Hand Therapy, 33*(1), 127–133. https://doi.org/10.1016/j.jht.2018.09.004

Pipicelli, J. G., Chinchalkar, S., Grewal, R., & Athwal, G. S. (2011). Rehabilitation considerations in the management of terrible triad injury to the elbow. *Techniques in Hand & Upper Extremity Surgery, 15*(4), 198–208. https://doi.org/10.1097/bth.0b013e31822911fd

Epilepsy
Engel-Yeger, B., Zlotnik, S., Ravid, S., & Shahar, E. (2014). Childhood-onset primary generalized epilepsy—Impacts on children's preferences for participation in out-of-school activities. *Epilepsy & Behavior, 34*, 105. https://doi.org/10.1016/j.yebeh.2014.02.021

Fracture: Humerus
Finley, W. P., & Van Lew, S. (2018). Occupational therapy for nonoperative four-part proximal humerus fracture: A case report. *American Journal of Occupational Therapy, 72*(3), Article 7203210010. https://doi.org/10.5014/ajot.2018.026963

von der Heyde, R. L. (2011). Occupational therapy interventions for shoulder conditions: A systematic review. *American Journal of Occupational Therapy, 65*(1), 16–23. https://doi.org/10.5014/ajot.2011.09184

Fragile X
Fragile X Clinical & Research Consortium. (2014). *Sensory processing and integration issues in Fragile X syndrome.*

Martin, G. E., Ausderau, K. K., Raspa, M., Bishop, E., Mallya, U., & Bailey, D. B., Jr. (2013). Therapy service use among individuals with fragile X syndrome: Findings from a US parent survey. *Journal of Intellectual Disability Research, 57*(9), 837–849. https://doi.org/10.1111/j.1365-2788.2012.01608.x

Grief and Loss
American Occupational Therapy Association. (2012). *Grief and loss: School mental health toolkit.*

Scaletti, R., & Hocking, C. (2010). Healing through story telling: An integrated approach for children experiencing grief and loss. *New Zealand Journal of Occupational Therapy, 37*(2), 66–71.

Hanson's Disease (Leprosy)
MacRae, C., Kopalakrishnan, S., Faust, L., Klowak, M., Showler, A., Klowak, S. A., & Boggild, A. K. (2018). Evaluation of safety tool for ambulatory leprosy patients at risk of adverse outcome. *Tropical Diseases, Travel Medicine and Vaccines, 4*, Article 1. https://doi.org/10.1186/s40794-018-0061-9

Hereditary Angioedema
Engel-Yeger, B., Farkas, H., Kivity, S., Veszeli, N., Kőhalmi, K. V., & Kessel, A. (2017). Health-related quality of life among children with hereditary angioedema. *Pediatric Allergy and Immunology, 28*(4), 370–376. https://doi.org/10.1111/pai.12712

Kessel, A., Farkas, H., Kivity, S., Veszeli, N., Kőhalmi, K. V., & Engel-Yeger, B. (2017). The relationship between anxiety and quality of life in children with hereditary angioedema. *Pediatric Allergy and Immunology, 28*(7), 692–698.

Infectious Encephalitis

Christie, S., Chan, V., Mollayeva, T., & Colantonio, A. (2016). Rehabilitation interventions in children and adults with infectious encephalitis: A systematic review protocol. *BMJ Open, 6,* Article e010754. https://doi.org/10.1136/bmjopen-2015-010754

Christie, S., Chan, V., Mollayeva, T., & Colantonio, A. (2018). Systematic review of rehabilitation intervention outcomes of adult and paediatric patients with infectious encephalitis. *BMJ Open, 8,* Article e015928. https://doi.org/10.1136/bmjopen-2017-015928

Inflammatory Bowel Disease

Laforest-Tanguay, E., & Lapointe, J. (2018). Impacts of inflammatory bowel disease on occupational performance and engagement: The potential role of occupational therapists. *Occupational Therapy Now, 20*(3), 18–20.

Intrauterine Spinal Cord Infarct

Felter, C., Neuland, E. E., Iuculano, S. C., & Dean, J. (2019). Interdisciplinary, intensive, activity-based treatment for intrauterine spinal cord infarct: A case report. *Topics in Spinal Cord Injury Rehabilitation, 25*(1), 97–103. https://doi.org/10.1310/sci18-00025

Kidney Disease

Farragher, J. F. (2017). "Nephrol-OT": Bridging the gap between occupational therapy and kidney disease care. *Occupational Therapy Now, 19*(6), 26–27.

Limb Lengthening

Hamdy, R. C., Montpetit, K., Aiona, M. D., MacKenzie, W. G., van Bosse, H. J. P., Narayanan, U., Raney, E. M., Chafetz, R. S., Thomas, S. E. S., Weir, S., Gregory, S., Yorgova, P., Takahashi, S., Rinaldi, M., Zhang, X., & Dahan-Oliel, N. (2016). Safety and efficacy of Botulinum Toxin A in children undergoing lower limb lengthening and deformity correction: Results of a double-blind, multicenter, randomized controlled trial. *Journal of Pediatric Orthopedics, 36*(1), 48–55. https://doi.org/10.1097/BPO.0000000000000398

Loneliness

Hirji, R. (2016). Let's get together: Fighting loneliness for a healthier society. *Occupational Therapy Now, 18*(5), 12.

Mechanical Ventilation

Needham, D. M., Korupolu, R., Zanni, J. M., Pradhan, P., Colantuoni, E., Palmer, J. B., Brower, R. G., & Fan, E. (2010). Early physical medicine and rehabilitation for patients with acute respiratory failure: A quality improvement project. *Archives of Physical Medicine and Rehabilitation, 91*(4), 536–542. https://doi.org/10.1016/j.apmr.2010.01.002

Pohlman, M. C., Schweickert, W. D., Pohlman, A. S., Nigos, C., Pawlik, A. J., Esbrook, C. L., Spears, L., Miller, M., Franczyk, M., Deprizio, D., Schmidt, G. A., Bowman, A., Barr, R., McCallister, K. Hall, J. B., & Kress, J. P. (2010). Feasibility of physical and occupational therapy beginning from initiation of mechanical ventilation. *Critical Care Medicine, 38*(11), 2089–2094. https://doi.org/10.1097/CCM.0b013e3181f270c3

Miscarriage/Pregnancy Loss

Hanish, K. K., Margulies, I., & Cogan, A. M. (2019). Evaluation of an occupation-based retreat for women after pregnancy or infant loss. *American Journal of Occupational Therapy, 73*(5), Article 7305345030. https://doi.org/10.5014/ajot.2019.034025

Watson, M., Jewell, V., & Smith, S. (2018). Journey interrupted: A phenomenological exploration of miscarriage. *Open Journal of Occupational Therapy, 6*(3), Article 7. https://doi.org/10.15453/2168-6408.1439

Mitochondrial Disorder

Lindenschot, M., de Groot, I. J. M., Koene, S., Satink, T., Steultjens, E. M. J., & Nijhuis-van der Sanden, M. W. G. (2018). Everyday activities for children with mitochondrial disorder: A retrospective review chart. *Occupational Therapy International, 2018,* Article 5716947. https:// doi.org/10.1155/2018/5716947

Mucopolysaccharidosis Type II
Amaral, I. A. B. S., Filho, R. L. D. O., Neto, J. A. D. R., & Reis, M. C. D. S. (2017). Assessment of functional capacity of teens who are mucopolysaccharidosis type II carriers. *Cadernos Brasileiros Terapia Ocupacional São Carolos, 25*(2), 297–303. http://dx.doi.org/10.4322/0104 -4931.ctoAO0799

Multiple System Atrophy (MSA; Shy-Drager Syndrome)
Cure PSP. (2016). *What every social worker, physical therapist, occupational therapist, speech-language pathologist should know about progressive supranuclear palsy (PSP), corticobasal degeneration (CBD), multiple system atrophy (MSA): A comprehensive guide to signs, symptoms and management strategies.* https://www.psp.org/wp-content/uploads/2016/08/ALLIED-HEALTH-BROCHURE _web.pdf

Multiple System Atrophy Trust. (2016). *Factsheet: A guide to multiple system atrophy for occupational therapists.*

Musician Injuries: General
Guptill, C. (2018). Musicians' health: A developing role for occupational therapists. *Occupational Therapy Now, 16*(6), 29–31.

Musician Injuries: Piano
Kaufman-Cohen, Y., Portnoy, S., Sopher, R., Mashiach, L., Baruch-Halaf, L., & Ratzon, N. (2018). The correlation between upper extremity musculoskeletal symptoms and joint kinematics, playing habits and hand span during playing among piano students. *PLOS ONE, 13*(12), Article e0208788. https://doi.org/10.1371/journal.pone.0208788

Oikawa, N., Tsubota, S., Chikenji, T., Chin, G., & Aoki, M. (2011). Wrist positioning and muscle activities in the wrist extensor and flexor during piano playing. *Hong Kong Journal of Occupational Therapy, 21*(1), 41–46. https://doi.org/10.1016/j.hkjot.2011.06.002

Neuralgic Amyotrophy
Ijspeert, J., Janssen, R. M. J., Murgia, A., Pisters, M. F., Cup, E. H. C., Groothuis, J. T., & van Alfen, N. (2013). Efficacy of a combined physical and occupational therapy intervention in patients with subacute neuralgic amyotrophy: A pilot study. *NeuroRehabilitation, 33*(4), 657–665. https://doi.org/10.3233/NRE-130993

Occupational Injuries and Diseases
Blas, A. J. T., Beltran, K. M. B., Martinez, P. G. V., & Yao, D. P. G. (2018). Enabling work: Occupational therapy interventions for persons with occupational injuries and diseases: A scoping review. *Journal of Occupational Rehabilitation, 28*(2), 201–214. https://doi.org/10.1007/ s10926-017-9732-z

Pierre-Robin Sequence
Lee, M., Ho, E. S., & Forrest, C. R. (2019). Pierre Robin Sequence: Cost-analysis and qualitative assessment of 89 patients at the hospital for sick children. *Plastic Surgery, 27*(1), 14–21. https:// doi.org/10.1177/2292550318767922

Stokes, M., Cook, E., Sanders, C., & Coker-Bolt, P. (2014). The case for early power mobility: Developmental outcomes for a toddler born with a rare neuromuscular disorder. *Technology Special Interest Section Quarterly, 24*(4), 1–3.

Plagiocephaly
Mortenson, P., Steinbok, P., & Smith, D. (2012). Deformational plagiocephaly and orthotic treatment: Indications and limitations. *Child's Nervous System, 28,* 1407–1412. https://doi.org/10 .1007/s00381-012-1755-3

Zachry, A. H., Nolan, V. G., Hand, S. B., & Klemm, S. A. (2017). Infant positioning, baby gear use, and cranial asymmetry. *Maternal and Child Health Journal, 21*, 2229–2236. https://doi .org/10.1007/s10995-017-2344-6

Pollicization

Lightdale-Miric, N., Mueske, N. M., Lawrence, E. L., Loiselle, J., Berggren, J., Dayanidhi, S., Stevanovic, M., Valero-Cuevas, F. J., & Wren, T. A. L. (2015). Long term functional outcomes after early childhood pollicization. *Journal of Hand Therapy, 28*(2), 158–166. https://doi.org/ 10.1016/j.jht.2014.11.003

Lightdale-Miric, N., Mueske, N. M., Dayanidhi, S., Loiselle, J., Berggren, J., Lawrence, E. L., Stevanovic, M., Valero-Cuevas, F. J., & Wren, T. A. L. (2015). Quantitative assessment of dynamic control fingertip forces after pollicization. *Gait & Posture, 41*(1), 1–6. https://doi.org/10.1016/ j.gaitpost.2014.08.012

Posterior Cortical Atrophy

Bier, N., El-Samra, A., Bottari, C., Vallet, G. T., Carignan, M., Paquette, G., Brambati, S., Demers, L., Génier-Marchand, D., & Rouleau, I. (2019). Posterior cortical atrophy: Impact on daily living activities and exploration of a cognitive rehabilitation approach. *Cogent Psychology, 6*(1), Article 1634911. https://doi.org/10.1080/23311908.2019.1634911

Posterior Reversible Encephalopathy Syndrome

Kadkol, M. S. (2013). A case review of perceptual deficit in PRES: Detailed perceptual evaluation is a key to definite goal achieving techniques. *Indian Journal of Physiotherapy and Occupational Therapy, 7*(3), 124–127. https://doi.org/10.5958/j.0973-5674.7.3.078

Progressive Supranuclear Palsy

Cure PSP. (2016). *What every social worker, physical therapist, occupational therapist, speech-language pathologist should know about progressive supranuclear palsy (PSP), corticobasal degeneration (CBD), multiple system atrophy (MSA): A comprehensive guide to signs, symptoms and management strategies.* https://www.psp.org/wp-content/uploads/2016/08/ALLIED-HEALTH-BROCHURE_web.pdf

Pulmonary/Lung Injury

Dinglas, V. D., Colantuoni, E., Ciesla, N., Mendez-Tellez, P. A., Shanholtz, C., & Needham, D. M. (2013). Occupational therapy for patients with acute lung injury: Factors associated with time to first intervention in the intensive care unit. *American Journal of Occupational Therapy, 67*(3), 355–362. https://doi.org/10.5014/ajot.2013.007807

Regulatory Sensory Processing Disorder

Jorge, J., de Witt, P. A., & Franzsen, D. (2013). The effect of a two-week sensory diet on fussy infants with regulatory sensory processing disorder. *South African Journal of Occupational Therapy, 43*(3), 28–34.

Replantation: Tendon

Deepak, G. (2011). A case report on the role of occupational therapy in revascularised and replanted surgical case of flexor tendon of hand. *Indian Journal of Physiotherapy and Occupational Therapy, 5*(4), 34–35.

Retinoblastoma

Sparrow, J., Brennan, R., Mao, S., Ness, K. K., Rodriguez-Galindo, C., Wilson, M., & Qaddoumi, I. (2016). Participation in an occupational therapy referral program for children with retinoblastoma. *Journal of Pediatric Rehabilitation Medicine, 9*(2), 117–124. https://doi.org/10.3233/ PRM-160372

Shoulder Injuries

Villafañe, J. H., Valdes, K., Anselmi, F., Pirali, C., & Negrini, S. (2015). The diagnostic accuracy of five tests for diagnosing partial-thickness tears of the supraspinatus tendon: A cohort study. *Journal of Hand Therapy, 28*(3), 247–252. https://doi.org/10.1016/j.jht.2015.01.011

von der Heyde, R. L. (2011). Occupational therapy interventions for shoulder conditions: A systematic review. *American Journal of Occupational Therapy, 65*(1), 16–23. https://doi.org/10.5014/ajot.2011.09184

Sports Injuries (See also Anterior Cruciate Ligament Reconstruction)

Shimizu, Y., Mutsuzaki, H., Tachibana, K., Tsunoda, K., Hotta, K., Fukaya, T., Ikeda, E., Yamazaki, M., & Wadano, Y. (2017). A survey of deep tissue injury in elite female wheelchair basketball players. *Journal of Back and Musculoskeletal Rehabilitation, 30*(3), 427–434. https://doi.org/10.3233/bmr-150457

Tendon Transfers

Kakinoki, R., Duncan, S. F. M., Ikeguchi, R., Ohta, S., Nankaku, M., Sakai, H., Noguchi, T., Kaizawa, Y., & Akagi, M. (2017). Motor and sensory cortical changes after contralateral cervical seventh nerve root (CC7) transfer in patients with brachial plexus injuries. *Journal of Hand Surgery (Asian-Pacific), 22*(2), 138–149. https://doi.org/10.1142/s0218810417500162

Thoracic Outlet Syndrome

Abdolrazaghi, H., Riyahi, A., Taghavi, M., Farshidmehr, P., & Mohammadbeigi, A. (2018). Concomitant neurogenic and vascular thoracic outlet syndrome due to multiple exostoses. *Annual of Cardiologic Anesthesia, 21*(1), 71–73. https://doi.org/10.4103/aca.ACA_119_17

Tourette Syndrome

Weisman, H., Parush, S., Apter, A., Fennig, S., Benaroya-Milshtein, N., & Steinberg, T. (2018). A study of sensory dysregulation in children with tic disorders. *Journal of Neural Transmission, 125*(7), 1077–1085. https://doi.org/10.1007/s00702-018-1858-4

Transplant

Bernardon, L., Gazarian, A., Petruzzo, P., Packham, T., Guillot, M., Guigal, V., Morelon, E., Pan, H., Dubernard, J.-M., Rizzo, C., Feugier, P., Streichenberger, T., Bincaz, L., Urien, J.-P., Mezzadri, G., Rousselon, T., Plotard, F., Seulin, C., Braye, F., Mojallal, A., Herzberg, G., Kanitakis, J., Abrahamyan, D., Kay, S., & Badet. L. (2015). Bilateral hand transplantation: Functional benefits assessment in five patients with a mean follow-up of 7.6 years (range 4–13 years). *Journal of Plastic, Reconstructive & Aesthetic Surgery, 68*(9), 1171–1183. https://doi.org/10.1016/j.bjps.2015.07.007

Hiemstra, L. E., Terblanche, L., & Adriaanse, B. (2015). Rehabilitation outcomes following autologous human stem cell transplantation in a chronic complete C4 tetraplegic—The first 12 months: A case report. *South African Journal of Occupational Therapy, 45*(2), 29–42. https://doi.org/10.17159/2310-3833/2015/v45n2a6

Tuberculosis and Multidrug-Resistant Tuberculosis

Firfirey, N., & Hess-April, L. (2014). A study to explore the occupational adaptation of adults with MDR-TB who undergo long-term hospitalization. *South African Journal of Occupational Therapy, 44*(3), 18–24.

Williams Syndrome

Wuang, Y. P., & Tsai, H. Y. (2017). Sensorimotor and visual perceptual functioning in school-aged children with Williams syndrome. *Journal of Intellectual Disability Research, 61*(4), 348–362. https://doi.org/10.1111/jir.12346

Wolfram Syndrome

Bumpus, E., Hershey, T., Doty, T., Ranck, S., Gronski, M., Urano, F., & Foster, E. R. (2018). Understanding activity participation among individuals with Wolfram syndrome. *British Journal of Occupational Therapy, 81*(6), 348–357. https://doi.org/10.1177/0308022618757182